THE JOURNAL OF PEDIATRICS

A MONTHLY JOURNAL DEVOTED TO THE PROBLEMS AND DISEASES OF INFANCY AND CHILDHOOD

Official Organ for The American Academy of Pediatrics

VOLUME 9

JULY—DECEMBER, 1936

ST. LOUIS

THE C. V. MOSBY COMPANY

1936

Printed in U. S. A.

Press of
The C. V. Mosby Company
St. Louis

66

The Journal of Pediatrics

Vol. 9 | July, 1936 | No. 1

Original Communications

THE EFFECT OF VITAMIN D ON LINEAR GROWTH IN INFANCY

Genevieve Stearns, Ph.D., P. C. Jeans, M.D., and
Verva Vandecar, R.N.
Iowa City, Iowa

THE influence of improved nutrition and environment on the rate of growth of school children has often been noted. Baldwin,[1] among others, demonstrated that children from better class homes grow at faster than the average rate. The more rapid growth was credited to better nutrition. His findings have been amply confirmed.[2] More recently increased rates of growth of average European school children have been reported[3] and the cause ascribed not only to diet, but also and to a greater degree to the increase in outdoor life and greater exposure of the body to sunlight.

In contrast to the numerous studies of growth of school children, the literature contains few reports concerning the effect of modern dietaries and mode of life on the rate of growth during infancy. Robertson[4] in 1916 compared the rate of growth of breast-fed British infants in England and in Australia, and considered the increased rate of growth of the Australian born infants as due to improved "environment." Sunlight certainly would be one of the most important environmental factors to be considered. Daniels and her associates[5] first pointed out that well infants given cod liver oil grow at a greater rate than infants similarly fed except that no cod liver oil was given. The increased growth was credited primarily to the greater vitamin D intake, and the conclusion was drawn that accepted standards of growth were too low. Both of the above studies concerned growth in weight only. Nelson[6] reported from this laboratory that infants given acidified whole milk feedings and ingesting one teaspoonful of cod liver oil daily were both longer and heavier than the accepted standards for their ages.

From the Department of Pediatrics, State University of Iowa.

This study was assisted by a grant from Mead Johnson and Company, Evansville, Indiana.

The average increase in length of well male infants during the first year of life has been variously given as from 19.8 (Quetelet[7]) to 25 cm. (von Pirquet[8]). Baldwin[9] in 1921, from a study of nearly 5,000 Iowa male infants, stated that the average Iowa male infant grows from 52.4 cm. at birth to 74.7 cm. at one year of age and that American infants were superior to French and German infants in height and weight during infancy. A length increase of 22 cm. during the first year of life is still a common standard for American male infants.[10]

During each of the past seven years a group of well male infants has been housed in our metabolism ward, particularly for the study of mineral metabolism. Careful records of growth and development have been kept, as well as the usual ward records. The type of feeding has remained practically constant, namely, cow's milk acidified or otherwise curded and with 6 per cent added carbohydrate, usually a dry dextrin-maltose preparation. Each infant has been given 30 c.c. of orange juice daily up to three months of age, and 60 c.c. daily subsequently. Sieved vegetables were included in the diet at five months of age, and sieved fruits at six months. For this group of studies, cereal was not included during the period discussed. When the vitamin D intake was unrestricted, an egg yolk a day was given to infants over four months of age. For infants whose vitamin D intakes were to be limited, ferric citrate solution was given instead of the egg.

It became obvious during the first year's study in 1930 that the rate of growth of each infant observed[11] exceeded the average rate of growth of Iowa infants as reported by Baldwin. A search was made for higher standards, and those published in 1929 by Kornfeld[12] were chosen. These standards were based on studies of American, British, and North and Central European infants—racial stocks prevalent in our own groups. While the Kornfeld standard rate of growth was greater than the Baldwin standard, the infants studied by us grew in length at a rate definitely more rapid than the Kornfeld standard rate, and maintained weights normal for their lengths according to that standard. This growth was achieved despite an epidemic of acute respiratory infection occurring during the study.

During the following three years, the groups of infants studied also showed the same increase in rate of growth as was observed in 1930. In the study of 1934 the intake of vitamin D was decreased from approximately 340 U.S.P. units daily to the amount which could be consumed by a baby given irradiated milk, namely, from 60 to 135 U.S.P. units daily. The intake of vitamin A was also decreased by this procedure. The infants of this study grew at almost exactly the standard (Kornfeld) rate of growth, although the other factors of the diet and care were the same as during the preceding years. At the close of the study in the spring the infants were put out in the sun, fully clothed, during a part of each sunny day. The rate of growth increased. Cod liver oil was then given in the amount of one teaspoonful daily, and the growth of the younger infants quickly attained the ward average. The two older infants showed increased growth, but not at the same rate as did the younger infants.

The following year the vitamin D intake of the group studied was obtained from milk containing a cod liver oil concentrate in the amount of 400 U.S.P. units to the quart (from 245 to 400 units ingested daily), or from 400 U.S.P. units daily as cod liver oil. The intakes of both vitamins D and A were thus increased, and again the growth rate of the infants increased above the Kornfeld standard. During the past year four infants have been given irradiated milk feedings permitting a vitamin D intake of 60 to 135 U.S.P. units daily and have maintained only an average rate of growth. The growth results obtained are thus readily duplicated by repetition of conditions.

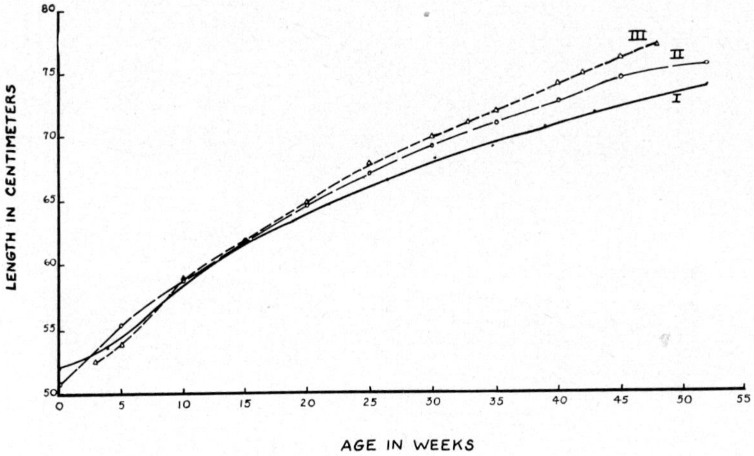

Chart 1.—*I,* average rate of linear growth of Iowa male infants, Baldwin, 1921. *II,* average rate of linear growth of male infants, Kornfeld, 1929. *III,* average rate of linear growth of thirty-six male infants given whole milk feedings and 340 U.S.P. units of vitamin D as cod liver oil daily.

The results of the seven years' observations are shown in the charts. The three curves of Chart 1 are: *I,* the average growth rate of Iowa infants as reported by Baldwin in 1921; *II,* the average rate of growth according to Kornfeld's standards of 1929; and *III,* the average rate of growth of thirty-six infants given the equivalent of one teaspoonful of cod liver oil daily (340 to 400 U.S.P. units of vitamin D). The average length of the infants whose growth is shown in Curve *III* was 0.5 cm. less than that of the other two groups at three weeks of age, but by the forty-eighth week this group averaged 77 cm. in length, in contrast to 75 cm. for the Kornfeld standard and 73 cm. for the Baldwin standard. The average rate of growth of the two groups of infants fed irradiated milk or its vitamin D equivalent (60 to 135 U.S.P. units of vitamin D daily) is almost identical with that of Curve *II,* faster than the growth of the average Iowa infant of 1921, but slower than that of the infants given the equivalent of a teaspoonful of cod liver oil. For purposes of comparison it may be stated that the standards recently reported by Stuart[13] for the growth of Boston infants are also nearly identical with the Kornfeld standard.

Chart 2 includes the same growth Curve *III* as is shown in Chart 1, namely, the rate of growth of infants given 340 or more U.S.P. units of vitamin D as cod liver oil daily (who will hereafter be designated as the high vitamin D group). The shaded portion and the light background lines indicate the average range and the normal limits, respectively, of the Kornfeld standard. Curves *I* and *II* show the average rates of growth of the two groups given a moderate amount of vitamin

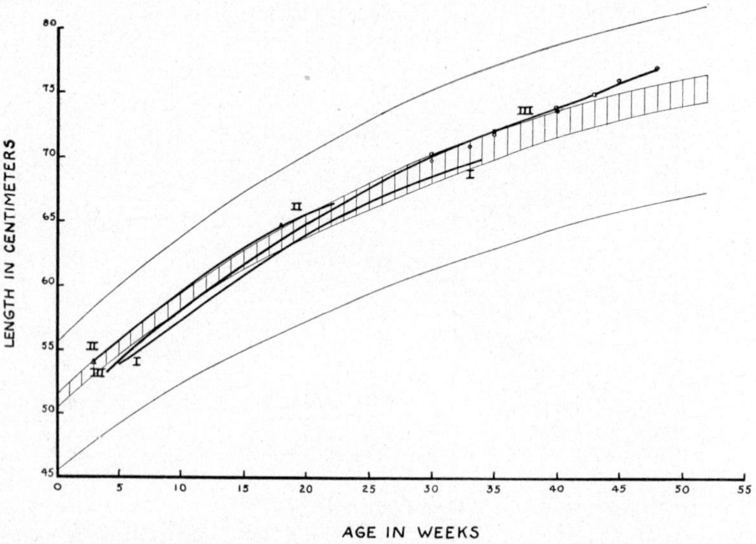

Chart 2.—*I*, average rate of linear growth of seven infants given irradiated milk or its vitamin D equivalent as cod liver oil or cod liver oil concentrate milk, ingesting from 60 to 135 U.S.P. units of vitamin D daily.

II, average rate of linear growth of four infants given irradiated milk (60 to 135 U.S.P. units of vitamin D daily).

III, same curve as *III*, Chart 1. In this and succeeding charts, the shaded portion and the light background lines indicate the average range and normal limits respectively of the Kornfeld standard.

D as irradiated milk (135 U.S.P. units to the quart) or its vitamin D equivalent in either cod liver oil or cod liver oil concentrate milk. The infants of Group II were larger at the beginning of the study than the infants of Group I. The infants of Group I were born in the winter, those of Group II in late summer. Curve *I* follows closely the lower line of the Kornfeld average range, and Curve *II* follows the upper line as closely. Both of these groups, therefore, may be considered as growing at the standard rate.

The infants of Group II, who were given irradiated milk as the only source of vitamin D, received from 60 to 135 U.S.P. units of vitamin

D daily and no additional vitamin A. The infants of Group I each received irradiated milk for from six to eight weeks of the study, and during the remainder of the period received the vitamin D equivalent as cod liver oil or cod liver oil concentrate milk, both of which provide additional vitamin A. These infants, therefore, during two-thirds of the study were receiving more vitamin A than the infants of Group II. The differences in growth rates between Group I and II are negligible. This indicates that vitamin D rather than vitamin A was the factor responsible for the increase in growth rate in Group III.

It seems logical to assume that in this study vitamin D is the chief factor affecting the rate of linear growth, for growth in length depends primarily on skeletal growth, and vitamin D, through its effect on mineral retentions, increases the amount of calcium salts available for

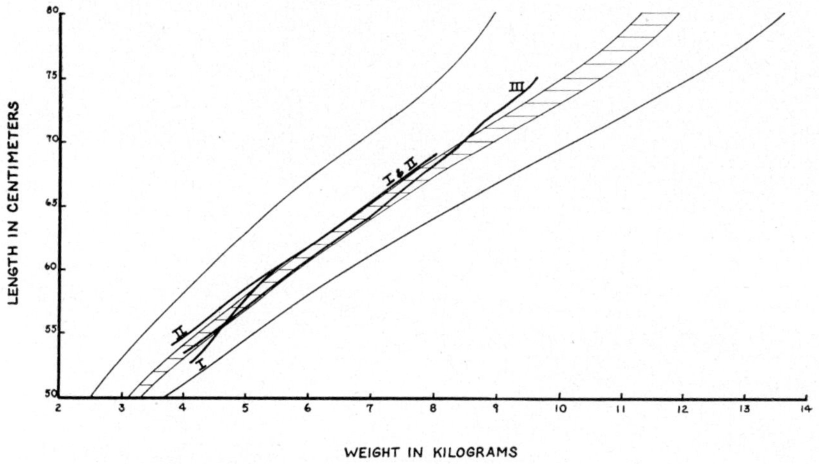

Chart 3.—Weight-length curves for the three groups of infants whose growth in length was shown in Chart 2.

The shaded portion and fine lines indicate the average range and normal limits of the Kornfeld weight-length standard.

the formation of new bone. Supporting this assumption is the fact that, although the milk intakes were the same in the three groups, the average quantities of calcium and phosphorus actually retained daily by the infants given one teaspoonful of cod liver oil a day were significantly greater than the mean daily retentions of calcium and phosphorus by infants given the moderate intake of vitamin D (135 unit milk).[14] The rate of growth of the group given high vitamin D (Curve *III*) was consistently greater throughout the entire period studied. At the beginning of the study, the infants of Group III were the same average size as those of Group I and 1.75 cm. shorter than the infants of Group II. At twenty-two weeks of age, the infants of Group III averaged only 0.5 cm. shorter than those of Group II and were more than 1 cm. longer than the infants of Group I. By thirty-four weeks of age, the difference between the growth rates of Groups I and III was more marked, as the growth rate of Group I showed a distinct slowing, while that of Group III continued to increase, making a difference of nearly 2 cm. in the average length of the two groups. At forty-eight weeks, the average length of the infants in Group III was 77 cm., 3.5 cm. greater than that expected from their size at the beginning of the study according to the Kornfeld standard.

The weight-length curves for these three groups of infants are shown in Chart 3. The shaded portions and fine lines again represent the average range and normal limits of the Kornfeld standards, and the curves are numbered as in Chart 2. It will be observed that the infants of all three groups tend to become somewhat slender but remain close to the average range.

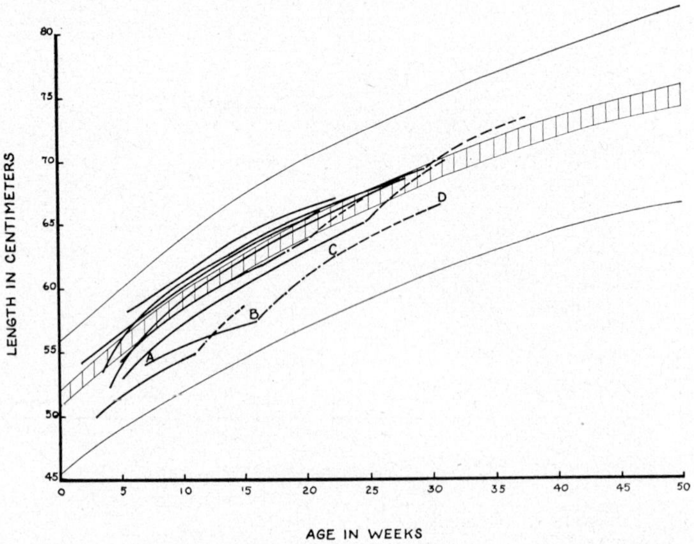

Chart 4.—Growth in length curves of individual infants with moderate vitamin D intake (60 to 135 U.S.P. units of vitamin D daily). Standards shown as in Chart 2.

Dot-dash lines indicate periods when infants received sunlight in addition to diet; broken lines indicate periods when both sunlight and cod liver oil were given.

Chart 4 depicts eight curves of growth in length of individual infants of the two groups given the moderate amount of vitamin D (60 to 135 U.S.P. units). The shaded portions and light lines indicate the average range and normal limits of the Kornfeld standard, as in Chart 2. The growth rate of a very short infant is compared with the slope of the lowest line of the standard range; that of a very tall infant with the uppermost standard line; the slope of the growth curves of the remainder is compared with that of the central average range. In this manner average rates are not biased by comparing the rate of growth of very large or very small infants with that of infants average in size at the beginning of the study. It will be observed that in general the growth curves of all the infants fed a moderate amount of vitamin D tend to parallel the lines of the standard. Two infants showed a greater than standard growth during early infancy, but by the tenth week of age the growth rate of both had definitely slowed. Growth of infants during the first weeks of life probably may be affected by the vitamin D intake of the mothers during the latter part of pregnancy.

The dot-dash lines of the growth curves indicate the periods during which the infant received additional sunlight, and the broken lines the periods when both sunlight and additional cod liver oil were given. For example, the line *AB* represents the growth of one infant given milk containing 135 U.S.P. units of vitamin D to the quart; *BC*, his growth on the same diet plus the added effect of sunlight; *CD*, the effect of one

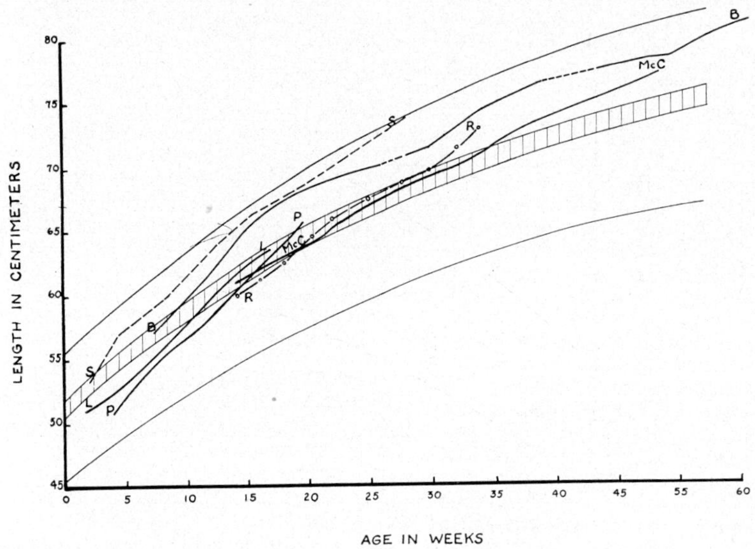

Chart 5.—Linear growth curves of individual infants given 340 U.S.P. units of vitamin D daily. Curve *S*, the growth rate of a breast-fed infant given 340 units of vitamin D daily; on curve *B*, the dotted portions show periods of illness.

teaspoonful of cod liver oil daily added to the regimen of the preceding period. This curve gives further evidence that for these babies vitamin D rather than vitamin A was the important factor and that probably the vitamin A ingestion was already adequate for growth without further additions.

Chart 5 records, in the same manner as Chart 4, the individual growth curves of infants given one teaspoonful of cod liver oil daily (340 or more U.S.P. units of vitamin D). These growth rates are typical of the group and were chosen to illustrate particularly the rates of growth of infants both small and large at the beginning of the study. The dotted curve *S* represents the growth rate of a baby kept under the same housing conditions as the others, but fed human milk and one teaspoonful of cod liver oil daily. This curve is not included in the averages, but it is shown here to illustrate the fact that more rapid growth is observed also with other types of feeding when the vitamin D intake is high. Curve *B* is of particular interest because it shows the effect of illness on the growth rate of an infant. This child, the fifth in the family, was of Scandinavian stock and was born of a mother with nephritis. He entered the ward at seven and one-half weeks of age and was of average length and weight. The infant was always unusually susceptible to respiratory infection. Minor respiratory infections are not noted on the growth curve. The first dotted portion of the curve denotes the period of a mild chickenpox infection, and the second dotted portion illustrates the effect of a severe illness, a laryngitis requiring tracheotomy, wherein the child was critically ill for a period of several days and moderately ill for a month or more. The growth rate was

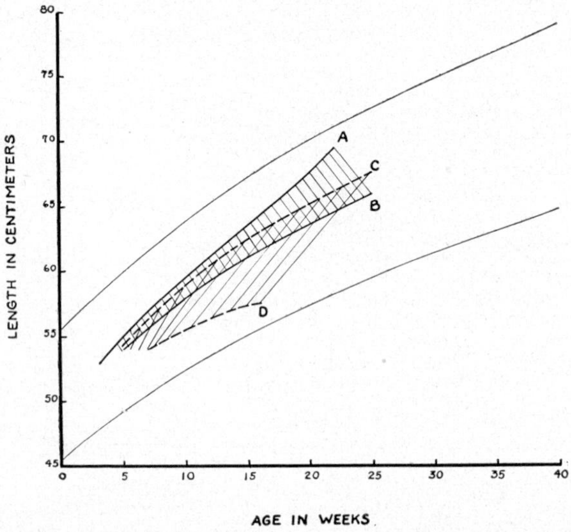

Chart 6.—Relative variability of growth rates with different intakes of vitamin D. The shaded portion between the two solid lines represents the range of growth rates exhibited by thirty-six infants given 340 units of vitamin D daily as cod liver oil; the portion between the two dotted lines, the range of growth rates shown by eleven infants given 60 to 135 units of vitamin D daily, as cod liver oil, cod liver oil concentrate milk, or irradiated milk.

definitely slowed for a period of nearly ten weeks, but later compensated by a rapid increase during the succeeding seven weeks. At seven weeks of age this baby was average in height, while at one year of age he was 5 cm. taller than the expected height by the Kornfeld standard, notwithstanding one severe and several minor illnesses. The remaining curves illustrate the rates of growth customarily observed with the dietary regimen used, namely, whole milk feedings and one teaspoonful of cod liver oil daily.

In Chart 6 are indicated the relative variability of growth rates that may be expected from the two dietary regimens under discussion, namely, moderate and high vitamin D. The shaded portion between the two solid lines represents the difference in growth rate, respectively, of the group given the larger amount of vitamin D (340 U.S.P. units daily); the portion between the two dotted curves represents similarly the range of growth rate among the infants given the moderate amount of vitamin D (135 unit milk or its equivalent).

The range in the group given the smaller amount of vitamin D is almost double that in the high vitamin D group, although the former group included less than half as many children as the latter. For convenience in comparison, the increases in length between seven and sixteen weeks and between sixteen and twenty-two weeks of age are stated. The most rapid growth from seven to sixteen weeks of age in the high vitamin D group was 7.4 cm., the slowest 6.1 cm., a difference of 21 per cent. The moderate vitamin D group varied from 6.8 to 3.5 cm. increase in length, a 94 per cent range. Between sixteen and twenty-two weeks of age the rate of growth slows in both groups. The most rapid growth in the moderate vitamin D group just equalled the slowest growth in the high vitamin D group, namely, 3 cm. The most rapid growth in the high vitamin D group was 5.3 cm.

Much discussion has been presented in the literature on the general subject of desirability of rapid or slow growth.[15] It seems to be customary to consider as normal whatever happens to be the prevailing rate. However, when one considers that the customs of modern life necessarily deprive the infant of sunlight and that the ingestion of cod liver oil or other source of vitamin D tends to bring the environment back to its original normal, it would seem that the rate of growth illustrated by the high vitamin D group is nearer the true normal than would be the growth of infants not so fed. The fact that the breast-fed baby, close-housed but given cod liver oil, grew at the same rapid rate may be taken as evidence in this direction.

The increased rates of growth of the Kornfeld and the Stuart standards over the earlier standards may readily be due to increased intake of vitamin D or exposure to sunlight, even though such alterations in regimen may have been casual. At the time when the Baldwin standards were prepared, it was not customary to give cod liver oil to well infants, and babies were more often shielded from sunlight than exposed to it. Since 1920 customs have altered materially in this regard. Standards compiled recently may include all grades of vitamin D (and A) intake, the resultant being a definite increase in growth rate, but not equal to the average growth rate when each infant studied receives ample cod liver oil.

SUMMARY

The rate of growth in length of infants given one teaspoonful of high grade cod liver oil (340 to 400 U.S.P. units of vitamin D daily) has been compared with the rate of linear growth of infants given the same type of diet, but with the source of vitamin D from irradiated milk

(60 to 135 U.S.P. units of vitamin D daily) or its vitamin D equivalent as cod liver oil or cod liver oil concentrate milk, and with standard growth rates reported in the literature.

A review of the growth standards shows that the rate of linear growth in infancy is increasing. Standards reported in 1929 and 1933 show rates of growth definitely increased over those of older standards.

Infants given 340 to 400 U.S.P. units of vitamin D daily grow at rates definitely more rapid than those of even the recent standards. Infants ingesting from 60 to 135 U.S.P. units of vitamin D daily grow at the same rate as the recent standards. Exposure to sunlight increased the rate of growth in the few infants in whom this measure was tried and who were receiving the lower of the two stated amounts of vitamin D.

The increased rate of linear growth is ascribed chiefly to the increased intake of vitamin D and its resultant effect on skeletal growth. Although the influence of vitamin A has not been entirely excluded, certain of the observations recorded indicate that vitamin A was not the limiting factor in the growth of the infants studied.

REFERENCES

1. Baldwin, B. T.: Physical Growth and School Progress, U. S. Bureau of Education, 1914, No. 10, Washington.
2. Gray, H.: Am. J. Dis. Child. **32**: 554, 1926.
3. Kornfeld, W.: Wien. klin. Wchnschr. **46**: 683, 1933.
   Koch, E. W.: Arch. f. soziale Hyg. u. Demeg **6**: 385, 1933-34 (abst. in Nutrition Abst. and Rev. **5**: 175, 1935).
4. Robertson, T. B.: Am. J. Physiol. **41**: 535, 1916.
5. Danie's, A. L., Hutton, M. K., Stearns, G., and Hejinian, L.: Am. J. Dis. Child. **37**: 1177, 1929.
6. Nelson, M. V.: Ibid. **39**: 701, 1930.
7. Quetelet: Quoted by Czerny-Keller, Des Kindes Ernährung, Leipzig, 1925, Franz Deuticke.
8. Von Pirquet, C.: Ztschr. f. Kinderh. **6**: 253, 1913.
9. Baldwin, B. T.: Physical Growth of Children, Birth to Maturity, University of Iowa Studies, Iowa City, 1921.
10. Holt, L. E., Jr., and McIntosh, R.: Diseases of Infancy and Childhood, ed. 10, New York, 1933, D. Appleton & Co.
11. Jeans, P. C., and Stearns, G.: Am. J. Dis. Child. **46**: 69, 1933.
12. Kornfeld, W.: Ztschr. f. Kinderh. **48**: 188, 1929-30.
13. Stuart, H. C.: J. Pediat. **5**: 194, 1934.
14. Jeans, P. C., and Stearns, G.: Proc. Soc. Exper. Biol. & Med. **31**: 1159, 1934; **32**: 1464, 1935.
    Stearns, G., and Jeans, P. C.: Proc. Am. Soc. Biol. Chem. **114**: c, 1936.
15. Wetzel, N. C.: J. Pediat. **4**: 465, 1934.
    Editorial, J. A. M. A. **104**: 1826, 1935.
    Sherman, H. C., and Booher, L. E.: J. Biol. Chem. **93**: 93, 1931.
    Campbell, H. L., Bessey, O. A., and Sherman, H. C.: J. Biol. Chem. **110**: 703, 1935.

THE PREMATURE INFANT

William W. Swanson, M.D., Vernon E. Lennarson, M.D., and
Fred L. Adair, M.D.
Chicago, Ill.

THIS study supplements the recent publication on institutional mortality of the newborn infant[1] and deals with the care and vital statistics of 752 premature infants in 10,660 consecutive births. Comparisons with similar data, published from other clinics, have been made on the basis of weight since this one measurement is at present the only uniform criterion of prematurity. In recent literature,[2, 3] specialized procedures have been stressed, which are of undoubted value in the care of premature infants but are beyond the reach of many clinicians. The data reported in this study are intended to show the results obtainable with readily available and simple measures.

In Table I the distribution of the 752 premature infants from the 10,660 consecutive births is shown according to three criteria: body weight, crown-to-heel length, and period of gestation. The 97 infants over 2,500 grams at birth have been included since they are considered by two of these three criteria to be prematurely born.[1] The 47 infants in the fourth group have been included for purposes of comparison with data using weight as the only criterion of prematurity.

Table I

Classification of 752* Premature Infants in 10,660 Consecutive Births

WT. IN GM. AT BIRTH	CROWN-HEEL LENGTH 47 CM. AND UNDER		CROWN-HEEL LENGTH OVER 47 CM.		TOTAL
	GESTATION 37 WK. AND UNDER	GESTATION OVER 37 WK.	GESTATION 37 WK. AND UNDER	GESTATION OVER 37 WK.	
1,000 and under	31				31
1,001 to 1,500	51				51
1,501 to 2,000	141	13	1		155
2,001 to 2,500	179	166	26	47	418
2,501 to 2,800	97				97
Total	499	179	27	47	752

*Fourteen premature infants were not included in this total since they were discharged to other institutions, eleven of the fourteen going to the Century of Progress.

In Table II are shown data from two clinics with respect to (1) the average initial weight loss, (2) the average time required to regain this weight loss, and (3) the average length of stay in the hospital. These findings are compared on the basis of weight. The data from the 752

From the Chicago Lying-In Hospital and the Departments of Obstetrics and Gynecology and the Department of Pediatrics, University of Chicago.

premature infants appear to show that a very small infant may regain birth weight in as short a time as the one born near term.

TABLE II

COMPARATIVE STATISTICS FROM PREMATURE STATIONS

	CHICAGO LYING-IN HOSPITAL*					SARAH MORRIS HOSPITAL†				
	NO. OF IN-FANTS	BIRTH WEIGHT 1,000 TO 1,500	1,501 TO 2,000	2,001 TO 2,500	2,501 TO 2,800	NO. OF IN-FANTS	1,000 TO 1,500	1,501 TO 2,000	2,001 TO 2,500	2,501 TO 3,000
Initial weight loss	15	96.2				77	98.0			
Average number of	118		120.4			251		173.8		
grams	393			147.2		290			178.1	
	92				210.7	31				231.8
Birth weight regained	15	8.2				77	18.6			
Average number of	118		9.4			251		14.4		
days	393			8.0		290			11.8	
	92				8.4	31				12.0
Stay in hospital	15	41.6				77	45.7			
Average number of	118		27.3			251		30.5		
days	393			13.4		290			19.9	
	92				12.5	31				16.8

*All infants under 2000 grams were given breast milk only.

†Includes infants born in homes and other hospitals and brought to Sarah Morris Hospital for subsequent care during years 1930 to and including 1933.

In Table III are shown the mortality rates for the various weight groups during the first twenty-four and forty-eight hours and then for weekly intervals. It should be emphasized in defense of this mortality finding that every premature infant, if only breathing for a few seconds, was recorded as a living birth. It should also be mentioned that of the 134 deaths, 53 died in the birth room and of the 81 infants who reached the nursery, 62 died within the first forty-eight hours.

TABLE III

MORTALITY DURING HOSPITAL RESIDENCE IN A GROUP OF 752 PREMATURE INFANTS

BIRTH WEIGHT IN GM.	NO.	NUMBER OF DEATHS: WITHIN 24 HR.	WITHIN 48 HR.	3-7 DAYS, INCLUSIVE	8-14 DAYS, INCLUSIVE	15 DAYS TO END OF RESIDENCE	TOTAL NUMBER OF DEATHS	MORTALITY PER CENT	INFANTS SURVIVING FIRST 48 HR. MORTALITY PER CENT
Under 1,000	31	29	1	1			31	100.0	100.0
1,001 to 1,500	51	27	2	5	1	1	36	70.6	31.8
1,501 to 2,000	155	27	5	2	2	1	37	23.8	4.1
2,001 to 2,500	418	16	3	5	1		25	6.0	1.5
2,501 to 2,800	97	5					5	5.2	0.0
Total	752	104	11	13	4	2	134	17.8	3.0

Considering the table as a whole, the total mortality of 17.8 per cent is as low as any found in the literature, and if it is permissible to exclude all deaths occurring within the first forty-eight hours, as thought justifiable by Blackfan and Yaglou and also by Hess, the mortality is less than 3 per cent.

Table IV summarizes the data showing the percentage of premature infants who were graduated from the Chicago Lying-In nurseries in the years from 1931 to 1935. It should be mentioned that no premature infants were received from homes or other hospitals.

TABLE IV

PERCENTAGE OF PREMATURE INFANTS GRADUATED

BIRTH WEIGHT IN GM.	NUMBER	GRADUATED		NUMBER SURVIVING FIRST 48 HR.	PER CENT GRADUATED OF INFANTS SURVIVING FIRST 48 HR.
		NUMBER	PER CENT		
1,000 and under	31	0	0	1	0
1,001 to 1,500	51	15	29.4	22	68.2
1,501 to 2,000	155	118	76.1	123	95.9
2,001 to 2,500	418	393	94.0	399	98.5
2,501 to 2,800	97	92	94.8	92	100.0
Totals	752	618	82.2	637	97.0

In Table V are listed the causes of death as revealed by necropsy findings and as judged by clinical signs. Neither upper respiratory infections nor serious digestive disorders played any prominent part in this mortality. A few infants at autopsy showed pneumonic involvement, but this finding was usually associated with atelectasis. The low incidence of infection may be due in part to the fact that not more than four premature infants were together in the same nursery at any one time.

TABLE V

CAUSES OF DEATH OF 134 PREMATURE INFANTS

CAUSE OF DEATH	LENGTH OF LIFE				TOTAL
	UNDER 1 DAY	2-7 DAYS INCLUSIVE	8-14 DAYS INCLUSIVE	15 DAYS TO END OF RESIDENCE	
Congenital weakness	64	11	1	0	76
Accidents of labor	14	9	0	1	24
Pneumonia	0	0	2	0	2
Atelectasis	3	0	0	0	3
Congenital syphilis	0	1	0	0	1
Malformations	9	3	1	1	14
Hemorrhage	0	0	0	0	0
Sepsis	1	0	0	0	1
Asphyxia	13	0	0	0	13
Accidental	0	0	0	0	0
Undetermined	0	0	0	0	0
Total	104	24	4	2	134

The care, hygiene, and nutrition of these 752 premature infants cannot be discussed in detail, but the principles of management will be outlined briefly. The extent to which specialized nursing care is required depends primarily upon the stage of prematurity. Conservation of heat is the first essential of good care and is accomplished by the use of a heat lamp immediately after delivery. The premature infant may either be covered with a garment of warmed flannel wool or, if the infant is very small, by a light covering of warmed cotton batting and transferred to a Nobel box type of incubator.[4] The regular carrying out of such routine procedures as weighing, bathing and taking of temperature often depends upon the infant's condition.

The most frequent complication occurring during delivery is asphyxia, and the younger the premature infant the more frequent is its incidence. The first step in the treatment of asphyxia is the removal of obstructing material, such as blood and mucus, from the oropharynx or trachea by a tracheal catheter. Pure oxygen or oxygen (95 per cent) and carbon dioxide (5 per cent) should be administered by mask until the color of the infant's skin indicates improvement.

It is often advisable to continue oxygen-carbon dioxide administrations for short periods (3 to 5 minutes) at one-hour intervals for days to forestall cyanotic attacks. The best method of resuscitation, if respiration should cease, is the gentle rhythmical compression of the thorax about 15 times per minute combined with the administration of oxygen and carbon dioxide. It is not always easy to determine the cause of cyanotic attacks frequently seen in premature infants. Often an attack occurs during or after a feeding. Apparently the effort of swallowing and distention of the stomach are contributory causes. Many premature infants suffer from various degrees of atelectasis after birth,[5] and, if this is extensive, it may predispose to cyanotic attacks. Other more serious causes of cyanosis, however, are congenital heart conditions and intracranial hemorrhage.

The handling of a premature infant during any procedure, such as feeding, the taking of the temperature, bathing, weighing, and the changing of the cotton pad or diaper, should be done with as little exposure as possible. Routinely the temperature is taken twice a day, the body is cleansed with olive oil, albolene, or baby oils every other day for two weeks and then every day, and the infant, if very small, is weighed twice a week and later every other day.

The maintenance of body temperature has in all instances been accomplished by the use of a Nobel box type of incubator containing only one heating element, a 40-watt lamp. The very small infants were in addition placed in a service room where the temperature ranged from 80° to 95° F. and where the humidity was high. As a rule, a very small infant is likely to have a somewhat subnormal temperature. If an attempt is made to maintain the premature infant at all times at the supposedly normal level of 98.6° F., decidedly unfavorable results may follow.[1]

Many factors enter into the consideration of feeding and sustaining the nutrition of the smaller premature infant. Proportionally the need of fluids and food is at least equal to that of the full-term infant. However, because of the immature stage of development the premature infant is neither ready nor able to ingest food and fluids in comparable amounts.

All of the 752 premature infants were started on breast milk which was given either by dropper, tube, or bottle. It became necessary in many instances, however, to change the food after a few weeks to a simple artificial formula of two-thirds cow's milk (evaporated or pasteurized) with a 5 per cent dextrin-containing carbohydrate. Feedings were started for most infants about four hours after birth and continued at three-hour intervals eight times during the day. Water was offered by dropper one hour before feeding as long as the milk intake was less than the normal fluid requirement, approximately one-sixth to one-eighth of the body weight. The amount of breast milk given varied with the infant's size. An infant weighing 1,000 gm. may be started on 2 c.c. of breast milk at each feeding; one weighing 1,500 gm., 4 to 8 c.c.; and one weighing 2,000 gm., 16 c.c. After the first few feedings, each alternate feeding may be increased from 1 c.c. to 4 c.c. every day or every other day. It must be emphasized that the amount of food or fluid readily taken will depend even more on the vitality than on the weight.

The very small premature infant can take only limited amounts of food at any one time. To increase the caloric intake but not the volume of the food, a teaspoonful of dryco may be added to every ounce of breast milk, or, if it is desired to increase the minerals and proteins, the formula may include one-third buttermilk or one-third skimmed lactic acid milk. An increase in the protein content of the food is important when the stools are loose or too frequent. In the present routine of feeding very little attention is paid to total calories. The idea that one should strive to give so many calories per pound or per kilogram has been overemphasized. The ideal sought is to feed each premature infant an amount productive of a consistent gain in weight. On such a schedule the birth weight may often be doubled in less than fifty days. A good average gain should be about 30 gm. a day. It is frequently found that premature infants have refractory periods when little or no gain in weight takes place. This growth inactivity or failure to gain weight is not due to an insufficiency of food or lack of care since a stimulant in the form of 10 to 20 c.c. of whole blood injected intramuscularly, preferably in the infant's buttocks, will start the growth impulse. This type of treatment was suggested some years ago by Dr. Blackfan and has been of material value in shortening the duration of the premature infant's residence in the hospital.

Three accessory food factors are given to those premature infants who remain longer than two weeks in the hospital. Iron in the form of ferric ammonium citrate, 1 drop of a 20 per cent solution, is added to each feeding by the end of the second week. Orange juice and cod liver oil are started in small amounts beginning with the fourth week and the dosage of each increased gradually until one ounce of the former and two teaspoonfuls of the latter are given before the end of the third month.

In the care of these 752 premature infants, the work has been carried on with a continually changing nursing personnel. From the standpoint of the nurse, this frequent rotation has definite advantages, but the vigilance of the staff must necessarily be increased.

SUMMARY

Statistical data and a brief summary of the institutional care of 752 premature infants are presented. The total mortality is 17.8 per cent. Excluding deaths occurring within forty-eight hours after birth, the mortality is less than 3 per cent.

REFERENCES

1. Swanson, Wm. W., Turner, A. R., and Adair, Fred L.: J. Pediat **7**: 516, 1935.
2. Blackfan, K. D., and Yaglou, C. P.: Am. J. Dis. Child. **46**: 1175, 1933.
3. Hess, J. H., Mohr, G. J., and Bartelme, P. F.: The Physical and Mental Growth of Prematurely Born Children, Chicago, 1934, University of Chicago Press, Ch. IV.
4. Parmelee, A. H.: Am. J. Dis. Child. **41**: 33, 1931.
5. Farber, Sidney, and Wilson, J. L.: Am. J. Dis. Child. **46**: 572, 1933.

MORTALITY AMONG PREMATURELY BORN INFANTS

Ethel C. Dunham, M.D.
Washington, D. C.

THE present high mortality among prematurely born infants constitutes a large part of the general problem of infant mortality in the United States today. At least half the deaths of infants in the first year occur in the first month of life, and of these neonatal deaths nearly half are caused by premature birth.

The infant mortality rate as a whole (infants under one year of age) declined from 1915* until 1933, when the decline gave place to a slight rise, which was followed by another slight rise in 1934. The mortality rate among infants under one month, however, declined much more slowly than that for infants under one year. The mortality rate from premature birth has declined only about half as much as the neonatal mortality rate and only about one-third as much as the infant mortality rate as a whole. The problem of reducing neonatal mortality is, to a great extent, a question of reducing mortality from premature birth.

The extent of the problem of premature birth in the United States can only be estimated. It is probable that there is considerable variation in different communities and different sections of the country and among births in hospitals and in homes. Woodbury[1] found among nearly 23,000 liveborn infants in eight cities that 5 per cent were born prematurely (after a gestation period of eight months or less). In New York State in 1933, 4 per cent of the live births were reported as premature.[2] Schwarz and Kohn[3] found among more than 11,000 infants born at home nearly 3 per cent who were regarded by them as premature because the birth weights were 2,500 gm. or less. On the latter basis recent hospital reports show between 6 and 7 per cent of births to be premature.

When considering how mortality among premature infants may be reduced further, it is desirable to analyze the factors that bring about premature birth, to inquire into the mortality rates and the causes of death among premature infants, to attempt to evaluate the efforts that have been made or are being made to lower this mortality, and to estimate the results achieved. In this paper the discussion of studies that have been made for these purposes will be limited mainly to those made in the United States.

The importance of premature birth as a factor in infant mortality has been referred to frequently over a period of many years in the medical literature of the United States and other countries. Investiga-

From the United States Department of Labor, Children's Bureau, Washington. D. C.
This paper was presented before the Seventh Pan American Child Congress, Mexico City, October 12, 1935.

*In 1915 the United States Birth Registration Area was established and since then comparable figures have been available from the Bureau of the Census.

tions on this subject made in the United States are far less numerous and, as a whole, less adequate than those made in other countries. Moreover, since investigators in the United States have, as a rule, used neither a uniform criterion of prematurity nor similar methods of analyzing their figures, comparison of results is not always possible.

Studies of causes of premature birth made so far have shown that in nearly half the cases investigated the causes of the premature birth were not determined. It is apparent, therefore, that further investigations on this subject are needed. Of the known causes of premature birth, that most frequently reported is multiple pregnancy. Other important causes, reported in varying frequency by different authors, are toxemias of pregnancy, syphilis, chronic diseases of the mother such as nephritis and heart disease, and bleeding due to placental abnormalities (placenta previa and premature separation of the placenta).

Although multiple pregnancy is considered the most frequent cause of premature birth, the mortality of infants in this group of cases is probably not very high, since many of them are not so premature as the weight alone would indicate. The toxemias of pregnancy, although apparently not preventable, can probably in many cases be modified in severity by proper prenatal care. In this way the need for induction of labor can often be prevented or delayed until the fetus has reached a viable period. Syphilis, it is hardly necessary to point out, is *the* outstanding preventable cause of premature birth. It is a fact, however, that even in the most enlightened communities syphilis is still reported as a frequent cause. When such conditions as severe cardiac or renal disease exist in a pregnant woman, prolongation of pregnancy may be impractical. Likewise, in certain other conditions, such as bleeding due to placental abnormalities, little can be done with the knowledge at present available to prevent premature birth.

Some causal influences that seem to affect the occurrence of premature births were pointed out in a Children's Bureau study of causes of infant mortality published in 1925.[1] It was shown that a higher proportion of premature births occurred among plural births than among single ones and among male infants than among female. The proportion was high among first infants, infants of young mothers, and infants born at short intervals after preceding births, and it was especially high among infants born to mothers employed away from home during pregnancy. The direct relationship, moreover, that the mother's health bears to prematurity was shown by the very high proportion (39 per cent) of premature births among infants born alive to mothers who died either at confinement or within one month thereafter.

In addition to further studies of the causes of premature birth, studies should be made of methods for prolonging pregnancy safely in the presence of complications, and the knowledge already available should be more generally applied in an effort to reduce further the incidence of premature birth.

There is great variation in reported mortality among premature infants and some question as to the best methods of caring for them.

A member of the Children's Bureau staff recently visited more than 100 hospitals in twenty-seven large cities of the United States to obtain a general idea of methods commonly used in the care of premature infants and of the results obtained. Although a great variety of methods of care were in use in the different hospitals, in only four had an evaluation of any method been made on the basis of morbidity or mortality. A number of the hospitals, however, later compiled their statistics and reported a mortality varying all the way from 18 to 94 per cent.

Reports published between 1921 and 1934 of studies of the mortality among premature infants, in which any infant having a birth weight of 2,500 gm. or less was classified as premature, show, for studies made in the United States, a mortality ranging from 27 to 77 per cent and, in European countries, from 13 to 55 per cent. Furthermore, recent studies, as yet unpublished, made in four large hospitals in the United States show a mortality between 25 and 34 per cent, averaging somewhat less than that given in the earlier reports.

In evaluating these mortality figures, however, a number of factors must be taken into consideration. All reports available have shown that when studied on the basis of birth weight, mortality is inversely proportional to the weight. For example, in the four hospitals already referred to the mortality for infants weighing less than 1,000 gm. at birth was high, varying between 93 and 100 per cent, whereas for those weighing between 2,000 and 2,500 gm. the mortality was low, varying between 6 and 14 per cent. The mortality for infants in two other intermediate weight groups decreased as the weight range increased. Comparisons of mortality among premature infants should be made only when the weights of the infants included in the groups to be compared fall within certain specified narrow ranges. Moreover, since the mortality for premature infants born at home and brought into hospitals for care is known to be higher as a rule than that for infants born in hospitals and cared for in the hospitals in which they are born, these two groups should be considered separately in evaluating results of care. As has been mentioned, multiple births also should be taken into consideration, as there is some evidence that, when birth weight is the criterion of prematurity, the mortality for premature twins is lower than that for single premature infants.

The extent of the efforts that have been made or are being made to reduce mortality among premature infants is difficult to determine, since, as has been pointed out, reports are not numerous and criteria of prematurity as well as methods of analyzing material have differed in the hands of various investigators; moreover, in reports advocating various methods of care of premature infants, it is only in rare instances that satisfactory statistical evidence of the results of care has been presented. Although birth weight is probably not the most accurate measure of prematurity, yet for clinical and statistical purposes the adoption of a birth weight of 2,500 gm. or less as the basis for the diagnosis of prematurity would be advantageous since it would set up a uniform standard. Adoption of this standard in the United States would permit comparisons with the results reported by foreign investigators, who have almost without exception used it.

The causes of *death* of premature infants are often difficult to determine, as is shown by the fact that "premature birth" alone is the cause most frequently reported. If pathologic and other laboratory studies were made in these cases, intracranial hemorrhage and septicemia would be found to account for the death of some of them. There is little doubt that premature infants are peculiarly susceptible to intracranial trauma during birth, and intracranial hemorrhage is one of the most important causes of death reported. Infection, particularly general septicemia, although frequently not reported as such because not recognized, is nevertheless another important cause of death. Special studies in which routine cultures of the blood were made of premature infants ill with obscure conditions have shown in a number of instances the presence of blood stream infection in the absence of the usual clinical evidences of it. Atelectasis, a condition that is of course physiologic during intrauterine existence, is also frequently reported as a cause of death, but probably should not be regarded as the primary cause in very immature infants but simply the result of immaturity. The absence of demonstrable pathology in many premature infants who die suggests that they may succumb through lack of certain hormones or other substances which in full-term infants are probably transferred from the mother by the placental route in the last weeks of pregnancy. Some clinical reports[4] tend to confirm these theories, and there is here a field for research, the results of which may offer a greater hope of bringing about reduction of mortality among infants of low birth weight than clinical methods have afforded as yet.

Certain fundamental rules for the care of premature infants have become firmly established through use, such as maintenance of normal body temperature, isolation in an effort to prevent infection, and treatment of asphyxial attacks. Methods of feeding the premature infant are not so well established, since some authorities advocate breast milk as the only food for these infants while others obtain what they consider equally favorable results with artificial feeding. Some advocate frequent feedings of small amounts; others infrequent feedings of somewhat larger amounts; some feed the premature infant only by bottle, medicine dropper, or Breck feeder, others only by gavage, while still others use combinations of these methods. The advocacy of such methods of treatment as inhalations of carbon dioxide or oxygen or both, parenteral administration of fluids, transfusions of blood, and so forth, varies greatly from clinic to clinic. All these questions will be greatly clarified when more accurate studies of results have been made.

Evaluation by statistical analysis of methods of care of premature infants has been made by a number of workers in this field. Hess,[5] for example, has shown a decrease in mortality over a period of twelve years in the Premature Infant Station of the Sarah Morris Hospital in Chicago. He attributes some of this decrease to the education of physicians and parents, which has resulted in an increase in the number of premature infants sent from the home to the hospital within the first twenty-four hours of birth, and some of it to the use of a special electrically heated "hand ambulance" which protects the infant from chilling during transportation. Blackfan and Yaglou[6] have presented statistical evidence of lowering of morbidity and mortality by the air-conditioning of the nursery so that certain temperature-humidity relationships were maintained. Clifford[7] has pointed out the value of roentgen ray demonstration of fetal development in utero and its practical application in lowering fetal mortality through control of the time at which pregnancy is terminated.

A vigorous city-wide campaign has recently been inaugurated in Chicago by Bundesen[8] to reduce the death rate from prematurity, which he found to be as low as 5 per thousand in some institutions but as high as 500 per thousand in others. The American Pediatric Society in 1934 appointed a committee which is studying the problems of neonatal mortality and morbidity, particularly when due to premature birth. The Children's Bureau, as part of its research program, has undertaken an intensive study of premature infants in an effort to develop methods that may reduce the high mortality now prevailing among these infants.

SUMMARY

Reduction of mortality among prematurely born infants constitutes a large part of the infant mortality problem in the United States today.

Since in a large proportion of cases the causes of premature birth are reported as "unknown," further efforts should be made to determine these causes. Moreover, information now available as to the causes of premature birth should be more generally applied in efforts to prolong pregnancy until the infant is mature enough to survive.

The causes of death of prematurely born infants are in at least half the cases reported as "unknown." Further investigations should be made, since the causes must be understood before attempts to lower mortality can be intelligently made.

The methods of care and treatment of prematurely born infants now in use should be evaluated on the basis of morbidity and mortality studies, and the methods found to be of value should be more widely applied. Since it is among infants of low birth weight that mortality is highest, further efforts should be made to develop special methods of caring for this group of infants.

It is only when the medical profession and the public become better aware of the problem of the prematurely born infant, and when they make concerted efforts to solve it, that mortality among these infants will be reduced to any great extent.

REFERENCES

1. Woodbury, Robert Morse: Causal Factors in Infant Mortality, Children's Bureau Publication, No. 142, 1925.
2. Personal communication to the author.
3. Schwarz, Herman, and Kohn, Jerome L.: Am. J. Dis. Child. **21**: 296, 1921.
4. Mügel, Gertrud: Monatschr. f. Geburtsh. u. Gynäk. **88**: 79, 1931.
5. Hess, Julius H., Mohr, George J., and Bartelme, Phyllis F.: The Physical and Mental Growth of Prematurely Born Children, Chicago, 1934, The University of Chicago Press, pp. 12-14.
6. Blackfan, Kenneth D., and Yaglou, Constantin P.: Am. J. Dis. Child. **46**: 1175, 1933.
7. Clifford, S. H.: J. A. M. A. **103**: 1117, 1934.
8. Am. J. Pub. Health **25**: 750, 1935.

THE PATHOGENIC SIGNIFICANCE OF "LATE LACTOSE-FERMENTING" COLI-LIKE BACILLI

LEROY D. FOTHERGILL, M.D., CECIL A. KRAKOWER, M.D., AND
DON FREEMAN, M.D.
BOSTON, MASS.

SEVERAL years ago one of us[1] reported the not infrequent occurrence of a heterogeneous group of gram-negative, late lactose- or non-lactose-fermenting bacilli, in the stools of infants suffering from summer diarrhea. No definite evidence was obtained that such organisms played an etiologic rôle in this syndrome although in an occasional infant the serum agglutinated the organism isolated from its stool. Since the question of pathogenicity of these organisms is obscure, it was felt justified to review our own experience of the last few years. It was felt that a combined bacteriologic, clinical, and pathologic study of those patients from whom such organisms were recovered might shed some light on this question.

It is difficult, if not impossible, to review the literature concerning this group of organisms with precision because of the lack of differential descriptive detail in many of the reports. Again, the confusing similarity between this group and the paratyphoid group makes a number of the descriptions inadequate.

Some consideration was given to these organisms during the World War in the course of bacteriologic and protozoologic studies of the feces of soldiers convalescing from dysentery and other enteric diseases. Dean, Adamson, Giles, and Williamson[2] studied 488 dysentery convalescents and in 77 instances found organisms that seem to belong to this group. They make no mention whether or not their strains were motile. Douglas[3] reported finding similar organisms in a small group of men who had contracted dysentery in Gallipoli. Fildes,[4] and Dobell, Gettings, Jepps, and Stephens[5] made similar observations on dysentery convalescents. Glynn and Robinson[6] in an intensive study of 2,360 convalescents from enteric disease report, "A non-motile, indol-positive bacillus producing acid and gas in glucose, mannite and maltose was the commonest non-lactose fermenter in the feces of enteritis convalescents and 'normals.' Bacilli like these, but also dulcite fermenters, occurred in 3.2 per cent of 'normals' and in 11 per cent of 'convalescents.'" These authors state further that "indol-positive, paratyphoid-like bacilli are probably very rarely pathogenic; one variety, however, has been found three times in the blood during life; they are often found in the feces of acute and convalescent enteritis cases and sometimes in normal feces."

From the Department of Pediatrics, the Department of Pathology, and the Department of Bacteriology and Immunology, Harvard Medical School, and the Infants' and the Children's Hospitals.

Since the World War a few reports have appeared concerning the presence of these organisms in stool cultures. Dudgeon[7] in 1926 reported on their occasional occurrence and thought that they might cause intestinal disorders. Fothergill[1] found them with considerable frequency in the stools of infants suffering from summer diarrhea. He believed that in some instances they may have been of etiologic importance. Johnston and her associates[8] also noted the occasional presence of such organisms in the feces of infants with summer diarrhea. Kriebel[9] isolated twenty-nine strains during the course of a study of the feces of food handlers in the various Harvard dining rooms. These were all healthy individuals.

In 1918 Bronfenbrenner and Davis[10] isolated similar organisms from food during a study of food poisoning. They made the important observation that, by frequent transfer and by increasing the percentage of lactose, these organisms could be adapted to ferment this carbohydrate. For this reason it seemed that the bacilli observed by them were closely related to the colon group.

It would appear from a review of the literature regarding the occurrence of these organisms in the intestinal tract that there is little or no evidence that they are of importance in the production of gastrointestinal symptoms or actual enteric infection. However, more direct evidence has been obtained that they may be pathogenic under special circumstances in the urinary tract. In a study of *B. coli* infections of the urinary tract Dudgeon, Wordley and Bawtree[11] refer to two cases of acute pyelocystitis from which slow lactose-fermenting bacilli were isolated. One of these terminated fatally. Later Dudgeon[12] reported a group of forty-nine cases of infection of the genitourinary tract due to these organisms. He felt that these infections were more severe and lasted longer than ordinary colon bacillus infections. On the other hand, ultimate complete recovery and freedom from organisms was more common. Positive blood cultures were not obtained. Dudgeon and Pulvertaft[13] subsequently reported a more detailed bacteriologic study of these urinary infections.

In Caldwell's study[14] slow lactose-fermenting bacilli were found in 9 per cent of 112 urine specimens. However, the cultural data, as presented, are not sufficient to convince the reader that all these organisms belonged to the particular group under discussion. There was no clear differentiation from members of the dispar group.

A number of investigators, particularly Dudgeon and Pulvertaft,[13] Fothergill,[1] Kennedy, Cummings, and Morrow,[15] and Kriebel,[9] have studied the cultural, biochemical, and serologic characteristics of this group. It will be pertinent briefly to review its outstanding biologic characteristics with special reference to classification.

It should be emphasized that these organisms are easily confused with the paratyphoid group. When fecal material or urine is plated on one of the differential lactose-containing plates, the nonlactose-fermenting type of colony is produced. Such colonies are essentially no different from those of typhoid, paratyphoid, or dysentery bacilli. When such colonies are picked to Russell's double sugar agar slants, they produce the typical ''paratyphoid'' reaction, i.e., an alkaline slant with acid and gas production in the butt of the tube. Further study, however, clearly differentiates these organisms from the paratyphoid group. The most striking reaction in this respect is the late fermentation of lactose. This sugar is fermented by the majority of strains after from two to fourteen days' incubation. Practically all of these strains form indol—a valuable differential reaction from the paratyphoid group. Motility is variable although the majority of strains are nonmotile. Most of the strains isolated from the cases described in this study were nonmotile. Further differentiation is obtained by agglutination. Such organisms are practically never agglutinated by the serums of the more common members of the paratyphoid group. If such agglutination does occur, it is only in very low dilution and never approaches the specific titer of such serums. These are the important general characteristics which permit one to separate these organisms from the paratyphoid bacilli.

Our own experience has shown that these bacteria form a very heterogeneous group,[1] both culturally and by cross-agglutination reactions. Kriebel was able to separate her twenty-nine strains into seven subdivisions on the basis of fermentation reactions. It is likely that more variants would have been found if more strains had been studied. Furthermore, we doubt if such grouping would be substantiated by a serologic study.

It is, of course, difficult to place these organisms into any scheme of classification. As a group they possess certain common characteristics which seem to separate them definitely from the well-known gram-negative intestinal bacilli. With respect to their cultural reactions they seem to occupy an intermediate taxonomic position between the paratyphoid and the colon aerogenes groups with, as Kriebel has suggested, a closer resemblance to the colon bacilli. Furthermore, as discussed below, they may be dissociation variants of one of these.

It will be recalled that Bronfenbrenner and Davis found that organisms, probably similar to those under discussion, could be adapted to ferment lactose, a fact which suggested to them close kinship to the colon group. Dudgeon and Pulvertaft were less successful in adapting their ''urine'' strains to lactose fermentation.

Dulaney[16] in 1928 studied the dissociation of *B. coli communis.* It was found that the S to R change, with distinct difference in the virulence of the variants, could be produced by aging provided that the ultimate reaction of the medium remained alkaline. Dissociation was inhibited by growth in a medium rendered acid by the utilization of sugars. With respect to the cultural reactions of these variants this author states, "A distinct difference, however, was found in the reactions which the stabilized R form gave on Endo plates and in Russell's double sugar tubes. While the S organism produced the typical acid reaction with characteristic metallic sheen on Endo plates, the R colonies remained colorless. On Russell's double sugar medium the S form soon gave the typical *B. coli* picture while, with the R organism, the slant either remained unchanged or developed very slowly a faint acid reaction." This study suggests that these late lactose-fermenting organisms might have been rough variants of the colon group.

Nungester and Anderson[17] published a contradictory report. They isolated a *B. coli*-like organism from an empyema of the gallbladder and studied its dissociation variants. They produced two forms, a rough variant which fermented lactose and an S variant which did not. The change from the nonlactose-fermenting S form to the lactose-fermenting R form was easily effected, whereas the opposite change was more difficult to produce. Kriebel found that continued growth of her strains in 5 per cent lactose solution resulted in varying degrees of dissociation into lactose-fermenting types. This suggested to her that she was dealing with dissociation variants of the colon group.

Another hypothesis that has been offered to explain the presence of these organisms in the stools of patients with diarrheal disease or in those of convalescents from such disease is that they may be normal inhabitants of the upper intestinal tract and are found in the stools only when the intestine is being rapidly emptied during a diarrheal state due to some other cause. In fact, Dudgeon[7] states, "In my experience slow lactose-fermenters are present in cultures of the feces obtained from the region of the caecum more frequently than from the lower bowel, at the few opportunities which have occurred during life."

In order to test this hypothesis, observations were made at necropsy on 38 patients from various levels of the bowel. The technic employed was as follows: After the intestine was freed from its mesentery, a small transverse cut was made with sterile scissors at the desired level. A sterile cotton swab was inserted through the opening and a small amount of liquid and solid material was obtained. This was emulsified in broth and immediately streaked on eosin methylene blue plates. After incubation, suspicious colonies were picked and carried through to final identification. Cultures were taken in this manner from the midduodenum, midjejunum, upper ileum, lower ileum, cecum, and sigmoid. There was no selection of cases. So far as possible, cultures were taken from consecutive autopsies regardless of the cause of death.

These organisms were recovered from 13 per cent of the cases. There was no significant difference in the frequency with which they were isolated from different levels of the intestinal tract. This would indicate that these organisms do not inhabit one level of the bowel more frequently than another. Furthermore, the gross frequency of positive results in this series was essentially the same as that obtained during the course of routine stool cultures.

During the past few years organisms belonging in this category have been isolated from 107 cases (excluding the above necropsy study). They were most frequently obtained from stool cultures. Occasionally they were isolated from urine and from purulent material such as appendicial abscess. There was no reason to suppose that these organisms were of significance in 94 of these cases. A few of the patients in this group had enteric disease due to known etiologic agents such as the typhoid or dysentery bacillus. In the remaining 13 cases they played a significant part in the production of disease. The individual patients are presented below. Necropsy findings are described for a few cases that present striking features. It is felt that an analysis of these cases may serve to clarify the question of the pathogenicity of the late lactose-fermenting gram-negative bacilli.

CASE 1.—M. C., a six-year-eleven-month-old girl, was admitted because of chronic pyuria. A late lactose-fermenting bacillus was recovered by culture from catheterized urine specimens.

CASE 2.—G. K., a three-year-ten-month-old boy, was brought to the hospital because of diarrhea and abdominal pain for four days and fever and vomiting of one day's duration. He was operated on for a ruptured appendix and localized peritonitis. Cultures of pus from the peritoneal cavity yielded a late lactose-fermenting bacillus, *B. coli,* and *B. pyocyaneus.*

CASE 3.—E. K., a five-year-old boy, was admitted to the hospital for operation for acute appendicitis with abscess formation. A pure culture of a late lactose-fermenting bacillus was obtained from pus from the peritoneal cavity.

CASE 4.—D. P., a one-year-old female infant, had been receiving treatment for congenital syphilis for several months. Intramuscular injections of sulpharsphenamine were being given in the gluteal region. She developed a deep abscess of one buttock, which was incised and drained. A pure culture of a late lactose-fermenting bacillus was cultivated from this pus.

CASE 5.—W. D., a male infant, aged six months, was admitted because of severe pyelonephritis. He was extremely ill for several weeks with a septic, swinging temperature. A late lactose-fermenting bacillus was recovered by blood culture. The same organism was obtained in pure culture from catheter specimens of urine. This patient's serum agglutinated this organism in a dilution of 1:1280.

CASE 6.—J. W., a twenty-month-old infant, was admitted to the hospital because of severe, acute pyelonephritis. A cystogram resulted in a bilateral reflex. The right ureter was tortuous and somewhat dilated. A late lactose-fermenting bacillus was recovered in pure culture from catheterized urine on two occasions.

CASE 7.—P. C., a seven-year-three-month-old girl, was brought to the hospital for operation for a ruptured acute appendix. Pus from the peritoneal cavity yielded a pure culture of a late lactose-fermenting bacillus.

In the above group of cases this organism played an important rôle in the production of disease. It should be pointed out that in these cases the type of local disease produced is identical with that commonly caused by the colon bacillus. In the following cases a description of the pathologic changes is included.

CASE 8.—B. D., a two and one-half-year-old girl was admitted to the hospital because of fever and pain in the left lower abdominal quadrant. Urinary frequency and urgency were additional complaints. Physical examination revealed a large mass in the region of the left kidney. A late lactose-fermenting bacillus was isolated in pure culture from a specimen of urine obtained by catheterization. Diagnosis of perinephritic abscess was made. At operation a large abscess was found surrounding the left kidney and extending down along the course of the left ureter. The kidney was small and largely destroyed. Pus oozed from its cortex. Cultures of the pus yielded *B. coli, B. alkaligenes,* and a late lactose-fermenting bacillus. Specimens of bladder urine obtained by catheter during the convalescent period yielded pure cultures of a late lactose-fermenting bacillus. Postoperative convalescence was normal except for continued pyuria.

The patient was readmitted a month after discharge because of continued pyuria. Retrograde pyelograms revealed a distended, sacculated, left ureteral stump. Cultures of bladder urine and fluid from the ureteral stump taken at this time yielded a pure culture of a late lactose-fermenting bacillus. Laparotomy was performed five days later and the ureteral stump removed. Cultures of abdominal fluid and fluid from the ureteral stump taken at operation yielded the same organism. A subsequent culture of bladder urine was still positive. Convalescence from this second operation was uneventful, and the patient has continued in good health.

Pathologic Examination (S-34-106).—The kidney was large. Small, elevated nodules, averaging 0.8 cm. in diameter, were scattered over the external surface. Some of these presented grayish white, necrotic centers with, in one instance, a cratered area. On section the pelvis and calyces occupied about three-quarters of the cut surface of the kidney. Their walls were greatly thickened and their mucosal aspects, grayish red in color. The remaining renal substance measured from 0.2 to 0.3 cm. in thickness. The usual markings were obliterated, and in the subcapsular zones there were about twelve small abscesses, 0.4 cm. in diameter, with dark red hemorrhagic borders. The wall of the ureter was greatly thickened.

Microscopically there was very little well-preserved renal substance. There were extensive necroses and hemorrhages, together with areas of suppuration. Closer to the pelvis, in the remaining cortical and medullary portions, the inflammatory process was of more chronic character with increase in fibrous tissue, tubular atrophy, hyalinization of glomeruli and the presence of many round cells and finely vacuolated monocytes. There was a fibrinopurulent exudate over the pelvic mucosal surface with underlying acute and chronic inflammatory changes, as well as here and there epithelial regeneration. The ureteral mucosa was, for the most part, ulcerated with an underlying thick zone of granulation tissue, extending into and involving the edematous muscular coat. The adventitia was thickened and edematous, with increase in fibrous tissue, perivascular lymphocytic infiltration, occasional thrombosed vessels and a fibrinous deposit on the outer surface in the process of being organized. In sections stained with Gram and Giemsa stains, rare organisms were seen, some of which were gram-negative rods.

The remaining ureteral stump measured 12 cm. in length. It was greatly dilated. The external surface was roughened and reddish gray in color. The ureteral wall was greatly thickened. Microscopically the mucosa was thrown into prominent thickened folds. The overlying, rather thickened, transitional epithelium was intact with, in the more superficial layers, hydropic cellular changes and occasional intercellular polymorphonuclears. The thickened mucosa was edematous with increase in fibrillar connective tissue, lymphocytic and plasma cell infiltration, and occasional lymphoid nodules. There was increased fibrous tissue throughout the muscular and adventitial coats. Dilated lymphatics, occasionally containing polymorphonuclears, were at times noted in these layers. No organisms were recognized in sections stained by Gram and Giemsa stains.

CASE 9.—Baby F., a six-day-old infant, was brought to the hospital because of twitchings and cyanotic attacks. Delivery was normal, without anesthesia, after a four-hour labor. The infant was cyanotic at birth and was resuscitated with difficulty. Two days before admission he became cyanotic and had frequent generalized convulsions. Physical examination was essentially negative except for slight stiffness of the neck. The clinical impression was that the patient had an intracranial hemorrhage. Lumbar puncture yielded xanthochromic cerebrospinal fluid that was otherwise not abnormal. The patient died six hours after admission.

Necropsy (A-35-16) was performed four and one-half hours postmortem. The body was well developed and nourished, measuring 54 cm. in length. There were no noteworthy external features. The peritoneal, pleural, and pericardial cavities were not remarkable. The umbilical vessels were patent and contained fluid blood.

The *heart* was not remarkable.

The *lungs* anteriorly were light pink, air containing, with a few emphysematous blebs. Posteriorly they were deep red with firm and airless zones. One of these in the posterior portion of the right upper lobe measured 3×2.5 cm. and presented dark red solid cut surfaces, from which bloody fluid could be scraped. A second, in the upper aspect of the right lower lobe, measured 1 cm. in diameter. There were several smaller ones throughout the left upper lobe which measured from 0.3 to 0.4 cm. in diameter, associated with scattered, soft, livid atelectatic areas. The bronchi and pulmonary vessels were not remarkable. Microscopically sections from the anterior portions of the lung presented fairly wide bronchioles, alveolar ducts, and infundibula with partially aerated or, less frequently, almost complete atelectatic alveoli. In some of the latter there were cornified epithelial cells, vernix, with occasional hyaline membranes, and rounded alveolar lining cells in part attached, and in part desquamated. Sections from the consolidated areas, on the other hand, revealed hemorrhagic extravasation into the alveoli, polymorphonuclear infiltration of bronchiolar walls with ulceration, and infiltration of the interlobular septums with red blood cells, fibrin, and polymorphonuclears.

The *spleen* weighed 8 gm. (normal weight, 9 gm.). It was soft in consistency. Sectioned surfaces were deep red with poorly defined corpuscular markings. Histologically there were numbers of reticular cells within the follicles presenting, in instances, evidence of phagocytosis. There were many monocytes scattered throughout the pulp with engulfed red blood cells in a number of them.

The *alimentary tract* was not remarkable except that in sections from the colon there were increased numbers of polymorphonuclears in the interglandular stroma, perivascularly in the submucosa, as well as within dilated lymphatics.

The *liver* weighed 144 gm. (normal weight 96 gm.). It was firm, reddish brown and speckled by minute, yellow areas. The cut surfaces were of similar appearance, smooth with somewhat rounded edges. Microscopically the liver cells were large and pale staining with moderate fatty infiltration (scharlach R) in some of the pericentral lobular zones. The sinusoids were moderately dilated with somewhat activated Kupffer cells.

The *kidneys* were not remarkable although in the microscopic sections there were brownish, fairly coarse, pigment granules and fine fatty droplets in Henle's limbs, together with fatty droplets in the epithelial cells of the collecting tubules and urates in some of their lumina.

The *thymus* weighed 2 gm. and histologically presented accidental involutional changes, with depletion of lymphocytes and increase in monocytes, as well as fairly marked, vascular congestion.

The *brain* weighed 435 gm. (normal weight 358 gm.). There was a small amount of subdural blood with a small tear in the right tentorium. The pial vessels over the surface of the brain were markedly congested, and there was some convolutional

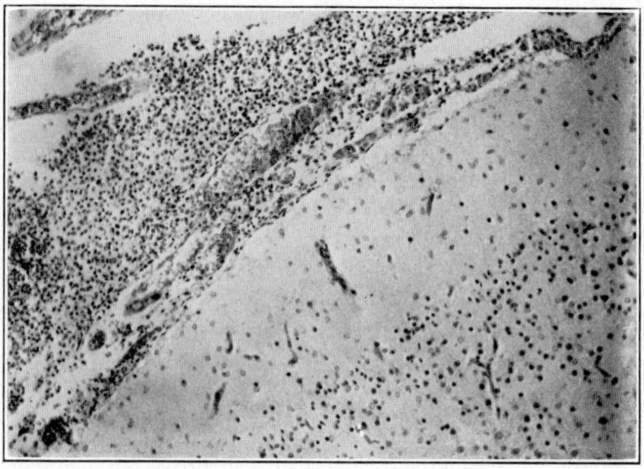

Fig. 1.—(Case 9.) Cerebral cortex with meningeal exudate (× 300). Hematoxylin and eosin.

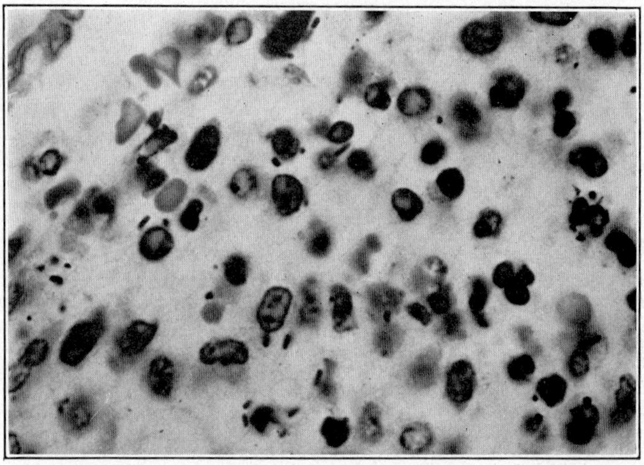

Fig. 2.—(Case 9.) As in Fig. 1, with higher magnification of the meninges. Bacterial rods are seen lying against, but largely within, polymorphonuclears and monocytes (×1175). Giemsa.

flattening. Histologically there was fairly diffuse and moderately marked meningeal infiltration with polymorphonuclears, lymphocytes, and monocytes. Except for edema and congestion, the brain tissue itself was not remarkable.

Both *middle ears* contained thick, yellow, purulent exudate.

The *bone marrow* was markedly congested with small foci of hematopoiesis, chiefly myeloid. There were no foci of necrosis.

In sections stained by Gram and Giemsa stains, one had no difficulty finding bacterial rods (gram-negative) in the blood vessels of the stomach, lung, spleen, adventitial vessels of the aorta, sinusoids of the liver, and in the organizing thrombus of the umbilical vein and in some of the cerebral vessels. Whereas in these the growth probably was in part postmortem, in the meninges there were numerous organisms with many of them within the cells of the exudate, so that there can be no doubt that they were intimately associated with the inflammatory process.

Postmortem bacteriologic cultures yielded a pure growth of a late lactose-fermenting bacillus from the heart's blood. This organism, together with *B. coli* and pneumococci, was recovered from the purulent material in the middle ears.

The *anatomic diagnoses* were acute meningitis, pulmonary atelectasis with acute bronchiolitis and alveolar hemorrhage, subdural hemorrhage (mild) with tentorial tear, and acute otitis media (bilateral), aspiration of amniotic sac contents.

CASE 10.—M. W., a five-day-old female infant, was admitted because of cyanosis and listlessness since birth. Delivery was normal at full term. She was inactive after birth and did not nurse well. Physical examination revealed a flabby, apathetic infant with marked, generalized cyanosis. She presented the facies and other characteristic signs of mongolian idiocy. The skin was dry and scaly. The cardiac dullness was markedly increased to the left, but no murmurs were heard. There was no improvement in the patient's condition. Death occurred on the fourth day after admission. The clinical diagnoses were mongolism and congenital heart disease.

Necropsy (A-31-76) was performed two and one-half hours postmortem. The body measured 46 cm. in length. Postmortem lividity was more marked than usual with generalized, slight, bluish discoloration of the skin of the entire body. The external features were mongoloid. There was flaked, white scaling of the skin over the thorax and abdomen, with a maculopapular rash over the neck and occipital region of the scalp. The papules were deep purplish in color, measured 2 mm. in diameter, and were covered, in some instances, by adherent crusts. The umbilical cord was dry and dark red. The surrounding skin margin was normal.

The peritoneal cavity contained from 25 to 50 c.c. of fibrinopurulent exudate.

The pericardial cavity contained 10 c.c. of similar exudate.

The pleural cavities were clear. The umbilical vein and hypogastric arteries contained fluid and clotted blood without evidence of any inflammatory involvement.

The *heart* weighed 22 gm. (normal weight 19 gm.). In addition to the pericardial exudate, there was an elliptical defect in the membranous interventricular septum, measuring 1.2×0.6 cm. There were no superimposed vegetations. The mitral and tricuspid valves were continuous through the defect with only two leaflets composing the latter. In the apex of the left ventricle there was a firm, dark, red, laminated thrombus, which measured 1.5×0.5 cm., adherent to the walls of the ventricle and septum. Microscopically there was a fibrinopurulent exudate overlying the pericardium. The latter was thickened, increasingly vascular and edematous with scattered polymorphonuclears, lymphocytes, and areas of hemorrhagic extravasation. There were several foci of necrosis and platelet thrombi within blood vessels where the swollen and rounded lining endothelial cells were necrotic. There were dilated lymphatics stuffed with polymorphonuclears. On the endocardial aspect in juxtaposition to the adherent thrombus, there were dilated and, in part, thrombosed intertrabecular recesses with very slight underlying myocardial reaction.

The *lungs* together weighed 50 gm. (normal weight 56 gm.). There were occasional pleural petechiae. Over the posterior portions of the lungs there were scattered, firm, dark red, nodular areas, from the sectioned aspects from which dark red fluid could be expressed. The bronchi were partially occluded by thick, hemorrhagic, mucopurulent exudate. Microscopically there were wide areas of atelectasis both with markedly congested alveolar septal capillaries, as well as less vascularized septums with pale, clear, lining alveolar cells. In these narrowed atelectatic alveoli there were desquamated pale alveolar cells, polymorphonuclears, some fibrin, rare keratinized epithelial cells, and hyaline membranes. The dark red areas were largely zones of wide hemorrhagic extravasation. The bronchioles were widened and contained in some instances fibrinopurulent exudate. The adventitial coats of the arterial vessels were thickened and edematous. The veins were moderately dilated with occasional mural thrombi. The lymphatics were dilated and contained red blood cells and often fibrinous thrombi.

The *spleen* weighed 7 gm. (normal weight 10 gm.). The pulp was firm and deep red. The corpuscles were scarcely visible. Histologically there were distorted, shrunken, nuclear forms about the periphery of the small follicles, with occasional eosinophiles. Throughout the congested pulp there were a number of large monocytes with either engulfed red blood cells or more often green pigmented spherules or granules. There were rare nucleated red blood cells and occasional blood-forming precursors. In the hilar region there were dilated lymphatics containing fibrin and polymorphonuclears.

The *alimentary tract* was not remarkable except for the esophagus where microscopically there were areas of necrosis and ulceration with underlying acute inflammatory reaction and vascular thrombosis. Similar foci of necrosis and suppuration were noted in the adventitial coat. In the small adjacent lymph nodes, there were widened sinusoids filled with monocytes, polymorphonuclears and red blood cells.

The *liver* weighed 90 gm. (normal weight 123 gm.). It was fairly firm in consistency and of grayish brown appearance. The lobular markings were well defined. Except for one focus of necrosis the sections of liver were not very remarkable microscopically. The Kupffer cells were moderately prominent, with bile pigment and red blood cells in some.

The *kidneys* were not remarkable except for uric acid deposits and moderately dilated calyces and pelves. The ureters were mildly dilated, and in the left one there were constricting points formed by folds of mucosa.

The *brain* was not removed.

The other organs grossly were in no way remarkable. Microscopically there were foci of necrosis with acute inflammatory reaction in peripancreatic, periadrenal, and perirenal tissues with involvement of the interlobular septums of the pancreas as well. The serosal tissues of the fallopian tubes were edematous with widely dilated lymphatics stuffed with purulent exudate. In the leptomeninges of the spinal cord there was a purulent exudate.

Most of the sections were stained by Gram and Giemsa stains with the following findings: Gram-negative rods both intra- and extracellularly within the pericardial necrotic foci and exudate, in the hilar lymphatics of the spleen, in the deeper layers of the esophageal ulcers, in the inflammatory foci of peripancreatic, periadrenal, and perirenal tissues, in the lymphatics of the fallopian tube, and in the exudate within the meninges of the spinal cord. Gram-positive cocci in diploid and chain formation were demonstrable only within the pulmonary exudate and in the surface layers of the esophageal ulcers. There were no demonstrable organisms in the agonal thrombus of the left ventricle.

Postmortem bacteriologic studies revealed a pure growth of a late lactose-fermenting bacillus in the heart's blood and in the pericardial and peritoneal exudate. The same organism, together with pneumococci and *Staphylococcus aureus*, was recovered from the lungs.

The *anatomical diagnoses* were congenital heart disease with interventricular septal defect, mural thrombus of the left ventricle, acute meningitis, acute pericarditis, acute peritonitis, bronchopneumonia, acute esophagitis, uric acid renal deposits, and dilatation of the renal pelves and ureters.

CASE 11.—P. L., a seven-day-old male infant, was brought to the hospital because of a rash of four days' duration. The patient was delivered normally at term. No immediate postnatal abnormalities were noted. Four days before admission a "blisterlike" lesion appeared on the chest. Other similar lesions appeared rapidly on the chest and abdomen. Two days before admission the patient

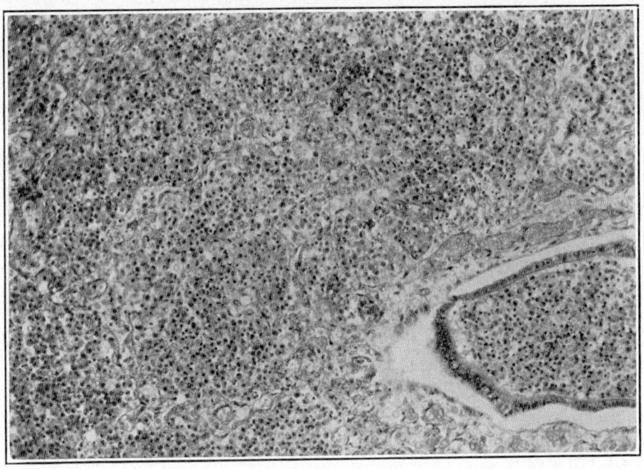

Fig. 3.—(Case 11.) Lung. The alveoli and adjacent bronchioles are filled with cellular exudate (× 300). Hematoxylin and eosin.

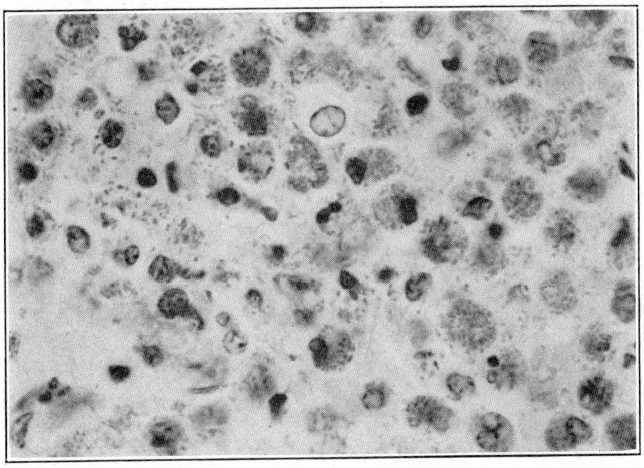

Fig. 4.—(Case 11.) As in Fig. 3. Myriads of bacterial rods within the cells of the alveolar exudate (× 1200). Giemsa.

developed a cough, rapid respirations, and poor color. Physical examination presented an acutely ill, cyanotic infant, breathing with rapid, labored respirations. There were numerous large, bullous lesions over the chest and abdomen. Examination of the lungs revealed evidences of bronchopneumonia. The liver and spleen were palpable. The umbilicus was red and moist. The patient failed rapidly with a gradual increase in cyanosis and respiratory distress. The clinical diagnoses were pemphigus neonatorum and bronchopneumonia.

Necropsy examination (A-33-51) was performed one hour postmortem. The body was well developed and well nourished, measuring 54 cm. in length. The skin was dry with marked desquamation over the lower portion of the abdomen. There were vesicular and bullous lesions, many containing purulent material, over the left cheek, entire left side of the neck, the left arm and wrist, two over the left chest, one medial to the right nipple, and one above the right axilla. The scrotum and buttocks were excoriated and reddened. The sacral spine was bifid for a distance of 2 cm. above the coccyx. The liver and spleen were enlarged and extended three fingerbreadths below the costal margins. The umbilical vessels and heart were not remarkable.

Pleural Cavities.—There were about 6 c.c. of opaque, gelatinous fluid in the left pleural cavity and about 4 c.c. of similar fluid in the right. In addition, the left lung was bound to the parietal chest wall by numerous fine, fibrinous adhesions.

Lungs.—Each weighed 66 gm. (normal weight 24 gm.). The visceral pleural surface of the left lung was slightly roughened with a layer of fibrin over the diaphragmatic aspect. The anterior margins of both lungs were reddish yellow and air containing. Elsewhere, the lungs were reddish purple and firm, particularly the right middle and left lower lobes. The cut surfaces of the latter lobes were dark red, and only a small amount of bloody fluid could be expressed from them. The bronchi contained a moderate amount of reddish, mucoid material, and their mucosal surfaces were slightly thickened and reddened. Microscopically there was an extensive and widespread bronchopneumonic process. The exudate was somewhat variable in character with predominantly large mononuclear cells in varied stages of degeneration, together with polymorphonuclears, occasional red blood cells, serum, and fibrin. The bronchioles were likewise filled with similar exudate with here and there an absence of surface epithelium. Perivascular lymphatics, interlobular septums and pleural tissues and lymphatics were to a variable degree infiltrated or filled with similar exudate. Many of the alveolar septal capillaries were thrombosed and there were mural thrombi in some of the interlobular septal veins. In some of the pneumonic areas there were early necroses containing clusters of bacteria which were clearly gram-negative rods. When stained by Gram and Giemsa stains, myriads of similar organisms, to the complete exclusion of coccal forms, were noted elsewhere, particularly within the large mononuclear cells. Staining with scharlach R revealed many fatty droplets within the cytoplasm of these larger cells. In the less involved portions of lung tissue, there were evidences of aspiration of amniotic fluid with demonstrable keratinized epithelial cells and vernix.

The *spleen* weighed 12 gm. (normal weight 9 gm.). It was soft in consistency and sectioned surfaces were dark red in color. Microscopically the follicles were small with considerable lymphocytic fragmentation. The pulp was congested, but there was no erythrophagocytosis.

The *liver* weighed 230 gm. (normal weight 96 gm.). It was moderately firm in consistency, dark purplish red with fine, yellow mottlings. Cut surfaces were yellowish with intervening translucent, reddish brown parenchyma. Lobular outlines were thereby demarcated. Microscopically there was mild central atrophy with moderate fatty infiltration (scharlach R). The peripheral lobular cells were well preserved. The Kupffer cells were active and, in some instances, brown pigmented.

Lymph Nodes.—Those of the mediastinum were enlarged, reddish purple in color, soft and edematous. Microscopically these presented greatly widened sinusoids, containing numbers of polymorphonuclears, red blood cells and fewer pale, large mononuclear cells. There were occasional small fibrinous thrombi with enmeshed polymorphonuclears. There was apparent depletion of lymphoid elements. The arterial vessels appeared thickened with prominent lining endothelial cells. About some of them there was an increased amount of loose fibrillar connective tissue. The mesenteric nodes were histologically mildly edematous and contained abundant well-preserved lymphoid tissue. In contrast to the mediastinal nodes, only the medullary sinusoids were widened and contained practically acellular lymph. The peripancreatic nodes presented changes similar to those of the mediastinum but less marked.

The *thymus* weighed 7 gm. Histologically there were marked accidental involutional changes with practically complete replacement of the cortical thymocytes by large, pale mononuclear cells.

Skin.—Histologically the epidermal cells underlying the bullae were swollen and hydropic. Similar swollen cells were not infrequently noted elsewhere in the noninvolved epidermis close to the basal cylindrical cell layer. There were occasional abscesses, either within a hair shaft or within the epidermis involving the orifice of one. The vessels of the papillary layer of the corium were widened and congested. There was a mild degree of edema throughout the corium with scattered lymphocytes and polymorphonuclears. Stained by Gram and Giemsa stains, there were many coccal forms and only infrequent rods within the abscesses.

Postmortem bacteriologic studies showed a pure culture of a late lactose-fermenting bacillus in the heart's blood, the right bronchus, a bulla in the left axilla and in stab cultures from the lungs—right middle and left lower lobes. Cultures of the exudate in the left pleural cavity yielded this organism together with *Staphylococcus aureus.* Both gram-positive cocci and gram-negative rods were seen in smears of the bullous contents.

The *anatomical diagnoses* were pemphigus neonatorum (bullous impetigo), bronchopneumonia, acute pleuritis (bilateral), acute lymphadenitis (mediastinal and peripancreatic), uric acid renal deposits, petechial hemorrhages (mucosa of urinary bladder and adrenal medulla), fatty infiltration of the liver and accidental involution of the thymus.

CASE 12.—J. H., a two-month-old female infant, with an irrelevant family and past history, was admitted because of jaundice and convulsions. Five days before admission the patient became pale and limp. The temperature was 103° F. The following day jaundice was noticed, and the patient had a generalized convulsion lasting three hours. Fever, increasing jaundice, and occasional convulsions continued until admission. On physical examination the patient was found to be moderately jaundiced. The abdomen was distended and presented shifting dullness and a pouting umbilicus. The liver and spleen were enlarged. The patient lived for eight days after admission. The leucocyte count varied between 41,000 and 72,000 cells per cubic millimeter. The urine was loaded with pus cells. On three occasions the blood culture was positive for a late lactose-fermenting bacillus. Death occurred on the eighth hospital day after a series of generalized convulsions.

Necropsy (A-33-70) was performed four and one-half-hours postmortem. The body measured 51 cm. in length and was poorly nourished. There was generalized jaundice. The abdomen was markedly distended. The liver edge was palpable 2.5 cm. and 3 cm. below the costal margin in the right nipple and midsternal lines, respectively. The spleen was palpable 2 cm. below the left costal margin. The peritoneal cavity contained 6 c.c. of clear, amber-colored fluid. The peritoneal surfaces were all smooth and glistening except for filmy adhesions between the anterolateral surface of the spleen and omentum. The kidneys were soft and very large; almost reaching the brim of the pelvis. There were no enlarged mesenteric or periaortic lymph nodes. The lymph glands of the mediastinum were enlarged, soft, and edematous, the largest measuring $0.6 \times 0.4 \times 0.3$ cm. The pleural and pericardial cavities were not remarkable. The umbilical vessels were obliterated. The heart was not remarkable except for mild hypertrophy and the presence of edematous, jaundiced epicardial tissues.

Lungs.—The right weighed 46 gm. (normal weight 32 gm.) and the left 38 gm. (normal weight 30 gm.). Anteriorly the lungs were pale, yellowish pink and air containing. Posteriorly they were dark purplish red in color, almost airless, with small, dark red, firm areas, the largest measuring 0.7 cm. in diameter. The cut surfaces presented appearances similar to those noted externally, and from the posterior portions a small amount of serosanguineous fluid could be expressed. The pulmonary vessels and bronchi were not remarkable. Microscopically sections from the posterior portions were characterized by a marked degree of lobular pneumonia. The exudate varied in different areas, being composed of serum, densely massed fibrin, polymorphonuclears, red blood cells, and large monocytes. In several instances there were hyaline membranes. The pleural and interlobular septums were edematous and contained dilated lymphatics with acellular lymph. In one instance there was interstitial emphysema. In less involved zones, the bronchioles were frequently filled with exudate, and their parietes were involved in the inflammatory process with extension to, and early ulceration of, the surface epithelium. The alveoli contained many large, pale, vacuolated monocytes and the alveolar septums were approximated and thickened by polymorphonuclear and monocytic infiltration. With Gram and Giemsa stains there were frequent clusters of bacterial rods, some intracellularly, with only rare coccal groups in diploïd and chain formation.

The *spleen* weighed 46 gm. (normal weight 13 gm.). It was firm in consistency, with dark reddish purple cut surfaces, presenting rather indistinct, irregular, gray, corpuscular markings. Histologically there was marked increase in numbers of cells in the pulp and sinusoids. These were in part lymphocytes and plasma cells with many immature cell forms and large actively phagocytic monocytes. The latter contained a moderate amount of hemosiderin, fatty droplets (scharlach R), and occasional clustered rods (Gram and Giemsa). There were frequent foci of hematopoiesis. The lining cells of the sinusoids were hypertrophied. In areas of the pulp there were increased numbers of polymorphonuclears.

The *gastrointestinal tract* was not remarkable.

The *liver* weighed 206 gm. (normal weight 136 gm.). It was firm in consistency and of pale brownish yellow color. The cut surfaces were similar in color with distinct markings. Histologically there was fairly marked periportal fatty infiltration (scharlach R) with considerable hemosiderin pigment both within liver cells and in enlarged Kupffer cells. There were occasional foci of necrosis with more frequent single-celled degeneration and necrosis. Frequent hematopoietic foci were noted in the sinusoids and occasionally in portal spaces. The reticular stroma in the periportal zones appeared edematous and increased in amount.

Each *kidney* weighed 53 gm. (normal weight 19 gm.). Externally, when the thin capsule had been stripped, one noted a finely irregular surface, reddish in color with pale yellow mottlings. The cut surfaces were pale, with poor demarcation between cortex and medulla. The calyces and pelves were deeply jaundiced, edematous and thickened (0.1 cm.). Microscopically there was a marked degree of pyelonephritis with purulent exudate within tubules, as well as to a lesser degree in the interstitial tissues. In the latter there were many lymphocytes, monocytes, some plasma cells, many young blood-forming precursors, and some definite foci of hematopoiesis. With Gram and Giemsa stains there were many rods, particularly within the lumen of the tubules, both free and intracellularly, with fewer numbers in the interstitial tissues. The pelvic tissues were thickened, markedly edematous and infiltrated by polymorphonuclears and monocytes. There were occasional hematopoietic foci. There were areas of epithelial metaplasia to that of a more squamous and keratinizing type.

The *ureters* and *bladder* were not remarkable.

Of the other organs there were, histologically, several small foci of necrosis in the adult cortex of the adrenal with involution in great part of the fetal cortex. In the medulla there were collections of cells of leucopoietic type and in the periadrenal fetal fat, perivascular foci of hematopoiesis. There was from mild to marked accidental involution of the thymus, with loss of the usual corticomedullary distinctness associated with depletion of lymphocytes, variable degrees of fibrosis, and infiltration with large pale vacuolated monocytes. A section of one lymph node revealed moderate lymphoid hyperplasia, some sinus endothelial proliferation and infrequent foci of leucopoietic cells. The bone marrow was chiefly leucopoietic. A small focus of polymorphonuclear infiltration was noted in a section of gasserian ganglion adjoining the dural aspect. The brain, spinal cord, thyroid, trachea, parathyroids and aorta were grossly and microscopically in no way unusual. Both middle ears contained serohemorrhagic exudate. The tympanic membranes were intact but slightly reddened. The mucosa of the mastoid antrums was moderately reddened.

Bacteriologic Examination.—A late lactose-fermenting bacillus was isolated from the heart's blood, left bronchus, ureter, left middle ear, ileum, and jejunum.

Anatomical Diagnoses.—Acute bronchopneumonia; pyelonephritis (bilateral, acute otitis media; hyperplastic splenitis; fatty infiltration of the liver with focal necroses; hematopoiesis, liver, spleen, kidney, adrenal; accidental involution of thymus; jaundice.

CASE 13.—B. C., a ten-week-old female, was admitted because of drowsiness, fever, and diarrhea of three days' duration. Physical examination revealed an acutely ill, listless, slightly cyanotic infant with no definite localizing signs of pathology. Following admission the patient continued to have diarrhea and ran a high, sustained fever. The urine was loaded with white cells. The course was progressively downhill and death occurred three days after admission.

Necropsy (A-32-31) was performed two and one-half hours postmortem. The body was fairly well developed but poorly nourished and measured 51 cm. in length. The serous cavities, unbilical vessels, and heart were not remarkable.

Lungs.—The right lung weighed 68 gm. (normal weight 35 gm.), and the left, 52 gm. (normal weight 30 gm.). The posterior portion of all lobes, particularly the lower, were firm, nodular and dark, purplish red in color. On section these areas were deep red, and from them thick, dark red fluid could be expressed. The anterior portions of the lungs were pink and air containing. The bronchi contained a small amount of blood-tinged, mucoid exudate. Histologically there was a diffuse exudative process, chiefly of seropurulent or fibrinopurulent character. There were also many large phagocytic mononuclear cells. The bronchioles contained a small amount of purulent exudate and some cellular débris. The interlobular septums were thickened, edematous and infiltrated largely with mononuclear cells. They contained dilated lymphatics filled with serous exudate. Some of the larger blood vessels were thrombosed. There were numerous gram-negative rods in the alveolar exudate, many within the large monocytes and some, apparently, in the alveolar septums (Gram and Giemsa stains). Only rare coccal clusters were seen.

The *spleen* was not enlarged. It was fairly firm in consistency. The pulp was dark red in color. Microscopically there were many large phagocytic cells in the pulp and sinusoids with moderate deposits of hemosiderin.

The *alimentary tract* was not remarkable except for the distal portion of the ileum where there were numerous grayish red Peyer's patches with occasional small, irregular, shallow ulcers from 1 to 2 mm. in diameter. The bases of these were flat and pale gray. The surrounding margins were not reddened. Histologically these ulcers extended to, or were deep to, the muscularis mucosae. The underlying reaction was proliferative in type, with fibrosis and perivascular and diffuse lymphocytic and monocytic infiltration. There was very little superficial exudate. An occasional thrombosed venule was encountered close to the ulcerated surface. In the submucosa, muscularis and serosa there were dilated lymphatics, containing lymphocytes and large pale degenerating monocytes. The serosa was thickened and edematous, increasingly vascular, with scattered monocytes and increased numbers of fibroblasts. The uninvolved portions of ileum presented a curious rounding of the blunted villar and interglandular surfaces. Both villi and interglandular tissues were quite cellular, more so in some areas than in others, but without acute inflammatory changes. Numerous gram-negative rods covered the surface of the ulcers but none could be recognized deeply (Gram and Giemsa stains).

The *liver* and *pancreas* were not remarkable.

Kidneys.—The right weighed 24 gm. (normal weight 20 gm.) and the left, 20 gm. (normal weight 19 gm.). Except for the lower pole of the left kidney, the perirenal tissues, capsule, and renal substance itself were not remarkable. In the former region there was scarcely any demarcation between cortex and medulla, the sectioned aspect appearing pale gray and edematous. The pelves were slightly dilated but free of exudate. Sections from the lower pole of the left kidney revealed extensive parenchymatous destruction, largely cortical, with several small abscesses and diffuse and heavy lymphocytic, monocytic, and polymorphonuclear infiltration. The tubules, in less involved areas, were compressed with epithelial

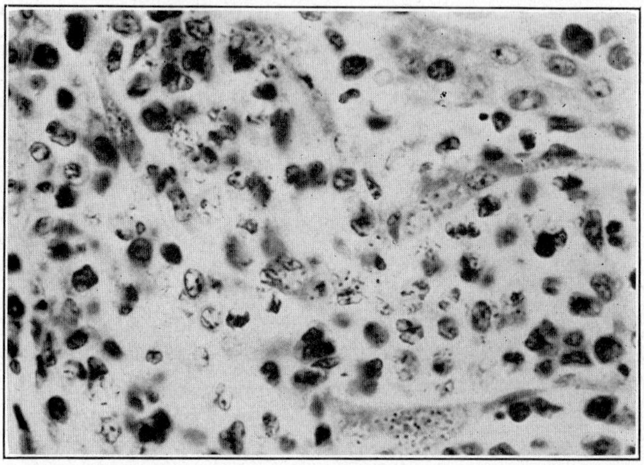

Fig. 5.—(Case 13.) Kidney. Bacterial rods within greatly enlarged and expanded tubular epithelial cells, also in the cells of the exudate interstitially and within the tubular lumen (×1225). Giemsa.

degenerative and regenerative changes and were filled with exudate similar to that in the interstitial tissues. Numerous gram-negative rods could be demonstrated both free in the lumen and interstitial tissues as well as intracellularly within monocytes and polymorphonuclears. In some instances the epithelial cells contained large numbers of these organisms and were thereby enlarged and expanded (Gram and Giemsa stains). The peripelvic tissues were edematous and very lightly infiltrated with lymphocytes and polymorphonuclears. The pelvic tissues were likewise mildly involved. The ureters and bladder were not remarkable.

The *costochondral rib junctions* were convex toward the metaphysis with general broadening in the ephiphyseal region. Microscopically there was irregular proliferation of cartilage with irregular penetration by rather poorly vascularized, but highly cellular and fibrillar marrow. The fibrous marrow extended for a short distance within the diaphysis and in it there were longitudinal and transverse trabeculae with fair osteoid deposition and some remaining central cartilage. Higher up in the shaft there was a series of transverse bars, not too well calcified. The periosteum was not remarkable. The chondral nutrient vessels were surrounded by an increased amount of cellular fibrillar connective tissue. The marrow was quite cellular and predominantly granulocytic. There were small foci of early necrosis. In the vertebral sections there was moderate histiocytic phagocytosis.

The *thymus* weighed 5 gm. and histologically presented accidental involution with large numbers of pale monocytes, actively phagocytic, and many eosinophilic myelocytes. One of the enlarged edematous nodes associated with the capsule of the thymus presented mild acute inflammatory changes. The peripheral sinus was dilated, containing polymorphonuclears and deposits of fibrin with, infrequently, the presence of a gram-negative rod (Gram and Giemsa stains). Elsewhere the node was edematous and congested, diffusely and lightly infiltrated with polymorphonuclears with increased numbers of littoral cells and monocytes.

Except for a mild inflammatory reaction in the epidural tissues of one section of spinal cord, the central nervous system was not remarkable.

Both middle ears contained a thin serous exudate.

Bacteriologic studies revealed a late lactose-fermenting bacillus in the heart's blood, right middle ear, left middle ear, ileum, and colon.

The *anatomical diagnoses* were chronic ulcerative enteritis, acute bronchopneumonia, pyelonephritis, acute lymphadenitis (mediastinal), rickets, accidental involution of the thymus, otitis media (bilateral).

DISCUSSION

It is of interest to note the variety of lesions caused by this organism as well as their character in the different age periods. In the youngest (Case 9) there was an overwhelming bacteremia with little localization. The organisms were found in the small blood vessels of many viscera, often accompanied by vascular congestion and in the lungs by alveolar hemorrhage. There was a frank meningitis, and the organisms could be demonstrated readily within the cells of the exudate.

In Case 10 there was again widespread bacterial dissemination, but here it was associated with many foci of inflammation, chiefly, however, in serous cavities, peritoneum and pericardium, as well as in the meninges.

In Case 11 the organisms were chiefly localized in the lungs where they were unquestionably the causal agent in the extensive and marked pneumonic process. Countless numbers of them were present largely within the cells of the exudate. The acute pleuritis and mediastinal lymphadenitis were accompaniments of the pneumonia. The bullous impetigo was probably incidental.

The above three infants were under ten days of age.

Case 12 (patient aged two months) presented evidences of a fairly long-standing septic process indicated by the poor nutritional state, the arrest of growth, the persistent extramedullary hematopoiesis and the enlarged, cellular spleen. The oldest lesion, in point of reaction, was the pyelonephritis. The pneumonia and otitis media were quite recent.

This apparent fact that the organisms might lodge in certain organs and give rise to a continued inflammatory process with subsequent wider dissemination is again borne out in Case 13 (patient aged two and one-half months). The ulcers of the ileum are clearly of long-standing duration, with the pyelonephritis of about the same or slightly shorter duration. Again in this case, as in the former, the pneumonia and otitis media were more terminal in character and were associated with a generalized septicemia.

In the older aged group of living patients these organisms were important causal agents of pyelonephritis in three, peritonitis associated with appendicitis in three, and an abscess of the buttocks in one.

In taking the 13 cases as a group, therefore, the incidence of specific lesions was as follows: 6 with pyelonephritis, 4 with peritonitis, 4 with pneumonia, 3 with otitis media, 2 with meningitis, and one each with pericarditis and pleuritis.

In these cases in early infancy, as Dr. Wolbach has frequently stressed, there is a striking resemblance to a disease in newborn calves, fully described in a series of papers by Theobald Smith and his associates.[18-21] Calves, deprived of colostrum, frequently develop diarrhea (scours), exudative arthritis, insterstitial nephritis, pneumonia, and omphalitis. Scours is caused by *B. coli.* It is associated primarily with the overgrowth of the organism in the lower small intestine with continued spread toward the duodenum, so that in advanced cases the mucosa may be carpeted by layers of colon bacilli extending from the duodenum to the ileocecal valve. Concomitant with this, in the earliest stages, there is wide dissemination so that the organisms can be cultured readily from the spleen, lungs, and kidneys. Histologically they are present in large numbers within dilated small blood vessels which, at times, may be thrombosed and accompanied by smaller or larger areas of hemorrhagic extravasation. In the later stages of the disease there is a frank inflammatory reaction with localization chiefly in the kidneys, joints, and lungs. In almost no instance is there intestinal ulceration. Although the mortality amongst calves with scours is high, some recover, and the lesions probably heal. The gray, patchy, renal lesions, the so-called *weisse Fleckniere* or *nephritis maculosa alba* in older animals are considered to be such healing or healed forms of nephritis.

This anatomic analogy between scours in calves and widespread colon bacillus infections in infants does not hold when the two species are compared immunologically. There is no striking evidence that the human infant derives maternal antibodies through the colostrum. In man the transfer of antibodies to the fetus occurs through the placenta by virtue of its greater permeability for such substances as compared to the bovine placenta.

In this group of cases it seems logical to assume that these late lactose-fermenting bacilli behaved like the colon bacillus, by virtue of their widespread distribution, multiple foci of suppuration, and predilection for the kidney. The pathologic findings in a series of cases of colon bacillus septicemia in newborn infants have been compared with the findings in these cases. They are essentially similar. It is well known that the colon bacillus produces lesions similar to those described here in the older age group.

As a result of this study, therefore, it is felt that this group of late lactose-fermenting bacilli is in no way different, in its pathogenic significance, from the colon bacillus. Under ordinary circumstances these organisms are normal inhabitants of the intestinal tract in a small percentage of individuals. When they are associated with the production of disease, it is under circumstances identical with those which might be associated with the colon bacillus.

While the problem of the exact biologic classification of this group is not settled, our study lends support to the opinion that they are either closely related to, or are variants of, the colon bacillus.

It should be reiterated that, from the point of view of bacteriologic diagnosis, these organisms are easily confused with the paratyphoid group. Elsewhere in this paper the differential characteristics have been discussed.

SUMMARY

The literature is reviewed concerning a group of late lactose-fermenting bacilli.

The biologic characteristics of these organisms are described and discussed.

A series of cases is described in which these organisms were of pathogenic significance. It is pointed out that in some cases they may invade widely and cause a variety of lesions entirely analogous to those occasionally caused by the colon bacillus.

REFERENCES

1. Fothergill, L. D.: J. Infect. Dis. **45**: 393, 1929.
2. Dean, H. R., Adamson, R. S., Giles, J. D., and Williamson, R.: J. Roy. Army M. Corps **28**: 428, 1917.
3. Douglas, S. R.: Medical Research Committee, Special Report Series, No. 6, 1917.
4. Fildes, P.: Medical Research Committee, Special Report Series, No. 6, 1917.
5. Dobell, C., Gettings, H. S., Jepps, M. W., and Stephens, J. B.: Medical Research Committee, Special Report Series, No. 15, 1918.
6. Glynn, E., and Robinson, A. L.: Medical Research Committee, Special Report Series, No. 7, 1918.
7. Dudgeon, L. S.: J. Hygiene **25**: 119, 1926.
8. Johnston, M. M., Brown, A., Tisdall, F. F., and Fraser, D. T.: Am. J. Dis. Child. **45**: 1, 1933.
9. Kriebel, R. M.: J. Bact. **27**: 357, 1934.
10. Bronfenbrenner, J., and Davis, C. R.: J. M. Research **39**: 33, 1918.
11. Dudgeon, L. S., Wordley, E., and Bawtree, F.: J. Hygiene **20**: 137, 1921.
12. Dudgeon, L. S.: J. Hygiene **22**: 348, 1924.
13. Dudgeon, L. S., and Pulvertaft, R. J. V.: J. Hygiene **26**: 285, 1927.
14. Caldwell, J. A.: J. Infect. Dis. **43**: 353, 1928.
15. Kennedy, J. A., Cummings, P. L., and Morrow, U. M.: J. Infect. Dis. **50**: 333, 1932.
16. Dulaney, A. D.: J. Infect. Dis. **42**: 574, 1928.
17. Nungester, W. J., and Anderson, S. A.: J. Infect. Dis. **49**: 455, 1931.
18. Smith, Theobald, and Little, R. B.: J. Exper. Med. **36**: 181, 1922.
19. Smith, Theobald, and Little, R. B.: J. Exper. Med. **36**: 453, 1922.
20. Smith, Theobald, and Orcutt, M. L.: J. Exper. Med. **41**: 89, 1925.
21. Smith, Theobald: J. Exper. Med. **41**: 413, 1925.

THE TREATMENT OF PERTUSSIS WITH AN INTRANASAL ANTIGEN

Preliminary Report

H. A. Slesinger, M.D.
Windber, Pa.

DURING the interval between May, 1935, and February, 1936, we treated twenty-four active cases of whooping cough in various stages of the disease by the intranasal administration of a soluble antigen prepared from the *Hemophilus pertussis.* The antigen consisted of a solution of soluble substances derived from recently isolated cultures of *Hemophilus pertussis* and represented the soluble protein of about 20,000 million organisms per cubic centimeter.

Method of Administration.—The patient was placed in the recumbent posture with the head held in a dependent position below the level of the body. Ten drops of the antigen were instilled in each nostril. The patient was kept in this position for two or three minutes in order to permit proper absorption. Treatments were usually given daily; in some cases they were given every second day. The total number of treatments varied from four to twelve.

ANALYSIS OF CASES

In addition to the twenty-four patients with whooping cough, 3 contact cases were treated prophylactically. Ten control cases were followed simultaneously, most of these being in the same families as the treated children. This gave us an opportunity to compare the severity of the untreated cases with those which were treated. Although the treatment was first instituted in May, 1935, most of the cases were treated during the interval of November to February when whooping cough is usually at its worst. The youngest patient was seven months old; the oldest was eleven years old.

Results.—The results were graded according to the degree of improvement. The following code is used in Table I in order to tabulate the degree of improvement.

"A"—Marked improvement. Definite decrease in the number and severity of paroxysms. Definite decrease in the duration of the illness. The average duration of the illness in this group was 15.1 days after the first treatment. The average duration of the illness from the date of onset was 25.7 days.

"B"—Moderate improvement. In this group there was a decrease in the number and severity of paroxysms, but there was no great de-

From the Department of Pediatrics, Berwind Clinic, Windber Hospital.

crease in the duration of the illness. The average duration after the first treatment was 20.7 days, and the average duration from the date of onset was 32.4 days.

"C"—Slight or no improvement. In this group there was either no improvement whatsoever or a questionable degree of improvement. In a few instances the treatment was begun late, and the improvement observed after several treatments may have been the result of a spontaneous improvement which often occurs during the fourth week of the illness. The average duration after the first treatment in this group was 23.5 days, and the average total duration from the date of onset was 34.7 days.

Using the above code the results in general, regardless of the type of case treated or the time at which treatment was begun, were as follows:

A—(Marked improvement)—11 cases..........45.8 per cent
B—(Moderate improvement)—7 cases..........29.2 per cent
C—(Slight or no improvement)—6 cases........25.0 per cent

It will thus be seen that definite improvement occurred in 75 per cent of the cases. It was possible to shorten the total duration of the disease to a minimum of 17 days and an average of 25 to 35 days depending upon the promptness of the treatment.

An analysis of Table I will show that results were more favorable when treatment was begun early. Results were particularly good in those cases in which treatment was started during the first 10 days. Eleven cases were treated within 10 days after the onset of the cough. The results showed 7 in Group A, 3 in Group B, and only 1 in Group C. Eight cases were treated between 11 and 19 days after the onset. Of these cases 4 were in Group A, 2 in B, and 2 in C. Out of a total of 5 cases treated after 20 days, only 1 fell in Group A; 1 was in Group B; and 3 were in Group C. This demonstrates clearly that treatment must be instituted early to obtain favorable results.

In some cases the results were quite striking. Cases 7 and 8 showed especially good results. Both of these patients had severe attacks before treatment was begun. Other members of the family in each case were used as untreated controls. In Case 7 the whoop completely disappeared after four treatments and in Case 8 after five treatments. They both continued to cough occasionally during the next 9 or 10 days. The control cases in both families had severe attacks and continued to have paroxysmal seizures of coughing for a total of six to eight weeks as compared with four weeks in the treated cases (the last 10 days of which the patients had only a mild cough). In several of the cases classed under Group A, the whoop and vomiting disappeared 6 or 7 days after treatment was begun. However, they continued to have a mild cough for some time afterward.

TABLE I

ACTIVE CASES TREATED WITH INTRANASAL ANTIGEN

CASE	AGE	DURATION OF ILLNESS BEFORE TREATMENT (DAYS)	NUMBER OF TREATMENTS	TYPE OF ATTACK BEFORE TREATMENT	RESULT			REMARKS
					DURATION OF COUGH AFTER FIRST TREATMENT (DAYS)	TOTAL DURATION OF COUGH (DAYS)	DEGREE OF IMPROVEMENT	
1. G. W.	3 yr.	7	5	Mild	10 Mild attack	17	A	Exposed to brother.
2. T. W.	1 yr.	6	5	Mild	14 Mild attack	20	A	Three other children in family were not treated. They had severe attacks lasting 6 to 8 weeks.
3. M. D.	3 yr.	14	5	Moderate	14	28	A	Marked improvement noted after 7 days.
4. P. D.	7 mo.	5	5	Mild	14	19	A	Marked improvement after 4 treatments.
5. M. P.	5 yr.	13	5	Severe	16	29	A	Improvement noted at end of 5 treatments.
6. A. Z.	5 yr.	10	9 (over 15-day period)	Severe	21	31	A	Severe case. Marked decrease in number and severity of paroxysms after 6 treatments.
7. M. O.	3 yr.	15	5	Severe	14	29	A	Whoop disappeared after 4 treatments.
8. L. H.	5 yr.	14	5	Severe	14	28	A	Whoop disappeared after 5 treatments. Two other untreated members of family were severe cases.
9. N. T.	7½ mo.	21	5	Severe	14	35	A	Marked improvement after 5 treatments.
10. D. B.	11 yr.	5	5	Mild very early	15	20	A	Very early case. Contact with sister.
11. P. P.	3 yr.	7	9 (over 12-day period)	Mild	20	27	A	Paroxysms were mild and infrequent. No vomiting.
12. R. B.	6 yr.	8	10 (over 14-day period)	Moderate	22	30	B	Paroxysms fewer in number and severity.

TABLE I—CONT'D

CASE	AGE	DURATION OF ILLNESS BEFORE TREATMENT (DAYS)	NUMBER OF TREATMENTS	TYPE OF ATTACK BEFORE TREATMENT	RESULT			REMARKS
					DURATION OF COUGH AFTER FIRST TREATMENT (DAYS)	TOTAL DURATION OF COUGH (DAYS)	DEGREE OF IMPROVEMENT	
13. B. H.	6 yr.	13	6	Severe	23	36	B	Paroxysms fewer in number and less severe.
14. S. W.	6 yr.	10	5	Severe	21	31	B	Moderate improvement. Attack shorter than usual but paroxysms severe.
15. R. H.	3 yr.	8	6	Severe	25	33	B	Moderate improvement.
16. J. S.	6 yr.	23	5	Severe	12	35	B	Treatment late.
17. R. H.	13 mo.	6	6	Severe	24	30	B	
18. M. D.	3 yr.	14	9	Severe	18	32	B	Improvement noted after 7 treatments.
19. B. B.	3 yr.	14	4	Severe	28	42	C	Very little improvement.
20. E. T.	15 mo.	24	4	Severe	21	45	C	Late case. No improvement.
21. W. W.	6 yr.	20	5	Severe	15	35	C	Slight improvement.
22. M. A.	2 yr.	19	12	Severe	28	40	C	Some improvement after 10 days. Had occasional paroxysms for 4 weeks.
23. E. O.	5 yr.	28	5	Severe, late	21	49	C	Some improvement at end of 1 week, but treatment was late, and this may have been spontaneous.
24. G. Z.	7 mo.	9	12 (over 16-day period)	Severe	28	37	C	Some decrease in number and severity of paroxysms but cough continued for 4 weeks.

TABLE II

RELATIONSHIP OF RESULTS TO THE TIME AT WHICH TREATMENT WAS STARTED

I. Cases treated within 10 days from onset of cough				11
Marked improvement	(A)	7	63.6%	
Moderate improvement	(B)	3	27.3%	
Slight or no improvement	(C)	1	9.1%	
II. Cases treated between 11 and 19 days from onset				8
Marked improvement	(A)	4	50%	
Moderate improvement	(B)	2	25%	
Slight or no improvement	(C)	2	25%	
III. Late cases (treated 20 or more days from onset)				5
Marked improvement	(A)	1	20%	
Moderate improvement	(B)	1	20%	
Slight or no improvement	(C)	3	60%	

In all of the cases the parents were requested to keep an accurate record of the number of paroxysms per day together with a description of the severity of the paroxysms and the number of attacks of vomiting which occurred. In most cases in Group A or B the paroxysms would diminish in number from fifteen to twenty per day to five or six per day after a few treatments. The number of attacks of vomiting would decrease. In most cases the paroxysms were milder. but in some they continued to be severe even though the number had decreased to five per day. In general, the parents stated that they felt that these children had milder attacks of whooping cough than neighbors' children who were untreated or than others of the family who were untreated.

Prophylaxis.—We are not in a position to make any definite statements about the value of this method of treatment as a prophylactic measure. Three contact cases were treated before any cough developed. All of these patients had intimate contact with other members of the family and were all over one year of age. Two developed a mild form of pertussis characterized by a short paroxysmal cough but not associated with any whoop or vomiting. The cough lasted from two to three weeks. The third patient did not develop any symptoms. It would, therefore, seem that this method of treatment may be of value in the prophylactic treatment of contact cases.

Controls.—Ten patients were used as untreated controls. Most of these children were in families in which other members were being treated. The average duration of the cough in this group was fifty days. The paroxysms were more frequent and more severe than those of the treated cases.

COMMENT

Vaccine therapy has been used in the treatment of whooping cough during the past twenty-five years. The type of vaccine, the method of administration, and the results have varied considerably. There has been considerable doubt about the rôle of the Bordet-Gengou bacillus in the etiology of pertussis. However, work during the past three years has corroborated the view that this bacillus is the direct cause of the disease. Madsen[1] employed a vaccine in the prophylaxis of the disease and reported good results. He used forty-eight-hour blood agar cultures—in a strength of 10,000 million bacilli per cubic centimeter. Three injections of 0.5, 0.7, and 1.0 c.c., respectively, were given at intervals of three to four days. He was able to prevent the disease in 458 out of 1,832 vaccinated children in the Faroe Islands; only 8 patients out of a total of 446 unvaccinated cases did not become infected. Sauer[2, 3] used a freshly prepared vaccine—with a strength of 10,000 million per cubic centimeter—giving a total of 7 to 8 c.c. in three weekly injections. He reported 169 definitely exposed patients over a period of seven years, none of whom developed typical whooping cough.

MacDonald and MacDonald[4] made some interesting observations on the etiology and prophylaxis of the disease. Four brothers were used in the experiment. Two brothers were vaccinated against whooping cough according to the method of Sauer; the other two were not vaccinated. Five months later the four boys were inoculated intranasally with a filtrate from a freshly prepared culture of *Hemophilus pertussis.* The two vaccinated boys remained free from symptoms; their cough plates were normal and their blood counts remained normal. The two who were not inoculated developed typical attacks of whooping cough.

All of these observations seem to establish definitely the *Hemophilus pertussis* as the cause of whooping cough and the value of large doses of vaccine for its prophylaxis. However, the value of vaccine in the active treatment of definitely established cases has been of questionable value. Sauer does not advise the use of his vaccine for treatment and states that three months are required for immunity to develop.

Any treatment which may shorten the course of whooping cough or alleviate the symptoms is certainly valuable. In 1933, Krueger, Nichols, and Frawley[5] described a method for preparation of a new pertussis antigen. Frawley, Stallings, and Nichols[6] used this antigen in the treatment of 165 active cases after the onset of symptoms. They reported good results in 69 per cent of the early cases and 45 per cent of the later cases. They used daily hypodermic injections of 0.1 c.c. increasing until 1.0 c.c. was given. Frawley[7] later recommended the use of much larger doses, using 5 c.c. twice daily, the total amount given varying from 25 to 122 c.c.

Zoeller and Ramon[8] in 1927 described an intranasal method of administering diphtheria toxoid with remarkable success. Friedman, Esserman, and Black[9] in 1934 described a method of immunizing children against scarlet fever by the intranasal instillation of scarlet fever toxin. They used this method in two groups of cases and reported complete immunity in 60 per cent and 71 per cent of these groups and partial immunity in many others.

An intranasal method of administering a pertussis antigen appealed to us for three reasons: (1) The treatment avoids the necessity of the use of the hypodermic needle to which the children and parents usually object. (2) It can be administered very easily by the mother. (3) There is complete freedom from reactions.

The antigen which we used was prepared by the laboratories of the Sharp & Dohme Company according to the following method:

The cultures of *Hemophilus pertussis* were grown on blood agar. They were then macerated in physiologic saline adjusted to pH 8.4. The insoluble residue was discarded, and the soluble protein was precipitated with acetone. The acetone precipitate, after removal of the acetone, was dissolved in physiologic salt solution to which a mercurial preservative had been added. The final product represented the soluble protein of about 20,000 million organisms per cubic centimeter.

We realize that the number of cases in this series is small. However, we feel that the high percentage of favorable results and the simplicity of the method of treatment definitely class this intranasal antigen as a valuable therapeutic procedure in the treatment of active cases of whooping cough.

SUMMARY

1. Twenty-four active cases of whooping cough were treated with an intranasal antigen.

2. Of this series 45.8 per cent showed marked improvement; 29.2 per cent showed moderate improvement; 25 per cent showed slight or no improvement.

3. The antigen was given daily or every second day for from four to twelve treatments.

4. It was used prophylactically in three cases: two patients developed mild attacks and one patient did not develop any symptoms.

5. The antigen can be administered with ease. There are no reactions, and the nasal mucosa is not irritated.

REFERENCES

1. Madsen, Thorvald: J. A. M. A. **101**: 187, 1933.
2. Sauer, Louis: J. A. M. A. **100**: 239, 1933.
3. Sauer, Louis: Am. J. Pub. Health **25**: 1226, 1935.
4. MacDonald, H., and MacDonald, E. J.: J. Infect. Dis. **53**: 328, 1933.
5. Krueger, A. P., Nichols, V. C., and Frawley, J. M.: Proc. Soc. Exper. Biol. & Med. **30**: 1097, 1933.
6. Frawley, J. M., Stallings, M., and Nichols, V. C.: J. Pediat. **4**: 179, 1934.
7. Frawley, J. M.: J. Pediat. **7**: 692, 1935.
8. Zoeller, C., and Ramon, G.: Présse med. **69**: 1049, 1927.
9. Friedman, E., Esserman, A. L., and Black, M. H.: J. Pediat. **5**: 505, 1934.

PROPHYLACTIC PERTUSSIS IMMUNIZATION

Eli Y. Shorr, M.D.
Brooklyn, N. Y.

The use of pertussis vaccine in the prevention of whooping cough was given added stimulus by the report of Sauer[1] in 1933 on a group of 500 children, followed over a period of five years. A total of 8 c.c. (1 c.c. equals 10 billion bacteria) of *Bacillus pertussis* vaccine was given in three weekly bilateral injections of 1, 1.5, and 1.5 c.c. At that time none of the injected children intimately or accidentally exposed had contracted whooping cough during the period of observation. In a later report[2] in November, 1935, a summary of his results, together with reports of thirty-three physicians in nineteen states using the Sauer vaccine and dosage, showed protection in 92 per cent of the vaccinated group.

These studies perhaps emphasize the importance of dosages larger than had previously been employed by Madson,[3] who reported his observations of two epidemics in the Faro Islands in 1924 and 1929. Using 22 billions as his dose in the 1929 epidemic, he found sixteen times as many severe cases and a mortality thirty-three times greater in the unvaccinated group, as compared with the vaccinated group. Further, 24.5 per cent of the vaccinated individuals did not contract the disease, as against 1.8 per cent in the unvaccinated group.

Shortly after Sauer's report in 1933 a study checking the effectiveness of larger doses of vaccine on a group of preschool children in a crowded lower east side section of Manhattan was started. A preliminary survey of 100 records of children enrolled in the Jacobi-Calhoun Pre-School Clinic of the Henry Street Visiting Nurses Association revealed an incidence of approximately 25 per cent of whooping cough in this district. We were interested not only in checking the efficacy of larger doses of Sauer vaccine, but also in evaluating prophylactically the efficacy of a toxin vaccine developed by Mishulow,[4] which was being distributed by the New York City Department of Health and which had been in general use therapeutically since 1930.

OUTLINE OF STUDY

1. Children of preschool age whose histories as to previous illnesses were known from birth were carefully selected. Whenever possible, in families of two or more children, half the number were left unvaccinated as controls. The selected children were all from a very densely populated and circumscribed district, where they were in daily and intimate contact with one another during the period of observation. About half the number attended the same nursery school.

2. A vaccine developed by Mishulow, containing 10 billion *Bacillus pertussis* organisms per cubic centimeter and small amounts of a toxic

substance capable of giving the Shwartzman phenomenon in rabbits, was used. This vaccine differs from the Sauer preparation in that stock strains of proved antigenicity, grown on infusion agar plus 25 to 30 per cent of normal animal blood, were used.

3. A comparison of the intramuscular, subcutaneous and intracutaneous methods of injecting the vaccine was attempted, to determine the best route of administration. The intracutaneous route was suggested by the work of Tuft, Yagle, and Rogers,[5] who found that this method in antityphoid vaccination gave the best results. Mishulow[6] in 1932 also found a delayed but higher agglutinin response to typhoid vaccination when given intracutaneously.

4. Studies of agglutinin response to pertussis vaccine were carried out on a small number. Bleedings were taken before injections, and one week, one month, two months, and three months after the completion of vaccination. This study was in the nature of a preliminary attempt to determine the type and duration of agglutinin response to vaccination. More elaborate and complete studies by Miss Mishulow will be published elsewhere.

5. White blood counts and differential counts were likewise made on this small group in an attempt to check the characteristic lymphocytosis reported by Sauer.

6. A small group was treated with the Sauer vaccine for comparative study.

7. A comparable group of children of preschool age was observed as controls, some receiving injections of sterile milk, which was diluted to the same opacity and injected in the same volume as the vaccine, the remaining controls receiving no injections of any type.

RESULTS

Table I indicates the results of prophylactic vaccination carried out on 74 children. It will be noted that the incidence of those definitely and intimately exposed is quite high—36.5 per cent over a period of thirty months from February, 1933, to August, 1935. The actual exposure, including accidental or casual exposures, must undoubtedly have been higher in such a district as this one.

Of those receiving the Mishulow vaccine, that is, 63 children, 10 developed whooping cough, an incidence of 15.8 per cent. Six of these cases were of not more than three weeks' duration and were without the characteristic whoop and vomiting. They might easily have gone undiagnosed except for the close observation made on these children.

It is to be noted further that 6 of the 10 developing pertussis came down within four months after vaccination, an arbitrary period established by Sauer as necessary for complete immunity to have developed. Four children of this group received small doses from 9 to 22 billions, including 2 who received the vaccine intracutaneously.

In the smaller group of 11 children receiving the Sauer vaccine, one child developed whooping cough 16 months after vaccination, an incidence of 9 per cent. He had received, however, a total of only 40 billion bacilli. The combined groups of 74 vaccinated children show an incidence of pertussis of 14.8 per cent.

TABLE I

VACCINE AND METHOD	TOTAL DOSAGE IN BILLIONS	NO. VACCINATED	DEFINITELY EXPOSED				NO. IN EACH GROUP
			NO.	DOSAGE IN BIL.	MONTHS AFTER VACCIN.	CHILDREN DEVELOPING PERTUSSIS	
Mishulow				79	17	–	0
10 bil.	77-88	7	3	79	4	–	
per c.c.				77	26	–	
				75	1	+ atypical	
	67-75	10	4	75	4	–	2
				73	24	+ atypical	
				70	5 & 21	–	
				66	1	+ atypical	
Intram.				65	1	–	
51				65	2 & 17	–	
	45-66	29	10	65	2	+ mod. severe	2
				60	24	–	
				55		–	
				50	On Vacc.	–	
				50	On Vacc.	–	
				46	3	–	
				45		–	
	12-35	5	2	18	22	+ severe	
				22	18	+ mod. severe	2
Subcut.				70	4	+ atypical	2
7	65-80	7	2	65	4	+ atypical	
Intrac.	9-10½	5	2	10	3	+ atypical	
5				9	7	+ mild	2
Sauer							
10 bil.							
per c.c.				70	4 & 6	–	0
Intram.	40-70	9	3	70	5	–	
9				40	16	+ mod. severe	1
Subcut.				65			
2	20-65	2	0	20			0

The intracutaneous route of administration was quickly abandoned because of the marked local reactions and the large number of injections necessary to give a total anywhere approaching the proposed dosage. The largest single injection given intracutaneously was 0.2 c.c., and the total amount did not exceed 1 c.c. in any child.

Reactions to the subcutaneous or intramuscular injections were never severe, consisting of redness, induration, and tenderness and occasionally a low-grade fever lasting for twenty-four to forty-eight hours. In the majority of the children, the reactions were limited to slight tenderness and induration at the site of injection.

We were unable to confirm the leucocytosis and lymphocytosis reported by Sauer. The blood counts were quite variable, ranging from

TABLE II

INTRAMUSCULAR VACCINATION

DOSAGE C.C.	AGE YR.	SERIAL NO.	NORMAL BLEEDING		AGGLUTINATION PERIOD AFTER VACCINATION WAS COMPLETED: 1 WEEK		2 WEEKS		1 MONTH		6-8 WEEKS		3-5 MONTHS		EX-POSED TO W. C.	DEVEL-OPED W. C.
			DATE	TITER	DATE	TITER	DATE	TITER	DATE	TITER	DATE	TITER	DATE	TITER		
			1933		1933		1933		1933		1933		1933			
6.9	3	S1	2/28	Neg.			5/16	1-80			6/13	1:40	9/19	1:40	+	No
7.9	3	S2	2/28	Neg.					5/2	1:30	6/20	1:8	8/2	1:20	+	No
8.0	3½	S6	3/28	Neg.					5/2	1:130	6/6	1:70	8/29	1:40	–	No
7.0	4	S7	3/28	Neg.	5/16	1:80					6/27	Neg.			+	No
8.0	3½	S8	3/28	Neg.	5/2	1:35			5/23	1:80	6/6	1:40	8/22	1:10	+	No
7.5	4	S9	4/4	Neg.					5/23	1:160	7/11	1:80	8/22	1:35	+	No
7.9	3½	S10	4/4	Neg.	5/16	1:120					6/20	1:75	8/1	1:60	+	No
7.5	3	S11	4/4	Neg.			5/31	Spec Lost							0	No
7.5	3	S18	3/7	Neg.	5/9	1:60									+	Mild
6.9	4	S15			4/18	Neg.	5/23	Spec Lost					7/25	1:30	+	No
6.3	3	S20	5/31	1-30									7/18	Neg.	+	No
Intracutaneous																
1.10	6	S3	3/6	Neg.	4/11	1:60					5/31	1:120	8/8	1:35	+	No
1.00	2½	S4	3/6	Neg.	5/9	1:60									+	Atyp.
0.90	3	S5	3/6	Neg.					5/9	1:40	6/13	1:40	8/29	1:120	+	Atyp.
1.25	3½	S12	4/4	Neg.	4/11	Neg.					5/31	1:40	7/25	1:15	+	No
1.05	3½	S13			4/11	Neg.							7/18	Neg.	0	No
Controls—Milk—Intramuscular																
7.5	5	S14	4/15	Neg.					5/23	Neg.	6/27	Neg.	8/29	1:8	0	No
7.5	3½	S16	4/25	Neg.	5/31	1:15							9/12	1:15	0	No
7.5	3	S17	4/25	1-8	5/31	1:8			6/20	Neg.			8/1	1:10	0	No

normal to an occasional leucocytosis as high as 15,000. There was, however, no uniformity in the blood counts to suggest a specific reaction. The counts were done at the same time bleedings for agglutinin studies were taken.

The agglutinin studies, as seen in Table II, although sparse, revealed in most instances an absence of agglutinins in the control bleedings with a consistent increase in the titers to as high as 1:160 one month after vaccination was completed, and an apparent falling off in the titer in the two- and three-month bleedings. This corresponds with the results obtained by Kristensen and Larsen[7] in complement fixation studies in which they found the highest complement fixation titers were obtained in the first two weeks after vaccination, with a rapid decrease in the titers thereafter. The agglutinin response to the vaccine when given intracutaneously was comparatively delayed but more sustained and reached a titer in two instances at the end of seven to twenty weeks of 1:120, which compares favorably with the highest titers found after 7 to 8 times the amount of vaccine given by the intramuscular route. The controls treated with milk diluted to the same opacity as the vaccine and given in the same way as the vaccine showed consistently negative or insignificantly low titers.

A control group of 72 children, aged two to six years, carefully selected from the same district, were followed for periods of five to nineteen months; 26 children of this group developed unquestionable whooping cough, giving an incidence of 36.1 per cent. The period of observation in this group was somewhat shorter than in the vaccinated group, which was followed as long as thirty months, and it is not unlikely that over a similar period the incidence might be even higher. Twenty-three of the 26 children in the control group developed whooping cough during a local epidemic from seven to nineteen months after observation was begun, only 3 coming down with whooping cough from one to three months after observation was started. No child was included in this group who had not been free from cough for at least one month from the time observation was begun. A comparison of the incidence of pertussis in the vaccinated and unvaccinated groups is shown in Table III.

TABLE III

	NO. OF CHILDREN	NO. OF CHILDREN DEVELOPING W. C.	PERCENTAGE
Controls	72	26	36.1
Mishulow Vaccine	63	10	15.8 } 14.8
Sauer Vaccine	11	1	9.0 } 14.8

DISCUSSION

The answer to the question as to the effectiveness of the prophylactic use of pertussis vaccine must wait on its use in a large series of cases properly controlled and followed for a sufficient period of time. The rather striking difference in the incidence of whooping cough in the vaccinated, as compared with the unvaccinated group, and the apparent amelioration of symptoms in 7 of the 11 children who did develop whooping cough certainly justify further wide-scale use of the vaccine. The exact dosage is not yet clearly established, although it appears that those receiving the highest doses were apparently completely protected, while those receiving less than 40 billions were likely to develop modified or moderately severe whooping cough.

Although the significance of agglutinins as an index of immunity is not established, it is interesting to note the response to vaccination. Assuming some relationship, it seems reasonable to believe from our studies that vaccinated children should be at least partially, if not entirely, protected against pertussis much earlier than the four-month period proposed by Sauer, and we have consequently included all cases developing after a period of one month or longer, following the completion of vaccination. This is obviously a more rigid test of a vaccine, but until the exact value of the presence of those antibodies which are measurable in the blood stream is established, the elapsed period necessary for complete immunization must remain uncertain.

The subcutaneous route of administration thus far appears to be the method of choice, and the larger doses can be easily given in three weekly bilateral injections of 1, 1.5, and 1.5 c.c. without fear of any untoward reactions. It is interesting to note the type of agglutinin response in those children who received the vaccine intracutaneously and the fact that even very small amounts given this way were able to modify the disease considerably in the two children who eventually developed whooping cough. Therefore, in spite of the rather marked local reactions, the use of the intracutaneous route either alone or combined with the subcutaneous administration should not be abandoned without further study.

On the basis of the reduction of incidence of whooping cough in the vaccinated group treated with the Mishulow[4] vaccine, it would appear that potent vaccines may be prepared of stock cultures. It has been found that pertussis cultures can be maintained in stock without loss of their original characteristics if they are grown under suitable conditions. Furthermore, Mishulow[6] reports a higher agglutinin response in a group of children injected with the toxin vaccine than in those who received the Sauer preparation. The advantage of such a vaccine for large-scale prophylactic use is important in that it eliminates the necessity for obtaining freshly isolated strains to be grown on culture media containing human blood.

SUMMARY

1. Of 74 children injected with the varying doses of pertussis vaccine and followed over a period of thirty months, 11 developed whooping cough, giving an incidence of 14.8 per cent.

2. A comparable number of controls (72) followed over a somewhat shorter period (nineteen months) showed an incidence of 36.1 per cent of whooping cough developing during this time.

3. The subcutaneous or intramuscular injection of pertussis vaccine in amounts of not less than 65 billion bacilli has apparently afforded complete protection of those children subsequently exposed or has resulted in a marked amelioration of symptoms in the few who developed whooping cough.

4. The intracutaneous route of administration, although associated with rather marked local reactions, gave an agglutinin response comparable in titer with that found in children receiving from seven to eight times as much subcutaneously or intramuscularly and even in small amounts (10 billions) was apparently able to modify the infection when it occurred.

5. The use of the Mishulow vaccine compares favorably with that of Sauer in its prophylactic effect and for large-scale prophylactic usage eliminates the necessity of obtaining freshly isolated strains to be grown on culture media containing human blood.

Miss Lucy Mishulow, of the Bureau of Laboratories, New York City Department of Health, supplied the vaccine and carried out the agglutination studies reported in this paper.

REFERENCES

1. Sauer, L.: J. A. M. A. **100**: 239, 1933.
2. Sauer, L.: Am. J. Pub. Health **25**: 1226, 1935.
3. Madson, T.: J. A. M. A. **101**: 187, 1933.
4. Mishulow, L., Mowry, I. W., and Scott, E. B.: J. Immunol. **19**: 227, 1930.
5. Tuft, L., Yagle, E. M.. and Rogers, S.: J. Infect. Dis. **50**: 98, 1932.
6. Mishulow, L.: To be published.
7. Kristensen, M., and Ahrend Larsen, L.: Compt. rend. Soc. de biol. **95**: 1110, 1926.

CALCIUM AND PHOSPHORUS METABOLISM IN A CASE OF INTRACTABLE RICKETS

WALTER J. HIGHMAN, JR., AND BENGT HAMILTON, M.D.
CHICAGO, ILL.

WITHIN recent years cases of late rickets which did not respond to ordinary antirachitic treatment have been described. Hess[1] reported on a patient to whom 1,600 drops of viosterol had to be given daily before satisfactory healing was obtained. In cases published by Shelling and Hopper[2] some of the patients required much larger doses of viosterol than are ordinarily given in order to obtain healing. We have had the opportunity to observe three cases of this kind, and in one of them we have made a study of the calcium and phosphorus metabolism.

In rickets an enlargement of the parathyroid glands has been reported,[3-7] and increased amount of parathyroid hormone have been found in the blood.[8] In two important respects, however, the calcium metabolism in rickets differs from that in hyperparathyroidism accompanying a tumor of the parathyroids: the serum calcium in rickets is either normal or, if tetany supervenes, lower than normal, while hypercalcemia is nearly always found in the disease caused by parathyroid tumor; and, second, the urinary output of calcium is normal in rickets[9] and is high in the presence of parathyroid tumor.[10] On the other hand, the rachitic metabolism is characterized by an increased excretion of phosphorus and sometimes, although to a lesser extent, calcium in the stools.[9]

In the presence of a parathyroid tumor, the hyperparathyroidism is, obviously, the primary cause of the disease of the bones. In rickets the rôle played by the hyperparathyroidism is not known, but it seems highly probable that it is a secondary phenomenon and not a primary factor. The question arises, however, whether in the type of case under discussion here, where the rachitic symptoms do not yield to ordinary treatment, the parathyroid glands may play a more important rôle in the development of the disease than in the ordinary case. If that were so, then one might expect to find also other symptoms of primary hyperparathyroidism, such as a high serum calcium and increased calcium output in the urine.

Our chief purpose in making this study was, then, to investigate whether the metabolism of calcium and phosphorus in this case was that usually associated with rickets, or whether it presented any other features, especially those of primary hyperparathyroidism.

From the Department of Pediatrics, University of Chicago.

METHODS

The basic diet (Diet 1) was low in calcium so that the endogenous calcium output might be approximately measured.[11] Diet 2 contained calcium and phosphorus in amounts calculated to be normal for an individual of this age. The patient received the test diets for three days or more before the collection of urine and stools was begun for each period. Each period was of six days' duration.

The composition of the food was calculated from the tables of Sherman,[12] Pattee[13] and the United States Department of Agriculture.[14] Occasional aliquots of the diets were analyzed to check the calculated values. According to our calculations, Diet 1 should contain 0.102 gm. of calcium per day, and our two analyses gave the content as 0.104 and 0.110. In Diet 2 the calculated value was 1.282 gm., the determined values 1.352 and 1.298 gm. Phosphorus in Diet 1: the calculated value was 0.850; the determined value, 0.862 gm. and 0.865 gm. In Diet 2 the calculated value of phosphorus was 1.563 gm.; the determined value, 1.554 and 1.598 gm. The nitrogen determinations gave similarly good checks with the calculated values.

Calcium was determined by the method of Fiske and Logan[15] slightly modified, phosphorus by the method of Fiske and Subbarow.[16] Both these determinations were made on the ash of stool, urine, and diet. Nitrogen was determined directly on urine, and on dried stool and diet by the method of Kjeldahl. The method of Hamilton and Schwartz[17, 18] was used for estimating the amount of parathyroid hormone in the blood.

HISTORY OF CASE

C. W., a white female child, was first seen in this clinic at the age of five years in 1931. The complaint then was marked bowing of the legs, which had first been noticed three years previously. She had been a full-term, breast-fed baby, and had cut her first teeth at eleven months and walked at eighteen months of age. Since the age of six months "she had received three teaspoons of cod liver oil daily." Presumably her development during the first two years of life had been fairly normal, and she had not been seriously ill at any time.

The bowing of the legs had first been noticed at the age of two years but had not been recognized as rickets at that time. On her first hospital visit all the long bones showed marked deformities; the roentgenogram showed typical rachitic changes in the epiphyses. A diagnosis of active rickets was made, and treatment was recommended (16 c.c. of phosphorized cod liver oil daily). After seven months of this treatment no improvement was noted, and the child was admitted to the hospital for study. The diagnosis of rickets was confirmed by biopsy, by determination of the serum phosphorus, and by further roentgenograms.

During the subsequent years, the child was constantly on antirachitic treatment in ordinary doses, but no definite improvement of the condition was ever observed. Operations were performed to correct the deformities of her legs, but these operations had no lasting result. During these years the serum phosphorus was determined ten times. The average value was 2.1 mg. per 100 c.c., with a minimum of 1.5, a maximum of 2.7 mg. per 100 c.c. The average of ten determinations of serum calcium was 10.3 mg. per 100 c.c., the minimum was 9.6, the maximum 11.2 mg. per 100 c.c.*

At no time were any symptoms observed indicating that the rachitic condition might be due to kidney disease. In November, 1934, the nonprotein nitrogen of the serum was 31 mg. per 100 c.c.; the phenolsulphonephthalein test gave 65 per cent recovery in two hours; and the concentration test showed a maximum concentration of 1.026. Renal rickets could, therefore, be ruled out.

Two tests for parathyroid hormone in the blood were made at this time. The rise in the rabbit's blood calcium was 0.40 mM on the first occasion, 0.60 mM on the

*Seven of the phosphorus determinations and seven of the calcium determinations were made during the period of metabolic study reported in this paper.

second (normal, not more than 0.30 mM). Both tests are definitely positive, indicating that more than normal amounts of parathyroid hormone were present in the patient's blood.

In December, 1934, she was admitted for the studies of calcium and phosphorus metabolism which are here reported. It may be mentioned that during the time this

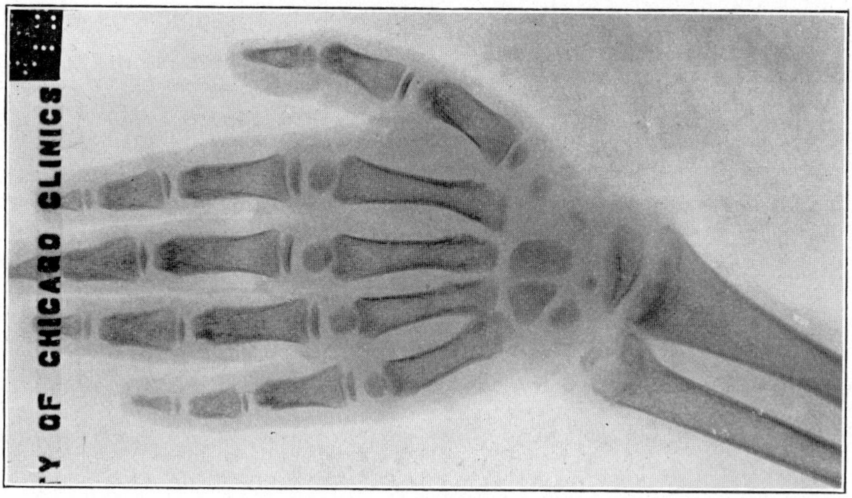

Fig. 1.—Roentgenogram of left wrist in April, 1931.

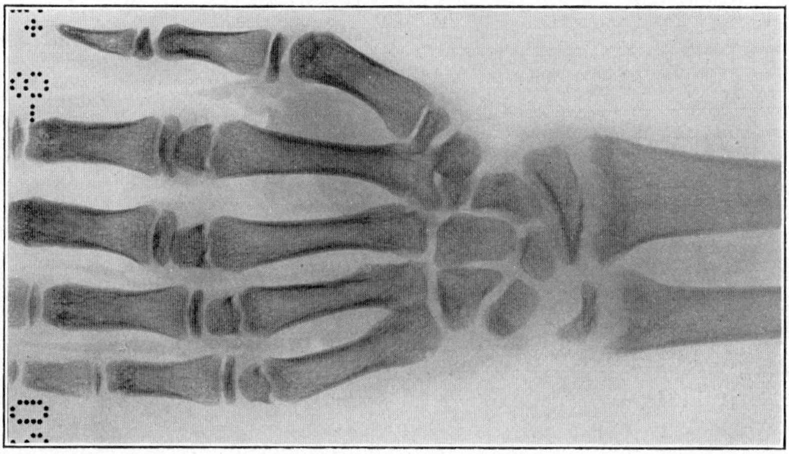

Fig. 2.—Roentgenogram of left wrist in August, 1935, after more than four years of antirachitic treatment. The rachitic changes are about equally marked as in the first film.

study has been in progress (Dec. 10, 1934, to Aug. 13, 1935), no definite improvement of the rachitic process has been observed either in the roentgenogram or the value for serum phosphorus.

DISCUSSION

Nitrogen Metabolism.—The child was in positive nitrogen balance throughout the study.

Calcium Metabolism.—The patient's output of calcium in the stools and urine on the low calcium diet (Diet 1, Table I) showed little difference from the figures given by Stearns, Oelke, and Boyd[19] for normal children and by Bauer, Albright, and Aub[11] for normal adults on a low calcium diet. The calculated balance of calcium (intake minus output) was slightly negative on the low calcium diet but tended to become positive when 30 drops of viosterol were given. Considering the fact, however, that the intake was calculated from tables, not determined by analysis, the only conclusion we feel justified in drawing is that there were neither any marked loss or gain of calcium on this diet. On the diet containing a normal amount of calcium, the daily balance became definitely positive.

It has already been mentioned that the serum calcium of this patient was consistently normal, and we may, therefore, conclude that in every respect in which it was tested, the calcium metabolism was normal. The excretion of calcium in the urine was not increased; although the amounts of parathyroid hormone in the blood were greater than normal, the case presented no features typical of primary hyperparathyroidism.

Phosphorus Metabolism.—On a low phosphorus intake the phosphorus balance was consistently and markedly negative. There was an improvement when viosterol (30 drops) or sodium glycerophosphate was given, but even after this improvement had taken place, the losses of phosphorus must be considered quite marked.

When a normal intake of phosphorus was given with the food (Diet 2, Table I), the phosphorus balance approached zero, and after the addition of 100 drops of viosterol to this diet small amounts of phosphorus were, apparently, retained.

Calculating the "absorption" of phosphorus, that is, the intake minus excretion in the stools, we find that on a low phosphorus diet without viosterol, and during early viosterol administration on this diet, more phosphorus left the intestine in the stools than entered it in the food. When the phosphorus intake was increased the "absorption" improved, but only when 100 drops of viosterol were given was this improvement sufficient to cause a retention of phosphorus.

The study of the phosphorus metabolism shows, then, that the phosphorus given with the food was not at all, or only poorly, utilized. In all probability the phosphorus was not absorbed from the intestinal tract, at least not in normal amounts. In favor of this assumption is the constantly low serum phosphorus and also the fact that sometimes larger amounts of phosphorus were excreted in the stools than the amounts ingested; some of the phosphorus entering the intestinal tract with the digestive juices was, obviously, lost to the body. It should be mentioned in this connection that the patient did not have any diarrhea; to the contrary, there was a marked tendency to constipation.

TABLE I

PERIOD AND DATES	REMARKS		CALCIUM GM./24 HR. OUTPUT	CALCIUM GM./24 HR. INTAKE	CALCIUM GM./24 HR. RETENTION	PHOSPHORUS GM./24 HR. OUTPUT	PHOSPHORUS GM./24 HR. INTAKE	PHOSPHORUS GM./24 HR. RETENTION	"ABSORPTION"
I		Stool	0.138			1.217			
12/10/34	Diet 1*	Urine	0.042			0.325			
12/16/34		Total	0.180	0.099	–0.081	1.542	0.804	–0.738	–0.413
II		Stool	0.081			1.080			
12/16/34	Diet 1 and 30 drops irradiated	Urine	0.037			0.323			
12/22/34	ergosterol	Total	0.118	0.102	–0.016	1.403	0.850	–0.553	–0.230
12/23/34 to 1/3/35 at home on normal diet and 30 drops irradiated ergosterol per day									
III		Stool	0.074			0.788			
1/ 7/35	Diet 1 and 30 drops irradiated	Urine	0.029			0.317			
1/13/35	ergosterol	Total	0.103	0.101	–0.002	1.105	0.843	–0.262	+0.055
IV		Stool	0.075			1.434			
1/22/35	Diet 1 and 100 c.c. 5 per cent	Urine	0.017			0.645			
1/28/35	sodium glycerophosphate	Total	0.092	0.102	+0.010	2.079	1.649	–0.430	+0.215
V		Stool	0.879			1.120			
2/3/35	Diet 2	Urine	0.028			0.554			
2/9/35		Total	0.907	1.282	+0.375	1.674	1.553	–0.121	+0.433
2/20/35 to 7/31/35 at home on normal diet and antirachitic treatment†									
VI		Stool	0.850			0.896			
8/ 7/35	Diet 2 and 100 drops irradiated	Urine	0.029			0.562			
8/13/35	ergosterol	Total	0.879	1.282	+0.403	1.458	1.563	+0.105	+0.667

*Because of a tendency to constipation, 0.5 c.c. of aromatic fluid extract of cascara was given daily.

†The patient was advised to take 100 drops of viosterol daily. For economic reasons the mother at times gave 3 teaspoonfuls of cod liver oil instead of the viosterol. At other times the patient was given free samples of various concentrated preparations of vitamin D. It is probable, however, that during all this period antirachitic treatment was given, most of the time in rather high doses.

The metabolism of this case is typical of rickets, in that the chief abnormality consists of marked losses of phosphorus in the stools. Quite atypical, however, is the very sluggish response of the phosphorus metabolism to the administration of vitamin D, and it seems possible that the underlying condition is an inability to utilize this vitamin.

SUMMARY

A girl ten years old had suffered from marked rickets at least since the age of two and was not benefited by antirachitic treatment in ordinary doses.

The metabolism of calcium and phosphorus in this case was typical of rickets and showed no similarity to that found in primary hyperparathyroidism. This rachitic metabolism did not, however, respond to the administration of vitamin D in the usual manner; an inability to utilize this vitamin might, therefore, be the cause of disease in this case.

REFERENCES

1. Hess, J. H.: Am. J. Dis. Child. **42**: 488, 1931.
2. Shelling, D. H., and Hopper, K. B.: Am. J. Dis. Child. **47**: 61, 1934.
3. Erdheim: Denkschr. d. k. Akad. d. Wissensch., Math.-naturw. Klasse, Wien **90**: 363, 1914.
4. Ritter, C.: Frankfurt. Ztschr. f. Path. **24**: 137, 1920.
5. Pappenheimer, A. M., and Minor, J.: J. M. Research **42**: 391, 1921.
6. Higgins, G. M., and Sheard, C.: Am. J. Physiol. **85**: 299, 1928.
7. Stoltenberg, L.: Norsk. Mag. f. Laegevidensk. **90**: 729, 1929.
8. Hamilton, B., and Schwartz, C.: Am. J. Dis. Child. **46**: 775, 1933.
9. Hess, A. F.: Rickets, Including Osteomalacia and Tetany, Philadelphia, 1929, Lea & Febiger.
10. Literature reviewed by Barr, D. P., and Bulger, H. A., Am. J. M. Sc. **179**: 449, 1930.
11. Bauer, W., Albright, F., and Aub, J.: J. Clin. Investigation **7**: 75, 1929.
12. Sherman, H. C.: Chemistry of Food and Nutrition, ed. 4, New York, 1932, The Macmillan Company.
13. Pattee, A. F.: Dietetics, Mount Vernon, N. Y., 1929.
14. U. S. Department of Agriculture, Bulletin No. 28, American Food Materials.
15. Fiske, C. H., and Logan, M.: J. Biol. Chem. **93**: 211, 1931.
16. Fiske, C. H., and Subbarow, Y.: J. Biol. Chem. **66**: 375, 1925.
17. Hamilton, B., and Schwartz, C.: J. Pharmacol. & Exper. Therap. **46**: 285, 1932.
18. Hamilton, B., and Highman, W. J., Jr.: J. Clin. Investigation **15**: 99, 1936.
19. Stearns, G., Oelke, M. J., and Boyd, J. D.: Am. J. Dis. Child. **42**: 88, 1931.

CARCINOMA OF THE ADRENAL CORTEX

A. A. Little, Jr., M.D., Houston, Texas

CARCINOMA of the adrenal cortex with its interesting symptom-complex, virilism, hirsuties, adiposity, and hypertension has been reported a number of times. Lehman[1] reported a case of adrenal tumor removed from an eleven-month-old infant in 1917, which was described as an undifferentiated tumor. Lightwood[2] recorded a case of an infant eighteen weeks old who at autopsy was found to have a carcinoma of the left suprarenal cortex. Van der Bogert[3] reported a case of a female, aged two years, with the symptom-complex of obesity, precocious development, hirsuties, voice changes, virilism, marked hypertrophy of the clitoris and external genitals, together with hypertension and cardiac enlargement. At operation a tumor mass, differentiated as a carcinoma, was removed from the left suprarenal gland. No autopsy was permitted. F. Graham Lecher,[4] in 1935, reported a case of carcinoma of the adrenal cortex in a woman thirty-five years of age, which showed all the cardinal and most of the occasional symptoms and signs recently ascribed by Cushing to an adenoma of the basophile cells of the anterior lobe of the pituitary. Hare, Ross, and Crooke[5] reported a similar case in a woman thirty-two years of age. An extensive search of the pituitary at postmortem failed to reveal any change either in the gross or microscopic sections.

The following is a report of a case presenting the interesting, complex-syndrome of virilism, hirsuties, adiposity, hypertrophy of the clitoris, precocious development, voice change, hypertension, muscular weakness, and convulsions.

The patient, a white female, aged seven and one-half years, was admitted to the pediatric service of the Jefferson Davis Hospital, Sept. 28, 1935, in a convulsive state.

She was the first child of young, healthy parents. There was no family history of mental or glandular disorders. There was no history of syphilis. Pregnancy was normal and delivery not unduly prolonged. There was no history of birth injury or injury in early childhood. She had had chickenpox, pertussis, and mumps. Her mental and structural development was normal for the first two years. When she was three and one-half years old, the parents noted that she was rather large for her age, development being more horizontal than vertical. At the age of four and one-half years hair began to appear on the body and face, and the habitus became that of the male. Pubic hair at this time was extensive, and there was hypertrophy of the external genitals. The voice deepened. Medical aid was sought at this time and treatment consisting of thyroid and whole ovary was followed by some regression of symptoms and signs. After about fifteen months of treatment there was a return of the symptoms; the family became despondent and discontinued treatment. The symptoms and signs progressed, and the child became more and more of the masculine type. On Sept. 27, 1935, the patient ate a large supper and awoke about 4 A.M. with severe abdominal cramps. Following this she went into a generalized convulsive state (her first convulsion), and was brought to the hospital, where she was placed on the ward. She could be aroused with some difficulty. The convulsions were controlled, and the study of the case was begun.

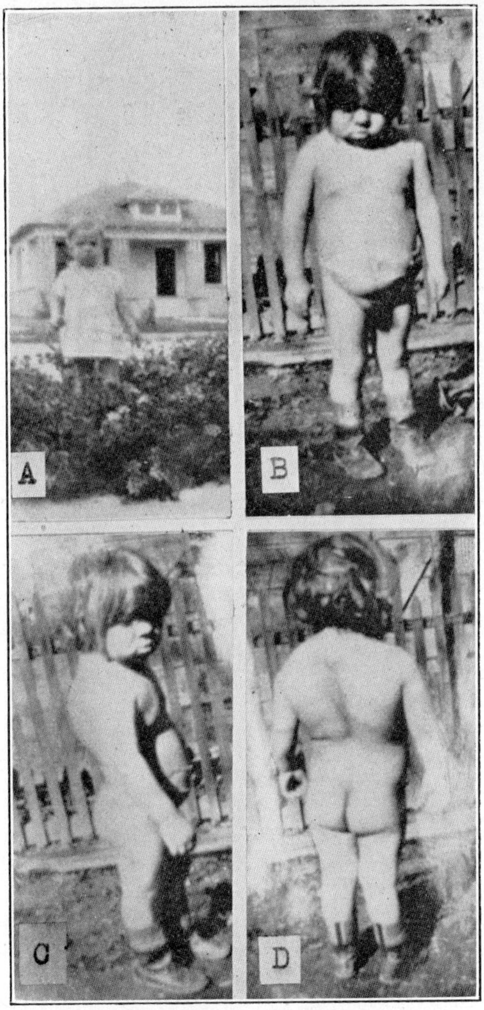

Fig. 1.—*A*, upper left, patient at the age of three years. *B*, upper right, patient at the age of four and one-half years, front view. *C*, lower left, patient at the age of four and one-half years, side view. *D*, lower right, patient at the age of four and one-half years, back view. Note broad shoulders, thick neck, narrow hips, and thin legs.

On examination the patient was a stocky, seven-and-one-half-year-old girl with adult habitus. The height was normal. The face thick, broad, and round, and the eyebrows were thick and bushy. There was a coarse growth of hair on the chin, throat, and upper lip. An aciniform eruption was present on the face. The voice was deep and resounding. The skull was thick, with heavy bones. The neck was short and thick. The shoulders were broad with the waist, the arms, and the legs,

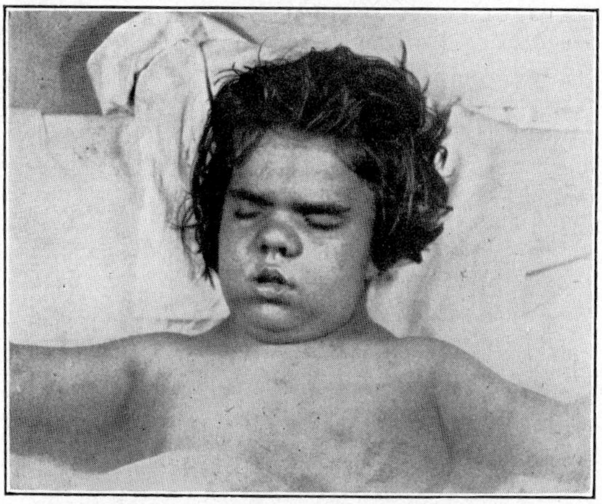

Fig. 2.—Patient at the age of seven and one-half years. Note the heavy hair, thick lips, bushy eyebrows, thick nose, and male type of breasts.

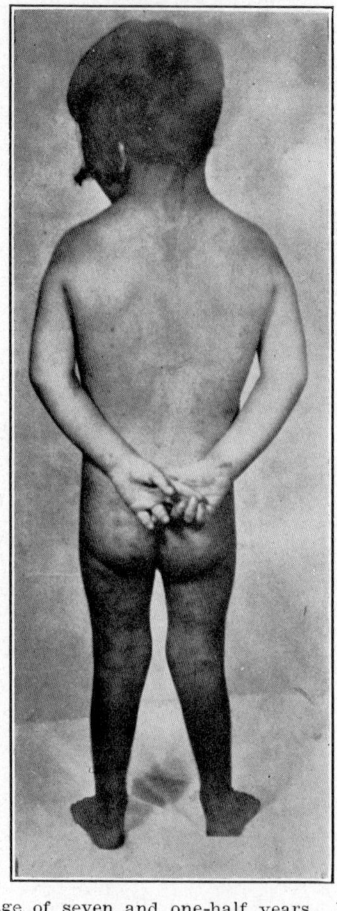

Fig. 3.—Patient at the age of seven and one-half years. Note the broad shoulders, narrow hips, thin legs, and the male type of torso.

thin. Fatty deposits were present around the neck and shoulders. There was extensive hirsuties and fully developed pubic hair.

The fundi of the eye were normal. The teeth showed no abnormalities. The tonsils were enlarged and cryptic and slightly inflamed, and the pharynx was mildly injected. The chest was short and wide with flat nipples resembling the male type. Areolar hair was present. Auscultation and percussion of the lungs were normal. The heart action was rapid. The blood pressure was 120/80, and there was moderate cardiac hypertrophy.

The abdominal wall was thick. No abnormal masses could be felt, nor was tenderness present. Pubic hair was fully developed, and there was a hypertrophy of the external genitals, with an abnormally developed clitoris. The clitoris was about 3 cm. long by 1 cm. thick, resembling the male penis. There was a normal female type urethra. The hymen was intact, and the vaginal orifice admitted one finger. Rectal examination was negative. Digital examination showed the uterus to be small.

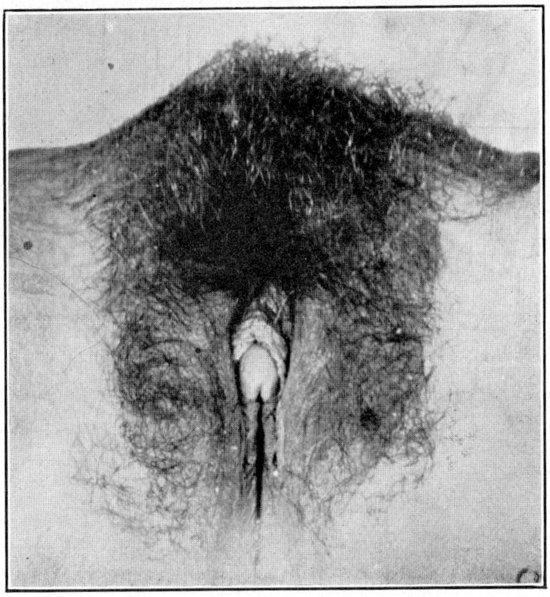

Fig. 4.—Hypertrophy of clitoris and external genitals. Note fully developed pubic hair.

The extremities were thin and resembled the male type. Reflexes were normal.

Laboratory Findings.—The hemoglobin content was 80 per cent; red blood cells were 3,500,000; leucocytes, 16,000; and differential count was normal. Urinalysis was normal except for a trace of albumin. The blood Wassermann was negative. Blood chemistry: sugar, 100 mg. per 100 c.c.; creatinin 1.0 mg.; urea nitrogen, 17.8 mg.; total nonprotein nitrogen, 38 mg.; phosphorus, 2.4 mg.; calcium, 8.6 mg. The spinal fluid was clear under no increase in pressure; cell count, 10; globulin, unincreased; Wassermann test, negative; mastic test, negative. Stool examination was negative. Sugar tolerance was lowered. Kidney function was normal. Aschheim-Zondek test was negative.

X-ray examination of the skull showed a normal sella turcica. The chest plates showed some cardiac enlargement, with hilar glandular involvement. The bones showed moderate osteoporosis with a more brittle appearance than normal. Flat plates of the abdomen showed an irregular, calcified mass in the upper left quadrant. Pyelograms showed a distortion of the calyces and pelvis of the left kidney.

No therapy was begun until all studies had been completed. On October 22 an indefinite mass was felt in the left upper quadrant with a moderate degree of tenderness. After a rather copious stool the mass disappeared, and the tenderness was relieved. Muscular weakness progressed to such a point that the patient became bedridden. While in the hospital she complained chiefly of headaches, abdominal pain, and general weakness. The blood pressure remained consistently high. Exploratory operation of the left kidney and suprarenal was advised, and the patient was posted for operation. Two days before the scheduled operation she developed hypostatic pneumonia and died seven days later.

Autopsy.—The body was opened in the midline, and the organs of the thorax and abdomen were examined. The right pleura was shiny and glistening. The left pleura was covered by a purulent exudate, and there was a pleural effusion of about 100 c.c. The lower lobes of both lungs showed a hypostatic pneumonia, the left lower lobe more involved than the right. Throughout the lobes of both lungs there were multiple metastatic nodules, varying in size from pinpoint to 1 cm. in diameter. The thyroid and parathyroid glands were normal. The heart was normal in size, shape, and position. The gastrointestinal tract was normal throughout. The liver was normal in size, shape, position, color, and consistency, but in the upper portion of the right lobe there was a metastatic nodule 3 cm. in diameter, which was apparently composed of the same tissue as the nodules down in the lungs. The right suprarenal gland was small and atrophic. The left suprarenal gland was involved in a large tumorous mass involving the whole left upper abdominal gutter. The mass was very nodular, measuring 15 by 13 by 5 cm., and was well encapsulated. On section the consistency was variable, some portions being soft and necrotic and others being firm. The color was reddish with yellowish streaks and areas. The mass did not invade the left kidney but was attached to it and pushed it down into the pelvis. On section both kidneys were apparently normal. The pituitary gland was normal in size, shape, and position, and the sella turcica was normal.

Microscopic sections from the adrenal growth showed a highly cellular structure. The cells were hyperchromatic and of irregular size with a considerable number of giant cells interspersed. The arrangement was diffuse, with strands of fibrous connective tissue intervening. The nuclei of the tumor cells were highly granular with many mitotic figures. The stroma was scant and consisted of a framework of fibrous connective tissue. Necrosis was rather marked and much diffuse hemorrhage was observed. The sections from the metastatic nodules of the lung and liver showed the same histologic picture as described above, except that the sections from nodules in the lungs showed many more capillaries filled with blood than did the adrenal growth and the nodules in the liver. Sections of the pituitary body showed normal cellular structure.

COMMENT

A case of carcinoma of the cortex of the suprarenal gland with metastasis to the liver and lungs is presented. The accompanying symptom-complex syndrome of virilism, hirsuties, adiposity, precocious development, voice change, hypertension, and hypertrophy of the clitoris and external genitals associated with hyperfunction of the adrenal gland has been reported a number of times. The function of the adrenal cortex remains shrouded in mystery. Animals without the cortex die. Whether hyperfunction or hyperexcretion of the hormones of the cortex of the suprarenal gland influences the function of the other glands of internal secretion is debatable. There are cases of adrenal adenomas which produce the symptoms described by Cushing and are attributed to adenomas of the basophile cells of the anterior lobe of the pituitary body.[6] In this case gross and microscopic sections of the pituitary failed to reveal any deviation from the normal. Sections of the ovary were normal for development. No abnormalities were found in the thymus, thyroid, parathyroid and pineal glands.

CONCLUSIONS

1. A case of carcinoma of the adrenal cortex, with a symptom-complex of virilism, hirsuties, adiposity, hypertrophy of the clitoris and external genitals, voice changes, hypertension, muscular weakness, and convulsions is presented.

2. The remaining glands of internal secretion were found to be normal.

REFERENCES

1. Lehman, E. P.: Ann. Surg. **95**: 473, 1932.
2. Lightwood, Reginald: Arch. Dis. Child. **7**: 37, 1932.
3. Van der Bogert, Frank: J. Pediat. **3**: 629, 1933.
4. Lecher, F. Graham: Quart. J. Med. **4**: 23, 1935.
5. Hare, Dorothy, Ross, J. M., and Crooke, A. C.: Lancet **2**: 118, 1935.
6. Loeb, Robert F.: J. A. M. A. **104**: 2177, 1935.

817 Holman Avenue

HEMORRHAGES COMPLICATING DEEP PHARYNGEAL INFECTION

Ira Frank, M.D., and Arthur F. Abt, M.D.
Chicago, Ill.

SEVERE arterial hemorrhage occurring as a complication of pharyngeal infections in childhood is usually of such sudden and dramatic occurrence that prompt and effective treatment is necessary to meet an emergency which has not been sufficiently stressed in the pediatric literature.

We have recently encountered four cases of this type, which we wish to report. Liston[1] in 1843 was probably the first to demonstrate that an abscess of the cervical region could erode the carotid artery. Gross[2] in 1871 collected cases of hemorrhage from the common carotid and internal carotid arteries caused by postscarlatinal cervical abscess.

Salinger and Pearlman[3] in 1933 were able to collect from the literature 231 instances of arterial and venous hemorrhage complicating peritonsillar, pharyngeal, parapharyngeal, and cervical abscesses. The types of abscess occurring in our patients were retro- or parapharyngeal, and the hemorrhage in all four cases was arterial. We shall, therefore, exclude from consideration other infections of the throat and neck and hemorrhage of venous origin. The hemorrhages with which we are concerned occurred as a result of erosion of important arteries due to pharyngeal infection and were not due to injury or incision of blood vessels as a direct result of a surgical procedure.

CASE REPORTS

Case 1.—T. S., a nine-year-old boy, was admitted to the hospital on April 30, 1923, because of difficulty in swallowing, slight dyspnea, marked left cervical adenitis, temperature of 104° F., and a rapid pulse.

Previous History.—The mother stated that the child had been well until ten days prior to admission, when he complained of slight chilliness, mild sore throat, and headache. The temperature at that time was only slightly elevated. The usual home remedies were employed without any improvement. These symptoms were followed by difficulty in swallowing and cervical adenitis. A diagnosis of a left-sided retropharyngeal abscess was then made, and the patient sent to the hospital for surgical care.

The child was admitted late at night, and, since there appeared to be no immediate indication for surgical interference, it was decided to wait until morning to make a more thorough examination. During the early morning hours the child suddenly began to bleed profusely from the mouth. The amount of blood was estimated at 300 c.c. He was immediately taken to the operating room. Inspection of the throat showed a soft fluctuating mass on the left side of the pharynx when the soft palate was retracted upward. A steady stream of bright red blood spurted from

From the Departments of Pediatrics, Northwestern University Medical School.

the mouth from the location of the bleeding vessel. We were of the opinion that the hemorrhage came from the ascending pharyngeal artery. Accordingly, under local anesthesia, the external carotid artery was ligated. The bleeding immediately ceased. At the time of this surgical experience, blood transfusion was not so universally used as a substitute for loss of blood due to a severe hemorrhage. This child made an uneventful recovery.

CASE 2.—N. C., a nine-year-old boy, was admitted to the hospital on Dec. 19, 1932, because of severe hemorrhage from the nose, throat, and right ear.

Previous History.—The illness of this patient began Dec. 10, 1932, with the usual symptoms accompanying an acute upper respiratory infection. Within a few days the child complained of a mild right-sided sore throat with pain radiating toward the right ear. Examination at this time was negative. A few days later an examination disclosed a slight edema of the posterior pillar of the fauces on the right, moderate right cervical adenitis, and a bulging of the right tympanic membrane, which, when incised, discharged mucopurulent secretion. The condition the next few days remained unchanged with the exception of the swelling in the throat, which became pronounced. On December 19, without any apparent change in the condition of the child, he had a sudden hemorrhage, blood pouring from his nose, throat, and right ear. He was immediately taken to the hospital. An examination of the throat showed a large blood clot in the nasopharynx. Under gas anesthesia, the right external carotid artery was ligated and a transfusion of 350 c.c. of whole blood was given. The temperature at this time was 103.6° F.; pulse, 130; blood pressure, 134/84. During the next few days no actual hemorrhage occurred, although definite oozing was evident from the throat.

On December 24, as the boy was sitting up, there occurred a sudden severe hemorrhage from the throat, the blood spurting beyond the foot of the bed. The patient became comatose, and his pulse was imperceptible. An intravenous injection of 100 c.c. of a 25 per cent glucose was immediately given, following which the patient regained consciousness. The child was again taken to the operating room and the previous incision was opened and the right common carotid artery was ligated. No anesthesia was used, and the patient rallied immediately. A transfusion of 250 c.c. of whole blood was given twelve hours later. There was no recurrence of bleeding. The patient made a complete recovery.

CASE 3.—C. S., a six-year-old girl, was admitted to the hospital because of a severe hemorrhage from the throat.

Previous History.—When first seen, this child was found to be suffering from a right-sided retropharyngeal abscess. The abscess was opened in the usual manner, with a blunt forceps and without difficulty or accident, considerable pus being evacuated. The following day the abscess seemed to be draining satisfactorily, consequently no attempt was made to reopen the cavity. The progress was so satisfactory that it was thought unnecessary to see the child again. Three days later we were notified by telephone that the child had just had a severe hemorrhage from the throat. The child was brought immediately to the hospital, and on her arrival taken to the operating room. Under gas anesthesia the right common carotid artery was ligated. The father proved to be a suitable donor, and the child was given a transfusion of 350 c.c. of blood. The next day, to our amazement, the child had another hemorrhage of 300 c.c. of blood. She was given another transfusion of 300 c.c. of whole blood from a professional donor. Repeated examination of the throat showed no bleeding point. For the next five days the child seemed to be progressing favorably; she took nourishment and appeared interested in her toys. During the night of the fifth day a very severe hemorrhage occurred—to quote the nurse, "The blood just seemed to pour from the mouth." The amount estimated was 400 c.c. The child was again taken to the operating room and the right external carotid artery was ligated. She was given another transfusion of 300 c.c. of whole blood. No further bleeding occurred.

CASE 4.—B. G., a five-year-old girl, was admitted to the hospital because of a sudden hemorrhage from the throat.

Previous History.—This child had been ill for ten days with an upper respiratory infection accompanied by a mild sore throat. After several days the general condition seemed to improve, but symptoms from the throat became more pronounced. The child refused nourishment because of pain on swallowing; she held her head rigidly, and a mild trismus developed. The physician in charge diagnosed a right-sided retropharyngeal abscess and made an unsuccessful attempt to open the abscess. Three days later while the child was resting, she suddenly began to bleed from the throat and lost in all about 100 c.c. of bright blood. She was immediately sent to the hospital, and inspection of the throat showed an abscess cavity on the right side of the pharynx, filled with coagulated blood. The opening into this cavity easily admitted the index finger and the transverse processes of the upper cervical vertebrae could be felt. Just below the angle of the jaw on the right side a swelling about the size of a pigeon's egg was palpable, which could easily be distinguished from the cervical glands present. It was tense, painless, and fluctuation could be elicited.

The history of the case—the spontaneous hemorrhage from the throat following a retropharyngeal abscess, the rather sudden appearance of the swelling in the right cervical region, and the abscess cavity in the pharynx filled with coagulated blood—indicated to us that an erosion of one of the major blood vessels of the neck with the formation of a false aneurysm had occurred. From our previous experience and the experience of others, we considered it in accordance with good surgical judgment to ligate the common carotid artery. Before doing this, however, we aspirated the swelling at the angle of the jaw and found it to contain fluid blood. Ligation of the common carotid artery caused this swelling to disappear, and no further bleeding occurred. The child was given a transfusion of 150 c.c. of whole blood, and recovery was uneventful.

It is of interest to note that all of the four patients here reported had had their tonsils and adenoids removed several years prior to the illness here recorded.

DISCUSSION

A brief anatomic description of the retro- and parapharyngeal spaces will aid in understanding the mechanism of these hemorrhages.

The retropharyngeal space lies anterior to the vertebral column and extends upward to the base of the skull and downward toward the posterior mediastinum. It lies between the pharynx in front and the vertebral column behind. It is enclosed anteriorly and posteriorly by two layers of fascia. It invests the superior constrictor of the pharynx and is continued forward on the buccinator muscle. Laterally it blends with the sheaths of the great vessels. There is a chain of lymph nodes on either side of the midline between the pharyngeal and prevertebral muscles. Each chain consists of a medial and lateral group of lymph nodes. The lateral group is always present in infants and young children, but it may be absent in adults. In early life the number of nodes may vary from three to ten and in adult life rarely more than one or two in the retropharyngeal space. A group of lymph nodes lies in close proximity to the internal carotid artery in the region where it enters the carotid canal. Therefore, an infection in the retropharyngeal space might easily involve this important vessel and, by producing erosion and false aneurysm, could cause rupture and hemorrhage from this artery. The retropharyngeal nodes receive efferent lymphatic vessels from the accessory sinuses of the nose, the nasal fossae, the pharynx, the larynx, and the middle ear. Thus an initial infection arising in any of these regions could be transmitted through the lymphatics to the retropharyngeal space.

The parapharyngeal space is the region of connective tissue which is separated medially from the tonsil by the constrictor muscles of the pharynx and the parapharyngeal fascia.[4] The lateral boundary is formed by internal pterygoid muscle, the ascending ramus of the lower jaw, and the capsule of the parotid. The space extends upward to the base of the skull and downward along the esophagus and larynx into the posterior mediastinum. It is filled with connective tissue and fat, as well as important vessels and nerves. Here are found the carotid artery, the internal jugular vein, the ninth to twelfth cranial nerves, and the sympathetic nerves. There is also a rich network of small veins and numerous lymphatic nodes.

Retropharyngeal or parapharyngeal abscess is usually secondary to an infection of the upper respiratory tract, such as nasopharyngitis, acute rhinitis, tonsillitis, sinusitis, and otitis media.[5] Abscesses of these spaces occur rarely during scarlet fever or measles, though they may complicate a severe erysipelas of the pharynx. They also may be caused by an injury to the pharyngeal wall or by perforation. It has been maintained that retropharyngeal abscess never occurs once the tonsils have been removed. The four patients here reported had their tonsils and adenoids removed several years prior to the acute illness here recorded. These abscesses need not, therefore, be preceded by tonsillar inflammation, and the initial infection may have originated in the nose, pharynx, sinuses, or ears, as probably occurred in our four patients.

A point of particular interest in the cases under discussion is the mechanism of the hemorrhages. In general, it is believed that blood vessels are protected against adjacent infection by an encasing fascial sheath. The protective mechanism is somewhat different if the infection attacks a vein instead of an artery. An infection eroding through the walls of a vein may cause thrombosis within its lumen, the venous walls being strengthened by a fibrinous deposit. Thus while the infection may erode the venous wall, hemorrhage will be unlikely if thrombosis has preceded perforation. The proximity of the internal and common carotid arteries to an infection occurring in the retro- or parapharyngeal spaces has been noted in the anatomical description of these regions. Should the infection penetrate the arterial sheath and directly involve the artery, an erosion of the arterial wall may occur, leading either directly to perforation and rupture of the artery, or to the development of a false aneurysm whose walls may eventually weaken with the result of hemorrhage. Direct perforation of the arterial wall may involve any of the arteries in the proximity of the infected area. The internal carotid artery, from its anatomical position, is most often involved. Less frequently one of the branches of the external carotid artery is involved, such as the ascending pharyngeal or the ascending palatine artery. Occasionally, however, the ascending pharyngeal artery may arise from the internal carotid, and anastomose with the ascending palatine artery arising from the external carotid. Such an anomaly would lead to difficulties in diagnosis and treatment.

DIAGNOSIS AND TREATMENT

The nature and source of the hemorrhage may be of aid in determining the vessel involved. A. B. le Mesurier[6] has pointed out that when swelling of the neck and a fullness of the pharynx precede a sudden diffuse hemorrhage from the ear, which cannot be controlled by packing, the internal carotid artery probably is involved. Brauer[7] has pointed out that spontaneous hemorrhage from the ear in the majority of cases in his experience has been due to a false aneurysm of the internal carotid artery and that erosion of the aneurysm has occurred either into the eustachian tube or into the external auditory canal by way of the parotid space. Case 2 here reported is most likely an example of this type of hemorrhage. Hemorrhage from the pharynx due to direct perforation or rupture of a false aneurysm of the internal carotid artery may be characterized by several minor hemorrhages which may be followed by a severe flow, or by a single fatal hemorrhage. In the severe type of hemorrhage the blood is not coughed up or vomited, but the bright red blood is projected from the mouth with great force. In our second case the nurse was standing at the foot of the bed before the patient's second severe hemorrhage. The boy was apparently resting quietly, when without warning he suddenly aroused and bright arterial blood gushed over the end of the bed and upon the nurse before she could move to his aid. Repeated severe hemorrhages are usually indicative of the erosion of a branch of the external carotid artery. Our Case 1 is probably an example of such a condition, as ligation of the external carotid artery arrested the hemorrhage. When infection and erosion have caused a false aneurysm of the internal carotid artery, a soft smooth swelling may be present in the pharynx, causing a mass behind the tonsillar fossae or a bulging forward of the lateral pharyngeal wall. These swellings may be semifluctuant, and occasionally a definite pulsation is noted. If severe hemorrhages as here described are not adequately treated, they will recur and cause death.

The treatment following an arterial hemorrhage complicating retropharyngeal or parapharyngeal infections demands prompt ligation of the vessel involved. If the character of the hemorrhage is severe and suggests perforation by erosion of the wall or formation of a false aneurysm of the internal carotid artery, the carotid sheath should be exposed and the common carotid artery ligated on the affected side. Ligation of the common carotid artery may produce serious consequences because of the sudden shutting off of the circulation to one-half of the brain. If the circulation could be slowly occluded, the dangers connected with ligation of the common carotid artery would be greatly lessened. However, the emergency following a severe hemorrhage demands that the artery be ligated at once. In regard to ligation of the internal carotid artery, it has been said that cerebral complications are more severe when this artery is tied than when the common carotid itself is tied because of the fact that any collateral circulation between the external and internal carotid arteries would thus be eliminated. Moreover, a more extensive dissection would be necessary in order to reach the internal carotid artery, involving an exposure of the bifurcation. If the bleeding is indicative of perforation of a branch of the external carotid artery, this vessel should be exposed and ligated. Supplementary treatment for severe loss of blood through hemorrhage, such as transfusion, use of acacia, or injection of glucose solution intravenously, and saline solutions administered by hypodermoclysis, should be given as indicated. Complications following ligation of the common carotid artery, such as hemiplegia, or multiple paralyses, convulsions, and other nervous manifestations produced by sudden loss of circulation to the brain, together with ocular and otitic symptoms in the patients who recover, may be of a permanent nature. It must be understood, therefore, that ligation of the common carotid artery is not without danger, but the desperate situation which confronts the surgeon permits him no choice; he must treat unhesitatingly the condition by ligation, when the indications for this procedure are as here stated. The common carotid artery was ligated in three, and the external carotid artery in one of the cases here presented, with no resulting complication, and we are convinced that the procedure was undoubtedly a life-saving measure.

SUMMARY

Four cases of severe arterial hemorrhage from the pharynx and middle ear, arising as a complication of retropharyngeal and parapharyngeal infections, are here reported; all of these patients recovered.

These infections originated from upper respiratory or ear infections; all of the four children here reported had previously had their tonsils removed. The erosion and the perforation of the large arteries of the neck by infection in the retropharyngeal and parapharyngeal spaces have been discussed.

Criteria for the diagnosis of the particular artery involved in the hemorrhage have been enumerated. When the bleeding has been from a branch of the external carotid artery, its ligation has been advised. In three instances of direct perforation of the arterial wall or of false aneurysm of the internal carotid artery, we have successfully ligated the common carotid artery, and in one instance in which perforation occurred in a branch of the external carotid artery, this vessel was also successfully ligated.

We have pointed out that this operation, while not without inherent danger, is imperatively indicated to prevent fatal hemorrhage.

REFERENCES

1. Liston, R.: Brit. & Foreign Med. Rev. **15**: 155, 1843.
2. Gross, S. W.: Am. J. M. Sc. **122**: 337, 1871.
3. Salinger, S., and Pearlman, S. J.: Arch. Otolaryng. **18**: 464, 1933.
4. Abt, Isaac A.: J. Pediat. **1**: 8, 1932.
5. Frank, I.: J. A. M. A. **77**: 517, 1921.
6. Le Mesurier, A. B.: Canad. M. A. J. **25**: 551, 1931.
7. Brauer, W.: Ztschr. f. Hals-, Nasen-, u. Ohrenh. **32**: 561, 1933

104 S. Michigan Avenue

A CASE OF GANGRENOUS VULVITIS WITH ASSOCIATED MOUTH AND RECTAL LESIONS IN A CHILD

William D. Deuell, M.D., and John F. Landon, M.D.
New York, N. Y.

Cases of gangrenous vulvitis are not unusual and have been frequently reported. In the majority of the cases, however, there has been no question concerning the etiology of the condition, either infectious conditions such as diphtheria, gonorrhea, and pneumonia, or blood dyscrasias, such as purpura and agranulocytic angina, being definitely responsible for the vulvar ulcerations. The case here reported, however, does not fall into any specific etiologic category and is presented because of its many unusual features, especially its occurence in a very young child. A careful review of the literature fails to reveal a single similar case reported.

K. F., a three-year-old white child, was admitted on Nov. 14, 1934, to the children's ward of Roosevelt Hospital, service of Dr. Philip Van Ingen. Her history was that of a head cold and cough of ten days' duration, and bleeding from the vagina and rectum for four days. The blood was bright red and appeared as a constant seepage. The child's past history was essentially negative; she had been delivered normally and spontaneously; the birth weight being 7 pounds; she had been bottle fed entirely.

The physical examination revealed an acutely ill child with frontal bossing of the head, a slight nasal discharge, coated tongue, and crusted lips. The tonsils and pharynx were red and injected. There was a slight impairment of the breath sounds over the left lung posteriorly and many coarse râles were heard over both sides. The vagina was filled with clotted blood. The labia majora were red, swollen, and excoriated. On admission there were no mouth lesions other than the excoriations of the lips.

A vaginoscopic examination showed a normal cervix with no bleeding from the uterus. Bloody mucus was present in the vagina, the blood apparently seeping from the vaginal mucous membrane. There were no ulcerations of the vaginal wall. Sigmoidoscopic examination revealed a normal mucosa of the sigmoid with engorgement of the hemorrhoidal veins and small ulcerations of the lower rectum.

On the fourth day after admission, numerous white plaques were seen in the mucous membranes of the mouth, which were buccal, sublingual, and lingual in distribution and which became necrotic. They were similar in appearance to the lesion of the vulva.

The laboratory work failed to reveal the common etiologic organisms of such ulcerations. Repeated nose and throat cultures were negative for diphtheria and hemolytic streptococci. Vaginal smears and cultures were negative for diphtheria and streptococci, with staphylococci predominating and a few gram-positive diplococci present. Smears from the sigmoid and lower rectum showed no Klebs-Loeffler bacilli, no predominating organisms; cultures taken during the proctoscopic examination grew minute gram-negative cocci and *B. pyocyaneus*. Smears from the membrane of the labia showed much fungus growth and white blood cells, and cultures revealed a minute gram-negative coccus. Smears from the mouth lesions were negative for diphtheria, Vincent's organisms, and fungi, only cocci being present.

The white blood cell count was 32,900 with 94 per cent polymorphonuclear leucocytes on admission, with similar counts on later occasions through the course of the disease.

The bleeding time was prolonged, being eighteen minutes by the finger-prick method. The platelets were abundant on the blood smear. The clotting time by the capillary tube method was four and one-half minutes.

Roentgenographic examination of the chest the day after admission showed accentuation of the hilum of both sides, more marked on the right, with no evidence of consolidation.

Course.—Throughout the hospital stay, the temperature remained practically normal with only slight rises to 100.2° F. following transfusion and before death. The pulse rate, however, was accelerated and during the second week remained over 120 per minute.

There was constant oozing of blood from the vagina and rectum. The red blood cell count fell rapidly despite transfusions of 200 c.c. on two occasions, becoming as low as 1,980,000 during the second week.

The lungs remained full of moist râles, and, although there was no rise of temperature, the patient developed a bronchopneumonia, pneumococcus Type IV being cultured from the blood on two occasions.

Throughout the illness the child consistently refused to eat and took fluids poorly.

The lesion of the vulva which appeared on admission as a congested indurative process of the labia majora with superficial excoriation, gradually developed a gray membrane extending into the lower part of the vagina and fourchet. This spread to the perineum and extended into the anus about ½ inch, at which point several engorged bleeding veins were seen with small ulcerations of the mucous membrane. The vulva itself became greatly edematous and swollen, and was painful and tender.

Local treatment of the vulva consisted of heat, diphtheria antitoxin spray, warm potassium permanganate dressings, and nupercaine ointment. There was moderate improvement of the lesion with regression of the necrotising process toward the end of the illness. Death occurred on the thirteenth day after the onset of the illness.

At autopsy the essential findings were those of the mouth, vulva, and lung. The mouth revealed multiple ulcerations and fissures, and the mucous membranes were covered with blood and pus. The vulva presented a dark purple surface, and there was a smooth ulceration encircling the urethra for a depth of one inch. The membrane noted during life had regressed.

All the lobes of the lungs were involved with masses of induration from 1 to 4 cm. in diameter. On section these appeared dry, granular, and purple.

The stomach contained considerable red blood. The small intestine appeared normal; the large intestine had a reddened mucosa, and on section of the sigmoid a considerable zone appeared shaggy because of numerous small shallow ulcerations, which were more pronounced toward the anus.

The vagina contained considerable fibrin. The anterior lip of the cervix was covered by red granulations and fibrin. The uterus was small and the cavity dry, with the tubes and ovaries normal in size and shape.

Microscopic examination of the lung showed the alveoli to be solidly infiltrated with polymorphonuclear leucocytes. With gram-staining many diplococci were found, ovoid in shape, often appearing in short chains of 2-3 pairs.

A section through the genitourinary organs included the uterus, vagina, and bladder. The endometrium was normal. The epithelium of the cervix was eroded and covered with red cells. The vaginal epithelium showed only moderate erosion with slight congestion of the underlying muscularis in the proximal part of the vaginal wall.

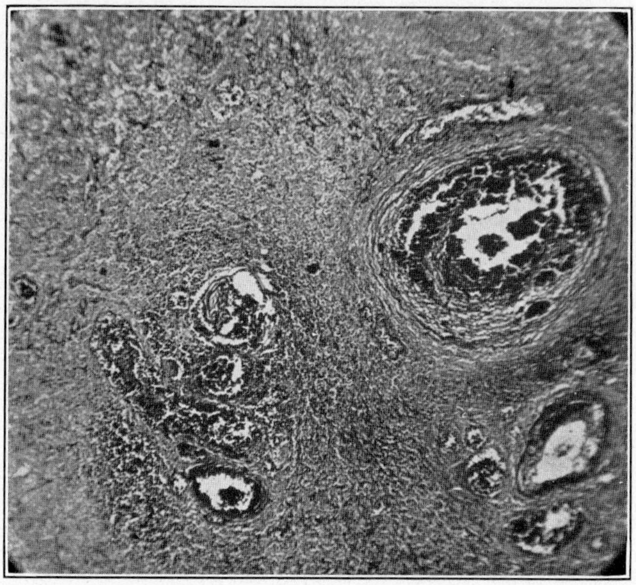

Fig. 1.—Section of the vulvar ulcer showing thrombosis of the vessels from a photomicrograph. (×60.)

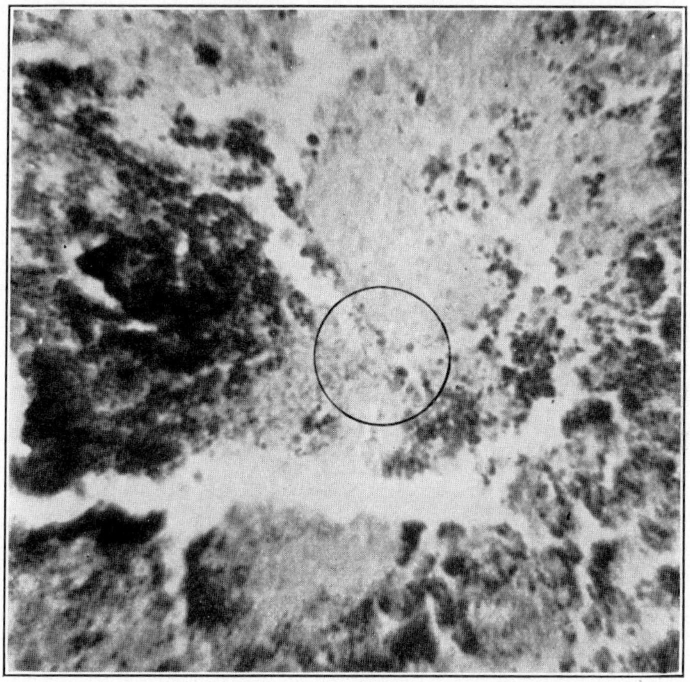

Fig. 2.—Section of the vulvar ulcer showing in the circle a clump of Gram-positive bacilli. (×1800.)

A section of the vulvar ulcer included the clitoris. On the surface the epithelium was markedly eroded. There were large masses of bacteria on the surface as well as in the glands, with massive necrosis of the superficial and deep tissues and extensive hemorrhagic and polymorphonuclear infiltration. Many of the blood vessels were thrombosed (Fig. 1). Bacterial staining showed a preponderance of gram-positive cocci which lay in large clusters as well as singly and in short chains throughout the area of necrosis. A small group of poorly defined, thin, gram-positive bacilli not unlike *B. crassus* was found lying deep in the necrotic tissue (Fig. 2).

DISCUSSION

The etiology of gangrenous ulceration of the vulva usually is not difficult to ascertain, the majority of cases being clearly associated with various vulvar infections, commonly diphtheria or septic or febrile conditions, such as scarlet fever, measles, bacillary dysentery, or typhus fever. It has been observed in cases of granulocytosis.

Wallfield and Litvak[1] reviewed the literature of 44 cases of diphtheritic vulvitis occurring before 1933; since that time there have been cases (reported by Cantrell[2]) associated with ulceration of the skin under the breast and lesions of the mouth and throat, and a case reported by Grant,[3] primary in the vagina with secondary lesions in the throat.

Gonorrheal vulvovaginitis has been known to develop ulcerations. Mention should also be made of acute phagedenic ulcers and the chronic ulcerations of tuberculosis and syphilis. These rarely, however, are confused with the acute gangrenous lesions.

Cases[4] have been reported of gangrenous vulvitis from which the fusiform bacillus and spirilla of Vincent have been obtained, but it is still a moot question whether this combination of organisms is the causative agent.

Two cases of vulvar infection by the pneumococcus have been reported, one by Dana Powell[5] in which there was extensive destruction of the vulva and surrounding tissues. In the other case reported by Trancu-Rainer,[6] there was marked congestion and edema, without ulceration.

The association of ulcers of the vulva with lesions of the mouth and throat is infrequent except in the instance of diphtheria, when on careful search the bacterium usually is isolated from the throat.

Rather an extensive literature has recently been built up on the subject "ulcus vulvae acutum" since the original paper of Lipschütz[7] in 1913 describing the association of this ulcer with mouth lesions and the finding of the *Bacillus crassus* as the etiologic factor. In 1932 Wien and Perlstein[8] reviewed twenty-nine cases of combined vulvar and mouth lesions and added a new one. Since that time cases have been reported by Matras,[9] Talalov[10] (two cases), Ziserman,[11] and Scherber[12] (two cases). This type of ulceration occurs in adults, the youngest reported patient being sixteen years old; they are chronic, recurring in nature; they involute spontaneously; and the *Bacillus crassus* is isolated from the vulvar lesions.

Lipschütz reported 51 cases in which the lesions occurred only on the vulva; since that time there have been many cases observed of the local lesion without accompanying mouth ulcerations.

The *Bacillus crassus* has not been isolated from the mouth ulcerations except by Talalov who also recovered them from axillary lesions. In nine cases reported by Wien and Perlstein and in subsequent cases of Matras and Talalov, the *Bacillus crassus* has been isolated from the vulva.

In the case presented, repeated cultures of the mouth and vulva failed to show any of the usual bacteria found in the past as the etiologic factor. It is believed that the Klebs-Loeffler baccillus would certainly have been recovered if it had been present. The definite regression and healing that took place in the lesions points decidedly away from diphtheria as the etiologic factor. In view of the pneumococcus pneumonia and septicemia this bacterium must be considered, but cultures from the lesion should have been recovered if present, nor were any seen on microscopic section. It seems reasonable to assume that the pneumococcus infection was secondary.

The presenting symptom of severe and continuous vaginal and rectal bleeding associated with prolonged bleeding time, normal clotting time, and abundant platelets places the case in the group of purpuras due to vascular dysfunction. It is an atypical purpura in that the bleeding is limited to the mucous membranes, no purpuric spots on the skin being noted throughout the child's illness. Purpuras have been described with bleeding limited to the mucous membranes without skin manifestations. Bleeding from the gums, vagina, and gastrointestinal tract have all been observed.[13] Gangrenous forms of purpura are extremely rare but do occur, reports being limited mainly to the older literature.[14, 15]

Agranulocytosis is definitely ruled out by the high degree of leucocytosis present.

We believe that the disease probably progressed as follows: Ulceration of the vulva and rectum due to bacteria normally saphrophytic occurred in a child with a hemorrhagic diathesis. The local process became gangrenous with erosion of blood vessels. Similar ulcerations appeared in the mouth. The profuse hemorrhage and toxemia lowered the general resistance of the child and pneumonia was contracted with a fatal termination.

SUMMARY

A case of ulcerative vulvitis in a child associated with mouth and anorectal lesions is presented. The possible etiologic factors are discussed, and a review of the literature is presented.

The authors are indebted to Dr. Grete Stohr for her kind assistance and to Dr. Lawrence Sophian for the autopsy report and the photomicrographs.

REFERENCES

1. Wallfield and Litvak: J. Pediat. **3**: 756, 1933.
2. Cantrell, R.: J. A. M. A. **102**: 1295, 1934.
3. Grant, J.: Brit. M. J. **1**: 1074, 1934.
4. Schnabl, E.: Dermat. Wchnschr. **85**: 1281, 1927.
5. Powell, D.: J. A. M. A. **64**: 1239, 1915.
6. Trancu-Rainer, M.: Zentralbl. f. Gynäk. **54**: 1356, 1930.
7. Lipschütz, B.: Dermatologische Studien, 25, 1933.
8. Wien and Perlstein: J. A. M. A. **98**: 461, 1932.
9. Matras, A.: Arch. f. Dermat. u. Syph. **166**: 491, 1932.
10. Talalov, D.: Arch. Dermat. and Syph. **30**: 510, 1934.
11. Ziserman, A.: J. A. M. A. **104**: 826, 1935.
12. Scherber, G.: Dermat. Wchnschr. **99**: 1553, 1934.
13. Christian: Oxford Loose Leaf Medicine **2**: 780, 1924.
    Junghans: Zentralbl. f. Gynäk. **58**: 1874.
    Idem: Arch. f. Gynäk. **149**: 515, 1932.
14. Charon, E.: Purpura foudroyant d'une forme anormale observé chez un enfant de trois ans, 1883.
15. Vechsler-Vérea, A.: Faculté de Médecine de Paris, Thèse, 1908-1909.

112 East Seventy-Fourth Street

INFANTILE VOMITING—ITS RELIEF BY X-RAY

Reginald A. Higgons, M.D., Theodore West, M.D., and
Margaret Duryee, B.S.
Port Chester, N. Y.

About five years ago a premature baby in our nursery had intractable vomiting from birth. Since this did not respond to any of the usual medical measures, the child became very dehydrated and jaundiced. On the third day of life an x-ray examination of the gastro-intestinal tract, following ingestion of a barium meal, showed no evidence of organic pathology of the stomach or duodenum and no gastric retention or retardation of emptying. We were greatly surprised to find that after the child's return to the nursery, the vomiting ceased entirely, and prompt recovery followed.

During the next five years we noted the same phenomenon repeated several times in vomiting babies, both after x-ray examinations for various reasons and after x-ray treatments of enlarged mediastinal shadows. The improvement in the gastric symptoms was so prompt and startling that it seemed logical to suppose that the x-ray, or the barium, or a combination of the two was responsible.

With this in mind, in May, 1935, we decided to record our experiences in any further cases, keeping careful clinical records. It was decided to try first the effect of atropine and luminal sodium and then, if the vomiting continued, to experiment with both the barium meal and the x-rays. Suffice to say that the barium alone apparently had no beneficial effect. If a child received barium and was then subjected to an x-ray examination, the vomiting was relieved. Because of this we decided that the essential part of the procedure was the x-rays. Since then we have used the x-ray alone whenever we did not feel that there was an organic pyloric or duodenal obstruction.

The value of radiation in the relief of vomiting is not original with us. In 1927 Peterson and Muller[1] suggested that the effect of x-rays was due to a nonspecific protein reaction which stimulates the sympathetic nervous system, thereby inhibiting the action of the vagus. Rodick[2] suggests that the x-rays act through the nerve roots and sympathetic ganglia. Barbour and his associate[4, 6, 8] have made the most extensive study of the beneficial effect of radiation of the upper chest upon the vomiting of children with pyloric stenosis. Rubin[7] noted relief of vomiting in children receiving radiation for enlargement of the thymus gland.

Read before the Medical Society of the County of Westchester, February 18, 1936.

Most of the patients reported, however, have had some organic pathologic condition, and the vomiting has been only a concomitant condition. We find no report of x-ray treatment of those young infants who suffer from disturbing vomiting without demonstrable organic pathology. Brush[3, 5] reports the use of repeated exposures of the abdomen to infra-red rays, as an aid in controlling this type of vomiting. Because of the frequency of this condition, we feel that our small series should be reported as a stimulus to others to carry this work further both in infants and in adults.

Our procedure now is as follows. The infant is first placed on a suitable type of formula if we feel that the existing feeding is not properly adapted to the case. Some are given atropine sulphate gr. $\frac{1}{1000}$, or luminal sodium gr. $\frac{1}{8}$, or both, before each feeding. If the vomiting is not relieved in from twenty-four to forty-eight hours, the case is then referred for x-ray therapy.

The amount of radiation necessary in these cases is very small. In the earlier cases, those which drew our attention to the matter, the only radiation received was that amount necessary for fluoroscopic examination of the stomach and for the making of one or two subsequent negatives.

In the cases now reported, we gave approximately 60 to 100 r. units over the dorsal spine and corresponding paravertebral area. The factors used are: 9 inch gap (115 kv.); 5 Ma.; 10 inch S.T. distance; 3 mm. aluminum filter; one to one and one-half minutes' time. (Case 2 was treated by grenz ray as described in the case report.)

If there is a definite improvement in symptoms, nothing further is done. If, however, the vomiting increases again after a period of improvement, the x-ray treatment is repeated. In no case have we found it necessary to administer more than two x-ray treatments.

With this technic we have been unusually successful in controlling those cases of severe, intractable vomiting after feedings, which are often the bane of the pediatrician's existence. It is our belief that the x-rays act in some manner upon the pylorospasm, which is the most probable cause of the vomiting in these cases. The effect may be through the dorsal nerve roots or ganglia, producing a reflex relaxation of the gastroduodenal musculature.

We now have complete records on ten vomiting infants treated in this way. Only one of these cases had a true hypertrophic pyloric stenosis. A brief résumé of each of these cases follows.

SUMMARY OF CASES

Case 1.—B. M., born normally May 25, 1935, weight 6 pounds 9 ounces, was in nursery for twelve days. The infant vomited a great deal both on breast feeding, whole milk formula, lactified formula, and routine thick cereal formula, with both bottle and tube feeding.

On the seventh day child had a gastrointestinal series which showed no obstruction and normal gastric emptying. The child vomited definitely less for thirty-six hours after taking the pictures. After thirty-six hours the vomiting became frequent again. On the twelfth day the child weighing 6 pounds 3 ounces and showing evidence of mild dehydration was transferred to the pediatric service.

The infant was fed on a lactified barley gruel mixture and continued to vomit after feedings; the weight remained stationary for five days. The infant given luminal sodium gr. 1/8 before feedings vomited less for the next week, and gained weight slowly. At 1 month of age the baby weighed 6 pounds 11 ounces and had been vomiting more. One x-ray treatment was then given on June 28, 1935.

Almost immediately the vomiting became greatly less, and the child gained 7 ounces in the next three days. The child then regurgitated a little for two days, then stopped vomiting entirely, and was discharged on July 17, 1935, weighing 8 pounds 4 ounces.

CASE 2.—K. T., born May 29, 1935, at Harbor Hospital, New York City, weight 6 pounds 6 ounces, vomited after practically every feeding for first two weeks. The infant was fed dryco and then a lactified evaporated milk formula. On June 14, 1935, the weight was 6 pounds 2 ounces.

The child then received three treatments of grenz ray at two-day intervals—two on the back, and one on the chest—10 cm. focus skin distance, 22 m. half absorption value in aluminum, 250 r. units per session.

The child immediately stopped vomiting and regurgitated very little. The weight began to increase on the same formula, and she weighed 6 pounds 13 ounces on discharge from the hospital on June 21, 1935.

This child has been followed since and has had no return of pylorospasm.

CASE 3.—J. C., born normally June 7, 1935, weight 8 pounds 11 ounces, was breast fed first six days with supplementary milk formula after first week. The infant vomited a great deal after feedings in the nursery. The child was discharged on twelfth day weighing 8 pounds 8 ounces.

After discharge the infant vomited after almost every feeding and cried a great deal. After readmission to the pediatric ward on June 27, 1935, the infant, weighing 8 pounds 8 ounces, was put on lactified evaporated milk formula, and still cried a great deal and regurgitated considerable milk after each feeding.

On July 1, 1935, a gastrointestinal series showed evidence of pylorospasm but no organic obstruction. The gastric emptying time was normal.

This child began to do better immediately following the gastrointestinal series. Vomiting decreased. The child cried much less and gained weight satisfactorily.

This child has been followed carefully to date and has continued to do well, with no return of pylorospasm.

CASE 4.—G. C., born July 21, 1935, delivery normal, weight 6 pounds 4 ounces, was not nursed but was fed weak milk dilutions. The infant vomited after almost every feeding. Gastric lavage before feeding showed retention of milk curds after four hours. On the sixth day the weight was 6 pounds.

One x-ray exposure was given on July 27, 1935. The child stopped vomiting immediately following the treatment and started to gain weight on the same formula and has done well since.

CASE 5.—E. C., was admitted to pediatric ward on August 15, 1935, at age of five-plus months. The history recorded a normal birth and a normal hospital period, birth weight of 7 pounds 3 ounces. The child had nursed irregularly, had gained weight satisfactorily, but had always vomited a great deal. He was seen once in the out-patient department at three months of age and was given one x-ray treatment.

The mother was advised concerning addition of solid foods to breast feeding and the child was not seen again until admission. The mother reported that there had been no improvement in vomiting following the x-ray therapy. Our social worker, however, reported that the home investigation showed the mother to be very negligent in her care of the child and that she never followed any orders accurately. The mother reported continued projectile vomiting.

On Aug. 10, 1935, child received second x-ray treatment and at the same time was removed to the grandmother's home and put in her care. No change was made in the feeding. The grandmother reported that during the five days at her home following the second x-ray treatment, the child never vomited and regurgitated only a little.

Child was admitted to the ward because of poor nutrition and anemia and also in order to observe the vomiting. During two weeks' stay in the hospital the child ate well, gained weight, and never vomited. He regurgitated occasionally during the first week but not at all during the last five days of his stay.

CASE 6.—B. D. was seen first July 27, 1935, at age of one month because of repeated vomiting after feedings with a great deal of gas and colic. She was put on a thick barley gruel feeding and given luminal sodium before feedings for several days without benefit.

On Aug. 1, 1935, she received one x-ray treatment, without any change in feeding or medication. On Aug. 6, 1935, the mother reported that the child had not vomited since treatment and had cried very little.

On Aug. 7, 1935, solid food was added in form of cereal and purée of vegetable, because of evidence of hunger. After the feeding of the solid food the child began vomiting again and cried a great deal with colic. Luminal sodium would relieve the colic and crying but did not stop the vomiting. The child was placed on simple evaporated milk formula without benefit.

On Aug. 16, 1935, she received second x-ray treatment and was admitted to pediatric ward for observation. She was put on an evaporated milk, beta lactose, and barley gruel formula. During the week in the hospital the child regurgitated very little, cried very little, and gained 7 ounces.

This child has been followed ever since and has done very well. She has always had a tendency to regurgitate some of her food but has had no more real vomiting or colic since the last x-ray treatment.

CASE 7.—B. V., born July 10, 1935, weight 7 pounds 14 ounces, nursed only five days and then was fed milk dilutions. She was discharged from the nursery on the tenth day weighing 7 pounds 12 ounces. Nursery records showed some vomiting but not severe.

After discharge from nursery the child began vomiting a great deal—after almost every feeding. She cried a great deal day and night and was tried on many different types of formula without benefit.

The child was admitted to pediatric ward on Aug. 27, 1935, weighing 9 pounds 3 ounces and was put on lactified evaporated milk formula. She vomited the first feeding taken and several subsequent feedings.

She was then given one x-ray treatment. The vomiting stopped immediately, and child took all her food well for next twenty-four hours. She had very little regurgitation but did cry considerably and was then given three doses of luminal sodium to quiet her.

She remained in the hospital for one week and gained 8 ounces. She regurgitated a little at times but did not vomit, crying very little.

This child has been followed since discharge, has done very well, and has had no return of pylorospasm.

CASE 8.—J. F., born normally Nov. 5, 1935, weight 8 pounds 4 ounces, nursed and was given supplementary feeding. He vomited after feedings from birth. The vomiting became projectile on the third day. When he was seen by us on sixth day, he weighed 7 pounds and showed considerable dehydration. He was put on a lactified formula, atropine sulphate and luminal, together with suitable measures to replace fluid loss.

Although the child did better, he continued to vomit considerably, with occasional projectile vomiting, until the tenth day. On Nov. 15, 1935, he was given one x-ray treatment.

The child stopped vomiting immediately following the x-ray treatment and gained 15 ounces in the next eight days on the same formula.

This child has been followed since discharge and has done very well with only very occasional mild vomiting and slight after-feeding regurgitation.

CASE 9.—M. J. was born Oct. 24, 1935, after difficult delivery of a face presentation, with the cord tight around the neck. Birth weight was 8 pounds 8 ounces. From birth she was bottle fed on milk dilutions with dextrimaltose. The child was seen first at the age of two and one-half months because of difficult feeding. She weighed 11 pounds and showed evidence of poor nutrition and flabby tissues. She was put on a formula of suitable strength of the same type and cereal gruel. After one week the child was admitted to the pediatric ward because of loss in weight and strength and refusal to nurse the bottle. She had taken only 6 ounces of the formula in the thirty-six hours preceding admission and was vomiting occasionally after feedings. On admission at two months and three weeks of age her weight was 10 pounds 11 ounces.

After admission the child was put on a lactified, evaporated milk formula and was fed by gavage. Immediately after assuring a complete filling of the stomach by gavage feeding, the child began to vomit after feedings. This vomiting soon became projectile in type and would occur several times each day. The child then received luminal sodium and atropine sulphate without any change in the vomiting. At the same time a bilateral myringotomy was performed to drain the middle ears, which had become infected, probably as a result of the vomiting.

After five days of repeated vomiting, the child was given one x-ray treatment. She immediately ceased vomiting although it was still necessary to feed her by gavage. The vomiting never returned, and eventually the child's appetite improved after a direct blood transfusion several days later.

The child has been followed since and has never again vomited or had any serious regurgitation after feedings, although it is still somewhat of a problem to make her eat sufficient food.

CASE 10.—D. N., whose birth history was irrelevant, was seen first at age of three months, weighing 9 pounds 5 ounces. This child had been followed in a welfare station continuously for the two months preceding admission. The net change in weight during this past two months was a loss of 5 ounces. The child had vomited projectily several times each day. He had been treated by both atropine sulphate and dietary measures without apparent benefit.

On admission he showed the typical picture of hypertrophic pyloric stenosis with malnutrition, visible gastric waves, palpable pyloric tumor, and small, infrequent, constipated stools.

He was first put on the standard thick cereal feeding, and given luminal sodium gr. $\frac{1}{8}$ and atropine sulphate gr. $\frac{1}{1000}$ before each feeding. After three days the dosage of atropine was doubled without benefit. On the fourth day he was given a standard barium meal from the x-ray department, but no negatives were made. This had no effect upon the vomiting, and gastric lavage four hours after feeding always showed a large amount of retention.

On the seventh day he received one x-ray treatment without any change in the feeding or medication. During the succeeding three days the child vomited only once, had large, soft, yellow stools, and gained 11 ounces in weight. During the following week he vomited only three times in spite of discontinuing the luminal.

He then did very well until the twenty-first day, when he again vomited several times and showed a small weight loss. He then received a second x-ray treatment. After this treatment all vomiting stopped although the pyloric tumor could still be felt, and the gastric waves could still be seen after feeding.

He was discharged on the thirtieth day in good condition and showing only occasional regurgitation. After discharge all medication was discontinued, and the child continued to do well. At six months of age he weighed 17 pounds 3 ounces, and the pyloric tumor was no longer palpable. He was then eating well and was on a regular intermediate mixed diet with straight milk.

SUMMARY

An analysis of the ten infants treated shows:

Onset of vomiting—birth in 5 cases, two weeks of age in 2 cases, and one month of age in 3 cases.

Loss of weight preceding treatment in 8 cases.

Relief of vomiting by formula change and medication—none in 7 cases, partial in 3 cases.

X-ray therapy administered from six to sixty-seven days after the onset of symptoms.

Result of first x-ray treatment—permanent relief of vomiting in 7 cases, temporary relief of vomiting in 2 cases, no relief of vomiting in 1 case.

Result of second x-ray treatment given in 3 cases was permanent relief of vomiting in all.

CONCLUSION

1. X-ray therapy is of definite value in the control of vomiting in infancy, whether due to hypertrophic pyloric stenosis or to functional pylorospasm.

REFERENCES

1. Peterson, W. F., and Muller, E. F.: Arch. Int. Med. **40**: 575, 1927.
2. Rodick, J. C.: New Orleans M. & S. J. **87**: 820, 1935.
3. Brush, Clinton E.: Physical Therap. **50**: 41, 1932.
4. Barbour, Orville: J. A. M. A. **97**: 455, 1931.
5. Brush, Clinton E.: Physical Therap. **49**: 1, 1931.
6. Barbour, Orville, and Connell, J. W.: Illinois M. J. **57**: 110, 1930.
7. Rubin, Mitchell I.: J. A. M. A. **90**: 1694, 1928.
8. Barbour, Orville: Arch. Pediat. **44**: 314, 1927.

264 King Street

EPIDEMIC VOMITING AND DIARRHEA

Roy M. Greenthal, M.D.
Milwaukee, Wis.

DURING the month of March, 1936, a considerable proportion of the residents of Milwaukee suffered from an illness characterized by vomiting. Diarrhea was associated with the vomiting in some instances, but in many there was constipation. The disease was quite familiar to the physicians of this community as they had recognized it as a clinical syndrome for many years, but the large number of individuals affected caused considerable comment and much discussion as to the nature and cause of this epidemic illness. It was thought that a clinical report might be of interest, as very little has been written about this disease. Zahorsky,[1] of St. Louis, in 1929, published a paper entitled "Hyperemesis Hiemis, or the Winter Vomiting Disease." He mentioned that he had observed this disease for the past thirty years and believed that it should occupy a distinct place in the nosology of children's diseases. His description resembles very much the condition observed in Milwaukee.

Nomenclature.—Many names have been used to designate this disease; it has been called stomach or gastric influenza, intestinal grip, epidemic gastroenteritis, winter vomiting disease, and epidemic vomiting and diarrhea. The last designation is the only one that can really be given to this illness at the present time, as there is no proof that it is a form of influenza or grip. It is probably gastritis or enteritis or both, but this has not been proved, as the illness is rarely fatal. Zahorsky's term, "Winter Vomiting Disease," is apt, but many outbreaks are seen in the spring and fall, and occasionally it may be observed in summer.

Symptomatology.—The disease affects infants, children, and adults, but only the symptomatology of infants and children will be described. It is certainly very rare in breast-fed infants and in infants under three months, but it may be seen even then. The onset during the last epidemic was very sudden and began with forceful vomiting, repeated frequently. After the stomach was empty, the vomitus consisted of thick stringy mucus. In some instances the vomitus was bile stained, and even small amounts of blood were seen mixed with the mucus. The vomiting continued for one to five days and then subsided. Relapses were frequent and were observed from two days to two weeks after the subsidence of the first attack.

Diarrhea was observed in some instances, but constipation was present more often during this epidemic. In previous years diarrhea was observed in most patients, sometimes with vomiting and at other times without vomiting. Another prominent symptom was abdominal pain. This was usually intermittent and spasmodic and occurred just before vomiting or defecation. Sometimes the abdominal pain was continuous and severe enough to cause the child to double up and thrash violently about the bed. The pain was usually referred to the upper abdomen, but often could not be localized.

At times there was a disquieting complaint of pain in the right lower quadrant, and it was comforting to know in some instances that children with pain in this region had had previous appendectomies. The general symptoms were prostration, anorexia, and a characteristic lethargy alternating with irritability. Recovery appeared complete after two or three days, but, as will be mentioned later, this recovery was more apparent than real with many children. Very rarely were there any symptoms of upper respiratory infection, such as nasal discharge, cough, or earache. Occasionally a head cold would precede the illness or follow it, but this was the exception. There was no permanent immunity.

Examination.—Many patients did not appear very ill. Others were prostrated and pale, with unhappy facial expressions and sunken eyes. A few appeared alarmingly toxic and dehydrated, especially after the illness had progressed a few days. There was a slight redness of the palpebral conjunctivae.

The tongue was dry and coated, with prominent red papillae. The tonsils were not inflamed, and there was no cervical adenopathy, but in many patients a slight faucial redness was observed. It was difficult to be sure that this was abnormal, and in some cases the throat was normal in all respects. The heart and lungs were always normal. The abdomen was sometimes slightly distended and sometimes sunken. On palpation peristaltic gurglings were often observed. There was never any evidence of spasm or rigidity, and the muscle walls were soft, except in certain instances in which the children resisted abdominal examination. The question of appendicitis was often considered and was a very important problem. Any definite tenderness or spasm in the right lower quadrant should rule out this epidemic vomiting disease. In most instances the patients were not exactly sure "just where it hurt" but complained bitterly of pain in the abdomen. The diarrheal stools were usually yellow in color. The odor of the stools was foul and putrefactive. There was rarely any excoriation of the buttocks. The diarrhea was considered to be putrefactive as distinguished from a fermentative diarrhea, in which the stools have a sour odor and produce extensive excoriation of the buttocks. Zahorsky writes that the microscopic examination of the stools in the winter vomiting disease rarely shows cells, but generally in summer diarrhea examination shows a massive cellular content of the stools.

The temperature at the onset of the illness was usually slightly elevated (99 to 100° F.). Some children developed a much higher temperature on the second day (102 to 104° F.), which subsided after one or two days.

Laboratory Examinations.—The urine was often normal. Some dehydrated patients had a concentrated urine with a trace of albumin. Acetone was rather commonly present, but very rarely was diacetic acid found. The microscopic examination was negative, except that a few casts might be found when the urine contained albumin. The blood count was not distinctive and was frequently within normal limits. A slight leucocytosis was present in a few cases. Leucopenia was not observed. Nothing unusual was found in the differential count. Zahorsky found the leucocyte count to range from 7,000 to 13,000 in his cases. Blood counts were not often required in this disease as seen in the home, but they were obtained from a few of the sicker patients. It was not considered necessary to investigate the question of acidosis or alkalosis although it is possible that severe vomiting with the loss of chlorides may have produced temporary alkalosis in some of the more severely ill patients.

Relapses and Second Attacks.—As has been mentioned, relapses were seen rather frequently. The patient would seem to have recovered from the vomiting and diarrhea, and then after a day or two or a week or two, the illness would recur. In previous years I had observed children who had several attacks during a period of weeks. When the illness reappeared after an interval of a week or ten days, it was a question whether the second attack was a relapse or reinfection. This question cannot be answered at this time, but I believe that in most instances it was a relapse. It would seem that there is a subacute stage which may follow the acute vomiting or diarrhea. There are children who have had this disease in the acute form and apparently recover. However, they are not well, in that they are tired and irritable and have poor color. There may be occasional vomiting, or they may have two or three loose stools daily which are light yellow in color and putrefactive in odor. There is a frequent complaint of colicky abdominal pain, often after food is eaten. These children may be relieved in a short time with a high carbohydrate and a low protein and fat diet. Untreated they recover completely after two or three weeks.

Treatment.—Since the disease is self-limited and nonfatal, recovery nearly always occurs. The severe vomiting is not relieved by any measure that I am familiar with. The best procedure would seem to be the giving of small amounts of liquids if the patient desires to drink. The liquids may consist of water, weak tea, carbonated beverages, cereal gruels, and fruit juices. I do not believe that milk or broth should be given. If the patient can abstain from food or water for a few hours, he will be relieved from his nausea more quickly. Drugs are of very little value. Sedatives or opiates may be of some use but are usually not given for fear that some serious abdominal disease, especially appendicitis, may be present. Heat to the abdomen is often very soothing to the patient. After the subsidence of the vomiting, a high carbohydrate diet is given for a few days. Milk, eggs, meats and soups are omitted. Starches and sugars are given freely.

The diarrhea usually responds promptly to this regime. The apple diet has been used in a few cases with diarrhea with very good results. Paregoric may be given for diarrhea and colicky pain after the illness has lasted for a few days and the diagnosis is certain, but as has been mentioned it is best not given at the onset.

If the patient is apparently well, a general diet is introduced gradually. Some children will relapse when milk is taken, and they are again given the high carbohydrate diet for a day or two. If the patient is seen in the subacute stage, he is placed on the high carbohydrate diet and in two or three days, his condition improves. The rationale of the high-carbohydrate, low-protein and low-fat diet is demonstrated chiefly in the treatment of diarrhea—the relapses often seen when the patient is given large amounts of proteins and fats after he is considered recovered—and in the beneficial effect of this diet in the subacute stage of this disease.

Etiology.—This is entirely in the realm of speculation at the present time. The disease is undoubtedly infectious and contagious and apparently has a short incubation period of one to three days. Whether the organism is a bacillus or a virus is unknown. Although it is apparently not associated with the common cold or acute respiratory infections seen during the winter months, some believe that the disease begins as a mild throat infection and the gastric and intestinal symptoms are complications. The drinking water has been accused, but the usual bacteriologic examinations do not agree with this theory. If this disease is due to a virus, it may not be demonstrated by the usual bacteriologic examinations. The occurrence of this illness in widely separated communities is also evidence against the contaminated water theory. It is very likely spread by direct contact, as it may be seen in infants who received nothing but sterile food and water. Zahorsky considers four theories: (1) frozen milk, (2) peculiar manifestation of influenza, (3) respiratory infection (common grip), (4) toxic substance in milk, cream, or butter, but does not accept any of these theories. It may be possible that this is a definite clinical entity with a specific causative agent, but at present we can only confess our ignorance of the etiology.

CONCLUSION

Epidemic vomiting and diarrhea has been described. The etiology is unknown. A high-carbohydrate, low-protein and low-fat diet, after a period of starvation, appears to be of benefit in the treatment.

REFERENCE

1. Zahorsky, John: Arch. Pediat. **46**: 391, 1929.

425 East Wisconsin Avenue

CONGENITAL OBSTRUCTIVE JAUNDICE

I. H. Kass, M.D., and F. P. Osgood, M.D.
Toledo, Ohio

THE question of jaundice due to congenital obstruction of the bile ducts is one essentially of the degree of obstruction. In most patients who live any length of time, a certain amount of bile is found in the gastrointestinal canal. With complete obliteration of all the ducts, the outcome is necessarily fatal and in the majority of such cases reported, fatal termination has occurred in several weeks or several months. The following case is presented because of the unusually long duration of life and the absence of hemorrhages in the presence of complete biliary obstruction.

Case reports of congenital obstructive jaundice have been reviewed by Lavenson,[1] Deaver,[2] Holmes,[3] Croswell,[4] Rosenberg and Judd,[5] Ladd,[6] Scriver,[7] Parsons and Hickman,[8] Cole and Whittle.[9] In Lavenson's series from the literature, there were only three patients out of sixty-two who lived longer than three months. Two of these three patients died before the age of nine months, and one died before the age of eleven months. Deaver[2] reported a child who attained the age of one year and twelve days. In this case the jaundice appeared at the age of six weeks, making the duration of obstructive jaundice, clinically, ten months, three weeks, and five days. Holmes,[3] in a large series of cases, showed that surgical intervention is doomed to failure in 84 per cent of patients because of anatomic anomalies in which sufficient structure was not present to permit of creation of a passageway for the bile to reach the intestinal tract, or because the degree of hepatitis present was so marked that the radicles of the intrahepatic bile ducts were so obstructed that an adequate external outlet for the bile was not apparently present.

REPORT OF CASE

Baby R. R., female, ten weeks old, was first seen on March 11, 1935. The presenting complaint was jaundice since birth.

Past History.—The family history was essentially negative. There were five other children living and in good health. The family history was negative for syphilis, tuberculosis, familial jaundice, or any chronic disease.

The birth weight was 7 pounds 10 ounces. The delivery was normal and spontaneous. The baby was breast fed and took her feedings well. Neither cod liver oil nor orange juice had been included in the patient's diet.

Present Illness.—A yellowish discoloration of the skin and mucous membranes was noted soon after birth. The jaundice became intense on the second day and continued to increase in severity. The gain in weight had been slow. The bowel movements had been regular with pasty and clay colored stools. The urine was a deep brown color. There had been no vomiting, diarrhea, fever, or hemorrhages.

From the Departments of Pediatrics and Surgery, Women's and Children's Hospital, Toledo.

Reported by courtesy of Dr. J. F. Frye.

Physical Examination.—The patient was a poorly nourished but active baby showing a striking deep yellowish discoloration of skin, sclerae, and mucous membranes. The skin was dry and inelastic. There was a loss of the normal muscle turgor. The head and neck showed no abnormalities. The heart and lungs were normal. The liver margin could be distinctly felt three fingerbreadths below the right costal margin. The liver edge was firm and smooth to the examining hand. The remainder of the examination was essentially negative. There were no hemorrhages visible. The infant's weight at time of examination was 8 pounds 4 ounces. The temperature was 98° F. (rectally).

Laboratory Findings.—The blood findings after the infant was admitted to the hospital showed: hemoglobin, 76 per cent; erythrocytes 3,480,000; leucocytes, 22,600; platelets, 288,000; polymorphonuclear neutrophiles, 53 per cent; lymphocytes, 40 per cent; mononuclears, 5 per cent; eosinophiles, 1 per cent; basophiles, 1 per cent. Urinalysis showed a specific gravity of 1.012, acid reaction, negative reactions for albumin and sugar, four-plus bile reaction, and amorphous urates in the sediment. The blood Wassermann test was negative. The bleeding time was 3 minutes; the clotting time was 4 minutes. The erythrocyte fragility test showed hemolysis beginning at 0.41 per cent sodium chloride with complete hemolysis at 0.28 per cent sodium chloride. The immediate direct van den Bergh reaction was positive. The icterus index was 71.

The feces were consistently clay colored and gave a negative reaction for the presence of bile.

Course.—In the hospital the infant was placed on a high carbohydrate diet and given liver extract (Armour) 30 drops, four times daily. Orance juice and cod liver oil were included in the diet. There was a slow gain in weight during the period of hospitalization. The feedings were well taken, and the bowel movements were regular. On the fourth day of hospitalization, a laparotomy was performed by one of us (F. O.) with the hope of finding a biliary obstruction that might be relieved by surgery.

Under ether anesthesia the abdomen was opened through an upper abdominal paramedian incision. The organs were all bile stained, and there was a small amount of free yellowish fluid in the peritoneal cavity in excess of normal. The liver was enlarged about 3 cm. below costal margin with a sharp edge, and numerous fibrous markings on the surface. On the under surface the gallbladder presented as a normal shaped viscus about the size of an unshelled almond. Exploration for ducts revealed complete absence of cystic, hepatic, and common ducts. There was a short fibrous cord at the end of the neck of the gallbladder which had no apparent connection with the structures in the region of the hepatic artery and portal vein. Aspiration of the gallbladder produced colorless mucus. A small piece of tissue was taken from the liver for biopsy. Bleeding during the operation was not excessive.

Biopsy section (Fig. 1) showed pale liver cells with prominent nuclei and yellow bile-stained cytoplasm. The cells appeared in normal arrangement but were compressed and overlapping. The entire lobular outline showed a contracted border. The interlobular tissue was increased in amount and showed extensive lymphocytic and leucocytic cellular infiltration. There was a multiplication of bile ducts, numerous biliary calculi, and thickened blood vessels. The diagnosis was obstructive cirrhosis of the liver.*

The patient was discharged from the hospital ten days after admission. Her general condition appeared somewhat improved. The weight was 8 pounds 10 ounces.

On Aug. 7, 1935, nearly five months after the abdominal exploration had been performed, the patient was again examined. The interval history revealed little in addition to the fact already known about the case. The child had maintained a fair degree of health but was less active. She took her feedings well and continued to

*Report by Dr. S. S. Hindman, pathologist.

show all the signs of a complete biliary obstruction. On examination she now showed a more intense jaundice. The child appeared irritable but at times was apathetic. The skin and mucous membranes were a deep greenish bronze color. There was a scattered fine papular eruption over the body and evidence of pruritus. The weight was 10 pounds 7 ounces. There were marked malnutrition, marked dehydration, and loss of normal tissue turgor. There was no evidence of hemorrhagic diathesis. The liver edge was firm and could be felt four fingerbreadths below the right costal margin. The spleen could not be palpated. The remainder of the examination was essentially unchanged. A stool specimen was clay colored and showed a negative test for the presence of bile. The urine was a deep brown color and showed a four-plus bile reaction but was otherwise negative. The regular seven-month dietary additions were prescribed. The continuance of a high carbohydrate diet and liver extract was advised.

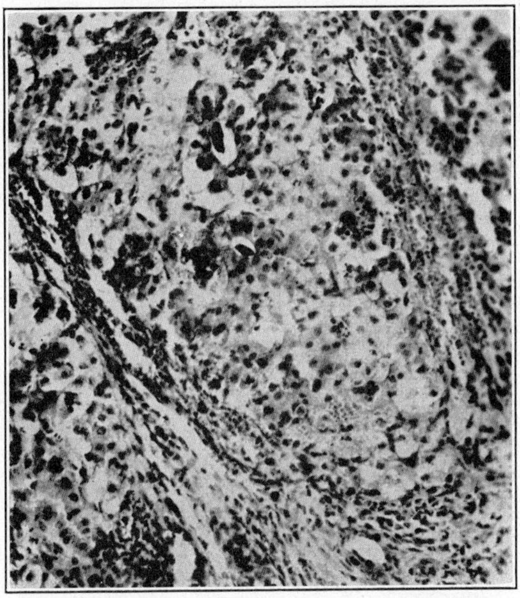

Fig. 1.—Biopsy from liver showing increase in interlobular tissue, multiplication of bile ducts, biliary calculi, and interlobular cellular infiltration.

Readmission to Hospital.—On Dec. 26, 1935, the patient was readmitted to the hospital intensely jaundiced and with bilateral bronchopneumonia. The liver was enlarged and could be felt two handbreadths below the right costal margin. The edge of the spleen could be palpated with some difficulty because of the marked abdominal distention. The physical and laboratory examinations were similar to the earlier reports of a complete biliary obstruction. The icterus index was 82 . The patient expired on the third day of hospitalization.

The essential findings at autopsy showed congenital obliteration of the cystic, hepatic, and common bile ducts; congenital obstructive cirrhosis of the liver; chronic passive congestion of the liver and spleen; bilateral bronchopneumonia.

The liver weighed 600 gm. The cut surface was a deep greenish red to reddish black color and was coarsely lobulated. The central veins were conspicuous, and there were prominent fibrous streaks throughout. The gallbladder was normal in size and shape, thin walled, and contained a small amount of thin flocculent fluid. Dissection showed that the cystic duct was a fibrous cord with no definite termination. Fibrous structures in the tissue around the hilus of the liver appeared to resemble ducts, but microscopic examinations did not show any definite duct structure.

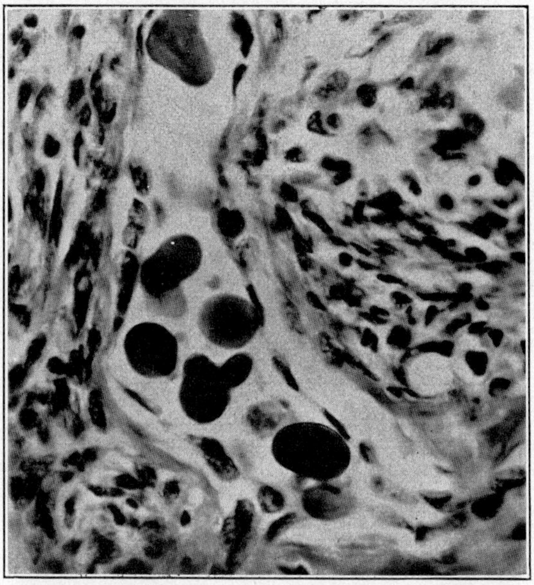

Fig. 2.—Section from liver obtained at postmortem showing marked interlobular fibrosis, increased interlobular cellular infiltration, and numerous biliary calculi.

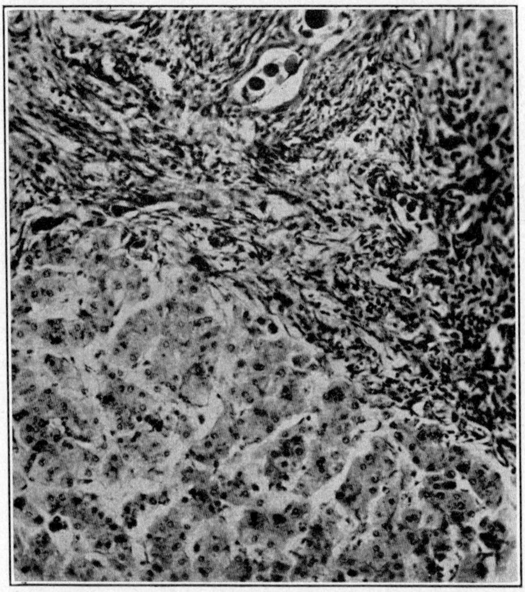

Fig. 3.—High power photomicrograph of liver section showing biliary calculi, numerous fibroblasts, and evidence of new connective tissue formation.

Microscopic examinations of sections of the liver (Figs. 2 and 3) showed a marked increase in interlobular tissue. The fibrosis was widespread. There were more and larger biliary calculi, many of which showed a distinct concentric formation. The lobules were smaller and more contracted than those observed in the biopsy specimen. There was a more marked cellular infiltration and a lesser degree of multiplication of bile ducts. The diagnosis was obstructive cirrhosis of the liver.

COMMENT

It has been generally agreed that a high carbohydrate diet aids in the protection of the damaged liver and reduces its metabolic work. Whipple, Opie, and others have shown that livers containing an abundance of glycogen are far less susceptible to certain toxic agents than glycogen-poor livers. Mann[10] has shown that dogs with completely obliterated biliary outflow will survive up to ten or thirteen months provided they have been maintained on a high carbohydrate diet. Such animals, however, will survive only a few months if maintained on meat diets. In the case reported, a high carbohydrate formula and supplementary foods high in carbohydrates were given.

A positive test for the presence of bile in the stools of complete biliary obstruction may occur. There is a possibility of bile-stained intestinal mucosa sloughing sufficiently to appear in the feces and to stain them.[5] The case reported at no time showed any evidence of the presence of bile in the intestinal canal. The findings at the time of the laparotomy and finally at autopsy conclusively showed a complete biliary obstruction and a nonfunctioning gallbladder due to congenital causes.

A review of the literature on congenital obstructive jaundice reveals that hemorrhagic manifestations appear in all cases. It is of interest to note that our patient showed no evidence of hemorrhage after being jaundiced nearly twelve months. Ottenberg[11] has pointed out that the subject of hemorrhagic diathesis in jaundice patients is at present in a very unsatisfactory state. No one has as yet discovered the real mechanism of the hemorrhagic tendency in jaundice.

SUMMARY

A case of congenital obstructive jaundice in a female child, dying at the age of eleven months and twenty-nine days of age, is reported. Exploratory laparotomy done when the patient was ten weeks old revealed a congenital obliteration of the cystic, hepatic, and common ducts, and a nonfunctioning gallbladder. Biopsy of the liver at the time of the laparotomy and pathologic changes in the liver at autopsy are described. The long duration of life in the case presented is ascribed in part, to the hepatogenic functions of organs other than the liver and to a high carbohydrate diet.

REFERENCES

1. Lavenson, R. S.: J. Med. Research **8:** 61, 1908.
2. Deaver, J. Montgomery: Am. J. Dis. Child. **46:** 356, 1933.
3. Holmes, J. B.: Am. J. Dis. Child. **11:** 405, 1916.
4. Croswell, C. V.: J. Tennessee State M. A. **27:** 316, 1934.
5. Rosenberg, Lester, and Judd, George: Arch. Surg. **8:** 2339, 1929.
6. Ladd, W. E.: J. A. M. A. **91:** 1082, 1928.
7. Scriver, B.: Canad. M. A. J. **27:** 517, 1932.
8. Parsons, L. G., and Hickman, Evelyn: Am. J. Dis. Child. **31:** 461, 1926.
9. Cole, Leslie, and Whittle, C. H.: Brit. J. Child. Dis. **26:** 258, 1929.
10. Mann, Frank: J. A. M. A. **104:** 371, 1935, and Personal Communications.
11. Ottenberg, Reuben: J. A. M. A. **104:** 1681, 1935.

316 MICHIGAN STREET

Critical Review

THE NEWBORN

Barnet E. Bonar, M.D.
Salt Lake City, Utah

IN PREVIOUS reviews[1, 2] it was pointed out that there was need for uniformity of definition of such terms as "live birth," "stillbirth," "prematurity," "viability" and "abortion," before authentic interpretations could be made of the statistics accumulated by various institutions or states. During the past year or two some progress has been made in this respect through the rather independent efforts of committees appointed by several national societies, chief among which have been the Committee on Child Health Relations of the American Academy of Pediatrics, the Committee on Neonatal Mortality and Morbidity of the American Pediatric Society, a subcommittee of the American Public Health Association, and the American Committee on Maternal Welfare. In general, then, there are three groups, the public health men, the obstetricians, and the pediatrists, working practically independently toward the same end. The intimacy between maternal and neonatal death rates, as evidenced by the stubbornness with which both resist attempts to reduce them, indicates the need for closer cooperation between obstetrician and pediatrist if the most satisfactory solution of the problem is to be brought about. For this reason it seems unfortunate, indeed, that the several groups cannot appoint representatives to serve upon a joint committee whose function shall be to correlate the ideas of these groups and to serve as a liaison between them. In this way uniform definitions can be formulated which will be of inestimable value in serving to standardize statistical reports coming from various parts of the country and thus make them more readily comparable. As it is now, there is such complete variance among the states in respect to the definitions mentioned above that statistics derived from these sources cannot be used for purposes of reliable comparison. For instance, in regard to the period of gestation to which a stillborn fetus must have advanced before a certificate is required, two states require that all products of conception must be reported, and two have no definite ruling (Delaware and New Hampshire). Most states require that stillbirths shall be reported from the fifth month on while some require reporting only from the seventh month on. Furthermore, in five states (Colorado, Connecticut, Illinois, Nebraska, New Jersey, and the District of Columbia) a stillbirth is reported as a stillbirth while in the remaining states a stillbirth must be reported as a birth and as a death.

If such comparisons are desired at present, it will be necessary to create in the various states agencies using an arbitrary standard irrespective of the statutory definitions of the individual state. Actually there is a vital need for some such expedient in order that a correct cross-section of conditions throughout the country may be obtained. As it is at present the most reliable information comes from large maternity hospitals in crowded centers of population. Such reports derived solely from the clinic type of patients are not representative because such patients are not representative of the nation. Again, statistics from such institutions where all patients are cared for by obstetricians depict a condition that does not maintain in the country at large, for it must be remembered that the great majority of confinements are handled by general practitioners. Thus of the approximately 2,160,000 live births in 1934 a little less than one-third (760,000) occurred in towns of 30,000 or over, where possibly there might be one or more obstetrician. Of this number probably not more than 20 per cent (150,000) were delivered by obstetricians. In the final rough analysis, then, it is apparent that probably not more than 15 per cent of the total deliveries in the United States were conducted by obstetricians. Therefore, it can be readily seen, that if an authentic picture of the true status of maternal and neonatal morbidity and mortality rates in the United States is desired new studies based upon new standards must be made. Studies of this nature are essential if procedures adaptable to the general practitioner, who delivers most of the babies, are to be evolved. Certainly methods used in maternity hospitals, while admirable in many respects, cannot be used always in general practice, and in some instances should be prohibited rather than urged. Advocation of the general adoption of some of these measures has, undoubtedly, been due to the inability of many teachers to realize that some of the obstetric maneuvers or methods of analgesia and anesthesia, which may be suitable to the well-regulated maternity hospital, cannot help but be harmful in the hands of those who have neither the skill nor armamentarium to carry them out in general practice. Until this is realized and there is a shift from the complicated to the simple type of procedure both the maternal and neonatal rates will fail to drop.

While reduction of the neonatal mortality rate cannot help but go hand in hand with any material reduction in the maternal mortality rate, it would seem a little more fitting if obstetricians were to consider the welfare of the newborn more specifically in conjunction with maternal welfare than is done at present. It is suggested, therefore, that the American Committee on Maternal Welfare should increase its membership to include those interested in neonatal welfare as well. The subordinate state committees of this organization could then serve more satisfactorily in these two closely related fields than if two separate committees were formed. Furthermore, such a state committee could readily cooperate with the Maternal and Child Health Program of the Social Security Act, perhaps in an advisory manner as is being done at present in Utah. In this way the duplication of time and effort of several committees could be dispensed with to the benefit of everyone concerned.

While a great deal is known regarding the gross mortality during the different age periods in man from birth on, such is not the case with the death rate during the intrauterine period and especially the early part of it. A few attempts have been made to estimate the mortality rate of the antenatal period, but, owing to the difficulty of obtaining accurately the abortion rate, the figures published are inaccurate and will continue to be largely speculative. In a large group of private patients Grier[3] found that the spontaneous abortion rate was 11 per cent and that over 16 per cent, or one out of six, of the mothers consulting him about confinement did not receive a live baby. Naturally these figures are not high enough but they are of value in pointing out that in an obstetric practice among mothers desiring babies the fetal mortality was startlingly high. Using a method which at best could not be more than speculative, Taussig[4] estimated that one in four pregnancies resulted in abortion with variations of from one to five in the rural districts to one to two and one-half in the urban districts. Pfaundler[5] has published a most interesting chart of the mortality from conception to the tenth month of postnatal life. This is perhaps one of the best interpretations of its kind in existence at the present time. This chart shows that during the first months of gestation the mortality rate is exceedingly high, dropping rapidly until at the fifth month it is at the same level as that of the neonatal period. After the fifth month the rate is much lower, approximating that found after the third month of postnatal life. During the first postnatal month, owing to the damaging effect of labor, there is a quick rise followed by a rapid drop. The various attempts to estimate the gross mortality rate from conception on brings out very clearly the fact that our knowledge about the mortality rate of the intrauterine period of life is indeed scant. It does fit in with the suggestion that it is highly probable that the conception rate is more or less static and that any fluctuation in the birth rate is governed by changes in the abortion rate.[6] In other words, our declining birth rate is not so much due to lack of fecundity as to the increase in abortions, to which must be added also the increased use of contraceptives.

Since it is practically impossible to determine the abortion rate, the national and state bureaus of vital statistics have of necessity scrupulously avoided this factor and their rates have been based upon the one denominator which can be ascertained with a close degree of accuracy, namely the number of live births. Infant deaths under one year of age including neonatal deaths and stillbirths are all computed from live births. While there is no doubt that this method is the only one to be used at the present time by such bureaus, nevertheless, it does not give a true picture of the gross fetal death rate. Special studies of smaller and more intimate groups are needed to help get a more accurate conception of the gross mortality rates. In many of the statistical reports published by different observers, the term "corrected mortality" is used. It is an unfortunate term which, save perhaps in exceptional instances, should be discarded for it tends to mislead the reader. Another criticism of many of the numerous reports is the failure upon the part of the author to make statistical interpretations. In all reports of this nature the significance of percentages should be calculated statistically and the tables should indicate that this has been done.

Realizing full well the present impossibility of vital statistic bureaus making computations except upon live births, the reviewer continues to feel the need for further research into the gross fetal mortality rate as computed from total births. What we desire to know after all is how many conceptions fail to produce live offsprings and the underlying causes of such failures. The true condition of affairs is masked when computations are based upon live births, and there is a tendency upon the part of all concerned to interest themselves little or not at all in the most obscure but greatest causes of intrauterine death. With this idea more or less in mind some attempts have recently been made to draw a base line of gross fetal mortality which could be used temporarily as a standard to go by. Clifford[7] has endeavored to do this by publishing the record of the Boston Lying-In Hospital for 60 years basing his rates upon the total number of births.

While it is desirable to study the gross mortality rate in this manner, it must be conceded that for the time being, at least, this cannot be achieved with any degree of success. Therefore, such endeavors should be attempted only as special studies and our maximum efforts should be spent upon trying to emphasize the necessity of uniformity in definitions and bases for statistical analyses.

The following outline is offered as a means by which uniformity can be brought about in classifying and recording mortality from conception through the neonatal period:

Mortality rate (per 1,000 live births).

1. For stillborn infants.
   a. Rate for abortions.
   b. Rate for prematurely born infants.
   c. Rate for full-term infants.
2. For liveborn infants (neonatal rate).
   a. Rate for prematurely born infants.
   b. Rate for full-term infants.

As a corollary to this, it is necessary to have a clear understanding of what the various terms mean. The following list of definitions has been evolved largely by a committee of the American Public Health Association and has been endorsed by the Committee on Neonatal Morbidity and Mortality of the American Pediatric Society:[8]

Live Birth.—A liveborn infant is one who shows "any evidence of life after complete birth." *Evidences of life* are breathing, action of the heart or movement of a voluntary muscle. *By birth or completion of birth* is meant the instant of complete separation of the entire body (not body in the restricted sense of trunk but the entire organism including the head, trunk and limbs) of the infant from the body of the mother whether or not the cord is cut or the placenta detached.[9]

Stillbirth.—A stillborn infant is one who shows no evidence of life (no breathing, no action of heart, no movement of voluntary muscle) after complete birth. Unless gestation has advanced to the fifth month the product of pregnancy need not be reported as a stillbirth.

Abortion.—An abortion is any product of conception of less than twenty-eight weeks' gestation, measuring 35 cm. (14 in.) or less and weighing less than 1500 gm. (3¼ pounds). The term "nonviable," which is ordinarily used to indicate a fetus of less than twenty-eight weeks' gestation, should probably be discarded since it has no particular significance statistically or otherwise.*

Premature Infant.—An infant with a birth weight of 5 pounds 8 ounces (2500 gm.) or less, a crown-heel length of 47 cm. (18 in.) or less and a gestation of thirty-seven weeks or less, should be considered immature and, by virtue of the fact that special handling is indicated, premature. Birth weight is the most important, and probably crown-heel length and the duration of gestation should be disregarded. In re-

*If this term is used, lower limits of duration of gestation, weight, and length would be better not only clinically but anatomically. Histologically the lungs of fetuses under twenty-four weeks show an insufficient amount of elastic tissue and the formation of aveoli has just begun[10, 11] so that the possibility of such fetuses living is, indeed, remote. Clinically 95 per cent of the infants weighing under 1000 gm. at birth die, and there have been reports of only five infants surviving birth weight under 700 gm. None of these has been 30 cm. long or less.[12, 13] In 10,000 consecutive births at the Chicago Lying-In Hospital no infant weighing under 800 gm. at birth survived twenty-four hours.[14]

porting premature studies, Ylppö's grouping, which has been more or less accepted the world over, is satisfactory: (1) under 1000 gm.; (2) 1000 to 1500 gm.; (3) 1501 to 2000 gm.; and (4) 2001-2500 gm. Any weight group may be split into subdivisions if the number of cases is sufficient. Infants should be grouped according to *birth weight*, not *admission weight*.

Neonatal Period.—This term should be used to designate the first thirty days of postnatal life.

It is hoped that in the near future some satisfactory group of definitions and some scheme of reporting the mortality during this particular span of life can be agreed upon. This accomplishment alone will serve as a great aid in ascertaining more definitely some of the obscure causes of prenatal, natal, and neonatal death. Until this is done the tremendous number of statistical reports that are continually being published will be largely worthless, at least from the standpoint of their value in making statistical comparisons. In repetition it seems advisable to emphasize again that in all reports the significance of percentages should be calculated statistically.

CONGENITAL DEFECTS

When one considers the tremendous rapidity with which cell multiplication takes place during the period from conception to maturity of the fetus, it seems surprising indeed that more gross abnormalities are not observed at birth. Not all fertilized ova are of good enough quality to survive the period of gestation. Thus, it has been estimated that as many as 25 per cent of these ova succumb during the early period of development.[15] Such episodes furnish an explanation for many of the cases of spontaneous abortion. The importance of quality is not limited to uterine life, for failure to survive after birth depends not inconsiderably upon the original quality of the egg. Eggs differ greatly in such qualities as endurance and capacity for growth, and many of these differences are hereditary. With so many endogenous and exogenous factors continually at work upon the maternal organism during pregnancy, damage to the primitive cells at an early period, undoubtedly, would result in a greater incidence of defects were not these cells endowed with certain inherent powers of which we know but little. The cells have the ability to multiply at a rapid but well-governed rate and to become differentiated into special types peculiar to the various organs. With differentiation, or specialization, seems to come inhibition of growth, and the earlier differentiation appears the sooner does growth of that particular structure cease. Embryonal tissue, likewise, has the innate power to flourish at the expense of its host if necessary—a parasitic or neoplastic characteristic. The entire process follows a definite organismic plan or pattern (heredity) which can, however, be influenced considerably by environmental factors. The end-product is the result of the interplay between the more constant hereditary factors and the environmental ones. While the power of adaptation is potentially greatest in the beginning of development, actually it is utilized only slightly at this period. In other words, the end-result of the power to adapt, adaptibility, is not great at this time. As a consequence, the intrauterine mortality, especially in the beginning is exceedingly high, and then gradually decreases as the organism becomes better able to adapt itself—a situation that is maintained more or less with few fluctuations until old age is reached. When the noxious influences are not too injurious, adaptation will take place and be facilitated by the distinct ability of fetal tissue to substitute, compensate, and regenerate, that is, its greater plastic capacity. Malformations are the result of such incidents.

By virtue of a deficiency in embryonal tissue of the necessary instruments or apparatus by which coordination between structures or organs occurs, circulatory and nervous systems, inflammation in the early stages of development does not react in the general or systemic way it does in the older organism and adult. There seems to be a failure of response to antigenic poisons which is carried over to some extent into the neonatal period. Thus, while these tissues are susceptible to infectious agents, their ability to react to them remains more or less localized and limited. In most instances this so-called immunity cannot be ascribed to the presence of antibodies, for they are definitely wanting in the fetus, but instead to the functioning of an entirely different mechanism. The increased resistance to generalized infection is the result of incompleteness of development, that is, of lack of ability of the tissues to exhibit a generalized inflammatory reaction in the presence of infection. The immune bodies that are sometimes found in the blood serum of the newborn are probably not transferred from the mother to the fetus by way of the placenta or breast milk but are formed independently in a manner perhaps somewhat similar to that which controls growth.[16] The recent investigations of McKahnn and Chu indicate that the placenta may be the spot at which immune bodies are formed.[17] It is probable, therefore, that natural or species immunity is after all not transferred from mother to child in the manner ordinarily assumed.

Numerous theories regarding the cause of some of the congenital abnormalities have been elaborated. Fetal inflammation years ago was considered one of the chief agents, and syphilis was given a place at the top of the list. With the advent of serologic procedures and methods of staining spirochetes in the tissues, our views about the part syphilis plays in the etiology of congenital malformations have changed considerably. The fact that it plays such an insignificant rôle in the causation of neonatal death or of prematurity seems to depreciate its importance in the etiology of fetal abnormalities, including congenital deafness.[18] In Clifford's report[7] comprising over 120,000 births, syphilis was credited with a death rate of only 0.52 per 1,000 births. Swanson and his coworkers[14] attributed to congenital syphilis only one death in 10,000 consecutive births. Cruickshank[19] was able to establish a definite diagnosis of congenital syphilis in but 0.75 per cent of 800 neonatal deaths. The actual part that infections of a nonspecific nature play in the development of fetal anomalies that cannot be linked with heredity is unknown. Perhaps they are more important than ordinarily thought to be the case. Certainly here is a much neglected problem.

The relationship between congenital abnormalities and maternal poisoning is not clear. The fact that the embryo is less resistant to the abortifacient poisons as well as to the heavy metals, iodine, phosphorus, and nicotine would tend to indicate that perhaps some anomalies might be the result of tissue damage by one or more of these poisons. However, if the injury were at all great, it is likely that early death of the embryo and abortion would occur. The same in all probability can be said of the possible damage to the embryo by the poisons in maternal toxemias. While the fetal mortality, including abortions, from the various toxemias has been found to be 30 per cent[20] and from maternal diabetes over 40 per cent,[21] there are no reports that either are related to the incidence of congenital anomalies. In view of the increased use of tobacco among women a good deal has been said about its effect upon the fetus. Setting aside purely personal prejudices, so far there has been little proof offered on one or the other side that moderate or even excessive smoking affects either fecundity or fetal mortality. Even the limited number of studies that have been made regarding the effect of nicotine poisoning upon the female reproductive organs of animals have not been particularly enlightening.[22] Certainly there is little unprejudiced evidence that even excessive use of tobacco by the pregnant woman has any relationship to the incidence of congenital anomalies. Nor would one expect much effect since an amount of nicotine or carbon monoxide in the maternal blood sufficient to damage the embryo would in all probability result in death and abortion. Sontag and Wallace[23] found that later in pregnancy cigaret smoking increased the fetal heart rate slightly. They did not remark about any subsequent effects upon the neonatal heart rate. Embryonal tissue is sometimes affected deleteriously by quinine with resulting death and expulsion of the product of conception. The drug has, likewise, been incriminated occasionally as a cause of late fetal death when used to induce labor.[24, 25, 26] Accumulation of quinine in the fetal tissues was ascribed as the cause of death. Taylor[27] has reported an increased incidence of congenital deafness among infants born in malaria-infested regions, where quinine is used in large doses. In a few other instances there was some evidence that quinine used for induction of labor might have caused deafness in the newborn.[28] The drug is thought to act selectively upon the auditory nerves. Although a great deal of inquiry has been made into the effect of alcoholism upon the progeny, the results of numerous experiments have varied considerably. The consensus of opinion at present seems to be that fertility is unaffected by alcohol. Alcohol also seems to be a selective agent which destroys the weaker or more susceptible fertilized germ cells and produces superiority on the part of the surviving ones.[29] Furthermore, there is no difference in the proportion of physical abnormalities between alcoholized and control stock.[30] Therefore, there is no experimental proof to show that alcohol is an idiokinetic poison nor is there much clinical evidence to show that alcohol can produce directly in the first generation mental defects which can be transmitted as such. It is probable that alcoholism is more often a result of mental deficiency than a cause of it.[31, 32]

The destructive effect of radium and roentgen rays upon fetal tissues has been the subject of considerable interest in the past few years. The rays seem to have a particular affinity for tissues of the central nervous system, irradiation frequently resulting in the birth of anencephalic monsters or infants manifesting various anomalies of the brain and its coverings. However, abnormalities of other parts of the body have been reported. Bagg[33] has produced experimentally limb abnormalities capable of hereditary transmission. Perhaps in the instance there is displacement of the genes—the translocation theory of Muller—by the bombardment of the chromosomes by the rays.[34] Since the rays are known to have more effect upon nuclei in the process of division, embryologic tissue with so few nuclei in the resting state is especially liable to damage. Arrest of development associated with the formation of blebs and hematomas seems to be the pathologic lesions produced.[15] Focal deficiencies of this sort might explain many malformations. When conception follows soon after irradiation, phenotypic and possibly genotypic injury may occur. When conception is subsequent to the end of the period of temporary amenorrhea caused by irradiation, no damage results.[35] Apparently the diagnostic use of roentgen rays does not have a deleterious effect upon the fetus, if used sparingly, but therapeutic irradiation after conception is so imminently dangerous to the fetus that it should be followed by abortion.[36]

Some observers have attributed certain fetal anomalies, especially those relating to the brain and spinal cord, to abnormalities of the amnion. Jansen[37] blamed pressure changes associated with shortness of the amniotic membrane for a number of these abnormalities as well as some forms of idiocy, especially the mongoloid type. So far this hypothesis has gained few supporters.

Peterson[38, 39] recently has attributed the origin of congenital anomalies to meteorologic causes, namely, variations in the barometric pressure occurring at an early period of embryologic development with a resulting disturbance of the oxidative-reductive mechanism and of the hydrogen ion concentration. This is somewhat similar to Stockard's theory[40] that an unfavorable temperature and oxygen supply affecting the fetal metabolic rate during critical phases of the development of an organ or part may account for some of the extreme degrees of fetal malformation. Peterson bases this theory upon the fact that there is a geographic increase in the incidence of certain anomalies which parallels the storm tracks of the United States. Murphy[41] was able to corroborate this in a study of congenital deformities in Philadelphia. In fact, his findings disagreed entirely with those of Peterson in that particular area.

Other factors, such as age of the mother and the number of children she has borne, seem to affect the incidence of congenitally malformed children. Murphy[42] found in a study of mothers who had at least one normal and one defective child that there were fewer defectives when the mothers were between the ages of twenty and twenty-five years. There was an increasing number of malformed children from year to year when the mothers were over thirty years old and the greatest number of defectives was born to mothers who were over forty years old. The ratio of defective children to normal children was three or more times greater after thirty years than before. In another study he and Maser[43] noted that the first four children in a family were less likely to be malformed than the subsequent progeny. These observations bring to mind the old view concerning exhaustion of germ plasm as an etiologic factor in the production of congenital abnormalities.

In general, it may be said of the various factors, mechanical, chemical, physical or otherwise, which may affect the germ cells or embryonal cells that they tend to lessen the power of adaption of these cells. By virtue of this there is an increased mortality rate, whether it is due to the primary disturbance or secondarily to a subsequent increased susceptibility to disease, and in turn through early death, race deterioration is prevented. To a considerable extent the preserving effects of our civilization work against this selective effort of nature to purify the race. With the exception of radiant energy there is little evidence to show that these other factors are truly teratogenic.[41] With Bagg's studies as a guide it may be possible in the near future to learn more about the numerous agents that underly the various developmental defects.

No doubt, nearly every physician has been confronted by the anxious parents of a malformed child with the question, "What are the chances of another defective child being born?" I wonder how many times the reply has been that lightning rarely strikes twice in the same place. According to a recent report Murphy,[45] who studied this particular question in a group of families in which there was at least one malformed child, found that such an answer was erroneous. He concluded that congenital defects serious enough to be recorded on birth certificates were approximately twenty-four times as likely to occur in families containing one congenitally malformed child as in the population at large. This problem brings up the subject of heredity.

HEREDITARY DEFECTS

The medical practitioner has been so thoroughly engrossed in the study of acquired, or what he considers acquired, disease that he has devoted but little attention to the rôle inheritance plays in some of these disorders. While he has recognized that there are individual differences in the ability of an organism to combat acquired disease and that susceptibility varies considerably in persons and families, he has been inclined to attribute these qualities chiefly to acquired factors, such as immunity. As a result of looking elsewhere, many conditions of a distinctly heritable nature have been overlooked and, if not, have engaged only cursory attention. There are several reasons why medical men have not been particularly interested in genetics. This science has gone along at such a rapid pace with its controversies and backtrackings that most of us, who have never taken as much as an elemental course in the subject, have had neither the fundamental knowledge nor the courage to attack such a chaotic and immense literature. The attempt of earlier geneticists to separate the inseparable factors, heredity and environment, and their tendency to emphasize the former perhaps at the expense of the latter has been responsible to some extent for the passiveness of the medical profession in respect to the hereditary aspect of disease. After all, the physician is primarily interested in the prevention and cure of disease, and the environmental or acquired forms have responded more satisfactorily to his efforts. In other words, the relative incurability of hereditary disease as it is known to him has been largely responsible for neglect of this field by the doctor. However, this attitude has been unfortunate, for it has limited the scope of medical practice and has not only hampered progress in medical diagnoses but also advancement in human genetical research. Genetics is such a complex subject, especially in relation to man, that there must be the closest cooperation between geneticists and physicians if any progress is to be made. Eventually this cooperation will come, for it is becoming increasingly more essential now for the doctor to interest himself in problems of heredity. The result of modern methods of hygiene and treatment has been to protect and preserve to a fertile age many individuals who years ago would have succumbed before this period was reached. Such contraselective characteristics of our civilization now tend "to preserve and accumulate abnormal mutations, whether visible defects or hidden physiological pecularities."[31] A good example of this is seen in diabetes which is recognized as an inheritable disease. Successful palliation of this disorder has permitted more diabetics to reach the child-bearing age and has transformed the diabetic woman into a fertile rather than a relatively sterile individual. Furthermore, it has resulted in a considerable reduction in both the maternal and fetal mortality rates of this group. Other examples of this nature point to the fact that in the future the increasing incidence of inheritable disease will of necessity create more interest in the racial and eugenic aspects of preventive medicine. Hence, the physician will be required to give more advice or information regarding the probability of a given trait being transmitted to the child, that is, a eugenic prognosis. This cannot be accomplished unless the medical curriculum is modified to include courses in genetics. These should be organized to supply the student with a working knowledge of genetics which will be applicable to clinical medicine.

In undertaking to ascertain the inheritance element in disease it will be found that this can be detected with striking clarity in some cases while in others it is more obscure and nebulous. There are well-known reasons for this. Man is a poor breeder and a slowly maturing animal so that the turnover of generations is only about three to the century. Pure strains are practically nonexistent owing to outbreeding, and experimental breeding is impossible. Family pedigrees are difficult to trace and are usually too meager to be of value in genetic analyses. One of the outstanding difficulties in tracing pedigrees is failure to realize that recessive traits may not be visible in several generations. Morgan[46] considers it rather hazardous to attempt to apply even the simpler rules of mendelian inheritance to man because of his complex genetic composition. The development of many inherited human characteristics depends to a large extent on the presence of modifying factors and on external environment for their expression. Such a complexity makes him disrespect the human as genetical material and question the simplicity with which some write of complicated processes of human inheritance.[47] Thus, one would infer that the physician in his admission of ignorance about human heredity is joined by only a few of his geneticist colleagues. The medical man has come in for no little criticism and ridicule by students of heredity because of his lack of genetic technic in dealing with an acknowledged complex problem in an animal that can neither be experimented with nor compared satisfactorily with others. Of necessity more devious routes must be taken to secure information of a sort that may be of a little value to the human race. For this reason some of the so-called archaic but "well-intended" efforts of the medical profession to classify man into gross physical types, constitutions, or diatheses, must be continued even though they are considered "so far in advance of our genetical information that the geneticist may be excused if he refuses to discuss them seriously."[46] If for nothing but humanitarian reasons, and after all medicine is not a cold mathematical science, these constitutional types which have been fostered by the continental writers[48] will continue to be used as diagnostic and prognostic aids until something more constructive is offered. In other words, groupings of this sort, which have existed in some form for centuries, have served the physician good stead and will be used by him until the geneticist can apply his experimental and biometric methods to human material. To some extent this method of approach is now being tried in some of the biologic institutes of Russia and Germany.[49] Robb,[50] in perusing medical literature, finds that the medical author does not give due credit to the recessive genes in etiology and decrys the use of the "ubiquitous label 'familial but not hereditary' " which has been used to convey the fact that the parents apparently show none of the abnormal traits exhibited by the offspring. He also notes that lethal and semilethal factors are rarely identified although the latter were responsible for 13 per cent of infant deaths in 1929 as compared with 1.5 per cent 40 years ago. These figures emphasize the increasing importance of the eugenic prognosis in medicine. The behavior of allelomorphs, likewise, does not seem to have been generally appreciated in medical writings. Criticisms of this nature should stimulate the medical profession to greater interest in genetics so that the little that has been found out about the human can be utilized to the fullest extent. So far, it does not seem to the reviewer that medical men in general have appreciated sufficiently the use that studies of twins can be put to in the evaluation of human heredity.

It has been observed, as mentioned above, that certain structural and physiologic characteristics are peculiar to the members of certain families.[51] Such traits or predispositions to them are primarily of a hereditary nature but are subject to environmental influences to an extent that at times they will tend to appear only when these environmental conditions are present. In order to correlate the numerous but confusing observations relative to this subject, an attempt has been made by some to classify roughly these gross physical states or types so that a better perspective may be had of man's tendency to react along certain clinicopathologic lines. This system of grouping has been of considerable value to the clinician in many ways, especially in respect to diagnosis, prognosis, and prophylaxis. Thus, it has helped the doctor to recognize disease in the making. It has made it easier for him to try to anticipate and forestall disease by entering, gropingly to be sure, a sort of prepathologic realm where minor variations or incipiencies develop into the potential and finally the recognizable disease state. In this way it gives him, at least, an opportunity to attempt to follow out the principle that the best treatment is prevention. Thus, the intimation that certain types of individuals react somewhat typically to certain environmental influences gives the physician a chance to be on the lookout for disease at a time when it can be more successfully treated or prevented. This grouping of individuals has helped to correlate much scattered information so that a better composite picture, for instance, of metabolic and hormonic disturbances, could be painted. It has been through this method that the subtle influence of the endocrines upon the individual has been brought out. It must be realized that this particular phase of medicine is merely a makeshift used to bridge over tremendous gaps in our knowledge. For this reason, there is little need to create an extensive and detailed classification as it would make the subject too complicated and really a comprehensive study of syndromes. At present the pediatrist can continue to utilize successfully in his practice some of the information gained by reading of the so-called archaic diatheses which have been included in pediatric texts for years: exudative, lymphatic, neuroarthritic, and spasmophilic. While the diathetic concept is beyond the pale of scientific preciseness demanded by pathologist and geneticist, for the clinician it still serves a definite purpose. The diatheses, or constitutions, should be considered as merely impressions based upon astute clinical observations which serve to assist the clinician temporarily until these impressions can be metamorphosed into biologic facts.

In the past few years geneticists have furnished physicians with abridged information about human inheritance. This has been of value in helping them to give more satisfactory eugenic prognoses and in interesting them in the accumulation of hereditary pedigrees. Several monographs worthy of reading have been published, most of which include interesting data about the more common diseases in man which seem to show fairly well-proved transmissibility. It must be remembered, however, that, while heredity may be demonstrated in a given disease, other factors should not be ignored. In fact, as has been emphasized before, heredity and environment must be considered inseparable, and the concept of the gene must include three components: the gene matter, situated in the chromosome; the relation to other genes, the genetic environment; and the external environment.[52] In giving genetic advice, "judgment should always be given with the reservation involved in the fact that genetics primarily deal with *probabilities*" [italics ours].[53]

Briefly the present-day conception of genetics is that the chromosomes form the basis of the mechanism of inheritance. They carry within themselves the genetic factors known as genes, which are likened to a string of beads the individual members of which represent the character determinants. Genes are relatively stable but on rare occasions may change, thus causing mutations. These factors usually work in conjunction with one another. When chromosomes subdivide, they split longitudinally so that the line of genes is split likewise, each daughter chromosome receiving exactly half of the original line. All characters are in pairs called allelomorphs (alternates) one of which is usually dominant and the other recessive. Thus, while the dominant characteristic may be the only one apparent in the individual, a recessive factor may be present. A recessive gene may be transmitted for generations before it meets a similar gene in another individual and the recessive character becomes visible. This process makes it difficult to trace heredity in humans. If an individual inherits the same gene from both his parents he is homozygous, or pure for that character. If he inherits a dominant and a recessive gene, then he is in a hybrid or heterozygous condition. In the inheritance of dominant characteristics the character appears in every generation. Some genes are dominant to one and recessive to another so that irregularity of reaction may appear. Homozygous dominants are rarely found. Heterozygous dominants usually marry normals so that half of the children will be of each type. When a heterozygous dominant marries a recessive, about half of the children will be of the recessive type. When two heterozygous dominants cross, about one-fourth of the children will be of the recessive type. In the human race, families are often so small that these ratios may not appear. The pedigree of recessive inheritance is different. It may be transmitted for generations before it meets the same gene in another individual. This is the danger in cousin marriages. Inbreeding accumulates recessive defects as well as dominant defects whether they be good or bad. When the genes are carried in the sex chromosomes they are said to be sex-linked. In such instances the characteristic is usually carried by the female and manifested in the male. Lethal factors, or genes, may prevent the development of the gamete or zygote by causing intrauterine death, which may occur early or late. Semilethal factors are likely to cause postnatal death. Lethal factors are recessive, appearing only when present in a homozygous condition.

Fertility.[54]—There is a significant correlation between the number of children born to women and to their mothers. Therefore, the heredity of fertility seems to be established.

Multiple Births.[55, 56-68]—The ratio between twins and single births is 1:85 and between triplets and single births 1:87.[2] Triplets occur once in 7,000 births. Heredity factors are of importance in twinning, both parents transmitting the tendency. It is recessive. Multiple births are more often girls than boys. Repetition of twins occurs about once in twenty times. Approximately 15 per cent of all women have the twinning tendency, so that in a given pregnancy the chance that one of these women will actually produce twins is 1:10.

Physical Characteristics.[57, 58]—Stature seems to be related to heredity. In tall families the normal offspring are characteristically tall, and in short families the reverse holds true. A slight regression may appear in the younger generations in tall families, but in short ones there is no increase. Thus, shortness seems to be due to positive or dominant factors that limit growth while the factors for tallness are probably recessive. Brown eye color is incompletely dominant to blue, several genes probably being involved. Blue eye color is recessive to brown but dominant to red (albinism). In general, the darker hair colors appear to be dominant over the lighter colors, as with skin colors. Red hair is apparently recessive.

Skin.—*Psoriasis* shows a definite hereditary character in a large number of cases. The common mode of inheritance is probably recessive, and, therefore, no more than one-fourth the children will be affected. Skipping of a generation is often observed. *Ichthyosis* is a variable inheritable trait conforming to several forms of inheritance. *Nevi* adhere chiefly to the dominant type, especially when on the cheek. *Albinism* is usually transmitted as a mendelian recessive trait. It has been estimated that in random mating there would be about one person in seventy carrying the gene for albinism. *Pattern baldness* is inherited from father to son as a dominant. When the woman transmits, it acts as a recessive. The condition is usually sex-limited. The pattern is usually constant in families and frequently the pattern can be outlined in the newborn.

Skeleton.—The *teeth* are subject to a number of inherited anomalies, the most common one being the absence of one or more. It appears to be both dominant and recessive. Studies of identical twins suggest that early decay may have sometimes a background of inheritance as does the time and order of their appearance of teeth. *Osteogenesis imperfecta* behaves as a mendelian dominant as probably does *achondroplasia* and *dysostosis cleidocranialis.* In such cases parenthood is inadvisable. *Cleft palate and cleft lip* shows an inheritable recessive tendency at times, but in many pedigrees it seems to be purely sporadic and accidental. The same may be said for *congenital dislocation of the hip. Clubfoot* in about one-half of the cases seems to have a hereditary background requiring a guarded prognosis as to the probabilities of the defect in the offspring. Eleven per cent of the offspring of normal persons mated with affected ones are found to be affected. *Flatfoot* is also reported to be largely inherited. *Polydactylism, syndactylism, and brachydactylism*[59-62] can occur in normal families as sporadic sports, but the group shows a striking hereditary character which usually acts as a dominant. A guarded eugenic prognosis must be given.

Eye.—Knowledge of the hereditary transmission of occular defects is unusually complete. *Refractive errors* manifest a hereditary tendency of a complicated type owing to the interplay of several factors. In the normal emmetrophic condition hereditary transmission seems to be dominant. *Myopia* frequently appears as a recessive or dominant character, and occasionally its transmission may be sex-linked. Consanguinity in parentage, therefore, definitely affects the incidence of myopia. It is the only refractive error serious enough in its implications to warrant attempts to limit its incidence in future generations. While abuse of the eyes plays a part, it cannot be considered the primary cause of the disorder. *Hypermetropia* of the milder type is dominant in character, while the high-grade type which is sometimes associated with cataract is usually recessive in character. *Astigmatism* is frequently an inherited error and like smaller errors of refraction is usually transmitted as a dominant. *Squint* shows inherited tendencies, but there seems to be no constancy about its behavior. *Retinitis pigmentosa* is definitely hereditary and, although acting as a dominant in most cases, may appear as a recessive occasionally. Transmission of other hereditary diseases of the retina is usually of a recessive nature. *Amaurotic family idiocy* seems to be transmitted as a recessive character and *congenital optic atrophy* as a dominant. *Congenital night blindness* may be inherited as either a dominant or recessive and in some instances it is sex-linked. *Color blindness* of the red-green type, which shows an incidence of 8 per cent in males and 0.5 per cent in females, is usually inherited as a typical male sex-linked character. It is recessive in the female. The rarer form, total color blindness, is transmitted as a recessive character. *Congenital cataract* is strongly hereditary being transmitted as a dominant character. Since 13 per cent of the inmates of blind schools have the disease, eugenic measures should be used to combat its production. *Infantile glaucoma (buphthalmos)* behaves as a recessive. *Congenital nystagmus* and *congenital ptosis* are usually found to be transmitted as dominant characters. Sex-linking may occur in the former.

Ear.—Deaf-mutism is inherited in about one-seventh of the cases as a mendelian recessive factor. It is more likely to appear in consanguineous marriages. When both parents are deaf-mutes, conception should be interdicted. If one parent suffers from the defect, and the other is normal and has a normal pedigree, the chance of deaf offspring is small although a few of these will be recessive to hereditary deaf-mutism. However, if the normal parent has a family history of deaf-mutism, about as high as 35 per cent of the resulting families will contain deaf-mutes. If both parents have normal hearing but come from a family with a tendency to the disease, the chance for deaf children is so high that conception should be prevented. *Otosclerosis* occurs frequently enough, one in two hundred, to engage the interest of many prospective parents. The disease is more common among females. There is a hereditary basis for the disease, but no uniform manner of transmission is found. When both parents come from affected stocks, the prospect for the children is bad. There is slightly less likelihood for otosclerosis in the offspring when the husband is deaf and his pedigree shows the disease than when the same situation prevails in the wife. When either parent is affected but the pedigrees of both are normal, the risk is less. It is often difficult to differentiate between otosclerosis and adventitious deafness in the pedigree.

Blood.—Blood groups are distinctly subject to heredity, but, owing to a peculiar condition known as multiple allelomorphism, hereditary transmission of these groups is not generally understood. In this instance the original recessive gene, which may be designated "O," is thought to have given rise to two dominant genes A and B. The groups are represented in the following way:[56]

Group	Genes
I	OO
II	AA or BO
III	BB or BO
IV	AB

Since both A and B are dominant to O either AA or AO will act alike and result in Group II. The same can be said for BB and BO in Group III. From this it is possible to understand why union between parents of blood Groups I and IV will result in offspring whose blood characteristics will not resemble that of either parent. The children's bloods will conform to either Group II or III. Such knowledge is of inestimable value in seeking donors because it may make it possible to eliminate many obviously unnecessary tests for compatibility. Diseases of the blood have been found to manifest striking inherited tendencies. *Hemophilia* is a sex-limited disorder which is transmitted only by females and manifested by males. With a carrier mother and a normal father 50 per cent of the sons will be affected, all the daughters should be normal, but 50 per cent should be carriers. With a normal mother and an affected father all the siblings should be normal, but all the daughters, carriers. It would be expected that one in 200 females should manifest the disease. Actually few if any do. This may be due to a lethal factor which kills the offspring *in utero*. From a eugenic standpoint only the unaffected males of a hemophilic family should be permitted to propagate. *Acholuric jaundice* or familial hemolytic anemia is inherited as a mendelian dominant as is *sickle-cell anemia*. There are a number of blood diseases which afflict several members of a family but about which there is an insufficient amount of authentic information regarding its transmissibility through successive generations. In this group belong familial icterus of the newborn, erythroblastosis, Gaucher's disease, and lipoid histiocytosis.

Nervous System.—Migraine is considered to be transmitted as a mendelian dominant, but, since the presence of exogenous factors play an important part in its production, inheritance studies are difficult to make. Apparently, even though a dominant, it can be transmitted by individuals who do not suffer the disease. *Huntington's chorea* is, likewise, inherited as a mendelian dominant. Nearly all the cases in the United States have been traced to three brothers who emigrated to this country in the seventeenth century.[63] Its behavior is that of a typical mendelian dominant uninfluenced by sex. It is clear that patients with the disease should not marry. Although *paralysis agitans* is usually sporadic, it may appear as either a dominant or recessive character. *Amaurotic family idiocy* is a vicious disorder showing evidence of being transmitted as a mendelian recessive. The genes are sublethal. It may also be classed as one of the abiotrophics. Brain[31] uses the term *hereditary ataxia* for a group of disorders having more or less common clinical features; *Friederick's ataxia* and *Marie's cerebellar ataxia* are the most common forms. The former usually operates as a simple dominant or recessive, but sometimes a more complicated inheritance seems to be present. Affected members may transmit the disorder to as high as 30 per cent of their offspring and apparently unaffected members, to 13 per cent. Children of affected parents are more likely to suffer the disease than those remotely related to an affected individual. *Peroneal muscular atrophy* may be transmitted as either a dominant or recessive which may be sex-linked. The *muscular dystrophies* seem to act in the same variable way and eugenic prognoses must not be made until the individual has passed the age at which symptoms usually appear in members of the family. In *myotonia congenita* inheritance seems to be a dominant. *Neurofibromatosis* appears to be inherited as a mendelian dominant, and, therefore, those free from the disease will not transmit it. *Spina bifida* is often inherited as a dominant trait. *Epilepsy*[69] may or may not be an inherited disease in about 50 per cent of the cases. Owing to the fact that, when the predisposition is present, it may take an additional factor such as an acquired cerebral lesion to initiate the symptoms, it is impossible to trace accurately the heredity of the disease. Multiple heritable factors rather than simple ones are probably present. The chances are about 1 to 10 that an epileptic will transmit the disease to its offspring, and transmission seems to be equal in both sexes. In the case of the *petit mal* form, the risk of inheritance is somewhat less.

In respect to the inheritance of mental disorders, there have been so many inadequately controlled studies, histories are so difficult to obtain, and the material itself is subject to such a great number of variable factors that positive statements about it are practically impossible to make. In general, it may be said that such disorders as schizophrenia and manic-depressive insanity are transmitted, and there is no reason to change the eugenic prognosis if these disorders have been recovered from. There is reason to believe that criminals, moral defectives, impulsive hysterics, severe hypochondriacs, obsessionals, and alcoholics are probably unsuitable progenitors.[31] Definite mental defectives are likewise unsuitable progenitors, and, when familial taints are present in both parents, transmission is likely. When there is a family history of mental deficiency on one side and of soundness on the other, transmission to the immediate offspring is not so likely. *Mongolism* is probably not transmissible. However, as has been mentioned before,[45] there is a greater chance for some form of malformation in subsequent children when a woman has produced one child with a gross abnormality. Further childbearing after the age of thirty-five in such women should not be encouraged.

Metabolic Disturbances.—Diabetes mellitus[64] shows definite hereditary tendencies in at least 25 per cent of the cases, but the mode of transmission is not sufficiently clear to state exactly the mendelian principle involved. Several genes may be involved. When there are numerous diabetics in the pedigree, there is a probability of transmission, and, if both sides are involved or the disease is present in every generation, dominance of the trait is suggested, and the chances of transmission are strong. The chances for a diabetic to beget an offspring with the tendency is high. With the modern method of treating diabetics the disease is not incompatible with subsequent economic efficiency. Since the fertility of the treated diabetic has been greatly increased and since the lethality of the disease from both the maternal and fetal standpoint has been substantially decreased, we are now faced with an increased incidence of diabetes in our population.[65] *Renal diabetes* appears to behave as a dominant character and such rare disorders as alkaptonuria, cystinuria, pentosuria, porphyrinuria, and steatorrhea are thought to be recessives.

Allergic Diseases.—There is rather definite evidence that the allergic tendency may be transmitted. However, since the incidence of the disturbance in families surpasses the expected proportions for mendelian inheritance, undoubtedly in many cases it is an acquired abnormality. Placental transmission has been reported.[66] It is thought, however, that inheritance can be explained in the majority of cases on the basis of mendelian dominance.[67] In 50 per cent of affected individuals the pedigrees will show the trait on one side, and in 20 per cent it will be found on both sides. In angioneurotic edema there seems to be a clear-cut dominance.

LETHAL FACTORS

While there is every reason to expect that lethal factors exist in man as well as animals and plants, direct evidence to substantiate this belief is difficult to obtain. Some but not all the monstrosities appearing at birth are probably of this origin, and perhaps some miscarriages are due to the action of lethal genes. Congenital ichthyosis seems to be a good example of a lethal factor at work. Sublethal genes are thought at times to be involved in the following conditions: xeroderma pigmentosa, osteogenesis imperfecta, glioma retinae, spinal progressive muscular paralysis, amaurotic family idiocy, spina bifida, hydrocephalus, cretinism, and mongolism. Unfortunately some of these are too viable in man. Since lethal factors exist only in the recessive state, except possibly for brachydactyly, it is very hard to get accurate information about them. As Mohr states, it is surprising that there is such a perfect coordination between the numerous genes that embryologic abnormalities are relatively infrequent.

From the foregoing brief résumé it can be seen that the present-day knowledge about human inheritance is meager and most unsatisfactory. This is due to the complexity of man's genetic make-up as well as to the difficulty in obtaining reliable pedigrees. In order to satisfy the statistical laws upon which genetics are based, it is necessary to deal in large numbers. Single pedigrees rarely do this. Furthermore, the data from pedigrees extending over many generations is unreliable not only because hearsay evidence must be relied on for the earlier generations, but also because diagnoses and diagnostic methods change. Pooled data from two-generation pedigrees, therefore, are much more reliable scientifically than data from a few pedigrees of many generations. The medical profession can be of infinite service in obtaining pedigrees for these pools, provided it learns how to take them properly. Pedigree blanks may be obtained from the Eugenics Record Office.

The method of dealing with the problem of heredity in the human differs from that in animals or plants. It is not possible to build a race free from defects, nor is it always desirable. For instance, it is better to eradicate an infectious disease by such public health measures as sanitation and individual immunization, e.g., typhoid, than to try to breed a race immune to the disease. Consanguineous marriages or inbreeding among tainted families as a means of localizing the disorder does not seem to be justifiable or possible. So far, sterilization of defectives has not met with much popular success. Such problems belong rather to the sociologist and the eugenist than the doctor. The little that can be accomplished, at present, must come through efforts to discourage procreation among hereditary defectives.

From a medical standpoint the greatest attention should be focused upon removing the external causes of disease and protecting against disease.

SUMMARY

1. Present-day lack of uniformity in definitions and bases for statistical analyses tends to prevent accumulation of accurate information about the underlying causes of fetal and neonatal deaths.

2. In an attempt to overcome such difficulties, an outline and group of definitions agreed upon by several organizations interested in the subject is herewith presented.

3. Some of the possible etiologic factors in the production of congenital defects are reviewed.

4. The brief résumé of the present status of human inheritance presented emphasizes the meagerness of our information about this complex subject.

5. The medical profession is urged to take greater interest in human genetics in order that more authentic information may be made available to geneticists and more satisfactory eugenic prognoses may be given to prospective parents.

REFERENCES

1. Bonar, B. E.: Problems of the Newborn, J. PEDIAT. **5:** 216, 1934.
2. Bonar, B. E.: The Newborn, J. PEDIAT. **7:** 99, 1935.
3. Grier, R. M.: Fetal Mortality, Am. J. Obst. & Gynec. **22:** 890, 1931.
4. Taussig, F. J.: Abortion and Its Relation to Maternal Mortality. To be published.
5. Pfaundler, M.: The Diseases of Children, Pfaundler and Schlossmann. English translation. Vol. 1, p. 34, Philadelphia, 1935, J. B. Lippincott Company.
6. Young, J.: Maternal Mortality and Maternal Mortality Rates, Am. J. Obst. & Gynec. **31:** 198, 1936.
7. Clifford, H.: A Study of Neonatal Mortality, J. PEDIAT. **8:** 367, 1936.
8. Special Report: Stillbirths, Am. Pub. Health A. Yearbook, 1935-36.
9. Manual of International Causes of Death, 1924, p. 379.
10. Feldman, W. M.: The Principles of Antenatal and Postnatal Child Psychology, New York, 1920, Longmans, Green & Company, p. 142.
11. Scammon, R. E.: Abt's Pediatrics **1:** 353, 1923, Philadelphia, W. B. Saunders Company.
12. Hess, J. H.: Premature and Congenitally Diseased Infants, Philadelphia and New York, 1922, Lea & Febiger, p. 364.
13. Hess, J. H., Mohr, G. J., and Bartelme, P. F.: The Physical and Mental Growth of Prematurely Born Children, Chicago, 1934, The University of Chicago Press, p. 221.
14. Swanson, W. W., Turner, A. R., and Adair, F. L.: Institutional Mortality of the Newborn, J. PEDIAT. **7:** 516, 1935.
15. Streeter, G. L.: Focal Deficiencies in Fetal Tissues and Their Relation to Intrauterine Amputation, Pub. No. 414, 1930, Carnegie Institute, Washington, D. C.
16. Musselmann, L. K.: Natural Immunity of the Newborn, Am. J. Obst. & Gynec. **8:** 45 and 141, 1924.
17. McKahnn, C. F., and Chu, F. T.: J. Infect. Dis. **52:** 268, 1923; and Tr. Am. Pediat. Soc. **45:** 65, 1933.
18. McCarty, V. W.: Otological Observations in the Congenitally Syphilitic Child, Tr. Am. Laryng. Rhin. & Otol. Soc. **38:** 479, 1932.
19. Cruickshank, J. N.: The Causes of Neonatal Death, M. Research Council. Special Report Ser. 145, London, 1930, H. M. Stationery Office.
20. Peckham, C. H.: Fetal Mortality in the Toxemias of Pregnancy, J. A. M. A. **101:** 1608, 1933.
21. Ronsheim, J.: Diabetes and Pregnancy, Am. J. Obst. & Gynec. **25:** 710, 1933.
22. Campbell, A. M.: The Effect of Excessive Cigarette Smoking on Maternal Health, Am. J. Obst. & Gynec. **31:** 502, 1936.
23. Sontag, L. W., and Wallace, R. F.: The Effect of Cigarette Smoking During Pregnancy on the Fetal Heart Rate, Am. J. Obst. & Gynec. **29:** 77, 1935.

24. Sadler, E. S., Dilling, W. J., and Gemmell, A. A.: Further Investigations Into the Death of the Child Following the Induction of Labor by Means of Quinine, J. Obst. & Gynaec. Brit. Emp. 37: 529, 1930.
25. Torland, T.: Fetal Mortality After Induction of Labor by Castor Oil and Quinine, J. A. M. A. 10: 1190, 1928.
26. King, E. L.: Does Quinine in the Induction of Labor Have a Deleterious Effect on the Fetus? J. A. M. A. 101: 1145, 1935.
27. Taylor, H. M.: Prenatal Medication as a Possible Etiologic Factor in Deafness of the New Born, Arch. Otolaryng. 20: 790, 1934.
28. Taylor, H. M.: Further Observations on Prenatal Medication as a Possible Etiologic Factor of Deafness in the Newborn, South. M. J. 28: 125, 1935.
29. Pearl, R.: The Effect of Parental Alcoholism and Certain Other Drug Intoxications Upon the Progeny, J. Exper. Zool. 22: 573, 1917.
30. Durham, F. M., and Woods, H. M.: Alcohol and Inheritance, M. Research Council, Special Report No. 168, 1932.
31. Blacker, C. P.: The Chances of Morbid Inheritance, Baltimore, 1934, William Wood & Company, p. 152.
32. Schmucker, S. C.: Heredity and Parenthood, New York, 1929, Macmillan Company, p. 118.
33. Bagg, H. J.: Hereditary Abnormalities of the Limbs, Their Origin and Transmission, Am. J. Anat. 43: 167, 1929.
34. Fitchet, S. M.: The Etiology of Congenital Hereditary Deformities, New England J. Med. 213: 164, 1935.
35. Miller, J. R., Corscaden, J. A., and Harrar, J. A.: The Effects of Radiation on the Human Offspring, Am. J. Obst. & Gynec. 31: 519, 1936.
36. Findlay, P.: Pelvic Irradiation in the Child-Bearing Woman, J. A. M. A. 95: 857, 1930.
37. Jansen, M.: Feebleness of Growth and Congenital Dwarfism, 1921, Oxford University Press.
38. Peterson, W. F.: The Distribution of Congenital Malformations in the United States, Am. J. Obst. & Gynec. 28: 70, 1934.
39. Peterson, W. F.: The Seasonal Trend in the Conception of Malformations, Ibid. 28: 445, 1934.
40. Stockard, C. R.: Developmental Rate and Structural Expression, Am. J. Anat. 28: 115, 1921.
41. Murphy, D. P.: The Month of Conception for 935 Malformed Individuals, Am. J. Obst. & Gynec. 31: 106, 1936.
42. Murphy, D. P.: Maternal Age at Conception of the Congenitally Malformed Child, Am. J. Dis. Child. 51: 1107, 1936.
43. Murphy, D. P., and Maser, M.: The Birth Order of Five Hundred and Eighty-Two Malformed Individuals, J. A. M. A. 105: 849, 1935.
44. Graves, G. W.: The Consideration of Genetic and Developmental Factors From the Pediatrist's Viewpoint, Arch. Pediat. 52: 649, 1935.
45. Murphy, D. P.: Congenital Defects, J. A. M. A. 106: 457, 1936.
46. Morgan, T. H.: The Relation of Genetics to Physiology and Medicine, Scientific Monthly 41: 5, 1935.
47. Morgan, T. H.: The Scientific Basis of Evolution, New York, 1932, W. W. Norton & Company, Inc.
48. Pende, N.: Constitutional Inadequacies, English Translation, Philadelphia, 1928, Lea & Febiger.
49. Muller, H. J.: Human Genetics in Russia, J. Hered. 26: 193, 1935.
50. Robb, R. C.: Discrepancies of Etiology in Ten Medical Text Books Now Used at Syracuse University, J. A. Am. M. Coll. 10: 295, 1935.
51. Draper, George: The Human Constitution, Philadelphia, 1924.
52. Hogben, L.: Nature and Nurture, New York, 1935, W. W. Norton & Company, Inc.
53. Mohr, O.: Heredity and Disease, New York, 1934, W. W. Norton & Company, Inc.
54. Fisher, R. A.: The Genetical Theory of Natural Selection, 1930, Oxford Press.
55. Brown, M. J.: Twinning in the Hebard Family, J. Hered. 26: 115, 1935.
56. Popenoe, P.: The Child's Heredity, Baltimore, 1929, Williams & Wilkins Company.
57. Davenport, C. R.: Inheritance of Stature, Genetics 1: 313, 1917.
58. Fantham, H. B., and Porter, A.: Inheritance of Stature Through Selection, J. Hered. 26: 377, 1935.
59. Branders, J. W.: Polydactylism as a Hereditary Character, J. A. M. A. 64: 1640, 1915.

60. Murphy, D. P.: Five Successive Generations of Webbed Finger Deformity, J. A. M. A. 84: 576, 1925.
61. Snyder, L. H.: Recessive Factor of Polydactylism in Man, J. Hered. 20: 73, 1929.
62. McClintic, B. S.: Five Generations of Polydactylism, J. Hered. 26: 141, 1935.
63. Davenport, C. B., and Weeks, D. F.: J. Nerv. & Ment. Dis. 38: 64, 1911.
64. Macklin, M. T.: Inherited Anomalies of Metabolism, J. Hered. 24: 349, 1033; and 25: 123, 1934.
65. Skipper, E.: Diabetes Mellitus and Pregnancy, Quart. J. Med. 2: 353, 1933.
66. Kuttner, A., and Ratner, B.: The Importance of Colostrum to the New Born Infant, Am. J. Dis. Child. 25: 414, 1923.
67. Smith, J. J., et al.: Occurrence of Hypersensitiveness or Allergy in Five Generations of One Family, Arch. Int. Med. 41: 472, 1928.
68. Davenport, C. B.: A Strain Producing Multiple Births, J. Hered. 10: 382, 1919.
69. Brain, W. R.: The Inheritance of Epilepsy, Quart. J. Med. 19: 299, 1926.

The following works have been consulted in the preparation of this review:

Abt, I.: Abt's Pediatrics, Vols. 1 and 2, Philadelphia, 1926, W. B. Saunders Company.
Blacker, C. P.: The Chances of Morbid Inheritance, Baltimore, 1934, William Wood & Company.
Cockayne, E. A.: Inherited Abnormalities of the Skin and Its Appendages, 1933, Oxford University Press.
Fisher, R. A.: The Genetical Theory of Natural Selection, 1930, Oxford University Press.
Hogben, L.: Nature and Nurture, New York, 1933, W. W. Norton & Company, Inc.
Mohr, O. L.: Heredity and Disease, New York, 1934, W. W. Norton & Company, Inc.
Morgan, T. H.: The Scientific Basis of Evolution, New York, 1932, W. W. Norton & Company, Inc.
Morgan, T. H.: The Theory of the Genes, New Haven, 1928, Yale University Press.
Pfaundler, M., and Schlossmann, A.: The Diseases of Children, English Translation, Peterman, Vols. 1 and 2, Philadelphia, 1935, J. B. Lippincott Company.
Popenoe, P.: The Child's Heredity, Baltimore, 1929, Williams & Wilkins Company.

9 EXCHANGE PLACE

American Academy of Pediatrics

Proceedings

SIXTH ANNUAL MEETING OF THE AMERICAN ACADEMY OF PEDIATRICS

KANSAS CITY, MAY 11 AND 12, 1936

Round Table Discussion on Prophylaxis and Treatment of Whooping Cough

Chairman: Dr. E. J. Huenekens, Minneapolis, Minn.

Assistants: Dr. W. L. Bradford, Rochester, N. Y.; Dr. J. M. Frawley, San Francisco, Calif.; and Dr. Louis W. Sauer, Evanston, Ill.

CHAIRMAN HUENEKENS.—This is the third successive year that pertussis has been a subject for round table discussion. The prophylaxis and the treatment of pertussis are decidedly live subjects and also it is difficult to arrive at satisfactory conclusion as to the value of the various measures prepared for its control, for the test of treatment both prophylactically and therapeutically must be judged largely on an empirical basis. Some of the questions we propose to discuss today are: (1) Can we produce active immunity against pertussis? (2) If so, how long does it persist? (3) Which vaccine, Madsen's, Sauer's, or Krueger's, is most effective? (4) What methods, other than vaccines, are available? (5) Are vaccines effective in treatment? Obviously, we cannot give the final answers to these questions today, but we can report progress.

While there can be no doubt that preventing whooping cough is more important than subduing it after it has occurred, nevertheless we must not permit our enthusiasm for prophylaxis to blind us to the need of considering treatment. I think that vaccine administered during the incubation period of the disease, or even during the early catarrhal stage, is of some therapeutic value. Madsen, of Copenhagen, says: "Most of the reports conclude that if given early in the catarrhal stage, the vaccine will have a good effect. This appears from the reports of most of the Danish officers of health, and also is the consensus of the Danish Pediatric Society." It must be conceded that judgment on the therapeutic value of the vaccine does not lead itself to statistical analysis. Statistics are only of value when a catagorical answer of yes or no can be given. When the answer must be given in degrees of improvement, statistics have relatively slight value. But even though the value of therapeutic effectiveness of vaccine is difficult to gauge, it does not follow that we can lightly dismiss it. The discussion in last year's round table conference encouraged the distinction that Sauer's vaccine is especially adopted for prophylaxis, while Krueger's vaccine is more effective for therapy. It would seem that the vaccine which is finally judged to be more effective in prophylaxis should also be better therapeutically and vice versa. A frank discussion of this subject would be a distinct contribution.

Another point which might be profitably considered is the contention that, during the four-month period while the child is developing his active immunity to pertussis, no other immunizations should be administered. One could imagine that a severe case of measles or scarlet fever with high fever and prostration might interfere with production of immunity by pertussis vaccine. But that the slow nonincapacitating immunization by diphtheria toxoid or pertussis vaccine should interfere with each other is rather a strain on our credulity.

These and any similar questions pertaining to the prophylaxis and treatment of pertussis should be discussed frankly here today.

I had asked Dr. Pearl Kendrick, Associate Director and Bacteriologist of the Michigan Department of Health, to assist in this round table discussion, but she is unable to be present. However, she has kindly permitted me to present the latest reports on her work here today.

"Since the latter part of 1932, a study of whooping cough has been in progress in Grand Rapids. The work has been outlined and certain bacteriological findings have been summarized in previous reports. In this paper we are reporting our findings to date in connection with our investigation of the value of *B. pertussis* vaccine in the prevention of whooping cough. Our study has not been carried on for a sufficient time nor do our results embrace sufficient numbers to warrant final conclusions. However, we believe they do contain sufficient of interest to justify a progress report.

"The vaccine used has been described.* Briefly, it is a once-washed 10,000 million per cubic centimeter suspension of *B. pertussis,* Phase 1 of Leslie and Gardner, grown on Bordet-Gengou medium enriched with 15 per cent sheep's blood. The organisms are killed with merthiolate 1:10,000 or phenol 0.5 per cent allowed to act at cold-room temperature for a week or more.

"The optimum dosage by no means has been determined. Sauer used more than three times as large a total dose of vaccine as Madsen—perhaps the most important difference between the procedures of these two authors. The fact that Sauer reports such excellent protection results calls attention to the need for considering the question of total amount of injected antigen. In most of our vaccine-treated individuals we have used a total quantity of vaccine close to that suggested by Sauer."

WHOOPING COUGH PREVENTION STUDY*

TOTAL IN STUDY APRIL 15, 1936—2,285

EXPOSURES AND CASES IN STUDY SERIES TO DATE, APRIL 15, 1936

KIND OF EXPOSURE HISTORY	VACCINE-INJECTED GROUP			CONTROL GROUP			TOTALS		
	EXPOSED	CASES		EXPOSED	CASES		EXPOSED	CASES	
		NUMBER	% OF EXPOSED		NUMBER	% OF EXPOSED		NUMBER	% OF EXPOSED
Definite	60	9	15.0	72	58	80.5	132	67	50.75
Indefinite	55	3	5.5	51	27	52.9	106	30	28.30
None	3	3	----	26	26	----	29	29	----
Totals	118	15	12.7	149	111	74.5	267	126	47.2
Per cent of total cases		11.9			88.1			100.0	

*From the Michigan Department of Health, Bureau of Laboratories, Western Michigan Division, Grand Rapids.

The Use of Immune Blood in Whooping Cough and Its Effect Upon Phagocytosis

W. L. Bradford, M.D.

Although recent evidence does not support a filtrable virus as the sole cause of whooping cough, further investigation to determine the value of immune blood as a prophylaxis for the exposed baby is justified. The reasons for this attitude

*Kendrick, Pearl, and Eldering, Grace: Progress Report in Pertussis Immunization, Am. J. Pub. Health, 26: 8, 1936.

are: (1) The immunizing power of vaccine in the very young infant is not yet known. (2) It is probable that very young infants do not respond favorably to antigenic stimulation. (3) In the exposed infant, the time interval may not permit proper active immunization. (4) There is evidence that immune serum neutralizes the skin-necrotizing substance of *H. pertussis* and to a certain extent protects animals against lethal dosages of virulent organisms.

Since 1931 we have been interested in the administration of immune adult blood and of convalescent serum to babies obliged to remain in family contact with cases of whooping cough.

During the interval from June 1, 1931, to Sept. 1, 1934, forty-four such infants were given this type of prophylaxis. The results, along with a review of the literature, were recently published.[1] In general, it seemed probable that immune blood was effective in the prevention and modification of the disease when given before the catarrhal symptoms appeared.

Since 1934, about twenty-five additional infants have been similarly treated. The results obtained in this second group were similar to those observed previously in the first group studied.

We have extended our investigation to ascertain if immune blood affects the degree of phagocytosis in the infant's blood against *H. pertussis.* The exact methods of study and the results obtained constitute the material for a future report.

In summarizing the work completed to date, the following may be said: (1) The addition of convalescent, or of immune adult serum, to a mixture of newborn's blood and a suspension of *H. pertussis,* markedly increases the susceptibility of the organisms to phagocytosis by the polymorphonuclears leucocytes of the newborn's blood. (2) When infants are given such serum or blood intramuscularly or intravenously, the opsonizing power of the serum is increased in the majority of instances. (3) The opsono-cytophagic power of the blood increases during the course of whooping cough as was shown by Kendrick.[2] (4) It was approximately three times as great in a group of children (twenty-two in number) who had previously had the disease as in a similar group of twenty-two children who had never suffered from whooping cough.

References

1. Bradford, W. L.: Am. J. Dis. Child. 50: 918, 1935.
2. Kendrick, Pearl: Personal communication.

A Note on the Use of Reinforced Convalescent or Hyperimmune Serum for Passive Immunization of Infants Exposed to Pertussis

Dr. Pearl Kendrick

Even though pertussis vaccine should prove to be an effective agent for the active immunization of young children, we still have unsolved the problem of specific immunization in the infant from birth to the age at which we start active immunization. And it is in this very young age group that the death rate due to pertussis is so extremely high. A specific means of protecting the exposed infant is needed.

Various references are to be found concerning the use of convalescent blood for passive immunization against pertussis. The literature on the subject is reviewed by Bradford[1] in connection with a report of his own experience. He believes that immune blood probably is effective in the prevention or modification of whooping cough if given before the catarrhal symptoms appear.

So far as we have been able to discover, there has been but one report of an attempt to use a reinforced convalescent serum, that is a hyperimmune serum. Jundell[2] used the serum from an adult who had received several injections of pertussis vaccine—a maximum total of 7.5 c.c. of a one billion per cubic centimeter suspension. The serum was given in the incubation or early stages of disease. The report included five cases which were considered mild in comparison with the primary cases in the family. While the data in his report are too few and indefinite to be judged by themselves, the underlying idea is worthy of trial.

Having obtained some inconclusive but suggestive results in exposed children following the use of convalescent serum from recently recovered donors, we decided to test hyperimmune serum as a possible means of preventing pertussis in exposed infants under one year—giving particular attention to the newborn baby in an infected family. An adult with a history of whooping cough in childhood was given a series of injections of a 10 billion per cubic centimeter suspension of *B. pertussis* vaccine, such as we are using in our immunization study.[3] The total quantity of vaccine has varied from 7.0 c.c. to as much as 20.0 c.c. over a period of time. The blood was collected about ten days after the last of a series of injections, and the processing of the serum included a final Mandler filtration. Each serum has shown agglutinins for *B. pertussis* and a very strong opsonic reaction. The dosage for the exposed infant has in general been 20 c.c.—10 c.c. as soon as possible after exposure was recognized and a second dose of 10 c.c. about ten days after the first, to cover the period of continued exposure.

To date we have completed histories for 22 infants under one year, 8 of them under one month. The exposure histories were definite in all, being familial in all but 3. Of these 22 infants, 17 were injected with serum, and 5 control babies received none. Of the 17 serum-injected infants, 11 were given the first dose of serum before symptoms of pertussis were recognizable, and 6 after symptoms had been present from one to eleven days. In the group of 11 serum-injected infants, pertussis did not develop in 9 of them, there was a light attack in one and a light to moderate attack in the other. The primary cases to which these 11 infants were exposed numbered 22, of which 8 were severe, 7 moderate, 6 light, and 1 very light. In the group of 6 infants injected with serum after symptoms were present, there were 1 light, 1 severe, and 4 moderate attacks of pertussis. Of the 7 primary cases to which these 6 had been exposed, 2 were severe and 5 were moderate.

It should be pointed out that the primary cases in the families with the serum-treated infants do not constitute true controls—they are in an older age group, and furthermore the real point to be controlled is the probable incidence of pertussis in the untreated, exposed infants. A pertinent question here is just what part the mother's immunity to pertussis plays in the protection of the newborn infant. The incidence of the disease in young infants as well as some unpublished results we have on opsonins in mothers and their infants would cast some doubt on the importance of the mother's immunity as a factor in the protection of the baby who has had an intimate exposure to pertussis. This point needs further study.

As true controls, we have to date only 5 infants who are in the same age group as the serum-injected children and have come to our attention during the study period. Two were newborn, 2 were eight weeks, and one was 6 months old. All were in families with one or more children in the early stages of whooping cough. Three of these control infants had severe attacks; two of them being critically ill. The fourth had a moderate attack, and the fifth escaped infection. In the last instance the mother made an effort to isolate the baby, and it is doubtful if the baby had an adequate exposure. The 8 primary cases to which the controls were exposed included 5 moderate and 1 severe, and 1 light, and 1 very light cases.

To summarize, we are beginning a study of the value of reinforced convalescent or hyperimmune serum for the prevention of pertussis in the exposed infant. We have in our series to date 22 under one year of age with definite history of exposure—17 who received serum and 5 control babies who did not. While the series obviously is too small to afford a basis for conclusion, it is encouraging to note that in the group of 11 exposed infants who received serum before the onset of symptoms, only 2 developed pertussis. We believe that the possibility of such a serum having a place in the prevention of pertussis in the exposed infant merits the attention of interested workers who have the facilities for testing the procedure.

References

1. Bradford, William L.: Use of Convalescent Blood in Whooping Cough, Am. J. Dis. Child. **50**: 918, 1935.
2. Jundell, I.: Has Specific Serum of Adults Any Value as a Remedy Against Whooping Cough? Acta Paediat. **15**: 1, 1934.
3. Kendrick, P., and Eldering G.: Progress Report on Pertussis Immunization, Am. J. Pub. Health **26**: 8, 1936.

Immunization With B. Pertussis Vaccine

(Progress Report)

L. W. Sauer, M.D.

Between 1928 and 1932, about 100 c.c. of vaccine were prepared at intervals of about two months, from five to seven hemolytic strains which had been isolated during the preceding weeks. The vaccine was refrigerated until used. About 200 fresh strains were used to make thirty-six lots of vaccine (1 c.c. = 10,000 million bacilli). In all, 394 selected, young nonimmune private patients were injected with a total of 7 to 8 c.c.[1] To date, 172 of them have been reported exposed, a total of 378 times. None is known to have contracted pertussis.

Since 1932, two laboratories have been authorized to prepare vaccine according to detailed specifications. For commercial reasons, several deviations from the original technic were necessary. The medium contains only 10 per cent human blood; the vaccine is not refrigerated while in transit; and the expiration date is one year. During the first two years, various Phase I strains were used for periods exceeding two months. The results are given in Table I.

TABLE I

IMMUNIZATION WITH AUTHORIZED COMMERCIAL VACCINE

		INJECTED*	EXPOSED		FAILED
Evanston health department (1933-)		865	68	16 familial, 52 outside	4
Private patients (1932-)		627	77	35 familial, 42 outside	6
Three orphanages (1932-)		252	57		6
"Cradle" infants (under 2 mo.)					
(1932-33)	6 c.c.	400	15	8 familial, 7 outside	6
(1934-)	8 c.c.	330	2		0
		2,474	219		22

*Children over three years of age now receive a total of 10 c.c. (1, 2, and 2 c.c. bilaterally).

If the 6 Cradle infants who contracted pertussis are excluded, only 16 of the 219 subsequently exposed children contracted the disease. It was light in 9, typical in 6, and severe in 1 child. Five of the children were more than three years of age when injected; 8 of the cases occurred in four households. An older infant, who contracted pertussis a year after injection, had received vaccine from the same lot as two older boys who developed the disease eighteen months after injection.

Seventy-four physicians in 24 states have reported their results; thirty-eight had written because they had one or more failures. A summary is given in Table II. It

TABLE II

RESULTS OF 74 PHYSICIANS IN 24 STATES

PHYSICIANS	INJECTED	EXPOSED	FAILED	
13	1,147	---*	0	
23	3,177	282	0	
15	2,068	133	15	(1 failure each)
12	1,089	67	24	(2 failures each)
3	656	45	9	(3 failures each)
4	471	29	16	(4 failures each)
2	229	11	10	(5 failures each)
1	309	72	8	
1	145	21	14	
74	9,291	660	96	

*No known exposures.

includes every reported failure. More than half occurred in children over three years of age when injected. The disease was light in many instances. Twelve physicians reported two, one reported three, and one reported four failures in a household. A physician in a city in the South reported 14 failures among 145 injected children; another physician in the same city used the same vaccine in 309 nonimmune children with 72 exposures and 8 failures. Several physicians wrote that their own children had been willfully, intimately, and repeatedly exposed more than four months after injection, without a failure.

Discussion.—Young children are very susceptible to pertussis. Because it is so prevalent, and often goes unrecognized throughout the most contagious stage, exposure is more frequent, intimate and repeated than smallpox, diphtheria, or scarlet fever. The immunizing power of an antigen depends upon its essential immunizing substance content at the time it is injected. Whether stock strains, kept under optimum conditions in the laboratory and grown on sheep's blood, will yield an antigen as potent as that made from five to seven recently isolated, hemolytic strains* will probably be decided within the next few years. The influence of intensive cultivation on the antigenicity of strains will receive further study. Little is known of such factors as heat, interrupted refrigeration,† and preservatives, on the stability of the immunizing fraction. Standardization of vaccine is not possible without a qualitative or quantitative test for this fraction. With no recognized test for immunity, occasional failures are quite inevitable. Agglutination and complement fixation tests have been proposed as guides in the selection of strains, also as an index of immunity conferred by vaccine. These tests are usually positive soon after the disease, also after the injection of vaccine into nonimmunes. In the latter, they are often positive before active immunity has been established. They become negative within a year or two after the disease or vaccine injection, i.e., when the humoral antibodies disappear. Immunity is more prolonged. Antigenicity is not identical with such antibacterial antibody response. Paterson, Bailey, and Waller[2] found that the intracutaneous injection of 0.1 c.c. of vaccine produces a positive skin test after the disease. A negative skin test in an immune individual becomes positive after the injection of 8 c.c. of vaccine. Whether this is an index of immunity has not yet been determined. If intimate exposures of children with negative tests prove them nonimmune, and similar exposures of children with positive tests prove them immune, the test will probably also be valuable as a biological test for the standardization of antigen. Intimate exposure to early pertussis remains the ultimate test of immunity. For the best results, vigilance is necessary in the selection of strains and in the preparation, preservation, and administration of the vaccine.

*In nearly four years, 141 freshly isolated strains have been sent to the one laboratory; in nearly three years, 117 fresh strains have been sent to the other.

†A chilled thermos food jar (½ pint) will keep cold vaccine cold for 24 hours.

References

1. Sauer, L.: Whooping Cough: A Study in Immunization, J. A. M. A. **100:** 239, 1933.
Immunization With Bacillus Pertussis Vaccine, Ibid. **101:** 1449, 1933.
2. Paterson, D., Bailey, R., Waller, R.: Control of Whooping Cough With Serum and Vaccine, Lancet **229:** 361, 1935.

Report on Krueger's Pertussis U.B.A. (Commercial)

J. M. Frawley, M.D.

Krueger's pertussis undenatured bacterial antigen has been used as a prophylactic agent before exposure, in prophylaxis after exposure, and therapeutically after coughing has begun.

1. As a prophylactic agent pertussis U.B.A. was given to two groups totalling 618 children. Five hundred and five children received 8.0 c.c., 113 received 12.0 c.c. Children in three groups who were subsequently exposed contracted whooping cough in a high percentage of cases, as shown in Table I.

Table I

Summary of Prophylactic Vaccination With Krueger's Pertussis U.B.A. (Commercial)

Dosage	No. of Children Vaccinated	Exposures		Developed Whooping Cough		Percentage of Failures
8 c.c.	505	Home	30	Mild	33	44.0
		School	68	Moderate	6	
			—	Severe	4	
		Total	98		—	
				Total	43	
12 c.c.	113	Home	9	Mild	6	47.6
		School	12	Moderate	1	
			—	Severe	3	
		Total	21		—	
				Total	10	

2. The published reports[1, 2, 3] on the use of pertussis U.B.A. as a prophylactic agent after exposure have been summarized by J. J. Miller.[4] The vaccine was used during the incubation period, in 98 cases; 50 per cent developed a cough. The cough in these cases was mild or atypical. It seems that the greatest benefit from pertussis U.B.A. is to be obtained when it is used in this manner.

3. The use of pertussis U.B.A. in treatment.

In a recent questionnaire replies were received from 162 pediatricians who had used pertussis U.B.A. in the treatment of over 3,700 cases of whooping cough. One hundred four (63 per cent) reported favorably.

However, in these cases no controls were used, and pertussis is a disease of such great variability that it is difficult to attribute good results to any particular agent unless there are adequate controls. Moreover, in many cases other agents besides pertussis U.B.A. were employed, e.g., sedatives, alternating doses of other vaccines, etc.

On the other hand, there is a definite feeling that in its present strength large doses should be employed (5 c.c. daily to children over one year of age, 2 c.c. to 5 c.c. to children less than one year) also that the best results are obtained when injections are begun either during the incubation period or the first day or two of coughing or else in the late stages after the disease has passed its peak. There is no certainty about the influence which may be expected when injections are begun during the height of the infection.

References

1. Frawley, J. M., Stallings, M., and Nichols, V. C.: J. PEDIAT. 4: 179, 1934.
2. Munns, G. F., and Aldrich, C. A.: J. PEDIAT. 5: 590, 1934.
3. Stallings, M., and Nichols, V. C.: Am. J. Dis. Child. 48: 1183, 1934.
4. Miller, J. J.: Report on Pertussis Undenatured Bacterial Antigen (Krueger) Given Before the Laboratory Section of the Am. Pub. Health Assn., Milwaukee, October, 1935.

GENERAL DISCUSSION

DR. TOM MITCHELL (MEMPHIS, TENN.) questioned Dr. Sauer as to his method of sterilization of syringes and needles.

DR. SAUER favors and uses only the method of dry sterilization in oven rather than boiling. He stores his sterile needles in gauze-packed test tubes.

DR. A. G. HELMICK (COLUMBUS, OHIO) asked Dr. Sauer whether artificial immunization for pertussis may not be greater than that of natural immunization.

DR. SAUER did not know.

DR. F. B. MINER (FLINT, MICH.).—Why distribute dosage in both arms?

DR. SAUER.—The dosage is distributed in both arms because the reactions appear milder. The first dosage of 2 c.c. can safely be given in one arm. Give the injections subcutaneously near the skin and not intramuscularly. It is desirable to feel a nodule from one to two weeks after injection.

DR. F. R. JANNEY (WAUWATOSA, WIS.) stated he has immunized more than 300 infants with Sauer's vaccine by injecting all of each dose in one arm instead of using both arms. He has seen no untoward effects.

DR. C. O. TERRELL (FORT WORTH, TEXAS) questioned Dr. Sauer as to why it is necessary to refrigerate his commercial vaccine.

DR. BRADFORD.—I have been greatly interested in the plea of Dr. Sauer for extreme precaution in the proper refrigeration of the vaccine, and, of course, subscribe to this idea, but I should naturally wonder why a commercial whooping cough vaccine should require greater precautions as regards refrigeration than does, let us say, a commercial typhoid vaccine.

DR. SAUER advises that the vaccine be kept in the refrigerator at all times. Failures of immunization have been noted in cases in which the vaccine used has been kept on the shelf in the home or in the physician's bag. When the physician does the immunization in the home, it is advisable to transport the vaccine in a half-pint vacuum food container.

CHAIRMAN HUENEKENS.—Where can this portable container be obtained?

DR. SAUER.—Either through your druggist or at a hardware store.

DR. TERRELL.—Is there any scientific reason why diphtheria toxin and pertussis vaccine cannot be given two or three weeks apart?

DR. SAUER.—As far as is known there is no contraindication for following diphtheria toxoid with the pertussis vaccine and vice versa. We allow four-month intervals between the pertussis inoculations, diphtheria toxoid, and smallpox vaccination. This is done so we can be sure one does not interfere with the other for statistical purposes. The pertussis vaccine should be given first usually around the sixth month. It is not necessary to hurry all these immunizations.

DR. GILBERT J. LEVY (MEMPHIS, TENN.) gives the vaccine between the fourth and eighth months.

DR. MURPHY immunizes with Sauer's vaccine not later than the fourth month.

DR. F. C. NEFF (KANSAS CITY, MO.) asked a question relative to the occurrence of second attacks of whooping cough.

DR. TERRELL stated he had had several cases in which mothers and nurses who had previously had whooping cough developed mild coughs while taking care of a child with whooping cough.

DR. BRADFORD.—In support of Dr. Neff's contention that second attacks of whooping cough may easily be missed, I should like to refer to a case recently observed in the private practice of Dr. Daniel Landau, in Rochester, in which the cough was very mild, lasting less than ten days; yet a typical Phase I organism was isolated by the cough-plate method. The attack was supposedly primary and occurred in a young boy exposed to known cases of whooping cough in his schoolroom. A more accurate method of determining immunity such as a dermal reaction would be of great assistance in such cases.

In connection with the remarks of Dr. Terrell concerning the incidence of whooping cough among mothers, the studies reported by Christensen are of interest in that he found that about 3 per cent of case contacts showed the presence of the bacillus on culture.

DR. SAUER stated that in his experience grandmothers were most frequently affected, mothers less often, and fathers rarely. He knows of only one case of recurrent whooping cough in childhood.

DR. TERRELL.—What are the best therapeutic measures? Results with vaccine as a therapeutic measure?

DR. SAUER.—The following three procedures are better than vaccines: (1) 25 per cent ether in olive oil inserted into the rectum with a catheter. One tablespoonful of this mixture two or three times daily is usually sufficient; (2) rest in bed one to two weeks; (3) avoidance of infections.

I cannot express an opinion relative to the value of vaccine given early. Some physicians give dosage at four-day intervals during the incubation and catarrhal stages. I do not believe any harm can be done with the vaccine; some individuals develop immune bodies in varying lengths of time from one to four months.

DR. TERRELL.—In twenty cases in which a vaccine was given at the beginning of exposure, all resulting cases were very mild.

DR. BRADFORD.—The favorable results obtained by Dr. Terrell from vaccine administered to the exposed child may in part be explained by the work of Kendrick who showed that an increase in the phagocytic power of the blood occurred as early as ten days after injection of vaccine.

CHAIRMAN HUENEKENS.—Vaccine gives partial immunity before the fourth month following inoculation so we should keep an open mind relative to the use of vaccine as a therapeutic agent. It should be used only during the incubation and catarrhal stages. I agree with measures outlined by Dr. Sauer.

DR. H. D. PYLE (SOUTH BEND, IND.).—What is the definite way of gauging dose of ether?

DR. SAUER.—It is best to give one tablespoonful of 25 per cent ether in olive oil regardless of age except in the older child, in whom a double dose can be used.

DR. TERRELL asked a question relative to therapeutic results of Krueger's endoantigen.

DR. PYLE, DR. THOMAS, AND DR. STRINGFIELD all reported definite benefit in over 50 per cent of their cases. Dosage of 2 c.c. was given at two-day intervals in from five to eight inoculations.

DR. O. L. STRINGFIELD, Recorder.
Stamford, Conn.

REPORT OF THE COMMITTEE ON HOSPITALS AND DISPENSARIES

Contagious Disease Hospitals

Part I

Chairman, Dr. Clifford G. Grulee; Secretary, Dr. George F. Munns; Dr. Murray H. Bass, Dr. Laurence R. DeBuys, Dr. Henry Dietrich, and Dr. Lewis Webb Hill.

THE first report in the following series will concern contagious disease hospitals found in Region III of the Academy of Pediatrics. Questionnaires were sent to thirty-eight institutions in this region which were listed as contagious disease hospitals. Thirty-five were returned, but among this number were several reports which indicated that the institutions would hardly be described by the name of contagious disease hospital. Perhaps ''pesthouse'' would be more suitable. The replies of some other hospitals were so incomplete that they were of no use to us in compiling this report. In other sections certain portions of the questionnaires were not filled out, hence as each section is discussed we shall indicate the number of hospitals which replied to that section.

Region III

Hospitals

Table I

KEY NO.	NAME
1	City Isolation Hospital, Colorado Springs, Colo.
2	Steel Memorial Hospital, Denver, Colo.
3	Municipal Contagious Disease Hospital, Chicago, Ill.
4	Evanston Hospital, Evanston, Ill.
5	City Contagious Hospital, LaSalle and Peru, Ill.
6	Fort Wayne and Allen County Isolation Hospital, Fort Wayne, Ind.
7	St. Anthony's Hospital, Contagious Section, Carroll, Iowa
8	City Isolation Hospital, Council Bluffs, Iowa
9	City Isolation Hospital, Grinnell, Iowa
10	City Isolation Hospital, Sioux City, Iowa
11	Herman Kiefer Hospital, Contagious Disease Division, Detroit, Mich.
12	Municipal Isolation Hospital, Grand Rapids, Mich.
13	Jackson County Contagious Hospital, Jackson, Mich.
14	Lansing City Hospital, Lansing, Mich.
15	Oakland County Contagious Hospital, Pontiac, Mich.
16	Port Huron Emergency Hospital, Port Huron, Mich.
17	Saginaw County Contagious Hospital, Saginaw, Mich.
18	Minneapolis General Hospital, Contagious Dept., Minneapolis, Minn.
19	Ancker Hospital, Contagious Department, St. Paul, Minn.
20	City Isolation Hospital, St. Louis, Mo.
21	Isolation Hospital, Lincoln, Neb.
22	Municipal Hospital for Contagious Diseases, Omaha, Neb.
23	Cincinnati General Hospital, Cincinnati, Ohio
24	Cleveland City Hospital, Contagious Hospital, Cleveland, Ohio
25	Quarantine Hospital, Dayton, Ohio
26	Municipal Hospital for Contagious Diseases, Toledo, Ohio
27	City Detention Hospital, Aberdeen, S. D.
28	City Detention Hospital, Sioux Falls, S. D.
29	Beloit Detention Hospital, Beloit, Wis.
30	City Isolation Hospital, Green Bay, Wis.
31	Detention Hospital, Janesville, Wis.
32	Isolation Hospital, Madison, Wis.
33	South View Hospital, Milwaukee, Wis.
34	Lincoln Memorial Hospital, Racine, Wis.
35	Isolation Hospital, Superior, Wis.

In general the form of the questionnaire is the same as that used by the committee in previously published reports concerning general and children's hospitals.

1. *Staff: Professional Staff—Attending Staff.*—Among 25 hospitals 11 report that ward patients are under the exclusive care of the attending staff. Nineteen report that all physicians in the community are permitted to send patients to the wards and treat them there. This disagreement in figures is probably accounted for by the custom of allowing only members of the staff to care for so-called service (free or semifree) cases which usually go to the wards, but a few private cases may also go to the wards, and their own physicians are allowed to care for them there. Only 12 replies were received concerning qualifications permitting nonstaff physicians to attend patients in the hospital. All of them require the attending man to be a licensed physician in good standing.

Information concerning attending physicians in the various specialties is best presented by Table II.

Among 20 hospitals which replied, the attending staff is full-time in 6, but among several of these (4) the claim was based on the fact that a resident physician or health officer was in charge. The attending staff was stated to be salaried in 11 instances, but in at least 7 instances this seemed to apply to only one man, and he in turn often was the city health commissioner.

TABLE II

	NUMBER OF REPLIES	HAVE SPECIALISTS ON ATTENDING STAFF	HOW MANY?	VISIT AT REGULAR INTERVALS IN?	ON CALL ONLY IN?
Pediatrics	16	13	2-8	5	8
Otolaryngology	18	16	1-5	5	10
Orthopedics	16	12	2-8	2	12
Ophthalmology	16	14	2-3	2	12
Oral surgery	14	9	1-2	2	11
Oral hygiene	14	8	1-2	2	10
Roentgenology	15	10	1-5	3	10
Pathology	15	12	1-4	3	10
Allergy	15	9	1	1	10
Surgery	17	15	2-15	2	13
Neurology	16	12	2-7	2	13
Psychiatry	16	12	2-5	1	11
Dermatology	15	12	1-5	3	13
Dentistry	14	10	1-4	4	10
Psychology	16	10	2-3	1	10

House Staff.—Twenty-five hospitals replied to this section of the questionnaire. Nine employ residents; 15 have no resident; 1 did not reply. In 6 institutions women are eligible for this position. Salaries are paid in 8 instances. These salaries vary from $30 per month to $900 per year. Four hospitals require a preliminary general interneship of one year. One hospital requires a previous experience of one year of general interneship and one year of work as assistant resident in contagious work. One requires two years of hospital experience including at least one year in pediatrics. In 2 instances the position is included as part of a general interneship, and 1 hospital employs a senior medical student in that capacity. The usual term of the service is one year except in 2 instances in which contagious service is part of a general interneship. The period is for six weeks in one and six months in the other. The resident has dispensary duties in only 4 instances.

Only 4 hospitals employ assistant residents. Women are eligible for this service in 2 hospitals. All pay the assistant resident a salary. All require previous experience consisting of one year of general interneship. The service is for one year in 2 hospitals, six months in 1, and ten weeks in another. Assistant residents have dispensary duties in 3 hospitals. Thirteen hospitals employ internes; 12 do not, the number varying from 1 to twelve. Six employ more than 2, one as many as 32, the next highest in order being 12, 8, and 6. Only 10 hospitals replied concerning eligibility of women for interneship. Women are eligible in 8 of these. Salaries are paid to internes in only 1 instance. Ten replied concerning qualifications for interneship. All require a degree from a Class A medical school. None require previous hospital experience. The length of the service varies from eight weeks to one year. One offers ten-day periods of service during the busy months.

Educational Activities.—These are presented in Table III.

Twenty-five hospitals replied to this section of the questionnaire. Among these only 7 are connected with medical schools. Clinics are given to medical students in 8, while ward rounds are offered for medical students by 10.

Special Information is presented in Table IV with summary.

Newly admitted patients are retained in observation wards in 10 hospitals. Two of these report that a cubicle system is used. Ten do not retain patients in an observation ward. Six did not reply. Nine report that patients are usually retained in an observation ward until the diagnosis is made or "as long as necessary." There were only 4 replies to the question concerning procedure before admission. Among 19 hospitals all but 1 take routine throat cultures for *B. diphtheria;* 1 takes cultures "as indicated." Thirteen culture routinely for *Streptococcus hemolyticus;* three, "when indicated." Routine vaginal smears are done in 14 "when indicated"; von Pirquet tests, in three; Wassermann or Kahn tests, in two; Schick and Dick tests, in seven and six, respectively. Routine blood counts are taken in 10. Urinalyses in 19, and routine history and physical examinations are done in 18 and 16, respectively.

Superintendent.—Nineteen hospitals replied to this section of the questionnaire which concerns the physical set-up of the hospitals. Seventeen of these hospitals are located in residential districts and 16 of these in better or middle-class districts. Only 1 is found in a tenement district. Five are located in factory districts and 3 in shop districts. All but 2 are not in noisy districts. These 2 report that there is noise from both factories and heavy traffic. Two are located on unpaved streets; the remainder report that the pavements near them are smooth.

Tables V and VI give the more interesting details concerning the physical organization, size, etc., of these hospitals.

Quickly summarizing these tables we find that some of these hospitals are quite large and many are small. Only 3 have 10 or more buildings while 15 have one or two. Some are old, dating from 1883, many are fairly modern. Only 3 were constructed prior to 1900. Most of these buildings are not large, 15 hospitals reporting that they have one or two floors. Among 24 hospitals only 13 are reported to be fireproof. Six report that they have fire stairs and 12 that they have outside fire escapes; 11 and 7 hospitals, respectively, do not reply to the latter 2 questions. "Cost of buildings" needs no comment except that wide variations here probably indicate size and modernity of the plants. Bed capacities among 22 hospitals which replied vary from 16 to 1,000. Eleven, or one-half, possess bed capacities of 50 or less, 8 have 100 or more. The 3 largest report 1,000, 681, and 500 bed capacities. The 3 smallest, 4, 10, and 10. Eleven report the number of cribs available. These vary from a number as low as 3 to as high as 228, the 3 highest being 228, 150, and 68, and the lowest 3, 4, and 6.

Of 15 hospitals which replied, 14 have wards. Six indicate that they have cubicles containing 1, 2, 3, or 4 beds. Seventeen exclude no type of contagious disease. Two exclude smallpox; one, erysipelas; one, measles, chickenpox, and pertussis; and one, tuberculosis, typhoid fever, and venereal disease.

Table III

Educational Activities

	Hospital connected with med. school	Clinics given med. students	Ward rounds or walks given for med. stud.	Clinics open to pract. phys.	No. and character	Ward rounds or walks open to pract. phys.	No. and character	Definite courses of postgrad. instruction	Limited number	Enrollment last year	This year	Length of course	Hours	Clinical conference for internes	How often	Path. conf. held for internes	How often	Medical library	No. volumes	Research facilities available to res. and house staff	Describe briefly	Research projects in communicable disease encouraged
1	no	no	no					no						yes	1 per mo.	yes	once a mo.	yes	38	clin.		yes—cases reported to med. journals
2	yes	yes	yes	no		no		no						yes	2 per wk.	yes	irregularly	yes	0	Av. lab. fac. for any res. (but not the best)		
3	no	no	yes	no		no		no						yes	no reg. time	yes	monthly	yes	100	ltd.		yes
4	yes	yes	yes	staff only				no						yes	weekly	yes	weekly	yes	3,100	ltd.		yes
7	no	no		no				no											0	no		no
8	no			no		no		no											0			
9	no	no	no	no		no		no											0			
10	no	no	no	no		no		no											0			
11	yes	yes	yes	yes	1 per wk. in early part of yr.	yes	as many as requested	yes	to all phys.	250	250	5 wk.	2 hr. per wk.	yes	biweekly	yes	weekly	yes		yes	private lab.	yes

Blank spaces in chart indicate that there was no reply.

TABLE III—CONT'D

12	no	no	no	no		yes		no														yes
14	no	no	no	no		no		no														no
15	no	no	no	no		no		no														
16	no	no	no	no		no		no														
17	no	no	no	no		no		no														
18	yes	yes	yes	occasionally		no		no						no		yes	weekly	yes	30	clin.		yes
19	yes	yes	yes	no		yes		no						yes	daily	yes	weekly	yes	journals only	clin.		not discouraged
20	no	yes	yes	yes	1 series of 5 clin.	yes	daily informal	no						yes	weekly	no		yes	10	yes	clin.	yes
21	no	no	no	no		no		no														
22	no	no	no	no		no		no						yes	as required	yes	as required	no	none	no		yes
23	yes	yes	yes	yes		yes		no						yes	weekly	yes	weekly	yes	40,000	yes	assigned def. prob.	yes
24	yes	yes	both	no		yes	twice w'kly	no						yes	weekly	yes	weekly	yes	4,000	yes	clin.	yes
31	no	no	no	no		no		no											none			no
32	no	no	no	no		no		no														no
33	no	no	yes	no		occasionally		no						yes	daily	yes	daily	yes	12			yes
35	no	no	no	no		no		no														no

TABLE IV

SPECIAL INFORMATION

	ARE CASES RETAINED IN OBSERV. WARD	HOW LONG MAY THEY BE KEPT	PROCEDURE BEFORE ADMISSION	THROAT CULTURE FOR B. DIPH.	THROAT CULTURE FOR HEM. STREP.	VAG. SMEARS FOR GONOCOCCI	VON PIRQUET OR MANTOUX	WASSERMANN OR KAHN	SCHICK TEST	DICK TEST	ROUTINE BLOOD COUNTS	URINALYSIS	HISTORY TAKEN	COMPLETE PHYS. MADE
1	Depends on case	As long as phys. desires	Diag. made by phys.	Yes	Yes	Yes	Yes by int.	Yes	Yes	Yes	At phys. request	Routine	Complete hist. kept	Yes
2	N.R.*	Indefinite	Phys. exam. & culture	Yes	Yes	Not unless indicated	No	Wass. only	No	No	Yes	Yes	Yes	Yes
3	None	Cubicle system used		Yes	Not always	Yes	No	Yes for adult scarlets	No	No	Yes	Yes	Yes	Yes
4	Until report from T.C. and vag. smear			Yes		Yes	No	No	No	No	Yes	Yes	Yes	Yes
7	N.R.			Yes	No	Yes	Occasionally	If indicated	Yes	Yes	Yes	Yes	Yes	Yes
8	None							No				Yes	Yes	Yes
9	None													
10	None													
11	Cubicle system	Until diag. is confirmed		Yes	Yes	Yes	When indicated	Yes	When indicated	When indicated	Yes	When indicated	Yes	Yes Vac. for smallpox

*N.R., no report.

TABLE IV—CONT'D

12	N.R.												
14	As long as nec.			Yes	Yes	Yes	No	No	No	No	No	Yes	No	No
15	Yes	3 days to 2 wk.		Yes	Yes	Yes	Yes	No	Yes	Yes	Yes	Yes	Yes	Yes
16	None			Yes	Yes	Yes	No	No	No	No	No	Yes	Yes	Phys. takes care
17	Until positive diag. is made	Not longer than neces-sary	Bath, sham-poo, physical	Yes	Yes	Yes	On sus-pected cases	When ordered	When ordered	When or-dered	When or-dered	Yes	Yes	Yes
18	N.R.	As long as nec.		Yes	Yes	Yes	No	No	Yes	No	Yes	Yes	Yes	Yes
19	N.R.			Yes	Yes	Yes	No	No	No	No	Yes	Yes	Yes	Yes
20	1 day	As long as nec.		Yes	No	No	If indi-cated	Yes	Yes	No	Yes	Yes	Yes	Yes
21	None													
22	N.R.			Yes	Yes	Yes	No	Yes	No	No	No	Yes	Yes	Yes
23	Cubicle			Yes	No	Yes	No	No	No	No	Yes	Yes	Yes	Yes
24	7-14 days	B. of H. release		Yes	Only if indi-cated	If in-dicated	Only in meas. B. & whoop. cough	If in-dicated	No	Yes	Where in-dicated	Yes	Yes	Yes
31	None			Yes	Yes	No	No	No	Yes	Yes	No	Yes	Yes	No
32	Long as nec.		3 cul-tures, nose and throat	Yes	Yes	No	No	No	No	No	No	Yes	Yes	Up to phys.
33	None			When indicated										
35	None			Yes	Yes	Yes	Avail-able	Yes	Yes	Yes	No	Yes	By phys.	Phys.

TABLE V

SUPERINTENDENT

	NO. OF BLDGS. IN PLANT	DATE OF CONSTRUCTION	DATE OF ADDITION	NUMBER OF FLOORS	FIREPROOF	FIRE STAIRS IN WALLS	OUTSIDE FIRE ESCAPE	COST OF BUILDINGS	BED CAPACITY	TOTAL NO. OF BEDS	CRIBS	BEDS	WARDS	CUBICLES	NO. BEDS IN EACH CUBICLE	EXCLUDE TYPE OF CONT. DIS.	TYPE
1	2	1918	None	3	Yes	Yes			16	16	3		4	None		Yes	Smallpox
2	5	1908	None	2	Partially		1		85	85	8	25	12	2			
3	7	1916 1919 1930		3 & 5	Yes	1	Yes	$2,082,000			228	200	34	4	2	Yes	Measles, erysipelas, smallpox, whooping cough, chickenpox
4	11	1898 1930		3 & 5	Yes		Yes			50	25	25		Yes	1		
7	1	1915	None	1	Semi					4	2	4	None			No	
8	1			2	No					10			2	None		No	
9	2	1919	None	4 & 2	Yes		Yes	90,000		15						No	
10	1			2	No	No	No		25	25							
11	11	1910 1911 1912 1913 1918 1922 1925 1928		2 3 4 7	Yes	Yes	Yes	8,000,000	500				7	Yes	1-4	No	

TABLE V—CONT'D

12	2	1910		1	No				50				4			No	
14	1	1921	1925	1	Semi	No	No	25,000	60	10	50					Yes	
15	2	1926		2	Yes	Yes	Yes	150,000		80	20	16	4			No	
16	1	1922		2	No	No	Yes	20,000		24	6	18				No	
17	1	1930		3	Yes		No	174,000	99				14	None		No	
18	6	1916		8	Yes		Yes	1,800,000	681				6	4	1	No	
19	12	1883 1927	1927	2-5	Yes	Semi	Yes		1,000	1,000						No	
20	4	1915 1926		2	Yes	No	No		250		150	100	8			No	
21										24						No	
22	1			3	No	Yes	Yes			40			3			Yes	
23	5	1915		2	Yes				150	150			7	5	3	No	
24	2	1910 1922		7	Yes	Yes		600,000	196	150			7	4	1	No	
31	1				No	No	No									No	
32	1	1923		3	Yes	Yes	Yes	150,000		54	4	50				No	
33	3	1911 1915 1919		2	Semi		Yes	586,310		250	68	25	18			Yes	Tuberculosis, typhoid fever, venereal disease
35	2	1896 1921		2 & 1	No	No	Yes	19,184		17		17				No	

Only 15 hospitals reply to the section concerning observation wards. Thirteen have them, that is, either wards, rooms, or cubicles. Two have none of these.

Contagious Diseases Wards.—Among 17 hospitals replying, 16 have wards (one or more) with a total bed capacity of 1,303 (Table VI). The number of beds in wards vary from 1 to 21. Five have cubicles, and 12 have private rooms with a total bed capacity of 317. Nineteen have sunlight, and 10 have outdoor porches. Children and adults are placed in the same wards in 10 hospitals. In several instances these cubicle systems are used on the wards.

TABLE VI

SUPERINTENDENT

CONTAGIOUS DISEASE WARDS

	NUMBER WARDS	NUMBER BEDS	NUMBER BEDS IN WARDS	CUBICLES	SEPARATE ROOMS	SUNLIGHT	OUTDOOR PORCHES	ADULTS AND CHILDREN IN SAME WARD
1	2	12	2 W. 4 Porches	None	2 semi-private	East & west	1	No
2	4	65	Varies			Yes	Yes	Yes
3						Yes	No	Yes
4		20		Yes		Yes	Yes	No
7	None							
8								
9	7	15	2-3			Yes	No	No
10								
11	7	500	15	115	115	Yes	Yes	No
12								
14	5	50	2-16		3	Yes	No	Yes
15	8	80	10		8	Yes	No	Yes
16		24	2		9	Yes	1	No
17	7	56		None	10		No	Occasionally
18	2	46	4-5	4, 4-5	20	Yes	Yes	Occasionally
19					20	Yes	Yes	No
20	8	20-40			48	Yes	8	Yes
21								
22	3	40	1-8		16	Yes	No	Yes
23	7	150	21	11-15		Yes	Yes	Yes
24	7	196	3-4	164	64	Yes	Yes	No
31	1	3			4	Yes	No	No
32	2	16	4			Yes	No	No
33						Yes	No	Yes
35						Yes	No	No

Admissions.—Admission figures for hospitals listed by number for the years 1932, 1933, and 1934 are presented in Table VII.

Admission figures clearly indicate that comparatively few of these institutions are large; only 6 report admission of 5,000 or more in any one year. Two of these admitted that many patients during only one year each, and one apparently confused contagious disease hospital admissions with total admissions to the general hospital of which it is a part. Eight hospitals during at least two of the three years concerned admitted 100 or fewer patients, and exactly one-half of the total number of hospitals which replied have fewer admissions for any one of the three years.

The percentages of deaths for all hospitals were 6.4, 6.3, and 5.6 for the years 1932, 1933, and 1934, respectively.

Both white and negro children are admitted to 22 hospitals of 23 which replied. Nine hospitals segregate white and negro patients. None of them limit the number of negro patients that may be admitted. However, the proportion in all but one is very small. This one reports 20 per cent.

An attempt was made to determine the number of available charity beds among these hospitals, but only 9 replied to this query. Two report ''all''; two, 90 per cent and 95 per cent; the remainder, 50, 150, 500, 681, and 1,000 beds, respectively. Replies to the question concerning ''pay beds'' were equally incomplete. Three reported none, these being the largest of all the hospitals and municipal institutions in each instance. There were only 4 replies to the question concerning the number of private rooms for children. Two have them; 2 do not; probably these are available in many of the hospitals but are not used for children only. There are facilities for accommodation of mothers in case they desire to stay in the hospital with sick children among nine hospitals.

Finances.—No hospital among the 23 institutions which replied derived funds from the state. Twenty of these derive their funds entirely from city or county or both. Two report that they are entirely supported by private contributions. No hospital reports income from an endowment or from the community chest.

The cost of running these hospitals, of course, varies with the size. The lowest cost reported was $500; the highest, $903,788 for the year 1934. Cost per patient per day varied among 16 hospitals which replied from $1.82 to $5.50.

Information requested concerning detailed costs such as, interest on investment, land, teachers' salaries, etc., was forthcoming in so few instances that no report can be made. Only 4 reported the average daily cost per patient for food. This sum varied from $0.58 to $2.89. Only 2 replies were received concerning cost of nursing and supplies.

In 13 hospitals the superintendent is a man, and in nine, a woman. In 10 instances the superintendent is a physician; in 6, a layman; and in 7, a registered nurse. In no instance do the superintendents have charge of the nurses' training school if one exists.

Nursing (General).—Among 25 hospitals which replied, 11 are affiliated with other hospitals for the purpose of special training in nursing. Eleven offer courses in contagious disease nursing technic. The length of the courses varies from three weeks to three months. Two courses are for four weeks, one for three weeks, the remainder are for two or three months. One offers a four-month postgraduate course. Fifteen hospitals employ only graduate nurses. Immunization of nurses to diphtheria is done in 23, to scarlet fever in 14, to smallpox in 23, and to typhoid fever in 8. Nurses contracted diphtheria (1934) in 2 hospitals (16 in 1, 2 in the other) and scarlet fever in 7 hospitals, the number affected being 2, 3, 13, 1, 3, 1, and 3, respectively. Other contagious diseases were contracted by nurses in 9 hospitals; these infections were usually German measles, measles, and mumps. One nurse contracted smallpox.

Training.—About half the hospitals failed to reply to questions concerning the number of day and night nurses on duty and the length of their assignments. Many of those which did reply interpreted the question ''length of assignment'' to mean ''period of time on the service'' rather than ''number of hours on duty each day.'' Hence figures for this portion of the questionnaire are most unsatisfactory and noninstructive and are omitted.

Operating Room.—Fifteen hospitals have at least 1 special operating room, and only 2 assign student nurses for duty there. These are assigned for a two- or three-month period. The number of operations performed during 1934 is reported by only 14 hospitals, and again one of these does not report figures for the contagious

Table VII
Attendance

	Patients Admitted			Patients Discharged			Died in Hospital			No. in Hosp. Open Fiscal Year	No. in Hosp. Close Fiscal Year	White and Colored Children
	1932	1933	1934	1932	1933	1934	1932	1933	1934			
1	78	58	126	71	64	126	8	4	16	3	3	Yes
2	632	650	706	625	468	636	32	14	22			Yes
3	3,154	3,832	4,405	2,923	3,669	4,238	130	119	152	333	348	Yes
4			5,857?			5,695?			117?	117?	162?	No
7	9	25	16							4	1-2	Yes
8	122	77	60				1	1	2			Yes
9	1	3	5	1	3	5	0	0	0	0	1	Yes
10	98	75	80				1	2	0			Yes
11	5,374	4,061	3,312	5,314	4,293	3,398	316	267	189	164	78	Yes
12	110	114	310	*119	109	303	*Included in 119	5	3	9	13	Yes
14	152	319	309	146	302	323	0	3	4	25	7	Yes
15	798	703	806		678		41	43	16	29	24	Yes
16	55	26	30	50	23	29	5	3	1	1	9	Yes
17	376	281	250	320	260	224	39	35	29	33	35	Yes
18	13,665	14,179	13,768	13,467	13,884	13,672	1,031	1,004	957	459	509	Yes
19	12,617	12,045	12,387	11,071	10,514	11,523	802	815	899	762	730	Yes
20	2,105	1,942	5,003			2,629	159	142	304	224	167	Yes
21		5	2		5	2		0	0			
22												
23	961	1,088	1,413	940	956	1,281	73	62	146	96	98	Yes
24	2,348	2,280	1,758	2,148	2,080	1,608	146	123	123	115	83	Yes
31			3			3			0	3	0	Yes
32	111	92	174			170			4	4	15	Yes
33	860	876	2,624	907	852	2,482	19	25	20	55	24	Yes
35	22	10	25	22	9	24	0	1	0	0	2	Yes
Total	43,648	42,741	53,629	38,124	38,169	48,371	2,803	2,698	3,004	2,436	2,499	

division alone. One hospital reports 5,271 operations, another, 331; a third, 269; the remainder, fewer than 100, and among the latter only one reports more than 50—in other words 10 had performed 50 or fewer operations.

Diet Kitchen.—Only 4 hospitals report that they have diet kitchens for infant foods. Four others use the diet kitchen of a general hospital of which the contagious division is a part. Only 3 report that student nurses work in these kitchens. Their period of service usually is from one to two weeks. Only 2 hospitals indicate that training is given in the preparation of children's diets. Fourteen did not reply.

Supervision.—Ten hospitals report that a head nurse is employed for each ward. Seventeen do not reply. As a rule, there is a proportion of one graduate assigned to each ward, and this proportion applies to night nurses as well, except in two instances in which only student nurses are used.

Nursing.—An effort to obtain information concerning the number of hours of instruction in contagious disease nursing was not very successful. Only 12 hospitals replied, and of these only 5 give a course of lectures in that subject. The courses vary from ten to thirty-two hours, and the instruction usually consists of both lectures and demonstrations. Courses are conducted by members of the medical staff. Only 3 hospitals indicate that demonstrations in contagious disease nursing are given. Only 3 offer postgraduate courses. In general, very little information was offered relative to training for contagious disease nursing, except by hospitals connected with medical schools.

Rather few hospitals replied to questions concerning cross-infections during year 1934. The information that was given is as follows:

Diphtheria: Eight replied; one hospital had 1 cross-infection; 1 had 3; and 6, none.

Scarlet fever: Eight replied; 3 had 2; 2 had 3; and 3 had none.

Measles: Eight replied; 1 had 50, 1 had 5, 2 had 1, and 4, none.

Pertussis: Eight replied; 1 had 1; 1 had 3; 1 had 2; and 5, none.

Chickenpox: Nine replied; 1 had 41; 1 had 23; 1 had 7; 1 had 5; 1 had 1; and 4, none.

Other diseases: Seven replied; 1 had 14; 1 had 13; 1 had 1, and 4, none.

Information concerning x-ray facilities is given in Table VIII.

Eleven hospitals indicate that they have neither an x-ray department nor diagnostic facilities. From one there was no reply. Only 1 hospital has a separate x-ray department, but 13 have available diagnostic facilities at any hour, day or night, and in 11 instances full-time technicians are available. Eight are equipped for high speed radiography with milliamperage as indicated in Table VIII. Ten are equipped for superficial radiography at the voltage indicated in the table. Only 4 are equipped for deep radiotherapy with voltage as indicated on chart. Thirteen have a fluoroscope, 10 can make stereoscopic plates and 10 have a portable x-ray machine. Internes do not do x-ray work in any of these hospitals. Ten among 15 hospitals which replied consider their x-ray facilities to be adequate. The x-ray department serves the dispensary in 6 hospitals and outside physicians in 9. However, we believe that many of these departments are located in general hospitals and serve the entire hospital including the contagious disease division. With this thought in mind, we believe that figures given for the number of x-ray plates, treatments, etc., during the last fiscal year are not confined to the contagious disease department alone and hence are not very illuminating as far as this report is concerned.

Laboratories (Pathologic, Clinical, Bacteriologic, and Serologic).—There was no reply from five hospitals among twenty-six from whom we received questionnaires, and, as usual, among the 21 there was a number which failed to reply to all questions.

Table VIII
X-Ray

	Is there an X-ray dept.?	Diagnostic facilities	No. full-time technicians	Facilities at any hour, day or night	What hours?	Equipped for high speed radiography	What milliamperage?	Equipped for superficial radiography	What voltage?	Equipped for deep radiotherapy	What voltage?	Fluoroscope	Make stereoscopic plates	Portable x-ray machine	Internes: Do x-ray work	Internes: Routine	Internes: Special	Are facilities adequate? If not, how?	Dept. serve disp.	Serve outside phys.	No. of x-ray plates last fiscal year	No. superficial treatments	No. deep therapy treatments
1	yes	yes	2	yes	all	mod.	100	yes	75	yes	180	yes	yes	yes	no	no	no	want higher Ma. for Radio-therapy & deep therapy		yes	2,779	13	57
2	Denver Hosp.	yes	3	yes		yes		no		no		yes	yes	yes	no			except therapy	yes	no	exposures 21,776	0	0
3		yes	0	yes		no		no		no		yes	no	no	no			yes	no	no	85	0	0
4		yes	3	yes	all	yes	100	yes	50–130	yes	180	yes	yes	yes	no	no	no	yes	yes	yes	Exams. 5,370		
7		yes	1	yes		yes	?	yes	?	no		yes	yes	yes	no	Intern.		new x-ray dept.	no disp.	yes	751 includes Gen.		
8	none																						
9		in Gen. Hosp.	yes	yes		?		yes		no		yes	no	no	no			yes	no	yes	170	0	0
10	No Reply																						
11		yes	4	yes		yes	80	yes	120	no		yes	yes	yes	no			yes	yes	yes, if patient is in hosp.	533	14	0
12		yes	1	yes		yes	100		peak kilo volts	no		yes	as nec.	no	no			yes			?	?	?
14		no																no					

TABLE VIII—CONTINUED

15	no																						
16	no																	for this work		yes			
17	no													brought in if nec.									
18		yes	2	yes	any			yes	140,-000	no		yes	yes	yes	no			no deep rad. equip.	yes	no	37,072	1,081	0
19		yes	4	yes		yes	100	radio-ther.	90–140	no		yes	yes	yes			con-fer-ences	yes	yes	no			
20		yes	1 half time	yes		no		yes	70 kilo volts 4 mps.	no		yes	no	no	no	no	no	yes	no	no	500	25	0
21	no																						
22	no																	no isola-tion beds, etc.		yes serums			
23		yes	yes	yes		yes	500	yes	130	yes	250	yes	yes	yes	no			yes	yes	yes	33,316	434	1167
24		yes	3	yes		yes	500	yes	100 kv	yes	200 kv	yes	yes	yes	no		Fluor-osc. &GU Rad.	yes	main x-ray, not conta-gious	yes limita-tion	600	occa-sion-ally	none
31	no																						
32	no																						
33	no																						
35	no																						

General.—There is a director in charge of laboratory work in 15 hospitals. In 2 the work is done by the state laboratory; in 2 others by the city laboratory. Only 9 have a full-time director in charge of laboratory work.

Pathological.—Six hospitals have a full-time director of the pathologic laboratory. Often the contagious work is also a responsibility of the pathological laboratory of a general hospital. Seven have part-time directors, and 6 have no director. Only 12 hospitals replied to the question concerning technicians. Among these all but 1 have full-time technicians. Internes work in the pathologic laboratory in only 4 instances, and these duties are of a routine or emergency nature. Among 15 which replied, 2 consider their facilities inadequate, and among 16 replying 10 have facilities for research.

Clinical.—Ten hospitals have full-time directors, and in 12 there are full-time technicians. Internes do laboratory work in 9 instances. It is usually of a routine nature. Blood chemistry work is available in 12 hospitals. In 3 it is not, and the remainder do not reply. Six have "fume hoods," 9 have colorimeters. Nine are able to do basal metabolism tests. Eight of these use a Sanborn machine. Thirteen consider their facilities adequate; 1 does not; the remainder do not reply. Only eleven have facilities for research work.

Bacteriologic.—Ten hospitals have full-time directors of the bacteriologic laboratory. Nine have part-time directors, the remainder failed to reply. Of 17 which replied, 14 employ full-time technicians. In 5 instances internes do some of the routine laboratory work. In no instance do they perform special work. All of 18 hospitals which replied have incubators, 17 are electric, 1 gas. Fifteen keep animals for experimental purposes, and 12 have facilities for research work.

Serologic.—Among 22 hospitals replying to this section, 14 have full- or part-time directors. In 8 instances there is a full-time director. Eleven have full-time technicians. The internes do work in the serologic laboratory in only 2 hospitals. Wassermanns are done in their own laboratory in 9 hospitals, Kahn tests in 10. Among 15 hospitals which replied, all consider their facilities adequate, and 12 report that they have facilities for research which in 2 instances are limited.

Miscellaneous.—Seven hospitals possess facilities for photography, and 3, for color photography. Motion picture photography is available in 2 instances. An electrocardiograph is available in only 9 hospitals.

Diet Kitchen.—Of 20 hospitals which replied, only 12 have trained dietitians in charge of the diet kitchen. Among these there are several whose training in dietetics seems rather sketchy. In one instance the contagious disease patients' diets seem to be in the hands of "one cook in a general hospital," and in another they are left to the tender mercies of a "maid" whose qualifications are "ordinary cooking." We hope not too ordinary. The dietitian has entire charge of the menu in most instances. Standard special diets are drawn up by the medical personnel in 8 instances, in 7 by cooperation of both dietitian and the physician in charge of the case, and in three by the dietitian.

Social Service.—Of 26 hospitals only 8 have social service departments. All of these have a full-time worker in charge of the department. Among 6 which replied, 4 indicated that the person in charge had had special previous training for that position. Six departments have more than 1 full-time worker. Respective numbers were reported as 2, 5, 7, 7, 10, and 10. In several instances we believe, however, that this department does not exclusively serve the contagious disease section, but functions for a general hospital of which the contagious disease hospital is a part.

Eight hospitals report that patients are investigated. This is done in the hospital by 4, in the home by 3, and both hospital and home by 4. Only 2 investigate all cases at the home, but 7 investigate all special cases at home.

In 5 instances a complete social history is taken on all cases. Two departments accept private pay cases. Social histories are filed with medical records in 5 instances, and an abstract is attached to the bedside notes in 2 instances. Among 10 hospitals which replied, 7 investigate the patient's ability to pay charges.

Among 10 hospitals which replied, 7 arrange for convalescent care, and 7 have institutions available for that care. Four hospitals have available foster homes and use them. Three consider that their facilities for convalescent care are not adequate.

Among 10 hospitals 3 follow-up cases after discharge; 5 do this if necessary. Social service assists in getting patients back for recall in 4 instances. Volunteer workers are used by 3 social service departments. The social service department is supported by hospital funds in 2, and the remainder do not reply.

In no instances is there a special lay committee in charge of the social service department.

General Information (1934).—Table IX reveals the number of cases of the more usual contagious diseases admitted to these hospitals during 1934, together with total deaths and the percentage death rate in all hospitals for each disease. Information was also requested concerning cases of other diseases admitted by the hospitals, but the replies are too diverse and varied to warrant charting.

Table IX reveals several figures of particular interest. For instance the mortality per cent for diphtheria and measles are nearly equal; the rate for pertussis is greater than either of these; and the rate for smallpox was zero, no deaths occurring among 56 cases. One may observe that the death rate for chickenpox is low, 0.67 per cent, but that this low rate is accounted for by 759 cases with no deaths, reported from one hospital alone. If the latter figures are omitted, the death rate in the other hospitals is 2.79 per cent or nearly four times the first figure. A grand total of only 1,762 cases of diphtheria admitted for the year 1934 seems to indicate that prophylactic procedures are gaining headway but need to be considerably more emphasized in the cities of the Middle West. Half of the cases of typhoid fever are reported from one hospital and half of the remaining number are evenly divided between the others. In other words 75 per cent of typhoid fever cases in contagious hospitals were found in three localities, namely, St. Louis, Sioux City, and Detroit. These figures of course do not necessarily mean that 75 per cent of all typhoid fever cases are found in these three localities. The fact that among 108 cases of amebic dysentery, 103 are reported by one hospital is accounted for by the Chicago epidemic. Also 25 of a total of 28 bacillary dysentery cases are reported from St. Paul, Minn.

Among other diseases listed under ''miscellaneous'' and admitted to these hospitals, we find the most frequent to be venereal disease, erysipelas, poliomyelitis, lethargic encephalitis, encephalitis, undulant fever, Vincent's angina, pneumonia, diphtheria carriers, furunculosis, septicemia, various forms of meningitis, toxic erythema, and streptococcic sore throat. A total number of 119 cases of poliomyelitis were admitted, about half of which were reported from Cleveland, Ohio. One hospital in St. Louis reported 346 cases of encephalitis, the reminder of the recent epidemic there. The mortality rate in that hospital was 22.2 per cent. Among 18 hospitals, 673 cases of erysipelas were admitted. The mortality rate was 13.34 per cent.

COMMENT

There is occasion for almost endless comment as one studies the reports concerning contagious hospitals of Region III. We shall not attempt a detailed discussion here for many conclusions are perfectly clear to anyone who is interested enough to study the detailed report. We merely wish to call attention to the more important facts which this and future reports will illuminate.

There are not many large contagious disease hospitals to be found in this region. We received reports from only nine which would be called large, and all of these, of

TABLE IX

GENERAL INFORMATION (1934)

	DIPHTHERIA		SCARLET FEVER		MEASLES		WHOOPING COUGH		SMALLPOX		CHICKENPOX		EPIDEMIC CEREBROSPINAL MENINGITIS		TYPHOID FEVER		AMEBIC DYSENTERY		BACILLARY DYSENTERY	
	CASES	DEATHS	CASES	DEATHS	CASES	DEATHS	CASES	DEATHS	CASES	DEATHS	CASES	DEATHS	CASES	DEATHS	CASES	DEATHS	CASES	DEATHS	CASES	DEATHS
1	4	1	20	2	5	0	6	0	0	0	1	0	1	0	1	0	2	0	0	0
2	No reply																			
3	225	17	3219	47	54	2	54	4	0	0	10	1	104	21	0	0	103	0	0	0
4	No reply																			
7	1		2		8								? 2*		1	1			2	1
8	16		22	2	13		1				1				1					
9			1		3															
10	29	0	17	0	23	0					2	0								
11	248	21	1931	22	81	3	130	21	0	0	40	1	14	4	21	2	1	0	1	0
12	2		311		1		1				1									
14	10	1	317	3	1	0														
15	17	1	581	7	72	0	598	7			759	0	2	0	17	0	2	0		

TABLE IX—CONT'D

16			20												2					
17	5	1	88	3	5	0	6	2	0	0	4	0	6†	4	20	5	0	0	0	0
18	257	8	102	3	18		16	6			18		7	7						
19	22	1	154	2	17	0	33	1	9	0	36	0	3	2	4	0			25	2
20	446	18	254	5	673	47	457	23	12	0	63	3			89	14				
21	1	0	1	0																
22	176	5	133	2					26					2						
23	197	22	524	19	171	23	114	33	0	0	34	0	51	30	1	0				
24	105	19	920	15	81	4	108	15	0	0	45	2	16	5	1	0				
31	1																			
32	2	0	113	2	13	0	1	0	1	0	4	0	1‡	1						
33	31	4	2432	9	10	0	18	1	2	0	8	0	7	3						
34	16	1	239	3	1	0			5	0	1	0								
35			18	0					1	0			1	0						
Totals	1762	120	11,419	146	1250	79	1543	113	56	0	1027	7	206	79	158	22	108	0	28	3
Deaths %	6.8		1.27		6.3		7.3		0		0.67		38.3		13.9		0		10.7	

*Epidemic?
†Suspected various types.
‡Not epidemic.

course, are to be found in the larger cities, specifically Chicago, Detroit, St. Paul, Minneapolis, Cincinnati, St. Louis, Denver, Cleveland, and Milwaukee. With the exception of Denver, we have received questionnaires from no more than one hospital in any city irrespective of size, and in most instances that is the only contagious hospital in that municipality. Naturally there is a marked difference in their respective sizes, between an institution located in Chicago, which serves several millions of people, and one found in Beloit, Wis., which serves a few thousand. Among the larger hospitals the organization is usually more efficient and complete, in reference to staff, laboratory, x-ray facilities, social service, and nursing services. This is to be expected, for smaller institutions cannot afford such a complete organization when their admission volume is relatively low. There are probably certain periods during the year in which there are no patients in many of the smaller institutions.

Nine hospitals are sufficiently large to have house staffs consisting of more than one physician. They employ resident physicians as well as internes and 5 have residents, assistant residents, and internes. Training requirements for these positions seem satisfactory in most instances, save 1 in which senior medical students are employed.

The contagious disease hospital is connected with a medical school or affords training to medical students or both in the following cities: Denver, Evanston, Ill., Detroit, Minneapolis, St. Paul, Cincinnati, Cleveland, St. Louis, and Chicago. Research work is practically limited to the larger hospitals. In 11 instances the hospitals have affiliations that afford training in contagious disease nursing. Some of the courses are too short to be of much value, but others are long enough to be invaluable. The number of nurses who contracted contagious diseases while working in any of the hospitals seems to us to be rather small which fact should speak favorably for efficient training in contagious nursing technic.

Some of the hospitals do not indicate that they have an operating room. We wonder what the procedure would be if an emergency operation should be necessary.

We should have liked more information concerning cross-infections in the respective hospitals, but many seemed reticent about giving it. Whether this was because they could not be proud of their record or simply had kept no accurate account of these mishaps, accidents, or whatever one may call them, we do not know.

X-ray facilities in many hospitals seem excellent; however, we were somewhat startled to discover that 11 report that there are no x-ray facilities. These again are quite small institutions, usually tax supported and the need for x-ray work is probably very infrequent, the consequent conclusion being that cost is too great to warrant the expenditure required when the need is not great. Similar situations are found in reference to various laboratory facilities and services. Although provisions for an efficient organization in all of these facilities in each hospital would appear to be and would really be a great extravagance in many instances, on the other hand, these services are often indispensable if one is to provide efficient medical care. Where they are not available, the patients' chances of recovery may often be seriously impaired. Private patients in these institutions probably can have almost any type of laboratory service if they are willing to pay for it; we wonder, however, if the free patient may not occasionally suffer because of its lack.

REPORT OF THE TREASURER

Statement of Receipts and Disbursements
June 1, 1935 to May 31, 1936

Balance, June 1, 1935					$ 4,489.72
Receipts:					
Initiation Fees				$ 5,670.50	
Dues				13,470.00	
Exhibits (1935)				1,320.00	
Interest on Bonds				206.25	
Miscellaneous				5.00	$20,671.75
					$25,161.47
Disbursements:					
Office					
Salaries					
Secretary	$5,000.00				
Stenographer	1,560.00				
Office Help	360.00				
		$6,920.00			
Rent		515.00			
Traveling Expense		466.86			
Printing and Stationery		554.72			
Postage		457.80			
Office Supplies and Equipment		102.70			
Insurance (Treasurer's Bond)		62.50			
Telephone and Telegrams		30.88			
Exchange and Tax on checks		51.05			
Miscellaneous		43.11	$ 9,204.62		
Subscriptions to Journal		4,635.00			
Annual Meeting (1935 and 1936)		3,157.01			
Purchase of Bonds—Bal. Payment		347.75			
Executive Board Meeting		665.38			
State Expense		389.03	$ 9,194.17		
Regional Expense:					
Region I		307.79			
Certificates		148.80			
II		49.45			
Certificates		80.80			
III		106.68			
Certificates		123.60			
IV		13.18			
Certificates		34.00			
II and III Meeting		134.85	$ 999.15		
Committees:					
Council on Pediatric Research		480.17			
Clinical Investigation and Scientific Research		96.50			
Hospital and Dispensaries		54.00	$ 630.67		$20,028.61
Balance, May 31, 1936					$ 5,132.86

Academy News

Dr. Francis Scott Smyth, of San Francisco, Calif., and Dr. Oscar M. Schloss, of New York City, have recently been made Fellows of the Academy.

Dr. William L. Buhrman of Chicago died on June 10, 1936.

News and Notes

The following men have been certified by the **American Board of Pediatrics** since the last report. The Board again desires to call attention to the increase of the fee to $30, effective Sept. 30, 1936.

Edward Saunders Babcock, Sacramento, Calif.
Edward Parsons Bagg, Holyoke, Mass.
Charles Williams Bailey, Spartanburg, S. C.
Wilford W. Barber, Denver, Colo.
F. Duncan Barnes, New Rochelle, N. Y.
B. J. Berger, Dallas, Texas
Joseph Brown Bilderback, Portland, Ore.
Frank Lee Bivings, Atlanta, Ga.
Crawford Bost, San Francisco, Calif.
Ralph Bowen, Oklahoma City, Okla.
Howard Wheaton Brayton, Hartford, Conn.
Leroy J. Butler, Winston-Salem, N. C.
Dever Smith Byard, New York, N. Y.
John Caffey, New York, N. Y.
Ernest R. Carlo, Fort Wayne, Ind.
Thomas F. Daniels, Baltimore, Md.
John Hart Davis, Cleveland, Ohio
Laurence Richard DeBuys, New Orleans, La.
Katharine Dodd, Nashville, Tenn.
Karl Wilhelm Ebeling, Baltimore, Md.
Ten Eyck Elmendorf, New York, N. Y.
Theodore O. Elterich, Pittsburgh, Pa.
Joseph Wm. Epstein, Cleveland, Ohio
Arthur L. Esserman, Denver, Colo.
Yates W. Faison, Charlotte, N. C.
William White Falkener, Newport News, Va.
Warren Conrad Fargo, Cleveland, Ohio
Lloyd King Felter, Cincinnati, Ohio
Edmund Boyd FitzGerald, Wollaston, Mass.
Morris Friedson, New York, N. Y.
Elias Freidus, Long Beach, N. Y.
Irving A. Frisch, New York, N. Y.
Thomas Bolling Gay, Atlanta, Ga.
John E. Gonce, Jr., Madison, Wis.
Julian Graubarth, New Orleans, La.
William Russell Graves, Memphis, Tenn.
Otto Grob, Detroit, Mich.
Bengt Hamilton, Chicago, Ill.
Ernest W. Hancock, Lincoln, Neb.
Arild Edsten Hansen, Minneapolis, Minn.
Joseph Linn Hetzel, Waterbury, Conn.
John William Holmes, Philadelphia, Pa.
Arthur G. Jacobs, Memphis, Tenn.
Lawrence R. Jacobus, Oakland, Calif.
Herman M. Jahr, Omaha, Neb.
Charles Kimball Johnson, Burlington, Vt.
William Wiley Jones, Denver, Colo.
Gustav Leonard Kaufmann, Chicago, Ill.
Samuel Eleazer Kohn, Milwaukee, Wis.
Edmund Griffin Lawler, Chicago, Ill.
J. Hugh Lewis, Wyandotte, Mich.
Harry L. F. Locke, Hartford, Conn.
Maud Loeber, New Orleans, La.
Walter D. Ludlum, Brooklyn, N. Y.
Robert A. Lyon, Cincinnati, Ohio.
Roderick J. McDonald, Jr., Denver, Colo.
Eugene T. McEnery, Chicago, Ill.

Rustin McIntosh, New York, N. Y.
Walter Caraway McKee, Chicago, Ill.
Edwin Clare McMullen, Pine Bluff, Ark.
Howard B. Mettel, Indianapolis, Ind.
Milo K. Miller, South Bend, Ind.
Louis D. Minsk, Chicago, Ill.
Clyde Moore, Omaha, Neb.
J. Harry Murphy, Omaha, Neb.
Frank C. Neff, Kansas City, Mo.
Samuel Okrent, Cincinnati, Ohio
William J. Orr, Buffalo, N. Y.
Joseph B. Pincus, Brooklyn, N. Y.
Samuel Fitzsimons Ravenel, Greensboro, N. C.
Hartzell Harrison Ray, San Mateo, Calif.
Benjamin B. Rittenberg, Philadelphia, Pa.
Robert Rosenthal, St. Paul, Minn.
Solomon H. Rubin, Boston, Mass.
George Richard Russell, Tulsa, Okla.
Albert L. Salomon, Oklahoma City, Okla.
William J. Scott, Detroit, Mich.
John A. Shaw, Fayetteville, N. C.
Floyd Reeves Smith, Pittsfield, Mass.
Joe T. Smith, Knoxville, Tenn.
Henry E. Stafford, Oakland, Calif.
Albert Valentine Stoesser, Minneapolis, Minn.
Lee Edwards Sutton, Jr., Richmond, Va.
Clifford Sweet, Oakland, Calif.
Carl Leonard Thenebe, Hartford, Conn.
Edward Arthur Wagner, Cincinnati, Ohio
Edward Taylor Wakeman, New Haven, Conn.
Alfred Hamlin Washburn, Denver, Colo.
Gustave F. Weinfeld, Ravinia, Ill.
William Weston, Jr., Columbia, S. C.
Herbert B. Wilcox, New York, N. Y.
Edward A. Wishropp, Detroit, Mich.
Charles H. York, Cleveland, Ohio
Stuart Welsh Adler, Albuquerque, N. M.
Ralph L. Cook, St. Louis, Mo.
Max Miles Ginsburg, Denver, Colo.
Aymer Morgan Hill, Grand Rapids, Mich.
Jasper Stewart Hunt, Charlotte, N. C.
W. Eugene Keiter, Kinston, N. C.
Thomas Myers Palmer, Jacksonville, Fla.
Meyer A. Perlstein, Chicago, Ill.
George Edwin Robertson, Omaha, Neb.
Byron Kenneth Rust, Indianapolis, Ind.
Martha Chandley Souter, Indianapolis, Ind.
Edward Lawrence Tuohy, Minneapolis, Minn.
Ralph Henry Verploeg, Denver, Colo.
Morris Greenberg, New York, N. Y.

At the 48th Annual Meeting of the **American Pediatric Society** at Bolton Landing on Lake George, N. Y., Dr. Henry F. Helmholz was elected president for the ensuing year. Dr. Frederic H. Bartlett, of New York City, was elected vice president. Dr. Hugh McCulloch, 325 N. Euclid Ave., St. Louis, Mo., was reelected secretary and treasurer. Dr. P. C. Jeans, Iowa City, Iowa, was chosen member of council. Dr. Heyworth N. Sanford was reelected recorder-editor. This meeting was held jointly with the **Canadian Society for the Study of Diseases of Children.** Following the meeting of the Societies, exercises were held for the dedication of the Carl Schurz-Abraham Jacobi Memorial Park at Bolton Landing. Bolton Landing was Dr. Jacobi's summer home. The Society had held a meeting at Bolton Landing in 1905 as the guest of Dr. Jacobi. Dr. Herbert Willy Meyer, of New York, showed motion pictures of Dr. Jacobi made at Bolton Landing shortly before his death.

At the annual meeting of the **Section on Pediatrics of the American Medical Association** in Kansas City, the following officers were elected for the ensuing year: chairman, Ralph M. Tyson, Philadelphia; vice chairman, Aldrich C. Crowe, Atlantic City; secretary, Albert D. Kaiser, Rochester, N. Y.

At the meeting of the **Society for Pediatric Research** in Atlantic City, Dr. Francis Scott Smyth, of San Francisco, Calif., was elected president. Dr. A. A. Weech, 3975 Broadway, New York City, was reelected secretary.

The **Virginia Pediatric Society** held its First Clinical Session on Friday morning, May 29, at the Medical College of Virginia, Richmond, Va. The morning session was devoted to a symposium on disorders of the respiratory tract in infancy and childhood. The leaders of this discussion were Dr. William P. McDowell, Dr. Samuel R. Newman, Dr. Frank D. Wilson, and Dr. W. B. McIlwane. Dr. A. C. Broders, clinical professor of pathology, Medical College of Virginia, discussed malignancy in children.

The afternoon session was devoted to a clinical pathological conference with discussion of papers by Dr. Paul Kimmelstiel, associate in pathology, and members of the pediatric staff, Medical College of Virginia.

The next meeting of the Society will be in October, 1936, at Staunton, Va., at the time of the meeting of the **Medical Society of Virginia.** Dr. J. B. Stone, 2042 Park Ave., Richmond, Va., is secretary of the Society.

The **Fourth International Pediatrics Congress** has been postponed and will probably be held the first week in April, 1937, in Rome, Italy.

Attention is again called to the fact that after September, 1936, certification by the **American Board of Pediatrics** will be by examination only. At this time also the fee for certification will be increased to $30. All pediatricians eligible for certification without examination should attend to this important matter at once.

The Journal of Pediatrics

Vol. 9 | August, 1936 | No. 2

Original Communications

TREATMENT OF NINETEEN CASES OF TYPHOID FEVER IN CHILDREN

With a Report on the Importance of Nonspecific Immunotransfusion Therapy

Karl Habel, M.D., and Walter J. Crocker, V.M.D.
Philadelphia, Pa.

THE purpose of this paper is to report the treatment of nineteen cases of typhoid fever in children under twelve years of age who were admitted to the Children's Department of the Philadelphia General Hospital during an epidemic of the disease, and particularly to record the rapid recovery of five very severe cases of typhoid fever in children following nonspecific immunotransfusion therapy.

In Philadelphia during June, 1935, an epidemic of typhoid fever resulted in the admission of ninety-two patients to the various hospitals of the city. Since all patients came from the same district, the Department of Public Health traced the source of infection to potato salad served at a picnic held within the city limits May 30.

Cultures of the drinking water at the picnic grounds were negative for typhoid bacilli. Two patients who had not attended the affair became ill after eating potato salad brought to them from the picnic by neighbors. Through this fact the carrier was identified as the individual who had prepared the salad.

ONSET AND SYMPTOMS

The nineteen children who were admitted to the Philadelphia General Hospital during the epidemic were definitely exposed at the same time, yet the incubation period varied from ten to twenty-three days. Fever was the first symptom noticed by the parents in most of the children. In the beginning fever was accompanied by no symptoms other than malaise and anorexia. In six individuals these three complaints were the only symptoms of importance during their illness before admission

From the Children's Department and Division of Clinical Pathology of the Laboratories of Philadelphia General Hospital.

Read before the Second Annual Meeting of Region I of the American Academy of Pediatrics, Philadelphia, Oct. 12, 1935.

to the hospital. Fainting or sudden dizziness, as the initial symptom, occurred in six female patients. As definite complaints anorexia occurred in eleven and malaise in eight patients. Of the cardinal symptoms headache was the most frequent, being present in ten cases, diarrhea in four, epistaxis in three, and melena in none.

PHYSICAL EXAMINATION

The physical findings were more classical and made the diagnosis quite definite in this series of patients. All individuals showed rose spots on admission or a few days later, and approximately half of them subsequently developed new crops of rose spots. Eighteen patients showed the typical appearance of the tongue. It was coated on the dorsum and clean on the edges and tip. Abdominal distention was present in thirteen individuals. It was slight in the majority and marked in only a few patients. The spleen was palpable in twelve instances. Anterior and posterior cervical lymphadenopathy was noticeable in four patients. There was generalized tenderness on abdominal palpation in three cases. Bronchitis and dicrotic pulse were each found in two instances.

LABORATORY FINDINGS

Laboratory proof of the disease was found in all of the patients. Blood cultures were positive for typhoid bacilli in fifteen individuals. Positive Widal reactions were obtained in the four cases which showed negative blood cultures. The Widal reactions varied greatly. The dilutions showing agglutination ranged from 0 to 1 to 1,280, although the patients were exposed at the same time and the Widal tests were done at the same stage of the disease. There was no correlation between the severity of the clinical symptoms and the grade of the Widal reactions.

Urine cultures were positive in only one patient, and all of the feces cultures were negative. Blood cultures and Widal tests could not be followed during the course of the disease, and urine and feces cultures were done only on admission and prior to discharge because of the large number of typhoid fever patients in both the adult and children's wards.

The leucocyte counts were low in most instances. The highest count was 15,400 in one patient while fifteen were below 10,000. The highest neutrophile count was 76 per cent, and twelve individuals showed a relative lymphocytosis.

COURSE

The course of the disease in this series of patients was mild in general. The degree of toxicity was graded from 1+ to 5+, based on the duration of fever, amount of abdominal distention, degree of malaise and anorexia, occurrence of vomiting and diarrhea and the extent of the hemogramic left shift. Degrees of toxicity were as follows:

4 patients 1+	4 patients 4+
4 patients 2+	1 patient 5+
6 patients 3+	

The manifestations of toxicity were present only while the fever continued, although several patients showed very few toxic signs even while running high continuous temperatures. The duration of fever after admission is, we believe, a fair indication of the distribution of the severity of the infection. Days of fever were:

6 patients	0-10 days	1 patient	30-40 days
10 patients	10-20 days	0 patient	40-50 days
1 patient	20-30 days	1 patient	50-60 days.

Four patients had relapses, and only one ended her illness by becoming a carrier.

The details of the hospital course of the more severe cases are considered under the heading of treatment.

TREATMENT

Nineteen children of approximately the same age, infected at the same source at the same time, offered an excellent opportunity for comparing results of different types of therapy. All patients were given the usual high caloric diet therapy.

Six patients were treated with a specific immune human serum intramuscularly, under the supervision of Dr. Stuart Mudd, of the University of Pennsylvania Hospital, and Dr. Aims McGuiness, of the Children's Hospital of Philadelphia, a detailed report of which they will probably present at a later time.

Briefly, the blood serum was obtained from adults who had been immunized ten days previously with the standard United States Army typhoid vaccine and was found to have an average titer of 1 to 300 by the Widal agglutination test. Patients showing various degrees of toxicity were selected, and the quantity and the frequency of administration of the serum were varied with different individuals. The clinical course of the disease showed no remarkable change following this form of therapy according to the opinions of these physicians and the physicians and nurses who were in charge of the six patients.

Five of the most severely infected children were given the nonspecific immunotransfusion therapy as outlined by Crocker, Valentine and Brody[1] in the Philadelphia General Hospital in 1932. The splendid results from the use of this therapy during the past three years in the treatment of septicemia, pneumonia[2-6] and other acute infections gave promise of equally good or more effective results in the treatment of typhoid fever.

The patients treated with nonspecific immunotransfusions were selected because of their high temperature, marked toxicity and wide left shift in the Schilling hemogram. All patients except R. D. (Case 4), who had a relapse, were quite toxic at the time of transfusion. Three of these were treated in the second week of the disease and three in the first few days of a relapse. All five patients had had positive blood cultures, and two of these had been positive within five days of receiving the transfusions. Following this treatment all patients showed immediate marked improvement as detailed in the case reports.

Modified Schilling hemograms[7] were used to control the therapy. An extensive left shift in the hemogram twenty-four or more hours after treatment indicated that further transfusions were needed, and a right shift after treatment indicated that no additional transfusions were necessary. Shiftograms or charts of sequential hemograms were used to follow the course of the disease. The vertical graph, or shiftograph on the shiftograms, is a graphic representation of the successive Schilling indices, and shows at a glance the shift to the right or left from day to day, as the process improves or retrogresses during the entire course of the disease.

PREPARATION OF THE DONOR

A suitable donor is selected according to general health, serology, typing, and cross agglutination. He is hospitalized and fifty million killed typhoid bacilli are given intravenously. The usual stock typhoid or mixed typhoid, paratyphoid A and B vaccine, one billion organisms per cubic centimeter, is used, of which $\frac{1}{20}$ c.c. is the dose. If the donor does not have a reaction within an hour, the dose is repeated. Usually within an hour after injection of the killed organisms, the donor has a chill followed by a rise in temperature to from 102 to 104° F. and leucocytosis up to 25,000. This reaction continues for an hour or more, but the temperature returns to normal within a few hours. Eight hours after the injection of typhoid vaccine the donor's blood is taken. It is given to the patient by the direct or indirect method in two transfusions of from 100 to 200 c.c. on two successive days. Five hundred cubic centimeters of blood are drawn from the donor and that which is not used in the first transfusion may be kept safely in the ice box for seventy-two hours.

RATIONALE OF THE TREATMENT

The fifty million killed typhoid organisms are given to the donor intravenously as a standard, safe and effective dose of foreign protein for the purpose of producing in him a foreign protein reaction. They stimulate the donor's cells to a maximum production of opsonins, or nonspecific immune bodies, in approximately eight hours. Crocker, Valentine, and Brody have shown that the opsonins are increased in this manner from fivefold to tenfold. The opsonins, or nonspecific immune bodies, are transferred from the donor to the patient as a form of passive immunity where they so affect the bacteria in the patient that his leucocytes may readily phagocytize them and thus reduce the intoxication.

The typhoid vaccine is not given to the donor with the idea of stimulating his cells to the production of specific antibodies against the typhoid bacilli, as precipitins, agglutinations or lysins, in a period of eight hours. This does not occur. All Widal reactions on the donor's serum eight hours after injection of the vaccine intravenously were negative for typhoid bacillus agglutinins. For this reason it is assumed that the other specific immune bodies, precipitins and lysins, are also absent, but further work along these lines is planned. On the basis of negative Widal reactions for specific typhoid agglutinins and a positive increase of opsonins or nonspecific immune bodies on the donor's blood eight hours after intravenous injection of fifty million killed typhoid organisms, this method is considered to be a nonspecific immunotransfusion therapy.

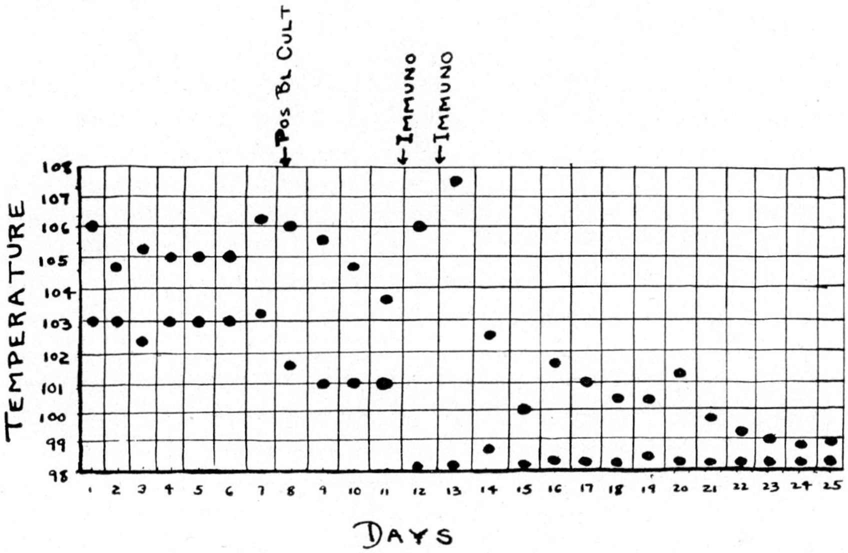

Chart 1.—Case 1. Markedly severe primary infection. Marked reaction after each of two nonspecific immunotransfusions with immediate improvement and subsequent recovery. In this and subsequent clinical charts the two readings for each day represent the highest and lowest temperatures during that day. *Immuno* indicates nonspecific immunotransfusion.

CASE REPORTS*

CASE 1.—A. B., a negro female, aged three years, was admitted July 12, 1935, with fever of two days' duration, vomiting, and loss of weight. Exposure was not known, and the onset was uncertain. She was very toxic with throat markedly inflamed, typical appearance of tongue, coarse râles throughout the chest and distention of abdomen. On July 13 the red blood cells were 4,340,000, white blood cells, 5,550; polymorphonuclears, 64 per cent; lymphocytes, 30 per cent; monocytes, 6 per cent. On July 15 rose spots developed; the Widal reaction was positive 1:640; and the blood culture was positive for typhoid. Treatment was symptomatic, and the patient continued to be very fretful, toxic, with a temperature of 103 to 106° F., abdomen markedly distended, and occasional vomiting and diarrhea. On July 23, the twelfth day of illness, with a multiple index of 104 in the Schilling

*These patients were admitted to the pediatric service of Wm. N. Bradley, M.D.

Date 1935	Day of illness	Pos. blood culture	Nonsp. Imm. Transf.	C.C. of blood	Grams hemoglobin	Red blood cells	White blood cells	Multiple index degrees of toxicity	Schilling index	Myelocytes	Juveniles	Stabs	Segmenters	Total neutrophiles	Lymphoblasts	Large lymphs	Intermediate lymphs	Small lymphs	Total lymphs	Monocytes	Eosinophiles	Basophiles	Segmenters cmm	Total neutrophiles cmm	Total lymphs cmm	Monocytes cmm
Date	Day	C	Tr	c.c.	Hb	RBC	WBC	MI	ShI	M	J	St	Sg	TN	Lb	L	I	S	TL	M	E	B	Sg	TN	TL	M
Normals					15.4	5.0	7500	1	1/16	0	0	4	64	68	0	5	1	20	26	4	2	0	4800	5000	2000	300
7-15	4	+			14.0	4.3	9400	59	3.7	0	0	60	16	76	0	6	0	4	10	14	0	0	1504	7144	940	1316
7-22	11				13.0	3.8	6450	176	11.0	0	0	44	4	48	2	4	0	40	46	6	0	0	248	2976	2944	384
7-23	12		1	90	13.0	3.7	6700	104	6.5	0	0	52	8	60	0	10	0	10	20	18	2	0	536	4020	1340	1206
7-24	13		2	100	13.0	3.6	7200	24	1.5	0	0	28	18	46	0	16	0	32	48	6	0	0	1296	3312	3456	432
7-25	14				13.0	3.4	8750	52	3.3	0	0	54	16	70	0	10	0	8	18	12	0	0	1392	6090	1586	1044
7-26	15				12.0	3.2	7150	64	4.0	0	0	40	10	50	0	20	0	20	40	10	0	0	710	3550	2840	710
7-27	16				12.0	3.2	5600	36	2.3	0	0	38	16	54	0	2	0	34	36	10	0	0	896	3024	2016	560
7-29	18				13.0	3.6	7700	24	1.5	0	0	28	18	46	0	26	0	12	38	16	0	0	1386	3542	2926	1232
8- 2	22				13.0	4.0	8100	17	1.1	0	0	22	20	42	0	4	0	48	52	6	0	0	1620	3402	4212	486
8- 8	28				14.0	4.2	7900	9	3/5	0	0	12	20	32	0	6	0	58	64	4	0	0	1580	2528	5056	316
8-14	34				14.0	4.2	7000	13	6/7	0	0	18	22	40	0	10	0	46	56	2	2	0	1540	2800	3920	112
8-16	36				14.0	4.3	10500	12	4/5	0	0	8	10	18	0	12	0	64	76	2	4	0	1050	1890	7980	210

Chart 2.—Case 1., A. B. Shiftogram of a case of typhoid fever illustrating wide alternating shifts to the left and right during the first twelve days of illness. On the twelfth day the first nonspecific immunotransfusion of 90 c.c. was given, which forced the shift to the right from a Schilling index of 6.5 to 1.5 or a multiple index of 104 to 24 or reduced the toxicity of the patient from 104 to 24 degrees in twenty-four hours. The second nonspecific immunotransfusion of 100 c.c. was given on the thirteenth day to reinforce the first. During the following forty-eight hours, the reaction between the opsonins of the nonspecific immunotransfusion and the toxins of the bacteria was in doubt, the shift extending to the left to a Schilling index of 4 and a multiple index of 64. On the fifteenth day the opsonins overcame the bacteria, and the shift was forced to the right to convalescence and recovery.

hemogram, the first nonspecific immunotransfusion of 90 c.c. was given. The patient had a chill, and the temperature rose to 106° F. The next day the second treatment was given and was followed by a chill and an elevation of temperature to 107.5° F. Improvement occurred quickly. Within twenty-four hours the multiple index dropped from 104 to 24 (normal multiple index, 1). The temperature dropped to normal within forty-eight hours, rising to 101° F. only twice during the next few days. The toxicity was greatly lessened, and in three days the abdominal distention had disappeared. Improvement continued until August 6, when the urine and the feces were negative for typhoid bacilli. The patient was discharged Aug. 22, 1935. This was the only patient not definitely associated with the epidemic of June, 1935.

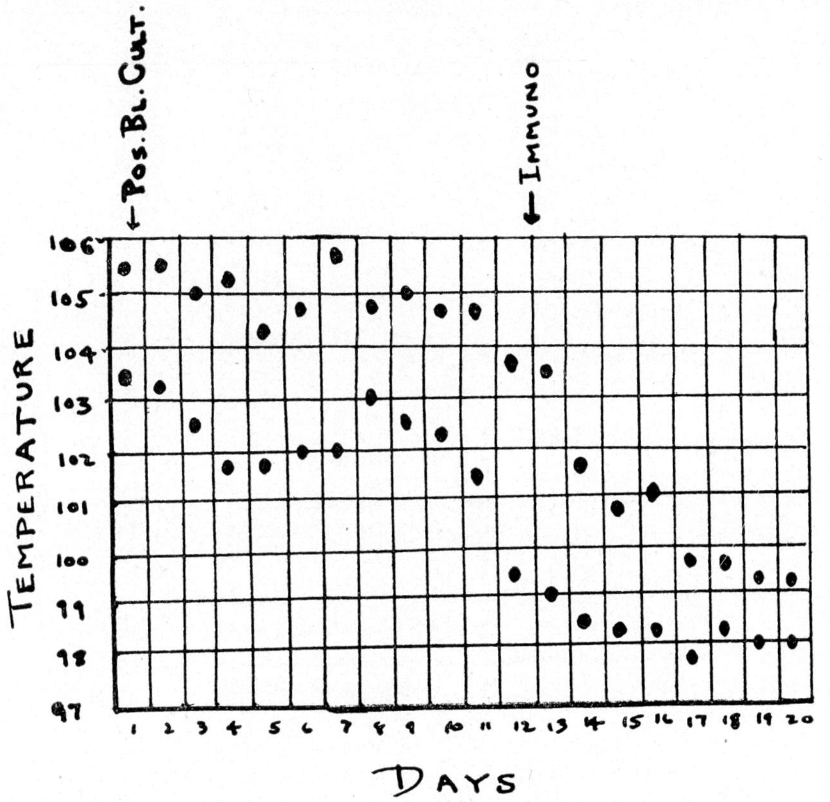

Chart 3.—Case 2. Moderately toxic primary infection with intestinal hemorrhage. One nonspecific immunotransfusion was followed by drop in temperature and recovery.

CASE 2.—T. H., white female, aged eight years, was exposed May 30, 1935; the onset was on June 19, with fever, dizziness, and anorexia. She was admitted June 24, in a toxic condition with rose spots, typical appearance of the tongue, nontransmitted apical systolic murmur, palpable spleen, and slight distention. On June 24 the red blood cells were 4,500,000 per cubic millimeter, white blood cells, 4,900; neutrophiles, 58 per cent; lymphocytes, 42 per cent; and the blood culture was positive for typhoid organisms. On June 27 the stools were bloody; the child was toxic and drowsy and was taking nourishment poorly, was vomiting frequently, and had slight abdominal distention. Temperature ranged between 103 and 105° F., becoming septic in type on July 5. One nonspecific immunotransfusion of 150 c.c. was

Date 1935	Day of illness	Pos Blood culture	Nonsp. Imm. Transf.	C.C. of blood	Hemoglobin	Red blood cells	White blood cells	Multiple index Degrees of toxicity	Schilling index	Myelocytes	Juveniles	Stabs	Segmenters	Total neutrophiles	Lymphoblasts	Large lymphs	Intermediate lymphs	Small lymphs	Total lymphs	Monocytes	Eosinophiles	Basophiles	Segmenters per cmm	Total neutrophiles cmm	Total lymphs cmm	Monocytes cmm
Date	Day	C	Tr	c.c.	Hb	RBC	WBC	MI	ShI	M	J	St	Sg	TN	Lb	L	I	S	TL	M	E	B	Sg	TN	TL	M
					15.4	5.0	7500	1	1/16	0	0	4	64	68	0	5	1	20	26	4	2	0	4800	5000	2000	300 Normals
SchI			33	30 27	24	21	18	15	12 9	6	3	1	½ 0													
6-24	1	+			15	5.0	4700	496	31.0	0	0	62	2	64	0	0	0	36	36	0	0	0	94	3008	1692	000
7- 4	11				8	3.0	5200	448	28.0	0	0	56	2	58	2	8	0	22	32	8	2	0	104	3016	1664	416
7- 6	13		1	150	8	3.0	4000	304	19.0	0	0	38	2	40	0	16	4	36	56	4	0	0	80	1600	2240	160
7- 7	14				9	3.1	4600	48	3.0	0	0	30	10	40	0	10	6	40	56	4	0	0	460	1840	2576	184
7- 9	16				10	3.4	5900	19	1.2	0	0	20	16	36	0	0	0	52	52	12	0	0	944	2124	3068	708
7-13	20				13	3.9	5400	12	3/4	0	0	6	8	14	0	14	0	72	86	0	0	0	432	756	4644	000
7-22	29				14	4.2	12600	17	1.1	0	0	22	20	42	0	8	0	42	50	8	0	0	2520	5292	6300	1008
7-26	33				14	4.2	12850	16	1.0	0	0	30	30	60	0	20	0	2	22	18	0	0	3840	7680	2816	2284
7-27	34				14	4.2	11800	10	2/3	0	0	16	22	38	0	30	0	20	50	12	0	0	2596	4484	5900	1416
7-29	36				14	4.3	13000	5	1/3	0	0	20	64	84	0	4	0	0	4	12	0	0	8320	10920	520	1560
8- 2	40				14	4.2	13000	10	2/3	0	2	20	34	56	0	18	0	22	40	4	0	0	4420	7280	5200	520
8- 8	46				14	4.5	10000	3	1/5	0	0	10	50	60	0	10	0	30	40	0	0	0	5000	6000	4000	000

Chart 4.—Case 2., T. H. Shiftogram of a case of typhoid fever illustrating a right shift to convalescence and recovery following one nonspecific immunotransfusion of 150 c.c. given July 6, 1935, on the thirteenth day of illness. Twenty-four hours after the transfusion the multiple index or degrees of toxicity dropped from 304 to 48, and the Schilling index, from 19 to 3. Slight alternating shifts to the left and right continued within convalescent limits to recovery. The shiftograph is a vertical graphic representation of the successive Schilling indices and shows the shift to the left or right at a glance.

given July 6, the thirteenth day of illness. No definite reaction followed, but the temperature became normal in four days with improvement in appetite and alertness and with disappearance of diarrhea and distention. At the same time the hemogram showed a shift to the right from a multiple index of 304 to 48 within forty-eight hours. The urine and the feces were negative July 19, and the patient was discharged Aug. 9, 1935.

Case 3.—V. A., white male, aged nine years, was exposed May 30, 1935; the onset was on June 16 with malaise, fever, anorexia, and diarrhea. He was admitted June 23 in a toxic condition, with rose spots, typical appearance of the tongue, bronchitis, dicrotic pulse, slight abdominal distention, palpable spleen, and moderate deafness in both ears. On June 23 the red blood cells numbered 5,100,000; white blood cells, 8,900; neutrophiles, 76 per cent; lymphocytes, 18 per cent; monocytes, 6 per cent. On June 24 the blood culture was positive for typhoid organisms, and the Widal reaction was positive 1:20. With symptomatic treatment the temperature ranged

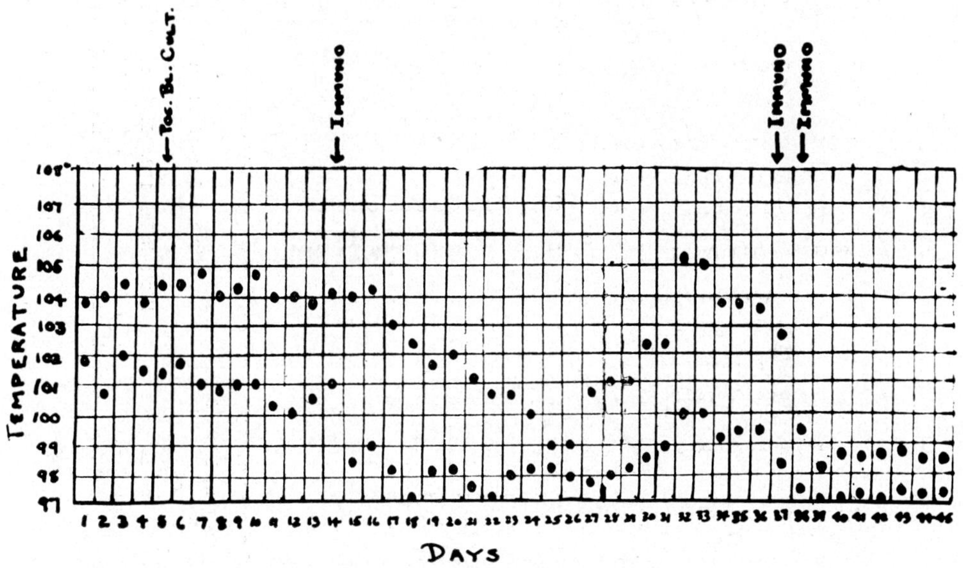

Chart 5.—Case 3. Severely toxic primary infection. One nonspecific immunotransfusion induced prompt symptomatic improvement but more gradual temperature drop. Recurrence followed by recovery after two additional nonspecific immunotransfusions.

from 101 to 105° F.; the patient was very toxic and irritable, had marked anorexia and moderate distention, and showed no signs of improvement. On the fourteenth day of illness, July 6, when the multiple index was 192, the first nonspecific immunotransfusion of 150 c.c. was given. There was no reaction, but the multiple index decreased to 32 within twenty-four hours, and the temperature became irregular and gradually defervesced to normal in nine days. The patient sat up and was no longer toxic or lethargic; his hearing was improved. This convalescence continued for approximately ten days when on the twenty-fourth day of illness, July 16, a relapse began. The temperature rose to 104° F. on July 27, with return of his previous toxicity and lethargy and a left shift in the hemogram from a multiple index of 12 to 128. On July 28 the second nonspecific immunotransfusion of 150 c.c. was given, followed by the third of 140 c.c. the next day. The temperature became normal in twenty-four hours, and the multiple index of the hemogram fell from 102 to 16. The urine and the feces were negative for typhoid organisms on August 6, and the patient was discharged Aug. 19, 1935.

Date 1935	Day of illness	Pos. blood culture	Nonsp. Imm. Transf.	C.C. of blood	Grams hemoglobin	Red blood cells	White blood cells	Multiple index Degrees of toxicity	Schilling index	Myelocytes	Juveniles	Stabs	Segmenters	Total neutrophiles	Lymphoblast	Large lymphs	Intermediate lymphs	Small lymphs	Total lymphs	Monocytes	Eosinophiles	Basophiles	Segmenters cmm	Total neutrophiles cmm	Totsl lymphs cmm	Monocytes cmm	
Date	Day	C	Tr	c.c.	Hb	RBC	WBC	MI	ShI	M	J	St	Sg	TN	Lb	L	I	S	TL	M	E	B	Sg	TN	TL	M	
					15.4	5.0	7500	1	1/16	0	0	4	64	68	0	5	1	20	26	4	2	0	4800	5000	2000	300	Normals
6-24	2	+			15	5.1	8900	155	9.7	0	0	78	8	86	2	2	0	10	14	0	0	0	712	7654	1246	000	
6-29	7				10	3.1	6000	208	13.0	0	0	80	6	86	4	2	2	6	14	0	0	0	516	5160	840	000	
7- 5	13				10	3.2	4200	48	3.0	0	0	60	20	80	0	8	0	12	20	0	0	0	840	3360	840	000	
7- 6	14		1	150	10	3.0	4500	192	12.0	0	0	72	6	78	0	6	0	16	22	0	0	0	270	3510	990	000	
7- 7	15				10	3.0	4300	32	2.0	0	0	40	20	60	0	12	0	18	30	8	2	0	860	2580	1290	344	
7- 9	17				10	3.0	4300	19	1.2	0	2	26	22	50	0	4	0	28	32	16	2	0	946	2159	1376	688	
7-11	19				12	3.4	3900	20	1.3	0	0	34	26	60	4	4	0	24	32	8	0	0	1014	2340	1248	312	
7-18	26				12	3.6	5000	12	3/4	0	0	34	40	74	0	16	2	6	24	2	0	0	2000	3700	1200	100	
7-22	30				13	4.3	8000	35	2.2	0	0	36	16	52	0	10	0	14	24	24	0	0	1280	4160	1920	1920	
7-24	32				13	4.3	7600	128	8.0	0	0	64	8	72	0	6	2	8	16	12	0	0	608	5472	1216	912	
7-28	36		2	150	13	4.2	8200	102	6.4	0	0	64	10	74	0	4	6	8	18	8	0	0	820	6068	1476	656	
7-29	37		3	150	13	4.4	11200	16	1.0	0	0	32	34	66	0	6	0	2	8	26	0	0	3808	7392	896	2912	
8- 2	41				13	4.3	10200	30	1.9	0	0	38	20	58	0	18	0	8	26	14	2	0	2040	5916	2652	1428	
8- 4	43				13	4.4	10400	14	7/8	0	0	30	34	64	0	8	2	24	34	1	1	0	3536	6656	3536	104	
8- 8	47				13	4.3	11300	24	1.5	0	0	36	22	58	0	12	0	28	40	0	2	0	2486	6554	4520	000	
8-14	53				13	4.4	9700	8	1/2	0	0	20	46	66	0	4	0	22	26	6	2	0	4462	6402	2522	582	
8-16	55				13	4.5	8400	10	2/3	0	2	24	36	62	0	10	0	20	30	4	2	2	3024	5208	2520	336	

Chart 6.—Case 3., V. A. Shiftogram of a case of typhoid fever illustrating wide alternating shifts to the left and right during the first thirteen days of illness. On the fourteenth day the first nonspecific immunotransfusion of 150 c.c. forced the shift right from a Schilling index of 12 to 2 and from a multiple index of 192 to 32, or reduced the toxicity from 192 to 32 degrees. The shift remained right for a period of eleven days, reaching the low multiple index of 12 on the twenty-sixth day of illness. On the twenty-sixth day a relapse began. The toxin forced the shift left during the next six days, reaching a Schilling index of 8 and a multiple index of 128 by the thirty-second day. The second nonspecific immunotransfusion was given four days later on the thirty-sixth day of illness, when the Schilling index was 6.4 and the multiple index 102. It forced the shift right in twenty-four hours to a Schilling index of 1 and a multiple index of 16, or reduced the toxicity of the patient from 102 to 16 degrees. The third nonspecific immunotransfusion was given the following day, the thirty-seventh day of illness, to reinforce the second. Together these treatments kept the shift right within convalescent limits and by overcoming the infection brought about recovery.

CASE 4.—R. D., white female, aged nine years, was exposed May 30, 1935. The onset was on June 10, with stiff neck, fever, headache, abdominal pain, and cough. She was admitted on June 22, with rose spots and typical appearance of tongue. On June 22 the red blood cells numbered 4,440,000; white blood cells, 10,200; neutrophiles, 54 per cent; lymphocytes, 42 per cent; and monocytes, 4 per cent. On June 24 the blood culture was positive for typhoid bacilli, and the Widal reaction was positive 1:320. With symptomatic treatment the temperature varied from 102 to 105.5° F., and there was moderate toxicity and abdominal distention. By July 4 the temperature became normal; the hemogramic shift went to the right to a multiple index of 8, and the patient was clinically well, remaining so for a week. On July 16 the temperature again rose, and the hemogramic shift started left in a relapse with a return of toxicity, drowsiness, and anorexia. By July 22 the temperature was 105° F.; the multiple index, 96; and the blood culture was again positive. The first nonspecific immunotransfusion of 150 c.c. was given on July 26 and was followed by

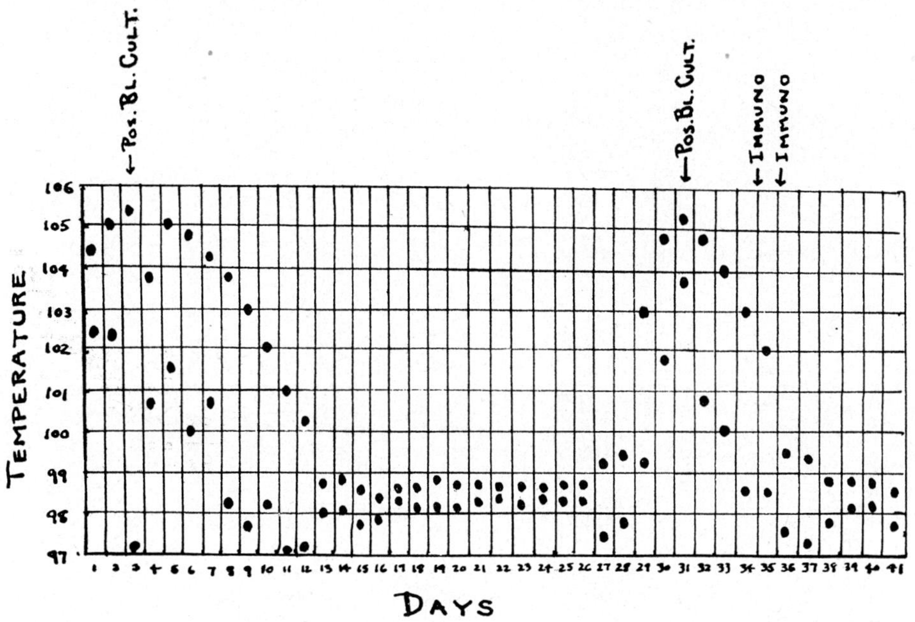

Chart 7.—Case 4. Moderately toxic patient in recurrence. Two nonspecific immunotransfusions followed by recovery.

a slight chill and a drop of the multiple index from 80 to 27 within twenty-four hours. The second nonspecific immunotransfusion of 150 c.c. was given the following day and caused a further drop in the multiple index from 27 to 16. Within the next twenty-four hours the temperature became normal; the signs of toxicity had disappeared; and the patient was clinically well. The urine and the feces were negative for typhoid bacilli on August 6, and the patient was discharged Aug. 17, 1935.

CASE 5.—J. F., white male, aged ten years, was exposed May 30, 1935; the onset was on June 15 with malaise, headache, anorexia, and epistaxis. He was admitted June 22 with tongue typical, spleen palpable and abdominal distention slight. On June 22 red blood cells numbered 5,140,000; white blood cells, 10,700; neutrophiles, 74 per cent; lymphocytes, 22 per cent, and monocytes, 4 per cent. The blood culture was positive for typhoid bacilli, and the Widal reaction was positive 1:80 on June 24. The patient rapidly became worse, the temperature remaining from 103 to 106° F.; he was very toxic and stuporous. Intravenous glucose and saline were used for sev-

Date 1935	Day of illness	Pos. blood culture	Nonsp. Imm. Transf.	C.C. of blood	Grams hemoglobin	Red blood cells	White blood cells	Multiple index Degrees of toxicity	Schilling index	Myelocytes	Juveniles	Stabs	Segmenters	Total neutrophiles	Lymphoblasts	Large lymphs	Intermediate lymphs	Small lymphs	Total lymphs	Monocytes	Eosinophiles	Basophiles	Segmenters cmm	Total neutrophiles cmm	Total lymphs cmm	Monocytes cmm	
Date	Day	C	Tr	c.c.	Hb	RBC	WBC	MI	ShI	M	J	St	Sg	Tn	Lb	L	I	S	TL	M	E	B	Sg	TN	TL	M	
					15.4	5.0	7500	1	1/16	0	0	4	64	68	0	5	1	20	26	4	2	0	4800	5000	2000	300	Normals
							Sh.I.	15	12	9	6	3 2	1½ 0														
6-24	3	+			14.0	4.4	10200	72	4.5	0	2	52	12	66	2	0	0	24	26	8	0	0	1224	6732	2652	816	
6-29	8				14.0	4.5	8200	64	4.0	0	0	48	12	60	4	12	4	16	36	4	0	0	984	4920	2952	328	
7- 2	11				14.0	4.4	8600	33	2.1	0	0	26	12	38	2	14	0	26	42	20	0	0	1036	3268	3612	1720	
7- 4	13				14.0	4.3	7600	8	1/2	0	0	20	40	60	0	6	0	30	36	4	0	0	3040	4560	2736	304	
7-10	20				14.0	4.2	7400	5	1/3	0	0	16	48	64	0	4	2	26	32	4	0	0	3552	4736	2368	296	
7-16	26				13.0	3.8	7100	6	2/5	0	0	20	50	70	0	2	0	24	26	4	0	0	3550	4970	1846	284	
7-22	32	+			13.0	3.8	8000	80	5.0	0	0	50	10	60	4	4	2	20	30	10	0	0	800	4800	2400	800	
7-25	35				13.0	3.7	7200	96	6.0	0	0	36	6	42	4	8	2	36	50	8	0	0	432	3024	3600	576	
7-26	36		1	150	13.0	3.7	10100	80	5.0	0	0	40	8	48	0	2	0	50	52	0	0	0	808	4848	5252	000	
7-27	37		2	150	13.0	3.6	6100	27	1.7	0	0	24	14	38	2	2	0	54	58	4	0	0	854	2318	3538	244	
7-28	38				13.0	3.8	10300	16	1.0	0	0	16	16	32	0	2	0	56	58	6	4	0	1648	3296	5974	618	
7-31	41				13.0	3.7	11800	17	1.1	0	0	18	16	34	2	46	0	16	64	2	0	0	1888	4012	7552	236	
8- 2	43				13.0	3.8	10600	12	3/4	0	0	18	22	40	0	2	0	40	42	18	0	0	2332	4240	4452	1908	
8-14	55				14.0	4.2	10000	16	1.0	0	0	20	20	40	0	12	0	42	54	4	2	0	2000	4000	5400	400	

Chart 8.—Case 4., R. D. Shiftogram of a patient with typhoid fever, illustrating a spontaneous right shift to convalescence after the first week of illness; a wide left shift indicating a relapse on the thirty-second day; two nonspecific immunotransfusions of 150 c.c. each on the thirty-sixth and thirty-seventh days, followed by a right shift to convalescence and recovery.

eral days; then tube feeding was started and continued for fifty-three days. Between June 25 and July 12 he received nine intramuscular injections of human specific immune serum, which produced no clinical improvement. Two ordinary blood transfusions had also been given with no effect on the clinical condition. On July 12 the

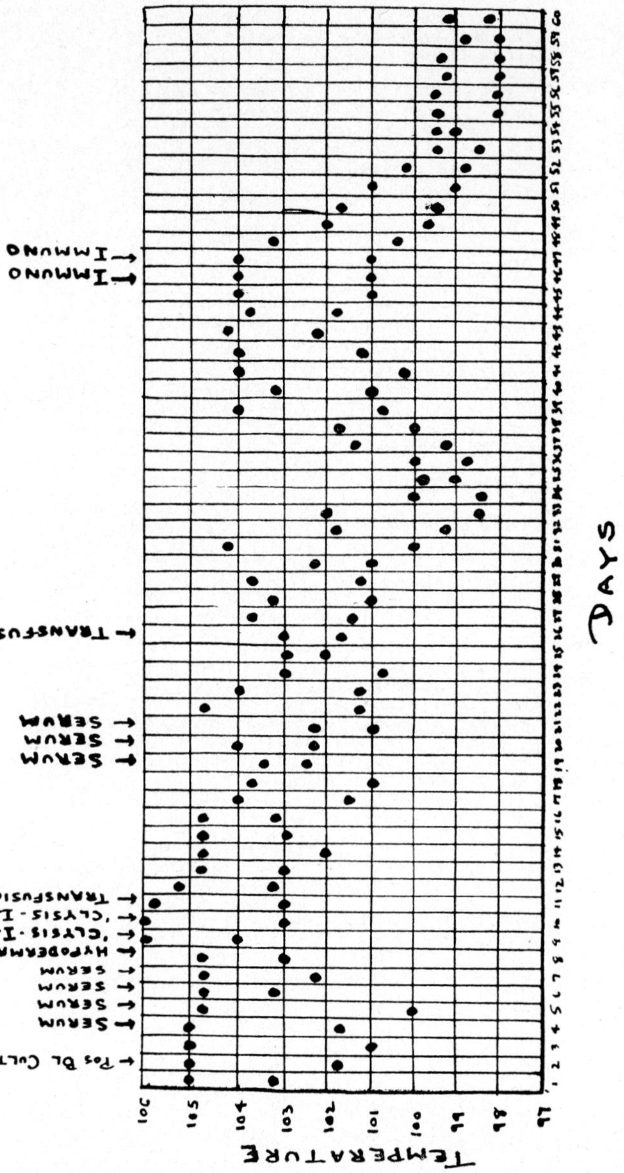

Chart 9.—Case 5. Severely toxic primary infection with temporary improvement followed by equally severe recurrence of symptoms. No response to various types of treatment until nonspecific immunotransfusions were given, which were followed by recovery. Transfusion refers to the ordinary type.

patient developed nuchal rigidity, positive Brudzinski reflex, ankle clonus, and bilateral positive Babinski reflex, but the spinal fluid cell count, smear, and culture were all negative. The hemogramic shift went left from 8 on July 12 to 70 on July 29. There was slight clinical improvement with a drop in temperature from July 21 until July 29, although he was still stuporous and required tube feeding. On July 29 the temperature rose to 104° F., and the multiple index to 70, with a return of the extremely toxic stuporous stage accompanied by marked diarrhea. On August 6 the

Date 1935	Day of illness	Pos. Blood culture	Nonsp. imm. Trans.	C.C. of blood	Grams hemoglobin	Red blood cells	White blood cells	Multiple index Degrees of toxicity	Schilling index	Myelocytes	Juveniles	Stabs	Segmenters	Total neutrophiles	Lymphoblasts	Large lymphs	Intermediate lymphs	Small lymphs	Total lymphs	Monocytes	Eosinophiles	Basophiles	Segmenters cmm	Total neutrophiles cmm	Total lymphos cmm	Monocytes cmm	
Date	Day	C	Tr	c.c.	Hb	RBC	WBC	MI	ShI	M	J	St	Sg	TN	Lb	L	I	S	TL	M	E	B	Sg	TN	TL	M	
					15.4	5.0	7500	1	1/16	0	0	4	64	68	0	5	0	20	26	4	2	0	4800	5000	2000	300	Normals
							ShI	15	12	9	6	3 2	1 1/2 0														
6-22	1				15.0	5.1	10200	40	2.5	0	0	50	20	70	0	10	0	10	20	10	0	0	2040	7140	2040	1020	
6-24	3	+			15.0	5.1	10700	27	1.7	0	0	48	28	76	0	8	0	6	14	10	0	0	2996	8132	1498	1070	
7- 2	11				13.0	3.8	7000	27	1.7	0	2	40	24	66	0	8	0	18	26	8	0	0	1680	4620	1820	560	
7- 5	14				13.0	3.7	9100	8	1/2	0	0	8	16	24	0	40	0	8	48	28	0	0	1456	2184	4368	2548	
7- 9	18				13.0	3.4	6200	10	2/3	0	0	26	38	64	2	2	0	2	6	30	0	0	2356	3968	372	1860	
7-11	20				10.0	2.5	9600	8	1/2	0	0	14	30	44	0	6	0	42	48	2	4	2	2880	4224	4608	192	
7-25	34				11.0	3.0	10850	16	1.0	0	0	24	22	46	0	30	0	8	38	16	0	0	2376	4968	4104	1728	
7-26	35				12.0	3.2	9000	40	2.5	0	2	28	12	42	4	16	0	18	38	20	0	0	1080	3780	3420	1800	
7-29	38				13.0	3.5	11400	70	4.4	0	6	56	14	76	0	6	0	6	12	12	0	0	1596	8664	1368	1368	
8- 6	46		1	215	13.0	3.8	9300	67	4.2	0	6	54	14	74	0	4	0	8	12	14	0	0	1302	6882	1116	1302	
8- 7	47		2	170	14.0	4.6	14700	36	2.3	0	0	46	20	66	0	16	0	14	30	4	0	0	2940	9702	4410	588	
8- 8	48				14.0	4.6	11200	33	2.1	0	0	48	22	70	0	6	0	16	22	8	0	0	2464	7840	2464	896	
8- 9	49				14.0	4.6	9500	38	2.4	0	0	34	14	48	0	0	0	42	42	6	2	2	1288	4416	3990	570	
8-10	50				14.0	4.8	8100	36	2.3	0	0	42	18	60	0	4	0	30	34	6	0	0	1458	4860	2754	486	
8-14	54				14.0	4.7	10100	38	2.4	0	0	34	14	48	0	6	0	42	48	4	0	0	1414	4848	4848	404	
8-16	56				14.0	4.7	7300	33	2.1	0	0	34	16	50	0	20	0	18	38	10	2	0	1168	3650	2774	730	
9- 9	80				15.0	4.9	12200	28	1.8	0	0	22	12	34	0	10	0	44	54	10	2	0	1464	4148	6588	1220	
9-11	82				15.0	4.9	10100	16	1.0	0	0	20	20	40	0	14	8	20	42	14	4	0	2020	4040	4242	1414	

Chart 10.—Case 5., J. F. Shiftogram of a patient with typhoid fever, illustrating a relapse on the thirty-eighth day as indicated by a left shift to a Schilling index of 4.4 and multiple index of 70. Two nonspecific immunotransfusions of 215 and 170 c.c. were given on the forty-sixth and forty-seventh days, forcing the shift sharply to the right from a multiple index of 67 to 33 and a Schilling index of 4.2 to 2.1 in forty-eight hours, where it wavered for a week and then shifted right to recovery.

first nonspecific immunotransfusion was given with no definite reaction, and it was repeated the next day, a total of 385 c.c. being given. Following these treatments, the temperature began to fall and reached normal in three days. The multiple index of the hemogram dropped from 67 to 33. Improvement was marked; stupor decreased; diarrhea disappeared; he took some food by mouth and talked rationally. Convalescence was then uninterrupted. The urine and the feces were negative August 20, and the patient was discharged Sept. 11, 1935.

DISCUSSION OF THE LITERATURE ON THE TREATMENT OF TYPHOID FEVER

The medical profession of this country for the past twenty-five years or more has been concerned with typhoid fever chiefly from the standpoint of its prevention. This work has been so successful that there have been but few epidemics large enough to offer opportunities for advancement in the treatment of the disease. The greatest improvement in typhoid fever therapy in this country was the introduction of the high caloric diet in place of the old time regimen of "starving the fever."

In Europe, on the other hand, there have been and still are fairly frequent epidemics, and in recent years much work has been done there in attempting to find a specific treatment for the disease. The following chemical and biological products have been used with varying degrees of success:

Drugs—neoarsphenamine, quinine bismuth iodide, alkalies, insulin, peptone intramuscularly, epinephrine, thymus extracts, sodium salicylate, amidopyrine, colloidal silver, strophanthin, barium chloride, atropine, sulphur, milk injections, salyrgan, methenamine, and mercurochrome.

Biologicals—antivirus, bacteriophage, Rodet's serum, autohemotherapy, typhoid vaccine (subcutaneous, intracutaneous, intravenous) antityphoid horse serum, and specific immunotransfusions.

The best results published on the treatment of typhoid fever have been with biologicals, especially with bacteriophage and specific immunotransfusions. The most extensive work with these methods has been done by the French clinicians. Bacteriophage was the earlier method. It was found to be of definite value by Manoussakis,[8] who reviewed work done by other Frenchmen with the same method. Its chief value was in carriers and in prolonged cases which were refractive to ordinary treatment.

More recent interest has been developed in the so-called specific immunotransfusions,* in which the donor has been a patient who has re-

*Our understanding of the types of transfusions to which we have referred is the following:

1. An ordinary transfusion is one in which the donor's blood is used in its natural state, with no special treatment of the donor before the transfusion. It may be given by the direct or indirect method.

2. A specific immunotransfusion[18] is one in which the donor has obtained a specific active immunity against the disease affecting the patient by having had and recovered from that disease or in which the donor is given an artificial active immunity by single or repeated subcutaneous or intramuscular injections of killed or attenuated organisms specific for the disease from which the patient is suffering.[8]

3. A nonspecific immunotransfusion is one in which the donor is given an intravenous injection of some foreign protein which causes a maximum increase in opsonins or nonspecific immune bodies in his serum in approximately eight hours. Fifty million killed typhoid or mixed typhoid and paratyphoid A and B organisms is a standard, safe, and effective dose of foreign protein.

covered from typhoid fever or someone who has been vaccinated against the disease within the year preceding the time of the transfusion. The original work in this field was done by Tzanck,[9] who with Tremolieres published a detailed report of ten cases so treated. Their studies have been confirmed by DeSize,[10] Villaret, Justin-Besançon and Desoille,[11] Roueche,[12] and Eschbach.[13] This type of therapy was also used in prolonged cases and in those requiring transfusion because of marked intestinal hemorrhage.

Grassat[14] in South Africa has used a specially prepared concentrated horse serum intramuscularly in 130 cases of typhoid fever with a drop in temperature to normal within five or six days and with clinical improvement. Spiropoulos[15] reports the use of typhoid vaccine given intravenously in fifty cases of typhoid fever with a resultant drop in temperature and with no after-effects.

Typhoid vaccine has been used subcutaneously by Crough[16] in patients already infected, but his conclusions were that to get a decrease in duration and severity of the disease the three immunizing doses must be given before the onset of symptoms. This obviously limits its use to those patients definitely known to have been exposed. Daily doses of typhoid vaccine detoxicated with formalin and phenol were given by Wherry, LeBlanc, Foshay, and Thomas[17] early in the disease with shortening of the course but no immediate results.

COMMENT

This series of patients has served the purpose of demonstrating the variability of the clinical picture of typhoid fever in children even when all extrinsic factors are similar, especially as regards the classical symptoms.

The diagnosis is easily established through laboratory methods after the disease is suggested by a history of prolonged fever with no other definite cause and the presence of a few characteristic physical signs. Those patients who showed only fever, malaise, and anorexia might not have been hospitalized or correctly diagnosed had not the parents been made "typhoid conscious" by the newspaper publicity given to the epidemic.

The mildness of the disease in the majority of these patients and their response to symptomatic medical treatment must not be misleading because typhoid fever in children can be a serious disease. Several children infected in this epidemic and admitted to other hospitals in the city died because of the overwhelming toxemia. Patient 5 is an example of the classical "typhoid state" occurring in a child.

It was the markedly toxic patients with continued high temperature, abdominal distention, apathy, stupor, and an alarming shift to the left in the Schilling hemogram to a multiple index close to 100 or above which induced us to seek a more effective form of therapy for this disease. The five patients receiving the nonspecific immunotransfusions ranged in toxicity from 2+ to 5+ and, clinically, included the sickest children on the ward. The charts clearly show the marked drop in temperature range and the extensive shift to the right in the hemograms after treatment in all five patients. Clinically, at the same time, their decrease in toxicity was shown by disappearance of lethargy, increase in appetite, lessening of diarrhea, and decrease of abdominal distention. Patient 3 suffered a relapse after a single nonspecific immunotransfusion but recovered quickly following two more similar treatments given on successive days.

The acutely ill patients responded as readily to this type of therapy whether treated in the early stages of the disease or after prolonged illness. Patients 1 and 4, who had had positive blood cultures a few days before receiving the nonspecific immunotransfusions, had the greatest reactions in the form of chill and elevation of temperature immediately after being given the blood, and they showed the most rapid improvement clinically. Usually patients do not have a temperature reaction following nonspecific immunotransfusions.

Ordinary blood transfusions have been used in the treatment of typhoid fever many times in the past but never with any apparent direct effect. There was not a sufficient number of severely infected patients in this series to afford controls in which ordinary transfusions might have been used. Patient 5, however, received two ordinary transfusions during the course of his illness, with no improvement, but convalesced quickly following two nonspecific immunotransfusions.

There were no deleterious effects noted in either the donor or patient during the use of this procedure, the elevated temperature reactions in the patient being easily controlled by tepid sponges.

Review of the literature on the treatment of typhoid fever revealed nothing which held great promise of immediate good results in the acute form of the disease or which could be prepared and given as quickly and conveniently, economically, and safely as nonspecific immunotransfusion therapy.

SUMMARY

1. An epidemic of typhoid fever is reported.

2. Nineteen children simultaneously infected were treated for typhoid fever.

3. All patients received high caloric diet therapy.

4. Six patients were treated with intramuscular injections of specific immune human serum with no marked effect.

5. Five very ill patients were given nonspecific immunotransfusion therapy with immediate marked improvement followed by recovery, this being the first time this form of treatment has been employed in typhoid fever.

6. The literature on the treatment of typhoid fever is discussed.

CONCLUSIONS

While this series of patients is too small to justify conclusions regarding the relative merits of the different forms of therapy employed it may, perhaps, suggest that the mild form of typhoid fever in children may be amenable to high caloric diet therapy, that specific immune human serum given intramuscularly may not be fairly judged on so few patients, and that nonspecific immunotransfusion therapy in typhoid fever in children deserves continued usage when opportunity occurs, as, we believe, it has given promise of being a very helpful form of treatment in this disease.

REFERENCES

1. Crocker, Walter J., Valentine, E. H., and Brody, W.: J. Lab. & Clin. Med. **20**: 482, 1935.
2. Colebrook, L., and Storer, E. J.: Lancet **2**: 1341, and 1394, 1923.
3. Wright, A. E.: Lancet **1**: 480, 1919.
4. Stephensen, R.: J. A. M. A. **100**: 100, 1933.
5. Kottke, E. E.: J. Iowa State M. Soc. **24**: 431, 1934.
6. Ersner, M. S., and Meyer, D.: Laryngoscope, May, 1934.
7. Crocker, Walter J., and Valentine, E. H.: J. Lab. & Clin. Med. **20**: 172, 1934.
8. Manoussakis, E.: J. de méd. de Paris **52**: 722, 1932.
9. Tremolieres, F., and Tzanck, A.: Bull. et mém. Soc. méd. d. Hôp. de Paris **54**: 1606, 1930.
10. De Size, S.: Clinique, Paris **29**: 155, 1934.
11. Villaret, M., Justin-besançon, L., and Desoille, H.: Progrès méd. December 26, p. 2350, 1931.
12. Roueche, H.: La Medicine **13**: 609, 1932.
13. Eschbach, M. E.: J. de méd. de Paris **53**: 528, 1933.
14. Grassat, E.: J. M. A. S. Africa **4**: 380, 1930.
15. Spiropoulos, N.: Arch. de Med. des Enfants, Paris **29**: 150, 1926.
16. Crough, J. H.: J. Med. **12**: 373, 1931.
17. Wherry, W. B., LeBlanc, T. J., Foshay, L., and Thomas, R.: J. Infect. Dis. **43**: 189, 1928.
18. Brody, W., and Crocker, Walter J.: J. A. M. A. **98**: 2191, 1932.

DYSENTERY BACILLEMIA

PHILLIP E. ROTHMAN, M.D.
LOS ANGELES, CALIF.

THE occurrence of a recent case of sepsis due to the dysentery bacillus has prompted this review of similar cases for the purpose of evaluating their clinical significance. For over a decade after the isolation of the dysentery bacillus, it was generally believed that the organism produced an infection strictly localized to the intestine and adjacent lymph glands. This opinion was originally stated by Shiga and reemphasized by Jochman as late as 1911. In the 1908 edition of Jordan's *General Bacteriology*[1] the following statement is made concerning the presence of the dysentery bacillus: "It is found at autopsy in the mesenteric glands, but, as a rule not in the spleen or other internal organs, nor does it occur in the blood or urine." In 1912 Darling and Bates[2] reported a case with a positive blood culture, and since then twelve additional cases have been recorded. Glynn[3] has pointed out that an analogous situation exists in the history of typhoid fever. He calls attention to Osler's statement in the first edition of his book in 1892 concerning the rarity of the typhoid bacillus in the blood. Subsequent investigations altered his opinion, and in the 1912 edition is the observation that the presence of the bacillus may be demonstrated in the blood of practically all cases. Undoubtedly more cases of dysentery sepsis have occurred than appear on record but not in sufficient number to make tenable this attempted analogy with typhoid fever.

The following case was observed at the Children's Hospital:

A white girl, aged two years, was admitted with a history of diarrhea of five days' duration. The past history contained no significant facts. The present illness began abruptly with fever and diarrhea. On the third day, blood appeared in the stools, which numbered six to eight a day. Her condition failed to improve, and on admission, two days later, she was moderately dehydrated and obviously ill. The history apparently justified a preliminary diagnosis of bacillary dysentery. It was noticed at this time that the cardiac pulsations were unusually forcible and the heart sounds increased in intensity. In the absence of evidence of organic heart disease, no special significance was attached to these findings. During the next two days, the temperature fluctuated between 101° and 106° F. Intravenous fluids and a blood transfusion were administered, and the usual dietary and hygienic measures were instituted. Although sepsis was not suspected, a blood culture was obtained on the day following admission, because the blood transfusion provided a favorable opportunity and because we were at a loss to explain the severity of the illness. The diarrhea was mild and no blood was observed in the stools. Two days after admission marked abdominal distention and facial edema were noted. The bladder was not distended although the nurses reported that no urine had been voided during the previous forty-eight hours. (Such reports are not always reliable as a child wearing diapers may void small quantities without detection.) The character of the radial pulse strongly suggested an elevation of blood pressure. The determi-

From the Children's Hospital.

nation first made at this time was 138 systolic over 70 diastolic. Attempts at catheterization were unsuccessful because of an anomalous opening of the urethra into the vagina. Because of this malformation, it was thought that additional abnormalities of the kidneys or urinary tract probably existed with a resulting terminal hypertension and renal failure. The patient became comatose a few hours preceding death on the eighth day of her illness.

Laboratory Reports.—Blood count (seventh day), hemoglobin, 38 per cent; red blood cells, 4,350,000; white blood cells, 30,800; polymorphonuclear cells, 92 per cent; lymphocytes, 3 per cent; monocytes, 4 per cent; premyelocytes, 1 per cent; neutrophiles contained toxic changes.

Nonprotein nitrogen (eighth day) was 55 mg. per 100 c.c.

Blood culture (seventh day) produced *B. dysenteriae* (Flexner). Growth was very slow and appeared after one week. Agglutination with a known antiserum was positive in a dilution of 1:640.

Culture from the large intestine at autopsy produced *B. dysenteriae* (Flexner). Agglutination in a dilution of 1:320 was secured only after transplants in veal infusion broth had been made for ten days.

Autopsy Report (Dr. C. M. Hyland).—The examination showed evidence of a generalized anasarca with small amounts of fluid in the peritoneal and pleural cavities. The large intestine showed prominent lymphoid follicles with edema and cellular infiltration of the mucosal stroma. In a few places the superficial portions of the mucosa had desquamated and the remaining mucosa beneath these areas gave evidence of early necrosis. No areas of marked ulceration were found. Strangely enough, similar changes were found in the small intestine and were slightly more prominent. The mesenteric lymph glands were enlarged. The kidney sections stained with hematoxylin and eosin showed swollen glomerular tufts with proliferation of the cells covering these tufts. The capillaries were engorged. Many of the convoluted tubules contained casts, and there was considerable destruction of the lining epithelium. No scar tissue was evident. Azan carmine stains showed in addition to the above lesions, a thickening of the basement membrane of the glomerular tufts. The picture was that of an acute nephritis involving principally the glomeruli. There were no abnormalities other than the anomalous opening of the urethra into the vagina. This apparently produced no obstruction to the flow of urine.

Final Diagnosis.—Bacillary dysentery, dysentery septicemia, acute nephritis with hypertension and renal failure.

Darling and Bates[2] described a patient observed in Panama. He was an adult negro, acutely ill with a temperature of 101° F., abdominal pain and a bloody diarrhea. There were marked tenderness over the colon and enlargement of the liver and spleen. The course was unusually severe and characterized by large hemorrhages from the bowel. The blood culture on the seventh day was positive for *B. dysenteriae* (Shiga), which was agglutinated in a dilution of 1:2,000. Death occurred on the tenth day of illness. Autopsy showed the usual diphtheritic inflammatory process from the rectum to the ileocecal valve with isolated gangrenous areas.

Kendall and Day[4] reported the case of a girl, aged five years, who was ill for three days with fever, obstinate vomiting, and bloody diarrhea. The illness was unusually severe and the patient markedly prostrated. The stool culture was positive for *B. dysenteriae* (Shiga). The blood culture obtained two days before death revealed *B. dysenteriae* (Shiga), paratyphoid beta, Morgan bacillus, *B. alkaligines,* and streptococci.

De Sautelle's patient,[5] the youngest on record, was a three-week-old breast-fed infant, ill for two days with a temperature of 105° F. The grandmother was ill with typhoid fever in the same house, and for that reason a blood culture was taken. This was positive for the dysentery organism (type not stated). The temperature remained high, and a watery diarrhea developed. After one week, a severe convulsion occurred, and spinal puncture revealed bloody fluid which on culture was positive for the dysentery bacillus. Death occurred shortly after the convulsion.

Ghon and Roman[6] reported five cases of dysentery sepsis in soldiers aged twenty to twenty-six years. All cases resembled mild typhoid. Typical diarrhea with blood and mucus was not present. Enlargement of the spleen occurred in three cases and an eruption similar to typhoid in two cases. The blood culture was positive for the "Y" dysentery organism in all cases on the third or fourth day of the disease. In one patient the urine culture was positive for Shiga organism. In only one individual was the stool culture positive.

Fränkel[7] reported a patient who presented a clinical picture suggestive of a mild but protracted case of typhoid. The strain cultured from the patient's blood agglutinated with the "Y" dysentery test serum in a dilution of 1:16,000.

Ledingham and Penfold's patient[8] had fever of five weeks' duration during which time *B. paratyphosus A* was recovered from the blood stream. An exacerbation occurred at the end of this period and a subsequent blood culture produced *B. dysenteriae* (Shiga). The patient had previously suffered with attacks of diarrhea and was considered a dysentery carrier. They believed that the intestinal lesion produced by the paratyphoid infection more readily permitted the dysentery organism to invade the blood stream. Recovery followed after twenty-three days, and during this time there was no return of blood or mucus in the dejecta.

TenBroeck's case[9] was a male infant, ill for two days, with marked prostration and a temperature of 105° F. Typhoid was suspected, and a blood culture was taken. *B. dysenteriae* (Flexner) was obtained on two occasions. Later the stools became typical of dysentery although repeated cultures were negative. The patient eventually recovered after a long illness.

Brünauer's patient[10] was a twenty-eight-year-old man, ill with fever, diarrhea, vomiting, and abdominal pain. The spleen was enlarged and a "typhoidlike" eruption was present. Blood culture on the twelfth day was positive for the "Y" dysentery. The course simulated typhoid and at the end of a month he was fever free.

Boyd[11] observed a patient while serving with the Salonika Force during the World War. The illness was of four days' duration and characterized by vomiting and bloody diarrhea. Blood and stool cultures produced the Flexner "Y" organism. The patient was sent back to the base, and no additional history was obtained. There were no symptoms that differed from the ordinary case of bacillary dysentery.

Through the courtesy of Dr. Arthur Black, the reports of three unpublished cases from the Peiping Union Medical College have been forwarded to me. The first case occurred in a Chinese male infant, aged one year, who was admitted with a history of a bloody diarrhea of four days' duration. The frequency of the bowel movements had progressively increased and amounted to about forty in a twenty-four-hour period. He was critically ill and markedly dehydrated. The temperature fluctuated between 39 and 40.4° C. The blood count on admission showed 5,540,000 red cells; hemoglobin, 14 gm., white blood cells, 30,450, with 80 per cent polymorphonuclear cells. Twelve hours before death the leucocytes numbered 45,500. One stool culture on the day of admission produced the Shiga organism. A blood culture obtained directly from the heart immediately postmortem also produced the Shiga organism.

The other two cases occurred in adults, and the records for a detailed report were not obtained from the general medical service. One patient was a Chinese male, aged thirty-two years, who died three days after an operation for an acute appendicitis. Blood culture, a day before death, produced *B. dysenteriae* of the mannite-fermenting group. The other case was a Chinese female, aged thirty-one years, admitted because of symptoms of sepsis following an induced abortion. Blood culture produced *B. dysenteriae* of the mannite-fermenting group. The patient recovered.

The following sentence from Dr. Black's communication is of interest: "In view of the fact that the number of cases of bacillary dysentery admitted to the hospital every year on all services ranges around three to four hundred with many times that number seen in the out-patient department, and, since the hospital has been open since 1922 with only these three cases, it is certainly clear that dysentery bacteremias are not common."

DISCUSSION

The similarity to mild typhoid of nine of the thirteen cases previously reported deserves comment. Several of these patients had splenic enlargement and a typhoidlike eruption. Severe diarrhea with blood and mucus was rarely present. The temperature curve and duration of illness were consistent with typhoid fever. The resemblance has led several authors to state that this clinical picture is characteristic of dysentery sepsis. A more plausible explanation suggested by Ledingham and Penfold is the possibility of a mixed infection. Their case was one due to *B. parathyphosus A* followed by an acute exacerbation due to the

Shiga organism. Some of the cases mentioned herein reported by European writers occurred in soldiers during the World War, and statistics collected by Wolko[12] in 1915 indicate the frequent occurrence of mixed typhoid and dysentery infections in the German and Austrian reserve hospitals. Unfortunately this very satisfactory explanation lacks complete serologic confirmation. The cases reported by Boyd, Kendall and Day, Darling and Bates, and the case of the infant described by Dr. Black conform to the usual picture of severe dysentery. DeSautelle's case is the only one that clinically suggests sepsis. Despite the paucity of clinical data in some of the above reports, it is permissible to conclude that the presence of the dysentery organism in the circulating blood fails to produce any characteristic signs or symptoms that would enable one to arrive at even a tentative diagnosis without the necessity of laboratory aid. Of the seventeen cases now on record, including my own, there were six deaths. The series is too small to be certain that the presence of sepsis increases the mortality. In regard to this point it is of interest that in the records of the Children's Hospital, the most fulminating type of dysentery, in which death occurs within twenty-four or forty-eight hours after the onset, has not been accompanied by sepsis. The presence of sepsis does apparently favor the occurrence of complications. This is evident in Elsworthy's case[13] of postdysentery arthritis. De Sautelle's case with meningeal involvement, Gunn's case[14] of pneumonia in which the dysentery organism was isolated, Brünauer's case with a thrombophlebitis of the left crural vein, and my case with an acute nephritis.

The relatively insignificant necropsy findings in some of the cases with sepsis has been discussed by several authors. The origin of the intestinal lesions, as proved many years ago by Flexner and Sweet,[15] is due to the act of elimination of the toxin by the intestinal mucosa and not by the direct effect of the bacteria upon the surface of the mucous membrane. Their experiments on the comparative toxicity of living, dead, and autolysed cultures showed that the separated toxin is more effective than the same quantity of poison contained within the living or dead bacilli. The presence of living organisms in the blood is in itself of only secondary significance in the production of intestinal lesions. The latter depend on the amount of liberated toxin and its excretion by successive acts of elimination through the intestinal wall.

There is on record a considerable amount of evidence to support the contention that the dysentery organism invades the blood stream more frequently than is ordinarily believed. Many observers have obtained pure cultures of the bacteria from the heart's blood, spleen, liver, or bile at autopsy in patients who died with bacillary dysentery. Instances of this nature are enumerated in the article by Ghon and Roman and also in the review by Davison.[16] Typical examples are contained in the reports of Gunn,[14] Caussade and Marbais,[17] Rosenthal,[18] and Baerthlein and Huwald.[19] These cases are subject to criticism as postmortem blood cultures are notoriously unreliable. Nevertheless, Gunn states definitely, "It is customary to accept a positive postmortem spleen culture, even in the case of motile bacteria, as evidence that a bacteremia had existed during life."

Positive cultures during life from the urine of male patients represent presumptive evidence of an existing bacteremia if one can exclude the possibility of contamination through feces. Brünauer has reported four cases, one of which occurred during convalescence from typhoid and another during a coexisting dysentery and paratyphoid infection. Fränkel observed one case in a series of thirty-six routine urine cultures.

The organism has been cultured from the joint fluid in a case of postdysentery arthritis by Elsworthy. In a somewhat similar case, Clifford[20] found dysentery agglutinins in the joint fluid of a boy with chronic arthritis although no history of an attack of dysentery could be obtained and cultures from the joint fluid and stools were negative.

Although cases of dysentery septicemia are undoubtedly overlooked, routine blood cultures have proved very disappointing. Dudgeon[21] and his coworkers made blood cultures on 145 cases of acute dysentery in Macedonia during the war but failed to recover the organism. Fränkel made 49 blood cultures and in only one case obtained a pure culture of the "Y" dysentery bacillus. Kessel,[22] at the Los Angeles County Hospital, made 60 blood cultures with completely negative results. TenBroeck made bacteriologic studies of various organs at autopsy in 14 cases of dysentery with negative results. These figures corroborate the prevailing opinion concerning the rarity of dysentery septicemia and emphasize that the presence of the organism in the peripheral blood is of no practical aid in diagnosis.

REFERENCES

1. Jordan, E. O.: General Bacteriology, Philadelphia, 1908, W. B. Saunders Co.
2. Darling, S. T., and Bates, L. B.: Am. J. M. Sc. **143**: 36, 1912.
3. Glynn, E., and others: Report upon 2,360 Enteritis "Convalescents" Received at Liverpool From Various Expeditionary Forces, Medical Research Committee Special Report Series No. 7, 1917.
4. Kendall, A. I., and Day, A. A.: Boston M. & S. J. **169**: 741, 1913.
5. De Sautelle, W. T.: J. A. M. A. **63**: 1853, 1914.
6. Ghon, A., and Roman, B.: Wien. klin. Wchnschr. No. 22, 579, 1915.
7. Fränkel, E.: Deutsche med. Wchnschr. **41**: 1182, 1915.
8. Ledingham, J. C. G., and Penfold, W. J.: Brit. M. J. **11**: 704, 1915.
9. TenBroeck, C.: Boston M. & S. J. **173**: 284, 1915.
10. Brünauer, S. R.: Wien. klin. Wchnschr. No. 5, 128, 1916.
11. Boyd, J. S. K.: Lancet **2**: 482, 1919.
12. Wolko, Karl: Wien. klin. Wchnschr. **9**: 236, 1915.
13. Elsworthy: Nelson Loose-Leaf Medicine **11**: 169, Part I, 1923.
14. Gunn, F. D.: Bull. Buffalo General Hosp. **4**: 3, 1926.
15. Flexner, S., and Sweet, J. E.: J. Exper. Med. **8**: 514, 1906.
16. Davison, W. C.: Medicine **1**: 389, 1922.
17. Caussade, G., and Marbais, S.: Bull. et mém. Soc. méd. d. hôp. de Paris, No. 7-8, 145, 1919 (cited by Boyd).
18. Rosenthal, L.: Deutsche med. Wchnschr. **6**: 98, 1903 (cited by Boyd).
19. Baerthlein, K., and Huwald, W.: Deutsche med. Wchnschr. **10**: 478, 1914.
20. Clifford, S. H.: Am. J. Dis. Child. **32**: 72, 1926.
21. Dudgeon, L. S.: A System of Bacteriology, Med. Research Council **4**: 201, 1929.
22. Kessel, J. F.: Personal communication.

3875 Wilshire Boulevard

SCLERODERMA

Report of a Case With Sclerodactylia and Hemiatrophy

Robert H. McCrackin, M.D.
Edea, Cameroun,
West Africa

Although cases of scleroderma, or hidebound skin, presenting the clinical picture of the adult type have been reported at all ages in life, from Cockayne's case[1] in a seven-month-old infant with scleroderma and sclerodactylia of the adult type with some fibrous myositis (of antenatal origin) to the commoner time for its occurrence during the later decades in life, it is a rare condition, particularly in children.

Some conception of the low incidence of scleroderma in children can be obtained from the fact that Dr. Howard Fox[2] went through the records of about 5,800 cases of miscellaneous diseases at the Nursery and Child's Hospital and found only one case of scleroderma. This case occurred in an infant, and since biopsy was not performed, he felt the condition could not possibly be differentiated from sclerema. He found that the records of about 75,000 skin diseases at the University of Bellevue Clinic contained only one case of scleroderma in a child, a boy, aged fourteen years, in whom the condition had been present since infancy.

DEFINITION AND ETIOLOGY

Scleroderma is described by Ormsby[3] as being a disorder characterized by induration of the skin in localized patches or diffuse areas frequently associated with atrophy and pigmentation. When the fingers are involved it is known as sclerodactylia. Two types occur fairly distinct as to distribution, the diffuse and the circumscribed, both types occasionally being seen in the same patient. As to age groups, two types are well differentiated, the so-called primary scleroderma occurring before birth and during the first two years of life, which is the more common up to the beginning of the period of the second dentition. In the later years of childhood the cases usually are of the adult type, the majority of all cases falling in the third and fourth decades of life. It occurs more commonly in the female sex, the proportion being 3 to 1. In sclerema neonatorum, with which scleroderma should not be confused, the sexes are equally liable. In Cockayne's tabulation of 102 cases in children under fourteen years of age, collected from the literature, there were 28 boys (29.2 per cent), 68 girls (70.8 per cent), and 6 in whom the sex was not specified.

Throughout most of the case studies which have been made, there is found to be a predominance of scleroderma in the Jewish race.

The exact etiology of scleroderma is still somewhat obscure although many contributing factors have been pointed to as precipitating the condition. Morphologic and functional changes of the endocrine glands, the thyroid in particular, have been said to play a part. This is based upon the disorders of the thyroid occurring in association with scleroderma such as hypertrophy, atrophy, sclerosis, and diminution of iodine content. The gland seems to be decreased in size more frequently than enlarged. The basal metabolic rate is variable in cases of scleroderma. It may be slightly lower than normal or higher or perfectly normal, but is usually within the normal limits. Roques,[4] in an analysis of thirty-one cases in which the state of the thyroid was mentioned, reported clinical modifications in the gland in twenty-two instances. The resemblance between myxedema and scleroderma has been frequently mentioned. The apparent success in the treatment of certain cases with the use of thyroid preparations probably accounts for a great deal of the blame's being placed upon a malfunctioning thyroid as the etiologic offender. At the present time, however, less confidence seems to be generally felt in this line of treatment unless there are definite symptoms of thyroid trouble.

Adrenal insufficiency has definitely been known to be present with scleroderma if not the causative factor in such cases as the one reported by Sequeira.[5] He describes a case of scleroderma in a twenty-four-year-old Polish Jewess with a hypotension of adrenal insufficiency. Scleroderma may also occur in association with Addison's disease.

The frequency with which calcium deposits are found in the soft tissues, particularly in the finger tips in sclerodactylia, and the fact that scleroderma may occur with a generalized calcinosis,[6] which cases may show improvement or cures following either a ketogenic diet or after parathyroidectomy, would indicate that hyperparathyroidism or some other parathyroid dysfunction may in some cases be the contributing factor, or an associated condition.

Scleroderma may follow various infectious diseases such as measles, tonsillitis, scarlet fever, diphtheria, pneumonia, and influenza. Trauma and exposure to cold appear to bring on certain cases. Emotional upsets, such as shock and grief, have been named as etiologic factors, as well as prolonged exposure to the sun's rays.

Scleroderma is found with relative frequency as an associated symptom of Raynaud's disease and, occasionally, of thrombo-angiitis obliterans.

Several observers have found a positive Wassermann reaction in a certain percentage of the cases inferring that syphilis may be a cause. Other observers find no larger percentage of sclerodermic patients with a positive Wassermann reaction than would be expected among the general population. However, the majority of syphilitic individuals with scleroderma show improvement or a clearing of the skin condition under antisyphilitic treatment.

Ayers[7] has found arsenic in the urine in a number of patients suffering from scleroderma suggesting that this process may be a manifestation of arsenic poisoning in these cases.

The general conception of the majority interested in this subject seems to be that scleroderma is an angiotrophoneurosis due to disturbance either in the peripheral or central nervous system. This view is borne out by the presence early in the course of the disease of the symptoms of erythema, occasionally of paresthesias or transient attacks of local cutaneous asphyxia, and later of pigmentation. The attacks of Raynaud's disease, which often precede sclerodactylia, are also in accord with this view. The areas of skin involvement often correspond to segmental areas either of the cutaneous nerves or over spinal areas. The atrophic involvement usually found in the adult type, as hemiatrophy of the face or of the whole body and the association with organic nervous diseases, such as tabes dorsalis, as does occur, would further indicate a nervous origin of scleroderma.

Cockayne suggests a very logical theory that, in patients suffering from disease of the ductless glands in the presence of scleroderma, the disease of the skin and the ductless glands are probably both due to a disorder of innervation, in which case all of the above mentioned endoctrine disturbances would have to be regarded as concurrent findings rather than causative factors. He is also of the opinion that the cases of diffuse scleroderma with sclerodactylia and often accompanied by myositis are more probably due to a local infection of the skin or of the skin and muscles. Nearly all of the cases of primary scleroderma from prenatal life on through early childhood are in this group, etiologically. In the later years of childhood the majority belong to the group which are most likely due to some derangement of the sympathetic system.

Poussepp and Rives[8] report a case of sclerodactylia with scleroderma which seems to bear out this theory of the condition's being due to a sympathetic upset. A girl with glandular tuberculosis and manifestations of sympathetic hypertonus, as exophthalmos, inversion of the oculocardiac reflex, and dilatation of the pupils, developed atrophy of the phalanges with joint lesions at the age of eight years. The skin became involved, showing areas of depigmentation, dilatation of the veins, and local warmth. Histologic examination showed the characteristic lesions of scleroderma. It seems theoretically plausible that these changes may have been induced by the tuberculosis virus, to which the sympathetic system is peculiarly sensitive.

Oliver[2] and Michael[9] both agree with Hoffmann's belief that sufferers from diffuse scleroderma have unstable vegetative constitutions. He based this theory on the lack of general reaction to epinephrine in thirteen cases of diffuse scleroderma and a lack of rise in the sugar curve after the administration of this drug. Controls in normal persons rarely acted in this manner. He believes that diffuse scleroderma may develop from shock, cold, trauma, syphilis, or other infections only in those who have an abnormal neuroendocrinologic mechanism.

SYMPTOMATOLOGY

Since the condition is characterized by circumscribed or diffuse hardening, rigidity, and immobility of the skin, the symptoms vary with the areas involved, and then largely on a mechanical basis, except where atrophic changes of the muscles have taken place.

Usually there are no subjective sensations prior to the cutaneous manifestations though there may be neuralgic and arthritic pains or paresthetic sensations as the first signs in certain cases, especially those involving the extremities, according to Dr. Ormsby. In diffuse scleroderma the process develops insidiously, as a rule beginning about the extremities, face, neck, or trunk, with merely a feeling of stiffness as the earliest subjective sign. In most cases the earliest cutaneous changes are either infiltration or a peculiar edema. When edema occurs as the first sign, it may or may not show also an erythema. The case herein reported is of the type showing edema without erythema as the first sign. There may be areas of telangiectasis. When scleroderma is fully developed, the skin feels leathery and cannot be picked up because it is bound down to the underlying structures, hence the synonym "hidebound skin." At first there is no color change, but later the areas become depigmented taking on still later a *café-au-lait* or an old ivory hue. Still later in the evolution of the process the lesions may be bronzed or definitely brown, prior to resolution. The skin involvement may spread slowly or rapidly, covering local areas or the entire body.

When the face is the site of involvement, expression lines are effaced. If the eye regions are involved, there will be difficulty in opening and closing the eyes. Mastication may be interfered with. In extensive chest involvement respiratory movement may be curtailed. Joints of the body may be bound as to impair motion.

When the hands are involved, there is produced sclerodactylia or claw hand. Here, as elsewhere, the joints themselves are not involved, but there is contraction and fixation of the flexors of the hand and wrist. In many cases the skin of the flexor surface of the forearm becomes bound down to the underlying tendons and muscles, which themselves seem sclerotic with the loss of their normal pliability and elasticity.

It is difficult to determine accurately just what proportion of the cases of scleroderma is complicated by sclerodactylia. Up until 1919 there were reported fifteen cases of scleroderma in which there was made special mention of an accompanying sclerodactylia. This hand condition is often considered as characteristic of one form of scleroderma, the diffuse, symmetrical, atrophic type. Therefore, there are undoubtedly many cases of scleroderma reported in which sclerodactylia has been in the picture but not pointed out, being regarded as an expected part of the process rather than an entity.

Following the stage of edema or infiltration, there occurs varying degrees of atrophy of the underlying structures. The atrophy which develops in the majority of the cases of the adult type is usually less extensive than the areas of preceding edema or infiltration. Cases have been reported of hemiatrophy of the face, an atrophy of an extremity, and even a hemiatrophy of the entire body. The edematous stage lasts from a few weeks to several months, after which time the edematous fluid is absorbed, the skin shrinks, and the atrophies make their appearance.

Cockayne, in his analysis of 102 cases in children collected from the literature, found that the commonest form of the disease in childhood is that with isolated plaques or bands of induration. Diffuse scleroderma with or without sclerodactylia and sclerodactylia alone is much rarer. He states further that more than one example of complete hemiatrophy with scleroderma of the atrophic half of the body has been encountered. This is the condition with which I am convinced we are dealing in our case. While the same course of events in the process is found in children with scleroderma, the course is more often acute, and severe atrophic forms are less frequently seen, even though Cockayne in his series found many which were severe and atrophic.

In the primary scleroderma of infancy areas of scleroderma appear, which spread for a time, often coalesce with others, then undergo resolution, and disappear. According to Dr. Ormsby, the skin in the areas may be normal in color, bluish or brownish red. The trunk, particularly the lower part posteriorly, and the extremities are the areas most commonly involved.

Other varieties of scleroderma are described, such as the above mentioned circumscribed scleroderma, or morphea, with the single or multiple discrete, firm, smooth patches, lines or bands, which are either elevated or depressed and surrounded by a violaceous halo, the involution of which may be followed by atrophy.

Morphea guttata, or white-spot disease, is discussed in most dermatology texts under scleroderma. The unusual thing about this eruption is the absence of color, the plaques being chalky white or snow white and the distribution being chiefly on the anterior surface of the chest and on the neck and shoulders. Occasionally they may occur on the arms, forearms, and other parts of the body.

PROGNOSIS

The outlook is variable. It is generally believed that the prognosis is very good in the primary scleroderma of infancy, the majority clearing up without residual findings. In children with the adult type the outlook is considered to be somewhat better than in adults, while some may terminate fatally by intercurrent infection. The process may stop at any time, and while the skin may soften and again return to its normal color, the sequelae depend upon the extent of the atrophic changes at the time of cessation of activity.

PATHOLOGY

The histologic study of the skin in the case of Atwater[10] is representative of the usual findings reported in scleroderma. The report is as follows: "The skin showed considerable thickening of corium, the connective tissue of which showed dense and, in places, hyaline collagen. The epidermis was of normal thickness and contained in the basal layer more than the average amount of brown pigment. Immediately beneath the epidermis the connective tissue was of much more delicate structure. The collagen bundles were small, loose textured, and there were occasional apparently active fibroblasts. The coil glands were normal. There were a few normal appearing hair follicles in the specimen."

The pathologic changes are usually described as being those of exudation and swelling around the sweat glands, hypertrophy of connective tissue followed by atrophy of the vessels and epidermoid structures. When the fingers are involved there is absorption and atrophy of bone.

X-RAY

Cases have been reported in which calcium concretions have been present in the fingertips in sclerodactylia and also in which generalized calcinosis with scleroderma[6] has been found. Atwater reviewed the cases of sclerodactylia reported with x-ray findings and reported his own case, finding that there is quite a typical appearance of atrophy, absorption, and eventually disappearance of the terminal phalanges, most commonly of the hands and sometimes of the feet. His own case showed a definite bone atrophy and absence of the tips of the terminal phalanges of the second to fifth fingers, inclusive.

Edeiken[11] reports three cases of scleroderma with sclerodactylia giving the x-ray findings. In these, all showed some absorption of the terminal phalanges, and two showed small calcareous concretions in the finger tips. He states that, while bone atrophy and absorption of the tips of the phalanges is common in Buerger's disease, Raynaud's disease, leprosy, and ainhum, as well as in sclerodactylia, from his own observations and a study of the literature he found that sclerodactylia is the only condition which will give the roentgenologic picture of calcareous deposits in the finger tips combined with bone absorption of the tips of the phalanges. These concretions are found to be composed of calcium carbonate and calcium phosphate and are densely opaque to x-rays.

In his article on calcinosis and scleroderma Kennedy[6] reports a case in a girl, aged six years, who was treated by ketogenic diet with good results. She came under "Type 2 Diffuse" in the following classification which he offers for cases of scleroderma with calcareous concretions.

Circumscribed

Type 1. The calcareous concretions of scleroderma *(en plaque)*.

Type 2. The calcareous concretions of scleroderma *(en bandes)*.

Diffuse

Type 1. Affecting women almost entirely (26 of 27 patients in reports found by Basch)—occurring as a rule in the course of Raynaud's disease and thyroovarian upset. The features are onset with a sclerodactylia, calcareous concretions with characteristic subcutaneous situation in the tissues of the digits, relative rarity of involvement of the muscles and skeleton, and slow evolution with relatively favorable prognosis.

Type 2. This group is characterized by the predilection for females. It is an affliction of the young, chiefly between the ages of eight and fifteen, designated by Basch,[12] whose work has been studied by Kennedy as chronic edematous scleroderma with "sclerotendonitis" and "scleromyositis" exhibiting calcification which localizes characteristically in the proximal portion of the extremities and trunk superficially and deep.

In the cases showing calcareous deposits, the blood calcium is usually normal or only slightly elevated.

TREATMENT

Many things have been tried in the treatment of scleroderma in the line of drugs, opotherapy, and, in recent times, surgery, with variable results. The most important single thing for the majority of patients would be the maintenance of nutrition and, if the patient is a child, growth, by a nutritious diet, cod liver oil, and perhaps iron tonic.

If there is found some condition associated with, or a definite underlying cause for, the scleroderma, this should certainly be treated, such as antiluetic treatment for those showing a positive Wassermann reaction, the treatment of hypothyroidism if it is present, or glandular therapy in cases showing signs of specific endocrine dysfunctions.

Many gland preparations have been used in times past. Roques reports success with thyroid administration in 63.7 per cent of the cases and states that this treatment should be begun early and should consist of small doses continued over a long period of time. The results with thyroid therapy are, in general, not striking enough to counterbalance the difficulty of evaluating results because of the fair percentage that clears up without it; thus this line of therapy does not hold the place that it did at one time in the treatment of scleroderma. In Roques' report suprarenal extract had been used with benefit in some cases. Pituitary extract had failed to show results in four cases in which it was tried. Testicular and ovarian extracts have been used almost without success. Schwerdt, in five cases of localized scleroderma, reports promising results with a mesenteric gland preparation.

Parathyroidectomy has been performed with good results; also sympathetic ganglionectomy has been coming into favor recently in certain selected cases.

Locally it is well to use massage; alternating hot and cold douches are of value in attempting to promote circulation and encourage resolution. In massaging the affected parts daily, inunctions of cod liver oil, lanolin, lard, vaseline, or slightly scented neat's-foot oil may be used (Ormsby). A small amount of ammoniated mercury or salicylic acid may be added.

Thorium X emanations incorporated in an ointment base containing eucerin has been used by Epstein.[13]

REPORT OF CASE

A. W., white female, aged five years and five months, was first seen by me in Chicago, on Jan. 4, 1936, with the major complaint of a flexion deformity of the fingers of the right hand and also numerous skin spots and areas of thickening with certain color changes, chiefly over the right half of the body.

The informant, the patient's father, gave the history that the first symptom to appear was the inability to open the hand which was discovered at play by an older brother on May 19, 1935. So far as the parents were able to determine, the condition of the hand when first noticed remained static until now, but the entire arm seemed to have become smaller during the past few months. In the process the third, fourth, and fifth fingers were the ones chiefly involved. The index finger could not be bent back as far as the corresponding finger of the left hand. The thumb was quite normal.

After some weeks there followed the appearance of depigmented areas over the anterior chest, the flexor surface of the right arm and forearm, the lower abdomen, beneath the right ramus of the jaw, and a small area over the right eye. There had been no redness or violaceous colored halos around the lesions at any time as described in morphea.

Then there appeared two plaques in the skin well described in the father's own words: "The white areas appeared in late July and August. We thought at first it was the way she had tanned in the sun. Then in September while massaging and soaking her arm in hot and cold water, we noticed a yellow skin spot on the inside of her right arm at just about the spot of the muscle (the medial aspect of the belly of the biceps). It seemed thick and leathery. Then we next noticed this same sort of a spot on her chest. It showed sort of shiny first in the sunlight; then it seemed to raise up as it is now. This spot spread over an area of 2 by 3 inches (5.08 by 7.62 cm.), not solid but spotted. The spots did not seem to appear where the white places were, except on the chest, which was more or less bleached out all over. This seemed to appear more on the right side, much more so, than on the left."

In December an uncle of the child first noticed that the right side of the patient's face was smaller than the left, particularly that the lower half seemed "more drawn up." This was preceded by the discoloration underneath the right margin of the jaw. At this time there were no lesions on the face except for the small spot on the forehead.

Just recently there has been a feeling, objectively, of thickness of the skin covering the anterior right thigh, without any color change.

There have been no subjective symptoms whatsoever in connection with these skin and muscular changes.

The past history did not vary from the story of a perfectly normal child. There was nothing relevant in the family history. The parents are both living and well. There have been three pregnancies, all of which were full term. The two brothers, aged sixteen and eleven years, were in good health. The patient has a normal birth history, weighing 7 pounds and 6 ounces (3.345 kg.). She weighed 15 pounds (6.804 kg.) at six months, 20 (9.072 kg.) at a year, and during the past year the weight has fluctuated between 33 and 35 pounds (14.968 and 15.876 kg.). She was breast fed for two months, and then was placed on a cow's milk-karo syrup formula. Orange juice and cod liver oil were started at one month and given regularly. There were two teeth at six months and ten days with an eruption of all the temporary teeth by the end of the second year. She was running "everywhere" at twelve and a half months and had quite a vocabulary at eighteen months.

Of the contagious diseases of childhood, the patient has had only measles (March, 1935.) She has not been vaccinated, nor has she had any other immunization. The surgical history was negative.

As to habits, the appetite was only fair; bowels were regular; patient slept well, seemed stable emotionally and had always been very active, preferring a romp outdoors to indoor confinement.

Physical Examination.—The physical examination revealed a thin but fairly well-developed white girl, who was cooperative and apparently happy, measuring 42½ inches (107.94 cm.) in height and weighing 35 pounds (15.876 kg.). Except for the sclerodermic and atrophic changes under discussion, the regional examination revealed nothing abnormal. The eyes reacted to light and accommodation. The ears and nose were normal. The teeth were in good condition with three fillings and with normal appearing gums and buccal mucosa. The tonsils were of medium size with no superficial evidence of being infected. The child breathed through the nose and spoke with the voice of one free from any nasal obstruction. There was no cervical lymph gland enlargement. The thyroid seemed to be of normal size. The heart was normal, and the lung fields were clear. There was no abdominal tenderness, and no abnormal masses were felt. The genitals were normal.

The distribution of the skin lesions was as follows: There was a small white spot over the right eye about a centimeter in diameter midway between the eyebrow and the hairline of the scalp. There was a band of sclerodermic involvement of the neck beneath the right ramus of the mandible and roughly parallel to it extending from the inferior tip of the lobe of the right ear with the circumference of the neck to the midline anteriorly at a point 1 inch (2.54 cm.) beneath the mental process and varying in width from ⅛ to ⅝ inches (3.17 to 15.85 mm.), elevated, indurated, and of an ivory color.

The most extensive and deepest involvement was that of the entire flexor surface of the right upper extremity. The skin of the palm and forearm (flexor surface) could not be picked up between the fingers. It had a firm feeling to the touch and seemed to be completely bound down to the underlying structures. The involvement of the arm was more in the form of a plaque which lay with the long axis of the

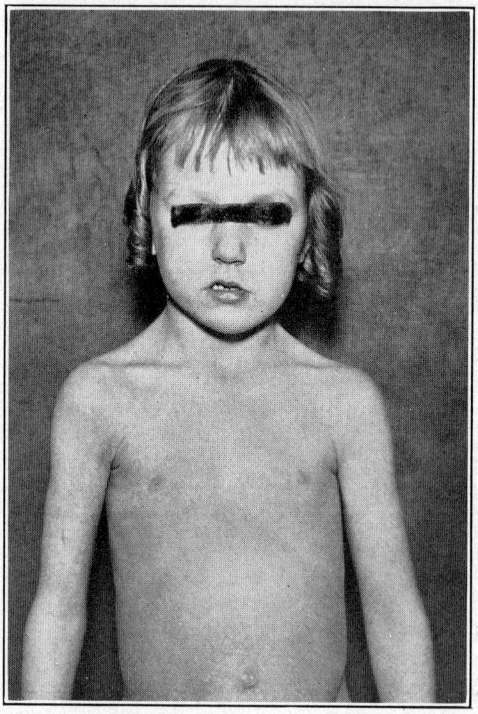

Fig. 1.—Case of scleroderma showing the hemiatrophy of the right side of face.

arm over the medial portion of the biceps muscle anteriorly to the inner margin, overlying the brachial artery. This plaque was elevated and measured ¾ by 2½ inches (1.9 by 6.35 cm.). This region was considerably warmer to the touch than the surrounding area. The color of these lesions on the arm and forearm could best be described as being a dirty yellow. Over the yellow areas, even more than the depigmented spots, the skin was intensely smooth and atrophic, there being no hairs or hair follicles that could be seen. There seemed to be no sensory changes in the affected areas.

The anterior chest region, in an area bounded roughly by the clavicles, the anterior axillary folds, and an imaginary transverse nipple line, inferiorly, was covered with areas of depigmentation varying in size from a pinhead to a half inch (12.70 mm.) with a tendency to become confluent and to form irregular larger areas. In the midsternal region with the long axis of the body there was an ivory-colored plaque similar to the one above described in every respect, oval in outline, and measuring ⅜ by 1¼ inches (0.95 by 3.17 cm.). Across the lower abdomen there were scattered discrete areas of depigmentation, more dense in the immediate suprapubic region.

Over the back and gluteal regions there were widely scattered small areas of depigmentation, most of them about 3 to 5 mm. in diameter.

The skin over the entire anterior surface of the right thigh extending from the right inguinal region to the patella had a very peculiar feeling when picked up in the hand. It seemed vaguely edematous or thickened without pitting on pressure. The color of the skin in this area was perfectly normal.

Attention to the atrophic changes revealed that the right side of the face from the midportion of the cheek downward was smaller than the left (Fig. 1). The right ala of the nose was smaller and described a slightly higher arch on that side. When the mouth was held in repose, there was visible a muscular inequality between the two halves of the mouth, with some deficiency about the right angle.

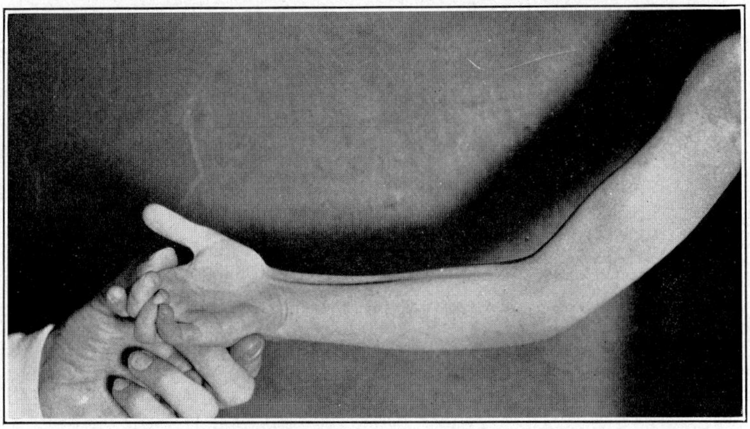

Fig. 2.—Sclerodactylia of the right hand showing the maximum extension possible.

The third, fourth, and fifth fingers of the right hand were flexed (Fig. 2) in about the position in which the hand is ordinarily carried in walking and could not be extended manually except by flexing the wrist, and then only partially. Upon attempts to extend the fingers the flexor tendons became prominent, showing that there was a definite shortening of this group of muscles and that, as usual in this condition, there was no joint involvement back of the difficulty. The active and passive movements of the index finger and thumb seemed normal, except that the former was somewhat more resistant to forceful extension than the corresponding finger of the left hand. There was a noticeable decrease in the size of the entire hand and forearm. The element of disuse could not enter here in view of the fact that the child had never favored the involved extremity in any way, writing and drawing with it quite as much as any right-handed child. When the arm was abducted, there was drawing of the anterior axillary fold due to skin shortening.

Course.—The patient was again seen three months later on April 8 and showed certain changes, some of progression and some of resolution of the process. Instead of the small white spot seen on first examination over the right eye there were two concentric arcs of scleroderma which seemed to be following cutaneous nerve branches. They were each ⅝ inch (15.85 mm.) wide and were situated 1 inch (2.54 cm.) apart. The longer of the two, situated laterally, began directly over the eye a half inch (12.70 mm.) above the eyebrow and curved upward and slightly outward extending ¾ of an inch (19.05 mm.) above the hairline. The other band extended from 1 inch (2.54 cm.) above the inner end of the eyebrow and likewise curved upward and outward ending ½ inch (12.70 mm.) above the hairline. There was a complete absence of hair where the ends of these bands extended into the scalp region. These areas were of the color of old ivory and showed atrophy of the underlying structures as evidenced by a definite depression along their entire course.

The condition of the hand seemed unchanged except that the index finger could not be extended quite so far as previously. The skin of the palm and of the forearm seemed definitely more pliable, particularly the upper two-thirds of the forearm.

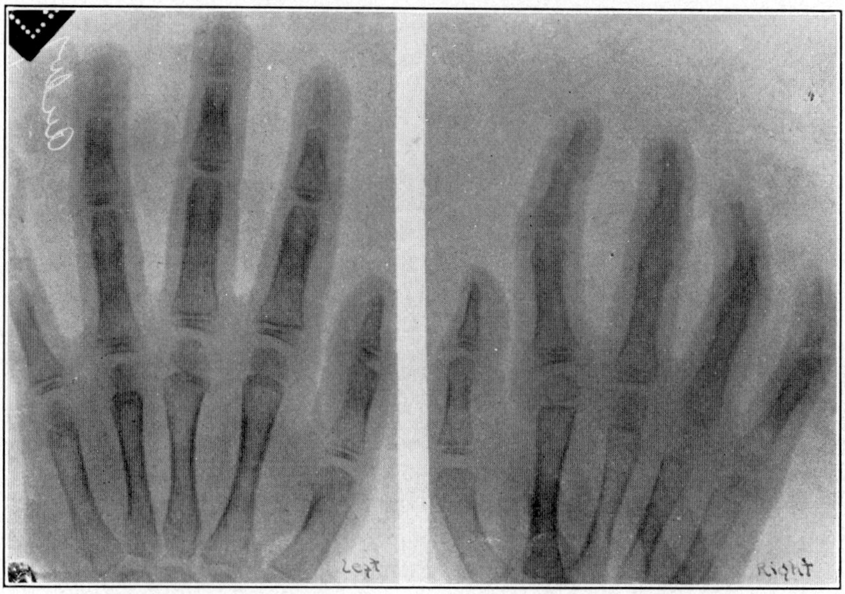

Fig. 3.—X-ray films of hands, sclerodactylia involvement of the right.

A new plaque had developed between the left nipple and the left sternal margin, oval in outline, and in a transverse direction measuring 1½ inches (3.81 cm.) with an average width of ½ inch (12.70 mm.). Another small plaque had developed in the region of the left biceps near the midpoint and medially.

The skin of the lower abdomen had returned to normal color except for a mottled area of depigmentation in the right lower quadrant about 1½ by 3 inches (3.81 by 7.62 cm.).

Since the last visit there developed an area of telangiectasis over the right scapula inferior to the scapular spine and extending medially to the midline.

The skin of the anterior thigh lost the feeling of thickness but has the flaky depigmentation spots which have been most noticeable over the trunk. The skin over the entire length of the tibia anteriorly was shiny and smooth. There was no marked change in pigmentation except from the edema. There was definite pitting of the skin when pressed against the tibia.

The circumferences taken of the extremities at corresponding levels show a definite soft tissue atrophy of the entire right upper extremity and of the right thigh. The measurements are as follows:

	Right	Left
Midarm	5⅝ in. (14.28 cm.)	6⅛ in. (15.56 cm.)
Midforearm	5¹⁄₁₆ in. (12.86 cm.)	5½ in. (13.97 cm.)
Wrist	4⅛ in. (10.48 cm.)	4⁷⁄₁₆ in. (11.27 cm.)
Palm	4¾ in. (12.06 cm.)	5 in. (12.70 cm.)
Thigh (at gluteal fold)	11 in. (27.94 cm.)	11½ in. (29.21 cm.)
Midthigh	10⅝ in. (26.98 cm.)	11 in. (27.94 cm.)
Suprapatellar region	8½ in. (21.59 cm.)	9 in. (22.86 cm.)
Calf	8⁷⁄₁₆ in. (21.43 cm.)	8¼ in. (20.95 cm.)
Ankle	5¾ in. (14.60 cm.)	5¾ in. (14.60 cm.)

It is interesting to note that the skin of the right thigh, having passed from the edematous stage to the atrophic, falls into the expected measurement relationship with the corresponding part, while the leg of the same extremity is in an earlier stage and, as a result, measures slightly more in circumference owing to the edema, than the normal left leg.

Laboratory Findings.—The laboratory study was made upon the second visit of the patient in April, 1936. Blood examination showed 80 per cent hemoglobin (Newcomer), 13.5 grams, with an erythrocyte count of 5,180,000. There was a total leucocyte count of 10,550 with a differential of polymorphonuclear leucocytes, 50 per cent, lymphocytes, 40 per cent, monocytes, 5 per cent and eosinophiles, 5 per cent. The urine was acid in reaction and negative throughout to both chemical and microscopic study. The blood calcium was 10.3 mg., and the phosphorus 4.3 mg. per cent.

X-Ray Findings.—The x-ray study was made by Dr. W. E. Anspach who reports:

"Films of both hands and other long bones, which include the greater portion of the trunk, fail to show x-ray evidence of calcium deposits in the soft tissues. The bones on the whole have normal texture and density, and there is only slight general loss of density of the bones of the affected right hand (Fig. 3) as compared with the normal left hand.

"The lung fields and heart appear to be within the limits of normal."

DISCUSSION AND SUMMARY

There has been presented in this paper a general discussion of the rare condition known as scleroderma, the adult type of which seems to be best explained upon the basis of an abnormal sympathetic endocrinologic mechanism and which is precipitated by such conditions as shock, cold, trauma, syphilis, acute infections, etc. There is the primary scleroderma, which occurs from prenatal life on through early childhood, but this is more probably due to a local infection of the skin. The case reported here is of the adult type of scleroderma in a child aged five years and five months, who presents, in addition to the skin lesions of scleroderma, a hemiatrophy of the body, or at least an atrophy of the right side of the face (including forehead, cheek, nose, and mouth), the right upper and the right lower extremities, and sclerodactylia of the right hand.

Out of as nearly a normal history as one often finds, measles is the only illness which might have precipitated the scleroderma; it is on the long list of causative factors to which the development of scleroderma has been attributed. This attack of measles preceded the onset of the sclerodermic process by eight weeks.

This case seems to be following the rule of this condition in that each case is a law unto itself, clearing up in areas while other regions continue on to atrophy of the underlying tissues. Just what the ultimate outcome will be it is very difficult to say.

REFERENCES

1. Cockayne, E. A.: Brit. J. Child. Dis. **13**: 225, 1916.
2. Oliver, E. L.: Arch. Dermat. & Syph. **25**: 72, 1932 (Reference also to Dr. Fox's discussion of paper).
3. Ormsby, O. S.: Diseases of the Skin, Philadelphia, 1934, Lea & Febiger Co.
4. Roques, E.: Ann. de Dermat. et de Syph. p. 393, July, 1910.
5. Sequeira, J. H.: Brit. J. Dermat. **34**: 124, 1922.
6. Kennedy, R. L. J.: J. Pediat. **1**: 667, 1932.
7. Ayers, S., Jr.: Arch. Dermat. & Syph. **2**: 747, 1920; ibid. **30**: 33, 1934.
8. Poussepp, L., and Rives, I.: Ann. de méd. **19**: 19, 1926.
9. Searle: South. M. J. **22**: 258, 1929 (Ref. to Michael's discussion).
10. Atwater, R. M.: Am. J. M. Sc. **158**: 29, 1919.
11. Edeiken, L.: Am. J. Roentgenol. **22**: 42, 1929.
12. Basch, Marianne: Le Syndrome de Thibierge-Weissenbach concretions calcaires des sclerodermies, Paris, 1931, Librairie Louis Arnette.
13. Epstein, S.: Arch. f. Dermat. u. Syph. **167**: 533, 1933.

L'Hôpital de Sakbayemé

TECHNICS FOR MEASURING INFANTS

HELEN L. DAWSON
IOWA CITY, IOWA

THERE seem to be nowhere in the literature adequate directions for measuring infants. This is a problem in which the mere definition of the particular measurement and the description of the instruments to be used are not sufficient, as anyone well knows who has attempted to apply to infants the measuring technics that are found in books of anthropometry. Such standard descriptions, while they are adequate for work on adults, leave much to be desired when they are applied to infants. In the few articles available, which give directions for measuring infants, the authors fail to mention the difficulties or to caution against some of the common posture factors which are found in this age period and which tend to introduce unnecessary errors into the data.

In this paper the author will describe the technics which are being used at present in measuring infants at the Iowa Child Welfare Research Station. An attempt will be made to anticipate some of the difficulties which may be encountered and to discuss some of the problems involved in measuring at this early age level. It is hoped that this paper, in which a statement of one method is given, will help to stimulate interest in the standardization of the technics at present being used in working with infants.

INSTRUMENTS

The various instruments that are used and the measurements that are taken with each one are listed below:

Measuring board for infants
- Crown-heel length
- Crown-rump length

Paper measuring scale
- Standing height
- Sitting height

Large sliding calipers
- Head length
- Head breadth
- Shoulder breadth (bideltoid)
- Chest breadth
- Chest depth
- Hip breadth (bi-iliac and bitrochanteric)
- Elbow breadth
- Knee breadth

Metal tape
- Head circumference
- Chest circumference
- Arm
- Forearm
- Thigh
- Calf

Fat calipers
- Chest front
- Chest back
- Arm front
- Arm back
- Suprascapular
- Suprailiac

Scales
- Weight

From the Iowa Child Welfare Research Station, State University of Iowa.

DESCRIPTIONS

The Measuring Board for Infants (Fig. 1*A*).—This board was designed by Dr. Bird T. Baldwin and was made in the manual training shop at the State University of Iowa.

> The scale is one meter in length, with an additional margin of 4.5 centimeters at the one end. The width is 20.5 centimeters, with standardized buttonwood millimeter scales on either side. The vertical plane for the head rest is 15 centimeters at its greatest height, and the sliding vertical plane is attached to a brass rod which moves freely in a brass groove in such a manner that the millimeter reading may be taken from either side. The board is made of inlaid walnut and buttonwood and the standards on which it rests when in contact with the table are covered with heavy felt. The scale is accurate and portable.*

In addition to the 15 cm. sliding vertical plane, it is necessary to have a second one, 8 cm. high, for very small children whose thighs are too short to allow the knees to flex properly when the 15 cm. plane is used. These two planes are interchangeable, and the one used will depend solely on the size of the subject.

Paper Measuring Scale.—This scale is the Baldwin modification of the Broca plane. In describing it Dr. Baldwin states:

> The plane consists of a strip of the best type of inextensible and unshrinkable paper, one meter long and twelve and a half centimeters broad, with the metric divisions on the right edge of the scale in centimeters and millimeters, and the English on the left edge in feet, inches and fifths of an inch, and with a margin on each side of the scale and also at the top and bottom.†

This scale is fixed to a stationary vertical board and is used for taking the height and sitting height measurements.

The Square.—The square, which has been constructed in the university carpentry shop, consists of two pieces of seasoned walnut, 18 cm. by 13 cm., joined at right angles. Within this angle and in the midplane a third piece of wood, in which an opening has been cut to serve as a handle, is joined to the two pieces mentioned above and serves to strengthen the square. It is used in taking both standing and sitting height. One surface of the square is held against the vertical measuring board and brought down until the other surface is in firm contact with the child's head. The reading is then taken from the measuring scale at the lower edge (angle) of the square (Fig. 1*B*).

The Bench.—The bench which is used in taking the sitting height has also been constructed in the university shop. The one suited to young children is 30 cm. high, 20 cm. wide, and 25 cm. long (Fig. 1*C*).

Large Sliding Calipers.—This instrument, also known as the Hrdlička compass, was made in Washington for the Iowa Child Welfare Research Station and was tested by the Bureau of Standards. It is light, durable, and accurate (Fig. 1*D*).

---

*Baldwin, Bird T.: The Physical Growth of Children From Birth to Maturity. Univ. Iowa Stud., Stud. in Child Welfare **1**: 18, 1921.

†Baldwin, Bird T.: The Physical Growth of Children From Birth to Maturity. Univ. Iowa Stud., Stud. in Child Welfare **1**: 15, 1921.

Metal Tape.—A steel tape graduated in millimeters is used.

Fat Calipers.—Special calipers, manufactured by the Kny-Scheerer Company, New York City, are used for taking measurements of the subcutaneous tissue (Fig. 1*E*).

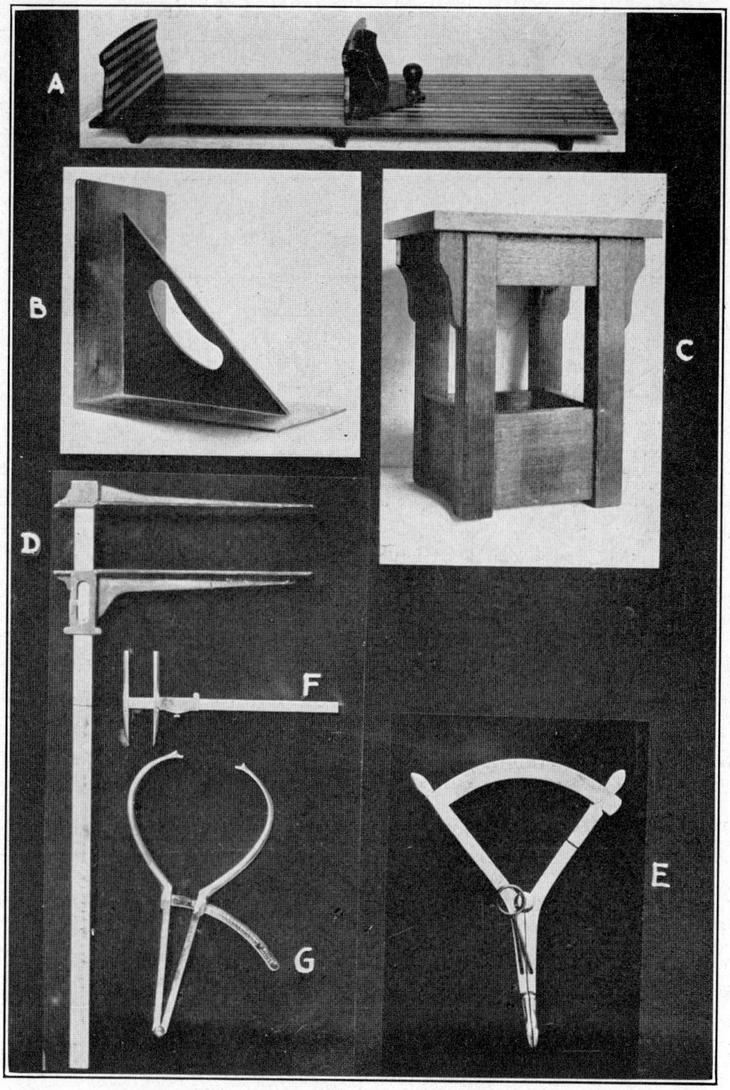

Fig. 1.

Scales.—Fairbanks scales which are graduated in both pounds and kilograms are used in taking the weight.

MEASURING TECHNICS

The technics described below are applicable to children from birth to three years of age. All measurements are taken with the infant nude, and in cases in which the measurement is taken on only one side of the body, the left side is always used. In working with children of this age the temperature of the room should be between 82 and 85° F.

Lengths

Crown-Heel (Fig. 2).—Age Range: From birth to two years, six months.

Instrument: Measuring board for infants.

Posture: Reclining; head in the Frankfort plane; head and body in a straight line; thighs and legs extended; feet flexed.

Technic: The subject lies on his back with the vertex of his head touching the stationary, vertical upright at the end of the measuring board. The legs are extended and the feet flexed. The movable, vertical upright is then brought up firmly two or three times in succession against the soles of the feet, and the reading is taken.

Comments: In measuring very young subjects, or older children who are not cooperative, an assistant will be found necessary to see that the head of the subject is in contact with the board and that the head and the body are in a straight line. The measurer places one hand on the child's knees in order to insure complete extension of the legs and with the free hand manipulates the sliding upright as indicated above.

In measuring very young children, who have not yet developed a lumbar curve, there will be difficulty in getting the legs extended. In complete extension of the legs a compensatory curve will be produced in the vertebral column. Since this procedure will be painful to the child, it should be done as rapidly as possible.

In older children, who are objecting to the position on the measuring board, the measurer must watch to see that the subject does not arch his back and shorten his total length in this manner. If he does, the condition may be corrected by flexing his thighs on his abdomen, then again extending the legs and measuring immediately.

Crown-Rump (Fig. 3).—Age Range: From birth to two years, six months.

Instrument: Measuring board for infants.

Posture: Reclining; head in the Frankfort plane; head and body in a straight line; thighs flexed so that the anterior surfaces of the thighs are at right angles to the horizontal base of the measuring board; legs flexed.

Technic: The subject lies on his back with the vertex of his head touching the stationary, vertical upright at the end of the measuring board. The thighs and legs are flexed and the movable, vertical upright is brought up two or three times in succession against the buttocks with a firm pressure, and the reading is taken.

Comments: Care should be taken that the thighs are flexed the right amount each time. In cases where the thighs are flexed more than

90 degrees, there will be a change in the curvature of the vertebral column; when the thighs are flexed less than 90 degrees the posterior parts of the thighs will interfere with the measuring. Both of these conditions will introduce an error into the measurement.

Standing Height (Fig. 4).—Age Range: From two through three years.

Fig. 2.

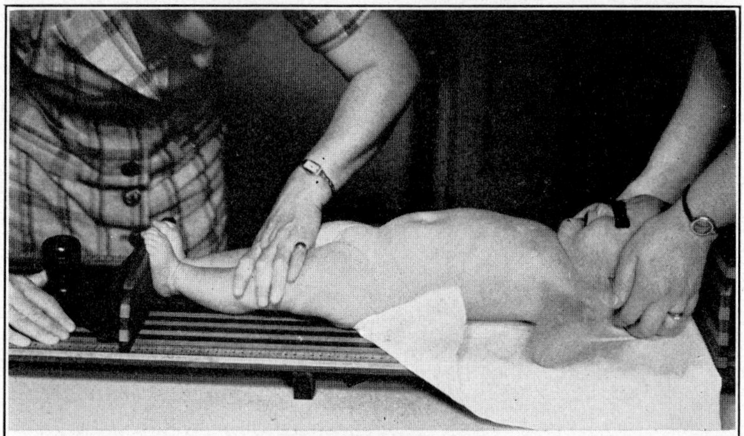

Fig. 3.

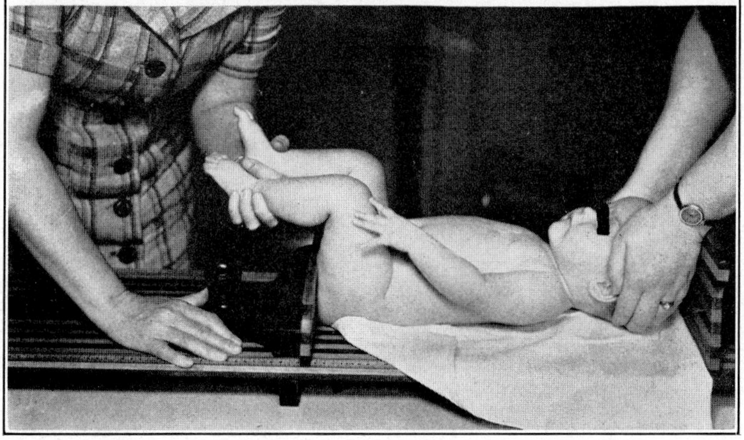

Instruments: Paper measuring scale (modification of the Broca plane) and square.

Posture: The subject stands erect, feet close together and flat on the floor. The back of the head, upper part of the back, buttocks, and heels should be in contact with the wall to which the measuring scale is attached. The arms hang at the sides in a natural position. The head is held in the Frankfort plane.

Technic: After placing the child in the correct position, the measurer holds the child's chin so as to maintain his head in the Frankfort plane. The square is held in the free hand and is brought firmly down against the head two or three times. Sufficient pressure is used to feel the impact of the skull. The reading is taken from the last position.

Comments: Unless they are closely watched, there is a tendency for young children to rise on their toes just as the measurer brings the square down against the head. The assistant should check to see that the child is standing with the feet flat on the floor and that the knees are straight.

Error may be introduced if the square is tipped either to right or left (in the sagittal plane). This may be avoided by lining up one edge of the square with the edge of the measuring scale.

Sitting Height (Fig. 5).—Age Range: From two years through three years.

Instruments: Paper measuring scale (modification of the Broca plane), square, and square or oblong bench with a horizontal seat.

Posture: Sitting position, with back of head, upper part of the back, and sacral region of the back in contact with the board on which the measuring scale is attached. Children whose feet will touch the floor should cross the ankles, spread the knees apart, and relax the legs. The head is in the Frankfort plane and the arms hang at the sides.

Technic: The subject sits on a horizontal and resisting seat in the above position. The back edge of the seat should be in contact with the vertical board to which the measuring scale is attached. The head is held in the Frankfort plane by the measurer who grasps the child's chin and holds it firmly. The measurer holds the square in his free hand and brings it down against the head two or three times, using sufficient pressure to enable him to feel the impact of the skull. The reading is taken from the last position.

Comments: There is a tendency for children (particularly older ones) to contract the gluteal muscles and thus increase the measurement of sitting height. This is easily avoided if the knees are spread apart, the ankles crossed, and the legs relaxed.

Care must be taken to see that the child is sitting as far back on the bench as possible (the back edge of the bench must be in contact with the vertical board on which the measuring scale is attached). At times children tend to slide forward on the bench into a position which will produce a curve in the vertebral column and thus give a smaller measure of sitting height.

Head Length.—Age Range: From birth through three years.

Instrument: Large sliding calipers.

Posture: Sitting or standing.

Technic: Children who are too young to follow directions and older ones who refuse to do so must have their heads held firmly during the measuring. The person assisting the measurer grasps the child's head at the base of the skull with one hand and with the other hand takes a firm hold on the chin. The chin is held in the palm of the hand with the thumb and the second and third fingers on opposite sides of the mandible. The fourth and fifth fingers are flexed under the chin to prevent the child from lowering his head. After the head has been stabilized in this manner, the measurer grasps the tip of the immovable blade of the calipers and places it just over the glabella. The tip of the movable blade is then brought into contact with the back of the child's head at the point which is farthest from the glabella and in the midline of the skull. The pressure used is very firm. The reading is taken several times to insure the accuracy of the measurement.

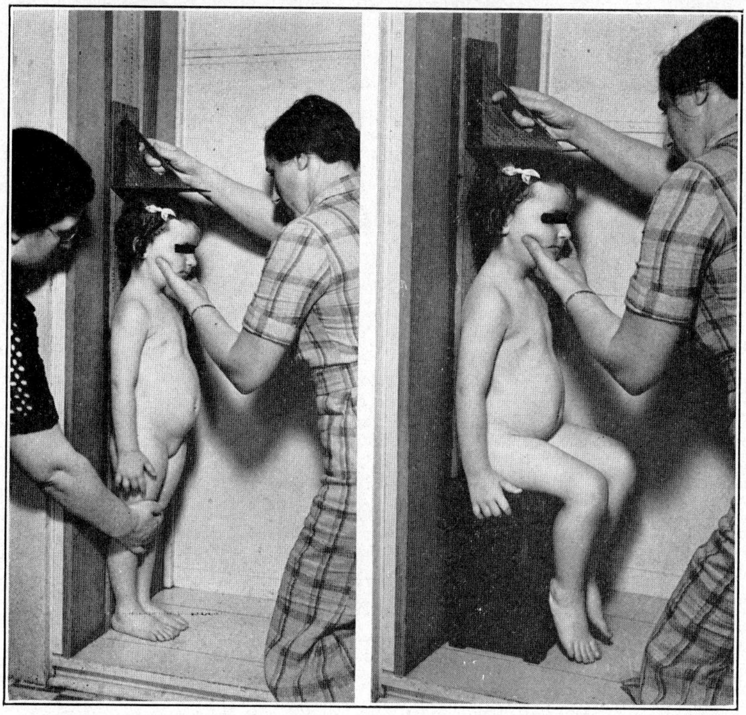

Fig. 4. Fig. 5.

Comments: Children between the ages of eight and eighteen months often object to having their heads held, and they may struggle to free themselves. If this occurs, the person holding the child must be very careful that the child does not jerk his head up and force the blade of the calipers into his face. Speed on the part of the measurer will help greatly.

Breadths

Head Breadth.—Age Range: From birth through three years.

Instrument: Large sliding calipers.

Posture: Sitting or standing.

Technic: When children are too young to follow directions or when older ones refuse to, the person holding the child places his hands (palms open) on either side of the child's head at a level with the ears and holds it firmly. Since this is a measure of the greatest transverse diameter of the skull, the measurer places the tips of the calipers just above the ears of the child, keeping the blades parallel, and using a firm pressure. He moves them forward and backward, repeating the above technic until he is positive that the maximum breadth has been measured.

Comment: In little girls where the hair ribbon or other similar device for fastening the hair interferes with the blades of the calipers, it should be removed and the blades allowed to come into contact with the head.

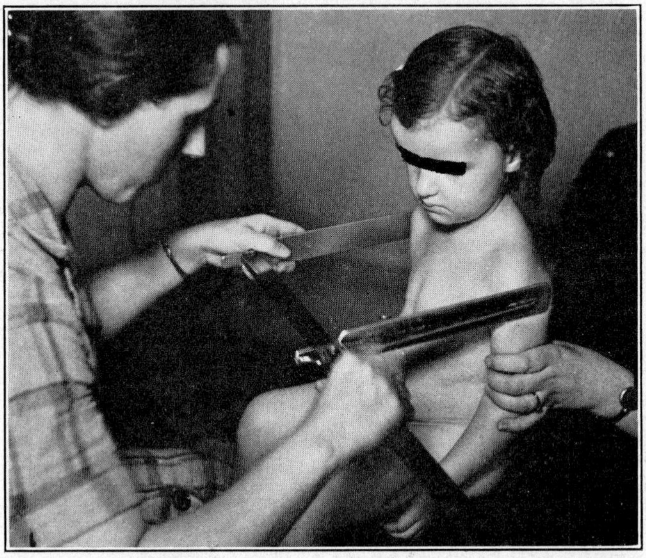

Fig. 6.

Shoulder Breadth (*Bideltoid*) (Fig. 6).—Age Range: From birth through three years.

Instrument: Large sliding calipers.

Posture: Sitting erect; with arms down and elbows held tightly against the sides of the body.

Technic: The tip of the immovable blade of the calipers is applied to the arm, over the deltoid muscle opposite the head of the humerus. The rod of the calipers should be in a horizontal plane at the same level as the heads of the humeri. The tip of the movable blade is brought against the opposite shoulder over the deltoid muscle. Firm pressure is used, and the reading is taken several times; the mean is recorded.

Comments: Shoulder measurements are the least reliable of any of the measures of growth. The shoulder girdle is loosely articulated and extremely mobile, and this, in addition to variability in posture, resistance of the individual who is being measured, and the amount of pressure used in measuring, tends to influence the measurement and to introduce errors. After experimentation with infants, the above combination of posture and technic was found to give the most reliable results.

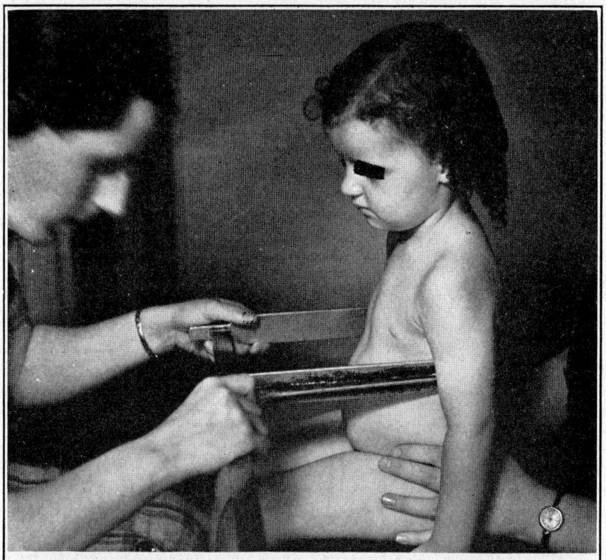

Fig. 7.

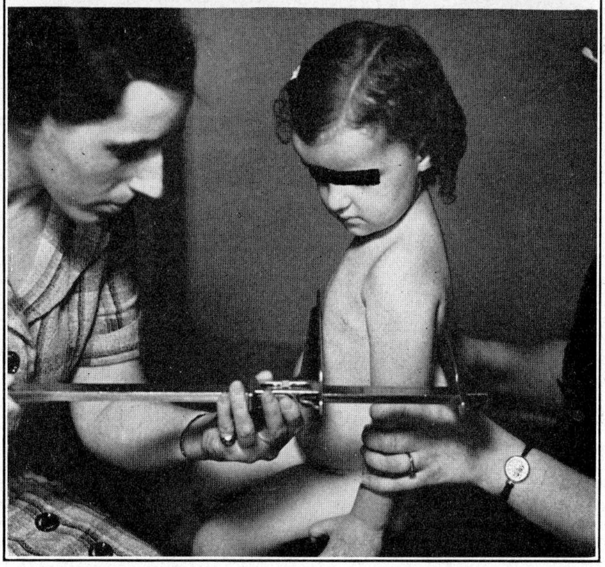

Fig. 8.

Care should be taken to see that children who object to being measured do not hunch their shoulders, for this will narrow the shoulder width.

If the blades of the calipers are warmed slightly, the infants will object less than if they are very cold.

Chest Breadth and Depth (Figs. 7 and 8).—Age Range: From birth through three years.

Instruments: Large sliding calipers.

Posture: Sitting; the trunk held erect with arms relaxed and hanging at the sides.

Technic: Breadth—The blades of the large calipers are applied to the sides of the chest at the level of the xiphoid process. The pressure should be firm and the reading taken several times as a check on the amount of pressure which is used.

Depth—The measurement of chest depth is taken at the level of the xiphoid process. One blade of the calipers is placed over the xiphoid process, and the other blade is applied to the back of the thorax, the instrument being held so that the plane of the blades is at right angles to the vertical axis of the thorax.

Comments: Since crying influences this measure, every effort is made to have the child quiet at the time the measurement is taken. Toys, particularly those that make noise, are found useful in attracting the child's attention. If it is impossible to quiet the child, the measurement should be taken, nevertheless, and a note made on the card that the child was crying.

Chest width and, to a greater extent, chest depth are influenced greatly by the position of the child. If the child is very young and is allowed to slump when sitting, the abdominal organs push up and the ribs spread apart. This is particularly true in infants in whom the ribs are still very pliable. In newborn infants the upright position with a straight back is maintained through the help of the person holding the child.

The blades of the calipers should be warmed slightly before they are used.

Hip Breadths (*Bi-iliac and Bitrochanteric*) (Figs. 9 and 10).—Age Range: From birth through three years.

Instrument: Large sliding calipers.

Posture: Reclining position until children are able to support their own weight with the help of the person holding them; from that time on they are measured standing. In both positions the body is straight, the legs are extended, and the feet are held close together.

Technic: Bi-iliac—The person measuring first locates the crests of the ilia by palpation; then the blades of the calipers are placed over the crests and are brought together with very firm pressure. This is done several times before the reading is taken in order to check the accuracy of the measure.

Bitrochanteric—The same technic is used in taking this measurement after the trochanters have first been located by palpation.

Comments: Care should be used in locating the points, and the blades of the instrument must be held parallel to one another and at right angles to the long axis of the body.

Children who are measured in the reclining position must have their thighs and legs fully extended.

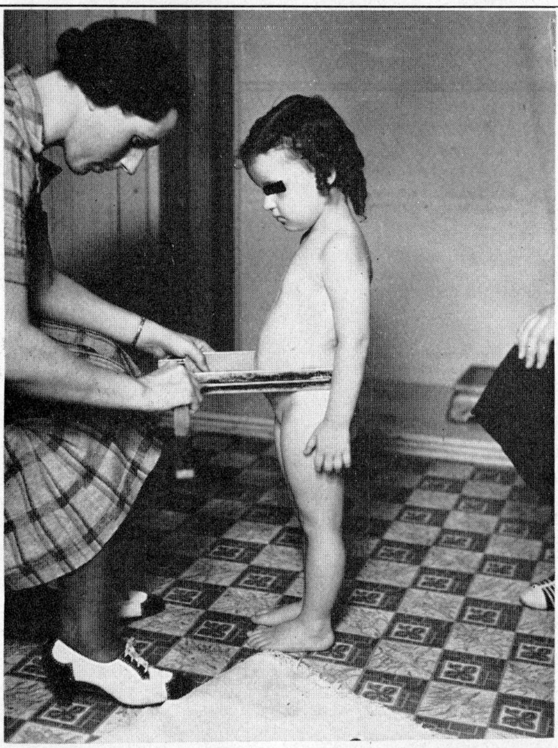

Fig. 9.

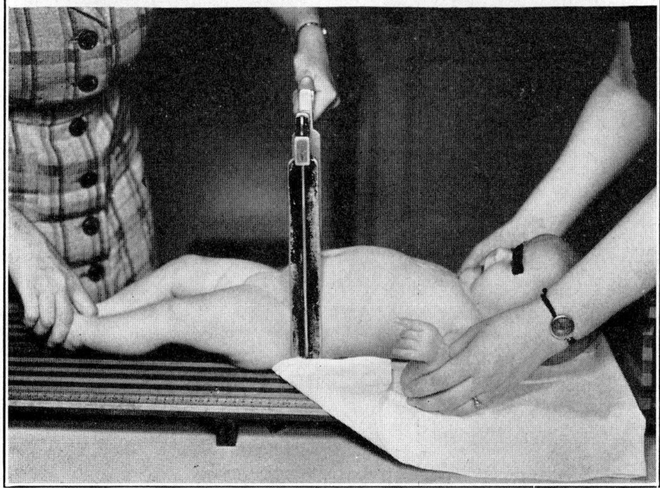

Fig. 10.

Joint Breadths (*Elbow and Knee*).—Age Range: From birth through three years.

Instrument: Large sliding calipers.

Posture: Elbow—The hand is in the supine position and the forearm is flexed until it forms about a 90 degree angle with the arm.

Knee—The sole of the foot should be parallel with the floor and the leg flexed on the thigh, forming about a 90 degree angle.

Technic: Elbow—The person holding the child grasps the left wrist, rotates the arm until the hand is in a supine position, then flexes the forearm. The measurer places the tips of the blades of the calipers on either side of the elbow so that the blades press upon the two epicondyles of the humerus. The pressure is very firm.

Knee—After the left leg has been flexed, the technic for measuring the knee is the same as that for the elbow. The tips of the blades of the calipers are placed over the two epicondyles of the femur.

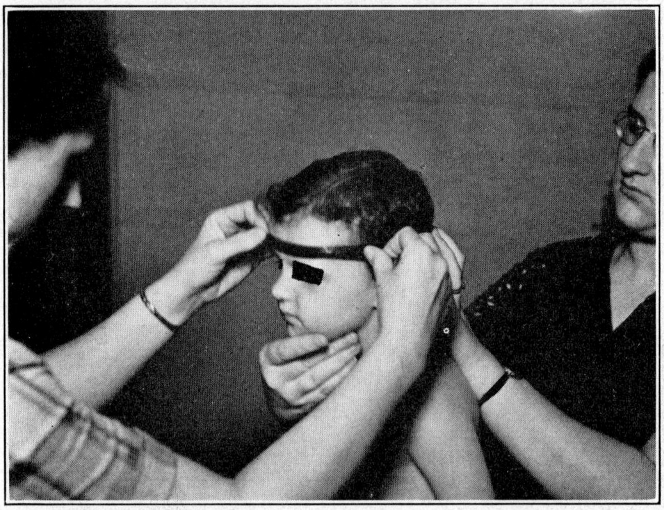

Fig. 11.

Comments: In measuring both the elbow and the knee it is important that these joints be flexed at the time the measurement is taken. If they are not, the muscles will cover the epicondyles and give an erroneously large measurement.

Circumferences

Head Circumference (Fig. 11).—Age Range: From birth through three years.

Instrument: Metal tape.

Posture: Sitting position with the head held erect.

Technic: First the tape is made into a circle with the two ends crossed and held by the measurer in such a manner that the circle can be made smaller by pulling on the free end of the tape. Enough of the tape is then released to make a circle which is larger than the child's head. The looped tape is slipped over the child's head, and the assistant adjusts the tape posteriorly over that part of the occiput which is farthest from the glabella. While the assistant holds the tape in place posteriorly, the measurer adjusts it anteriorly above the supraorbital ridges, draws it tight, and reads the measurement.

Comments: When the infant objects to this measurement and struggles to free himself, the person holding him must be careful that the tape does not slip from the desired place, as he is responsible for keeping the tape in the right position posteriorly. It may be necessary for the person holding the child to place one hand under his chin in order to stabilize the head.

Chest Circumference.—Age Range: From birth through three years.

Instrument: Metal tape.

Posture: Sitting; lumbar region of the back straight or slightly concave anteriorly; arms relaxed and hanging at the sides; head held erect.

Technic: The measurer slips the tape around the child's chest and the measure is taken at the level of the xiphoid process. The pressure is such that the tape firmly contacts the skin, but only enough pressure is used to indent the skin very slightly. The extremes of inspiration and expiration are noted and the average recorded.

Comments: If the child is crying at the time the measurement is taken, the measurer holds the tape so that it can follow the movements of the chest wall during expansion and contraction which result from crying. Increase and decrease in size are carefully noted for a short period and the average of the extreme measures is then recorded.

Changes in the position of the head will result in a change in chest size; therefore the position of the head should be carefully checked.

Girths of Extremities (Fig. 12).—Age Range: From birth through three years.

Instrument: Metal tape.

Posture: Extremity extended.

Technic: All measurements are taken on the left side. The person holding the child keeps the extremity which is being measured extended. The measurer places the tape around the arm, forearm, thigh, or calf at the level indicated below. The pressure used is such that the tape merely contacts the skin firmly.

Level of Measurement for Arm—The tape is placed around the arm at a level that would bisect the midpoint of the biceps muscle transversely.

Level of Measurement for Forearm—The level is just below the elbow (the greatest circumference of the forearm).

Level of Measurement for Thigh—The tape encircles the thigh at the level of the gluteal fold.

Level of Measurement for Calf—The circumference is taken over the fleshiest part of the calf.

Comments: If the child's skin is moist, care must be taken to see that the tape does not stick to the skin and give an erroneous measure.

Fig. 12.

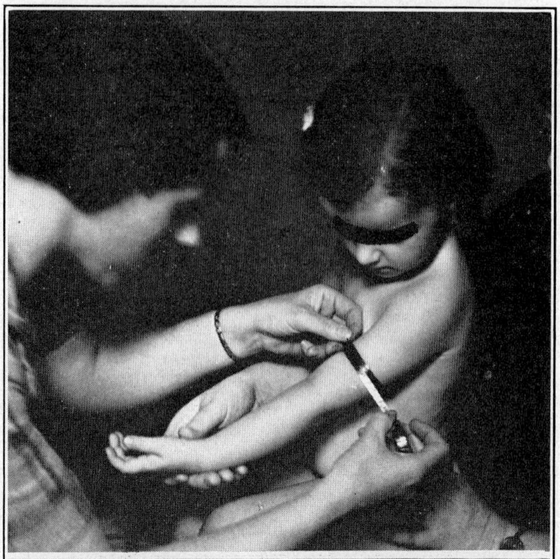

Fig. 13.

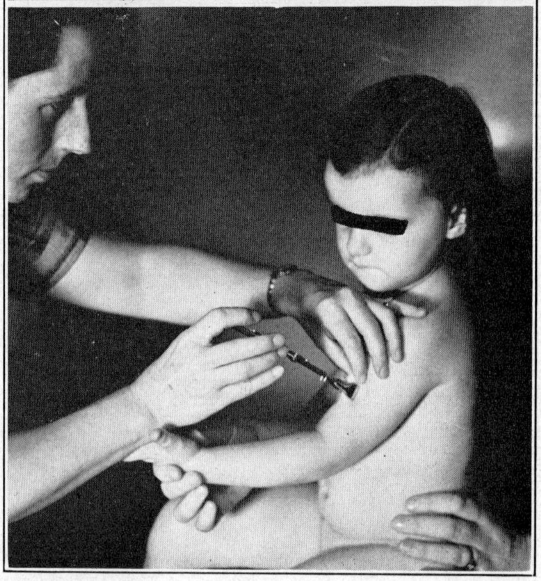

Measurements of Skin and Subcutaneous Tissue (Fig. 13).—Locations for measuring the skin and subcutaneous tissue are:

Arm (front)—This measurement is taken on the front of the left arm over the belly of the biceps muscle.

Arm (back)—The measurement is taken on the back of the left arm, opposite the location for measuring arm front.

Chest (front)—This measurement is taken on the left side about midway between the axillary line and the midline of the body and on a level with the seventh rib.

Chest (back)—This measurement is taken on the left side of the back, opposite the location for measuring chest front.

Suprascapular—The measurement is taken over the middle third of the spine of the scapula.

Suprailiac—This measurement is taken on the left side just above the crest of the ilium in the midaxillary line.

Age Range: Birth through three years.

Instrument: Fat calipers.

Posture: Sitting.

Technic: The measurer grasps the calipers in the right hand so that the movable arm is on the thumb side. The ball of the thumb is on the movable arm above the calibrated arc; the first and second fingers rest on top of the arc; and the other fingers remain on the outside of the stationary arm. With the thumb and forefinger of the left hand the measurer pinches up a double layer of the skin and subcutaneous tissue at the place of measurement, taking care not to include any of the underlying muscle. The long axis of the pinched-up tissue should run parallel to the long axis of the extremity of the body. The pinch should be taken by pressing inward with the ends of the fingers and at the same time pressing downward. The jaws of the calipers are opened wide enough to include this double layer of tissue and are pressed down over it to one side of the fingers; then the jaws are released, and the reading is taken from the calibrated arc. The fingers should retain their hold on the pinched-up skin and subcutaneous tissue with only enough pressure to prevent the tissue from slipping from between the blades. The measurement is taken several times before final recording to insure accuracy.

Comments: The pinched-up tissue over which the blades of the calipers are placed should represent a complete double layer of skin and subcutaneous tissue; none of the underlying muscle layer should be included.

WEIGHT

The weight is taken without clothing.

DISCUSSION

In conclusion, it may be well to mention briefly a few things of general interest in carrying out an infant-measuring program.

Because of the great variation in age of children being measured, it has been found that the measuring program could be carried on most efficiently with a minimum of three persons for the staff. This number includes one person who does the measuring, a second to hold the child, and a third person to record the data. It is advisable that the first two people be trained to do the measuring, in which case they may take turns holding and measuring the infants. Where this is done and where the study is such that the same child returns periodically for measurements, it is suggested that the same person measure the child each time he comes.

The parent of the child is not allowed in the room during the measuring (with very few exceptions), but sits outside the room and observes the procedure through an observation window made in the door. This regulation was adopted after having first tried permitting the mother in the room during the measuring.

The room should be of moderate size, well lighted, and equipped with ventilating and heating facilities that are easily controlled. A small closet is necessary in which to keep the instruments. The furniture will include two tables, one on which the measuring board is placed and the other for the small instruments and for the convenience of the recorder. In addition the room will contain the scales, the vertical board with the paper measuring scale attached, and the measuring bench, several large chairs, and at least one small chair for the children. A clothes hamper is necessary since the children are laid on diapers when they are placed in the scales and on the measuring board, and these are changed for each child. The instruments and the board are wiped with an alcohol sponge after each child is measured.

Toys are an important and useful part of the equipment for the measuring room. They should be selected with the idea of getting things which will appeal to children over the entire age range. Rattles and rubber dolls or animals that make a noise are useful in diverting the attention of young children. In the older ages some simple toys of bright color which can be used in building are most entertaining. All toys should be large enough so the children cannot get them in their mouths, and the paint should be of some harmless material.

TUBEROUS SCLEROSIS: ENCEPHALOGRAPHIC INTERPRETATION

Russell N. DeJong, M.D.
Ann Arbor, Mich.

TUBEROUS sclerosis is a disease characterized by congenital abnormalities in certain tissues of ectodermal origin, especially the nervous system, skin, and retina. Due to the coexistent involvement ot the nervous system and the skin, the condition is frequently spoken of as a neurocutaneous syndrome or as a congenital ectodermosis with associated nervous system involvement.[1] Certain of the visceral organs are occasionally involved as well. The disease is usually seen in children, and it is characterized clinically by a triad of symptoms consisting of retarded mental development, convulsive attacks, and so-called sebaceous adenomas. The term epiloia has also been suggested for this syndrome.[2, 3]

The cutaneous changes are of importance in the clinical recognition of the disease. They are characterized by multiple papular or nodular lesions which are most frequently distributed symmetrically, in a butterfly arrangement, over the bridge of the nose, the nasolabial folds, and the malar eminences. The individual lesion is spoken of as a sebaceous adenoma or a ''nevus multiplex'' of Pringle,[4] and it varies from yellowish pink to reddish brown in color, and from the size of a millet seed to that of a pea. Because of the fact that in most cases these lesions are not an adenomatous or hyperplastic condition of the sebaceous glands, but rather are lesions which belong to the nevoid group of disorders and consist of hyperplastic connective and vascular tissues, the use of the term nevus might be more justifiable.[5] The lesions, both from their appearance and their distribution, closely resemble those seen in acne rosacea. In addition to the involvement of the face, one occasionally sees skin manifestations over the back, shoulders, and the lumbosacral region. These resemble the lesions found in multiple neurofibromatosis,[6] and they may be of the following types: changes in pigmentation, areas of fibrous, hyperplastic skin of the type known as shagreen, nevi, or sessile, or pedunculated polyps.

The pathologic changes in the central nervous system in tuberous sclerosis are quite characteristic, and the clinical symptomatology is no doubt dependent upon the location of the changes. The brain is often small and hard, and pearly white to yellowish gray nodules may be found in the cortex, throughout the brain tissue, and in the ependymal

From the Department of Neurology, University Hospital, University of Michigan.

lining of the ventricles. These nodules vary in size and are seen most frequently in the frontal lobes, being rare in the brain stem and cerebellum.[7] When present within the ventricles the lesions give the appearance of bunches of grapes or "candle gutterings"[6] hanging down from the upper surface of the ventricles. Histologically these tumorlike accumulations are composed of large atypical cells surrounded by a dense glial network.[8] Certain of the large cells resemble giant nerve cells; others are thought to be primitive glial elements.[9] It has been suggested that these structures represent embryonal cells of the spongioblastic and neurcytic varieties which have failed to differentiate.[10] In addition to the skin and nervous system abnormalities, one may find tumorlike structures in the retina or the eyeball. The retinal tumors are of glial or vascular origin and have been referred to by Van der Hoeve as phakomata.[11, 12] Certain of the viscera, especially the heart, kidneys, pancreas, and liver, may contain cystic tumors or myomas.

The earliest recognition of the pathologic changes found in tuberous sclerosis was possibly that of von Recklinghausen (1862), who found sclerotic areas in the brain and myomas in the heart of a newborn child.[13] Credit for the first description of the syndrome is usually given to Bourneville, who in 1880 demonstrated islets of hypertrophic sclerosis over the cerebral hemispheres of a three-year-old girl with epilepsy, arrested physical development, hemiplegia, idiocy, and "acne rosacea" of the face.[14] Since then numerous descriptions of the clinical symptomatology and the pathologic changes in tuberous sclerosis have been reported in the literature. However, there are only three reports of pneumographic studies in tuberous sclerosis, and in none of these cases is the diagnosis incontrovertible. Stewart and Bauer have reported a case diagnosed as tuberous sclerosis in which the ventriculogram showed only dilatation of the lateral ventricles;[15] the patient did not have skin changes or tumors of the viscera. Postmortem examination of the brain showed diffuse hardening of the right cerebral hemisphere, which was felt to be a large area of tuberous sclerosis. A case with many congenital abnormalities such as cleft palate and cleft lip, but without sebaceous adenomas or recognized visceral involvement, was reported by Berkwitz and Rigler.[16] The encephalogram demonstrated bizarre deformities of the lateral ventricles, indicating gross cerebral abnormalities. Drake has reported a case without sebaceous adenomas or retinal tumors in which encephalographic studies showed three small discrete masses of calcification in the left occipital area and a similar single spot of calcification in the right cerebrum.[17] There was bulging of the right thalamus into the right lateral ventricle, and the basilar cisterns and subarachnoid channels were increased in size. The following case is of interest because it demonstrates encephalographic changes, similar to those found in Drake's case, in a patient in whom the clinical diagnosis of tuberous sclerosis is quite definite.

REPORT OF CASE

C. G., an eight-year-old boy, was brought to the University Hospital because he failed to show normal mental development. His birth and early developmental history were normal, but he had been slow to walk and talk, and during the two years that he had gone to school he had shown little progress. At the age of one year he had had a convulsion which had lasted an hour and a half. Since this time convulsions had occurred whenever the patient had a fever. A facial eruption had gradually appeared since the age of four. There was no family history of mental retardation, convulsions, or of similar skin disorders.

The patient was a well-developed and well-nourished boy, but he was obviously retarded mentally. On the face were many reddish brown papular lesions which

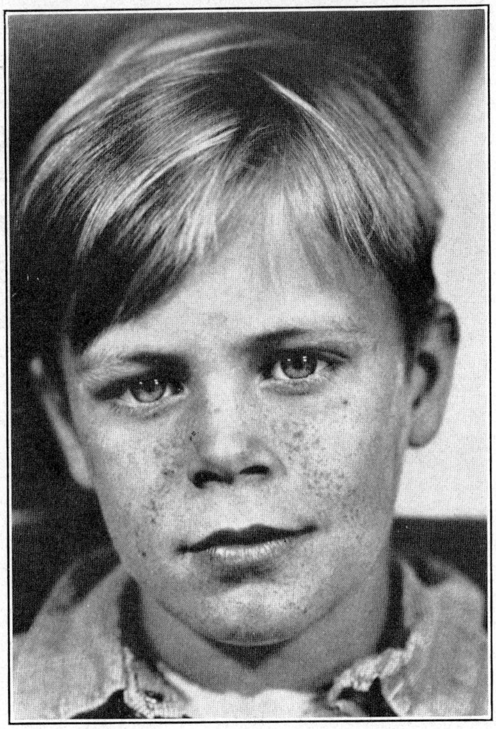

Fig. 1.—So-called sebaceous adenomas present on the face in a butterfly distribution.

were present in a butterfly distribution over the bridge of the nose and the nasolabial region (Fig. 1). The lesions were of a rather brilliant erythematous color and varied from the size of a pinhead to the size of a glass-headed pin. They were soft, and there was no superimposed scaling. Some of them appeared to be confluent. On the back in the lumbar and sacral regions were lesions of a somewhat different type (Fig. 2). There was one nonpedunculated polypoid area 1½ in. by ¾ in. in diameter; this was smooth and soft, but there were superimposed papules and nodules. There were more masses of papules and nodules which tended to become confluent. These varied in color, and some were erythematous, some pink, and a few were white. There were three small, irregular, depigmented areas on the back, one on the right buttock, and one over the right hip. Some small nodules were also seen in the intergluteal fold. The general physical examination showed no other abnormalities. Examination of the fundi oculi showed blurring of the disk margins with striations running out into the surrounding retina. There was a raised white lesion with a slightly yellowish tinge lying on the temporal side of the left disk. This appeared to be made up of a large number of small globular bodies. There was no evidence of inflammatory change, and the vessels were normal.

The neurologic examination showed, in addition to the above mentioned findings, some overactivity of the tendon reflexes, especially on the left. There was a moderately positive Babinski sign on the left, and Oppenheim's signs were positive bilaterally. There was no definite ataxia or dysmetria, although the patient's muscular coordination was inadequate, and he carried out skilled acts poorly. There

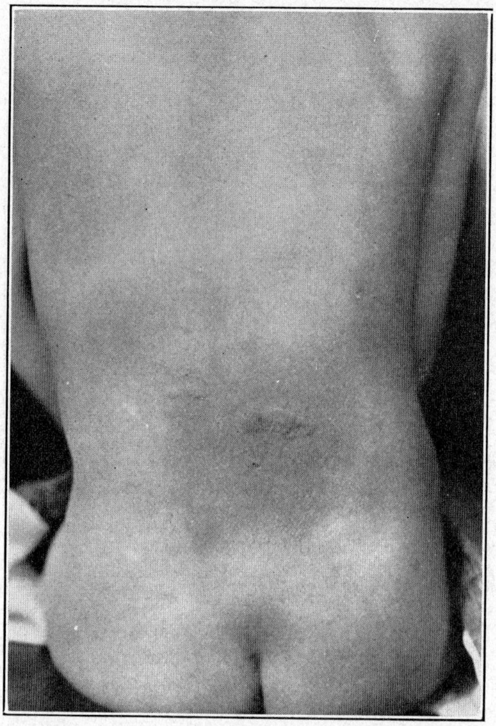

Fig. 2.—Polypoid and papulonodular lesions in the lumbosacral region.

was marked impairment of speech. The patient was jovial and appeared to be alert. He was very restless, and his attention was limited. A mental test recorded an intelligence quotient of 48. He failed especially in tests for memory, comprehension, and manual dexterity. Laboratory examinations on the blood and urine, including the blood Kahn test and nonprotein nitrogen, glucose, calcium and phosphorus determinations, were reported as being within the limits of normal. A skin tuberculin test gave negative results. The spinal fluid showed normal cytology, a total protein of 38 mg. per 100 c.c., and a three-plus globulin reaction. The colloidal gold curve was 0111100000.

Stereoscopic roentgen ray studies of the skull showed multiple calcium deposits in the brain tissue (Fig. 3). These were present on both sides of the midline but were more prominent on the right, and they were situated in the region of the superior margin of the third ventricle and above the pituitary fossa. The largest of these deposits, as projected, was not over ¼ inch in diameter. There were no signs of increased intracranial pressure. An encephalogram was made, and 105 c.c. of cerebrospinal fluid were withdrawn and replaced by air (Fig. 4). The right lateral ventricle was found to be definitely larger than the left. There appeared to be soft

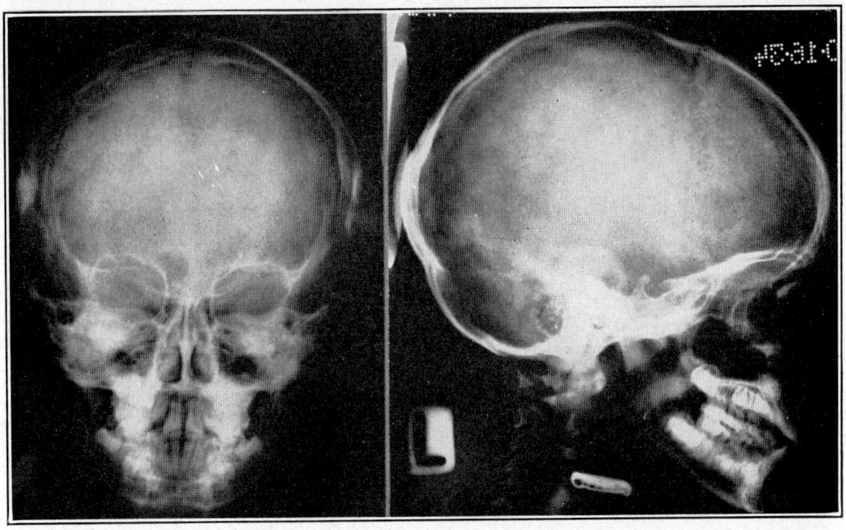

Fig. 3.—Anteroposterior and lateral roentgen ray studies of the skull showing calcium deposits within the brain tissue.

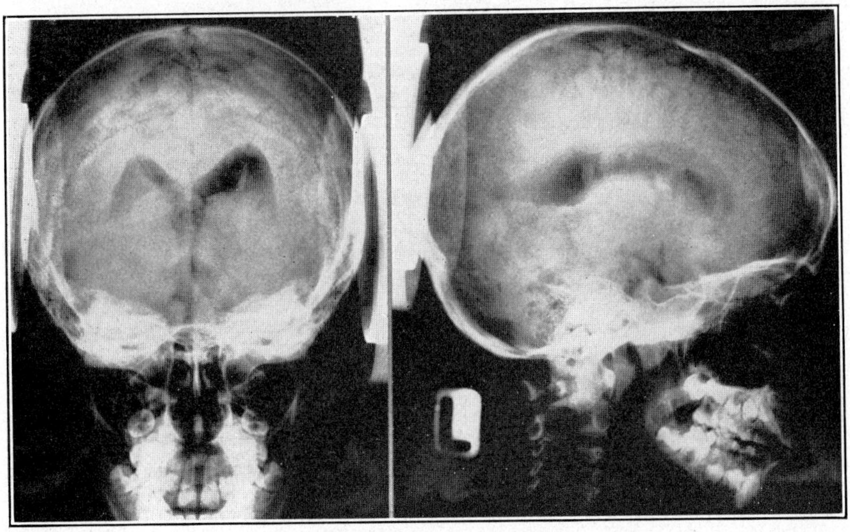

Fig. 4.—Encephalographic studies showing soft tissue masses and areas of calcification within the ventricles.

tissue proliferation along the floor of each lateral ventricle extending posteriorly from the region of the foramen of Monro. There were soft tissue tags extending into the posterior portion of the body of each lateral ventricle. These were felt to represent hyperplastic choroid plexus or other proliferated soft tissues. The larger calcium deposits noted in the skull films appeared to be in the region of the right foramen of Monro. A rounded soft tissue shadow containing some calcium was seen to protrude down into the upper half of the third ventricle. The aqueduct and fourth ventricle did not appear to be abnormal, and approximately normal amounts of air were present in the basilar cisterns and the subarachnoid channels.

CONCLUSIONS AND SUMMARY

Tuberous sclerosis is a congenital disorder of certain ectodermal tissues, and it is characterized clinically by mental retardation, convulsive attacks, and so-called sebaceous adenomas. A case has been reported which shows that the characteristic sclerotic areas in the cerebrum and within the cerebral ventricles may be demonstrated by roentgenography and encephalography.

REFERENCES

1. Yakovlev, Paul I., and Guthrie, Riley H.: Arch. Neurol. & Psychiat. **26**: 1145, 1931.
2. Sherlock, E. B.: The Feeble-Minded, London, 1911, Macmillan and Company, pp. 241-243.
3. Brain, W. R., and Strauss, E. B.: Recent Advances in Neurology, Philadelphia, 1929, P. Blakiston's Son and Company, p. 348.
4. Yakovlev, Paul I.: Congenital Ectodermoses, in The Practitioner's Library of Medicine and Surgery, New York and London, 1936, D. Appleton-Century Company, Vol. 9, pp. 754-758.
5. Schwarz, Herman, and Abramson, Harold: J. Pediat. **3**: 586, 1933.
6. Critchley, Macdonald, and Earl, C. J. C.: Brain **55**: 311, 1932.
7. Hassin, George B.: Histopathology of the Peripheral and Central Nervous Systems, Baltimore, 1933, William Wood & Company, pp. 326-328.
8. Bielschowsky, Max.: J. f. Psychol. u. Neurol. **30**: 167, 1924.
9. Globus, J. H.: Malformation in the Central Nervous System, in Penfield, Wilder, Cytology and Cellular Pathology of the Nervous System, New York, 1932, Paul B. Hoeber, Inc., pp. 1150-1166.
10. Grinker, Roy R.: Neurology, Springfield, Ill., 1934, Charles C. Thomas, p. 931.
11. Van der Hoeve, J.: Tr. Ophth. Soc. U. Kingdom **43**: 534, 1923.
    Idem: Tr. Ophth. Soc. U. Kingdom **52**: 380, 1932.
12. Gottlieb, J. S., and Lavine, G. R.: Arch. Neurol. & Psychiat. **33**: 379, 1935.
13. Von Recklinghausen, F.: Monatschr. f. Geburtsh. u. Frauenkr. **20**: 1, 1862.
14. Bourneville: Arch. de neurol. **1**: 81, 1880.
15. Stewart, H. L., and Bauer, E. L.: Arch. Path. **14**: 799, 1932.
16. Berkwitz, N. J., and Rigler, L. G.: Arch. Neurol. & Psychiat. **34**: 833, 1935.
17. Drake, R. L.: Arch. Neurol. & Psychiat. **34**: 681, 1935.

PEDIATRIC DIAGNOSIS

WILBURT C. DAVISON, M.D.
DURHAM, N. C.

FREQUENTLY it is said, and perhaps with truth, that physicians today are not as keen diagnosticians as were those of the last generation. There are at least three possible reasons for this: (1) Most students have been taught by excellent older clinicians, who through long experience in quizzing patients and thumping chests, have learned to weigh essential symptoms and signs so quickly that they often seemed to make "snap diagnoses"; (2) with the crowding of the curriculum by additional courses in the newer specialties and in laboratory aids, there is a tendency to neglect fundamental training in history taking and physical diagnosis; and (3) many medical school courses in physical diagnosis are limited to percussion and auscultation of the thorax and do not include the diagnostic problems of the other portions of the body or an adequate consideration of children.[1] Students trained under the usual present methods emulate their preceptors and try to make similarly rapid diagnoses, which frequently are wrong. As a result, many young physicians spend more energy defending their "snap diagnoses" than would have been consumed in obtaining a careful history and doing a painstakingly accurate physical examination. There is no royal road to diagnosis; for every correct one made by quick impressions, there are a dozen which can be obtained only after a careful study of the information obtained by the methods shown in Table I.

TABLE I

METHODS OF EXAMINATION

METHODS	DIAGNOSIS
History	Pain and its location; diet
Inspection	General diseases
Palpation	Surgical diseases
Percussion	Chest diseases
Auscultation	Chest diseases
Laboratory tests	Infectious and metabolic diseases

A wealth of information can be collected by the careful application of these methods. One hundred fifty-nine different symptoms and signs can be elicited by a careful history and physical examination, and the results of the laboratory tests indicated in Table II will supply additional helpful knowledge. Certain of these tests should be done rou-

From the Department of Pediatrics, Duke University School of Medicine, and Duke Hospital, Durham, N. C.

Presented before the Texas Pediatric Society, San Antonio, Nov. 13, 1934, by Dr. A. P. Bloxsom.

tinely. A Wassermann test should be performed on every child examined, regardless of clinical or social condition, and not alone on those children suspected of having syphilis. Certainly for every case of syphilis in children diagnosed by clinical signs, five are discovered by routine Wassermann tests. An intradermal tuberculin test which is negative will, with rare exceptions, eliminate the possibility of tuberculosis, while, if it is positive, an x-ray film usually will demonstrate whether the disease process is active or quiescent.[2]

These data often must be studied and restudied like clues in a detective story, for, after all, symptoms and signs are clues which may be caused by several diseases, all but one of which must be eliminated by the further study of the patient's other symptoms and often by the use of laboratory methods. For example, ten different symptoms and signs,

TABLE II

LABORATORY TESTS

LABORATORY TESTS	DIAGNOSIS
Routine tests	
Tuberculin	Tuberculosis
Wassermann	Syphilis
Urinalysis	Nephritis, pyuria, diabetes
Hemoglobin	Anemia
Blood smear	Leucemia, purpura
Special tests	
Xray	Chest diseases, fractures
Blood chemistry	Metabolic diseases
Blood cultures	Systemic infections
Throat cultures and smears	Stomatitis, diphtheria
Stool cultures and smears	Dysentery, typhoid fever, parasites
Urine cultures	Pyuria, typhoid fever
Vaginal smears and hanging drop preparations	Gonorrhea, trichomonas vaginitis

which may be caused by any one of one hundred and thirteen different pediatric diseases, can be detected by a careful inspection of the patient, and eight signs, caused by eighty-eight diseases, can be elicited by palpation, percussion, etc. A cross-reference table like a road map mileage chart would be ideal, but it is impractical; three of us tried arranging the one hundred fifty-nine pediatric symptoms and signs and the sixty-five laboratory tests into tables to facilitate the diagnosis of the three hundred seven diseases of children, but, except in a very limited way, the results usually were of no assistance. A similar attempt has been made to use this comparative method in adult diagnosis.[3] Clinical diagnosis, in the absence of specific tests, is an estimation, often subconscious, of probabilities, based upon experience, and any tabulation of the relative frequency of symptoms and signs must be corrected by judgment and observation.[4] This judgment and observation, of course, can be obtained only by experience, but, if a physician is assiduous in eliciting a wealth of symptoms and signs, these other attributes to diagnostic ability eventually will be added unto him. The difficulty, of course, is remembering all or most of the diseases which may cause that particular symptom. For instance, ninety-five different conditions may produce vomiting in children, and any one of seventy-six diseases may be responsible for abdominal pain.[5] A printed "ready reminder" list of them should be available for consultation, not with the idea of making a cross-reference differential diagnosis, but merely as a list of possibilities which should not be overlooked. If a physician's mind were sufficiently "encyclopedic" to remember all of these possibilities without a reminder, the chances are that his brain would not be adequately analytical to utilize this information in making a diagnosis. A book or list can jog the memory on possibilities, but it cannot do a physician's thinking for him.

Obviously a discussion of all of these symptoms and signs is impractical here, so eight have been selected as examples. *Headaches* in children may be caused by sixty-seven diseases or conditions. To consider the complete differential diagnosis of all of them in arriving at a decision probably is absurd, but, if a physician before making a final diagnosis in a child who complains of headaches will at least read the list, he often will save himself and the patient much embarrassment and occasionally will correct an erroneous "snap diagnosis." As a rule, a student or physician notices the patient's most obvious symptoms and recalls that they occur in a certain disease, but frequently he forgets that these same symptoms may be present in several diseases. An erroneous diagnosis often is the result. For instance, if the patient has a headache, is nauseated, is mentally dull, and has fever, the student or physician may think of typhoid fever and not remember that these same symptoms also are characteristic of meningococcus meningitis. Obviously if the patient has meningitis, his chances of recovery are not increased by a delayed diagnosis, for they depend upon prompt recognition and vigorous serum therapy. A list serves as a ready reminder of easily forgotten possibilities, which if they are at least recalled to memory can be confirmed or eliminated by searching for additional symptoms and signs or by various laboratory procedures.

Children are too often sentenced to weeks or months in bed because a physician or a school nurse has heard a *cardiac murmur*. The majority of rapidly growing children have definitely audible heart murmurs, but true cardiac disease, both congenital and acquired, occurs in less than 2 per cent of them.[6] Obviously a glance at Table III may suggest to a physician the need of additional study of the patient's other symptoms before condemning the child to bed and completely demoralizing the family. Many pediatric and parental neuroses are caused by hasty and erroneous diagnosis of heart disease. Cardiac murmurs, of course, are of some importance but not nearly so much as are the measurement of heart size, the cardiac functional capacity, symptoms of decompensation, x-ray pictures of the chest, blood pressure determinations, electrocardiograms, and last but not least the effect of respiration on the murmur, as most functional murmurs disappear at the height of full inspiration. The cardiac size usually is increased if the murmur is due to heart disease. The murmur of any individual's heart generally can be correctly diagnosed if the physician will study a list such as Table III so that he will be reminded of several possibilities and then carefully weigh *all* of the factors concerned.

TABLE III

HEART MURMURS

LOCATION	TIME	DIAGNOSIS
Apex	Systole	Functional
Apex	Systole	Mitral insufficiency
Apex	Diastole	Functional
Apex	Diastole	Mitral stenosis
Base	Systole	Functional
Base	Systole	Pulmonary stenosis
Base	Systole	Aortic stenosis
Base	Diastole	Aortic insufficiency
Base	Continuous	Patent ductus
Sternum	Systole	Patent septum
Sternum	Systole	Tricuspid insufficiency

Albuminuria is another symptom which to some physicians suggests only "Bright's disease" with a grave prognosis. That conditions other than nephritis cause albuminuria can be seen in Table IV. Occasionally it is very embarrassing to see a child who has nothing but orthostatic albuminuria yet has been kept in bed for months on an erroneous diagnosis of nephritis. Because the physician had not considered orthostatic albuminuria, he had not compared day and night urine specimens and had not found that the night specimen was free of albumin. The parents, of course, must be told that the child is well and except for the

TABLE IV

CAUSES OF ALBUMINURIA[7]

CONDITION	ESTIMATED CASE DISTRIBUTION (IN PER CENT)
Glomerular nephritis (acute, subacute and chronic hemorrhagic, exudative, purpuric)	59
Orthostatic albuminuria (lordotic)	20
Pyuria (pyelitis, pyelonephritis)	16
Tubular nephritis (acute and chronic nephrosis)	3
Interstitial nephritis (chronic nephritis with infantilism)	1
Paroxysmal hemoglobinuria	1

need of corrective exercises and physiotherapy to remove his lordosis, he can attend school and play as other children. However, when they ask the reason for this sudden change of instructions from complete bed rest to freedom from restraint, should they be informed that their former physician cured his patient or that because he did not consider all of the possible causes of albuminuria, he was mistaken in his diagnosis and that the child need not have been invalided? That question is raised too frequently to be amusing. After orthostatic albuminuria has been eliminated, the differentiation of the other forms of albuminuria is not difficult: red blood cells in the urine indicate glomerular damage; the presence of pus cells in clumps in the urine is diagnostic of pyuria; albuminuria with edema but without hematuria is characteristic of tubular nephritis, etc.

Convulsions occur in many childhood conditions, but a lumbar puncture, which should be performed on every child who has neurologic symptoms, and a glance at Table V frequently will suggest a tentative diagnosis which, of course, must be confirmed or eliminated by further study. If the patient has *meningitis,* the earlier adequate serotherapy is started, the better are the results.

TABLE V

SPINAL FLUID EXAMINATION

APPEARANCE	CELL COUNT	ORGANISM	DIAGNOSIS
Clear	10-1,000	Acid-fast bacilli	Tuberculous meningitis (33%)*
		None	Meningismus Poliomyelitis Encephalitis (lead, lethargic, etc.) Mumps or syphilitic meningitis Brain abscess or tumor
Turbid	1,000-5,000	Gram-negative cocci	Meningococcus meningitis (30%)
		Gram-negative bacilli	Influenzal meningitis (13%) Brucella meningitis
		Gram-positive cocci	Pneumococcus meningitis (12%) Streptococcus meningitis (7%) Staphylococcus meningitis (0.5%)

*Figure in parentheses indicates percentage of cases in children under two years of age due to that particular organism.[8]

Thus far, this discussion has been limited to the use of tables and lists as reminders of all of the diseases which may cause a particular symptom, but occasionally the tabular listing and comparison of all of the patient's symptoms and signs may lead to a diagnosis. For example, the differentiation of the several causes of *ataxia,* which after all is only a symptom and not a disease entity, is greatly facilitated if some such aid is used. A complete history and a careful physical examination are necessary, and clinical judgment, of course, is needed to evaluate the various symptoms and signs; but, unless all of them are compared, an erroneous diagnosis is frequent. When the proper technic is patiently pursued, the diagnosis usually makes itself.

The same observations apply to *muscular weakness* and the *myopathies.* Weakness is a common complaint, and "snap diagnoses" often can be exceedingly harmful to the patient. Bed rest and diet instead of "building-up exercises" are needed if the child has tuberculosis, and psychiatric care and a change of environment, if the child is neurotic. Even a casual study and tabulation of the patient's other symptoms may suggest some forgotten possibility.

Finally, it is important to divide the 307 pediatric diseases into the 83 which are curable and the 224 from which the patients usually recover or succumb regardless of therapy.[5] Accurate and prompt diagnosis should be stressed in the first group and the latter diseases should not be considered until all possibility of the presence of one of the curable conditions is eliminated.

CONCLUSIONS

1. A careful history and a complete physical examination always are necessary before even a tentative diagnosis is attempted.
2. All of the information available and every indication for further studies should be intelligently considered before a diagnosis can be established.
3. Symptoms and signs are clues which may be caused by several diseases, all but one of which must be eliminated by further study of the patient's other symptoms, and often by laboratory methods, before the correct diagnosis can be made.
4. "Snap" and often erroneous diagnoses can be avoided by a study of lists of all of the diseases which cause any particular symptom.
5. The presence or absence of a curable disease should be decided before considering the possibility of conditions for which adequate therapy is not available.
6. The art of arriving at a correct diagnosis is, or should be, based upon at least three processes: (a) remembering to obtain as many bits of evidence as possible, (b) recalling as many conditions as possible which will cause these symptoms, and (c) evaluating this material.

REFERENCES

1. Ruffin, J. M.: J. A. Am. M. Coll. **10:** 292, 1935.
2. Davison, W. C.: J. Pediat. **3:** 64, 1933.
3. Kitchens, W. L.: Clin. Med. & Surg. **39:** 360, 1932.
   Idem: Definite Diagnosis in General Practice, Philadelphia, 1934, W. B. Saunders Co.
4. McIntosh, R.: J. A. Am. M. Coll. **8:** 227, 1933.
5. Davison, W. C.: The Compleat Pediatrician, Durham, N. C., 1934, Duke University Press.
6. Davison, W. C.: South Med. & Surg. **90:** 342, 1928.
7. Hill, L. W.: Am. J. Dis. Child. **17:** 270, 1919.
8. Ward, H. K., and Fothergill, L. D.: Am. J. Dis. Child. **43:** 873, 1932.

OMPHALITIS IN THE NEWBORN

John W. Chamberlain, M.D.
Boston, Mass.

INTRODUCTION

Infection of the umbilicus in the newborn was one of the most important causes of death among infants before the days of asepsis. Cullen[1] writes, "Until the advent of asepsis, myriads of children succumbed to umbilical infection within a few days or a few weeks after birth." Today the disease is seen frequently enough and is of sufficient import to warrant more attention than has been paid it in recent literature.

During the last half of the nineteenth century, there appeared several reports of epidemics of "erysipelas" and "gangrene" of the umbilicus. These were summarized by Audion[2] (1901) in an excellent paper and more recently have been reviewed in detail by Cullen. It was recognized that there was some relationship between puerperal fever and umbilical infection, and between the latter and the secondary lesions which make it so serious; it was not until the work of Pasteur and Lister that this relationship was understood. In spite of this understanding and the aseptic and antiseptic precautions taken at the time of delivery and for the first two or three weeks thereafter, umbilical infections still occur. In certain communities, parts of China for instance, where street dust is used as dusting powder for the cord, it is estimated (Reed)* that 50 per cent of newborn infants die of umbilical infection even today. In more civilized communities the incidence of fatal sequelae in the cases that do occur is sufficiently great to merit serious consideration of the disease by obstetrician, pediatrician, and surgeon.

ANATOMY

Most of the pathology of the umbilicus, other than infection, is directly related to the embryology of the region and is a manifestation of arrested or abnormal development. Infection and its sequelae, on the other hand, are directly related to the normal anatomy and the physiologic changes taking place at the time of delivery and directly thereafter.

Up to the moment the cord is clamped or tied, the infant's blood is circulating through the two umbilical arteries and the umbilical vein. It will be recalled that the former are continuous at the umbilicus with the hypogastric arteries which rise from the internal iliac arteries in the pelvis, course along the back of the anterior abdominal wall on either side of the bladder, and converge to meet each other at the umbilicus.

From the Surgical Service, Children's Hospital and the Infants' Hospital.
*Quoted from Rice.

The umbilical vein (really the left umbilical vein) enters the abdomen at the umbilicus and passes upward as the free margin of the falciform ligament of the liver to the under surface of the latter. Here it gives off several branches and then, at the transverse fissure, divides into two branches. The larger joins the portal vein and enters the right lobe of the liver; the smaller continues upward as the ductus venosus to empty into the inferior vena cava. The fact that both the hypogastric arteries and umbilical vein are separated from the abdominal cavity only by a layer of peritoneum and a thin irregular layer of areolar tissue is an important anatomic relationship. Thus benign-appearing omphalitis or hypogastric arteritis may, by extending only a very short distance, become a fatal peritonitis.

The cutaneous lymphatics of the umbilical region (Cuneo and Marcillini, 1901) drain downward and outward to both inguinal regions. Lymph vessels arising just above the umbilicus drain upward and outward to both pectoral regions. The deeper lymphatics communicate with those of the fascial sheaths at the various levels.

When the umbilical cord is tied and cut, circulation of blood through the umbilical veins is permanently interrupted. The arteries become obliterated and project as the lateral umbilical ligaments. The vein and ductus venosus become obliterated and persist as the ligamentum teres and ligamentum venosum, respectively.

The nature of the process of obliteration and the time consumed are also of considerable importance because of their bearing on the spread of infection. Obliteration of the lumen of the vessels probably begins with partial emptying of the lumen and corresponding collapse of the vessel wall. It continues with the formation of a clot, its organization, and especially with a gradual proliferation of the subintimal layer of the vessel wall. The time consumed in the process is usually stated to be about five days. Study of autopsy material at the Children's Hospital reveals that the time consumed is from twenty to fifty days.* In other words, a lumen containing unorganized blood clot may be demonstrated not only with the microscope but with the naked eye during this time (Fig. 1). Final transformation of the vessels into fibrous cords requires a much longer time. Direct spread of organisms from an infected umbilicus via the vessels to the blood stream is thus facilitated for a much longer time than usually thought possible.

While the vessels are being obliterated, the cord is drying and separating. At the junction of the cord with the umbilicus, the skin is reflected onto the cord for a variable distance. As the cord dries, the ring of skin becomes smaller, so that by the time the cord separates, the raw surface which would otherwise be present is covered with a thin layer of skin and scar tissue. Probably a small area of clean granulation tissue should not be considered abnormal. Should the cord, for some reason,

*Farber, S.: Personal communication.

separate prematurely there would be left a larger raw, granulating surface in which would be incorporated the practically open ends of the partially obliterated umbilical vessels.

ETIOLOGY

Sepsis of the umbilical structures may be due to saprophytic or pathogenic organisms, or both. The liability to invasion of pathogenic organisms is increased by the presence of and reaction to saprophytic organisms since the latter delay separation of the cord and healing of the umbilical wound (Audion).

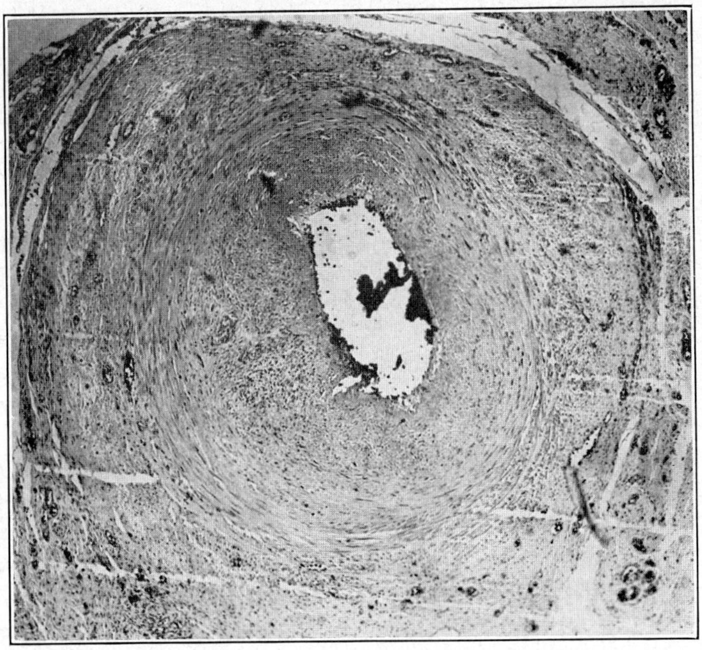

Fig. 1.—Low power (x60) photomicrograph of a hypogastric artery from a patient who died of dysentery and terminal bronchopneumonia at three and one-half weeks of age.

Bacterial invasion may occur intrapartum or postpartum. For many years it was thought that the birth canal did not contain pathogenic organisms, but it is now known that it frequently does. This is especially true when there have been frequent vaginal examinations during labor. It is not surprising, therefore, that Adair,[3] in a small series of cases, was able to recover pathogenic organisms from the surface of the cord and periumbilical region in 20 per cent of the cases studied. Premature rupture of the membranes and prolonged labor following this provides another route for intrapartum invasion with pathogenic organisms. Creadick[4] studied the umbilical cord in two thousand consecutive cases in which the infants weighed more than 1,800 gm. (4.2 pounds). Forty-three of these showed leucocytic infiltration (with polymorphonuclear and mononuclear cells) of the vessel walls and adjacent connective tissue. Usually the vein and sometimes the arteries were involved. Fourteen of these forty-three infants died, and in ten death was attributed to intrapartum infection.

Creadick pointed out that there were three possible sources of infection of the contents of the pregnant uterus: (1) by way of the maternal blood stream, (2) by way of the fallopian tubes, and (3) transamniotic, usually following premature rupture of the membranes. Sections through the insertion of the cord on the placenta showed branches of the umbilical vein involved in an inflammatory reaction in every one of the forty-three cases. In thirty-eight of these cases, the course of the reaction was traced backward into the subamniotic connective tissue. Premature rupture of the membranes occurred in twenty-six, and duration of labor was prolonged in twenty-five of the cases.

Siddall[5] more recently studied the association of inflammation of the umbilical cord with stillborn and premature infants. He found a much higher incidence of inflammation in the cords of these infants than in those delivered at term. In the cases he studied, however, the prognosis for the child was not affected by the presence of the inflammation.

While there may be an occasional case of fatal omphalitis due to intrapartum infection, by far the great majority of cases undoubtedly arise from postpartum contamination, from the scissors used to cut the cord, the material used to tie it, the hands of the doctor or nurse, or from the dressing.

Streptococcus hemolyticus and *Staphylococcus aureus* are the organisms most frequently recovered from the local lesion or blood stream. *Staphylococcus albus*, *B. coli* and pneumococcus are occasionally the infecting organism. In four hundred seven autopsies performed at the Hospital for Sick Children in Toronto (Wheeler),[6] there were nine cases of umbilical infection. *Streptococcus hemolyticus* was the infecting organism in four cases, *Staphylococcus aureus* in three cases, pneumococcus in one case, and *Streptococcus mucosus capsulatus* in one case.

TYPES OF LESIONS

Infection of the umbilicus may manifest itself in a variety of ways depending on the nature of the infecting organism and the degree to which the umbilical and periumbilical structures are involved. For purposes of classification, Audion considered the cord, the umbilical wound or scar, and the umbilical vessels separately and in this way derived three catalogues of pathologic states:

1. Infection of the cord.
2. Infection of the umbilical wound.
   a. Blennorrhea, simple ulcer, granuloma.
   b. Fungus, malignant ulcer, gangrene, erysipelas, periumbilical lymphangitis.

3. Infection of the umbilical vessels.

It is obvious that one or several of the above pathologic states may be present in the same patient and that the most serious type of lesion may show the least or nothing at all on gross examination.

As far as ordinary gross examination is concerned, we need consider no more than four types of lesion: blennorrhea ("moist umbilicus"), phlegmon, ulcer, and infection of the umbilical vessels. The important thing to remember is that no matter what type of lesion appears to be present, it should be considered serious, and the prognosis should be guarded.

In the days of epidemic omphalitis, the local lesions were frequently very similar in character. In the sporadic cases now seen, the more benign lesions are similar, but the severe lesions vary markedly in appearance so that, just as there is no characteristic symptomatology, there is no one typical lesion.

By far the most frequently seen lesion is the benign-appearing, small, moist, granulating area in the middle of the umbilical wound with a slight mucoid or mucopurulent discharge. In the ten-year period covered by this report, one hundred forty-three cases were seen and treated in the Out-Patient Department of the Children's Hospital, usually with prompt healing. The more severe lesions are characterized by varying amounts of purulent discharge with or without palpable thickening of the hypogastric arteries and patency of the latter as demonstrated by probing, and by varying degrees of cellulitis and lymphangitis of the periumbilical tissues. In such cases, there is redness, swelling and induration which may remain localized or which may extend peripherally, particularly downward to the inguinal regions, thighs, and scrotum. A third, now infrequently seen, severe lesion is the malignant spreading ulcer with progressive discoloration, softening, and sloughing of tissue. This lesion may start at the umbilicus or may arise elsewhere on the anterior abdominal wall or chest wall due probably to migration of the infecting organisms from the umbilicus via the lymphatics.

In our experience the fatal cases have most often shown clinically a slight to moderate purulent discharge with or without evidence of slight periumbilical inflammation. Death has been due to blood stream invasion with consequent multiple metastatic lesions in bones, joints, and viscera, or to peritonitis, arising from direct extension of the umbilical infection.

SYMPTOMATOLOGY

In concluding his discussion of umbilical infection in the newborn, Cullen (1916) states, "In every instance of illness in a newborn infant it should be the rule to inspect and, if necessary, reinspect the navel." This statement suggests the lack of specificity of the presenting symptoms. It is difficult to draw the line between mild out-patient department cases and house cases. It is significant, however, that whereas in the former the only complaint may be "moist navel" or failure of the umbilicus to heal, in the latter the complaints may seem at first wholly unrelated to the umbilicus. Usually, however, on direct questioning it will be learned that, in addition to the general symptoms, the infant's navel has never been completely healed or that it has been discharging pus for a varying length of time.

The general symptoms depend, of course, on the nature and site of the secondary lesions. In fatal cases, there is usually a septicemia; this may result in multiple soft tissue abscess formation, multiple osteomyelitis, brain abscess, pneumonia, empyema, and other metastatic lesions. Frequently there is a peritonitis. Symptoms and signs will vary accordingly. In the nine cases reported by Wheeler, five had peritonitis, two had septicemia without localized lesions, one had multiple abscess formation, and one had thrombosis of the hypogastric and iliac arteries and abdominal aorta.

TREATMENT

The treatment of omphalitis consists in cleansing the umbilical regions with soap and alcohol and in the repeated local application of wet dressings, usually of boric acid, hexylresorcinol, or magnesium sulphate solution. Occasionally alcohol dressings are used. Redundant granulation tissue is touched with silver nitrate. In the great majority of cases, this simple treatment results in rapid clearing up of the infection and complete healing of the umbilicus.

If there is extension of the infection into the hypogastric arteries with demonstrable abscess formation, incision and drainage is done, as there is rarely adequate drainage through the open end of these vessels. Pressure over the abscess will usually result in the appearance of a small amount of pus somewhere in the umbilical depression. At this point a probe and then a grooved director are inserted and passed downward into the abscess cavity. With the director as a guide, the abscess is then incised from above downward. Use of the grooved director is an essential precaution because of the proximity of the peritoneal cavity.

Treatment of the secondary or metastatic lesions is symptomatic and supportive. Abscesses are poulticed, incised, and drained as they develop; cellulitis is treated with cold magnesium sulphate compresses; and the spreading ulcers with wet dressings, heliotherapy and débridement. Parenteral fluids and blood transfusions are given when indicated.

There are far too many infants who arrive at the hospital too late to respond to any sort of treatment. These are the infants with blood stream infection and peritonitis, meningitis, or multiple abscesses, who get progressively worse and die within two or three to thirty-six hours after entry.

That the most promising treatment of omphalitis is prophylactic it is scarcely necessary to mention. Yet it is largely to point out the serious consequences of carelessness in tying, cutting, and dressing the umbilical cord that this paper is written.

SUMMARY OF CASES

During the ten-year period 1925 to 1934, inclusive, 74 patients with omphalitis were admitted to the wards of the Children's and the Infants' Hospitals. In 23 instances the omphalitis was incidental and not the primary reason for the hospitalization of the patient. It cleared up rapidly in those patients who did not die of other causes. In one of four fatal cases of intracranial hemorrhage with incidental omphalitis, there was postmortem evidence of an acute hypogastric arteritis, and in a fatal case of agranulocytosis there was terminal peritonitis which may have been secondary to the omphalitis; microscopic examination revealed a bilateral hypogastric arteritis.

Of the remaining 51 patients, 30 were males and 21 females. Thirty-three died, a mortality rate of 65 per cent. It should be pointed out that this is not the mortality rate of omphalitis, but rather of those cases in which the severity of the omphalitis or secondary lesions made admission to the hospital advisable. Various organisms were recovered from either the blood stream, umbilical discharge, or abscesses in 26 of the fatal and 12 of the nonfatal cases (Table I). It is noteworthy that *Streptococcus hemolyticus* alone was the infecting agent in 15 of the 26 fatal cases in which the organism was known and that either *Streptococcus hemolyticus* or *Staphylococcus aureus*, or both, were involved in all but 4 of these 26 fatal cases.

TABLE I

ORGANISM	FATAL CASES	NONFATAL CASES	TOTAL
Streptococcus hemolyticus	15	4	19
Staphylococcus aureus	5	5	10
Streptococcus hemolyticus and *Staphylococcus aureus*	2	1	3
Staphylococcus aureus and *B. coli*	1	1	2
Pneumococcus	1	1	1
Staphylococcus albus	0	1	1
Pneumococcus and Flexner bacillus	1	0	1
Staphylococcus aureus, Streptococcus viridans and *B. coli*	1	0	1
Unknown	7	6	13
Totals	33	18	51

The ages of the patients on admission varied considerably, the majority being between one and three weeks (Table II). It is a point of interest that all of 9 patients who were admitted to the Infants' Hospital between the fifteenth and twenty-first days of age and 6 of the 8 admitted to the Children's Hospital in the same age period died.

As might be expected, the most common complaint and positive finding was a purulent discharge or crusting of the umbilicus. This was

TABLE II

AGES	FATAL CASES	NONFATAL CASES	TOTAL
1 to 3 weeks	24	9	33
Less than 1 week	3	3	6
More than 3 weeks	6	6	12
	—	—	—
Totals	33	18	51

noted in 34 patients. In 25 instances there was redness and swelling of the umbilicus, 15 with purulent discharge. Cyanosis was noted or complained of on entry in 10 of the Infants' Hospital cases; 5 of them were premature infants. There were 15 cases with soft tissue abscesses, usually with other more serious lesions such as meningitis, peritonitis, or multiple osteomyelitis. A common complaint and finding was a tensely swollen and tympanitic abdomen. This usually indicated peritonitis, of which there were 15 cases. It was the most frequent complication and was invariably fatal. Cellulitis or erysipelas of the anterior abdominal wall was the next most frequent complication, occurring in 12 patients. In 8 instances the process extended to the external genitals. There were only 3 cases of osteomyelitis and 2 cases of extensive ulcer. One or both hypogastrics were incised and drained in 4 infants, two of whom recovered. Evidence of hemorrhagic disease of the newborn was noted in 3 instances before the onset of the omphalitis, and in 2 of these cases the cord was retied one or more times.

The course of the disease process in the fatal cases varied considerably, but in the cases of peritonitis especially, it was very rapid, about half of these patients dying within twenty-four hours after entry.

The importance of examining the umbilicus carefully in any infant with an unexplained septic process is brought out by the fact that in 4 of the above fatal cases, the omphalitis, or source of infection from which the patient died, was unsuspected clinically.

REFERENCES

1. Cullen, T. S.: The Umbilicus and Its Diseases, Philadelphia, 1916.
2. Audion, P.: Thesis, Paris, 1901. Gaz. de hôp., Paris **73**: 629, 1900.
3. Adair, F. L.: J. A. M. A. **61**: 537, 1913.
4. Creadick, A. N.: Surg. Gynec. Obst. **30**: 278, 1920.
5. Siddall, R. S.: Am. J. Obst. & Gynec. **14**: 192, 1927.
6. Wheeler, E. J.: Canad. M. A. J. **11**: 532, 1921.

ADDITIONAL REFERENCES

Friedlander, Axel: Acta paediat. **6**: 431, 1927.
Werthemann, A.: Schweiz. med. Wchnschr. **57**: 609, 1927.
Neuhaus, H.: Monatschr. f. Kinderh. **36**: 266, 1927.
Rice, G. E.: Colorado Med. **24**: 14, 1927.
Laurinsick, A.: Pediatria **32**: 1022, 1924.
Weitzman, C. C.: Am. J. Obst. & Gynec. **26**: 117, 1933.
Nordgren, R.: Acta pediat. **14**: 202, 1932.
Cumston, C. G.: New York M. J. **81**: 81, 1905.
Hinsdale, G.: Am. J. M. Sc. **118**: 280, 1899.
Lambert, S. M.: Med. News, New York **70**: 557, 1897.
Carstens, J. H. G.: Maandschr. v. kindergeneesk **2**: 538, 1933.
Wiesner, K.: Ztschr. f. Kinderh. **48**: 305, 1929.

THE INFLUENCE OF BREAST AND ARTIFICIAL FEEDING ON INFANTILE ECZEMA

CLIFFORD G. GRULEE, M.D., AND HEYWORTH N. SANFORD, M.D.
CHICAGO, ILL.

THERE is probably no subject in pediatrics that has received so much attention in the last few years as that of infantile eczema. Both external and internal factors have been studied, and some advances have been made in its treatment. We believe, however, that the effect of diet on these infants, once so stressed, has been largely lost sight of recently. For this reason the following study was made.

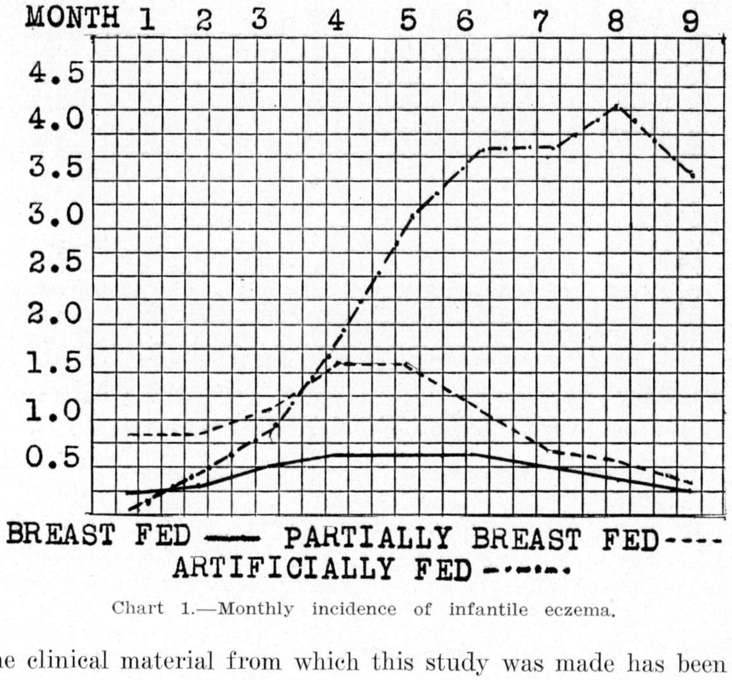

Chart 1.—Monthly incidence of infantile eczema.

The clinical material from which this study was made has been previously discussed.[1] The 20,061 babies represented in this study represent a five-year period in which each infant was fully followed.

An infant was considered as suffering from infantile eczema if there were any lesions on the face or body at the time of examination. This does not include "cradle cap." None of these infants received any treatment except the discontinuance of soap and water to the skin and the use of olive oil only for cleansing purposes. None of the feedings were changed in any way. In the artificially fed infants, 1.5 ounces of

From the Department of Pediatrics Rush Medical College, and the Infant Welfare Society of Chicago.

boiled cow's milk and 0.1 ounce of cane sugar per pound body weight were used. In all infants cod liver oil, orange juice, cereals, and vegetables were added to the diet.

In the total number of cases recorded, there were twice as many babies with infantile eczema in the partially breast-fed group as in the breast-fed group and seven times as many in the artificially fed group as in the breast-fed group. Another interesting fact is that, while in all groups the numbers are almost the same for the first three months, thereafter there is a rapid increase in the artificially fed group without any particular decrease at the end of the nine-month period; on the other hand, in both the completely breast-fed infants and the partially breast-fed infants the incidence of infantile eczema increases until the sixth month and then decreases markedly through the ninth month.

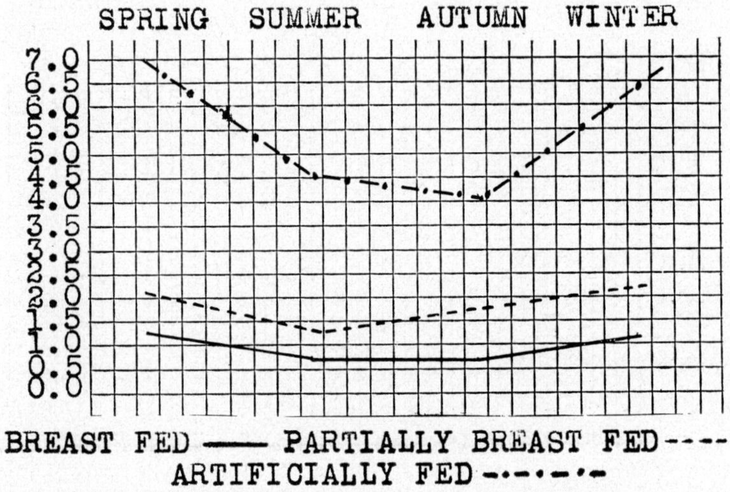

Chart 2.—Seasonal incidence of infantile eczema.

It may be argued that our feeding for the artificially fed babies is not an ideal one for the eczematous infant. This we will not deny. Our idea in the Infant Welfare Society is to keep up the infant's nutrition in spite of the effect it may have on the skin. In any case our greatest incidence in any month (the eighth) in the artificially fed babies was less than one in twenty (4.6 per cent), which we believe compares quite favorably with the usual incidence in private practice.

In the comparison of the seasonal incidence, the same proportion is shown. As to the general seasonal incidence, nothing new is added. In all groups the incidence is greatest in the spring and winter and lowest in the summer and autumn.

CONCLUSIONS

The general incidence of infantile eczema is lowest in the breast-fed infants. In the partially breast-fed it is twice as frequent as in the breast-fed infants and in the artificially fed infants, seven times as great.

In the monthly incidence both those infants entirely breast-fed and those partially breast fed show an increase to the sixth month and then a rapid decrease through the ninth month. The artificially fed infants

RESULTS

TABLE I.

AGE IN MONTHS

MONTH	1	2	3	4	5	6	7	8	9
*Breast-fed infants (number)	1	9	47	60	63	63	43	27	18
Percentage	0	0.1	0.5	0.7	0.7	0.7	0.5	0.3	0.2
Partially breast-fed infants (number)	7	74	96	106	109	100	73	54	40
Percentage	0.8	0.8	1.1	1.7	1.7	1.1	0.8	0.6	0.4
Artificially fed infants (number)	0	8	14	30	54	71	71	79	61
Percentage	0.0	0.4	0.8	1.7	3.2	4.2	4.2	4.6	3.5

*The total number of breast-fed infants in this series was 9,749; the partially breast-fed, 8,605; and the artificially fed, 1,7.07.

TABLE II.

SEASONAL INCIDENCE

	SPRING	SUMMER	AUTUMN	WINTER
Breast-fed infants (number)	113	60	59	99
Percentage	1.3	0.8	0.7	1.1
Partially breast-fed infants (number)	187	126	149	197
Percentage	2.1	1.4	1.7	2.3
Artificially fed infants (number)	122	78	72	116
Percentage	7.0	4.6	4.2	6.8

continue to show an increase until the eighth month and only a slight decline in the ninth month.

In the seasonal incidence all groups are increased in the winter and spring and decreased in the summer and autumn.

REFERENCE

1. Grulee, C. G., Sanford, H. N., and Herron, P. H.: J. A. M. A. **103**: 735, 1934.

636 CHURCH STREET, EVANSTON, ILL.
952 NORTH MICHIGAN AVENUE, CHICAGO.

A CAPILLARY RESISTANCE TEST AND ITS RELATION TO VITAMINS C AND D

C. B. WELD, M.D.
TORONTO, ONTARIO

NO precise method is yet established by which we can determine the optimal amounts of vitamin C required by humans. In a rough way the amounts necessary to prevent actual scurvy from developing are known, but, even if enough be present to prevent scurvy, it is possible that there may be insufficient to preserve optimal health conditions.

Among the various manifestations of scurvy the hemorrhagic tendency has been suggested as that most useful for detecting latent or subclinical cases. The hemorrhages are due to an increased permeability of capillaries, and several workers have suggested the use of the capillary resistance test to diagnose latent scurvy. For example, Hess and Fish[3] in 1914 developed the method of Rumpel[1] (1909), and Leede in 1911, reported that *most* cases of scurvy were positive but emphasized that the test was not specific for scurvy. In 1930 Göthlin[4] of Sweden standardized a technic and applied it to a large number of Swedish school children and adults. He established normal standards and concluded that 18 per cent of the school children were undernourished in regard to vitamin C. His method, however, may take half an hour or more to perform and is so uncomfortable to the subject that it is difficult to apply to young children. In 1907 Hecht[5] suggested a simpler method, involving the use of a suction cup instead of venous congestion as a means of putting stress upon the capillaries. Da Silva Mello used it in 1929, and in 1933 Dalldorf[6] used this method in a survey of 250 convalescent hospital patients who were receiving an excellent diet and of 50 adult and 50 children members of families in poor circumstances. These family groups were shown to have a somewhat lower capillary resistance than the hospital group. The capillary fragility of the children improved after admission to a preventorium. He has also reported prompt improvement of capillary resistance following administration of ascorbic (cevitamic) acid.

We hoped that some such method might be useful to us in detecting early or mild cases of vitamin C deficiency, and hence be of service in determining the optimal vitamin C content of the diet. We first applied Dalldorf's technic (in which the lowest degree of suction necessary to produce any petechiae, in a cup 1 cm. in diameter applied to the skin

From the wards and laboratories of the Hospital for Sick Children and the Department of Paediatrics, University of Toronto, under the direction of Alan Brown, M.D., F.R.C.P.(C.).

of the outer aspect of the upper arm for one minute, determines the threshold) to a group of normal individuals. This consisted of members of the laboratory staff, and convalescent cases in the hospital. The ages of the children ranged from four to fourteen years, the infants being under two years of age. All were receiving adequate amounts of vitamin C in the diet. In the cases of the infants the skin of the abdomen was used instead of that of the upper arm, though in several instances the arms were tested as well, with similar results. The results are given in Table I, from which it will be seen that in the cases of the children and adult groups much variation in the threshold of capillary resistance is found.

TABLE I

NORMAL SUBJECTS			
THRESHOLD AT WHICH PETECHIAE ARE PRODUCED (CM. HG)	INFANTS NUMBER OF SUBJECTS	CHILDREN NUMBER	ADULTS NUMBER
Over 50	18	23	9
50-40	6	22	7
35-25	–	12	4
20-15	–	6	2
10	–	–	1

Of the 85 children and adult subjects, 32 gave no petechiae even at 50 cm. of mercury suction, but the thresholds of 23 were 35 cm. of mercury or below and of these, 9 gave petechiae at 20 cm. of mercury or less. Of the 24 infants, however, only 6 gave any petechiae at 40 cm. of mercury suction, and none at lower levels. One would conclude, therefore, that infants show a greater capillary resistance than older children or adults.

Permission was granted by the Provincial Department of Health to determine the capillary resistances of a group of adult patients in a hospital, both on the ordinary hospital regimen and after supplementing their diet with tomato juice. These subjects were all fairly normal physically and were all receiving the same diet which is low in vitamin C. The group therefore should be particularly suitable for a survey of this type. A typical day's ration was as follows:

Breakfast: Cereal with milk and sugar; bread, butter and jam; coffee and milk (pasteurized).

Dinner: Split pea soup; meat pie, turnips and potatoes; bread; sago pudding, tea and milk.

Supper: Vegetable soup; bread and butter; preserved rhubarb and cake; tea and milk.

The only constant source of vitamin C is the daily portion of potato. The other vegetable in the instance given (turnip) would also be a source, but this vegetable is not a daily portion. About twice a week a cabbage salad is included in the menu for one meal.

Two groups of such subjects have been investigated. To the first, in the winter of 1934, each man was given 2 ounces of tomato juice daily for one week as supplement to the diet between capillary resistance estimations. In the second investigation a different group, conducted in the summer of 1935, each man was given 4 ounces of tomato juice daily for nearly three weeks. The larger dosage of tomato juice was given to meet the criticism that possibly in the first series an insufficient amount had been given. The tomato juice was found by analysis to contain an average of 17 mg. ascorbic acid per 100 c.c. During the summer the institutional diet contained perhaps three salads a week instead of the previous two, but fresh fruits were rarely given, and the diet would still be considered low in vitamin C. However, during the three weeks of tomato juice administration to this summer series, fresh tomatoes flooded the market, and the patients were given them freely. More than the 4 ounces of tomato juice calculated upon was therefore given; but, as this should merely accentuate any differences found in the capillary resistances, the conclusions are strengthened and not invalidated.

The results of these series are given in Table II in which the distribution of the subjects according to their threshold of capillary resistance is shown.

TABLE II

THRESHOLD AT WHICH PETECHIAE ARE PRODUCED (CM. HG)	NUMBER OF SUBJECTS			
	WINTER SERIES		SUMMER SERIES	
	BEFORE "C"	AFTER "C" 2 OZ. TOMATO JUICE DAILY FOR 1 WK.	BEFORE "C"	AFTER "C" 4 OZ. TOMATO JUICE DAILY FOR 3 WK.
Over 50	3	2	1	1
50-45	1	1	2	5
40-35	5	12	6	8
30-25	22	18	15	7
20-15	8	7	12	16
10	2	1	5	4
Total	41	41	41	41

It will be seen that the spread or distribution of the patients among the different threshold levels is not strikingly influenced by the added vitamin C. One would conclude indeed that the vitamin probably did not appreciably affect the capillary resistance. However, to further explore these results they have been arranged differently in Table III in which are recorded the numbers of subjects who showed a change in threshold following the administration of tomato juice.

It will be seen from these figures that of the winter series 11 subjects showed a greater capillary resistance after tomato juice while 9 showed lower capillary resistance, and the threshold of 21 was unchanged. Similarly, of the summer series, 13 showed an improved capillary resistance, but 11 showed a diminished resistance, and 17 showed no change.

TABLE III

SERIES	CHANGE IN THRESHOLD BETWEEN TESTS	THRESHOLD AT FIRST TEST (CM. HG) OVER 50-40	35-25	20-10	TOTAL SUBJECTS
Winter	Increase	0	6	5	11
	Unchanged	6	10	5	21
	Decrease	3	6	0	9
Summer	Increase	3	5	5	13
	Unchanged	3	5	9	17
	Decrease	3	5	3	11

In this table, too, the possibility is explored that only those subjects showing a rather low capillary resistance might show an improvement following vitamin C administration. If the winter series alone is considered, suggestion of this is seen, but, after including the summer series which incidentally were given much more tomato juice, this result becomes much less striking. Little evidence, therefore, is given by the results shown in this table to suggest an improvement of capillary resistance consequent upon administration of vitamin C.

Through the courtesy of Dr. McHenry, of the School of Hygiene, University of Toronto, we have also been able to ascertain the ascorbic acid content of the urine (fasting specimens) of some of these patients on the days of the capillary resistance determinations. Twenty patients of the summer series were investigated in this way, and the results given

TABLE IV

CORRELATION BETWEEN ASCORBIC ACID CONTENT OF URINE AND CAPILLARY RESISTANCE (SUMMER SERIES)

CASE	BEFORE "C"		AFTER "C"	
	ASCORBIC ACID (MG. %)	THRESHOLD (CM. HG)	ASCORBIC ACID (MG. %)	THRESHOLD (CM. HG)
1	0.5	50	0.3	40
2	0.6	30	1.0	30
3	0.7	25	1.1	20
4	0.7	30	0.9	35
5	0.8	25	1.2	35
6	0.9	20	1.9	30
7	1.0	40	0.9	25
8	1.0	20	0.9	20
9	1.1	30	1.4	40
10	1.1	20	0.8	20
11	1.1	20	0.7	10
12	1.2	10	1.1	25
13	1.3	20	1.4	20
14	1.3	50	1.9	50
15	1.4	10	0.7	20
16	1.5	25	1.3	30
17	1.5	30	1.3	20
18	1.5	20	1.3	10
19	1.7	25	1.4	25
20	2.1	40	1.3	40
Average	1.15	27.0	1.14	27.3

in Table IV in which the individual figures of the ascorbic acid content of the urine and the capillary resistance thresholds are placed side by side.

These results show no correlation whatever between the urine and capillary figures. Furthermore, the administration of tomato juice has had no effect upon these figures, the average ascorbic acid content of the urines and the average capillary resistance remaining unchanged.

While these investigations were being carried on we were fortunate in being able to observe ten infants with abnormally low vitamin C intake. Four of these were not scorbutic but had had no known source of vitamin C for two months or more; all four had a normal capillary resistance. The other six had scurvy, and in only one of these was the capillary resistance definitely low. Two were severe cases; one gave petechiae at the very low level of 3 cm. of mercury suction, while the threshold of the other was 40 cm. of mercury. The third was diagnosed on the basis of type of beading, x-ray findings, and history of no orange juice. The diet, however, was deficient in other ways as well, and the child was severely anemic and underweight. Orange juice promptly cleared up the irritability, during which time the capillary resistance threshold fell to 30 cm. of mercury. The fourth case was diagnosed on the basis of tenderness, beading, and x-ray, and was cleared up by the addition of orange juice to the diet, but the mother insisted that the child had always received the juice of an orange every day. The fifth case presented definite evidence of scurvy which, however, was showing x-ray evidence of healing (calcification of subperiosteal hemorrhages). Orange juice had been given prior to admission. The sixth case showed bleeding from the gums, slight scorbutic beading of ribs, tenderness about knees, and irritability, and was promptly cleared up with orange juice. The x-ray findings, however, were barely suggestive of scurvy.

It must be concluded therefore that in infants gross deficiency of vitamin C in the diet, even to the extent of scurvy development, does not necessarily result in a low capillary resistance. On the other hand, in adults a very low capillary resistance may be present even though ample amounts of vitamin C are being ingested. Since this paper was written, but before it was sent for publication, Abt and his coworkers[7] have reported a relation between diet and the reduced ascorbic acid content of the blood. They were, however, unable to correlate the vitamin C level of diet of the ascorbic acid level of the blood with the capillary resistances of their subjects. Hawley, Stephens and Anderson[8] have been unable to correlate the ascorbic acid content of the blood with the diet level of vitamin C, and they state that the capillary resistance does not parallel either of these factors.

During the course of these investigations, my own capillary resistance was found to be consistently low. As a final test before concluding that the dietary level of vitamin C had no relation to the capillary resistance, I took an added 8 ounces of freshly expressed orange juice daily for six weeks without making any other change in my diet or mode of life. No change in the capillary resistance occurred, the threshold of suction at which petechiae were obtained remaining at 30 cm. of mercury. However, shortly after this I went on a summer vacation and on my return found that no petechiae could be elicited even at 50 cm. of mercury suction. This remarkable increase in the capillary resistance lasted for more than two months before returning to the original value. A similar improvement was noted twice during the autumn, each time following a golf game and persisting only a few days.

In view of these observations, it was decided to determine the effect of irradiation with a mercury arc quartz lamp and of administration of viosterol upon the capillary resistance. Eleven subjects whose resistance was low enough to be susceptible of improvement were irradiated

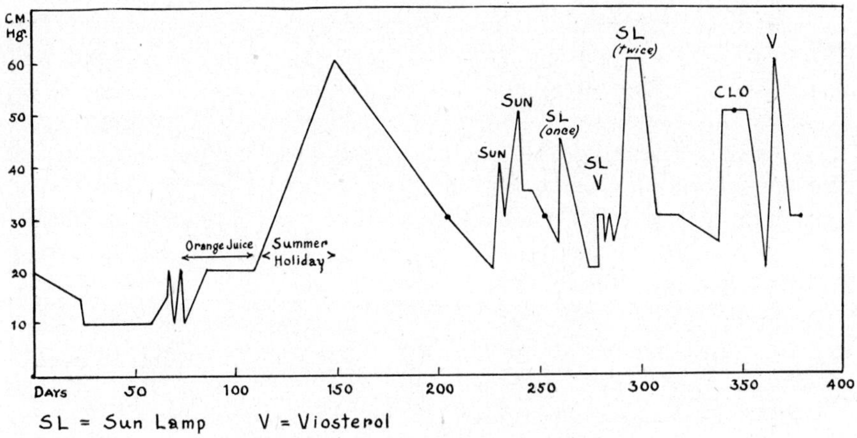

Fig. 1.—Capillary resistance thresholds.

or given viosterol for short periods of time. In three of the individuals observations could be made over a protracted period, and several courses of treatment were given. These individuals were laboratory workers, while the other subjects were convalescent children in the wards of the hospital, who were nearly ready for discharge. In all but one of the eleven subjects the irradiation and the viosterol treatments promptly resulted in a striking improvement in the capillary fragility, the improvement occurring usually within twenty-four hours. The dosage of viosterol given to the children was 10 drops daily for three or four days while in some instances rather larger doses were given to the adults. In no case were large enough doses given to make one think of overdosage effects. So far as the irradiation is concerned, the children were stripped except for a loin cloth and exposed prone and supine for 15 to 30 seconds in each position. This caused no glow or flushing to be apparent six hours after exposure. The adults were stripped to the waist only and the dosage aimed at was just sufficient to cause a feeling of warmth to become perceptible six or eight hours after exposure, but to leave no traces whatever the next morning. There was never any burn produced.

The details and results of the three laboratory subjects will now be discussed. One of these is the only one of the eleven who failed to respond to viosterol or irradiation as did the others. Her very fair skin necessitated only short exposures to the lamp, and even so some desquamation resulted. In two of the three series of lamp treatments her capillary resistance was diminished, a brisk rise being noted on the other occasion. Her response to viosterol too was irregular, a doubtful improvement being noted on one occasion and a definite reduction on another. She failed to show an increased threshold with orange juice, eight ounces being given daily for a week. Another of these subjects was myself, the results being given in Fig. 1. The first part of the

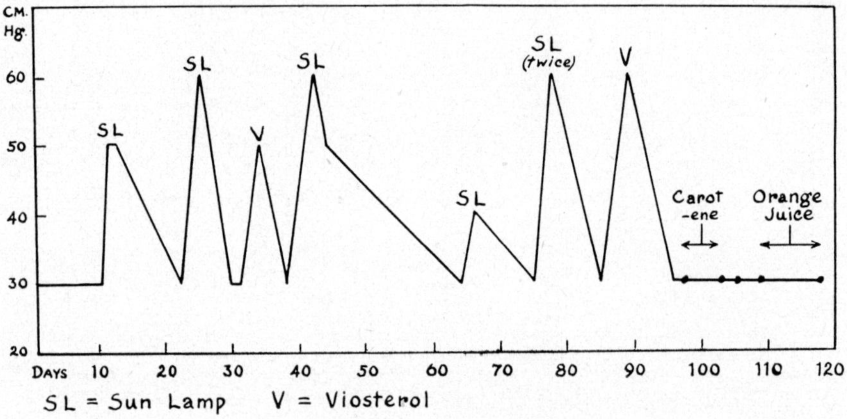

Fig. 2.—Capillary resistance thresholds.

curve has already been discussed, in which no response was obtained to orange juice, but a striking response was noted as a result of the summer holiday and the golf games. Equally definite improvements in capillary resistance occurred after sun lamp irradiation, after a single dose of 16 c.c. 10-D cod liver oil, and after 20 drops of viosterol daily over three days. The third of these subjects showed a remarkably consistent normal threshold at 30 cm. of mercury. His results are shown in Fig. 2. In all five instances in which he was irradiated he showed a striking rise in his threshold which then returned to its original level. Similar results followed the administration of viosterol, which was given twice, two doses of 10 drops each being given on the first occasion and three doses of 50 drops each on the second occasion. He failed to show any change in his capillary fragility to carotene or to orange juice administration. Eight ounces of orange juice were given daily for a week, and carotene equivalent to 40 c.c. cod liver oil was given in three doses.

In these results the striking feature is not only the response to the irradiation or viosterol but the return to the previous level and the repeatable nature of the observations. As each subject forms his own control, one is not depending upon statistical calculations to prove the point.

SUMMARY

The capillary resistance method of Dalldorf has been applied to a number of normal individuals and a great variation in their responses found. Young children tend to have a higher resistance than older children or adults. No improvement in the capillary resistance following administration of tomato juice was observed in a group of eighty adults. These were in an institution, their diet was well controlled, and it was one low in vitamin C. Several children suffering from scurvy or known to have had no source of vitamin C for weeks were found to have normal resistances. In ten of eleven subjects viosterol in moderate doses or irradiation with an ultraviolet lamp promptly raised the capillary resistance.

CONCLUSIONS

The capillary resistance determination is not a useful means of determining the state of nutrition with regard to vitamin C. Vitamin D is a more effective agent than vitamin C in increasing the capillary resistances.

REFERENCES

1. Rumpel: München. med. Wchnschr. **56**: 1404, 1909.
2. Leede, C.: München. med. Wchnschr. **58**: 293, 1911.
3. Hess, A. F., and Fish, M.: Am. J. Dis. Child. **8**: 386, 1914.
4. Göthlin, G. F.: Skandinav. Arch. f. Physiol. **61**: 225, 1931.
5. Hecht, A. F.: Jahrb. f. Kinderh. **65**: 113, 1907.
6. Dalldorf, G.: Am. J. Dis. Child. **46**: 794, 1933.
7. Abt, A. F., Farmer, C. I., and Epstein, I. M.: J. Pediat. **8**: 1, 1936.
8. Hawley, E. E., Stephens, D. J., and Anderson, G.: J. Nutrition **11**: 135, 1936.

RHEUMATIC INVOLVEMENT OF THE APPENDIX

Alexander T. Martin, M.D., and Samuel L. Ellenberg, M.D.
New York, N. Y.

PHYSICIANS of our modern era are beginning to appreciate a fact which was well known and quite freely commented upon by the medical reporters of other days, namely, the widespread distribution of the rheumatic process and its many bizarre and devious symptoms and manifestations. The older literature abounds with illustrations of rheumatism involving practically every structure in the body with the peculiar result that succeeding writers, exasperated with this extreme point of view, shifted in the opposite direction and commented very little on this malady—leaving it for present-day writers to rediscover gradually and to call attention again to the various manifestations of this rheumatic state.

Within recent years, little comment has been aroused relative to the involvement of the heart, joints, brain, pleura, and blood vessels by the rheumatic virus, whereas involvement of the appendix and the peritoneum is still viewed with considerable skepticism by a good many modern writers. Present-day textbooks of medicine fail almost entirely to consider the possibility of a peritoneal invasion by rheumatic fever and are in complete accord on the invulnerability of the abdominal structures to the rheumatic virus.

Although as early as 1880 Lambin concluded that acute rheumatism can localize itself anywhere in the digestive tract, the clinical entity of rheumatic appendicitis has not been given very much credence. In 1930 Giraldi, after reviewing the literature on abdominal symptoms in rheumatism, concluded that "in some instances acute rheumatism may give rise to abdominal symptoms simulating appendicitis, but at present there is no warrant for the use of the term rheumatic appendicitis."

As late as 1934 Guptill in discussing the differential diagnosis of abdominal manifestations of acute rheumatic fever from acute appendicitis also felt that there was no gross or macroscopic evidence that rheumatic involvement of the appendix occurs. However, within recent years careful examination of pathologic material from rheumatic fever patients has resulted in a slow accumulation of evidence which indicates there may be definite rheumatic involvement in certain cases.

The following case is reported as illustrating the belief that rheumatic involvement of the appendix can take place.

A. B., a colored lad, aged eleven years, was admitted to the Children's Surgical Ward of Lincoln Hospital April 30, 1935, with a history of pain in the epigastrium, which had begun two days previously and later had radiated to

From the Pediatric Service of Lincoln Hospital.

the right lower quadrant where it persisted and remained localized. There was no accompanying nausea, vomiting, or diarrhea, no cough, no pain in the chest, but anorexia was present from the onset of symptoms. The past history did not reveal any previous attack, but the patient had had measles, mumps, and pertussis, and a tonsil and adenoid operation was performed a year ago at the hospital. Physical examination disclosed a well-developed and moderately nourished lad, not appearing very acutely ill, although he had a temperature of 102.4° F., pulse, 100; respiration, 26. His ears, nose, and throat were negative; lungs, clear. The heart was not enlarged, had a regular rhythm, sounds of good quality, no murmur; P 2 > A 2; his blood pressure was 140/85. The abdomen moved freely with respiration; there was no skin hyperesthesia. Spasticity, tenderness, and rebound tenderness were present in right lower quadrant, most marked over McBurney's point. Rectal examination showed tenderness on the right but no masses.

Laboratory Findings.—The urine was negative; white blood cells numbered 12,000; 70 per cent segmented and 26 per cent unsegmented polymorphs; 4 per cent lymphocytes; red blood cells, 4,900,000; Wassermann reaction, negative. The blood chemistry was normal. A diagnosis of acute appendicitis was made, and the patient was operated on shortly after. "An appendix 3 inches long with a serosal coat much injected was removed after being freed from some bands which bound it down. No free fluid was found in peritoneal cavity."

On the second day postoperative, patient began to run a temperature which varied between 103 and 104° F. The patient had no complaints; the abdomen was soft; and there was no apparent cause for the temperature—the urinalysis was essentially negative except for a very faint trace of albumin. On the seventh day postoperative patient still had a temperature, but he appeared comfortable; the throat was not injected; the lungs were clear; the abdomen was soft, there were no masses. Rectal examination showed slight tenderness on the right, and a systolic murmur appeared at the apex, but the heart rate and rhythm were regular. The white blood cells numbered 9,300; polymorphs, 84 per cent; lymphocytes, 13 per cent; monocytes, 3 per cent. The sedimentation rate was rapid, the blood settling 26 mm. in twenty minutes (modified Cutler method).

The following day a pediatric consultation was requested in view of the suspicion that the persistent postoperative temperature of 103 to 104° F., unaccounted for by anything in the abdomen, with a pulse rate from 90 to 110 and the development of a systolic murmur and a rapid sedimentation time plus a negative x-ray plate for a possible pneumonic focus, pointed to a rheumatic process. The pediatric service agreed in suspecting an abdominal manifestation of rheumatic fever and advised the use of salicylates as a therapeutic measure.

Of interest is the pathologic report which came back approximately at the time the belief that the patient was suffering from an unusual manifestation of rheumatic fever was gaining ground. Dr. Chester R. Brown, the pathologist, reported the following: "Specimen consists of an appendix measuring 6½ × 1 cm. with mild serosal injection present. *Microscopic.*—Slides reveal a peculiar hyalinization and a thickening of the serosa. Submucosal fibrosis is marked. The latter and the muscular layer, also, show peculiar areas of hyaline or fibrinoid degeneration. Submucosa infiltrated with lymphocytes and some plasma cells—no polynucleoses. Mucosa hyperplastic and hemorrhagic and presents marked lymphatic hyperplasia. Any evidence of rheumatism?"

The past history of the patient was now carefully checked for a history of any previous rheumatic episode or early rheumatic manifestation, but none was found. The family history was also essentially negative.

On May 11 the systolic murmur grew in intensity and was transmitted to the axilla while a short presystolic rumble also made its appearance at the apex. Examination of the heart on May 14 showed enlargement of the left border, a marked sinus arrhythmia, a soft systolic murmur to the left of sternum with a rough systolic and diastolic murmur over the aortic area transmitted to the neck; no thrill or shocks were noted. Typical Corrigan pulse. Blood pressure was 134/48.

With the administration of salicylates the temperature promptly came down to normal, and the convalescence of the child was uneventful. The sedimentation rate continued to be rapid for a time, and then began to show some subsidence on June 16, 1935, and continued going down very gradually until the time of discharge on July 11, 1935. Electrocardiograms taken on May 28 and June 26 were essentially normal, while x-ray films of the heart showed slight enlargement of the cardiac shadow.

DISCUSSION

The clinical course of this case coupled with the pathologic report makes one consider very seriously the clinical and pathologic entity of a rheumatic appendicitis. Graham and Paul[4] in 1926 pointed the way to a serious consideration of the possibility of the rheumatic involvement of peritoneal structures by their highly instructive postmortem study of eighteen cases of rheumatic fever in which they were able to demonstrate a definite inflammatory condition of the peritoneal structures in some of the cases.

In 1930 Paul[5] demonstrated through the postmortem study of a patient who had rheumatic polyarthritis, endocarditis, pericarditis, pleurisy, and pain in the right side that peritoneal lesions were present, closely resembling both grossly and histologically, coexistent pleural and pericardial lesions which were of a typical rheumatic nature.

In 1933 Coburn[6] offered a valuable contribution to the pathologic study of rheumatism. He demonstrated that during the initial cycle of a rheumatic attack, hemorrhagic lesions without distinctive histologic structure were prominent and that this cycle was also characterized by vasodilatation, swelling of the endothelium, necrosis of the collagen fibers, infiltration with various wandering cells, and the absence of detectable microorganisms. Included in his study were two cases of involvement of peritoneal structures. In one the vermiform appendix showed subserous hemorrhages; the subserosal vessels were slightly dilated in the distal half; and some clotted blood was attached to the serosal surface of the proximal half, while one or two small ecchymoses were seen in the submucosa. In the second case the appendix was found to be hemorrhagic and the histologic examination revealed a partially broken down blood clot in the lumen without evidence of inflammation; sections of the appendix showed the architecture replaced by fibrofatty tissue, and superimposed on this was an acute hemorrhagic picture with marked hemorrhagic exudate in the lumen.

Judging from the reports in the literature where there has been apparent involvement of the peritoneum or the appendix in rheumatic patients, it would seem that Coburn's observations are well founded since it is invariably mentioned, in those cases in which operation was performed for abdominal symptoms, that hyperemia, edema, and infiltration of the peritoneum and subperitoneal tissues and clear fluid were found while the appendix usually was edematous and injected, with a variable amount of inflammatory reaction.

Giraldi's[1] review of the literature on this subject reveals that the etiologic relationship between acute rheumatism and acute appendicitis was frequently commented upon by the older writers. Sir James Grant[7] in 1893 and I. Burney Yeo[8] in 1894 reported cases of appendicitis which they attributed to rheumatism. Haig[42] also reported several cases of perityphlitis which he regarded as rheumatic and gouty in nature and successfully treated them with salicylates. Of all the English writers, Sutherland[9] seemed most convinced of the rheumatic origin of appendicitis. Finney and Hamburger[10] reported three interesting cases as examples of the relationship between the two diseases. Moffett and Rodgers[11] described two cases in which they regarded the abdominal symptoms as part of the rheumatic infection, and not as a genuine appendicitis, and Grenet[12] was convinced that acute rheumatism may be ushered in by a pseudoappendicular syndrome. Kelly and Hurdon[13] concluded that clinical evidence is in favor of an intimate relation between appendicitis and acute rheumatism. Nothnagel[14] offered the interesting theory that some cases of appendicitis begin as a rheumatic inflammation and subsequently become infected with other microorganisms. However, in contrast to these opinions Giraldi quotes Edwards, Poynton, and Morris as not attaching importance to rheumatism as a cause of appendicitis.

From our knowledge of the fact that rheumatism has a predilection for the lymphoid tissues—as for example the frequent involvement of the tonsils—we ought not to be surprised if the appendix is involved. Bland Sutton[18] called the vermiform appendix the "tonsil of the abdomen" when discussing the anatomy of this vestigial structure, laying stress on its richness in lymphoid tissue.

It is to be admitted that the diagnosis of rheumatic appendicitis is a difficult one to make. Our case, in common with most of the cases reported in the literature, did not give any clue as to its possible rheumatic origin until about four or five days after the onset of symptoms, when the development of a carditis pointed to the etiologic factor. It has been noted by other authors that the abdominal symptoms are preceded or followed in a few days by arthritic or myocardial manifestations but are not coexistent with them.

Guptill[3] in discussing the differential diagnosis of abdominal manifestations of acute rheumatic fever from acute appendicitis offers the following helpful points: (1) vomiting is less frequent in rheumatism. (2) A history of sore throat coincident or directly preceding acute rheumatic fever is often elicited in 30 to 40 per cent of the cases. (3) In acute appendicitis muscular spasm corresponds in extent with abdominal tenderness. (4) Jesierski[43] has noted miosis of the left eye from pressure in the ileocecal region in appendicitis. (5) Livingston claims that in

86 per cent of the cases of acute appendicitis prior to perforation there is a definite triangle in the right lower quadrant of hypersensitiveness of the tissues of the abdominal wall to pinching. (6) Yaguda[20] reports a constant increase in the percentage of immature polymorphonuclear cells in appendicitis consistent with the degree of suppuration.

As will readily be understood, no absolute rule can be set up for the treatment of these cases. When abdominal symptoms referable to the appendiceal region develop in an individual who gives a history of rheumatism or presents evidence of an old rheumatic condition, or who is passing through an acute attack of rheumatic fever, it is the policy of wisdom to treat such a patient expectantly with salicylates. These ought to allay the symptoms promptly. If a therapeutic response is not obtained within twenty-four hours of the administration of salicylates, an appendectomy or exploratory laparotomy is in order, for the literature does record cases of suppurative appendicitis developing in patients already suffering from rheumatic fever, tonsillitis, or upper respiratory infections. In cases in which neither a history nor physical evidence of rheumatism is obtained and reasonable doubt is entertained as to the diagnosis, operative interference is the treatment of choice since the diagnosis of rheumatic appendicitis or peritonitis is still too uncertain at the present time to justify consideration of any treatment other than operation. Although the lesions found in most cases of rheumatic peritonitis or rheumatic involvement of the appendix may not be of a serious enough nature to justify surgical interference, nevertheless they are of value in focusing attention on the gastrointestinal tract as a possible source of information regarding the pathogenesis of rheumatic fever.

CONCLUSIONS

1. A case is reported which helps to support the serious consideration of a rheumatic involvement of the appendix.

2. The pathology exhibited by the appendices removed from rheumatic individuals usually shows vasodilatation, necrosis of the collagen fibers, infiltration of various wandering cells and hemorrhages and, therefore, seems to correspond to the hemorrhagic lesions without distinctive histologic structure to which Coburn called attention as being predominant in the initial cycle of a rheumatic attack.

3. The diagnosis of rheumatic appendicitis is difficult to make at times but should be considered in any patient presenting signs and symptoms referable to the appendiceal region and giving a history of rheumatic fever or showing any of the manifestations of rheumatism.

4. The abdominal symptoms in rheumatism are usually followed in a few days by arthritic or cardiac manifestations but are not coexistent with them.

5. The treatment in an individual patient will depend upon whether a diagnosis of rheumatic involvement of the appendix can be made defi-

nitely. If this diagnosis is made, salicylates are indicated. If any doubt exists as to the diagnosis, or if the therapeutic response to salicylates is not obtained within twenty-four hours, surgical interference is the treatment of choice.

REFERENCES

1. Giraldi, J. J. J.: Arch. Dis. Child. **5**: 379, 1930.
2. Lambin, C.: Thèse de Paris, 1880.
3. Guptill, P.: Ann. Surg. **99**: 650, 1934.
4. Graham, R. S., and Paul, J. R.: Bull. Ayer Clin. Lab., Pennsylvania Hosp. **10**: 44, 1926.
5. Paul, J. R.: Bull. Ayer Clinic Lab., Pennsylvania Hosp. **2**: 9, 1930.
6. Coburn, A. F.: Am. J. Dis. Child. **45**: 933, 1933.
7. Grant, Sir J.: M. Rec. **2**: 609, 1893.
8. Yeo, I. B.: Brit. M. J. **1**: 1289, 1894.
9. Sutherland, G. A.: **2**: 457, 1895.
10. Finney, J. M., and Hamburger, L. P.: Am. Med. **2**: 941, 1901.
11. Moffett, R., and Rodgers, M.: Arch. Pediat. **41**: 431, 1924.
12. Grenet, H.: Progrès med. **1**: 422, 1925.
13. Kelly, H., and Hurdon, E.: Vermiform Appendix and Its Diseases, p. 381, 1905.
14. Nothnagel, H.: Encycl. Pract. Med., p. 837, 1904.
15. Edwards, W. A.: Am. Med. **3**: 595, 1902.
16. Poynton, F., and Weil, M. P.: Researches in Rheumatism, p. 359, 1913.
17. Morris, R. T.: Lectures on Appendicitis, p. 16, 1899.
18. Bland Sutton, J.: Lancet. **1**: 545, 1891.
19. Livingston, E. M.: Arch. Surg. **13**: 630, 1926.
20. Yaguda, A.: Am. J. Clin. Path. **1**: 39, 1931.
21. Jardine, J. H.: Brit. M. J. **2**: 943, 1931.
22. Geissinger, J. D.: J. A. M. A. **94**: 1427, 1930.
23. Hyman, A. S.: J. A. M. A. **94**: 1782, 1930.
24. Tallerman, K. H.: Brit. M. J. **2**: 844, 1931.
25. Auvray, M.: Bull. et mém. Soc. nat. de chir. **56**: 548, 1930.
26. Feure, M.: Bull. Soc. de pédiat. de Paris **28**: 492, 1930.
27. Costedoat: Bull. et mém. Soc. méd. d. hôp. de Paris, 532, 1353, 1929.
28. Meltzer, S.: Canad. M. A. J. **15**: 705, 1925.
29. Klinge, F.: Virchows Arch. f. path. Anat. **279**: 1, 1930.
30. Carmichael, F. A.: J. Kansas M. Soc. **33**: 363, 1932.
31. Wood, F. C., and Eliason, E. L.: Am. J. M. Sc. **181**: 482, 1931.
32. Rhea, L. J.: Am. J. Path. **9**: 719, 1933.
33. Leob, R. F.: M. Clin. North America **14**: 1539, 1931.
34. Schroeder, M. J., and Boas, E. P.: M. J. & Rec. **134**: 422, 1931.
35. Pearson, S. V.: Brit. M. J. **6**: 1120, 1904.
36. Von Glahn, W. C., and Pappenheimer, A. M.: Am. J. Path. **2**: 235, 1926; **3**: 583, 1927.
37. Klotz, O.: Tr. A. Am. Physicians **27**: 181, 1912.
38. MacCallum, W. G.: Bull. Johns Hopkins Hosp. **35**: 329, 1924.
39. Graff, S.: Deutsche med. Wchnschr. **56**: 603, 1930.
40. Shaw, A. F. B.: Arch. Dis. Child. **4**: 155, 1929.
41. McIntosh, R., and Wood, C. L.: Am. J. Dis. Child. **49**: 835, 1935.
42. Haig, A.: Practitioner **1**: 17, 1893.
43. Veritti, F.: Rassegna de chir. terap. e. sc. af. **29**: 163, 1930.

107 East Eighty-Fifth Street
250 West Twenty-First Street

TREATMENT OF GONORRHEAL VAGINITIS IN CHILDHOOD WITH ESTROGENIC SUBSTANCES

Margaret A. Limper, M.D., and Ethel E. Hieronymus, M.D.
Louisville, Ky.

FOLLOWING Allen's[1] experimental work on the effect of estrogenic substances on the vaginal epithelium of immature monkeys, Lewis[2] introduced the use of theelin in the treatment of gonorrheal vaginitis in children. Workers who had become discouraged with the results obtained with older types of treatment welcomed the innovation, and since the publication of Lewis' work in 1933 there have appeared in the literature seven reports,[3-9] dealing with 122 cases treated with various preparations of the estrogenic principle (Table I). In general, the results have been favorable, but there have been exceptions. The results reported with theelin have been uniformly favorable. Huberman and Israeloff[4] reported good results with an ethylene glycol solution of amniotin subcutaneously; Witherspoon,[9] using similar doses of the same substance, found desquamating epithelial cells but did not obtain a single cure. TeLinde and Brawner[8] did not observe the conversion of the immature to the adult type of vaginal epithelium with this substance and concluded that the one cure in this series was a coincidence; they obtained 77 per cent of cures with an oily solution of amniotin subcutaneously, and 100 per cent of cures with amniotin suppositories. With regard to oral treatment, Goldberg and his coworkers[7] concluded from a small series treated with amniotin that the results do not differ materially from those by hypodermic injection, although the dosage in units was larger. Nabarro and Signy,[5] using menformon, obtained fair results with oral administration. They advocate giving a large initial dose of the preparation intramuscularly and following this with oral administration; they used local treatment in conjunction with hormone therapy, but, on the whole, their results seem less favorable than those reported with the use of other preparations of the estrogenic principle. In contrast to these favorable reports of the oral method of treatment, TeLinde and Brawner concluded that amniotin administered orally is of no value.

The problems with which the various workers have been confronted are: (1) the possibility of harmful effects resulting from the administration of estrogenic substances to the child; (2) the optimum dosage for effective therapy; and (3) the duration of treatment after the smears have become negative.

From the Departments of Pediatrics and Gynecology, University of Louisville School of Medicine.

TABLE I

SUMMARY OF LITERATURE ON ESTROGENIC TREATMENT OF VAGINITIS

AUTHOR	PREPARATION USED	ROUTE OF ADMINISTRATION	NO. OF CASES	RESULTS
Lewis	Aqueous theelin	Subcutaneous	8	5 permanent cures 2 recurrences 1 reinfection (?)
Brown	Aqueous theelin	Subcutaneous	7	All cured
Huberman and Israeloff	Ethylene glycol Solution amniotin	Subcutaneous	5	All cured
	Amniotin oral	Oral	1	Cured
Nabarro and Signy	Menformon	Oral and intramuscular	20	6 permanent cures 14 relapses, all successfully retreated
Reading	Aqueous theelin	Intramuscular	2	All cured
	Theelin in oil	Intramuscular	6	
Goldberg et al.	Amniotin oral	Oral	6	All cured
	Ethylene glycol Solution amniotin	Subcutaneous	9	7 permanent cures 2 recurrences
	Combined	Oral and subcutaneous	1	Cured
TeLinde and Brawner	Amniotin oral	Oral	6	1 cured
	Ethylene glycol Solution amniotin	Subcutaneous	11	1 cured 1 recurrence
	Amniotin in oil	Subcutaneous	18	5 recurrences 13 permanent cures
	Amniotin suppositories	Vaginal	12	12 permanent cures
Witherspoon	Ethylene glycol Solution amniotin	Subcutaneous	10	None cured

With regard to the first of these questions, Huberman and Israeloff[4] showed that amniotin has no cumulative action, as is evidenced by the constant presence of this product in the urine of the children receiving treatment, and that, while the renal threshold of the estrogenic substance varies in different individuals, the amount of the substance in the urine is directly proportional to the intensity of treatment. Hartman,[10] working with monkeys, showed that the threshold for vaginal bleeding was far below that at which estrous changes occur in the uterus and ovaries and believed that although the hormone might induce a temporary inhibition of growth changes in the ovarian follicles, this effect is transient, and produces no permanent damage to the ovaries. Allen and Diddle[11] have recently made measurements on the ovaries and uteri of monkeys before and after comparatively large doses of theelin and examined the follicles afterward. Although there was some inhibition of the growth of the larger follicles, they concluded that this was not sufficient to interfere with normal function. In his earlier work with monkeys, Allen[1] had found that involution of the structures affected occurred within a few weeks after the hormone was discontinued. In the clinical application of these substances, vaginal bleeding has not been noted in any of the cases. Abdominal pain occurred after the injections in a number of cases. Turgescence of the labia, some hypertrophy of the breasts, and the appearance of a few scattered pubic hairs were also noted in quite a number of instances. Lewis,[2] Goldberg and coworkers,[7] and TeLinde and Brawner[8] found that several weeks after the cessation of treatment, biopsies from the vaginal mucosa showed a regression to the infantile type. It is of some interest, however, that several of the workers observed that in the treatment of recurrences after hormone therapy some months previously, smaller doses were required for a cure than in the original treatment.

The accumulated evidence is against any permanent harmful effects from the administration of estrogenic substances to young girls; the final answer to the question, however, should probably await observations on the treated cases after puberty. It would seem desirable to limit the treatment to the smallest dosage and the shortest duration that will give consistently good results.

There is considerable variation in the dosage and duration of treatment recommended by various authors. Goldberg and his coworkers employed 100 to 400 rat units of amniotin orally, and an average of 50 to 150 rat units hypodermically for periods of 8 to 120 days. TeLinde and Brawner concluded that daily 100 rat unit doses of the oily preparation of amniotin subcutaneously were as effective as larger doses; in the children who were permanently cured with this preparation, treatment was continued on an average of twelve days after the smears had become permanently negative. Mazer[12] is using 1,000 rat unit doses of progynon-B every other day for a period of eight weeks.

Our material consists of twenty-seven cases, of which all except three were dismissed after hormone therapy (Table II); one of the latter is still under treatment for a recurrence. A number of other patients had some hormone therapy, but they came in irregularly or discontinued treatment without obtaining a cure. In the year that we have conducted our vaginitis clinic, we have also dismissed as cured five patients with other types of therapy, mostly local instillations of silver nitrate ointment, supplemented in a few instances with injections of gonococcus filtrate or antigen. These cures were effected in three, four, eight, nine, and ten months, respectively.

Our first patients were treated with small doses (50 to 100 rat units) of an ethylene glycol solution of amniotin subcutaneously three times a week. The doses were small partly because our funds were very much limited and also because we knew very little about the optimum dosage clinically. As will be seen from Table II, Patients 1 and 3 were apparently cured with only 500 and 400 rat units, respectively. Patient 3 has remained well for one year. Patient 6 continued to show positive smears with a similar dosage and was cured with larger amounts of amniotin in oil. Patient 2 had a recurrence, or possibly a reinfection, after an apparent cure with 1,050 rat units. We are listing Patient 8 as having a recurrence, but she probably was not cured with 500 rat units in spite of five negative smears, for her mother told us afterward that the discharge never cleared up entirely.

After treating a few patients with an oily preparation of amniotin, we began using progynon-B as a source of the estrogenic principle. Upon the suggestion of Dr. Charles Mazer, of Philadelphia, we increased our dosage considerably. He had been using 1,000 rat units every other day. We decided to experiment with half this dosage, and since the oily preparation is absorbed and excreted slowly, we felt that three- or four-day intervals between injections would probably be satisfactory. We have followed the reaction of the vaginal epithelium by instilling into the vagina one or two dropperfuls of saline, and examining the washings microscopically. After from four to six injections the discharge appears caseous rather than purulent. Microscopically, pus cells begin to disappear, while large clumps of epithelial cells appear, some of which can be seen to be definitely cornified. With a few exceptions, the smears were permanently negative after two to four weeks of treatment. We found that this effect could be obtained by twice weekly injections of the oily preparation of the estrogenic principle. Recently, we have reduced our dosage to 300 rat units, and our results are comparable to those obtained with 500 rat unit doses.

Our plan is to continue treatment of these patients for four weeks after their smears become permanently negative, or for a total of eight weeks. In those children whose smears become negative after ten days or two weeks, it is probably safe to reduce the period of treatment to

Table II

Summary of 27 Cases of Gonorrheal Vaginitis in Childhood Treated With Estrogenic Substances

CASE	AGE IN YEARS	DURATION OF DISEASE	DOSAGE OF ESTROGENIC SUBSTANCE	TOTAL AMOUNT	DURATION OF TREATMENT IN DAYS	NO. CONSECUTIVE NEG. SMEARS BEFORE DISMISSAL	COMMENT
1	3	2 wk.	50 R.U. E.G.A.* x 10	500 R.U.	25	5	Checked after 6 wk.
2	6	3 mo.	50 R.U. E.G.A. x 12 100 R.U. E.G.A. x 5	1,100 R.U.	37	5	Followed by recurrence
			250 R.U. O.A. x 8 125 R.U. O.A. x 8	3,000 R.U.	51	7	Negative after 7 mo.
3	10	4 wk.	100 R.U. E.G.A. x 5	400 R.U.	60	7	Negative for 1 yr.
4	5	2 mo.	125 R.U. O.A. x 6 250 R.U. O.A. x 3	1,500 R.U.			
			500 R.U. P.B. x 7	3,500 R.U.	115	8	Checked after 1 mo.
5	6	1 yr.	125 R.U. O.A. x 12 250 R.U. O.A. x 2	2,000 R.U.	42	8	Followed 2 mo.
6	7	6 wk.	100 R.U. E.G.A. x 14 50 R.U. E.G.A. x 8	1,800 R.U.			
			125 R.U. O.A. x 4 250 R.U. O.A. x 7	2,250 R.U.	105	9	Checked after 3 mo.
7	1¼	2 wk.	125 R.U. O.A. x 5 100 R.U. once 250 R.U. O.A. x 2	1,225 R.U.			
			500 R.U. P.B. x 11	5,500 R.U.	56	8	Checked after 3 mo.
8	7	6 mo.	100 R.U. O.A. x 5	500 R.U.	10	5	Followed by recurrence
			500 R.U. P.B. x 10	5,000 R.U.	32	7	Negative after 1 mo.
9	6	18 days	500 R.U. P.B. x 19	9,500 R.U.	63	7	Checked after 1 mo.

*Key to table: E.G.A., ethylene glycol solution—amniotin
O.A., amniotin in oil
P.B., progynon-B in oil
F.M., folliculin menformon.

TABLE II—CONT'D

CASE	AGE IN YEARS	DURATION OF DISEASE	DOSAGE OF ESTROGENIC SUBSTANCE	TOTAL AMOUNT	DURATION OF TREATMENT IN DAYS	NO. CONSECUTIVE NEG. SMEARS BEFORE DISMISSAL	COMMENT
10	6	?	1,000 I.U. F.M. x 4 1,500 I.U. F.M. x 2 2,000 I.U. F.M. x 9	25,000 I.U.			
			250 R.U. O.A. x 6 125 R.U. O.A. once	1,875 R.U.	57	5	Smears negative after 47 days
11	8	?	125 R.U. O.A. x 10 250 R.U. O.A. x 3	2,500 R.U.			
			500 R.U. P.B. x 21	10,500 R.U.	80	9	Not checked
12	7	6 mo.	500 R.U. P.B. x 10	5,000 R.U.	53	7	Followed by recurrence
			300 R.U. P.B. x 8	2,400 R.U.	52	8	Checked after 2 mo.
13	2½	Chronic	500 R.U. P.B. x 9	4,500 R.U.	29	11	Not checked
14	4	2½ mo.	500 R.U. P.B. x 13	6,500 R.U.	33	10	Followed 3 mo.
15	6	?	1,000 I.U. F.M. x 31 2,000 I.U. F.M. x 25	81,000 I.U.	60	None	Left hospital with positive smear
16	7	1 mo.	500 R.U. P.B. x 8 250 R.U. P.B. once	4,250 R.U.	29	7	Followed 5 mo.
17	2	?	500 R.U. P.B. x 9 300 R.U. P.B. x 2	5,100 R.U.	36	8	Followed 2 mo.
18	9	4 yr.	500 R.U. P.B. x 7 300 R.U. P.B. x 8	5,900 R.U.	50	11	Smears negative after 2 wk. treatment Checked after 6 wk.
19	4	7 days	500 R.U. P.B. x 6 250 R.U. P.B. x 1 300 R.U. P.B. x 10	6,250 R.U.	60	7	Smears negative after 4 wk. treatment Checked after 1 mo.

Table II—Cont'd

CASE	AGE IN YEARS	DURATION OF DISEASE	DOSAGE OF ESTROGENIC SUBSTANCE	TOTAL AMOUNT	DURATION OF TREATMENT IN DAYS	NO. CONSECUTIVE NEG. SMEARS BEFORE DISMISSAL	COMMENT
20†	6	3 days	500 R.U. P.B. x 6 250 R.U. P.B. x 1 300 R.U. P.B. x 11	9,050 R.U.	88	6	Followed by recurrence after 2 days
			300 R.U. P.B. x 8	2,400 R.U.	35	9	Negative after 2 wk. follow-up
21	7	7 days	500 R.U. P.B. x 9 300 R.U. P.B. x 7	6,700 R.U.	57	11	Smears negative after 2 wk. treatment
22	9	10 mo.	500 R.U. P.B. once 300 R.U. P.B. x 12	4,100 R.U.	80	9	Smears negative after 4 wk.
23	8	8 mo.	500 R.U. P.B. x 6 300 R.U. P.B. x 7	5,100 R.U.	57	10	Smears negative after 2 wk. treatment
24	6	17 mo.	300 R.U. P.B. x 14	4,200 R.U.	54	10	Negative after 4 days' treatment
25	3	8 days	300 R.U. P.B. x 13 400 R.U. P.B. once	4,300 R.U.	67	8	Negative after 4 wk. treatment Checked after 6 wk.
26	2	13 days	300 R.U. P.B. x 15 400 R.U. P.B. once	4,900 R.U.	63	6	Smear negative after 36 days' treatment
27	5	2 mo.	500 R.U. P.B. x 5 300 R.U. P.B. x 8	4,900 R.U.	56	Pos.	Not dismissed

†Discharged as cured since completion of this article.

six weeks. The minimum number of negative smears for dismissal is five, and we attempt to check again six weeks after treatment has been completed. Many of our earlier patients had had unsuccessful local therapy before estrogenic treatment was begun. The only local treatment used in conjunction with hormone therapy has been external cleansing for the patient's comfort, and, in a few cases in which irritation was marked, sitz baths have been recommended for a period of a week or ten days.

As will be seen from Table II, 24 of the 27 cases may be regarded as having obtained cures from hormone therapy. One of the failures (Case 15) was in a patient treated with folliculin menformon. Our experience with this preparation was limited, but we believe it is less effective than the other two substances used. Patient 27 discontinued treatment of her own accord after thirteen injections over a period of eight weeks, with a positive smear on her last visit to the clinic. The recurrences in Cases 2 and 8 have been referred to above. Under our present routine of therapy, we have had two recurrences. Patient 20 required eight weeks of treatment before the smears became negative. She was treated for two weeks after the smears became permanently negative but developed a recurrence after thirty-eight days. She is at present under treatment for the recurrence. Patient 12 came in so irregularly for treatment that it is uncertain whether she had a recurrence or simply a "false cure." We have not calculated the average dosage or the average duration of treatment because most of the longer periods of treatment have been in patients who came in irregularly for injections. Our social service work has been inadequate, and we have been unable to follow these cases as closely as we would like.

Our giving the oily preparations of the hormone intramuscularly probably accounts for the fact that we do not observe the pain TeLinde and Brawner describe as associated with the subcutaneous injection of amniotin in oil. A 20 gauge needle is used, and the injections are given into the gluteal muscles on alternate sides. After the needle has been introduced, there is no complaint of pain, and there is no soreness during the period of absorption. We buy the progynon-B in concentrated form, and dilute it with oil of sesame so that 0.1 c.c. contains 100 rat units of the hormone; the total volume of each injection is therefore small.

Because of limited funds, we have been unable to use suppositories in treating any of our patients. TeLinde and Brawner obtained 100 per cent cures by this method and only 77 per cent cures in the patients treated with amniotin in oil. Because they found that less of the hormone was required for a cure when the suppository method was used, and since there were no breast changes with this method, they concluded that there is some local action which takes place as a result of an increased concentration of the drug in the pelvic tissues. The method is certainly worthy of further trial and study.

Hypertrophy of the genitals or of the breasts was not observed in any of our patients. One patient developed a minute cyst of the nipple, and a few patients developed a few scattered pubic hairs. Several of the patients treated with subcutaneous amniotin developed skin eruptions which may have been due to the injections.

SUMMARY

1. In four cases of gonorrheal vaginitis treated with an ethylene glycol solution of amniotin, there were two permanent cures and two recurrences.

2. With oily solutions of amniotin or of progynon-B administered intramuscularly twice weekly, conversion from the infantile to the adult type of vaginal mucosa was observed, and cures were obtained in all except two cases.

3. One patient treated with folliculin menformon daily for sixty days failed to respond to treatment.

4. No harmful effects as a result of injections were observed.

We wish to thank Dr. J. A. Kennedy and the Bacteriology Department for their cooperation, Dr. Hugh R. Leavell, City Health Director, for his financial support, and the members of the Social Service Department for their assistance.

REFERENCES

1. Allen, Edgar: J. Morphol. **46**: 479, 1928.
2. Lewis, R. M.: Am. J. Obst. & Gynec. **26**: 593, 1933.
3. Brown, J.: J. A. M. A. **102**: 1293, 1934.
4. Huberman, J., and Israeloff, H. H.: J. A. M. A. **103**: 18, 1934.
5. Nabarro, D., and Signy, A. G.: Lancet **1**: 604, 1935.
6. Reading, B.: South. M. J. **28**: 464, 1935.
7. Goldberg, L. E., Minier, C. L., and Smith, E. L.: J. Pediat. **7**: 401, 1935.
8. TeLinde, R. W., and Brawner, J. N.: Am. J. Obst. & Gynec. **30**: 512, 1935.
9. Witherspoon, J. T.: Am. J. Dis. Child. **50**: 913, 1935.
10. Hartman, C. G.: Am. J. Physiol. **95**: 662, 1930.
11. Allen, E., and Diddle, A. W.: Am. J. Obst. & Gynec. **29**: 553, 1935.
12. Mazer, C.: Personal communication, November, 1935.

American Academy of Pediatrics

Proceedings

SIXTH ANNUAL MEETING OF THE AMERICAN ACADEMY OF PEDIATRICS

KANSAS CITY, MISSOURI, MAY 11 AND 12, 1936

Round Table Discussion on Appendicitis

Chairman: Dr. Albert H. Montgomery, Chicago.

Assistant: Dr. Joseph Brennemann, Chicago.

CHAIRMAN MONTGOMERY.—It probably seems incongruous to you to have a surgeon head a round table discussion of this kind. However, when my colleague, Dr. Joseph Brennemann, kindly consented to participate in the discussion I thought that perhaps our experience extending over fifteen years in which we have seen together about 1,000 cases of appendicitis in children might give us some ideas that would be interesting for a discussion of this topic. I trust that our impressions and yours may be helpful in promoting a clearer understanding of this rather common disease in children and in reducing the unjustifiable mortality which prevails at present.

It is a strange commentary on modern medicine that a disease like appendicitis with which we have been rather familiar for fifty years and of which our knowledge of the etiology, pathology, symptoms, diagnosis, and treatment is rather complete, should show a rise instead of a decline in the mortality statistics. It is very timely, therefore, for those of us who are called upon to treat abdominal conditions in children to take stock of our present knowledge and see if we cannot in some way prevent a fatal termination in the patients that are afflicted with this disease.

In order to promote a logical discussion of this subject it would seem appropriate to me to call upon a man who can give you the impressions of the pediatrician who sees these patients first and on whom rests the burden of making a correct diagnosis and advising prompt and proper treatment.

Appendicitis in Children

Joseph Brennemann, M.D., Chicago

In the last fifteen years we have had nearly 1,000 cases of appendicitis at the Children's Memorial Hospital. The medical and surgical departments cooperate very closely and sympathetically and Dr. Montgomery and I have seen most of these cases and have mulled over an equal, or larger, number of abdominal conditions that called for confirmation or exclusion of a possible diagnosis of appendicitis. It seemed to both of us that the main discussion should begin with a presentation of the subject as it attacks the first line of defense, the pediatrician and the general practitioner. We all know that the one important point in treatment and resulting prognosis is an early diagnosis. The surgeon sees relatively few cases first hand. He is usually called in to confirm the diagnosis and to treat the patient after he has been seen by someone else. The pediatrician and the general practitioner see many more patients with abdominal pain not due to appendicitis than due to that condition. They must, therefore, not only be able to recognize the disease when present, but even much more often, to exclude it. The diagnosis is by no means always easy, or carefree, even by those with a large experience in a charity hospital where such cases are enormously more frequent than in a busy pediatric or general practice. This is also evident in the frequency with which appendicitis is diagnosed when it is not present, and also not diagnosed as such when it is present. The difficulty that is inevitable in the medical diagnosis of abdominal conditions of which pain and tenderness are a part is, however, a minor contribution to the unfortunate fact that the mortality and serious morbidity of appendicitis are still higher than the conditions would warrant under favorable circumstances. In spite of the fact that we are usefully informed as to the etiology and quite fully informed as to the morbid anatomy, symptomatology and ideal treatment, the mortality and serious morbidity are not decreasing, and probably will not for some time to come. The major factor in this deplorable condition seems evident. The appendix is an insignificant little organ, if one may call it so, that is important only because of its location. When inflamed it causes relatively little pain early, the all-important tenderness is not sought for, and there is little fever. The laity are apt to estimate the seriousness of a disease by the degree of pain and the height of the temperature. They will call a physician for a colic, or for a banal throat infection with a fairly high fever, and will interpret a case of appendicitis as a mere "stomach ache" or "intestinal upset." The almost inevitable vomiting clinches the interpretation and from time immemorial one or more cathartics are supposed to be prescribed when there is any abdominal, stomach, or bowel trouble. This situation is almost the rule in our experience. A doctor is finally called in at the end of twenty-four or forty-eight hours, or longer, the appendix has now ruptured and the mortality and serious morbidity have gone from near zero to 5 or 10 per cent. The prognosis of appendicitis is, therefore, more dependent on the intelligence and alertness of the parents than on any other one factor. For that reason statistics of results in private and charity practice are not comparable—are even misleading. It is evident, too, that a major factor in prophylaxis is lay education, a difficult problem.

The etiology of appendicitis is probably not to be found in a single factor and there is, as a result, some difference of opinion. The surgeon who usually sees only the local condition is naturally impressed by the presence of a fecalith, kinking, narrowing, bands, adhesions, even pinworms, and so leans toward an enterogenous or mechanical causation. The pediatrician, who examines the throat in every patient and is cognizant of the fact that the lymphoid tissue of the appendix so closely resembles that of the tonsils that the former has been spoken of as the abdominal tonsil and appendicitis as abdominal angina, so frequently finds a throat infection as a forerunner of appendicitis that he feels very confident that such infections have a very definite etiologic relationship to appendiceal inflammation. One can hardly expect the surgeon to be interested in, or properly interpret, a throat. Appendicitis has been seen many times to follow measles, scarlet fever, and other infections, and may possibly be more frequent with infections of the throat only because they are so much more frequent than all others combined. It is interesting in this connection to recall that Evans, among students in the University of Wisconsin, reported eight times as many cases of appendicitis during periods of grippy epidemics as in nonepidemic times.

The cardinal symptoms of appendicitis are pain and tenderness in the abdomen, vomiting, and a low temperature. As I said before, the appendix is a relatively little organ and one cannot expect either much pain or fever when it is inflamed and uncomplicated. If there is very severe pain, it speaks against appendicitis; not always, as we learned from a recent patient who apparently had excruciating pain. It was one of those exceptions that emphasizes the rule. A high fever speaks against an early, uncomplicated appendicitis, and the cause can usually be found elsewhere, usually in the throat or in the lungs. I recall a patient that I saw in consultation, with a temperature of 105.6° F., and just coming out of a third convulsion. He had a throat infection and an otitis media—but also a point of tenderness in the lower right quadrant of the abdomen. I emphasized the fact that the appendix should be watched. The next morning the temperature had sunk to the usual appendiceal level, there was still local tenderness, but the condition was interpreted as improved, not by myself, because the fever was lower. Two days later the child was brought to the hospital with a ruptured appendix, by another physician.

As in the adult, the pain usually starts in the epigastrium or about the umbilicus, and soon migrates to the region that is involved. In this it differs with the far more important sign of tenderness, the one significant and unfailing sign, which is always at the point of involvement. If there is early diffuse tenderness, it speaks against appendicitis—again, not always. Inasmuch as the appendix may occupy various positions, especially the part that is acutely inflamed, this tenderness, while usually at or near McBurney's point, may be high or in the flank in retrocecal appendicitis, low down near Poupart's ligament, or even on the left side. We had a child with the pain and tenderness on the left side because of a complete situs inversus; several in which the inflamed tip of the appendix lay across the midline and the point of tenderness was to the left of the left border of the left rectus muscle. Because of tenderness, it is sometimes of diagnostic value to bear in mind that colicky pain from any cause invites pressure, while inflammation brings out defense against pressure.

Rebound tenderness is stressed by some examiners. It has never seemed to me of determining significance in diagnosis. *I think it cannot be emphasized too heavily that the one important sign of early appendicitis is tenderness at one point, in the proper clinical setting.* It is not pathognomonic, however.

Rigidity is an important sign if present, but must not be looked upon as a desideratum. Early there may be none. A little later there is always a voluntary defense against the pain of pressure. When the rigidity becomes involuntary, instant and boardlike to any degree of pressure, peritonitis has supervened.

Except under certain conditions I do not feel that rectal examination is indicated in children. It is an extremely unpleasant procedure, a bad thing in itself unless necessary, and this often overshadows any information that may be obtained if that is not more easily and usefully elicited by external examination. It is of distinct value in determining purely objective conditions, such as a mass in late appendicitis or as a postoperative complication, especially if there is a question as to whether an abscess is pointing in that direction.

Vomiting is almost unfailing—but not quite. It has some diagnostic value—negative rather than positive. I have the impression that surgeons value it too highly because they are not as familiar with the fact, as we are, that young children vomit with nearly every infection.

The leucocyte count has a predilection for somewhere between 15,000 and 20,000 —but must never alone be considered of determining diagnostic value. We have seen it all the way from 5,000 to 30,000, or more. A very low count has often a bad prognosis—a very high count may, or may not have. An increase or a decrease in the white blood count is, on the other hand, of a great deal of significance as to progress in a doubtful or possibly receding case.

There is a point in the examination that I think bears emphasis. It is, of course, axiomatic that the examining hand must be warm, laid on flat, that the pressure must be gentle and must proceed from the unaffected to the affected side. I have an impression that the experienced surgeon is more gentle in his examination than is the pediatrician, or general practitioner, not to mention the interne, because he is more concretely familiar with the morbid anatomy and the potential danger of kneading an appendix that is about to rupture. The point that I want to stress is that it is not only useless, as a rule, but may also be misleading to keep asking with each poke whether this place hurts, or that one, etc. Far more reliable and certain information can be obtained by merely watching the child's face, or noting some expression of defense such as a squirm or a motion of the hand toward the tender spot. A wince is more decisive than a "yes" or a "no" and even a child that is appendicitis-conscious may dissemble by words, rarely by actions.

So far I have discussed only the earlier stages of appendicitis. In a way they run a fairly constant course and the diagnosis is usually easy. As a rule they run a day or even two without alarming symptoms. Only rarely does one see a fulminating case. And yet one came to us recently with a ruptured, gangrenous appendix in a child who was actively playing and apparently symptom-free six hours before.

Following the early course one of three things happens:

1. The symptoms and signs disappear and the inflammation recedes. This is not uncommon. If there is an undoubted recession it is probably best not to operate at the time, but to advise a later operation because of the probability of a recurrence.

2. The appendix ruptures and there is a spreading peritonitis. This calls for operation at any time.

3. The appendix does, or does not, rupture and a well-defined, sharply circumscribed mass ensues. These patients, as usually seen on the third or fourth day of the disease, do not appear alarmingly sick—often have a sort of convalescent look about them. We have seen a good many such cases and both Dr. Montgomery and I feel very strongly that they should not be operated upon at the time, and we have never regretted it. They must, of course, be watched closely and in a hospital. We have seen masses as big as my fist recede completely and rather quickly. They should always be operated later, not less than a month, preferably longer, after the complete disappearance of the mass.

Dr. Montgomery will discuss the treatment in detail, but I couldn't resist saying as much as I did from the pediatric standpoint.

We come, finally, from our standpoint, to the all important matter of diagnosis. Once made, the treatment usually follows naturally. In both of these points I cannot share the optimism and complacency of a pediatric friend who said, anent this discussion: "What is there to it? You make the diagnosis and then have them operated." We somehow still have plenty of trouble and once in a while we make a mistake—one way or the other. We never hide behind an "injected appendix"—we expect a certain small number of errors in diagnosis.

Probably the largest source of diagnostic unhappiness is the child who has a pain in the abdomen that one does not feel justified in ascribing to appendicitis. They are much more common in practice than is appendicitis. I am skeptical about indigestion and gas pains and if there is such an entity as spastic colon in childhood, it has been above the threshold of my diagnostic acumen. I have a suspicion that the allergists have allocated most of these pains to their special field. Maybe they belong there. To me they are still a mystery.

Pneumonia occasionally, but rarely should, leads to an error in diagnosis. The pain of the accompanying pleurisy is usually below the diaphragm—much more rarely in the corresponding shoulder. The general appearance, the high fever, the flaring alae nasae, the expiratory grunt, the rapid respiration, the flushed face and the high leucocytic count rarely leave any doubt. Bearing in mind that suppression of breath sounds is the earliest sign of lobar pneumonia may help. It unfortunately occurs, too, in appendicitis, though in less degree. A roentgenogram is usually decisive and should never be omitted if in doubt and if obtainable. It must be remembered, however, that both conditions may be present. Much that has been said applies also to pleurisy itself and even to acute pericarditis.

The late Carnet, of Philadelphia, wrote extensively on the frequency with which intercostal neuralgia was confused with appendicitis. In the former the tenderness was said to be superficial—in the latter, deep. If, after tensing the abdominal muscles, the tenderness persisted he attributed it to intercostal neuralgia; if not, to appendicits. I was always skeptical about his observations until I unexpectedly visited him at his hospital. He showed me several that seemed convincing.

Gallstones and renal colic hardly enter into the picture.

Pyuria is more often weighed in the balance by the surgeon than by the pediatrician. Probably the commonest cause of a transient pyuria is an upper respiratory tract infection and appendicitis may be present from the same source. Pyuria should not exclude appendicitis. The surgeons tell us that pyuria may result from contact of a ureter with an acutely inflamed appendix. I have never been able to diagnose that condition.

So-called primary peritonitis is often impossible to differentiate from a late appendicitis with spreading peritonitis. The differentiation is important because operation is indicated in the latter and probably contraindicated in the former. If there is a history of pain and tenderness in the right lower quadrant at the beginning of the disease, or if it still predominates in that region, one naturally leans toward the diagnosis of a spreading peritonitis following appendicitis. As a rule the differentiation is not difficult. In primary peritonitis the child is usually very sick from the start and there is pain and exquisite tenderness over the whole abdomen from the very beginning. I am inclined to think that we have been overcautious in not resorting more often to diagnostic puncture as proposed by Denzer fifteen years ago and again emphasized in the June, 1936, number of the JOURNAL OF PEDIATRICS.

A right-sided twisted ovarian pedicle with strangulation may closely simulate appendicitis. Dr. Montgomery once made the diagnosis from the nature of a mass felt per rectum. I have advised him not to try it again! A very high leucocyte count is characteristic and of considerable diagnostic value. One of our patients had a count of 80,000, and led the interne, who had recently had a gynecological service, to suggest the diagnosis from that observation. Fortunately, operation is indicated in both cases.

A perforating or inflamed Meckel's diverticulum can hardly be differentiated from appendicitis unless there is a coincidental hemorrhage from the intestines. A diverticulitis, in the usual sense, I have never encountered.

One of the most frequent and puzzling conditions that call for differentiation is the abdominal pain that occurs with such diseases as measles, scarlet fever, pneumonia, and, more frequently than with any other, upper respiratory tract infections. A child entered the ward acutely sick with a strong suspicion of appendicitis. We delayed because she was too sick and had too high a fever for appendicitis. The next morning she presented the picture of a florid scarlet fever. On this point it is rather unavoidable not to inject a personal matter. Some years ago (1921)

I wrote a paper on ''The Abdominal Pain of Throat Infections,'' in which I reported the frequent occurrence of pain in the abdomen, in fact two types of pain, with upper respiratory tract infections. One of these usually occurs early, is transient, has a colicky, neuritic quality, is practically always restricted to the region of the umbilicus and suggests a referred origin. The other usually occurs a little later, is more dull, diffuse and persistent, is not restricted to any one locality but is probably found more often in the lower right quadrant and is accompanied by tenderness somewhat less marked than that of appendicitis. There is every reason to believe that the latter type is due to mesenteric lymphadenitis. Such glands are not infrequently found at operation for appendicitis, erroneously diagnosed, as well as at necropsies of patients dying of grippy infections. I have known of several instances in which they have ruptured, making a differentiation from appendicitis impossible except at operation. Following the publication of that paper apparently a number of people had read at least the title, not the conclusions, because I saw several cases of appendicitis in consultation in which the diagnosis was missed because the child had an evident throat infection. I then went back over the last ten cases of appendicitis I had seen in practice and found that nine of them had such evidences of an immediately preceding, or present, throat infection, as tonsillitis, mastoiditis, otitis media, grippe, pneumonia, cough, etc. One child seen in consultation had a severe throat infection and a tender distended abdomen. It was my impression that the child had a throat infection, a right lower lobe pneumonia, a ruptured appendix and a general peritonitis. My impression was questioned, a blood transfusion (!) was given and further treatment was put off to await the result of an x-ray examination on the following morning. The necropsy that afternoon confirmed the fact that all of the things that had been suspected can follow, or accompany, an initial infection in the throat. So I wrote another paper with the purposely clumsy title of ''The Abdominal Pain of Throat Infections, and Appendicitis'' (1927) pointing out the unquestionably frequent association of the two conditions. This idea is not new, and I have already quoted Evans' experience at the University of Wisconsin. I am convinced that more than 50 per cent of the cases of appendicitis are secondary to infections in the throat. Because of the above experience I am anxious to leave this final impression: If clinical evidence in a child points to appendicitis and the child has at present, or had an immediately preceding, throat infection, lean toward rather than away from the diagnosis of appendicitis—or better still wholly disregard the throat.

CHAIRMAN MONTGOMERY.—Speaking from the standpoint of the surgeon, I wish to ask your attention to the anatomy of the appendix for I feel that it has a definite bearing on the clinical aspects of appendicitis as we see it in children. In infants the appendix is a cone-shaped affair with an open, wide mouth that permits free emptying into the cecum. This explains very clearly why obstruction does not occur in the organ and as a consequence, appendicitis is very rare at this age. When we recognize that most appendicitis occurs at the tip or distal portion of the organ or at the side of a fecolith, scar, constricting band, or twist, it seems very definite that primarily appendicitis is caused by something that obstructs the emptying of this blind tube. In children past the age of infancy such findings at operation are very common. Even when we do not find a definite obstruction there is often a kink of the appendix caused by a short mesentery which may not produce a definite appendicitis but may cause attacks of appendiceal colic.

Another anatomical point in connection with the clinical picture is the indefinite location of the appendix. In most instances, of course, it will be located in the right lower quadrant of the abdomen, hanging over the brim of the pelvis or pointing upward toward the spleen. When it is in the pelvis, the tip may rest on the left side of the mesentery and if an abscess forms it may produce a mass on the left side of the abdomen. In other cases the appendix is without a mesentery and rests behind the peritoneum in the retrocecal portion. In such cases the point of maximum tenderness will be on the right side posteriorly toward the loin. An inflamed appendix in that location is apt to produce a spreading cellulitis if it ruptures and prove fatal by extending retroperitoneally. Again, anatomically, the colon may not rotate completely and the appendix may be situated high up in the right side near the gallbladder. High abdominal pain and tenderness and occasionally a mild jaundice may produce a very confusing clinical picture in such cases. In rare instances the appendix may be located in the left lower quadrant of the abdomen with or without a situs transversus of the other organs. In that position it may simulate very much the picture of diverticulitis which is practically unknown in children but common in adults.

Coming now to the symptoms, it should be emphasized that the entire clinical picture is usually composed of symptoms of a mild degree which are entirely out of proportion to the seriousness of the condition. The pain is usually colicky but rarely of a severe type. Vomiting is generally present, but not often repeated and may be entirely absent. Nausea, however, is practically always constant. Localized tenderness is probably the most reliable sign and should always be carefully looked for. It is most marked over the site of the inflamed appendix and is the best guide for the surgeon in his search for the pathology. Rigidity in my experience has not been present nearly as often in children as in adults, but a slight degree of muscular fixation over the point of tenderness is a very important and suggestive sign which may be revealed by careful palpation.

I do not believe the blood examination has the relative value that most diagnosticians give to it. A polynuclear leucocytosis of 15,000 or 20,000 is usually present but a leucocytosis above that figure should suggest the probability of a pneumonia or some other trouble. On the other hand, a leucopenia is of considerable importance in ruling out such conditions as typhoid fever, measles and influenza. In any event, the absence or presence of a leucocytosis should not be the deciding factor when all other signs and symptoms point to appendicitis.

When we come to the differential diagnosis, there is a large number of conditions that must be taken into consideration. Some of these are very easily ruled out but certain ones may be rather difficult. The main thing for the diagnostician is to keep in mind all of the pathological conditions that cause abdominal pain and be sure that they are ruled out as definitely as possible before making a final diagnosis. It is well known that in children chest conditions such as pericarditis, pleurisy and pneumonia frequently cause pain which is referred to the abdomen, often accompanied by abdominal tenderness and rigidity. A careful physical examination and an x-ray film of the chest will usually be sufficient to settle the diagnosis. Lymphadenitis of the mesentery glands has frequently been a cause of diagnostic error in our cases. Where bovine tuberculosis is present in a community an x-ray film of the abdomen may show calcified glands. Otherwise the clinical picture is so similar to that of appendicitis that I know of no way in which a definite diagnosis can be made. In such instances we have always felt that it was better to err on the side of safety and open the abdomen as none of these children have had any bad effects from the exploratory laparotomy.

Another rather confusing condition is the inflammation that often occurs in patients who have a Meckel's diverticulum. Some observers say that the tenderness in this condition is most marked a little below and just to the right or left of the umbilicus, but the clinical picture in general is so much like that of appendicitis that a differential diagnosis is usually impossible. However, as the treatment of both conditions is essentially the same, the question of a definite diagnosis is only of academic interest. If at operation the appendix appears to be normal the surgeon should not forget to look carefully for a Meckel's diverticulum. By doing so he may solve his diagnostic problem and save his patient.

Tuberculosis of the spine may cause abdominal pain from the pressure on the nerves. A simple examination of the back for Pott's disease will usually clear up this question. Although pyelitis in girls frequently causes abdominal pain, the temperature and the leucocyte count are usually much higher and the patients are more toxic than is usually noted in appendicitis. Pus, of course, is present in the urine, but this may occur also in appendicitis if the tip of the inflamed appendix rests against the right ureter, and if there is any doubt about the matter an operative exposure of the appendix is the only safe course to follow. As a rule, conditions of the pelvic organs in girls do not often come into question. Tuberculous infections are very rare, but occasionally the pedicle of an ovarian cyst may become twisted and give a clinical picture that is rather suggestive of appendicitis. In one such case we were able to make a correct differentiation by means of a bimanual examination of the pelvis in the presence of a high leucocyte count. The onset of menstruation in girls at the age of puberty may be accompanied by sharp abdominal pain, but the general signs of appendicitis will be absent.

In peritonitis due to the streptococcus or pneumococcus which we see not infrequently in children the patients are usually more toxic than they are with appendicitis and the abdominal tenderness and rigidity are usually rather marked over the lower half of the abdomen. A differential diagnosis is often impossible to make and because of this we have felt that it was better to open the abdomen rather than to overlook a possible appendicitis.

Lymphadenitis affecting the iliac glands occurs not infrequently with tenderness low down in the abdomen. These patients often exhibit a tendency to fixation of the hip and a swelling may be present just above Poupart's ligament due to pus forming under the iliac fascia. There is a number of other conditions, of course, that occasionally have to be considered in the differential diagnosis, but I have tried to bring out the important and common ones that have given rise to confusion in our cases.

The treatment of appendicitis has been a matter of discussion for many years. I think we all agree that cases seen in the first twenty-four to forty-eight hours should be treated by operation at the earliest possible moment. There is a difference of opinion, however, as to what should be done when the disease has been present for a longer period of time. In our clinical experience we have encountered a number of patients who are not seen until this latter stage, and in this group we feel that if we can palpate a mass in the abdomen it is better to use conservative measures such as rest, subcutaneous fluids, hot applications, and no food by mouth. Nature is evidently trying to localize the process in these cases and an operation may cause a spreading of the infection and do more harm than good. During our conservative regime we watch these masses carefully. Many of them disappear completely after a few days and the patient's general condition gradually approaches normal. We advise such patients to return to the clinic after six or eight weeks for an appendectomy. If the abdominal mass instead of receding gradually increases in size, an abscess is evidently present and surgical drainage is advisable when the exact site of the pus is evident. However, in these later cases if the signs of appendicitis are present and no abdominal mass is palpable, we feel that localization has not taken place and that operative treatment is advisable at the earliest possible moment.

The complications that may arise in association with appendicitis are numerous and they frequently involve the diagnosis if they begin to appear within twenty-four to forty-eight hours after the onset of the attack. A careful palpation may reveal a mass in the right lower quadrant which is evidently an effort on the part of nature to localize the infection to the region of the appendix. Pathologically, it is made up of the omentum and the adjacent coils of small bowel which become adherent to the appendix and very often to the parietal peritoneum. In the course of time this inflammatory mass may go on to abscess formation or it may entirely disappear. Watchful expectancy in such cases is usually wise and advisable. An ileus or intestinal obstruction is very apt to occur in an appendix that is situated between the ileum and the ascending colon. The possibility of this complication should be thought of when the appendix is found in this location at the time of operation. A prophylactic enterostomy made by placing a tube in the ileum will prevent any serious effects of this complication.

Peritonitis is, of course, the most frequent and serious complication of this disease. In many cases it begins gradually as a spreading process which can usually be recognized by the increased area of tenderness and rigidity in the lower abdomen together with a rise in the temperature and a more toxic generalized condition. An immediate operation to remove the source of the spreading infection is indicated. When the peritonitis has become generalized, rupture of the appendix has usually taken place and the clinical picture is very evident. In such cases a rapid simple operation to remove the appendix and institute drainage should be done. However, in the most severe cases where the patient is moribund, an immediate operation would possibly be fatal and a conservative treatment should be employed for about twenty-four hours. By this means some of these very bad cases can be improved sufficiently in twelve or twenty-four hours so as to withstand the strain of an operation.

Subphrenic abscesses in children usually come from infection which spreads up along the right colon gutter from the appendix. It is a late complication and unless it is thought of and carefully looked for, it may not be recognized. Whenever a patient continues to have a fever for some days after the appendiceal operation, the possibility of a collection of pus between the diaphragm and the liver should come into question. Immobility and elevation of the diaphragm in a fluoroscopic examination is very suggestive. The careful use of the exploratory needle followed by an immediate operation to promote drainage is indicated.

In a number of cases where an elevation of temperature and other signs of sepsis persist after operation, a pelvic abscess is the most likely complication. Abdominal and rectal palpation will usually show the presence of an inflammatory mass. Many of these abscesses will rupture into the rectum and evacuate spontaneously and they should be given an opportunity to do so. Otherwise surgical drainage should be established at the point where the pus seems to be most superficial. Fecal fistulas occur rather frequently in cases where a tube has been placed in the wound for drainage, but these fistulas usually close as the wound granulates and do not require any surgical treatment.

GENERAL DISCUSSION

DR. BRENNEMAN.—I want to emphasize that there is often a bad delay because some doctors put too much importance in the blood count. Cases of mesenteric gland involvement are very interesting. A good many of them are associated with upper respiratory infections. Dr. Montgomery mentioned subdiaphragmatic abscesses from a ruptured appendix. I do not recall seeing any of these until the last four or five years, but during this period we have had an epidemic of them.

CHAIRMAN MONTGOMERY.—They are not frequent but should be considered.

DR. BRENNEMANN.—This abscess often contains air. I have seen Dr. Montgomery take an aspirating needle and poke around through the back until he finally locates the pus. This looks dangerous to me but I know of no harm ever resulting from this procedure.

Another problem is seen in young girls with abdominal pain who are about to menstruate.

DR. B. FEINBERG (PROVIDENCE, R. I.).—No mention of intussusception has been made as a complication of appendicitis or as a difficulty in differential diagnosis. One out of four acute abdomens I have seen has been due to obstruction. One case was a boy eight years old who developed an intussusception due to to a polyposis. Another case had had an upper respiratory infection for two or three days, then a localized pain in the usual area and presented a picture of a beginning acidosis. The white count was 5,000. At operation a normal appendix was found and an intussusception. In my experience very few cases of intussusception have had bloody stools, but have been diagnosed because of the characteristic pain.

CHAIRMAN MONTGOMERY.—Dr. Feinberg has had a very unique experience with his cases of intussusception because that number of cases at those upper ages is most unusual. Ninety per cent of intussusceptions occur under two years of age. This usually does not present much of a problem. In my experience in cases over three or four years of age, I see hundreds of cases of appendicitis to every intussusception. There are usually other conditions present such as polyposis in cases of intussusception in older children.

DR. FEINBERG.—In my locality, we divide our cases into two groups. They are acute abdomens or not acute, that is, there are those which should be opened immediately and those which should be considered conservatively. There is the problem of streptococcal and pneumococcal peritonitis.

CHAIRMAN MONTGOMERY.—The difficulty with pneumococcal and streptococcal cases is to know what is going on. The average results are just about as good with conservative management as with radical. There is the possible value of using a needle to aspirate some abdominal fluid to determine the organism present. The diagnosis of a ruptured graafian follicle which has been confused with appendicitis is usually made by the surgeon.

DR. BRENNEMANN.—Henoch's purpura might be confusing but usually in this condition the purpura develops early, thus making clear the diagnosis.

DR. SIMPSON (BIRMINGHAM, ALA.).—What about the symptoms of an ileitis which may be confusing? There may be an abscess formation up along the ileum.

CHAIRMAN MONTGOMERY.—Experimental work has shown that this is usually associated with a mesenteric adenitis and a regional ileitis.

DR. M. C. SOUTER (INDIANAPOLIS).—I have seen three cases recently which presented the picture of appendicitis, but on opening the abdomen the appendix was found normal and there was a mesenteric adenitis. These cases were all under four years of age. I did notice that the pain seemed more diffuse rather than localized in all three cases.

DR. BRENNEMANN.—An early diffuse pain is not usually sufficient for a diagnosis of appendicitis. What the case might be in infants, I do not know because I do not believe that we have any cases under one year of age.

DR. B. K. RUST (INDIANAPOLIS).—I have had one case of an infant, aged four months, who had a sudden onset of paroxysmal pain and I suspected an intussusception from the history. I was able to begin my examination while the infant was asleep and felt fairly certain that no tumor was present, but I did find very definite and marked tenderness directly at McBurney's point. The infant began vomiting about four hours later. There was just a slight elevation in temperature and a white count of 12,000. The abdomen was opened eighteen hours after the onset of pain and an extremely gangrenous appendix was removed, which was pronounced extreme by the pathologist. Marked point tenderness was about my only lead in this case.

DR. J. B. BILDERBACK (PORTLAND, OREGON).—Pyuria is confusing in these cases, and why does it occur?

CHAIRMAN MONTGOMERY.—This is due to the close association of the tip of the appendix with the ureter. Never mind the pus if the case looks like an appendicitis.

DR. BILDERBACK.—I have seen appendicitis increase when there are many cases of chickenpox, measles and other contagious diseases.

CHAIRMAN MONTGOMERY.—This is true.

DR. RUST.—What anesthetic do you prefer in the cases of severe upper respiratory infections where you consider it also advisable to do an appendectomy?

CHAIRMAN MONTGOMERY.—I use a local anesthetic with whatever amount of ethylene gas is necessary to get relaxation.

DR. J. R. LEMMON (AMARILLO, TEXAS).—I have been interested in the difference between the incidence of appendicitis in the Americans as compared to the Chinese, Japanese and Filipinos. I do not remember seeing intussusception or appendicitis in thousands of patients from these races until after we had an epidemic of influenza, and then we had quite a few cases of appendicitis. I have seen that here, too. Is there a relationship?

CHAIRMAN MONTGOMERY.—There seems to be for we have noticed from year to year how with epidemics of upper respiratory infections there will be at one time numerous mastoids, or at other times a tendency for nephritis to develop, and then another epidemic will produce many cases of appendicitis following these respiratory infections.

DR. BRENNEMANN.—This specificity in various epidemics undoubtedly occurs. The work in Wisconsin must be considered where over a period of six years approximately 6,000 students were closely followed. It was found that there were eight times the number of cases of appendicitis occurring along with upper respiratory infections as compared to those without an upper respiratory infection. In case of suspected appendicitis we depend more on pain for diagnosis than muscular rigidity. When we find muscular rigidity, there is already peritoneal irritation. The appendix does not make much pain. I have known of a few cases in which abdominal glands have broken down and brought on a peritonitis. I do not think we can decide from the organisms found in the appendix what the original etiology was. We have found Levine tubes to be life-savers in peritonitis.

DR. C. F. SAWYER (CHICAGO).—We recognize two types of the disease, the infective and the obstructive. Either may occur alone early in the disease. In the infective type I do not believe that in older people 50 per cent come from infections in other parts of the body, as has been the opinion of Dr. Brennemann. In the obstructive type there is a lot more pain than in the purely infective type. The pediatrician's batting average is much superior to that of general practitioners.

The mortality rate is high and is increasing. I agree with Dr. Montgomery that those cases with an abdominal mass should be left alone. Also in our experience the mortality rate of those surgeons who come into the hospital from the outside is two and one-half times that of the surgeons on the staff of the hospital.

DR. F. S. CLARKE (OMAHA, NEBRASKA).—What is your attitude toward those cases which have been given castor oil on the third or fourth day?

CHAIRMAN MONTGOMERY.—A spreading peritonitis should be operated upon at once. A mass should be treated conservatively.

DR. CLARKE.—Do you remove the appendix if you operate during peritonitis?

CHAIRMAN MONTGOMERY.—Yes, if it can be easily removed.

DR. PERCIVAL NICHOLSON (ARDMORE, PA.).—In my experience most surgeons are too conservative in the treatment of early appendicitis; they do not operate soon enough. Do you get much aid from your pathologists, as a result of their pathological examinations of appendices?

CHAIRMAN MONTGOMERY.—I wonder if there is such a thing as chronic appendicitis. I do not believe there is. Of course I operate upon interval appendices.

DR. J. N. LANDE (SIOUX CITY, IOWA).—I had one case where an abscess drained out through the rectum. I wondered if it might be a case of suppurative glands, such as has been referred to.

DR. JOHN AULL (KANSAS CITY, MISSOURI).—I have always felt that acute appendicitis in children is nearly always secondary to an upper respiratory infection, just as is the case with acute catarrhal jaundice. I think perhaps one reason why our mortality rate is rising is that too many operations are performed because of vomiting and abdominal pain due to the onset of some other acute infection. To me vomiting does not even suggest appendicitis. Abdominal pain makes me think of the appendix. Tenderness on pressure strongly suggests appendicitis, but I depend chiefly upon muscular rigidity for my diagnosis and more particularly slight differences in muscular rigidity on the two sides.

DR. GUSTAV LIPPMANN (ST. LOUIS, MISSOURI).—We should teach students when to look for appendicitis; abdominal pain without diarrhea and with low fever should be considered appendicitis or peritonitis until it is proved otherwise.

DR. T. F. HUMPHREY (XENIA, OHIO).—Appendicitis, at times, comes definitely in epidemics. When these epidemics come on, there is much respiratory infection at the time.

DR. BRENNEMANN.—More than 50 per cent have a respiratory thing back of them. Notice the striking difference of opinion here between those men in pediatrics and the surgeons. We look at this thing from different viewpoints.

DR. A. F. SALOMON (OKLAHOMA CITY).—I had two patients operated upon for appendicitis in whom a ruptured graafian follicle was found.

CHAIRMAN MONTGOMERY.—I have operated upon some also when menstruation was beginning. These cases are perplexing.

DR. ROBERT E. CUMMINGS (CHICAGO).—I had three cases of appendicitis following chickenpox.

DR. J. H. DAVIS (CLEVELAND, OHIO).—Dr. Brennemann, what can you tell us about the relation of skin hyperesthesia to appendicitis?

DR. BRENNEMANN.—To me it does not mean anything.

CHAIRMAN MONTGOMERY.—I operated upon one allergic patient and found a normal appendix. Also in diabetes we may have severe abdominal pain.

DR. SAWYER.—What is the significance of these abdominal glands? Many times the appendix is definitely involved.

DR. BRENNEMANN.—I think it is a difficult thing to know the difference between normal and abnormal lymph glands.

DR. M. R. WOODWARD (SHERMAN, TEXAS).—I use barbiturates per rectum to quiet a child from one to three years of age who cries when the doctor attempts to make an examination.

CHAIRMAN MONTGOMERY.—Light anesthesia is advisable in these cases.

CLOSING REMARKS.—In closing this discussion I wish to say that I think we have all profited by the frank exchange of opinions in which everyone present has participated. I think you will agree with me that we all have a duty to perform in cutting down the present death rate from appendicitis in children. The pediatrician and the family doctor must realize and understand the importance of making a diagnosis at the earliest possible moment and they must consider the possibility of an inflamed appendix in every case of abdominal pain.

The surgeon who comes into the picture a little later must not only be able to diagnose appendicitis but must also be on the alert for the complications and various clinical conditions that the disease may present at this time. His judgment is probably more important than his technical skill. It is very apt to be founded upon his experience as Dr. Sawyer has said, and some of the deaths from this disease are undoubtedly due to operations performed by men with too little knowledge or experience in surgery. While time is an importance factor in the average case of appendicitis it is not such a grave emergency as to require operation at the hands of the first man available. The little extra time required to get a good experienced surgeon will probably be to the best interest of the patient in the long run.

Finally, we all have a duty as members of the medical profession to instruct and advise the public in regard to appendicitis so that we may obtain intelligent cooperation from the parents who, after all, must be regarded as the first line of defense.

DR. JOHN AULL, KANSAS CITY, MO.
DR. BYRON K. RUST, INDIANAPOLIS, IND.
Reporters.

SIXTH ANNUAL MEETING OF THE AMERICAN ACADEMY OF PEDIATRICS

KANSAS CITY, MO., MAY 11, 1936

Panel Discussion on Cyanosis in the Newborn

Chairman: Dr. A. Graeme Mitchell, Cincinnati.

Assistants: Dr. Fred L. Adair, Chicago; Dr. Barnet E. Bonar, Salt Lake City; Dr. Glenn E. Cullen, Cincinnati; Dr. Nicholas J. Eastman, Baltimore.

CHAIRMAN MITCHELL.—I am sure there are those in this audience who are quite certain that they know as much about this subject as those who are to participate in this panel discussion. I really hope that some of you know a little more.

We decided a while ago that the title of our discussion was somewhat confusing. In the first place, we should define in the beginning what a newborn infant is. Most of us in the panel decided we should discuss this subject of cyanosis and asphyxia in infants up to two weeks of age, because we wanted to say something about the late effects of asphyxia. We also felt that we were discussing something with which, in the final analysis, the general practitioner had a good deal to do. However, the obstetrician and pediatrician and probably also the biochemist must tell him some of the things to be done. In order to accomplish all this, we felt we should first, if possible, say what we do know or do not know about the causes of cyanosis and asphyxia both from the clinical point of view and from the point of view of the mechanism of their production.

There are certain confusing terms, which have been widely used, such, for example, as "acarbia." What does that mean? Some one has just handed me the latest edition of *Time*. In its column on medicine, it was reported that 400 stillborn babies were made to breathe by injecting a drug called alphalobelin into the vein of the umbilical cord when held upside down. It is not stated whether the cord was held upside down or whether it was the baby.

Apparently it is intimated that most of us have been negligent and have allowed many babies to die because we have not used the wonderful drug about which *Time* tells us.

There are many problems which we would like to elucidate and we must at least make the attempt. In order to do this, perhaps we should ask questions. Those which we considered were sent around to the various members of the committee and were about as follows:

1. What are the various causes of asphyxia and cyanosis in the newborn?

2. What is the mechanism of their production and does this differ when resulting from the several causes?

3. What starts the respiratory effort?

4. What is the value and what are the dangers of some of the methods employed in resuscitation? For example, does cutaneous stimulation do good and should it be employed? If so, under what circumstances?

5. What is the value of the tracheal catheter and is its use to be recommended for the general practitioner?

6. What is the status of inhalation of CO_2?

7. What are the advantages and disadvantages of various types of infant resuscitators and respirators?

I think that we might attempt, more or less informally in the beginning, to ask and answer some of these questions. We are not going to be formal. We have decided not to be particularly polite but to interrupt each other whenever we wish.

I shall ask Doctor Adair to start the discussion of this subject. Perhaps he would like to tell some of the causes of cyanosis or asphyxia in the newborn.

DR. FRED L. ADAIR.—Dr. Mitchell has referred to cyanosis in the baby which occurs in the first two weeks after birth, but we know it makes a lot of difference how mature the baby is when it is born. Obstetricians realize that some of their difficulties with the gaseous exchange of babies originate in utero before onset of labor, and a great many of the complications which lead to suffocation and asphyxiation in the baby arise during labor.

Among the factors affecting premature babies there are: the incomplete development of the lungs and their circulatory mechanism; the development of diseases and disorders which interfere with the gaseous exchange in the lungs after birth; and the failure of development of the neuromuscular mechanism which has to do with the establishment of respiration and is not manifested until after birth.

But, undoubtedly, the respiratory mechanism, as Doctor Eastman will conclusively demonstrate, operates in utero. The neuromuscular mechanism is functioning before birth but respiration is not established. Other complications which have to be considered are those that affect the gaseous exchange, the extraneous conditions which affect the lungs in various ways, and perhaps, that which affects the central nervous system and interferes with the neuromuscular mechanism.

I feel that probably intracranial bleeding and lacerations of the dural membranes are the best evidence we have of intracranial injury, but I believe there are a good many cases of intracranial injury which lead to the death of infants which are not manifested by evidence of either laceration or hemorrhage.

CHAIRMAN MITCHELL.—So far, we have gained an idea of some of the causes of asphyxia with which there is cyanosis in some instances. We have not been told what we are going to do about these different conditions, but there is a suggestion that there are dissimilar treatments for the several types of asphyxia and cyanosis. I wonder whether Doctor Bonar has anything to add to this classification, or whether he wishes to add other causes, and perhaps he might even give us some idea of what he does about these different types of asphyxia.

DR. BARNET E. BONAR.—I think we could more easily comprehend this vast subject if we made a diagrammatic scheme or outline of the mechanism of anoxemia. By the way, I think we should consider this whole subject as one of anoxemia rather than cyanosis or asphyxia. According to my figures, roughly about 85 per cent of all deaths in infants are associated to some extent with cyanosis or anoxemia in some form.

TABLE I

ANOXEMIA IN NEONATAL DEATHS

Congenital debility (including prematurity)	90%
Pneumonia	100%
Birth injuries	95%
Atelectasis	100%
Congenital abnormalities	50%

In respect to the following outline of the mechanism of anoxemia in the newborn, I might say that I am not speaking of the intrauterine forms of anoxemia, although if we were to consider the placenta as the lungs in utero we could follow this same outline easily.

TABLE II

MECHANISM OF NEONATAL ANOXEMIA

Respiratory System	Pulmonary Ventilation	Upper Air Passages	— Obstruction
		Lungs	— Faulty Distention
	Arterial Exchange	Alveolar Wall	— Decreased Permeability
		Hemoglobin	— Defective Hemoglobin
Circulatory System	Transportation	Heart	— Defective Force
		Vessels	— Defective Circulation
	Tissue Exchange	Capillaries	— Stagnation
		Tissues	— Defective Exchange
Central Nervous System	Medullary Centers	Respiratory Cardiac Vasomotor	— Depression

Under the heading, respiratory system, pulmonary ventilation must be considered first. Naturally, we have to have normal air passages if an adequate amount of air is to get to the lungs. As far as the lungs are concerned, they must be properly distended if the organism is to reserve sufficient oxygen. Now, when we come to the next heading, the arterial exchange of the gases, the alveolar wall must be permeable in order that the proper gaseous exchange may occur. Under arterial exchange we must also consider the quality and amount of hemoglobin for not only must there be enough hemoglobin but also the hemoglobin must not be bound with some gas that is given off with great difficulty, such as carbon monoxide. However, in the newborn infant hemoglobin disturbances are found rarely.

The circulatory system in this outline may be divided into the transportation system, the heart and vessels, and that portion having to do with the tissue exchange of gases, the capillaries and tissues. Normal heart action must be maintained and the circulation of blood must not be interfered with. Otherwise, some of the symptoms found in asphyxia or cyanosis may appear. The vessels must be normal and the two systems, connected with the right and left sides of the heart, must not have abnormal communications which interfere with the oxygen supply to the tissues. For instance, if venous-arterial shunts or unaerated shunts are present we have difficulty for then the vessels carry improperly oxygenated blood to the tissues. In the tissues, changes occur which, I think, Doctor Cullen can tell you more about than I. The return of blood to the heart must be sufficiently satisfactory to prevent stagnation and asphyxiation of the tissues. The venous pressure must not be too great or stagnation will occur and the tissue exchanges will be interfered with.

Finally, there is the nervous system which, of course, has to do with the medullary centers, respiratory, cardiac and vasomotor. Under the various and several conditions encountered during and after birth, we often find these centers depressed and their depression in turn disturbs the normal functioning of the other systems that are outlined here.

From the next table (Table III) we can really consider the sites at which the normal interchange of gases may be broken up, that is, the actual contributing causes to cyanosis. All the instances of interference to the pulmonary ventilation through obstruction of the air passages may be divided into intrinsic or extrinsic causes producing pressure or obstruction from within or from without. These may be the result of foreign material such as mucus or amniotic sac contents, injury,

Table III

Extrauterine Causes of Neonatal Anoxemia

Obstructed Air Passages	Internal	Foreign Material Trauma Congenital Abnormalities Infection
	External	Congenital Abnormalities Tumors
Faulty Alveolar Distention	Internal	Atelectasis Occlusion Collapse Rupture Emphysema
	External	Weak Musculature Intrapleural Pressure Congenital Abnormalities
Decreased Alveolar Permeability	—	Pneumonosis Edema Exudate Hyalin
Defective Hemoglobin	—	Anemia Reduced Hemoglobin
Defective Cardiac Force	—	Failure
Defective Circulation	Unaerated Shunts	Cardiac Respiratory Peripheral
	Obstruction	Trauma Infection Congenital Abnormalities
	Vasodilation	Shock Chilling
Depressed Medullary Centers	Intracranial Pressure	
	Chemical	Toxins Drugs Ch
	Shock	Anesthesia Trauma

congenital abnormalities, infection or tumors. While external causes such as an enlarged thymus or an infection of the tissues in the neck may be sufficient to cause interference with the passage of air into the lungs, most instances of obstruction are found within the various parts of the upper respiratory tract itself, mucus, congenital abnormalities or tumors.

Under the next heading is faulty distention of the alveoli. This comes about principally, I believe, through immaturity of the fetus whether it be prematurity or the so-called congenital disability due to the toxemias of pregnancy or some other maternal disease. Immaturity itself favors faulty distention, either from inability of the alveoli to open up because of cohesion of the alveolar walls, atelectasis, or weakness of the respiratory muscles. Among the internal causes of faulty distention must be mentioned also occlusion with mucus or amniotic sac contents with alveolar collapse, rupture or alveoli which may occur from insufflation, or overdistention of some portions of the lung with subsequent inability of the adjacent alveoli to distend. Aside from weak musculature, intrapleural pressure from extravasation of blood or pleural transudates may be an external cause of faulty alveolar distention. Sometimes, however, as Doctor Adair has said, there are other extrinsic factors, mainly congenital abnormalities, such as eventration of the diaphragm, diaphragmatic hernia, or absence of some of the external muscles of respiration.

As far as the alveolar wall is concerned, we occasionally find an interference at this point, either through a fibrinous exudate or an edema of the wall which will not permit the gases to be interchanged, or as Rosenthal has spoken of occasionally, a hyaline membrane. This is found to have developed in some individuals, and when present, permeability is greatly interfered with.

We rarely see a deficiency in the hemoglobin of the newborn infant. Usually there is a sufficient amount of hemoglobin at birth and rarely is there such a thing as carbon monoxide poisoning or other abnormal combinations of hemoglobin.

Heart failure often develops from some of the causes I have mentioned, but as a primary cause of cyanosis it is rare. It is a late effect, a good example being found in the heart failure that occurs in the asphyxial crisis.

When we have an unventilated area of lung as in partial atelectasis, one of two things happens. Either the blood will go through the unaerated portion or it will be shut off from the involved area. If it goes through the undistended portion of lung, it will not take up oxygen, of course, and we have an unaerated shunt of venous blood to the arterial side. That is frequently a cause of some of the symptoms of asphyxia. But there is another thing that may happen at this particular point. The peripheral resistance in the lung will increase the pressure in the pulmonary blood vessel and cause something seldom mentioned, but which I think should be; namely, an increased pressure in the right heart with reopening of the foramen ovale and probably the ductus arteriosus. Peripheral shunts, such as the rare arteriovenous communications, may also interfere with the normal circulatory function.

Under the heading, obstruction, are listed briefly the several causes of more localized cyanoses. Trauma and infection usually produce only transient cyanosis through vascular dilatation, vasomotor paralysis causing stagnation in the capillaries with improper exchange of gases in the tissues. Congenital abnormalities, such as tumors, at times cause stagnation and cyanosis of a more permanent nature.

I think, under medullary centers, we might briefly mention intracranial pressure in which there occurs anemia of the brain from pressure upon it. This may be due to intracranial hemorrhage, depressed fractures, edema from trauma, tumors or hydrocephalus. Depression of the medullary centers may also occur from vasomotor paralysis, from chilling or following shock which is either a true vasomotor paralysis or possibly histamine shock from tissue injury.

Chemically, the medullary centers occasionally may be depressed as the result of toxins as in the neonatal infections. However, the most common chemical cause is the various drugs and inhalants used for reducing pain during delivery of the child.

CHAIRMAN MITCHELL.—Doctor Eastman, as you all know, has had a great deal of experience with this particular subject of asphyxia in the newborn, and has also done some significant work in relation to the causation and mechanism of the production of asphyxia and cyanosis and what ought to be done about it.

One of the questions I am hoping Doctor Eastman may answer or give some idea about is:

Why do these infants start to breathe or why do they not start to breathe after birth in those cases in which there is not obvious obstruction or something of that sort? Apparently the idea of most people who have attempted to make these babies breathe is that they are starting some new mechanism at birth. I think Doctor Eastman has some ideas about this, and I am going to ask him to discuss this particular phase of the subject.

DR. NICHOLAS J. EASTMAN.—While discussing these various causes of asphyxia neonatorum, it would seem worth while to consider for a few minutes, as Dr. Mitchell suggested, what happens normally in the few minutes after birth. What occurs in the absence of these interfering factors in the system of pulmonary ventilation? This, of course, brings up the question of the onset of respiration at birth. This subject has received an immense amount of attention, but it suffices to say here that theories based on physical stimulation as well as theories based on chemical stimulation fail to explain adequately the onset of respiration at birth.

Since the time of Ahlfeld in 1881, it has been suspected that fetuses make respiratory movements rhythmically in utero. This would seem logical and biologically sound since other organs such as the liver, kidneys, and heart function in utero, and it would seem singular if a system as important as that of pulmonary ventilation should suddenly start to function without previous preparation. While Ahlfeld thought these movements occurred, it was not until the present year that Snyder and Rosenfeld of our institution in Baltimore demonstrated them experimentally in rabbits, dogs, cats, guinea pigs, and monkeys. They are at present, I believe, able to demonstrate them through the abdominal wall in the human being.

I should like to present some motion pictures this afternoon showing these movements and at the same time emphasize the fact that this is not my work but that of Franklin F. Snyder, Associate Professor of Obstetrics at Johns Hopkins, and Morris Rosenfeld, Instructor in Pharmacology at the same institution.

They took rabbits at full-term pregnancy and under local novocaine severed the spinal cord to produce anesthesia of the lower limbs and abdomen, submerging the animal except the head in a bath of Ringer's solution at thirty-eight degrees. They then opened the abdomen under the Ringer's solution, exposed the pregnant horns of the uterus, and observed through the intact uterine wall these respiratory movements.

It is of interest to see occasionally as many as three fetuses breathing in utero at different rates, a circumstance which is difficult to correlate with any theory of the chemical onset of respiration at birth. In connection with such chemical theories, I should also like to call attention to the fact that at low cervical Cesarean section, performed under local infiltration anesthesia, it is possible to make a small incision in the lower part of the uterus, turn the baby around anteriorly and see it cry in utero. This again is a circumstance which is difficult to correlate with any chemical theory of the onset of respiration.

If a tracheal cannula is introduced into a rabbit and various gas mixtures given, it is found that they have a very definite effect upon these respiratory movements. When the uterine horn is incised and the rabbit fetus allowed to escape into the saline or Ringer's solution surrounding it, the placenta remaining intact, the fetus rolls about on the maternal abdomen and makes respiratory movements for an hour or two. It then can be taken out of the bath and breathes and develops quite normally. In the moving picture we will show one of the rabbit fetuses under the Ringer's solution crawling around and breathing readily under the fluid.

CHAIRMAN MITCHELL.—Doctor Eastman, do these animals inhale any of the fluid?

DR. EASTMAN.—That is a question which is usually asked but it is very difficult to make any definite reply at the present time since further work is necessary.

DR. BONAR.—Can these movements be seen in the human?

DR. EASTMAN.—Doctor Snyder is working at that now. Ahlfeld put a tambour on the abdomen of pregnant women and made tracings of these movements, but subsequent attempts to corroborate this work have been unsuccessful. It is necessary to sit down and watch by the hour and that has not been done since the time of Ahlfeld.

I want to devote a minute or two to the practical significance of this viewpoint of the onset of respiration. It seems to me that it throws a greater burden upon the obstetrician. It is no longer his task to initiate the onset of respiration at birth by trying to simulate some complex chemical mechanism which is not well understood. On the other hand, it becomes the duty of the obstetrician to preserve a very delicate mechanism which is already in existence but which is easily disrupted. He will be more careful in the use of drugs which may have a harmful effect upon the fetus and which, as Doctor Snyder and Doctor Rosenfeld have shown, interfere with these movements. He will be cautious, in certain cases, in the use of barbiturates. He will possibly lessen his dosage of quinine; he will be careful in the employment of gas-oxygen anesthesia and will not raise the concentration above a 90:10 mixture, because concentrations of nitrous-oxide-oxygen stronger than 90:10 invariably produce marked anoxemia of the fetus and in experimental animals stop these movements. He will be more careful to prevent intracranial injury and forthwith the problem of asphyxia neonatorum becomes one more of prophylaxis, of helping these movements, which are already in existence, to continue.

CHAIRMAN MITCHELL.—It is a matter of history and record that Doctor Cullen has differed with Doctor Yandell Henderson in some of his ideas. Some time soon in this discussion we must discuss two or three things in the practical application of medicine in children who have asphyxia or cyanosis. I wonder what we have to think about the use of certain respirators, whether they are physiologic in their action, whether they do harm or good and who should use them. Also we have to discuss the matter of the use of inhalation. Should we give these infants oxygen or give oxygen and CO_2, and in what strength and under what conditions?

Doctor Henderson has said, "If you go to any biochemist he will say, 'this is just an acidosis and you cannot treat acidosis with carbon dioxide.'" I might ask Doctor Cullen how about that.

DR. GLENN E. CULLEN.—It seems to me, Mr. Chairman, that that remark puts the biochemist very much on the spot. I cannot help but feel that in the attempt to discuss the abnormal biochemical or physiological conditions that have to do with cyanosis in the newborn, too little attention has been paid to the determination of the immediate problem. In this discussion, then, Mr. Chairman, let us separate sharply the conditions that exist in the initial asphyxia of the newborn and those which develop after delivery. Let us then differentiate between the treatment of the newborn child who suffers from lack of respiration, and the treatment which should be used when difficulties in respiration develop in the succeeding day or days. In searching the literature for information for this discussion, I have not found any other work as complete and convincing as that of Doctor Eastman. His work makes it clear that the immediate physiological need in the initial asphyxia at birth is oxygen. His work also shows that with the almost complete lack of oxygen there is, of course, definite change in the acid-base balance, and that with this change there is an unusually high tension of carbon dioxide already existing in the body. The immediate treatment, then, certainly centers around any method which will supply the oxygen to the tissues of these children. Since the CO_2 tension is already high, there would seem to be no need to increase further this high CO_2 tension in order to stimulate breathing. However, it does not follow that because there is already a high CO_2 tension the giving of a still higher CO_2 tension would not stimulate respiration or would be dangerous, because in the acidosis which occurs after ether anesthesia, the CO_2 tension, which is normally 45 mm. CO_2, goes up to 55 or 60 mm. CO_2 and yet the giving of sufficient CO_2 to increase the tension still further does result in a respiratory stimulus.

The possibility of damage from the use of CO_2 in stimulating respiration when it is really needed, seems to me to have an analogy in other conditions often met with in pediatrics. When a child is suffering from an alimentary irritation, we do not hesitate to temporarily deprive the child of food until we can get the alimentary tract back into a condition to handle food. The same is true of carbon dioxide. If a respiratory center for any reason, whether it be lack of oxygen or drug, has become insensitive to the stimulation which exists in that child's body, it would seem entirely logical to increase temporarily the stimulant by the administration of rather high CO_2 concentration. As soon as this initial stimulant has started respiration, it is then, of course, desirable to reduce the extra stimulation.

The answer to this question in this case is not one of reasoning but one of experimental evidence and I should like to ask Doctor Eastman if in those children, where he knows from analysis that the CO_2 tension is already 55 or 60, does he get as good results with oxygen alone as with oxygen plus CO_2?

DR. EASTMAN.—The question which Doctor Cullen raises brings one to the problem that has concerned a great many obstetricians and pediatricians in recent years, namely, whether carbon dioxide is the ideal stimulant to respiration at birth. For a great many years, Doctor Yandell Henderson has insisted on carbon dioxide. As a result of some studies that were begun in 1929 and which have been carried on since, I have accumulated certain evidence upon which I venture to take issue with Doctor Henderson. For the purpose of being brief, I have summarized this information on one lantern slide, which shows the oxygen content, the lactic acid content, the carbon dioxide tension, and the pH in various conditions at birth. It will be seen that the carbon dioxide tension in severe asphyxia is already extremely high and more carbon dioxide would seem not only superfluous but also possibly dangerous.

When we turn to the other question which Doctor Cullen mentioned, we have a different situation. We get away from the peculiar circumstances which exist immediately after delivery; and in the baby a few hours old, oxygen associated with carbon dioxide is probably logical since then, it seems to me, conditions are altered.

CHAIRMAN MITCHELL.—Could this be translated into the statement that in the newborn infants with asphyxia you do not need to give carbon dioxide under any conditions?

DR. EASTMAN.—If I may be permitted to do so, I should like to limit my statements to failure of respiration at birth, a condition with which after all the obstetrician is most directly associated and with which he has had the most experience. There I feel that carbon dioxide does not have a logical place and when given in mixtures of from 7 to 10 per cent, as is frequently done, may not only be superfluous but may prove harmful.

DR. CULLEN.—There is still one point, Doctor Eastman, that is not quite clear from what you have said. With those children where the CO_2 tension is 55 or 60, do you get as good results with oxygen alone as with CO_2 and oxygen?

DR. EASTMAN.—Clinically, it is very difficult to evaluate various gas mixtures. Often a baby is simply laid down and nothing is done to it because the condition of the mother demands immediate attention. Usually the baby starts to breathe perfectly well. It would require an enormous series of cases of asphyxia neonatorum to demonstrate definitely the most efficacious gases for initiating respiration at birth. I have not used carbon dioxide in excess of 4 per cent in the treatment of asphyxia neonatorum. I say 4 per cent because that is the concentration of carbon dioxide in the exhaled air, and I have often employed exhaled air in the treatment of this condition. However, that mixture can scarcely be considered stimulative.

DR. CULLEN.—Doctor Eastman's observation makes it necessary for us to think of the initial asphyxia at birth as primarily an oxygen lack and to plan future studies and treatment on that basis. Before we discuss the other division of our topic, the conditions that develop after birth, I should attempt to meet the criticism of the biochemist quoted by our Chairman from Dr. Yandell Henderson. I am very sorry that Doctor Henderson is not here so that the questions which he has raised in his many articles could be discussed with him. I should like to make clear how much admiration I have for Doctor Henderson's vigorous campaign for a logical method of resuscitation. There is no question that he should get the credit for introducing, universally, the use of carbon dioxide for carbon monoxide poisoning and for establishing a rational and proper administration of carbon dioxide and oxygen in this type of poisoning. He should also get credit for stimulating obstetricians and pediatricians to a more serious study of the problems of respiration of the newborn; but in giving him this credit we cannot refrain from insisting that the problems of respiration in the newborn are not questions of carbon dioxide only. These problems involve the interrelationship of carbon dioxide and of oxygen and of the whole electrolyte equilibrium of the fluids of the body and I think I am fair in saying that in his enthusiasm for the use of carbon dioxide, Doctor Henderson has lost sight of the physiology of respiration as a whole. He has introduced a term "acarbia," which I will not attempt to define for I think the concept incorrect, with the result of confusing the whole question of normal acid-base equilibrium of the body. My mission, today, is to attempt to make clear that in discussing respiratory distress we must consider the entire mechanism of respiration. This mechanism includes the absorption of oxygen by the lungs, the carriage of it by the blood to the capillaries, and the acceptance of it by the tissues. It includes the metabolism of oxygen to carbon dioxide, the neutralization of the carbon dioxide by sodium and potassium ions, the transportation of CO_2 as bicarbonate to the lungs, and the elimination of the carbon dioxide from the lungs by the reverse of the mechanism by which oxygen is absorbed. This mechanism involves to a great extent the change in the acid nature of hemoglobin with oxygenation and deoxygenation which, in ordinary respiration, accounts for 90 per cent of the transport of carbon dioxide from the tissues. One would think from Dr. Yandell Henderson's discussions that the only respiratory stimulant is carbon dioxide and that the alkalies in the body move back and forth from tissue to blood in some mysterious manner. This question has been studied for many years and most of us, who have been interested in chemical physiology of the blood, have thought that it is fairly well determined that it did not make any difference whether carbon dioxide or lactic acid or hydrogen ion was the immediate cause of this stimulus to the respiratory center so long as there was a change in the reaction of the fluid bathing the cells of the respiratory center. I have been using the term ''acid-base balance'' in an attempt to dodge the words ''acidosis'' and ''alkalosis.'' If it were possible for any one biochemist or physiologist to attain sufficient prestige or persuasiveness to remove the terms ''acidosis'' and ''alkalosis'' from present-day usage and to have the conditions which these terms should represent expressed in terms of acid-base balance, that man could die happy, knowing he had done something for medicine. Since that is probably not possible, we can only keep on attempting to use these terms intelligently. To do that we must recognize that the acid and alkaline constituents of body fluid exist in equilibrium which varies in the normal individual between two very definite, well-established limits. When there is an excess of normal acids, such as carbon dioxide or lactic acid, or when there are sufficient amounts of abnormal acids, such as occur with faulty metabolism of the fat in diabetes, we have a condition which may be termed ''acidosis.'' This may be measured in terms of lowered CO_2 content or of increased hydrogen ion concentration or of both. Whenever there is an excess of alkali in relation to acid either due to ingestion of abnormal amounts of alkali or to loss of acid in the system, as in vomiting, or to lowered tension of carbon dioxide as in excessive ventilation, the acid-base balance is disturbed toward the alkaline side and we have a condition of ''alkalosis.'' It is not safe, however, to use these terms unless we express the condition in a quantitative manner precisely as we state in a febrile condition the extent of temperature change. The continued use in a careless manner of the term ''acidosis'' to describe a condition where there are ketone substances in the urine or when some one has an upset stomach cannot be deplored or condemned too much. Further, I cannot overemphasize one of the fundamental points of view which has developed in studying such condition in young children. That is, it is not possible for even the best clinicians to determine by ordinary clinical observation whether or not a child, and especially an infant, has an ''acidosis'' or ''alkalosis.'' This is much more true for pediatric medicine than for adult medicine. After many years of cooperation with medical colleagues in various hospitals, I thought I could tell, fairly accurately, whether or not an adult was suffering from acidosis or alkalosis. Now, however, I know from experience in the Children's Hospital in Cincinnati (and I think you will admit that we have some fairly good clinicians there) that none of us can tell, without an examination of the blood, the condition of the acid-base balance of the blood. Still more important, even if by luck we make a correct guess as to which abnormality, if any, exists, we cannot with any safety prescribe adequate treatment without quantitative data upon which to base our theory.

When we once get this clear-cut and really simple concept of acidosis and alkalosis ingrained in the medical consciousness, then we can logically discuss whether or not the conditions in which we are now interested involve these disturbances of acid-base balance. There is no question at all that there is much more actual alkalosis, in the correct use of the term, in infants and young children than has been thought to exist. We have seen many children referred to us as problems of acidosis which, in reality, were acutely ill with an alkalosis, and we have been able to treat many of them with most happy results. But we would never have dared to treat a child with an acute alkalosis unless we knew by careful analysis exactly how severe was the condition. In other words, we have no right to treat any condition as a disturbed acid-base equilibrium unless we know that there is such a disturbance and we have no right to treat with specific therapy unless we can treat on a quantitative basis.

I hope some of you will stop and ask yourselves if you really know what you are saying before you again use the term ''alkalosis'' or ''acidosis'' or prescribe treatment for such a supposed condition.

CHAIRMAN MITCHELL.—Recently we have heard a good deal of criticism of some of the older methods of resuscitation where the newborn was played football with for a while. I wonder whether we had not better have some discussion of that. What about the matter of turning the baby upside down in relation to the possibility of increasing the danger of intracranial hemorrhage? Can those methods which have been used so widely for so many years actually do harm? The statement has been made, for example, that cutaneous stimulation does these babies no good. Clinically, it seems to do so under certain conditions if there is obstruction. What about tracheal catheter? Is that something we could or could not use? What is your experience, Doctor Adair?

DR. ADAIR.—For many years I have used oxygen and since coming to Chicago from Minneapolis have tried out various mixtures of carbon dioxide and oxygen clinically. Personally, I am convinced from clinical observation that Doctor Eastman is correct in his conclusions from experimental work. But I would also like to emphasize again and again the fact that many of these babies who do not breathe properly have something else radically wrong with them.

In order to convince you of that, I would like to give some data based on autopsy experience with practically one thousand cases in which 103 babies were born alive, where there was a heart beating and yet it was not possible to establish respiration. There was evidence of birth trauma present in forty-nine; a major anomaly in twenty-two; prematurity under seven months in three; atelectasis in four; four not diagnosed, with sixteen cases of suffocation and aspiration in which no other cause was found.

To summarize briefly my opinion relative to resuscitation, I would say it is important first to remove mucus, amniotic fluid, etc., from nasal and pharyngeal passages so that air may enter easily and obstruction of bronchi and alveoli does not occur. This may be done by holding the infant by the feet with head dependent, supporting the shoulders, and either milking out the content of the trachea and mouth or gently sucking it out with a tracheal catheter or bulb suction. When a baby once starts to breathe and the reflex action is established, there is little danger of aspiration into the trachea or bronchi.

The second main objective is to initiate respiration by artificial methods, various measures of cutaneous stimulation, snapping the nose or perhaps the mouth in the absence of something better, or gently rubbing the back with a rough cloth or something of that kind to stimulate respiration in the milder cases; the overcoming of anoxemia with oxygen; and (questionable) the stimulation of the respiratory center with CO_2 and oxygen. Proper temperature of the baby must be maintained while respiration is being established.

I should like to emphasize the importance of maintaining the proper temperature from the moment of birth on, and second, the importance of the frequent administration of oxygen. I should like also to emphasize again the necessity of using gentle procedure so that no additional lesion is produced or any existing one exaggerated and no additional trauma is created.

CHAIRMAN MITCHELL.—Would you say something about the use of infant respirators?

DR. ADAIR.—We have tried a number of different infant respirators. We have usually been so well satisfied and have relied so much upon the simpler procedures we have used that we hesitate to change. Also, although we have tried respirators on a series of cases, we are a little afraid of some of them, especially in teaching our students and internes certain of these methods, because we feel some of them are intrinsically dangerous. Furthermore, many of our students and many of our internes who go through our institutions are going to practice obstetrics where such an apparatus is not going to be available, both in the home and in hospitals which are not equipped with it. We think the simpler the procedure the better.

I might say that in some cases we have simply used the tracheal catheter with a Y-shaped tube connected with the oxygen tank and have allowed the flow of oxygen to come in with intermittent pressure over the free end of the tube, thus alternately injecting and releasing the oxygen. It is a simple device that can be controlled with this simple valvelike action so that pressure does not become excessive.

There is a very real danger of traumatizing babies from the introduction of instruments into the trachea, a danger of producing expansion with rupture of the alveoli of the lungs and danger of forcing material which may have been aspirated into the trachea or bronchi to a lower level in the lungs.

CHAIRMAN MITCHELL.—I think, Doctor Bonar, you have figures which show that 85 per cent of babies are stillborn in homes where the various types of apparatus are not available. A question which has been sent up here is: Can you tell us something more about the matter of anesthetics or analgesia, the matter of morphine, for example, and other things given to the mother? What effect do these have? It has been intimated they may have a direct effect.

DR. BONAR.—As Doctor Eastman has shown, there is no doubt but what morphine has a detrimental effect on the respiratory center of the newborn infant, and the barbital series in general have the same effect. We must be cautious in the use of these preparations and if we must use them, we should have the patient under continuous observation in order to be prepared to care for an asphyxiated baby in case of delivery before the anticipated time.

I think Dunham and Clifford have shown it is safe to use morphine or dilaudid up to three hours before delivery without any particularly deleterious effect upon the infant. But we do not always know whether the patient is going to wait for three hours, and if she does not there is impending danger of asphyxia. If that happens, one should immediately be prepared ahead of time, that is, be ready for an asphyxiated child.

One could not discuss the subject of anesthesia in childbirth in the two and one-half minutes allotted by the chairman. I feel we have been treading on dangerous ground in respect to these preparations. I think it pernicious, this habit that some men have of trying one of these drugs in a small series of cases and rushing into print to state that it is safe for the mother and that the baby is not asphyxiated. So far we have had no good criterion to determine whether or not the baby is asphyxiated. I think the work of Shute regarding the clinical manifestations of narcosis in the newborn is one of the best I have seen in this respect. All obstetricians should read it. Another pernicious habit is that of some men connected with well-manned and well-equipped lying-in hospitals advocating for general use some of these preparations which, after all, demand closer attention than can usually be paid the patient during labor in less sumptuous hospitals or in the home. Measures of this sort cannot be labeled innocuous for they all carry some hazard to both mother and child.

Furthermore, we have no simple clinical criterion as to when a child is free from anoxemia. In this respect I am not speaking of children immediately after birth but later on, that is, in the early days of life when pulmonary ventilation should be increased in extent.

Is it not possible that some of the anesthesias and analgesias may cause trouble through mild depression of the respiratory tract with subsequent faulty ventilation over a period of time? That is a question I cannot answer but I have always felt there is that danger and that brings up the question of the late effects of anoxemia in the child. I have agreed with Doctor Eastman for several years that the child at birth is acidotic. I think that comes about naturally through an increased amount of carbon dioxide in the blood. Once respiration has been established in a partially ventilated lung, it may develop the so-called physiologic shallow breathing which may wash out carbon dioxide and possibly produce what we might call an alkalemia.

In those particular cases where there is a high carbon dioxide content of the blood, it seems to me there is little indication for carbon dioxide but in those cases, the few that we might have, where there is a deficiency in the carbon dioxide in the blood it might be possible to help respiration by the use of carbon dioxide and oxygen.

Doctor Mitchell has asked what to do in the home or that group handled by the general practitioner. It seems to me there is a rule of thumb he can work out that is simple and does not need any fanciful equipment. If the patient is in a hospital, try oxygen first and if it does not succeed, try carbon dioxide and oxygen. There is no harm in it and if it helps out more than the oxygen, use the carbon dioxide oxygen mixture.

In the home other measures may be necessary. So far as insufflation is concerned, I think perhaps the mouth-to-mouth breathing could be better protected. It is dangerous from the point of view of distention of the alveoli. In using the Mackenzie mask, which is very small, the operator blows into the mask and the air is reduced in pressure so it will not be dangerous to the child, that is, the air will not overdistend the alveoli. At the same time, there is an opportunity in that instrument for the use of a little aromatic spirits of ammonia. This is an easy way for the physician to give oxygen and carbon dioxide. If he does not want to give carbon dioxide he can open his mouth, fill it with air, and blow into the mask without breathing out.

Tracheal catheterization is dangerous and I cannot feel that it can be used by every one as it will not be used properly in many instances. I noticed recently in the *Journal of the American Medical Association* an article about the use of the Flagg instrument. The writers of that article mention the fact that they have had a few injured babies. In a few the larynx has become edematous. I do not think the average person would be capable of using that instrument safely. It is not easy to insert a tracheal catheter into the trachea and since they are made of linen and are stiff, they can traumatize the larynx. The other method of modified mouth-to-mouth breathing would probably be satisfactory in the majority of instances and certainly more adaptable and safer for home conditions.

In regard to turning the baby upside down, I have never felt it necessary to do this. When the baby is turned upside down, we increase the brain volume and pressure, and one should be very cautious about doing this. I think it far better to first aspirate the mucus with a soft-nosed rubber bulb or ear syringe, which, by the way, is better than the mechanical aspirator for the negative pressure is about right and not too great. After the mucus has been aspirated the infant's head may be lowered a little.

CHAIRMAN MITCHELL.—Doctor Cullen, in your discussion of the chemical factors associated with asphyxia at birth, you did not go on to the cyanosis that develops after birth.

DR. CULLEN.—It is apparent that all of us are in agreement with Doctor Eastman in regard to the importance of the use of oxygen for asphyxia and cyanosis at birth. We cannot say for the cyanosis which develops after birth that the only disturbance is one of acid-base balance. Even though we may find such a disturbance, experience has taught us that changes of acid-base balance are not usually primary causes of abnormal conditions but are secondary. Further, even when we recognize that abnormal acid-base conditions exist which should be treated in order to prevent consequences that may be more serious than the initial condition, we should not become so enthusiastic about finding one abnormal condition that we forget that there are probably other equally important abnormalities. We must search for an understanding of the complete story. So, in these conditions of cyanosis which have developed in children after birth, and in which probably the most outstanding symptom is that of respiratory distress, we must realize that we may have an accumulation of difficulties such as slightly impaired circulation, a low temperature, a slight hemorrhage, or slight amount of fluids or other débris in the lungs, any one of which in itself may not be sufficiently severe to cause acute respiratory distress but which, operating together, have a cumulative effect that is dangerous.

No discussion of abnormal chemical conditions of the body in the newborn could be complete without mentioning two fundamental differences between the newborn and the adult human. The first of these is that the water mechanism of the infant's tissue is much more labile than in the adult and that loss of tissue fluid from any cause may bring about much more serious damage to the tissue than does a proportional loss of fluid in the adult. The second factor is that time is of much more importance in children than in adults.

It may seem naïve for me to emphasize these two points to an audience of pediatricians, but let me remind you that in general the application of fundamental physiologic chemical facts to children are based upon observations and experiments mainly carried out with normal adult human beings or upon adult laboratory animals. Although I do not know yet how to gather facts that can be expressed in sound mathematical terms, I am sure that when we carry over our experimences of abnormal acid-base conditions in the adult to children, we must add to other considerations that of time. For example, an acidosis not severe enough to injure permanently an adult even though it persists for a considerable period of time, may cause permanent damage to a child within a few hours.

CHAIRMAN MITCHELL.—I have the duty of trying to summarize what has been stated. It seems to me we have got two or three things fairly clear. In the first place, we cannot use the terms "asphyxia" and "cyanosis" as symptoms without qualifications any more than we can the term "edema." These may also be symptoms of different disturbances. Asphyxia and cyanosis in the newborn may be caused by a number of different things, which could perhaps be divided into the extrauterine and intrauterine groups. Certainly, we must first find, if possible, whether there is some mechanical obstructive factor. We have to think definitely of some of the other causes which need a different type of treatment. For example, intracranial hemorrhage puts a different aspect on the subject treatment of cyanosis.

I think that the obstetrician told us that one of the first procedures was to look for obstruction in the air passages, which frequently is caused by accumulation of secretion or mucus in the nose or throat. Those should be removed before attempting to do anything else. We must be careful not to use too much force, because this may possibly do the infant harm.

Probably, some of the older methods did more harm than good and they should be discarded, although I gather from the discussion and from reading that the obstetricians themselves are not willing to give up entirely some of the more gentle methods of artificial respiration.

I think that the work Doctor Eastman has shown us makes us think that after all we are not attempting to establish something new in respiration but rather attempting to assist something which is physiologic and automatic. Perhaps having done that, we do not need to do much more. Doctor Eastman makes the statement that often the best thing that can happen to the baby is that everyone else is too busy to bother about it so that it may have the opportunity to breathe itself.

I do not feel that there has been sufficient emphasis concerning the factor of giving anesthesia to the mother, which Doctor Bonar has stressed in this discussion. A matter which has not been touched upon is alphalobelin. I think Doctor Eastman agrees with Alan Moncrieff's published opinion that it is a very dangerous drug and it might be possible that we will find the article in *Time* to be entirely wrong.

DR. EASTMAN.—I have seen two deaths following injection of this drug, both preceded by convulsive seizures. The first one I thought was a coincidence but the second I felt was more than this.

CHAIRMAN MITCHELL.—We all agree that there is a difference in the treatment of asphyxia at birth and of respiratory distress that develops after birth.

I do not know how to summarize the matter of whether we should or should not use inhalation of carbon dioxide with oxygen. It seems clear that in the asphyxia at birth oxygen, either pure or as air, is most important. For the respiratory distress that develops after birth, it would appear that CO_2 may, in some instances, be of great value, since CO_2, judicially used in these cases, is probably not harmful and the logical procedure would be to give the infant the chance to show whether or not CO_2 benefits him. We certainly cannot now consider that the question is other than in the experimental stage and I cannot see how we can ignore Doctor Cullen's insistence that we determine the condition of acid-base balance before we treat for supposed acid-base disturbances.

In speaking for the group participating in this discussion, I think it fair to state that although we have not been able to answer finally the many questions that have been brought out we all have a much clearer concept of these various problems and their interrelation than we had before.

Academy News

The next annual meeting of the Academy will be held at the Waldorf-Astoria Hotel, New York City, June 3, 4, and 5, 1937.

Michigan Meeting, July 17, 1936

The Michigan Members of the Academy met July 17, 1936, at the Detroit Boat Club on Belle Isle, Detroit, Michigan, for dinner and the summer meeting. Twenty-two of the forty-five members in Michigan were present, with especially good representation of the out-state members.

Dr. Lillian Smith, one of the Michigan Members, who is Director of Maternal Welfare and Public Health Nursing of the State Department of Health, outlined the proposed program for the utilization of Federal Funds in Michigan under the Social Securities Act—Sections IV and V.

Dr. T. B. Cooley opened the discussion of the program. Dr. L. Fernald Foster, a member of the committee representing the Michigan Members of the Academy and also chairman of the Public Relations Committee of the Michigan State Medical Society, outlined the sentiment of the profession and discussed some of the problems involved.

After a lengthy discussion, the program as outlined by Dr. Smith with the additional suggestions and recommendations of the members, particularly with reference to the importance of providing postgraduate teaching in the areas to be covered by the program, was endorsed.

The Committee on Postgraduate Education through its chairman, Dr. J. Johnston, reported the success of the second annual three-day postgraduate course given in April in Detroit. Sixty-six physicians from Michigan, Ohio, and the Province of Ontario attended. Two-thirds of this group came from an area of more than thirty miles distance from Detroit.

Dr. Fred Miner discussed the advisability of the Michigan Members adopting a resolution requesting the State Medical Society to adopt the report of the Committee of the Academy covering prophylactic immunization.

It was reported that in all counties of the state in which members of the Academy resided, at least one member of the Academy was represented on the Medical Filter Committees appointed by the Judges of Probate to assist in the administration of the Afflicted Child Act.

The next meeting of the Michigan Members of the Academy will be held September 23, 1936 at Detroit at the time of the Annual Meeting of the Michigan State Medical Society.

News and Notes

Dr. Robert A. Strong, Professor of Pediatrics, Tulane University, began a course of lectures in Pediatrics on July 6, 1936, at Clarksdale, Mississippi. This course of lectures is open to physicians of Mississippi and is to be given in different sections over the state. It consists of five lectures a week on important phases of Pediatric practice.

These lectures are sponsored by the Mississippi State Medical Association, the State Hospital Association, and the State Board of Health; also, by Tulane University School of Medicine and the Graduate School of Medicine. The Mississippi State Pediatric Society has approved these lectures and is heartily cooperating with the other organizations. The following committee on Postgraduate Medical Education is in charge of the course. Dr. Harvey F. Garrison, President, Mississippi State Medical Association; Dr. J. W. Lipscomb, President, Mississippi State Board of Health; Dr. Felix J. Underwood, Mississippi State Health Officer; Dr. H. W. Kostmayer, Dean, Tulane University Graduate School of Medicine; Dr. C. C. Bass, Dean, Tulane University School of Medicine; Dr. Leon S. Lippincott, Secretary, Mississippi State Hospital Association and Dr. W. H. Anderson, Editor, *Mississippi Doctor,* official organ of the Mississippi State Medical Association.

At the meeting of the **Mississippi State Pediatric Society** which was held in Jackson, the following officers for 1936-1937 were elected:

Dr. Harvey F. Garrison, Jackson, Miss., President
Dr. John K. Bullock, Jackson, Miss., Vice-President
Dr. Guy C. Jarratt, Vicksburg, Miss., Secretary-Treasurer

Final notice is given by the **American Board of Pediatrics** to all pediatricians who wish to be certified by the Board, who belong in Group I, that after September 1 an examination will be required of all applicants in this group. This group consists of physicians who have been engaged in Pediatrics for ten or more years and are subject to certification without examination. Also, the fee for certification advances from $20.00 to $30.00 on the above date for all applicants, no matter to what group they belong. If you have not already made application, attend to this matter at once.

The Journal of Pediatrics

Vol. 9 SEPTEMBER, 1936 No. 3

Original Communications

MEDITERRANEAN DISEASE—THALASSEMIA (ERYTHROBLASTIC ANEMIA OF COOLEY)

Associated Pigment Abnormalities Simulating Hemochromatosis

G. H. Whipple, M.D., and W. L. Bradford, M.D.
Rochester, N. Y.

THIS interesting disease presents three important abnormalities together characterizing a syndrome which may be designated "Mediterranean disease." The anemia alone is not a diagnostic factor and is usually associated with a progressive splenomegaly. The bone changes alone are not diagnostic, as very similar changes have been reported in sickle-cell anemia[21, 9] and hemolytic jaundice.[19, 6] The pigment abnormalities are of fundamental importance but alone do not make the diagnosis as we may find exactly similar pigment deposits in adult cases of hemochromatosis.

The disease is also limited to the people who live about the Mediterranean—Italians, Greeks, Syrians, Armenians—and shows a strong familial tendency. We have reported the disease in identical male twins, and, if one would explain such coincidences on the probabilities of chance, it is necessary to indulge in astronomical figures. Obviously there is some *inherited defect* which is responsible for the total abnormality involving hemopoietic tissues, bone growth, and pigment metabolism.

We reported in detail four years ago the clinical and autopsy findings in a typical case of this disease.[22] As the *pigment abnormalities* there described had not been noted in other published reports, we could not stress the importance of these findings. We now report in detail three more cases with complete autopsy reports. We have had opportunity to study certain organ tissues from two other cases kindly sent us by Dr. T. B. Cooley. All this material gives us reasonable security in our belief that the *pigment deposits are just as characteristic of this*

From the Departments of Pathology and Pediatrics, the University of Rochester School of Medicine and Dentistry.

Presented in abstract before the American Pediatric Society, June 11-13, 1936, Lake George, N. Y.

disease complex as are any other factors. The pigment abnormalities simulate hemochromatosis in the adult and are remarkably uniform. Iron-containing pigment is abundant in liver, pancreas, lymph glands, gastric mucosa, thyroid, and adrenals. The same pigment is usually demonstrable in Brunner's glands, salivary and mucous glands, parathyroids, hypophysis, heart muscle, kidney tubules, spleen, and bone marrow. Pigments normally present in the body—for example the reticular zone of the adrenal, the epidermis, the choroid plexus and the interstitial cells of the testis—are as a rule increased in amount in these cases.

This disease presents a uniform *clinical picture* consisting of a progressive anemia beginning usually during the first two years of life and terminating in death in most instances before adolescence. The blood picture, though not distinctive, is uniform and is characterized by marked irregularity in the size and shape of the red cell, fragmentation, and erythroblastosis. All stages of erythropoiesis may be seen in the peripheral blood. The hemoglobin distribution within the matured red cell may be very irregular. After splenectomy showers of nucleated red cells always occur.

Definite *retardation of growth* results. In Case 8 (E. S.) only two carpal centers of ossification were found at four years while her normal twin sister had four.

As the disease progresses, the typical mongoloid features develop, probably because of bone changes. In certain cases the icterus index of the blood is slightly elevated but lends little support to the idea formerly entertained, that the disease is due to hemolysis.

Enlargement of the spleen is proportionally greater than that of the liver, but, when the former is removed, the latter seems to increase in size.

To this group of clinical features the addition of the interesting abnormalities which occur in the bones, the unusual pigment disturbances, and the racial and familial distribution completes a characteristic syndrome.

LITERATURE

It is not necessary to review the literature of this disease as this has been done adequately in recent papers by Baty, Blackfan and Diamond,[1] Parsons and Hawksley,[13] and Yaguda.[23] Yaguda suggests that the erythroblastosis of the newborn be classified with this disease as described by Cooley, but we can see no merit to this suggestion and feel that it would only lead to confusion. Cooley did a great service when he defined clearly the clinical syndrome designated by him as "erythroblastic anemia" and separated it from a group of unrelated anemias and splenomegalies. The erythroblastoses of the newborn have only one thing in common with this disease *(thalassemia)*, but they are not racial, nor do they show bone and pigment abnormalities.

Anemia and erythroblastosis in these children is not sufficient alone to make the diagnosis, as Bennett, Hunter and Vaughan[2] have reported an identical blood picture in adult celiac disease or idiopathic steatorrhea. This anemia, however, yields to iron therapy.

It has also been pointed out by Baty, Blackfan and Diamond[1] that the marrow changes found in these children *(thalassemia)* are similar to the marrow histology of pernicious anemia during relapse. Their report gives admirable illustrations of marrow and spleen histology. We have been impressed with the *variety of changes* which may be found in the marrow and spleen in our material. Possibly the picture may vary

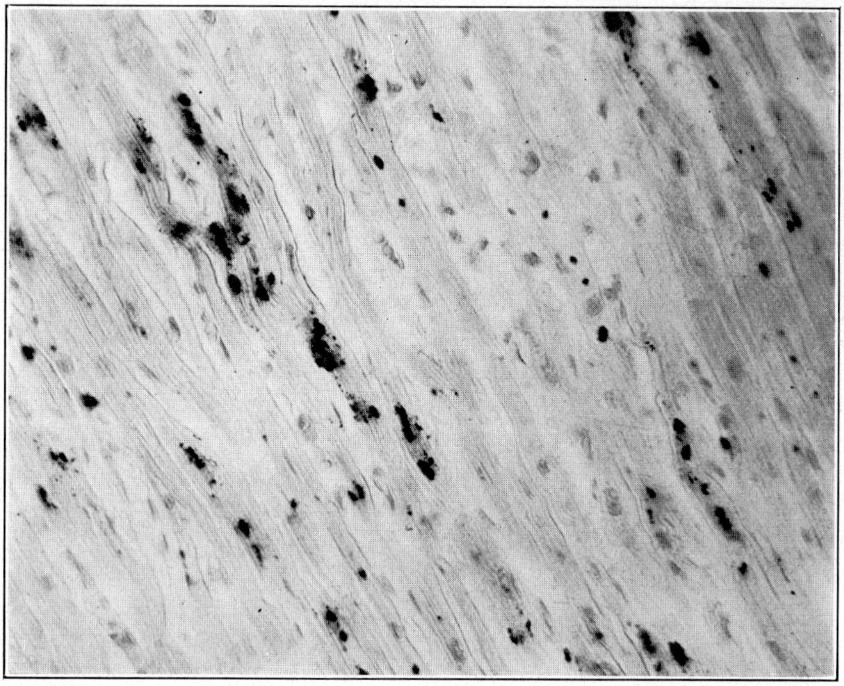

Fig. 1.—Case 4. Photomicrograph of heart muscle showing black grains of iron-containing pigment (magnification ×425).

somewhat depending upon the stage of the disease which happens to be represented. Both spleen and marrow may show chronic states of hyperplasia in which stroma and "foam cells"[22] may dominate the picture in contrast to the active cellular stages often illustrated.[1] These "foam cells" have been noted by others,[7] and at least in one case led to the diagnosis of Gaucher's disease from an examination of spleen alone.[12]

GENERAL PATHOLOGY OF THALASSEMIA

This is a composite picture of the autopsies studied by us. The mongoloid features are usually definite. General edema is quite common and may be related at least in part to the anemia. The fluid in the serous cavities may be of a yellow color but usually shows no urobilin and no bile pigment. The anemia is probably also responsible for the fatty changes noted in the liver, heart, and kidney.

Heart may be enlarged, is pale and decidedly brown in color. Fine fat droplets and excess pigment are found in the heart muscle cells. Some of the pigment is lipochrome and some gives a strong test for iron (Fig. 1). This iron staining pigment is not always present.

Lungs usually show edema and perhaps bronchopneumonia.

Liver is enlarged and shows a deep buff or bronze color. The surface is smooth, and the lobulation is regular. The liver cells show fat droplets usually conspicuous in the center of the lobules. The liver cells are filled with a fine granular yellow pigment, most of which gives a strong test for iron. This pigment is more abundant in the marginal half of the lobule. *Chemical analyses* show about ten times the amount of iron found in normal liver tissue. The pigment is found almost wholly in the hepatic epithelium and not at all in the biliary duct epithelium. Kupffer cells show some pigment which is usually noniron containing. Marrow cells in small nests may be found in some cases in the capillaries of the liver lobules. Gallbladder mucosa may show a brown color because of granular yellow pigment in the mucosa and the submucosa, and it is negative for iron.

Pancreas may be very distinctive grossly and presents a deep buff or bronze color. It is of normal size and is not indurated. The acinar cells may be very rich in granular yellow *pigment* much of which reacts to iron stains (refer to our first paper[22] for illustrations). This pigment is found only rarely in the epithelium of the islets but is commonly more abundant in the acini close to the islets. This distribution may be related to vascular supply.

Serous and Mucous Glands.—The mucous glands of the pharynx and trachea as well as the salivary glands usually show pigmentation, and much of this pigment reacts strongly with iron stains.

Gastrointestinal Tract.—The *stomach* in gross may show a deep pigmentation, often confused with postmortem staining. The acinar epithelium in this mucosa may be very rich in a yellow granular pigment which stains for iron. The chief cells and not the acid cells contain most of this pigment (refer to our first paper for illustrations[22]). Duodenum, jejunum, ileum, and colon show no iron-staining pigment in their mucosa, but *Brunner's glands* in the duodenum often do contain iron-staining pigment granules in the epithelium. The smooth muscle of the intestinal tract does not show deposits of pigment.

Genitourinary Tract.—*Kidneys* are a little enlarged and pale. There is usually a brownish color noted. Pigment is found in the epithelium of some tubules but not in others. Henle's tubules are often outlined by this pigment deposit (Fig. 2), some of which stains for iron and some not. Glomeruli, stroma, and collecting tubules are usually normal. Fat stains show a good many fat droplets in the convoluted tubular epithelium. A few casts are often present. *Bladder* is usually pale

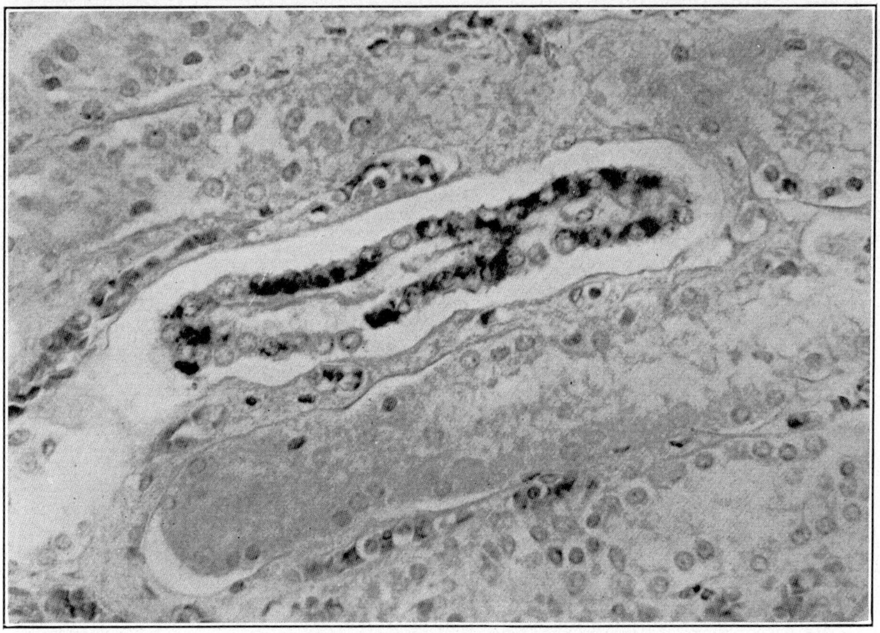

Fig. 2.—Case 4. Photomicrograph of kidney tubular epithelium containing black grains of iron-staining pigment (magnification ×425).

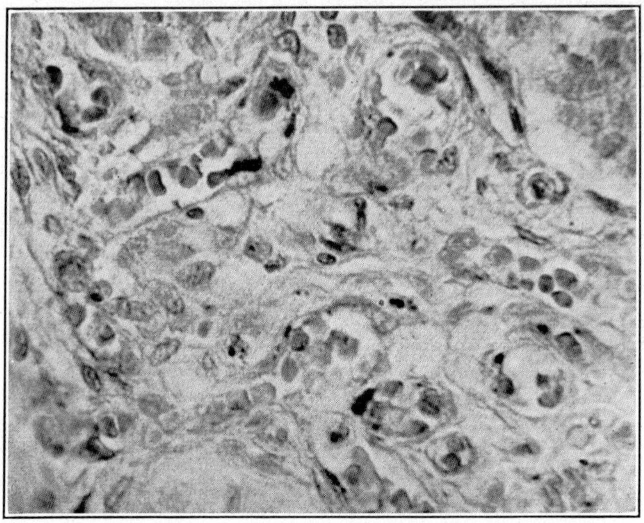

Fig. 3.—Case 5. Photomicrograph of testis with fine black grains of iron-containing pigment in the endothelium of several capillaries (magnification ×700).

and normal. The prostate is usually normal and nonpigmented but the immature acini in some cases may show lipochrome. *Testis* shows a deep brown color in gross and much pigment in sections. Coarse granular pigment, which is negative for iron, is found in the interstitial tissue. Fine pigment grains rich in iron are often found in the capillary endothelium of the testis (Fig. 3) but the immature seminiferous tubules usually contain no pigment. Ovarian tissue shows nothing of interest.

Spleen is always much enlarged and may approximate one-half the size of the liver. It may show infarcts and adhesions. The gross picture suggests a chronic process; the organ is firm and hard and presents a sharp cut surface which is not velvety, suggesting much connective

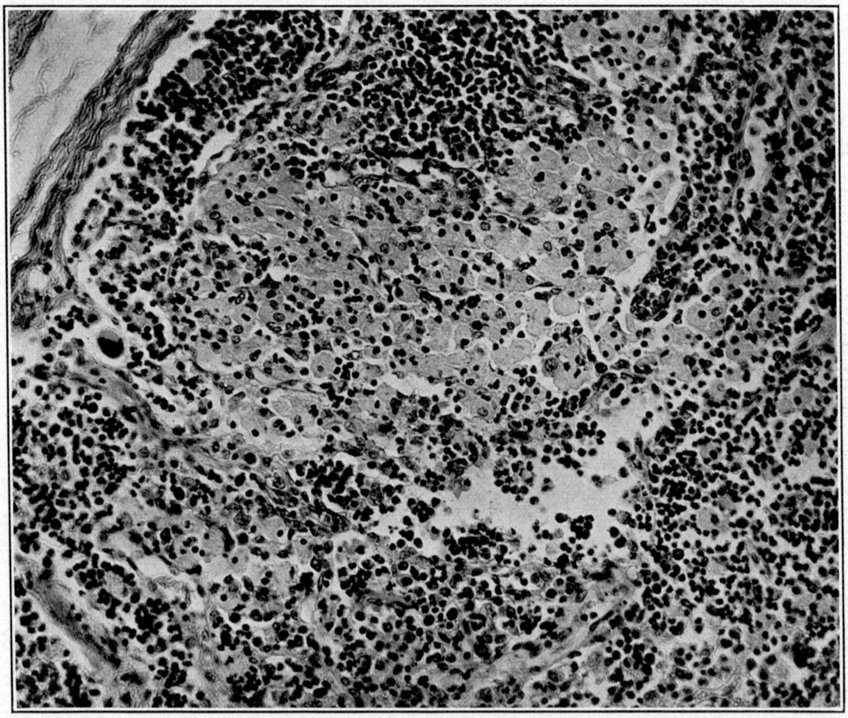

Fig. 4.—Case 3. Photomicrograph of retroperitoneal lymph gland which shows metaplasia: megakaryocyte (left), myelocytes (below), and foam cells (center), as well as normal lymphocytes (above), and gland capsule (left) (magnification ×300).

tissue increase. The histology varies with the stage of the disease, its rapidity of progress, and probably many other factors. The *lack of pigment* is conspicuous, and the spleen contains little iron in contrast to the liver and pancreas. *Chemical analyses* show less iron than normal (15 to 30 mg. per 100 gm. of fresh tissue). There is evidence of metaplasia and marrow activity in some areas of the spleen, with myelocytes, nucleated red cells, and megakaryocytes. Other parts may show accumulation of foam cells and great stroma increase. These foam cells at best give a faint pink color with fat stains. The malpighian corpuscles are approximately normal but may be small. The trabeculae may show hyaline changes and in such areas often show deposits of iron and calcium.

Lymphatic Tissue.—The lymph glands are usually much enlarged and may have a definite pink color or again a definite brown color like the liver. This includes cervical, bronchial, retroperitoneal, and mesenteric glands. *Pigment* is a conspicuous feature and is abundant in the gland sinuses as though coming into the gland from tissues outside of the gland. Much of it stains strongly for iron, but the larger pigment granules often do not stain for iron. Some may give a positive stain for hemo-

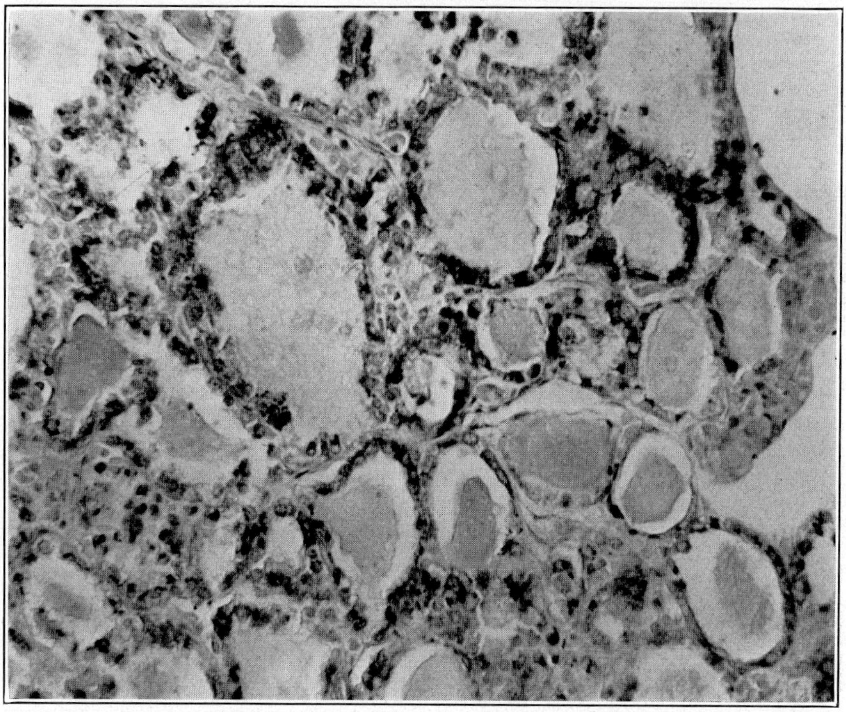

Fig. 5.—Case 5. Photomicrograph of thyroid. The alveolar epithelium is filled with black grains of iron-staining pigment (magnification ×365).

fuscin. Marrow metaplasia is seen in a few glands, and we may observe nests of myelocytes, nucleated red cells, and megakaryocytes. Foam cells are found in some lymph glands (Fig. 4). The germinal follicles are usually normal and appear active, but occasionally we observe a granule of iron-staining pigment in these cells. The solitary follicles and Peyer's patches of the intestine are usually normal. Only rarely is a cell noted containing a few granules of iron-staining pigment.

Thymus shows moderate regressive changes but no pigment deposits.

Blood Vessels.—Some of the moderate sized arterioles of the lungs, kidney, and mesentery may show accumulation of fine yellow granules of iron-free pigment in the smooth muscle layers. *Endothelium* may contain iron-staining and iron-free pigment in the capillaries of the spleen, testis, thyroid, liver, lymph glands, and striated muscle.

Ductless Glands.—Thyroid is always strongly pigmented and in gross presents a deep brown color. The acinar epithelium is rich in fine yellow pigment granules which give a strong test for iron (Fig. 5). No pigment is found in the colloid. The general structure appears normal, and the epithelium is well preserved. *Parathyroids* are usually normal but in some cases present a small amount of fine pigment granules

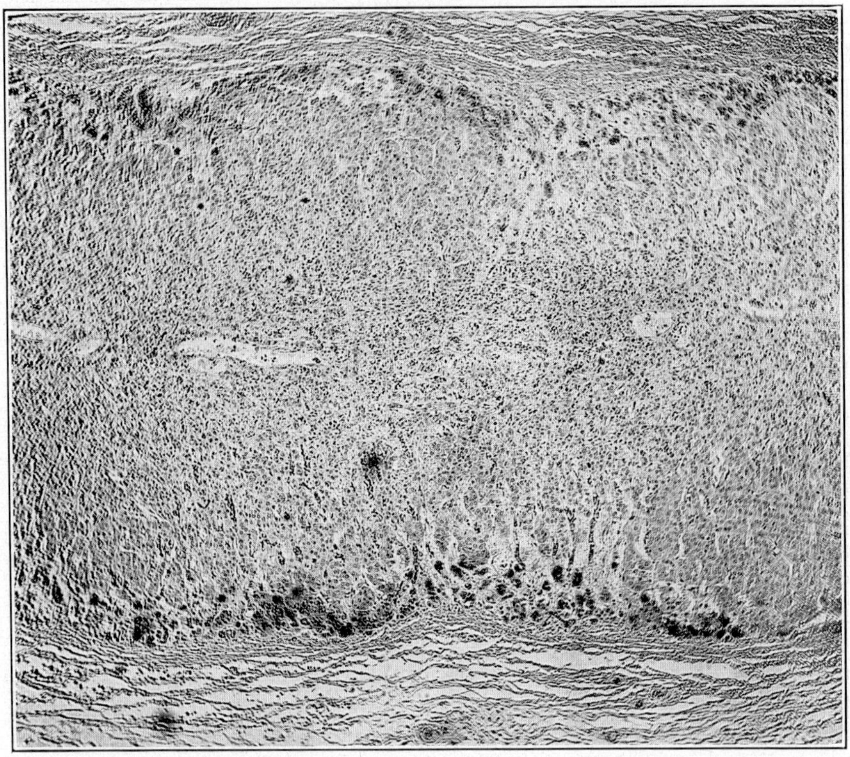

Fig. 6.—Case 5. Photomicrograph of adrenal cortex with iron-staining pigment as black granules in the glomerular zone only (magnification ×70).

which stain for iron in the cell protoplasm. *Adrenals* as a rule are smaller than normal and show a thin highly pigmented cortex. Iron-staining pigment is abundant in the glomerular zone (Fig. 6) and finely granular noniron-staining pigment is abundant in the reticular zone of the cortex. The medulla is normal.

Hypophysis may be somewhat pigmented and sometimes shows iron-staining pigment in the glandular portion. The general structure is normal. *Skin* is somewhat pigmented in gross, but in these races the skin is rather dark. There may be a little increase of yellow pigment in the basal cell layer of the skin, but we have never observed any iron-staining pigment in this area. *Muscles* show no abnormal pigmentation except the heart (Fig. 1). The striated skeletal muscles are rather paler than normal and show no evidence of pigment except rarely in the endothelium of capillaries a granule of iron-staining pigment.

Bones and Marrow.—The changes in the *bone* are of two types: an *atrophy* of the bone trabeculae and shafts of various bones and a *proliferation* of new bone of rather delicate structure in association with the characteristic thickening of the calvarium, which shows peculiar radial markings in the x-ray film. The ribs as a rule show this same proliferation which causes a fusiform thickening in the rib shaft usually close to the tubercle and not extending much beyond the axillary line.

Marrow changes have been described frequently and pictured by us[22] and others.[1] There is a great marrow hyperplasia as in primary anemia, and the parent stem cells of the marrow are very abundant. Nucleated red cells are numerous. Myelocytes of all types are numerous. Megakaryocytes are numerous and normal. Phagocytes are present in goodly numbers and many contain hemosiderin in small amounts. The foam cells may occur in small or large islands, and there may be in places some fibrosis of the marrow.

CASE 3.—(No. 19247.) J. S., an Italian boy, was born Oct. 29, 1928, and died Oct. 31, 1933. The clinical record in detailed chronologic order from birth until Oct. 6, 1931, was published in our first report.[22] Since it has been possible to study this case in detail throughout life, the remainder of the clinical course is described in similar manner below.

The sixth admission (Oct. 6 to Oct. 31, 1931) was when the boy was three years old.

October 6: The blood count was as follows: red cells, 2,600,000; white cells, 33,600; hemoglobin, 30 per cent. The differential count was as follows: polymorphonuclears, 37.5; eosinophiles, 0.5; lymphocytes, 59; mononuclears, 3. A smear showed marked anisocytosis, poikilocytosis, some basic stipling, a few Howell-Jolly bodies, and many nucleated red cells (258 per hundred white cells).

Roentgenograms of the skull and upper extremities suggested that the bone changes had increased since the last examination on June 24, 1930.

October 7: The blood uric acid was 4.0 mg. per 100 c.c.; the plant pigments, 0.088 mg. per 100 c.c.

October 8: The following measurements were found; circumference of head, 52.5 cm.; circumference of chest, 49.5 cm.; circumference of abdomen, 37.5 cm.

Stool examination was normal.

Urine examination was normal.

During this admission parathormone was given to note the effect upon the blood calcium. A basal metabolism test was done. The determined heat production was 10 per cent above the expected heat production for a three-year-old child.

October 9: The blood calcium was 10.4 mg. per 100 c.c.; the blood phosphorus was 4.4 mg. per 100 c.c.

One minim of parathormone was injected daily for three days, at the end of which time the calcium was 9.6 mg. The dosage was increased to 2 minims per day for three days. The calcium was then 10.8 mg. It was further increased to 3 minims daily for three days, and a final calcium value of 10.8 mg. was obtained.

Nov. 3, 1931 to March 23, 1932: The patient returned to the out-patient department ten times.

November 4: The weight was 13.2 kg. An acute respiratory infection was present. The blood examination revealed hemoglobin, 55 per cent; red blood cells, 2,900,000. Treatment: spleen extract was ordered to be given by mouth.

November 27: The body weight was then 12.4 kg. Blood examination revealed hemoglobin 45 per cent; red cells, 4,500,000. There was a severe cough without fever.

December 11: The cough was better. The body weight was 12.4 kg. Blood examination revealed hemoglobin, 40 per cent; red blood cells, 3,040,000.

January 8, 1932: The body weight was 12.6 kg. The general condition remained the same. Blood examination showed hemoglobin, 48 per cent; red blood cells, 2,680,000.

January 22: The blood pressure was systolic, 102; diastolic, 78. Examination of the blood showed the hemoglobin was 48 per cent. Since Oct. 21, 1931, the patient had been receiving secondary spleen extract. Today he was placed on a mixture of the secondary and of the pernicious anemia fraction of spleen, the dosage being 4 teaspoonfuls daily.

February 1: A recent head cold still existed.

February 26: Blood examination showed the hemoglobin to be 50 per cent; the red blood cells, 3,410,000.

March 11: The patient weighed 12.8 kg. The hemoglobin was 52 per cent; the red blood cells, 3,280,000.

Seventh admission was from March 23 to April 6. Blood examination showed hemoglobin, 55 per cent; red blood cells, 3,120,000; white blood cells, 48,000. The differential count showed; polymorphonuclears, 37; eosinophiles, 5; basophiles, 1; lymphocytes, 47; mononuclears, 7; degenerate cells, 8; nucleated red cells, 79 per hundred white cells.

The smear showed very marked changes in the size and shape of the red cells. Polychromatophilia, basophilia, stipling, and numerous shadow cells were found. The platelets were plentiful.

March 25: A sugar tolerance test was performed. Thirty grams of glucose were given by mouth. The following values were obtained:

Fasting:	78 mg. per 100 c.c.
½ hr.:	98 mg. per 100 c.c.
1½ hr.:	84 mg. per 100 c.c.
2½ hr.:	91 mg. per 100 c.c.
4½ hr.:	98 mg. per 100 c.c.

April 1: The plant pigments of the blood were 0.035 mg. per 100 c.c. The vitamin A content was found to be 13 units per 100 c.c.

April 4: A roentgenogram of the skull showed a definite increase of thickness, particularly in the posterior portion. Radial striations were more marked.

April 6: A sugar tolerance test was repeated. Thirty grams of glucose were given by mouth, with the following results:

Fasting:	71 mg. per 100 c.c.
½ hr.:	89 mg. per 100 c.c.
1 hr.:	91 mg. per 100 c.c.
2 hr.:	84 mg. per 100 c.c.
3 hr.:	75 mg. per 100 c.c.
4 hr.:	69 mg. per 100 c.c.

During this stay in the hospital, 10 c.c. of cortin were given daily by intramuscular injections for a period of ten days. No favorable effect upon the blood count was observed.

April 20 to June 7: Nine visits to the pediatric out-patient were made.

April 20: The weight was 13 kg.

The hemoglobin content of the blood was 52 per cent; the red blood cells, 3,500,000; the white blood cells, 35,000.

May 1: The urinary sediment examined according to the method of Rous[15] revealed no evidence of urinary siderosis such as occurs in hemochromatosis. Extralin (Lilly) (5.5 gm. = 200 gm. of liver digested with stomach) was started in doses of 2 teaspoonfuls daily.

May 18: The hemoglobin was 50 per cent.

Extralin (Lilly) (0.125 c.c. intramuscularly) was given. It was continued for several injections as follows:

May 21:	0.25 c.c.
May 24:	0.5 c.c.
May 28:	0.75 c.c.
May 31:	1.0 c.c.
June 4:	1.25 c.c.
June 7:	1.5 c.c.

Eighth Admission (June 12 to June 28): The patient was admitted because of swelling of both parotids with edema of face: diagnosis, mumps.

The blood examination revealed: hemoglobin, 5 gm.; red blood cells, 3,000,000; white blood cells, 7,400; polymorphonuclears, 37 per cent; lymphocytes, 52 per cent; mononuclears, 11 per cent; nucleated red blood cells, 7 per hundred white cells.

June 16: During convalescence a sugar tolerance curve was obtained after 25 c.c. of a 50 per cent solution of glucose were given intravenously (12.5 gm. or approximately 1 gm. of glucose per kilogram of body weight). The following values were obtained:

Fasting:	64 mg. per 100 c.c.
½ hr.:	187 mg. per 100 c.c.
1 hr.:	130 mg. per 100 c.c.
1½ hr.:	77 mg. per 100 c.c.
2 hr.:	48 mg. per 100 c.c.
3 hr.:	56 mg. per 100 c.c.

June 18: The blood serum proteins were 7.85 per cent by the refractometer method.

June 26: An x-ray examination of the skull revealed findings similar to those observed on April 4, 1932.

July 12 to December 13: Thirteen visits were made to the out-patient department.

July 12: The weight was 13.4 kg. He had been receiving fetal liver extract in dosages of 2 teaspoonfuls daily since June 28.

August 8: The blood counts were found to be hemoglobin, 46 per cent; red blood cells, 2,690,000; white blood cells, 16,000. There were 108 nucleated red cells per hundred white cells.

August 29: The plasma phosphotase was found to be 8.7 units.

September 19: A study of the blood by wet preparations for sickling failed to reveal such a tendency.

October 13: The patient fell and produced a fracture of the lower third of the left fibula. A plaster cast was applied.

October 18: The blood calcium was 10.8 mg. per 100 c.c.; the blood phosphorus, 3.8 mg. per 100 c.c.

Bone marrow extract (1 teaspoonful daily) was commenced. The blood hemoglobin was 38 per cent; the red blood cells, 3,660,000; the white blood cells, 42,250. The Schlesinger test on the urine revealed no evidence of urobilogen.

November 11: An x-ray of the left tibia revealed some new bone formations at the site of the recent fracture.

November 15: The hemoglobin value was 42 per cent; the red blood count, 3,000,000. Wet preparations of blood again revealed no evidence of sickling; marked fragmentation was now observed, however.

Ninth Admission (December 13 to December 16): The patient was brought in this time for special studies. The body measurements were length, 97 cm.; circumference of the head, 55.5 cm.; circumference of the chest, 51.0 cm.; circumference of the abdomen, 46.0 cm.

December 15: Blood volume studies were made by Dr. Alberto Hurtado. We are indebted to him for the following report:

Age, four and one-half years; body weight, 14 kg.
Red cells, 3,330,000
Reticulated red blood cells, 18.4 per cent
Hematocrit—red blood cell percentage, 25.0 per cent
Hematocrit—plasma percentage, 72.8 per cent
Mean corpuscular volume, 75 cubic microns
Mean corpuscular hemoglobin, 19.6 micromicrograms
Mean corpuscular hemoglobin concentration, 26.1 per cent
Total plasma volume, 767 c.c.
Total plasma volume per kilogram body weight, 54.8 c.c. (average, 50 cubic centimeters)
Total blood volume, 1,053 c.c.
Total blood volume per kilogram body weight, 75.2 c.c. (average, 72 c.c.)
Red blood cell volume, 263 c.c.
Red blood cell volume per kilogram body weight, 18.8 c.c. (average, 22 c.c.)
Hemoglobin per hundred cubic centimeters of blood, 6.53 gm.
Total circulating hemoglobin, 69 gm.
Total circulating hemoglobin per kilogram of body weight, 4.92 gm.
Blood viscosity, 4.0 (normal 4-4.5)

December 16: Determination of the blood lipids resulted in the following values:

Total lipids	586 mg. per 100 c.c.
Cholesterol	148 mg. per 100 c.c.
Fatty acids	438 mg. per 100 c.c.
Lecithin	179 mg. per 100 c.c.
Residual fat	245 mg. per 100 c.c.

December 17: The stool fat was 38 per cent of dry weight (normal, about 33 per cent).

January 17, 1933 to October 13, 1933: Nineteen visits to the out-patient department were made.

January 17: An acute upper respiratory infection existed. The hemoglobin was 41 per cent, the red blood cells, 2,630,000.

February 14: The weight was 13.8 kg. Bile (ox gall, Lilly), 5 grains twice daily, was now tried as a form of therapy. The blood showed hemoglobin, 42 per cent; red blood cells, 2,520,000; white blood cells, 64,000.

February 28: Blood examination revealed hemoglobin, 35 per cent; red blood cells, 2,450,000.

April 25: The hemoglobin was 38 per cent (6.6 gm.), and the red blood cells, 2,370,000.

Thymus extract, 2 grains three times daily (1 grain = 8 gm. fresh thymus), was started.

May 23: The hemoglobin was found to be 37 per cent (6 gm.), and the red blood cells numbered 3,700,000.

July 18: Swelling of the eyelids and enlarged cervical nodes were observed. The cardiac murmur had become more rough. The rate was rapid.

August 15: Ventriculin and dilute hydrochloric acid were prescribed.

September 5: The hemoglobin was now 37 per cent (5.7 gm.); red blood cells, 2,580,000. Lextron (Lilly), 1 teaspoonful three times daily, was started.

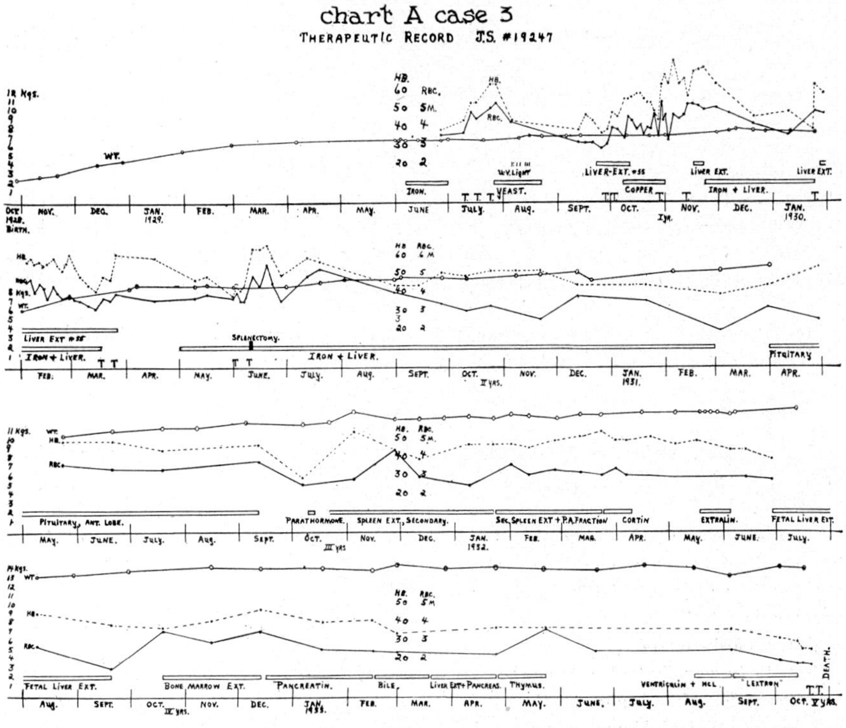

Chart A.—Case 3. Explanation of dosages. *Iron,* saccharated ferrous carbonate 0.3 gm. t.i.d.; *u-v. light,* ultraviolet rays, six treatments; *yeast,* one-half teaspoonful t.i.d.; *liver extract,* No. 55, one-half ampule daily (50 gm. liver); *copper,* 2 c.c. of 0.5 per cent solution of copper sulphate daily (0.02 gm.); *T,* blood transfusion, fifteen (total, 2020 c.c.); *iron and liver,* iron as above, liver daily in diet; *splenectomy; pituitary,* anterior lobe, 0.13 gm. t.i.d.; *parathormone,* 3 minims daily for nine days; *spleen extract,* secondary, one teaspoonful b.i.d.; *spleen extract, secondary with P. A. fraction,* four teaspoonfuls daily; *cortin* (adrenal cortex extract), 5 c.c. b.i.d. for 10 days; *extralin,* 0.125 to 1.5 c.c. daily, intramuscularly; *fetal liver extract,* two teaspoonfuls daily (150 gm. of fresh whole fetal liver); *bone marrow extract,* one teaspoonful b.i.d.; *pancreatin,* one teaspoonful daily; *bile,* 0.65 gm. daily; *liver extract* with *pancreas,* two teaspoonfuls daily; *thymus extract,* 2 grains t.i.d. (1 grain=8 gm. of fresh thymus); *ventriculin,* one teaspoonful b.i.d.; *lextron,* one teaspoonful t.i.d.

October 3: The heart was obviously enlarged. The hemoglobin was 32 per cent (4.8 gm.); red blood cells, 1,950,000; white blood cells, 30,600.

Tenth and Final Admission (Oct. 13, 1933 to Oct. 31, 1933): The patient was readmitted to the hospital because of progressive weakness, edema, and cardiac dilatation.

October 13: Blood examination showed: hemoglobin, 30 per cent (3.7 gm.); red blood cells, 1,840,000; white blood cells, 33,000. The body measurements were as follows: length, 97 cm.; circumference of head, 58 cm.; circumference of chest, 51.5 cm.; circumference of abdomen, 52 cm.

The blood typing, according to the Moss system, was found to be Group III.

October 14: The red cell volume was 14.3 per cent.

The total serum proteins were 7.29 per cent; albumin, 3.33 per cent; globulin, 3.38 per cent.

Blood lipid studies now revealed:

Total lipids	585 mg. per 100 c.c.
Phospholipid	85 mg. per 100 c.c.
Residual fat	404 mg. per 100 c.c.
Fatty acids	505 mg. per 100 c.c.

The electrocardiographic report was as follows: P-R interval, 0.15 sec.; QRS., 0.06 sec.; rate, 126; S-A tachycardia; right ventricular preponderance.

October 21: A blood culture remained sterile.

In the urine a trace of albumin and occasional casts were found.

It was evident that during this final admission the patient's condition was rapidly becoming worse.

October 29: Râles were heard throughout both lung bases, the heart dilated further, and death occurred on Oct. 31, 1933. There was some evidence of a gastrointestinal infection during the latter days of life. A stool culture at this time revealed a gram-negative bacillus belonging to the paratyphoid A group.

The clinical diagnosis was Mediterranean anemia, pericardial effusion, bronchopneumonia terminal.

AUTOPSY

J. S., white, male, aged five years, A-2414. The child died Oct. 31, 1933, at 5:30 A.M. Autopsy was performed by one of us (G. H. W.) the same day at 9:30 A.M.

Anatomic Diagnosis.—Anemia with hyperplasia of hemopoietic tissue. Abnormalities of the bony skeleton. *Pigmentation* of viscera, lymph glands, gastric mucosa, and ductless glands. Fatty degeneration of myocardium and liver. Slight bronchopneumonia. Subcutaneous edema. Hydropericardium. Laparotomy wound (splenectomy). *Thalassemia.*

The *body* was that of a somewhat emaciated Italian boy, five years old, measuring 100 cm. in length. Rigor mortis was well established. There was an old scar in the left half of the abdomen, running along the inner surface of the rectus for a distance of about 10 cm. and then laterally for a distance of about 8 cm. (splenectomy). The dorsa of the feet showed pitting edema. There was considerable edema of the face, particularly the eyelids and scalp. The eyes were completely closed by this edema. The head appeared very large. The *skin* seemed to show no abnormal pigmentation. Histologically the skin showed pigment in its basal cell layer, but its amount was not unusual, and it gave no stain for iron. The sweat glands contained no pigment. On incision, the subcutaneous fat was scant in amount and of a rather brownish yellow color. The striated muscles were decidedly pale and somewhat atrophic. The abdominal cavity contained no free fluid. There were old adhesions beneath the operative wound. The bladder contained a good deal of urine. The liver protruded several centimeters below the costal margin and was much enlarged. The spleen was absent. No accessory spleen was found. The thorax had a normal contour, and there was no evidence of beading or deformity due to rickets. The mediastinum showed very little fat. Both pleural cavities were free of fluid. The lungs were voluminous. The pericardial cavity contained a considerable amount of clear lemon yellow fluid, about 70 to 80 cc.; no bile pigment nor urobilin was present in this fluid. The pericardial surfaces were all smooth, and there was no apparent cause for this accumulation of fluid in this cavity whereas all the other cavities were free of fluid.

The *thymus* was atrophic although it extended over the parietal pericardium for a distance of 2 to 3 cm. The thymus had a definite yellowish brown pigmentation but was very thin. The lobes were clearly marked out. Histologically the thymus showed aplasia and no deposits of pigment.

Heart weighed 160 gm. It was of normal size. The epicardium was smooth and glistening. The epicardial fat was not abundant. All cavities of the heart contained tenacious, gelatinous clots, obviously rich in fibrin. The intima throughout all cavities was smooth and normal. The myocardium of the right ventricle was a little pale, but the myocardium of the left ventricle showed a typical mottling or tigering associated with anemia and fatty degeneration. Histologically the heart muscle fibers contained a good deal of yellow granular pigment resembling the usual lipochrome pigment and commonly situated at the poles of the nuclei. Some of this pigment gave a strong reaction for iron (Fig. 1). Fine fat droplets in muscle fibers were readily stained.

Lungs.—The left lung weighed 100 gm.; the right, 140 gm. Both lungs were voluminous and similar in every respect. The bronchi contained a little mucus. The bronchial lymph glands were enlarged and somewhat pigmented, but of a definite reddish tint as though hyperplastic. One or two of them measured at least 1 or 2 cm. in diameter. The pulmonary vessels were negative. Cut section in general was a pale pinkish gray color, and the tissue was air containing. A few dark, reddish pink areas gave the impression of recent consolidation. These areas occurred here and there, some in the upper and others in the lower lobes. Histologic sections showed acute bronchitis, edema and early bronchopneumonia.

Spleen was previously removed and described by us.[22] This spleen showed the cellular type of reaction (probably early stage) as contrasted with the other spleen reported in the same paper. Pigment was fairly abundant, and some of it gave a positive test for iron.

Gastrointestinal Tract.—The esophagus was pale. The fundus of the stomach showed an intact mucosa. It had a definite golden brown tint, the mucosa being obviously pigmented and the smooth muscle very pale. The mucosa close to the pylorus was pale and smooth, unpigmented. The pylorus was normal. The duodenum appeared normal and unpigmented as was the small intestine. Peyer's patches in the ileum were somewhat enlarged but did not measure over 1 to 2 mm. in thickness. They might have been slightly pigmented, but they did not have the reddish color of the mesenteric lymph glands and appeared to differ sharply from the body lymph gland tissue in this respect. The appendix was normal. The large bowel showed a pale, nonpigmented mucosa and easily seen but not enlarged solitary follicles. The rectum was normal. Histologically the stomach showed a normal structure but for pigment granules in the epithelium of the acini deep in the mucosa (see earlier paper[22] for illustration, *Fig. 3*). This pigment gave a strong test for iron and was found in the chief cells not in the acid cells. This pigment was not found in the mucosa of the duodenum. Brunner's glands showed a little pigment which gave a faint stain for iron. The mucosa of the jejunum and ileum was normal and pigment-free, but Peyer's patches showed small amounts of yellow granular pigment. Some of this might stain for iron. Appendix showed a slight inflammatory reaction. Colon showed normal mucosa and solitary follicles with no pigment.

Pancreas was a little enlarged and rather firm. The lobulation was regular. It had the color of maple sugar, a deep buff color as noted in the other cases. Histologic sections showed much pigment in the pancreatic acinar cells particularly adjacent to islets but not in the islet epithelium. This pigment all gave a strong blue reaction to the iron stain. Many acini were free from iron deposits, and some contained fine granules only, but many contained large coarse pigment granules, and some epithelium appeared to be degenerating because of large pigment deposits. There was no increase in stroma (see characteristic illustrations in our first paper,[22] *Figs. 4 and 5*).

Liver weighed 810 gm. It was definitely enlarged. The capsule was transparent, and through it could be seen the deep reddish brown parenchyma. This appearance was identical with the other cases of this type and indicated considerable pigment deposit. The consistency of the liver was normal. Lobulation was regular. There was some central yellowish tinting of the dark brownish color of the lobules. The *gallbladder* contained rather thin, brownish bile. The mucosa of the gallbladder had a pale brown tint after washing. The biliary passages were pale and normal elsewhere. There was bile present in the duodenum. *Chemical analysis* of the liver parenchyma showed 292 mg. Fe per 100 gm. fresh tissue. Histologic sections showed heavy pigment deposits in the hepatic epithelium particularly in the marginal half of each lobule. This pigment in the marginal half of the lobule gave a positive iron stain, but in the central half the pigment did not stain strongly for iron. The granular pigment was conspicuous in the Kupffer cells and did not stain for iron. The central half of the lobules showed large fat droplets in the liver cells and occasional focal necroses. There were no marrow cells seen in the lobules, but about the bile ducts were occasional nests of mononuclear cells. The *gallbladder* showed pigment granules in the epithelium and also in the submucosa especially at the crests of the folds. This pigment was negative by iron stains.

Kidneys.—The left kidney weighed 120 gm.; the right 120 gm. They were perhaps somewhat enlarged. The capsules stripped off easily, leaving a pale brown surface. On section the cortex measured 6 mm. in thickness. The striations were perfectly regular. Cut section seemed to have a definite pale brown pigmentation throughout. The glomeruli were hard to see. The pyramids were very pale. The pelves were normal. Chemical analysis of the kidney parenchyma showed 3.9 mg. Fe per 100 gm. fresh tissue, which is a low normal content. Histologic sections showed normal glomeruli and stroma. Many of the convoluted tubules showed epithelium which contained fine or coarse pigment granules which did not stain for iron. Occasionally one found a tubule which contained in its epithelium fine pigment granules giving a positive stain for iron (Fig. 2). The patchy distribution of this pigment was difficult to understand, but it explained the brown color of the renal cortex noted in gross. Casts were present in a few tubules.

Pelvic Organs.—The prostate was small and pale and appeared to be normal grossly. Histologically there was no pigment. The bladder mucosa was pale and nonpigmented. The epididymes were pale and white. *Testes* were definitely pigmented and showed a dark brown color. Histologically the *testis* showed much coarsely granular yellow brown pigment in the interstitial tissue. This pigment did not stain for iron nor hemofuscin. The immature tubules showed no pigment, nor did the endothelium of the blood vessels and capillaries.

Ductless Glands.—The *adrenals* were perhaps a little smaller than normal. They were normal in outline and measured 3.5 × 2 × .75 cm. On section the outer part of the cortex was thin, yellow, and opaque in contrast to the thicker inner brown portion. The medulla, where it appeared, was a pale milky color. The cortex seemed to have a definite brown pigmentation. Histologic sections showed small amounts of an iron-containing pigment in the cells of the glomerular zone of the cortex (compare Fig. 6 from another case). There was much pigment that did not stain for iron. Fat stains showed abundant fat droplets in the cortical cells. The structures in general were normal.

The *thyroid* appeared to be of normal size. It was removed after injection of formalin. It had the usual reddish brown color, but the brown was a little more conspicuous than in the normal thyroid. Lobulation was normal. The *parathyroids* were difficult to find. Histologic sections showed large amounts of iron-staining pigment in the majority of the acinar epithelial cells in the thyroid. No pigment appeared in the colloid (see Fig. 5). There was no fibrosis. Parathyroids (two) appeared to be normal and showed no pigment.

The *hypophysis* was definitely small and the sella turcica shallow. The stalk was well marked. It was pale. Histologic sections showed no pigment and a normal structure.

Vascular system was perfectly smooth and elastic throughout all large vessels. Tenacious clots could be pulled from a great many of the veins, even from the coronary veins. *Striated skeletal muscles* were normal and contained no pigment.

Lymphatic System.—The absence of the spleen might account in part for the enlargement of the lymph glands, which was a conspicuous feature in the autopsy. The lymph glands in the mediastinum and about the bronchi had an appearance much like that of the spleen. Enlarged lymph glands in the neck and retroperitoneal region might have this reddish tint but again might have a conspicuous reddish brown color. Some of the larger ones measured from 1 to 1.5 cm. in long diameter. They appeared to be rather moist and somewhat congested, although it was more the appearance of blood in the sinuses than of congestion of the capillaries of the gland. The lymph glands about the pancreas were conspicuously enlarged; some of them were brown in color, while others had a slight greenish brown cast, perhaps this pigment being added from the liver and pancreas. The lymph glands in the fan of the mesentery and along the large bowel were conspicuously enlarged. Most of these were of a distinct reddish color or had a reddish brown staining against the pale watery fat. Histologic sections showed much uniformity. The architecture was well preserved, and there was no chronic inflammation and fibrosis. The germinal follicles were large, active looking and nonpigmented. The sinusoids were filled with fluid and wandering cells. Red blood cells were numerous in many sections. *Pigment* was conspicuous, and much of it gave a positive iron stain. Some of the large pigment grains were a bright yellow and might give a positive stain for hemofuscin, but much of the pigment gave no reaction to any specific stains. Marrow metaplasia was noted occasionally, and some sections showed large nests of myelocytes, nucleated red cells and megakaryocytes. Occasional nests of foam cells, as described in spleen and marrow, were found (Fig. 4).

Skeletal System.—The skull cap was greatly thickened, and, when the scalp was turned back, it presented a definite mulberry color as though bone marrow was just beneath the periosteum. The *calvarium* was enormously thickened, the thickness ranging from a fraction of a centimeter up to 2 cm. In places the radial markings due to bone spicules and showing in the x-ray stood out clearly. The bone marrow between these trabeculae had a definite chocolate red color. This change seemed to involve all parts of the calvarium, tapering off to the thin temporal bones. In spite of the fact that this bone looked rather soft and porous, it contained a good deal of structural bone and could not be cut with the knife. The base of the skull appeared to be normal. All of the venous sinuses were clear and contained tenacious postmortem clots. The *ribs* were enlarged in places, as described in other cases, but this fusiform enlargement did not involve the portions of the ribs close to the costochondral junctions but the part of the rib close to the tubercle. This has been described in other clinics. This was particularly true in the upper six or eight ribs. The lower three ribs showed involvement of the inner two-thirds. It appeared that the bone marrow filled all the spaces and really replaced most of the outer bony shell, filling up all spaces right up to the periosteum. In spite of this, the rib cut with some difficulty although it had not the toughness of normal rib.

The rib marrow had the same chocolate, dark red color as noted in the calvarium. *Chemical analysis* of the rib showed 33.5 mg. Fe per 100 gm. fresh weight, which is within normal limits. The bones of the *vertebrae* showed the same colored bone marrow, and the trabeculae were inconspicuous; the bones cut with only moderate difficulty, indicating definite thinning of the trabeculae. The shaft of the femur in its middle third was greatly thinned, measuring 1 mm. in thickness. All of the space inside of this shell was filled with dark cellular, chocolate, red bone marrow, but there was no deposit of this marrow between the periosteum and the shaft. Histologically the bony trabeculae were thinned, but there was no apparent overactivity of the osteoclasts. In the ribs the red marrow was found between the shaft and the periosteum, and in the calvarium the marrow actually invaded crevices in the periosteum. The *red marrow* presented a considerable variety in ribs, vertebrae, long bones, and calvarium. The marrow was very cellular, and few fat cells remained anywhere. Nests of parent marrow cells were conspicuous as were nucleated red cells and myelocytes. Phagocytes were found in moderate numbers, and some contained iron staining pigment. Megakaryocytes appeared in goodly numbers. Some parts of the marrow showed some fibrosis, and there were islands of foam cells, which might attain a considerable size. These groups of foam cells were usually in the marginal portion of the bone and close to trabeculae. This change was illustrated in our first paper,[22] *Fig. 7.*

Brain weighed 1280 gm. The dura was not thickened nor pigmented but was somewhat adherent to the calvarium. The pia arachnoid over the brain was delicate, and the brain appeared quite pale and normal in all respects. On section the brain was normal, and the choroid plexus was not pigmented.

CASE 4.—Auburn City Hospital (Dr. C. H. Maxwell), No. 9272.

History.—M. D., an Italian boy, five years and ten months old, developed an acute upper respiratory infection on Jan. 17, 1932. When examined, he was found to be extremely ill. The temperature was 104° F. The respirations were rapid. The pulse was rapid and weak. He was markedly anemic. The skin was of dull yellowish tint. The head revealed some bossing, but only suggestive mongoloid features were observed.

The heart was somewhat enlarged. A loud blowing systolic murmur was audible over the entire precordium. Many crepitant râles were heard over the lung bases. The percussion note was unimpaired. The abdomen was distended and ascites was present. The spleen reached the crest of the ilium. The liver was palpated four fingerbreadths below the costal margin. The legs were edematous. He grew rapidly worse and expired on the fourth day of illness.

The past history revealed that birth had been of a normal spontaneous type. The birth weight was 4 pounds. He was one of twins, the other child weighing 5 pounds at birth. He was breast fed for two months, then was given a formula for eighteen months. Development was slow. He walked and said simple words at eighteen months. The first tooth erupted at fourteen months. He gained weight slowly and took food poorly.

The liver and the spleen were found to be enlarged while he was still a small infant. He had been in the Auburn City Hospital on three different occasions for the treatment of anemia, poor appetite, mild respiratory infections, mumps, nosebleeds, and other minor conditions. During one of these admissions (Jan. 21, 1931) it was noted that the facial expression was sad and pale. Edema of eye lids existed. The teeth were good. The tongue was coated. The tonsils were slightly enlarged. The head circumference at this time was 47 cm.; the chest, 56 cm. The lungs were normal. The heart was enlarged with the apex in the seventh intercostal space. A loud systolic murmur was heard. The abdomen was large and protuberant with prominent superficial veins. The spleen was very large and hard.

The father and mother and ten other siblings constituted the family. A twin brother and a two-year-old brother suffered from the same type of anemia. There was no evidence of other types of familial illness within the family.

The observations on the blood are reported in Table I.

TABLE I

DATE	HEMOGLOBIN (%)	RED CELLS	WHITE CELLS	POLYMORPHONUCLEARS (%)	LYMPHOCYTES (%)	MONONUCLEARS (%)	NUCLEATED RED CELLS PER HUNDRED WHITE CELLS
1/27/31	33	2,680	57,300	51	37	6	115
3/25/31	46	2,480	44,600	55	41	3	130
4/ 2/31	40	3,700	10,300	40	49	7	20
7/24/31	35	2,690	14,150	51	44	5	43

The stained smears revealed marked variations in the size and shape of the red blood cells. The platelets appeared plentiful.

The icteric index was 9 units. Fragility of the erythrocytes to hypotonic salt solution showed hemolysis to begin at the concentration of 0.30 per cent and was complete at 0.20 per cent. The urine was dark in color and showed a trace of albumin.

AUTOPSY

M. D., Italian, male, aged five years, A-1728. The child died Jan. 20, 1932, at 10:00 P.M. Autopsy was performed by one of us (G.H.W.) Jan. 21, 1932, at 10:00 A.M.

Anatomic Diagnosis.—Anemia, with hyperplasia of hemopoietic tissue. *Pigmentation* of viscera, ductless glands and lymph of glands. Abnormalities of bony skeleton. Enlarged liver and spleen. Infarcts of spleen. Hypoplasia of adrenals. Organizing bronchopneumonia and edema of lungs. Fatty degeneration of liver and myocardium. *Thalassemia.*

The body was that of an Italian boy, 42 inches tall. Rigor mortis was slight. Livor mortis was absent. The skin had a peculiar pigmentation, somewhat the color of a Chinese. The face had a definite mongolian cast, and the frontal bosses were slightly conspicuous. The hair was black and curly, the eyes, brown. The pupils were equal. The thorax was symmetrical; the abdomen, greatly distended. No hemorrhages were observed over the skin. The subcutaneous fat was scant and pale yellow in color. The striated muscles over the thorax and abdomen were decidedly pale and watery appearing. There was some subcutaneous edema over the lower legs. The peritoneal cavity contained a great excess (probably about 1000 c.c.) of clear, lemon yellow fluid. The surfaces were everywhere smooth and moist. No hemorrhages were noted. The omentum showed very little fat. It was normally disposed. The liver extended well below the costal margin. The lymph glands were everywhere conspicuous. The bladder was full of clear urine. Both pleural cavities were clear. The lungs were voluminous. The pericardial cavity contained a considerable excess of lemon yellow fluid. The pericardial surfaces were smooth.

The *thymus* showed two lobes, coming down to the base of the heart, measuring 2 and 4 cm. in length by 1.5 to 2 cm. across, and about 0.5 cm. in thickness. The tissue was normal histologically, and no pigment was noted.

Heart weighed 71 gm. It was about normal size for a child of this age. The epicardial surfaces were normal. The epicardial fat was scant. The endocardium and valves throughout were normal. The right ventricle contained well-formed antemortem clots. The chambers were dilated. The myocardium was pale reddish brown in color with perhaps more brown pigmentation than normal. There was no mottling with fat, but the muscle was distinctly pale. Histologically the heart sections showed edema. There was much pigment in the heart cells at the poles of the nuclei. This pigment was in fine grains and much, but not all, of it gave a strong test for iron (Fig. 1).

Lungs.—The left weighed 170 gm.; the right, 226 gm. They presented an identical picture. The glands at the hilum were conspicuous, and most of them were moist and pink, but some contained coal pigment. The bronchi contained a smooth velvety mucosa and were filled with frothy serum. The vessels were normal. On section, the lung tissue was very wet and dripped fluid. In places the lung tissue looked glassy and semitranslucent because of this fluid. Other areas were pale and normal. Posteriorly in the lower lobe was a definite area of bronchopneumonia, measuring 3 or 4 cm. in its greatest diameter. Here the lung tissue was gray, granular, and moist. Histologic sections showed the usual picture of a bronchopneumonia but with early organization in some areas. There was much edema but no abnormal pigment.

Spleen weighed 420 gm. It was enormously enlarged, measuring about 15 cm. in its long axis. There were adhesions over its anterior surface. The capsule in general was transparent, but there were irregular areas of opacity showing beneath the capsule, some of which lay beneath the adhesions mentioned. These *infarcts* presented a very irregular border, separating the opaque tissue from the normal splenic pulp. Some of these borders showed a greenish translucency, suggestive of many wandering cells. The larger infarcts measured 2 cm. in their long dimension. Some of these infarcts were indefinite as to outline, merging into the splenic pulp. These were less opaque than the others described. They made up perhaps one-seventh of the total bulk of the spleen. Section elsewhere showed a uniform fibrous spleen, presenting a glassy cut surface. The organ was very rubbery. There was no exceptional pigmentation. The cut section was a dull pinkish red. The connective tissue was obviously much increased and the malpighian bodies were obscured. Trabeculae were inconspicuous, because of the diffuse connective tissue increase. *Chemical analysis* showed 16 mg. iron per 100 gm. fresh weight which was less than normal or a low normal amount. Histologic sections of this spleen, in contrast to that in Case 3, showed a much more chronic process. There was much more fibrosis of the pulp, and the various pulp cells were obscured. Pigment in moderate amounts was seen in phagocytes and endothelial cells of the sinusoids. Some of this pigment gave an iron stain. The trabeculae might show occasional deposits of iron and calcium. Malpighian corpuscles were small and hard to find. There was little marrow metaplasia. The infarcts presented the usual picture.

Gastrointestinal Tract.—The esophagus was normal. The *stomach* contained partially digested food and was coated with mucus. Its mucosa had a definite brownish tint which was most marked in the cardia and faded close to the pylorus to a very pale brown. No hemorrhages were noted. The pylorus was normal. The *duodenum* showed only a very faint tint of brown. The jejunum shows a nonpigmented mucosa. The solitary follicles were easily seen and measured about 1 mm. in diameter. In the ileum the solitary follicles were conspicuous, some of them measuring about 2 mm. in diameter. Peyer's patches were rather conspicuous, and the follicles were easily made out. The appendix showed some postmortem slaty staining. The large bowel showed scattered solitary follicles, 1 to 2 mm. in diameter. No pigmentation was noted. There were no ulcers. Histologic sections showed abundant iron-staining pigment in the acinar cells of the gastric mucosa. The chief cells contained most of this pigment, but the acid cells did contain some fine pigment granules. The muscle coats contained no pigment. Duodenum contained no pigment in its mucosa but *Brunner's glands* contained liberal amounts of fine granular yellow pigment which stained for iron. Jejunum, ileum, and colon showed no pigment in mucosa or muscle coats. Peyer's patches and solitary lymph follicles showed an occasional granule of iron-staining pigment contained in a phagocyte. This was a replica of Case 3.

Liver weighed 1175 gm. It was enlarged. It was very deeply pigmented, having a dark buff color. The capsule was smooth, and through it the lobules could readily be seen. The consistency was normal. The architecture was regular. The lobules showed a peripheral translucent brown zone and a central opaque yellow spot which was undoubtedly fat. There was no increase in the periportal tissue. The pigmentation of the organ was as definite as is observed in hemochromatosis. *Chemical analysis* showed 114 mg. iron and 22 mg. copper per 100 gm. of fresh tissue. The *gall bladder* contained a little yellow bile and showed postmortem staining. The mucosa was perfectly smooth and normal. Histologic sections showed abundant large fat droplets in the center of the *liver* lobules. These central liver cells contained little pigment, and much of it did not stain for iron. Kupffer cells contained relatively little pigment, and most of this did not give an iron stain. The marginal liver cells close to the portal tissues contained heavy deposits of a yellow pigment containing iron. There were occasional nests of marrow cells in the capillary spaces in the liver lobules—an evident marrow metaplasia of moderate grade. Perhaps this change might compensate somewhat for the lack of marrow metaplasia in the fibrous spleen in this case. *Gallbladder* mucosa showed no pigment.

Pancreas was about normal in size and quite firm in consistency but very deeply bronzed—as dark as the liver—a dark maple sugar color. The lobules were distinct. The stroma was slightly edematous. Histologic sections showed a pancreas which was a replica of that gland in Case 3 and need not be described.

Kidneys.—Each weighed 100 gm. They were slightly enlarged. The capsule stripped readily leaving a very pale surface which had a faint brownish yellow color. On section the cortex was about 5 mm. in thickness. The striations were well preserved. The contrast between the brown cortex and the pinkish gray pyramids was conspicuous. The pelves and ureters were normal. Histologic sections showed normal structures. There were abundant fat droplets in the epithelium of the convoluted tubules. Pigment deposits were infrequent but picked out occasional tubules where they might be conspicuous. Henle's tubules were often involved. Some of this pigment stained for iron (Fig. 2).

Pelvic Organs.—The bladder was normal. No pigmentation was noted. The *prostate* was very small. Histologically it was normal, and no pigment was found. The *testes* were infantile in type. On section they presented a pale brownish color. Histologic sections showed the usual peculiar distribution of pigment. The immature tubules in the testis showed no pigment, but the interstitial tissue showed some yellow coarse pigment which contained no iron. In the endothelium of the capillaries were a few fine pigment grains which stained for iron. Epididymis was normal. The striated voluntary *muscle* was pale and moist in gross. Histologically the muscle fibers were normal. A few capillaries were found in which endothelial cells contained fine granules of iron-staining pigment. The blood vessels appeared perfectly normal. There was no pigment noted in the walls of arterioles in various organs and tissues.

Adrenals were distinctly smaller than normal and hypoplastic. The right measured 10 to 15 by 3 mm. The medulla was conspicuous. The cortex was very thin, measuring less than 1 mm. in thickness and showed a slight amount of brown pigment. The other adrenal presented about the same appearance. Histologically this adrenal was a replica of that in Case 3 (Fig. 6).

The *thyroid* was small. On section it showed a dark brown color. Colloid was obviously present. There was no question about the increase in the brown pigmentation. Histologic sections showed a very large amount of iron-staining pigment

(Fig. 5). Practically every epithelial cell in every acinus contained these fine pigment granules which were located in the colloid side of each cell but not in the colloid. The thyroid was very cellular and poor in colloid which stained faintly. There was no increase in stroma.

The *hypophysis* was normal in gross and showed some brown pigmentation. Histologically the structures of the hypophysis were normal. A few grains of pigment were seen in the protoplasm of the acidophile cells, and some of this stained sharply for iron.

Lymphatic System.—The lymph glands about the pancreas were large, a dull pink in color, and moist. Some of them contained a good deal of brown pigment, and others looked much like the spleen. The larger ones measured 1 cm. in diameter, and a great many smaller ones 2 to 4 to 6 mm. in diameter found close to the spleen, about the duodenum, and in the gastrohepatic omentum. The mesenteric glands were all conspicuous. They were a very faint pinkish gray color with a slight brownish tint and were moist and swollen. Some measured over 1 cm. in diameter. Conspicuous lymph glands were noticed in the thorax. Some of them appeared pink and moist; others appeared to contain brown pigment, and still others, a mixture of brown pigment and a little coal pigment. The retroperitoneal glands had the same general appearance but contained more of the brown pigment. Histologically these various lymph glands presented the same findings as described in Case 3. Metaplasia was conspicuous in some sections, and true bone marrow activity was seen. Foam cells appeared rarely but were often noted in association with the marrow cells (see Fig. 4). Phagocytes were frequent and some contained many red cells as well as pigment. The lymph glands appeared to be as active as the spleen in this case.

Bone Marrow.—The ribs did not show any unusual thickenings. On section, the bone marrow had a definite rusty red color. It was uniform. The bodies of the lumbar vertebrae showed a dark brownish red marrow thoughout. These bones contained delicate bony trabeculae. The shaft of the *femur* appeared to be definitely thin and was quite easily cut and split. The bone marrow was dark brownish red in color and cellular throughout. Histologic sections showed that this *marrow* was exactly like that described in Case 3, and by other observers. Phagocytes containing iron-staining pigment and even red cells were found occasionally but were not conspicuous. Foam cells were observed in small clusters but were less conspicuous than usual. The marrow hyperplasia was observed between the rib shaft and periosteum.

Brain weighed 1200 gm. Section through the calvarium showed it to be thin and normal except over the frontal region where the outer and inner tables were separated for a distance of about 8 or 9 mm. There was present characteristic bony hyperplasia in this region. A similar change was seen over the occipital region but was less conspicuous. The meninges were all clear, moist and normal. The brain appeared normal on section. The pineal gland appeared to be normal. The *choroid plexuses* showed a definite rusty brown pigmentation. The choroid histologically contained a good deal of coarsely granular yellow pigment staining negatively for iron within phagocytes in the areolar tissue below the epithelium of the plexus. A little of the same sort of pigment was noted in the epithelium. No hemosiderin was found.

CASE 5.—No. 22501 (Dr. J. M. Parker).

History.—John S., an Italian boy two and one-half years old, was admitted to the Strong Memorial Hospital on June 8, 1930.

At one year of age the patient developed an acute upper respiratory infection with fever. A mass, which the physician identified as an enlarged spleen, was noticed at this time by the mother. Pallor, weakness, and failure to gain weight developed soon and led to his admission to the hospital.

The birth, which was normal, followed a full-term pregnancy. The weight was 9½ pounds. He was breast fed for nine months and was then placed upon the usual infant diet. Cod liver oil was not given until he was two years old, and orange juice was given irregularly during infancy.

Dentition, speech, and muscular development were normal.

Frequent head colds, pneumonia at six months, and measles at two years had occurred.

The father, forty-two years old, the mother, thirty-six years old, and a brother, six years old, were normal.

Physical Findings.—Essential features were the prominent bosses of the head and facies suggestive of the mongoloid type. Pallor and puffiness of the eyelids and cheeks were present. The tonsils and cervical lymph nodes were enlarged. The heart was slightly enlarged and revealed a soft systolic murmur. The abdomen was prominent and contained a markedly enlarged, hard spleen which extended to the iliac crest. The liver border was palpated from three to four fingerbreadths below the costal margin.

Laboratory Findings.—Blood examination showed hemoglobin, 48 per cent; red blood cells, 2,960,000; white blood cells, 19,840. Only a few nucleated red cells were present, but the morphology of the cells was identical with that usually seen in Mediterranean anemia. The blood calcium was 8.5 mg. per 100 c.c.; phosphorus, 5.3 mg. per 100 c.c.; plasma protein, 8.7 per cent; serum chlorides, 485 mg.; non-protein nitrogen, 96.3 mg. The blood lipids showed: plasma, total lipids, 550 mg. per cent; cholesterol, 112; fatty acids, 438.

The urine contained 18 to 25 red blood cells per high powered field, and a few hyaline and granular casts.

The clinical impression was Mediterranean anemia, and it was suggested that the hematuria was the result of acute nephritis.

Course.—After an intravenous blood transfusion, the patient returned to the private care of Dr. J. M. Parker, to whom we are indebted for the opportunity to study the case in detail.

During the period from April, 1933, to July 4, 1934, when death occurred at the age of seven and one-half years, the patient was admitted upon three occasions to the Rochester General Hospital, where further observations were made and several blood transfusions were given.

Edema with pericardial and peritoneal effusions developed during the latter months of life. The weight increased from 55.5 pounds to 68 pounds during the last month.

Representative blood counts were:

April 27, 1933 (First admission): hemoglobin, 37 per cent; red blood cells, 1,580,000; white blood cells, 8550; neutrophiles, 14; mononuclears, 62; many nucleated red blood cells.

May 27, 1933 (one week before death): red blood cells, 3,580,000; white blood cells, 6,450; neutrophiles, 51 (juvenile forms, 5; stabs, 11; segmented forms, 35); mononuclears, 49; nucleated red blood cells, 31 per 100 white cells.

Hemolysis to hypotonic salt solutions began at the concentration of 0.42 per cent and was complete at 0.28 per cent (normal control, 0.42 to 0.32 per cent).

The x-ray studies of the long bones revealed thinning of the cortex and coarse trabeculation near the diaphyseal end. The bones of the vault showed marked porosity with thinning of both tables and with new bone laid down at right angles to the outer table.

AUTOPSY

John S., aged seven years, Italian parents; No. 89659. Autopsy was performed at the Rochester General Hospital by Dr. Istvan Gaspar. We are indebted to Dr. Gaspar for materials and permission to report this case.

Anatomical Diagnosis.—*Anemia* with hyperplasia of hemopoietic tissues. Splenomegaly. *Pigmentation* of viscera, ductless glands and lymph glands. Abnormalities of bony skeleton. Hypoplasia of adrenal glands. Fatty degeneration of heart and liver. Bronchopneumonia. General anasarca. *Thalassemia.*

The *body* was that of a young white boy showing excessive generalized anasarca. His eyelids, cheeks, lips, and neck were markedly edematous. Gums were anemic. Post mortem lividity was evidenced in the region of the neck and pelvis. About the face and the neck some petechial hemorrhages were noted, some of which were confluent. Scrotum and dependent portions were very edematous. The skin was of a yellowish icteric hue. *Abdomen* was distended and dome shaped. On incision a yellowish turbid fluid gushed out. No indication of peritonitis was seen. Approximately 4000 c.c. of this fluid was present. The pleural cavities were filled with fluid, yellowish in color and turbid in character. The right pleural cavity contained 200 c.c., the left contained 500 c.c. No adhesions of the pleura were noted. The pericardial sac was dilated and contained from 400 to 450 c.c. of transparent fluid. No inflammation of pericardium was seen.

Heart was hypertrophied, weighing 270 gm. Right ventricle was from 8 to 9 mm. thick, left ventricle, 11 mm. Myocardium was pale in color. Valvular constituents were normal. Histologic sections showed normal muscle fibers with little pigment at the poles of the nuclei. Only rarely did one see a pigment granule which stained for iron.

Lungs.—The right and left were of essentially the same character. Grossly no evidence of inflammation was seen. The left lung weighed 175 gm., the right lung, 240 gm. Histologically there were small areas of bronchopneumonia, some of which were of the interstitial type. Some phagocytes in the alveoli contained pigment which stained for iron. Occasional mucous glands in the mucosa of large bronchi contained pigment, some of which was hemosiderin. This pigment in the epithelium of the glands was largely in the central half of the acini close to the lumen. The blood vessels showed no pigment in the muscle coats.

Spleen was tremendously enlarged and weighed 800 gm. Externally it was of a bluish green color. The cut section was a dark red. Histologic sections gave a picture midway between the very cellular spleen (Case 3) and the chronic fibrous spleen (Case 4). There was considerable increase in interstitial stroma, and the sinusoids stood out conspicuously. The trabeculae were conspicuous, and occasionally one found deposits of hemosiderin in the crevices of the trabeculae. Hemosiderin was not readily found but was present in occasional phagocytes and rarely in endothelial cells of the sinusoids. Other yellow pigment giving negative stains for iron was found in occasional cells. The *marrow* cells were well represented, and one found many small nests of parent stem cells, abundant myelocytes, and nucleated red cells. Megakaryocytes were rare. Malpighian bodies were very small and inconspicuous. *Chemical analyses* showed 30 mg. iron per 100 gm. of fresh tissue, not far from a normal value, for the spleen.

Lymph Nodes.—The peribronchial, peritracheal, mesenteric, and mediastinal nodes were much enlarged and dark brown in color. Histologic sections showed increase in stroma in these lymph glands. Edema was conspicuous and the sinuses often contained red cells as well as wandering cells. Hemosiderin and iron-free pigment were present in many glands usually in phagocytes. Marrow cells were found in some glands but not in all. The lymph germinal follicles appeared active and normal.

Liver was markedly enlarged and of a peculiar brownish hue, and it weighed 2550 gm. The *gallbladder* contained a yellow brown colored bile which stained the mucosa brown. The bile ducts were normal. *Chemical analyses* showed a very high content of iron—395 mg. per 100 gm. of fresh tissue. Histologic sections showed an unusually heavy deposit of hemosiderin in the liver cells in the margin of the lobules. Some liver cells were so filled with hemosiderin as to show evidence of degeneration, and in fact there was some stroma increase in the portal tissues, which increase was probably related to this pigment deposit, as is seen in hemochromatosis. The Kupffer cells contained little pigment, and this was usually negative for iron. The bile ducts were normal, and bile canaliculi contained no pigment. There was some marrow metaplasia with scattered nests of marrow cells within dilated capillaries. The liver cells in the centers of the lobules appeared relatively normal and contained only a little hemosiderin.

The *stomach* mucosa showed nothing except postmortem autolysis. The *intestines* showed redness, cyanosis, and edema in the region of the duodenum and jejunum. Histologic sections showed a heavy deposit of hemosiderin in the acini cells of the gastric mucosa. There was postmortem autolysis. Duodenum showed a light deposit of hemosiderin in Brunner's glands and occasional granules of hemosiderin in the stroma of the tips of the villi.

Pancreas weighed 30 gm., and was of a peculiar yellowish brown coloration. Histologically there was postmortem autolysis, but a heavy deposit of hemosiderin was evident at a glance. Most of the hemosiderin was within acinar epithelium and in acini close to the islets. Occasionally an islet showed a few grains of hemosiderin within its epithelium.

Kidneys were definitely enlarged. The capsules stripped with ease. There was no deposition of pigment. Right kidney weighed 280 gm., left, 210 gm. *Chemical analyses* showed normal values for the kidney—4.6 mg. iron per 100 gm. of fresh tissue. Histologic sections showed normal structures. Occasional tubules showed a deposit of hemosiderin in the epithelium (Fig. 2). Other tubules showed a yellow pigment which was iron free. *Testis* histologically showed the usual pigmentation. Iron-free pigment was abundant in the interstitial tissue and appeared in large yellow granules. It also appeared in fine grains in the epithelium of a very few acini. Hemosiderin appeared in fine grains within the endothelium of many capillaries (Fig. 3).

Suprarenals were atrophic, the capsule thinned, and pigmentation increased. Histologically the glomerular zone of the cortex showed abundant deposit of hemosiderin within the adrenal epithelium (Fig. 6). Other tissues were normal.

Thyroid.—Externally the gland was of normal appearance. The pyramidal lobe was well developed and plainly visible on dissection. No manifest pathology was seen grossly. Histologically the picture was like that described in Cases 3 and 4. Fine granules of hemosiderin were abundant in the epithelium of the acini (Fig. 5).

The *vascular system* was normal in gross. Histologically many arterioles in the mesentery and kidneys showed a finely granular yellow pigment negative for iron in the smooth muscle coats. Many arterioles in the thyroid, adrenal, and mesentery contained some granules close to the elastica interna which stained for iron, and in some vessels the elastica interna in places took a deep blue iron stain.

Bone marrow was considerably increased and was of a peculiar brownish red hue. The color resembled somewhat that of the bone marrow in pernicious anemia. The bone shafts were considerably thinned. Portions of the ribs and the right femur presented similar pathology. Histologic sections were in general like those from Case 3. Hemosiderin was not abundant, but granules were found in phagocytes and occasional endothelial cells. Foam cells were rarely seen. The usual cellular hyperplasia was conspicuous.

CASE 6.—(M—i) This histologic material was sent to us through the courtesy of Dr. T. B. Cooley and supplements the material described above.

Heart.—Stains for iron were unsatisfactory.

Thymus showed aplasia but no pigment.

Spleen showed only a slight stroma increase and a cellular pulp. The malpighian bodies were normal. Iron-staining pigment was fairly abundant in phagocytes. There was relatively little marrow metaplasia in the single section studied.

Lymph glands showed abundant pigment, some of which gave a positive stain for iron.

Liver showed a heavy deposit of yellow pigment, most of which gave a positive iron stain. This pigment was very largely within the liver cells, but a little appeared in the Kupffer cells. There was a definite increase of wandering cells in the portal tissue.

Pancreas showed a heavy deposit of iron-staining pigment in the epithelial cells of the acini. Rarely a little hemosiderin was found in the islet epithelium.

Kidney showed no hemosiderin but some yellow granular pigment in the epithelium of a few tubules.

Marrow showed the usual picture of hyperplasia. Occasional foam cells were observed, and fibrosis was noted in some sections.

CASE 7.—(P—e) This histologic material was sent to us through the courtesy of Dr. T. B. Cooley.

Heart showed negative iron stains.

Thymus showed aplasia but no pigment.

Spleen in general was rather cellular, but the section was unsatisfactory.

Lymph glands examined contained only a little pigment.

Liver showed a heavy pigment deposit within the liver cells, especially in the margins of the lobules. Much of this pigment was noted in the Kupffer cells. Scattered focal hyaline necroses were found.

Pancreas presented the usual pigmentation with hemosiderin. There seemed to be a moderate increase in stroma.

Adrenal showed a faint stain for iron in the glomerular zone (compare Fig. 6).

Marrow showed the usual hyperplasia. There were sizeable islands of foam cells noted here and there as well as a little fibrosis.

CASE 8.—(No. 57332.) *History.*—E. S., an Italian girl, four years old, was born Feb. 5, 1932, by breech delivery after a twin sister, M. S., had been delivered spontaneously by vertex presentation. The obstetric record indicated that they were single ovum twins, only one placenta having been described. Nevertheless, the physical features are now so dissimilar (Fig. 7) that they are considered not to be identical twins. At birth the measurements were: length, 49 cm.; head circumference, 32 cm.; chest circumference, 31 cm.; weight, 2270 gm. On the twelfth day the weight was 2810 gm. Breathing was spontaneous. At the time of discharge from the nursery nothing abnormal was noted except that she was undersized.

When she was eight months old, pallor was noted. She became less active and more pale until eighteen months of age, when a lump was noticed in the left upper part of the abdomen. At nineteen months she was admitted to the pediatric service of the Rochester General Hospital and there received eleven transfusions during a period of nine months. Copper and iron were also administered.

At two and one-half years of age, she was admitted to the pediatric service of the Strong Memorial Hospital on July 30, 1934.

The first tooth appeared at five months. She sat at ten months, talked at one year, and walked at two years. She had not gained control of the bladder at two and one-half years.

The feeding had been normal. With the exception of an occasional cold, no infections had occurred.

The father, forty-nine years of age, and the mother, thirty-five years of age, were well. Three children, a girl eight years old, one six years old, and a boy five years old, were normal. The twin sister was normal and at the age of four years had a normal blood picture.

Physical Findings.—At the time of admission (two and one-half years of age), the patient was definitely undersized. The head, chest, and abdominal circum-

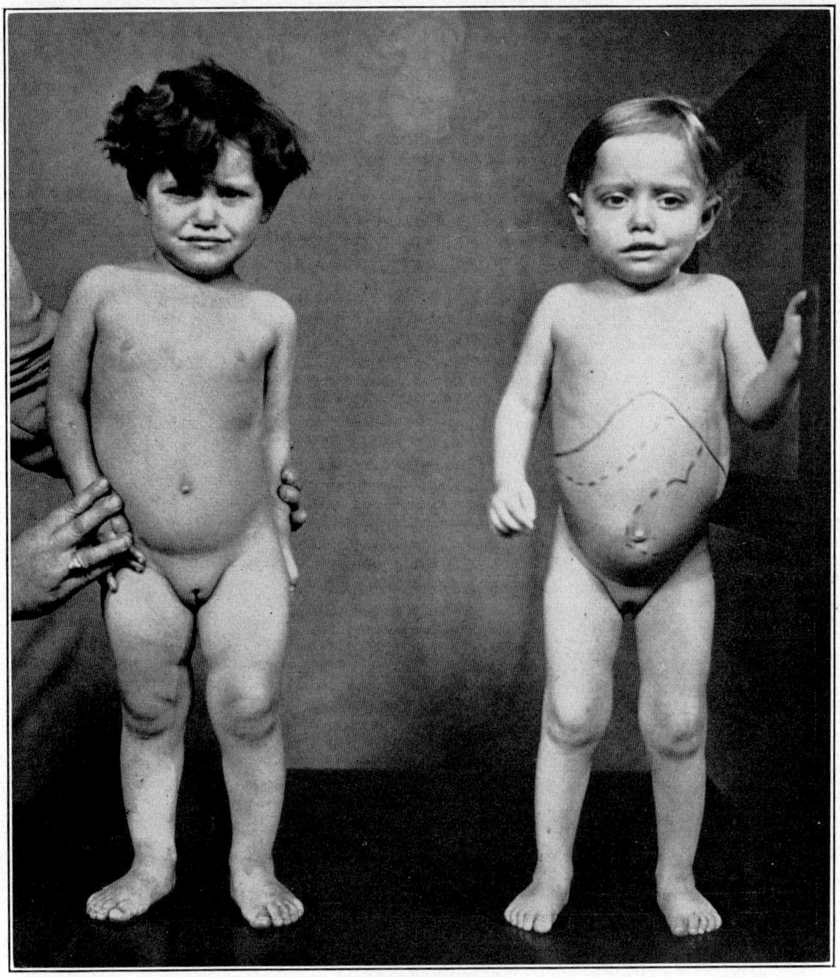

Fig. 7.—Case 8. Normal and abnormal twin sisters.

ferences were 45, 48.5, and 50 cm., respectively. The length was 80 cm., and the weight, 8.5 kg. The temperature, pulse, and respiratory rates were 38° C., 138, and 22, respectively. The patient was pale. The abdomen was distended, and the liver and spleen were enlarged. The heart was slightly enlarged, and a soft, systolic murmur was audible. The fact was suggestive of the mongoloid type (Fig. 7).

Course.—From the age of nineteen months until the present time (four years), careful observations of the blood were made, particularly in relationship to experi-

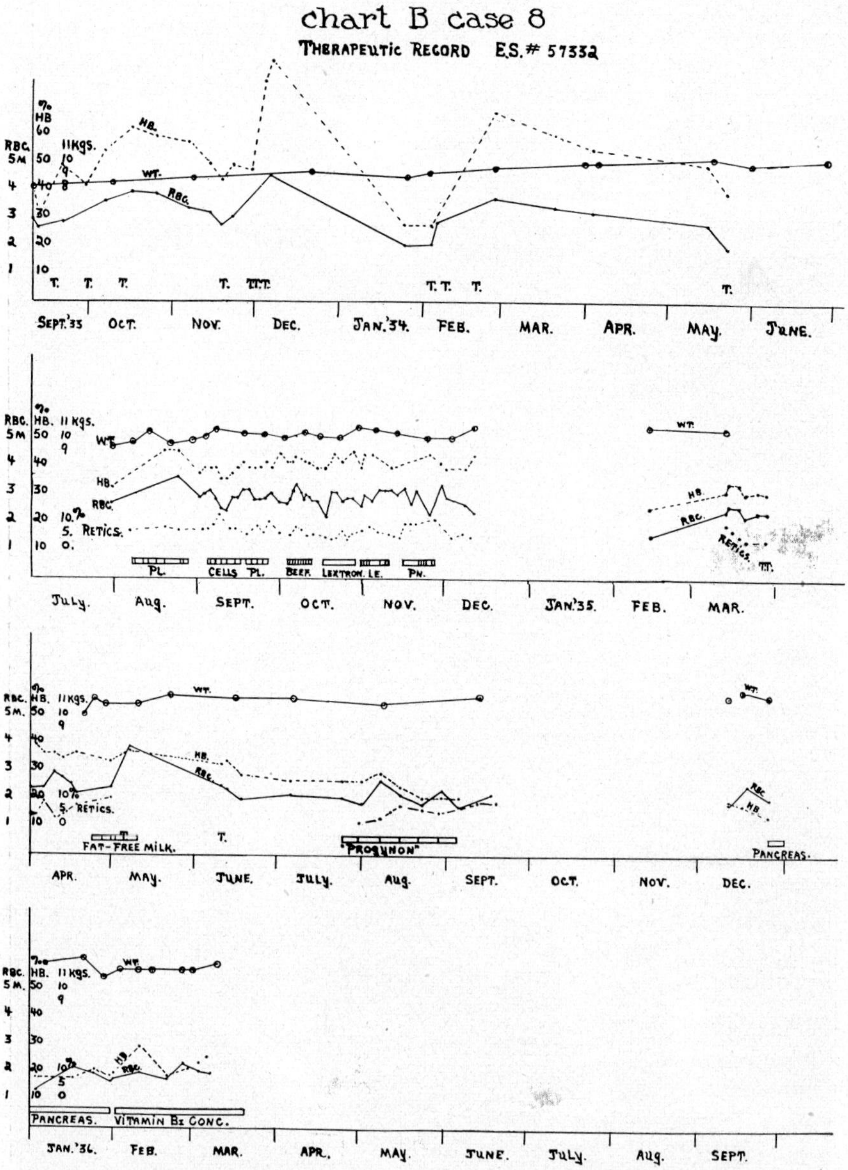

Chart B.—Case 8. Explanation of dosages. *T*, transfusions of citrated blood given intravenously, 50 to 150 c.c.; *PL*, alcohol extract of blood plasma, 5 to 10 c.c. intramuscularly, 9 injections; *cells*, extract of blood cells, 5 c.c. intramuscularly, 7 injections; *PL*, alcohol extract of blood plasma, 5 c.c. intramuscularly, 5 injections; *beef*, 50 gm. of beef muscle incubated with normal human gastric juice, prepared by the method of Castle; *lextron* (Lilly), one teaspoonful t.i.d.; *LE*, liver extract (Lederle), 1 c.c.=33 gm. of liver substance, 8 injections; *PN*, pentnucleotide, 2.5 c.c. intramuscularly, 7 injections; *fat-free milk*, 5 intramuscular injections of 0.5, 1.0, 2.0, 3.0, and 4.0 c.c., respectively; *progynon*, intramuscularly, 7 weekly injections of estrogenic preparation (progynon-B, Schering Corporation), 1 c.c.=2,000 R.U. or 10,000 international units; *pancreas*, fresh, raw, beef pancreas ground, two teaspoonfuls every 2 hours daily; *vitamin B_1 concentrate* (Merck) 1 to 3 mg. daily.

mental therapy (Chart B). Among other studies made, the following may be informative: blood lipids: plasma—cholesterol, 125 mg. per 100 c.c.; total lipids, 594; phospholipids, 159; fatty acids, 469; residual fat, 300; red cell phospholipids, 366. These values are within normal limits.

Vitamin A absorption tests revealed the normal values as follows: fasting, 12 units vitamin A per 100 c.c. After 2 c.c. of haliver oil were administered, values were as follows: 2 hours, 35 units; 4 hours, 250 units; 6 hours, 286 units; 9 hours, 113 units; 12 hours, 119 units; 24 hours, 65 units. The b'ood calcium was 9.2 mg. per 100 c.c.; blood phosphorus, 4.4 mg. per 100 c.c.

Blood volume studies were made by Dr. Nolan L. Kaltreider, to whom we are indebted for the following information:

Body weight, 10.8 kg.
Red cell count, 2,300,000
Reticulated red cells, 6.0 per cent
Hematocrit-red cell percentage, 13.9 per cent
Hematocrit-plasma percentage, 86.1 per cent
Mean corpuscular volume, 60.5 cubic microns
Mean corpuscular hemoglobin, 16.6 micromicrograms
Mean corpuscular hemoglobin concentration, 29.4 per cent
Total plasma volume, 673 c.c.
Total plasma volume per kilogram, 62.3 c.c. (normal, 50 c.c.)
Total blood volume, 782 c.c.
Total blood volume per kilogram, 72.4 c.c. (normal, 72 c.c.)
Red blood cell volume, 109 c.c.
Red blood cell volume per kilogram, 10.1 c.c. (normal, 22 c.c.)
Hemoglobin per 100 c.c. blood, 3.82 gm.
Total circulatory hemoglobin, 29.87 gm.
Total circulatory hemoglobin per kilogram, 2.77 gm.
Blood viscosity, 2.3 (normal, 4-4.5)

DISCUSSION

Since the important work of Cooley, the clinical recognition of this type of anemia is no longer difficult. The blood picture is not entirely characteristic, however, because some of the features are duplicated in the blood of other conditions.

Observations on the morphology of the blood have confirmed the findings of Cooley[5] concerning the marked degree of fragmentation. Attempts to correlate hematocrit studies with cell measurements have been made.[3] In two cases a tendency to macrocytosis occurred particularly after splenectomy. A similar observation has recently been made in cases of hemolytic jaundice after this operation.[14] There was also evidence that in certain cases of *thalassemia* the red cell is thinner than normal.

Retarded growth, with a delay in carpal ossification, in certain cases, and sugar tolerance curves of the type obtained in Case 3 are features seen also in celiac disease. One does not find, however, the characteristic increase in the fat content of the stools in *thalassemia*. Moreover, in Case 8, the vitamin A absorption curve is normal as compared with the low curve usually found in celiac disease.

In our cases the blood lipids have been essentially normal. In Case 8 and in one other case not reported here, slight increases in the phospholipid content of the red cells were found. Perhaps blood which contains many young cells is comparable with other growing tissues[18] known to have an increased phospholipid content.

In Cases 3 and 8, it will be noted that in each instance the total plasma volume and total blood volume per kilogram of body weight, as determined by the dye method, were normal. As might be expected, the red cell volume per kilogram of body weight was reduced, being only one-half normal in Case 8.

Because the pigment distribution in this disease resembles that in hemochromatosis, attempts were made to demonstrate urinary siderosis. Only an occasional iron-laden kidney epithelial cell was demonstrated in the urinary sediment.

Experimental Therapy.—Our attempts at experimental therapy have been mainly empirical. Our study of the anatomic material has led us to try substances which might supply material with which to build hemoglobin or cells. We have also tried certain glandular products. The hypoplasia of the adrenal cortex suggested the use of cortin. Although the results are entirely negative to date, we believe certain substances have been given sufficiently adequate trials to justify a report.

In Charts A and B, records of the experimental therapy used in Cases 3 and 8, respectively, are presented. The red cell count, hemoglobin values and the weight of the patient are shown by curves, beneath which is shown the time and duration that each therapeutic substance was used.

The therapeutic record in Case 3 (Chart A) is interesting because it covers his entire life from the time of diagnosis at seven months until death at five years. Of particular interest is the fact that repeated transfusions, splenectomy, the feeding of copper, of iron, and of various liver and spleen fractions have given negative results. Of the other substances tried, it seems certain that cortin (obtained through the courtesy of Dr. F. A. Hartmann, of Buffalo, N. Y.) and extralin were each given satisfactory trials. The oral administrations of such substances as anterior lobe, pituitary, thymus, and bone marrow extracts may represent inadequate tests. Extracts of these substances suitable for injection should, of course, be given a trial.

In Case 8 (E. S.) (Chart B) the parenteral injection of plasma and of cell extracts prepared according to the method of Josephs,[8] a potent liver extract preparation, and pentnucleotide have been adequately tested. The plasma and cell extracts were prepared for our use through the courtesy of Dr. S. W. Clausen. Except for a slight reticulocyte response to the cell extract and to pentnucleotide, no favorable results were obtained. Predigested beef prepared by the method of Castle[4] was also given an adequate trial in this patient without a response. Again this patient illustrates the temporary improvement expected from blood transfusion.

The *marrow* hyperplasia is a conspicuous feature of this disease, and in some respects it resembles the marrow of pernicious anemia. In both we have great hyperplasia of the marrow, which is unable to turn out adequate numbers of mature red cells but does flood the blood stream with immature and atypical red cells. One diseased marrow reacts to liver feeding but the other does not. However, one can scarcely avoid the thought[22] that the hyperplastic marrow in these children may be due to the *lack of something*—a deficiency state—as is surely true for pernicious anemia. These cases also may show nests of foam cells in marrow and spleen similar to the cells observed in Gaucher's disease. *Marrow metaplasia* with nests of myelocytes, nucleated red cells, and megakaryocytes may be noted in the spleen in most cases and in the liver and some lymph glands in some cases.

The changes noted in the *bony skeleton* are of some interest and by many writers are explained on the basis of marrow hyperplasia alone. We cannot agree with this belief and prefer to think of these peculiar lesions in the skull, ribs, and long bones as due to some metabolic factor. In other words, we prefer to think of these bone changes as of the order of those recorded in scurvy or acromegaly in which vitamins or ductless glands are concerned. Marrow hyperplasia in pernicious anemia or leucemia may be extreme and of long duration but does not give the bone abnormalities reported in this Mediterranean disease. Furthermore similar bone abnormalities have been noted in sickle-cell anemia and hemolytic jaundice, but the marrow changes in those diseases are of a different character.

The *pigment abnormalities* are conspicuous in this disease and follow accurately the pattern of pigment distribution in hemochromatosis. We[22] pointed out this similarity, but we cannot agree with Mallory[10] that this disease is "hemochromatosis in the child." This Mediterranean disease unlike hemochromatosis is racial, is associated with a progressive chronic anemia, splenomegaly, and characteristic bone abnormalities. We do not propose to join in the debate relative to copper as the cause of liver cirrhosis and hemochromatosis,[17] but we do feel that these cases of *thalassemia* give no support to this thesis and actually exclude copper as a cause of this particular pigmentary abnormality. If copper is the cause of the pigmentation of the viscera, then it is also the cause of the bone abnormalities and the peculiar anemia with splenomegaly, as these conditions always develop together in the same child. Also copper must injure especially the Mediterranean people and trail families like a bloodhound. It does not seem necessary to pursue the argument.

Pigments as they appear in tissues present difficulties of analysis, and this question has been reviewed recently by Nachtnebel.[11] Some pigments probably are of dietary origin, and many others come from hemoglobin. Others are thought to be related to fat metabolism (lipofuscin and lipochrome). One can at least differentiate the yellow granular pigments into those giving a positive staining reaction for iron (hemosiderin) and those giving no iron reaction (hemofuscin, lipofuscin, lipochrome, etc.). Sheldon[17] concludes that hemofuscin is more nearly related to the melanins.

It is usually assumed that hemosiderin is related to blood destruction, but in hemochromatosis it seems difficult to accept this mechanism. Sprunt[20] was the first to point out that in hemochromatosis there was no increased blood destruction, and he suggested that hemochromatosis was due to a fundamental disturbance of the pigment metabolism. With this assumption we can record all the peculiarities of pigment deposit and abnormalities of hemochromatosis without forcing a relationship to hemoglobin destruction. The same thing may apply to the pigment abnormalities of *thalassemia,* although in this disease we do have a definite blood abnormality. The pattern of pigment distribution in hemochromatosis and *thalassemia* is almost identical; therefore the inevitable conclusion follows that the blood disturbance probably is not responsible for the pigment abnormalities in *thalassemia.*

The pigment deposits found in *hemolytic jaundice* are of interest in this connection. In long-continued cases we may find some pigment deposits in heart, pancreas, thyroid, and gastric mucosa, but the pigment deposits in spleen and liver are very different. In hemolytic jaundice the spleen shows great amounts of iron contained in the endothelial cells of the sinusoids, and the liver shows much of the iron-containing pigment in the Kupffer cells, an entirely different distribution from that recorded in *thalassemia.* The kidney, which shows little hemosiderin in *thalassemia,* is very heavily pigmented in hemolytic icterus. The experiments of Rous and Oliver[16] with long-continued injection of citrated blood in rabbits are of interest and present the same general picture as hemolytic icterus.

Pigment distribution in organs and cells is of some interest and, as relating to hemochromatosis, has been tabulated by Sheldon.[17] This pigment distribution is practically identical in *thalassemia.* One is struck with the observations that the gastric mucosa presents much hemosiderin which is present in the epithelium of the deep acini, particularly in the chief cells and rarely in the acid cells. Sharply at the pylorus the mucosa becomes hemosiderin-free, and pigment appears in Brunner's glands. The mucosa of the small and large intestine is free of hemosiderin except for occasional granules in phagocytes.

As we stated in our first paper, we dislike the name ''erythroblastic anemia'' given by Cooley, who was responsible for the recognition of the clinical syndrome. As the disease is limited to races of people living about the Mediterranean Sea, we suggested ''thalassemia'' as a preferable term derived from Θάλασσα, the Greek word for the ''great sea''—designating in their writings the Mediterranean Sea.

SUMMARY

This disease is due to some racial, inherited defect which is responsible for the abnormalities of the hemopoietic tissues (of the order of pernicious anemia), the bone changes (of the order of acromegaly), and the pigment abnormalities (practically identical with hemochromatosis). This suggests a deficiency state which may be remediable when completely understood and gives adequate grounds for a variety of therapeutic tests.

We record in detail the complete autopsy findings in three new cases of this disease and partial autopsy findings in two others. We believe the pigment deposits in these cases (simulating hemochromatosis) are as characteristic of this disease as are the recorded abnormalities of the hemopoietic system and bony skeleton.

The anemia may be classified as microcytic and hypochromic. Macrocytosis and thinning of the cells occurred in two cases after splenectomy. In two cases (Cases 3 and 8) the total blood volume and the plasma volume were found to be normal, while the red cell volume was decreased. Wet preparations revealed marked fragmentation but no tendency to sickle.

The following therapeutic measures, which we believe have been adequately tested, failed to modify the clinical picture: blood transfusions, plasma and cell extracts, primary or secondary anemia liver extracts, fetal liver extract, spleen extract, raw pancreas, adrenal cortex extract (cortin), estrogenic substance (progynon), vitamin B_1 concentrate, iron, and copper.

REFERENCES

1. Baty, J. M., Blackfan, K. D., and Diamond, L. K.: Am. J. Dis. Child. **43**: 667, 1932.
2. Bennett, T. I., Hunter, D., and Vaughan, J. M.: Quart. J. Med. **1**: 603, 1932.
3. Bradford, W. L., and Dye, Jane: J. Pediat. **9**: 312, 1936.
4. Castle, W. B., Townsend, W. C., and Heath, C. H.: Am. J. M. Sc. **180**: 305. 1930.
5. Cooley, T. B., and Lee, P.: J. Pediat. **3**: 55, 1933.
6. Friedman, L. J.: Am. J. Roentgenol. **20**: 440, 1928.
7. Fries, J. H., Duhan, E., and Shair, H. M.: J. Pediat. **2**: 487, 1933.
8. Josephs, H. W.: Am. J. Dis. Child. **48**: 932, 1934.
9. LeWald, L. T.: Radiology **18**: 792, 1932.
10. Mallory, F. B.: Tr. A. Am. Physicians **50**: 14, 1935.
11. Nachtnebel, E.: Am. J. Path. **9**: 261, 1933.
12. Parker, D. W.: New England J. Med. **208**: 1147, 1933.
13. Parsons, L. G., and Hawksley, J. C.: Arch. Dis. Child. **8**: 184, 1933.
14. Paxton, W. T. W.: Arch. Dis. Child. **10**: 421, 1935.
15. Rous, P.: J. Exper. Med. **28**: 645, 1918.
16. Rous, P., and Oliver, J.: J. Exper. Med. **28**: 629, 1918.
17. Sheldon, J. H.: Haemochromatosis, London, 1935, Oxford Univ. Press.
18. Sinclair, R. G.: J. Biol. Chem. **88**: 575, 1930.
19. Snelling, C. E., and Brown, A.: J. Pediat. **8**: 330, 1936.
20. Sprunt, T. P.: Arch. Int. Med. **8**: 75, 1911.
21. Vogt, E. C., and Diamond, L. K.: Am. J. Roentgenol. **23**: 625, 1930.
22. Whipple, G. H., and Bradford, W. L.: Am. J. Dis. Child. **44**: 336, 1932.
23. Yaguda, A.: Am. J. Clin. Path. **5**: 266, 1935.

OBSERVATIONS ON THE MORPHOLOGY OF THE ERYTHROCYTES IN MEDITERRANEAN DISEASE—THALASSEMIA

(Erythroblastic Anemia of Cooley)

William L. Bradford, M.D., and Jane Dye
Rochester, N. Y.

THE distinguishing features of the blood in Mediterranean anemia have been well described by Kato and Downey.[1] Marked irregularity in the size and shape of the red cells, fragmentation, and the comparatively large number of nucleated red cells in the circulating blood, particularly after splenectomy, are the essential findings. Irregularity in the distribution of hemoglobin within the matured erythrocyte is also found.

Hematocrit studies have indicated that the anemia in this disease may be classified as microcytic-hypochromic in type. Because of the extreme degree of fragmentation often encountered, Cooley[2] has suggested that incorrect results may be obtained by hematocrit studies. For this reason we have extended our observations to include comparison of the values obtained by the hematocrit with those found by direct measurement of the cells.

Hematocrit values and cell diameter curves have been determined in eight cases observed in the pediatric department of the Strong Memorial Hospital and in the out-patient department. All of the children were of Italian descent.

METHOD

Five cubic centimeters of venous blood were placed in bottles containing exactly 5 mg. of potassium oxalate, and from these samples red cell counts and hemoglobin determinations were made with certified equipment. The hematocrit readings were determined in Wintrobe tubes after centrifugalization for thirty minutes at 4,000 revolutions per minute.

The frequency of distribution of the cell diameters was determined by the method of Price-Jones.[3] A description of the ocular micrometer used was previously given by McCann and Dye.[4] All of the cell measurements were made by one individual (J. D.). To test our method further, a smear was examined by Dr. Price-Jones and the distribution curve kindly submitted by him was found to be practically identical with the duplicate made by one of us (J. D.).

The volume index was calculated according to the method of Capps[5]: the number of cubic centimeters of packed cells in percentage of normal divided by the number of red cells in percentage of the normal.

From the Departments of Pediatrics and Medicine, University of Rochester School of Medicine and Dentistry.

The saturation index was determined by dividing the number of grams of hemoglobin per 100 c.c. of blood in percentage of normal by the number of cubic centimeters of packed cells per 100 c.c. of blood.

The thickness of the red cell was estimated by use of the three-dimension chart of Von Boros,[6] for calculating the thickness of the erythrocyte from the diameter and the volume.

The diameter-thickness ratio which best expresses the absolute thickness of the cell was calculated by dividing the mean diameter by the thickness.

The volume thickness index was determined according to the method of Haden.[7] For this purpose the nomogram described by Warburg[8] was used.

DISCUSSION OF RESULTS

Wet preparations revealed a marked degree of fragmentation. Knob-like projections were observed to form and to break off from the erythrocytes with regularity. One obtained the impression that many of these calls were leaflike and that they were thinner than normal erythrocytes.

Because Mediterranean anemia as well as sickle-cell anemia is racial and familial, and is characterized by similar bone changes, and since the sickle-cell type has been described in a Greek[9] as well as in an Italian[10] child, it seemed important to observe the blood carefully for the sickling phenomenon. This was studied in fresh and in carbon-dioxide treated blood at varying degrees of temperature, but no evidence of sickling was noted.

The results of the hematocrit observations are shown in Table I.* From these measurements it is apparent that the mean corpuscular volume is either normal or reduced. The combination of a decreased mean corpuscular volume and an increased mean-cell diameter (in the case of J. S.) suggests a cell thinner than normal. This is further shown to be true by the calculated cell thickness and the diminished volume thickness index.

If, as Haden[11] has shown, the volume thickness index is directly related to the fragility of the cells, we would not expect an hemolytic tendency to exist with a diminished volume thickness index. In the case of J. S., the resistance of the red cells to hypotonic salt solutions was found to be normal.

The same condition of an apparent thinning of the cells occurred in the case of T. Z. It is interesting that in these two cases (J. S. and T. Z.) the macrocytosis became evident after splenectomy had been performed. Paxton[12] has recently reported the occurrence of increased cell diameter in cases of familial acholuric jaundice after removal of the spleen.

*In the preceding paper J. S., aged eighteen months, is Case 3; J. S., aged seven years, is Case 5; while E. S., aged nineteen months, is Case 8.

TABLE I

MEASUREMENTS OF THE ERYTHROCYTES IN MEDITERRANEAN ANEMIA

PATIENT	AGE	DATE	RED CELLS (MILLIONS)	HEMOGLOBIN (GM. PER 100 C.C.)	HEMATOCRIT (C.C. OF CELLS PER 100)	VOLUME INDEX	SATURATION INDEX	MEAN CORPUSCULAR VOLUME (CUBIC MICRONS)	MEAN CORPUSCULAR HEMOGLOBIN (MICRO-MICROGRAMS)	MEAN CORPUSCULAR HEMOGLOBIN CONCENTRATION (PER CENT)	CELL MEASUREMENTS: MEAN DIAMETER (MICRONS)	CELL MEASUREMENTS: STANDARD DEVIATION (MICRONS)	CELL MEASUREMENTS: COEFFICIENT OF VARIATION (PER CENT)	CELL THICKNESS (MICRONS)	DIAMETER THICKNESS RATIO	VOLUME THICKNESS INDEX	INTERVAL SINCE LAST TRANSFUSION	DESIGNATION OF DISTRIBUTION CURVE (ON CHART 1)
Normal			*4.50*	*13.0*	*39.5*	*1.0*	*1.0*	*88*	*30*	*33*	*7.349*	*0.483*	*6.723*	*2.1*	*3.5:1*	*1.0*		
J. S.	18 mo.	5/31/30									5.849	1.169	19.9				68 days	A. J. S. ♂ 18 mo.
		6/11/30									6.610	1.084	16.4				2 days	B. J. S. ♂ 18 mo.
		12/ 5/32	3.30	6.5	25.0	0.86	0.79	75	19.6	26.1							29 mo.	Splenectomy 7/9/30
		5/23/33	3.70	5.4	25.0	0.77	0.65	67.5	14.7	21.6	8.073	1.789	22.0	1.35	5.9:1	0.66	34 mo.	C.
		6/20/33	3.23	6.6	25.0	0.87	0.81	78.1	20.6	26.4	8.330	2.182	26.2	1.45	5.7:1	0.71	35 mo.	
		8/15/33	3.28	7.2	22.5	0.78	0.96	68.6	21.9	32.0	8.421	2.046	24.2	1.25	6.7:1	0.60	37 mo.	
		10/ 3/33	1.88	3.5	14.3	0.88	0.75	76.0	18.6	24.4	7.647	1.900	24.9	1.70	4.5:1	0.90	39 mo.	D.
T. Z.	3½ yr.	6/26/33	2.60	5.0	18.7	0.81	0.81	72.0	19.2	26.7	6.268	1.010	16.1	2.30	3.1:1	1.50	13 days	A. T. Z. ♀ 3 yr.
		8/10/33	3.68	9.8	34.3	1.01	0.86	93.2	26.6	28.5	7.766	0.946	12.2	2.00	3.8:1	1.02	17 days	B. Splenectomy 7/24/33
		2/11/34	2.70	6.1	25.0	1.05	0.74	92.8	22.7	24.6	7.573	1.354	17.8	2.08	3.6:1	1.09	79 days	C.
		6/20/34	1.77	4.0	17.4	1.12	0.70	98.0	22.8	22.9	8.473	1.818	21.4	1.80	4.7:1	0.86	87 days	D.

TABLE I—CONT'D

PATIENT	AGE	DATE	RED CELLS	HEMOGLOBIN	HEMATOCRIT	VOLUME INDEX	SATURATION INDEX	MEAN CORPUSCULAR VOLUME	MEAN CORPUSCULAR HEMOGLOBIN	MEAN CORPUSCULAR HEMOGLOBIN CONCENTRATION	CELL MEASUREMENTS: MEAN DIAMETER	CELL MEASUREMENTS: STANDARD DEVIATION	CELL MEASUREMENTS: COEFFICIENT OF VARIATION	CELL THICKNESS	DIAMETER THICKNESS RATIO	VOLUME THICKNESS INDEX	INTERVAL SINCE LAST TRANSFUSION	DESIGNATION OF DISTRIBUTION CURVE
			(MILLIONS)	(GM. PER 100 C.C.)	(C.C. OF CELLS PER 100)			(CUBIC MICRONS)	(MICRO-MICROGRAMS)	(PER CENT)	(MICRONS)	(MICRONS)	(PER CENT)	(MICRONS)				(ON CHART 1)
E. S.	19 mo.	9/11/33	2.56	4.3	17.0	0.75	0.73	66.0	16.8	25.3							none	
		9/12/33	2.90	5.2	19.6	0.76	0.82	67.4	17.9	26.5	6.517	1.315	20.1	2.05	3.1:1	1.27	none	A. E. S. ♀ 19 mo.
		2/ 2/34	1.90	4.5	16.5	1.00	0.81	66.0	28.0	27.3	6.722	1.092	16.2	1.90	3.5:1	1.12	62 days	B.
		5/22/34									6.809	1.186	17.7				171 days	C.
		7/30/34	2.74	4.5	19.6	0.80	0.72	71.5	16.4	23.0							69 days	
		11/20/34	3.28	6.5	20.9	0.72	0.94	63.7	19.8	31.1	6.206	1.106	18.0	2.15	2.8:1	1.35	182 days	D.
		4/ 3/36	2.61	4.2	14.5	0.64	0.87	55.5	16.1	29.0	6.469	1.183	18.2	1.73	3.8:1	0.93	10 mo.	
P. G.	2 yr.	2/ 4/31	2.96	5.0	17.8	0.69	0.86	60.1	17.8	28.2	6.111	1.237	20.2	2.07	3.0:1	1.36	none	P. G. ♂ 2 yr.
R. M.	2 yr.	6/20/32	3.10	5.8	19.0	0.69	0.93	60.0	19.0	30.5	6.212	1.337	21.5	2.00	3.1:1	1.31	100 days	R. M. ♀ 2 yr.
J. S.	7 yr.	2/ 2/34	3.15	7.4	25.0	0.90	0.90	79.0	23.5	29.6	6.806	0.965	11.2	2.20	3.0:1	1.13	6 days	J. S. ♂ 7 yr.
B. D.	18 mo.	8/10/33									6.649	0.572	8.6					B. D. ♂ 18 mo.
J. D.	5 yr.	8/10/33									7.437	1.398	18.8					J. D. ♂ 5 yr.

In the cases, E. S., P. G., R. M., and J. S., microcytic curves were found, and the volume thickness index was either normal or slightly increased. None of this group had undergone splenectomy. Further observations on the cell morphology in relationship to splenectomy in this condition would be of interest.

The distribution curves (Chart 1) in general reveal wide bases and increased coefficients of variation. A similar Price-Jones curve was described by Moncrieff and Whitby[13] in a Greek child. This report is said to be the first of thalassemia from England.

It will be noted from observation of Table I that blood transfusions preceded some of the studies. That a recent transfusion would ma-

chart 1

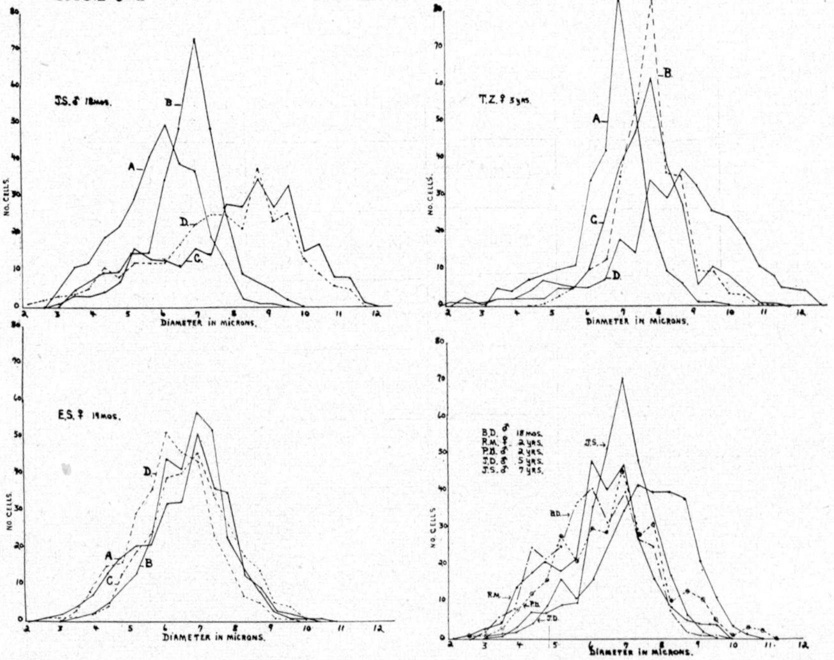

Chart 1.—Showing the frequency of the distribution of the cell diameters in eight cases of Mediterranean disease. In J. S. and T. Z. the tendency toward macrocytosis occurred after splenectomy.

terially change the results is admitted. How long such an influence would persist is not apparent because the life of transfused cells in this condition is not definitely known. Using the method of Ashby,[14] Edgar and Boisvert[15] have found from observations made in this clinic that transfused cells are no longer demonstrable after an interval of thirty to thirty-five days.

SUMMARY

Hematocrit studies in six cases and cell diameter measurements in eight cases of Mediterranean anemia (type of Cooley) have been made.

In all instances the evidence suggested an hypocythemic microcytic and hypochromic anemia.

In two cases the combination of decreased cell volume and increased mean cell diameter, along with decreased thickness of the cell, occurred after removal of the spleen.

Distribution curves usually showed wide bases and increased coefficients of variation.

The study of wet preparations confirmed the findings of Cooley and Lee that fragmentation of the erythrocytes is very marked. The phenomenon of sickling was not observed.

REFERENCES

1. Kato, K., and Downey, H.: Folia haemat. **50:** 55, 1933.
2. Cooley, T.: Discussion of paper by Dr. George M. Guest: Am. J. Dis. Child. **48:** 929, 1934.
3. Price-Jones, Cecil: Red Blood Cell Diameters, London, England, 1933, Oxford University Press.
4. McCann, W. S., and Dye, J.: Ann. Int. Med. **4:** 918, 1931.
5. Capps, J. A.: J. M. Research **10:** 367, 1903-4.
6. Von Boros, J.: Ergeb. d. inn. Med. u Kinderh. **42:** 635, 1932.
7. Haden, R. L.: J. Lab. & Clin. Med. **20:** 567, 1935.
8. Warburg, E. J.: Acta med. Scandinav. **66:** 187, 1927.
9. Cooley, T. B., and Lee, P.: Am. J. Dis. Child. **33:** 103, 1929.
10. Laws, Carl: Sickle-Cell Anemia in a Child of Italian Parentage, Paper read before the Section on Pediatrics, 129th Annual Meeting of the Medical Society of the State of New York, May 15, 1935.
11. Haden, R. L.: Am. J. M. Sc. **188:** 441, 1934.
12. Paxton, W. T. W.: Arch. Dis. Child. **10:** 421, 1935.
13. Moncrieff, A., and Whitby, L. E. H.: Lancet **2:** 648, 1934.
14. Ashby, Winifred: J. Exper. Med. **29:** 267, 1919.
15. Edgar, K., and Boisvert, P.: Personal communication.

INTRAVASCULAR CLOTTING IN ABANDONED FETAL CHANNELS IN THE NEWBORN

W. A. MULHERIN, M.D., AND JOSEPH KRAFKA, JR., M.D.
AUGUSTA, GA.

INCREASED coagulation time, polycythemia, hemolysis, and bilirubinemia in the newborn are associated phenomena which present a problem of both a practical and theoretical significance. One of us has dealt previously with one aspect of this problem in a study of reticulocytes in the newborn (Krafka). In a search for the *raison d'être,* the investigation was extended to include the question of a correlation with the closing time of abandoned fetal vascular channels and the time of dropping of the cord. Gradually the hypothesis developed that these phenomena constituted in part or in whole a rational protective mechanism which prevented thrombus formation, since the thrombi, should they form, would serve as an embolic threat during this critical period of life.

Satisfactory tests of such an hypothesis are elusive, but we offer, as a preliminary approach, the following methods and results.

METHODS

Long umbilical cords were left intact on newborn infants. At specified times new double ligatures were placed near the end of the cord; the peripheral pieces were cut off and fixed immediately in 10 per cent neutral formalin or in alcohol. Successive pieces were removed at intervals of one and one-half hours, four hours, twelve hours, and forty-eight hours after birth. Cords dropping off normally on the fourth day were also fixed. Sections were cut in paraffin or celloidin and stained with hematoxylin and eosin, Mallory's triple stain, or Weigert's fibrin stain. By way of control, we have studied the clots in severed umbilical cords in which the general observation is made that clots will eventually form and in which the fibrin appears either fibrinous, granular or hyaline.

Nature of the So-called Clot in the Intact Vein.—One and one-half hours after delivery, a thin halo of pale eosinophilic, homogeneous substance occurs firmly adherent to the endothelium of the vein. This is approximately 20 mu wide. Well-preserved discrete erythrocytes and occasional leucocytes lie superficial to this zone with only a rare cell incorporated in it. No fibrin is present. There is no evidence of a reaction on the part of the endothelium.

From the Departments of Pediatrics and Anatomy, University of Georgia School of Medicine.

Presented before The American Pediatric Society, Lake George, New York, May 11 to 13, 1936.

Such a clot, if it can be called a clot, has been described as a "hyaline clot." The nature of the homogeneous substance has been discussed by Welch, Aschoff, and MacCallum. They consider it to be made up of platelets in such close apposition that their borders are no longer visible. The hyaline clot has been interpreted as due to agglutination of erythrocytes, but in this instance, while the homogeneous substance is present, there is no evidence of a firm adherence of the red cells one to another.

There is no great addition to the width of this hyaline zone at the end of twelve or twenty-four hours. At forty-eight hours there is some evidence of hemolysis, but fibrin is still absent.

Even in the cord which has dropped, the so-called clot still shows the same characters, although the endothelium and media show marked degenerative changes. No fibrin is present. There is no organization of the clot such as produced by invasive connective tissue cells, connective tissue fibers or invading capillaries. Of course, organization would hardly be expected since it is thought to be initiated in the adult at about the tenth day. True clotting does not take place in the intact umbilical vein.

DISCUSSION

These observations are in accord with those of many investigators who have noted the absence of true clot in the abandoned fetal vascular channels. Meyer states that the intraabdominal portion of the umbilical vein contains unclotted blood in the sheep. He found red cells in a fair state of preservation in the dog at the end of the seventh week. Pöllot and other investigators have noted the absence of clot in the ductus arteriosus. Scammon in discussing the mechanism of closure of the ductus arteriosus states that less than 1 per cent show a clot at autopsy. Even in these instances, the nature of the clots is not established since they may be associated with infection at various other sites, as will be discussed below. Strassman (cited by Melka, 1926) believes that thrombosis of the ductus arteriosus is always pathologic. There are, however, some writers who still accept the theory of the closure of fetal channels by thrombus formation (Wiggers, Haberda). Meyer, Shaeffer, and Melka have dealt conclusively with this problem and have shown that the obliteration of the channels is brought about by contraction, infiltration of the intima, and obliteration of the lumen by connective tissue of the elastic type.

A casual review of the clinical literature is at first hand contradictory to the opinion that thrombosis of the fetal vessels does not occur. There are frequent references to cases of thrombosis of the aorta, sinus thrombosis, etc., in infancy. Careful study of these cases shows, however, that thrombosis is associated with infection at other sites, such as umbilical infection, fibrinous pneumonia, etc. Moschcowitz cites a case of death on the tenth day with thrombosis of the aorta following streptococcus infection of the umbilical vein. Hedinger's patient died on the fifteenth day with gangrene of both feet and a putrid coagulum in the umbilical vein. Rothstein's patient died on the thirteenth day with thrombosis of the aorta, no gross external inflammatory changes but a staphylococcus infection in a thrombus in the umbilical vein. Limper and Miller cite a case in which the cord dropped normally on the seventh day; dry gangrene of the legs followed; and at autopsy the aorta was found occluded by a thrombus. The umbilicus showed infection. Wheler presents a case with black feet on the tenth day from a thrombus ¼ inch below the entrance of the mesenteric artery. Cultures showed pneumococcus.

We present two cases from the records of the Pathology Department of the University of Georgia School of Medicine:

Case 34,171.—Child died on the eighth day with infection of the right hand; suppurative infection of the umbilical stump; thrombophlebitis of the umbilical vein and septic infarcts.

Case 30,125.—Child died on the twelfth day with thrombosis of the pulmonary and renal veins, associated with rachischisis and a suppurative meningitis.

Even the so-called marasmatic clots are exceedingly rare in infancy and occur associated with infections. Blackfan lists three cases in infancy, the youngest child, twelve days old, with "associated with a scalp infection."

Thrombosis and embolism are not conditions of infancy. Cases due to infection, in which fibrin formation is excessive, are rare, an opinion supported by Byers and Hass from their study of sinus thrombosis.

We find one exception to generalization that thrombi do not form except when infection exists. Bettinger presents a case of a child dying on the tenth day with a thrombus of the ductus arteriosus (ductus Botalli). There were no clinical signs except cyanosis and spasm. Suspected cerebral hemorrhage associated with a precipitate delivery was not shown at autopsy. There was no apparent infection. Despite this one case, the conclusion seems to be justified that intravascular clotting in abandoned fetal channels does not occur, and we may next pass to a search for a rational explanation as to why it does not occur.

Many studies have shown an increased coagulation time in the infant. (Rodda, Lucas and associates). This period lasts approximately ten to fifteen days—well beyond the normal limits of the functional abandonment of the various fetal channels. Scammon and Norris have shown that in 2 per cent the ductus arteriosus is completely obliterated at from eight to fifteen days. In 18 per cent the ductus venosus is no longer patent at from eight to fifteen days. While complete obliteration in the remainder of cases may extend well into the first year, functional abandonment of the various channels is practically simultaneous with birth. Flow through these vessels then is practically nil, and flow is one of the four main factors postulated by Aschoff as necessary for the growth of thrombi by accretion of new platelets.

Hydrodynamics, however, are not the main factors involved since fibrinous coagulation fails to occur in the same way that it fails to occur between two ligatures placed on either artery or vein unless the ligatures are septic (Fourmestreux). Included erythrocytes remain discrete and intact or are hemolyzed and absorbed. There is no organization of clot as may occur in the adult. This is in keeping with the observed fact that extravasations into the brain, due to birth injuries, show no fibrin and are rarely organized. Levinson and Saphir have emphasized this point when they state that 9 per cent of all newborn show hemorrhage but very few show permanent defects resulting therefrom.

It will also be noted that increased coagulation time extends well beyond the normal limits for the time of the dropping of the cord. The latter event occurs generally on the fourth or fifth day and rarely as late as the fifteenth, unless infection exists. We believe that the conclusion is justified that increased coagulation time noted in infancy is not incidental but that it exists as a part of the mechanism which provides against thrombus formation during the period when the abandonment of fetal channels would constitute a serious embolic threat.

Many studies have been instituted in an attempt to associate increased coagulation time with the marked hemolysis and bilirubinemia noted in the first ten days of life. Mitchell reports an indirect van den Bergh in all children under fourteen days of age. Bonar claims that the icterus index reaches the birth level at the end of the twelfth day. Lucas and his coworkers claim that the bilirubinemia increases as the coagulation time increases. The degree of jaundice, however, has no essential part in the mechanism but is purely incidental. Ylppö has reviewed the various theories responsible for the cause of the bilirubinemia. It is generally considered normal although it may become pathologic.

Regarding the mechanism of clotting in the infant, Whipple has shown an increase in antithrombin. Lucas has pointed out the fact that the blood of the newborn shows no defect in retraction of clot in vitro and that no fibrinolysis occurs. The number of platelets are normal (Leslie and Sanford). Gelston reviewed the subject in 1921. Lucas thinks that the prolonged coagulation time is due to a platelet defect as in hemophilia. It is also generally held that bile pigments are marked anticoagulants, and hence the delayed clotting is due to the bilirubinemia since calcium is rendered inert by the bile pigments (Whipple).

Whether or not we accept this conclusion, the bilirubinemia of infancy appears to be not a part of a pathological process, but a part of the normal mechanism (either cause or effect) which prevents thrombus formation during the critical period of vascular adjustment associated with birth.

The hypothesis here offered correlates a whole series of hitherto obscure and isolated events: (1) increased coagulation time; (2) bilirubinemia; (3) time of dropping of the cord; (4) time of abandonment of the fetal vascular channels; (5) absence of thrombi in such channels; and (6) absence of emboli except when infection exists. It affords a rational theoretical protective mechanism against the dangers of embolism during the period when the vascular bed is subject to the greatest amount of normal physiological insult.

REFERENCES

Aschoff, L.: Arch. Int. Med. **12**: 503, 1913.
Bettinger, H.: Centralbl. f. allg. Path. u. path. Anat. **54**: 287, 1932.
Blackfan, K. D.: Abt's Pediatrics **7**: 411, 1924, Saunders & Co.
Bonar, B. E.: Am. J. Dis. Child. **50**: 1143, 1935.
Byers, L. K., and Hass, G. M.: Am. J. Dis. Child. **45**: 1161, 1933.
Fourmestreux, A.: Arch. gén. de. chir. **1**: 515, 1907.
Gelston, C. F.: Am. J. Dis. Child. **22**: 351, 1921.
Haberda, A.: Die fötalen Kreislaufwege des Neugeborenen, Wien, 1896.
Hedinger, C.: Cor.-Bl. f. schweiz. Aerzte. **37**: 521, 1907.
Krafka, Joseph, Jr.: Folia haemat. **43**: 318, 1931.
Leslie, E. I., and Sanford, H. N.: Am. J. Dis. Child. **51**: 590, 1936.
Levinson, A., and Saphir, O.: Am. J. Dis. Child. **45**: 973, 1933.
Limper, M. A., and Miller, A. J.: Am. J. Dis. Child. **50**: 1216, 1935.
Lucas, W. P., Dearing, B. F., Hoobler, H. P., Cox, A., Jones, M. K., Smyth, F. S.: Am. J. Dis. Child. **22**: 525, 1921.
MacCallum, W. G.: Textbook of Pathology, Philadelphia, 1916, Saunders & Co.
Melka, J.: Anat. Anz. **111**: 348, 1926.
Meyer, A. W.: Am. J. Anat. **16**: 477, 1914.
Mitchell, J. McK.: Am. J. Dis. Child. **36**: 486, 1928.
Moschcowitz, E.: Proc. New York Path. Soc. **14**: 21, 1914.
Pöllot, W.: Histologisches Bau und Rückbildung des ductus Botali (Heidelberg), 1909.
Rodda, F. C.: Am. J. Dis. Child. **19**: 269, 1920.
Rothstein, J. L.: Am. J. Dis. Child. **49**: 1578, 1934.
Scammon, R. E.: Abt's Pediatrics **1**: 387, 1923.
Scammon, R. E., and Norris, E. H.: Anat. Rec. **15**: 165, 1918.
Shaeffer, J. P.: J. Exper. Med. **19**: 129, 1914.
Welch, W. H.: Allbutt's System of Medicine **6**: 697, 1910, The Macmillan Company.
Wells, G. H.: Chemical Pathology, Philadelphia, 1914, Saunders & Co.
Wheler, E.: Canad. M. A. J. **11**: 532, 1921.
Whipple, G.: Arch. Int. Med. **12**: 617, 1913.
Wiggers, C. J.: Abt's Pediatrics **4**: 198, 1923.
Ylppö, A.: Ztschr. f. Kinderh. **8**: 208, 1913.

AN OUTLINE OF THE PEDIATRIST'S RELATION TO MENTAL HYGIENE

C. A. Aldrich, M.D., Winnetka, Ill., and Borden S. Veeder, M.D., St. Louis, Mo.

IN SPITE of, or perhaps because of, the growing literature about mental hygiene in childhood, there is still considerable confusion as to the relative function of pediatrists and psychiatrists in this field. We quite agree with the viewpoint expressed last year before this Society by Dr. Crothers, that the "care of the whole child" is too large an order for any one man. In the present set-up the care of children must be participated in by physicians, nurses, psychiatrists, school-teachers, and all others whose businesses in life bring them in contact with children, the parents assuming the ultimate responsibility. We feel, however, that in his use of the term "whole child" he somewhat misinterpreted pediatric opinion in the matter, as we know of none who think that the entire responsibility for the welfare of children should rest in the physician's hands. Those who have stressed the importance of mental hygiene, education, and community life in the field of pediatrics have done so because they have felt that the children's specialist must look upon the child as a whole, not simply as a physical organism, and because they have been sensitive to the importance of environmental factors aside from disease as influences upon growth and development. It is a matter of fact that the "whole child" is influenced profoundly by the pediatrist, whether or not he intends to impress himself outside of the physical sphere.

In view of the rather loose discussions in recent years, it has seemed to us that a more explicit definition of the actual function of physicians in mental hygiene is needed. It is the purpose of this paper to present in outline form what may be considered proper fields of endeavor for the pediatrist.

We would immediately insist that in dealing with the problem as it exists today, the major effort of the pediatrist should be preventive. Physicans might be so well trained that they could treat serious psychiatric problems efficiently, but, since the rank and file are not so trained today, it would be an obvious error to advocate their assumption of this important service. The situation in the field of prevention, however, is entirely different. The pediatrist is the only physician who sees many children at a time in their lives when prophylaxis is applicable. Because of his unique opportunity and because preventive measures are

Presented before the annual meeting of the American Pediatric Society, Bolton Landing, N. Y., June 11-13, 1936.

not difficult technically, the children's specialist may reasonably be expected to undertake this most important task, during infancy and early childhood at least. Either he must accept this responsibility intelligently, or the whole matter will be relegated to chance.

In order to make their influence felt most forcefully, there should be unity in ideals and in technic so that physicians can present a more united front than is possible at present. Such unity can only be attained after careful consultation between representatives of the groups most interested, physicians, psychiatrists, and educators. The following outline is intended to list, merely, the subjects which seem most important to us.

I. Predominantly Physical Topics With Psychological Effects.

A. Habit formation. In some cases a transfer of subcortical reflexes to cortical control. The optimum age for training in each case must be considered.

1. Appetite.
2. Sleep.
3. Bowel and bladder control.
4. Physical skills.
5. Play.
6. Personal hygiene.

B. Associations with ill children. Bedside technic, pain, fear of doctor, suggestion, etc.

1. Treatment of disease.
2. Physically handicapped.
3. Fatigue.

C. Mental subnormalities on a physical basis. Possibilities for care at home and in schools.

1. Mongolism, cretinism, microcephaly, etc.
2. Brain injuries, hemorrhage, trauma, inflammation, etc.

D. Functional disturbances on a physical basis. Educational opportunities and our advice.

1. Reading and speech difficulties due to mixed cerebral dominance.

II. Predominantly Psychologic Topics With Physical Effects.

A. Emotions. Important in habit formation and personality development.

1. Fear.
2. Love.
3. Anger.
4. Hate.
5. Sorrow.

B. Conventionally unacceptable habits. The physician's opportunity in prevention and early treatment.

1. Lying.
2. Stealing.
3. Masturbation.
4. Thumbsucking.
5. Stammering.
6. Nail biting.
7. Tics.
8. Disturbed sleep.
9. Daydreaming.
10. Heterosexual activities.
11. Disorderliness and uncleanliness.
12. Temper tantrums.

C. Relation to society. From birth the physician must understand the complexity of the child's problem.

1. Negativism.
2. Pathologic attachment to mother and nurse.
3. Antisocial behavior.

D. Intellectual attainment. Physician must be able to give an approximate opinion.

1. Precocity.
2. Mental retardation.

E. Motor states. Physician must recognize types in order to fit individual into environment.

1. Hypermotility.
2. Hypomotility.

F. Adolescence. Understanding of major psychologic processes at this time.

III. Environmental Factors Modifying Development.

A. Education. Of major importance in physical and personality development.

1. Parent.
2. Nurse or nursemaid.
3. Physician.
4. Child's school.

B. Relation to other children in family. May be the cause of abnormal behavior in children.

C. Playmates.

D. Socio-economic factors. Perhaps the most important modern consideration in physical and mental health.

A discussion of all of these items would obviously require a text. However, in order to illustrate, we are selecting a few subjects for brief expansion.

It will require but few words before this Society to demonstrate that the child who has been so handled in relation to eating that he emerges from infancy with a pronounced aversion for food has suffered severe psychic trauma. Regardless of the cause of his anorexia or of the methods that have been used, such a child has been deprived of one of the basic pleasures of life. Good mental hygiene does not include such deprivation in its plan. But, serious as this aspect of the problem may be, it often becomes a minor consideration in the tense situations which too frequently arise. Children are still being browbeaten, threatened, and even literally forced and whipped into eating. Others are so pampered in efforts to secure ingestion of food that they become veritable tyrants in the family life. The bad psychic effects produced by these situations are too obvious to require elaboration. Any competent psychiatrist recognizes that such backgrounds are major causes of psychologic difficulties in older children and adults. It is the experience of the authors that anorexia is easily preventable except in rare instances of chronic physical disease; hence its prevalence is a direct challenge to us, an urgent demand that prophylactic measures be applied more widely.

Negativism is another type of abnormal mental reaction frequently encountered in developing children. In a sense it is the product of the child's awareness of his own individuality times the violence of external forces applied against it. Our attitude toward the child strongly influences these external forces. It is an easy matter for the pediatrist to recognize, even in early infancy, the type of baby who will be particularly resistant to coercion. The parents of such infants should be taught a tolerant attitude toward the growth and development of their babies so that they may learn to recognize in this exaggerated defense mechanism a trait which may be of extreme value to the individual later on and so that they may be reasonable in their early efforts at education. It should be explained to all parents that children face a tremendous task in developing from almost entirely egocentric animals at birth into quite reasonable members of society by two years of age. They should be shown that it is the function of adults to smooth the way rather than to make it more difficult by lack of respect for the child's individuality. It is our experience that the negativistic type of child is infinitely more worth while than his conforming neighbor, for the reason that he values himself more highly. In the prevalence of unhappiness in this type of patient, the pediatrist must recognize an appeal for preventive endeavor.

As an example of what we mean by the pediatrist's rôle in prevention, we may cite as an illustration mixed cerebral dominance. While this outline was being discussed between us, one of us was called to see a five-year-old child with a cold. The cold was of no importance, but it was noted that the child was uncertain as to which hand to use in drawing. On going deeper into the matter, it was found the child could spell her name by picking letters from blocks but wrote her name forward or backward, the direction seeming to make little difference to her. Thus a serious fault was accidentally discovered and proper measures outlined as to her training and education—even to a change in the choice of schools which the parents had selected, on account of the methods used in teaching reading. Thus a purely "medical visit" for a condition of little and transitory importance led to the discovery of a serious condition and, we hope, to a plan which will in all probability avoid serious maladjustment in a few years. It was not our function to reeducate and retrain the child, but to plan a system of education and training which would avoid difficulties arising from mixed cerebral dominance. Experience has shown that when such a condition is unrecognized, early educational difficulties are almost sure to arise and that these frequently end in behavior problems which require the psychiatrist in their treatment.

All the items listed in the outline could be considered in a similar manner. The intelligence of our response to the call for prevention will be, in a measure, dependent upon our respect for and knowledge of the physical and mental growth and development of children.

THE PRESENCE OF THE MENINGOCOCCUS IN THE NASOPHARYNX OF NORMAL INDIVIDUALS, AND THE BACTERICIDAL PROPERTY OF BLOOD AGAINST THE MENINGOCOCCUS

NELLES SILVERTHORNE, M.B.
TORONTO, ONTARIO

DURING epidemics of meningococcic meningitis many authors have reported high contact carrier rates. However, the presence of carriers has also been found during interepidemic periods. In 1931 Cameron[1] demonstrated four carriers in a group of twenty-nine persons swabbed, all of whom were in the same building. None of these individuals had been in contact with cases of meningitis. One of these individuals was still found to be a carrier one year later. In 1934 Rake[2] discovered carriers of the meningococcus in healthy individuals. Dudley and Brennan[3] in 1935 found a non-contact carrier rate as high as 60 per cent in a naval and military population.

As these observations are of practical importance to the pediatrician, during the past two years we have studied the carrier rate in a noncontact population. As it is also relevant to assess the importance of certain immune reactions in the blood of individuals who may be harboring strains of the meningococcus, we have investigated the bactericidal property of the blood of normal individuals and of noncontact carriers against various strains of meningococci.

TECHNIC

West tube swabs were taken of the posterior nasopharynx, planted, and spread on dextrose blood agar plates. The plates were incubated at 37° C. for twenty-four to forty-eight hours, and colonies were picked and examined microscopically. Cultures of these colonies were planted in carbohydrate media containing dextrose, maltose, and saccharose. A suspension of each culture was tested with polyvalent antimeningococcus serum. All strains isolated were found to be gram-negative diplococci and produced acid in dextrose and maltose but not in saccharose. They agglutinated with polyvalent antimeningococcus serum.

RESULTS

Previous to the present study we had isolated meningococci from 16 carriers in a group of 125 medical students. During the last two

---

From the wards and laboratories of the Hospital for Sick Children, the Department of Paediatrics and the Connaught Laboratories, University of Toronto.

Presented before the Forty-Eighth Annual Meeting of the American Pediatric Society in joint session with the Canadian Society for the Study of Diseases of Children, at Bolton Landing, N. Y., June 11-13, 1936.

years of this study, 63 healthy adults mainly physicians and technicians were swabbed at approximately monthly intervals. In all, 1,227 swabs were taken over the two-year period. No less than 243 were positive for the meningococcus. The percentage of the total positive swabs taken was 19.8. The monthly percentage of positive individuals varied between 16 and 28, with an average of 20. For the two-year period, of the 63 healthy adults tested, no less than 26, or 41 per cent, showed the presence of the meningococcus in the nasopharynx at one time or another. In these 26 individuals, 11 were shown to be harboring the meningococcus fairly persistently. Thirteen carried the meningococcus intermittently, and in 2 instances cultures of the meningococcus were obtained on only one occasion. It was also noted that there was either a complete absence or a marked reduction in the colonies of meningococci when swabs were taken during an acute upper respiratory infection in any given individual. These findings are in general agreement with those reported by Rake.[2]

In 1934 Silverthorne and Fraser[4] demonstrated that samples of blood from many adults contained bactericidal power to a recently isolated strain of the meningococcus. Other adults and infants failed to manifest this property in their blood. These authors further showed that two infants with meningitis possessed relatively little or no bactericidal power in samples of their blood at the onset of the disease, but developed it after recovery. It was also shown that strains of meningococci vary in their ability to thrive in a sample of blood containing no bactericidal power when measured against a "virulent" spinal fluid strain. A "virulent" strain is one that is lethal to mice in the more diluted suspensions in the mouse-mucin test.[7] These findings furnish one with two facts, first, that strains of meningococci vary in their power to "invade" a nonbactericidal sample of human blood and, second, that individuals possess varying amounts of the bactericidal principle in their blood against virulent meningococci. In 1935 we[5] found that the bactericidal principle was present in serum or plasma and depended on the presence of complement for its action. We also demonstrated the specificity of the bactericidal power of blood against the meningococcus and were able to produce this property in the blood of guinea pigs by vaccination with recently isolated virulent cerebrospinal fluid strains. Recently, we[6] have explored and extended some of these observations. The relation of the bactericidal power of blood to the virulence of the microorganism has been studied. Using as a control test a previously known nonbactericidal sample of blood, and a virulent recently isolated cerebrospinal fluid strain of the meningococcus, we demonstrated that samples of blood from five carriers were bactericidal to this virulent strain and to each of the five carrier strains. One might suppose from these findings that carriers possess bactericidal property in their blood which has been developed due to the continued presence of the meningococcus in their nasopharynx. Most of the samples of blood from carriers which were tested possessed this property to certain virulent spinal fluid strains. We also demonstrated that the power of meningococci to invade a nonbactericidal sample of blood was, in general, parallel to the virulence of strains as judged on the basis of the mouse-mucin test of Miller. By the use of the mouse-mucin test and the bactericidal test, eleven noncontact carrier strains were examined. Three of these proved to be as virulent as any of the recently isolated spinal fluid strains, and the remaining eight strains proved to be avirulent. In later studies, strains both from spinal fluid and noncontact carriers were found to be in a "midposition" in respect of virulence, and one spinal fluid strain was avirulent as judged by the results of these tests. This latter finding may be due to the lack of the rapid subculturing on suitable media of this strain before being received. Samples of blood obtained from two of the three carriers of virulent nasopharyngeal strains had marked bactericidal power to their respective strains; the third was not tested.

CONCLUSIONS

1. A total of 1,227 swabs were taken from 63 normal healthy adults over a two-year period; 19.8 per cent of these were positive for the meningococcus.

2. Sixty-three individuals were swabbed at approximately monthly intervals. On these monthly examinations the number of positive individuals varied from 16 to 28 per cent. No less than 41 per cent of the group of 63 were positive at one time or another during the two-year period. Eleven individuals were persistent, 13 intermittent, and 2 transient carriers.

3. Eleven noncontact carrier strains were examined by the bactericidal and mouse-mucin tests; 3 of these strains were found to be virulent, and 8 were found to be avirulent.

4. Carriers of the meningococcus possess bactericidal power in their blood to their respective strains whether these strains are virulent or avirulent. Also, samples of blood from carriers possess bactericidal power to certain virulent cerebrospinal fluid strains.

5. The determination of the virulence of strains of meningococci by means of the mouse-mucin and bactericidal tests may serve as a useful means of selecting strains for the preparation of therapeutic serum.

REFERENCES

1. Cameron, D. W.: Tr. Roy Soc. Canad., Sec. V. **9**: 97, 1931.
2. Rake, G.: J. Exper. Med. **59**: 553, 1934.
3. Dudley, S. F., and Brennan, J. R.: J. Hyg. **34**: 525, 1935.
4. Silverthorne, N., and Fraser, D. T.: Brit. J. Exper. Path. **15**: 362, 1934.
5. Silverthorne, N., and Fraser, D. T.: J. Immunol. **29**: 6, 1935.
6. Silverthorne, N., and Fraser, D. T.: (In press.)
7. Miller, C. P.: Science **78**: 340, 1933.

MEDIASTINAL LYMPHOSARCOMAS IN CHILDHOOD

F. W. Wiglesworth, M.D., A. E. Childe, M.D., and
Alton Goldbloom, M.D.
Montreal, Canada

INTRODUCTION

TO THE pediatrician malignant tumors of childhood bring to mind the Wilms' tumors of the kidney, the retinoblastomas of the eye, the neuroblastomas of the adrenals, and lymphosarcomas. The latter are usually associated with the intestinal and cervical tumors rather than the mediastinal group. However, the mediastinal lymphosarcomas are the commonest form of massive mediastinal enlargement in children (Cooke[1]) and perhaps the commonest form of lymphosarcoma. In six hundred fifty autopsies over a six-year period at the Children's Memorial Hospital there were only four cases of malignant tumors of lymphoid tissue. Two were mediastinal, and of the other two, one was situated in the cervical glands and the other in the lymphoid tissue of the ileum. In this paper we wish to present the clinical, roentgenologic, and pathologic findings in three cases of mediastinal lymphosarcoma. These cases appear to be of sufficient interest and rarity to be worth while reporting.

CASE I: CLINICAL AND LABORATORY NOTES

J. K. (Case 692-36), aged six years, was admitted to the Medical Service of the Children's Memorial Hospital on Jan. 8, 1936.

Complaints.—Lethargy and anorexia.

History.—The child had been seen one month previously by his physician when nothing remarkable was found in the physical examination of the chest. Two days before admission his physician was called to see him for the above complaints and found flatness over the entire chest, front and back, with displacement of the heart and trachea to the left. There was no respiratory distress. In the absence of fever, a tentative diagnosis of tuberculous pleurisy with effusion was made. The child was admitted to the hospital where the tuberculin test was found to be negative.

Several attempts at thoracentesis gave no results.

White blood cells numbered 8,050; polymorphonuclear leucocytes, 55 per cent; lymphocytes, 40 per cent; eosinophiles, 1 per cent; monocytes, 3 per cent; basophiles, 1 per cent. The urine was normal.

Roentgenologic Findings.—A chest film taken on admission revealed increased density throughout the right chest, associated with slight displacement of the heart and trachea to the left. Very little mediastinal enlargement was demonstrated (Fig. 1). A lateral view showed that the increased density was situated in the anterior part of the right chest, and that it was bounded posteriorly by a discrete convex

From the Children's Memorial Hospital.

Presented before a joint meeting of the American Pediatric Society and the Canadian Society for the Study of Diseases of Children. Bolton Landing, N. Y., June 12, 1936.

border (Fig. 2). There was also evidence of a small amount of free fluid in the right pleural cavity. Calcification was visible in the region of the right hilus, and a small calcified area, apparently a Ghon tubercle, was present, fairly well lateral in the lung, opposite the third interspace anteriorly. Fluoroscopic examination showed the displacement of the heart and trachea to be greater during expiration than during inspiration.

Fig. 1. Fig. 2.

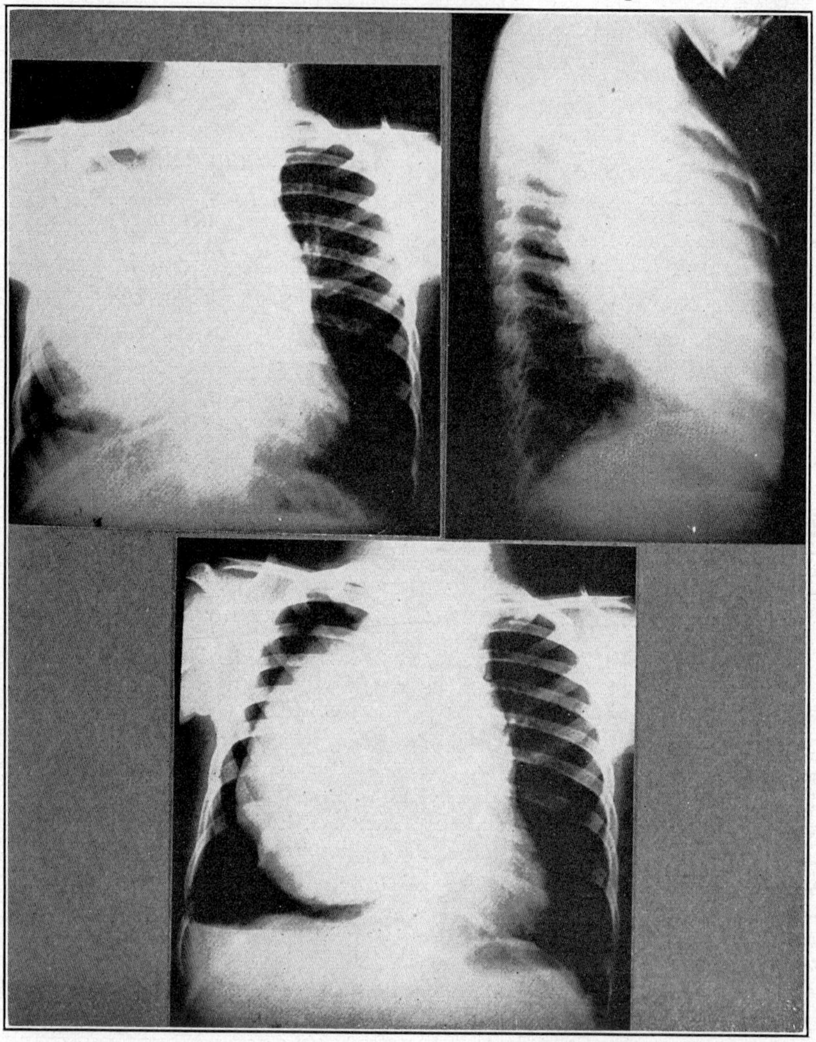

Fig. 3.

Fig. 1.—Case 1. Radiograph of chest on admission, showing right-sided increased density, and slight displacement of heart and trachea to left. The original film reveals calcification.

Fig. 2.—Case 1. Lateral view of chest on admission. The increased density is situated anteriorly.

Fig. 3.—Case 1. Appearance of chest following right-sided pneumothorax.

Reexamination of the chest one week later following the introduction of 80 c.c. of air into the right pleural cavity confirmed the presence of a small amount of free fluid on the right side. It also showed a large dense mass occupying the anterior portion of the right chest. This mass measured approximately 8 by 13 cm. in diameter and its margins were quite discrete (Fig. 3).

The roentgenologic findings suggested a diagnosis of mediastinal tumor. Dr. F. A. C. Scrimger, surgeon-in-chief to the hospital, who saw the child in consultation, advised its removal. Operation was performed Jan. 17, 1936, under avertin and gas. The following is the operation report:

"One came upon a large, solid, tumor mass. It was up against the chest wall. The tumor was densely adherent to the lung, the whole of which was collapsed due to pressure of the tumor and was displaced laterally and posteriorly. The tumor itself was about the size of two fists and was encapsulated, the capsule being adherent to the chest wall and to the lung itself. A pedicle was felt which ran to the mediastinum. This was freed, thus liberating the tumor which was delivered into the wound. The pedicle of the tumor was then cut and removed. The tumor itself, on cutting into it, consisted of semisolid material and resembled grossly a sarcoma. Following removal of the tumor, the patient's condition appeared very poor, respiration stopping and the pulse growing very feeble. The lungs, however, were expanded artificially by means of a bag and intratracheal tube, and respiration was resumed after about five minutes. The child's condition then became poor, and, although artificial respiration was resorted to, he died before leaving the operating table."

Pathologic Findings.—Gross: The specimen, which was removed surgically, consisted of a large, somewhat pyramid-shaped mass weighing 470 gm. It measured 14 cm. from base to apex, 14 cm. in diameter at the base and 7 cm. in diameter at the apex. The capsule consisted of a thin veil of tissue in which there were areas of marked thickening. The point of excision could be seen as a break in the capsule through which tumor substance protruded. The cut surface presented a uniform yellowish white encephaloid appearance. A few, small, scattered hemorrhages were present throughout the tumor, and centrally there were streaks of bright yellow. A few indefinite septums radiated centrally for a short distance from the periphery.

The autopsy (A-36-9) was performed four hours after death and was limited to the removal of the thoracic and abdominal organs through the surgical incision. For this reason the relationship of the various viscera could not be accurately ascertained.

At the cephalic end of the mediastinum a stub of tumor tissue was found, to which the mass removed surgically had been attached. On the left side of the trachea in this region, there was a flat piece of tissue which grossly appeared to be the left lobe of the thymus. The paratracheal lymph nodes on both sides were enlarged to twice their normal size, were discrete and obviously infiltrated with neoplastic tissue. Both lungs were collapsed and congested. In the anterolateral portion of the upper lobe of the right lung, there was a subpleural, encapsulated, calcified nodule 0.3 cm. in diameter. Grossly this was a Ghon tubercle. In the hilus of the right lung there was a large caseous partially calcified lymph gland adherent to a neighboring bronchus. The remainder of the hilar glands on both sides was normal. No gross lesion could be seen in the left lung. Both pleural cavities were normal.

The anterior pericardium about the root of the aorta showed several large, thin, plaquelike masses extending down from the mediastinum. The pericardial sac contained a normal amount of fluid which, as far as could be made out, was not hemorrhagic. The tumor did not extend behind the pericardium.

The liver weighed 548 gm. as compared with the normal 642 gm. It showed no gross change. The spleen weighed 78 gm. (normal 58 gm.). The cut surface of the spleen was bright red and somewhat soft with the lymphoid nodules standing out prominently. The gastrointestinal tract showed no change except for a marked prominence of the submucosal lymphoid tissue in the region of the ileocecal junction. The mesenteric and the retroperitoneal lymph glands, the myocardium, and the kidneys were normal.

Microscopic: Tissues were fixed in Zenker formol and formalin, embedded in paraffin and stained by differential methods. The sections from the surgical specimen showed most of the essential features of the tumor. They presented a strikingly uniform picture consisting of sheets of medium sized lymphocytic cells dotted at irregular intervals by larger pale staining cells (Fig. 4).

Some sections showed wide collagenous septums with finer strands branching off from these. They bore a distinct resemblance to the septums of the normal thymus gland. In one area, just beneath the capsule, were several small lobules separated by wide strands of connective tissue. These contained Hassall's corpuscles and were undoubtedly thymic tissue. The lobules were, however, completely replaced by tumor cells, which did not invade the surrounding connective tissue (Fig. 5).

Examination of a large series of sections showed the presence of a few normal and atrophic Hassall's corpuscles throughout the tumor. Many of these had almost completely disappeared, apparently as a result of invasion by the surrounding tumor

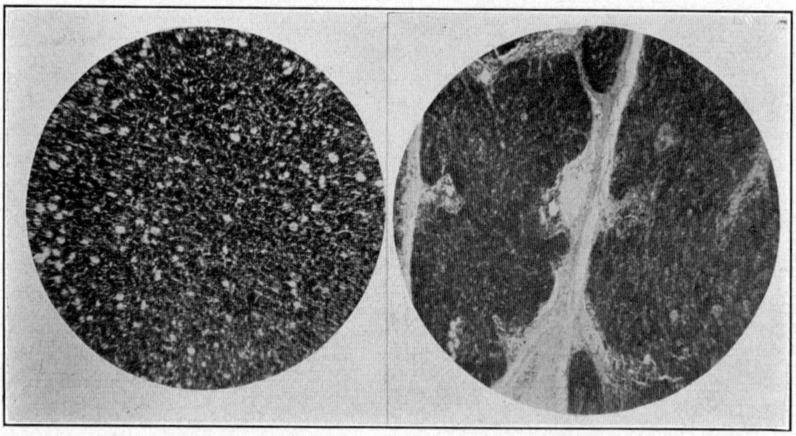

Fig. 4. Fig. 5.

Fig. 4.—Case 1. Low power photomicrograph showing tumor cells. Dotted at irregular intervals are pale staining reticular cells. Hemalum, erythrosin, and saffron stain.

Fig. 5.—Case 1. Low power photomicrograph showing thymic lobules at the periphery of the surgical specimen replaced by tumor cells which do not invade the trabeculae. Several pale staining Hassall's corpuscles can be seen surrounded by malignant cells. Hemalum, erythrosin, and saffron stain.

cells. The presence of fairly numerous eosinophilic leucocytes also served to identify this tissue as being originally thymus. The tumor cells themselves were of the medium-sized lymphocytic type. The nucleus was round, large, and more vesicular than the small lymphocyte, and contained a good deal of deeply staining chromatin, the amount of which varied somewhat from cell to cell (Fig. 6). The majority of the cells showed no visible cytoplasm, but a few had a narrow strip of nongranular, basophilic cytoplasm at one pole. There was, as a rule, one, but sometimes two, acidophilic nucleoli.

The most interesting feature of the sections was the presence of groups of closely packed cells which under low magnification gave the impression of staining more deeply than the remainder of the tumor cells. On oil-immersion examination, they appeared to have no cytoplasm, and their nuclei were actually larger and more vesicular than the type cell of the tumor. The depth of staining was due to their being so tightly packed. Mitotic figures in these foci were very numerous as compared with the rest of the tumor (Fig. 7). There was a gradual transition in differentiation from the primitive cell areas into the surrounding more differentiated, more loosely packed tumor cells. These areas lay mostly beneath the capsule or in close contact with the collagenous septums. Like the germinal centers of the lymph nodes, they contained relatively few reticulum fibers as compared with the remainder of the tumor. As will be seen later, in the left lobe of the thymus, these primitive cell areas were the actively growing foci of the tumor.

The peculiar pale cells noted under low power magnification (Figs. 4 and 6) were round or branched, were wedged between the lymphocytes, and had nuclei which were mostly round or oval with scanty fine chromatin granules and one nucleolus, although many were pyknotic. The cytoplasm was acidophilic and contained numerous tiny vacuoles and a few basophilic granules. These cells, which were separated from each other by tumor cells, were numerous in some areas and scarce in others. They were present in both the primitive and differentiated cell areas. The vacuoles contained neutral fat droplets as shown by the scharlach R stain. These cells were obviously not fat cells, showed no evidence of activity, and

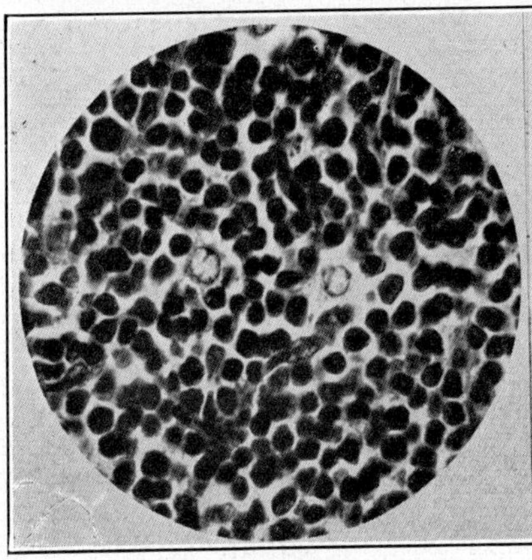

Fig. 6.

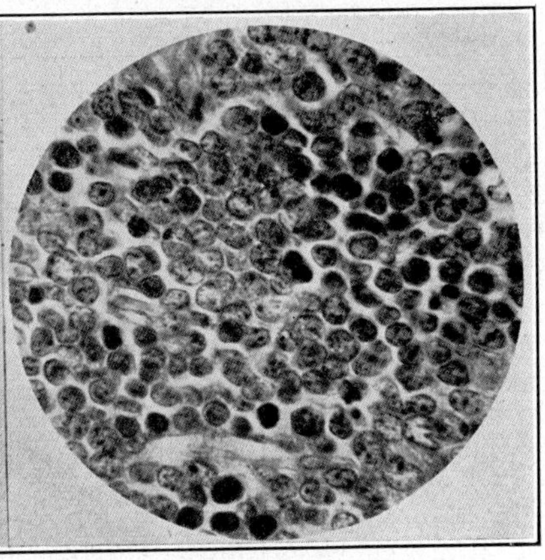

Fig. 7.

Fig. 6.—Case 1. Oil immersion photomicrograph of tumor cells. Stain used does not demonstrate the vesicular appearance of the nuclei. Note the two reticular cells in the center of the picture. Compare this photograph with Fig. 7. Iron hematoxylin, Ponceau fuchsin, aniline blue stain.

Fig. 7.—Case 1. Same magnification and section as Fig. 6. This shows the cells of the primitive cell areas. Note the size, the vesicular character of the nuclei, and the numerous mitotic figures as compared with Fig. 6. Iron hematoxylin, Ponceau fuchsin, aniline blue stain.

did not appear to be taking any part in the tumor process. They were, in fact, the reticular cells of the thymus and appeared to be degenerating, as shown by the fatty droplets in the cytoplasm and the pyknotic nuclei.

In the sections of the tumor from the postmortem, the cell type was essentially the same as that in the surgical specimen referred to above. The mass on the left side of the trachea was in part thymus. Although it was extensively infiltrated by tumor cells, it had retained its lobulated structure, and the cortex and medulla could be distinctly made out. Besides a few Hassall's corpuscles in the medulla, these two were differentiated by the presence of numerous primitive cell areas in the cortex (Fig. 8), exactly similar to those seen in the surgical specimen. The medulla contained only the differentiated type of tumor cell. The same gradation between the two areas was present as was seen in the surgical specimen.

It would seem that the neoplastic process had originated in the cortex with subsequent involvement and replacement of the medulla by the lymphosarcomatous process. The capsule of the left lobe was slightly infiltrated but was intact, except at one point where the tumor had broken through it and extended into the surrounding connective tissue.

Laidlaw's reticulum stain of the sections from the left lobe of the thymus showed a slight but definite increase in reticulum. This, in the normal thymic tissue, is very scanty and is mostly situated about blood vessels with almost none of the cortex. As in the normal gland, the reticulum was coarse both in the left lobe and in the main mass of the tumor in the right lobe.

The plaques noted grossly in connection with the parietal pericardium contained tumor cells. The inner surface of the pericardium was indicated by an irregular deposit of fibrin and red blood cells and an occasional cell of the serosal type. The opposite aspect of these plaques showed a thin collagenous layer, which was thymic capsule, for just within it was a zone of primitive tumor cells, similar to those previously described. The inner half of the plaque contained loosely arranged tumor cells and capillaries with a few strands of elastic tissue. These latter were probably remnants of the elastic tissue of the parietal pericardium. This section

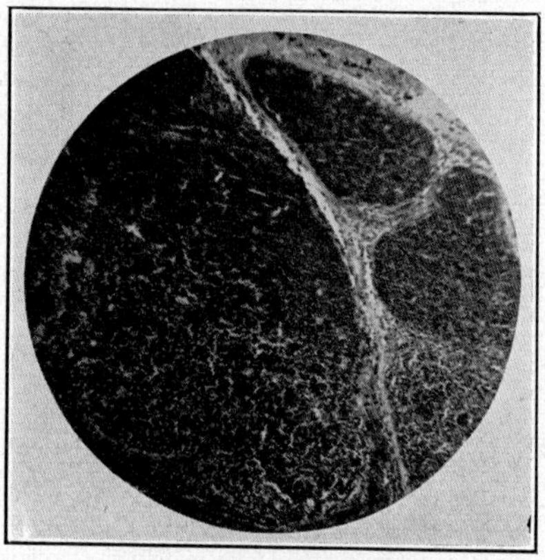

Fig. 8.—Low power photomicrograph of capsule, cortex and medulla of the left lobe of the thymus. Note the densely staining primitive cell areas (for cell character, Fig. 7) in the cortex (top of photograph). Hemalum, erythrosin, and saffron stain.

clearly illustrates the reason for the early involvement of the parietal pericardium in thymic lymphosarcomas. It is a result of the involvement of that part of the thymus which normally overlaps the parietal pericardium about the root of the aorta. The frequent occurrence of hemorrhagic pericardial effusion in thymic tumors is explained by the extension of tumor cells from the overlying thymus into the parietal pericardium.

The hilar lymph nodes of the lungs were normal. Most of the lung tissue was atelectatic and congested. The pleura of the right lung showed focal microscopic involvement by tumor cells associated with hemorrhages. This invasion was probably due to direct contact with the overlying tumor. A few bronchi in both lungs were infiltrated with small lymphocytes and plasma cells indicating mild peribronchitis. Many groups of alveoli and even small lobules showed a mild lipoid pneumonia. The alveolar walls were thickened, infiltrated by small lymphocytes and had an epithelial-like lining. This lymphocytic infiltration appeared to be inflammatory rather than neoplastic, as the cells were small, stained deeply, and showed no mitotic figures or nucleoli. The alveoli were filled with vacuolated macrophages.

The caseous gland in the right hilar region was encapsulated and partially calcified. It showed no definite histologic evidence of tuberculosis beyond an occasional Langerhan type of giant cell. The calcified lesion in the upper lobe of the right lung was encapsulated by a dense fibrous tissue wall and was apparently a healed primary tuberculous focus.

The lymph nodes of the mediastinum were largely replaced by sarcomatous cells, but their architecture was distinct and a few primary and secondary nodules were present. There was a mass on the right side of the trachea which was probably thymus, as it showed a few indefinite Hassall's corpuscles, reticular cells and eosinophilic leucocytes. The neighboring connective tissues were extenively infiltrated by tumor cells, as contrasted to the tissues about the lymph nodes which showed relatively little involvement. The arterial walls were intact, whereas the venous walls had been invaded by the tumor cells. As will be seen later, this vascular invasion had occurred to a greater degree in the second case.

The mesenteric lymph nodes, the grossly hyperplastic lymphoid tissue of the cecum and ileum and their associated lymph glands showed no change that could be called neoplastic. The lymph glands about the upper abdominal aorta were normal with one exception. This latter was no larger than the others but was completely replaced by sarcoma cells. The capsule was not invaded, and there was no increase in the reticulum, but these fibers were widely separated by tumor cells. Except for this fact which seemed to favor metastatic invasion, it was impossible to say whether this isolated lymph node neoplasia was part of a systemic process or a purely metastatic involvement. The superficial lymph nodes due to autopsy restrictions could not be examined.

The liver, the kidneys, the adrenals, and the pancreas were free from tumor. The malpighian corpuscles of the spleen were clearly defined and contained well-developed germinal centers. The red pulp was markedly congested and contained cells of the lymphoid series with a few neutrophilic and eosinophilic polymorphonuclear cells. There was no suggestion of a leucemic process.

The bone marrow of the costochondral junction showed definite changes which gave rise to some controversy in their interpretation. Under low magnification, the marrow was seen to be unusually cellular due to the presence of numerous deeply staining cells either scattered diffusely through the marrow or arranged in small foci. The deeper staining cells consisted of a dense staining nucleus with a fair amount of basophilic cytoplasm about it. These were erythroblasts and were associated with a few polychromatophile erythroblasts and normoblasts. Most of this cell activity appeared to be erythroblastic.

Comparison with the costochondral junction of a six-year-old child who died of a congenital cerebral lesion showed a marked similarity between the two sections but there was greater cellular activity in the tumor case. Nevertheless, there were cells present which closely resembled lymphocytes in that they had almost no cytoplasm and fairly dense nuclei with nucleoli. These looked more like small lymphocytes than neoplastic cells. However, a few similar cells could be seen in sections from ribs of normal cases. The myeloid elements appeared to be normal. The slides from the costochondral junction were shown to a number of pathologists, of whom all but one believed it to be erythroblastic. One considered that the marrow might be sarcomatous. We believe it to be erythroblastic.

Diagnosis.—Primary lymphosarcoma of the thymus gland with involvement of the mediastinal lymph nodes, the parietal pericardium, right pleura, and one small retroperitoneal lymph node. Erythroblastic activity of bone marrow.

CASE II: CLINICAL AND LABORATORY FINDINGS

B. C. (Case 3096-35), aged eleven years, was admitted to the Medical Service of the Children's Memorial Hospital on March 6, 1935.

Complaints.—Malaise for two weeks following a respiratory infection. Easy fatigability, disturbed sleep, and nervousness.

Past History.—At one year she weighed 22 pounds. Following pneumonia at one year of age she developed celiac disease and was treated at various clinics. She had had measles and chickenpox. At the age of five years she weighed 25 pounds. She did not walk until five years of age.

Family History.—Her father died seven years ago of tuberculosis. A brother, aged thirteen years, has a positive Mantoux reaction.

Examination on Admission.—The examination on admission showed the child was surprisingly well developed and well nourished. She showed no signs of discomfort. There were signs of fluid in the left chest with displacement of the heart and trachea to the right. Temperature was 99.8° F.; pulse, 85; respirations, 22. Red blood cells numbered 4,420,000; white blood cells, 12,000; hemoglobin, 80 per cent; and the differential count was as follows: Polymorphonuclear leucocytes, 30 per cent; lymphocytes, 61 per cent; eosinophiles, 2 per cent; monocytes, 3 per cent; myelocytes, 4 per cent.

The Mantoux test was positive.

March 7: Left chest was aspirated, and 700 c.c. of reddish brown fluid was obtained. This fluid on smear showed differential counts of 90 per cent large lymphocytes with 10 per cent polymorphonuclears. Inoculated guinea pigs died of generalized tuberculosis. Between March 7 and April 2 she received four blood transfusions, which, however, did not control a progressive anemia; by April 10 the blood count was as follows: Red blood cells, 1,400,000; white blood cells, 23,000; hemoglobin, 30 per cent.

April 17: Red blood cells, 2,080,000; white blood cells, 18,400.

April 21: White blood cells, 19,800.

April 24: Red blood cells, 2,180,000; white blood cells, 88,050; platelets, 30,000; reticulocytes, 2.3 per cent, hemoglobin, 40 per cent.

The differential count of leucocytes was as follows: Neutrophile polymorphonuclears, 24 per cent; lymphocytes, 4 per cent; eosinophiles, 1 per cent; myelocytes, 2 per cent; metamyelocytes, 3 per cent; myeloblasts, 33 per cent; and unclassified, 33 per cent. (These were probably myeloblasts, but lacked the characteristic nucleolus.)

Goodpasture's stain showed 78 per cent of the white cells to be oxidase negative.

Later, in view of the autopsy findings, these cells cannot be interpreted as myeloblasts, but rather as primitive lymphocytes. The lack of gradation of these cells into adult cells of the granular series is in favor of this. The nuclei of these cells were vesicular as compared to the normal blood lymphocyte, and many contained nucleoli, thus resembling the tumor cells.

The spleen became at this time just palpable, while the axillary glands appeared to be slightly enlarged to palpation. A small nodular mass was felt at the left costal margin, which was thought to be enlarged abdominal glands.

On May 1 she developed generalized purpura and died on May 3.

Roentgenologic Findings.—A radiograph of the chest taken on March 7, 1935, revealed definite displacement of the heart and trachea to the right, and an extensive collection of fluid in the left pleural cavity. A bubble of air was present at the left apex, this film having been made following the aspiration of a small amount of pleural fluid, and resultant leakage of air. No lung detail could be seen on the left side, with the exception of a dense area which occupied the medial portion of the left apex above the fluid level (Fig. 9).

Examination on April 1, 1935, revealed slightly more marked displacement of the heart and trachea to the right, and showed that the left chest was completely dense. Examinations at frequent intervals showed gradually increasing cardiac displacement and showed that the left chest remained opaque.

The final examination on April 29, 1935, was made in the upright position, following the introduction of a small amount of air into the left pleural cavity. This air did not travel up higher than the fourth interspace anteriorly. The heart and trachea were tremendously displaced to the right (Fig. 10).

When this child was first admitted to the hospital, the presence of signs of fluid in the chest, together with a history of exposure to a tuberculous father and the finding of a strongly positive Mantoux reaction, naturally led to an initial diagnosis of tuberculous pleurisy with effusion. The first demonstration of bloody pleural fluid, however, made one pause and give serious consideration to a diagnosis of thoracic neoplasm.

Pathologic Findings.—Gross: The autopsy (A-35-42) was performed sixteen hours after death. There were numerous subcutaneous petechial hemorrhages over the abdomen and chest. The superficial lymph nodes were not enlarged. To the

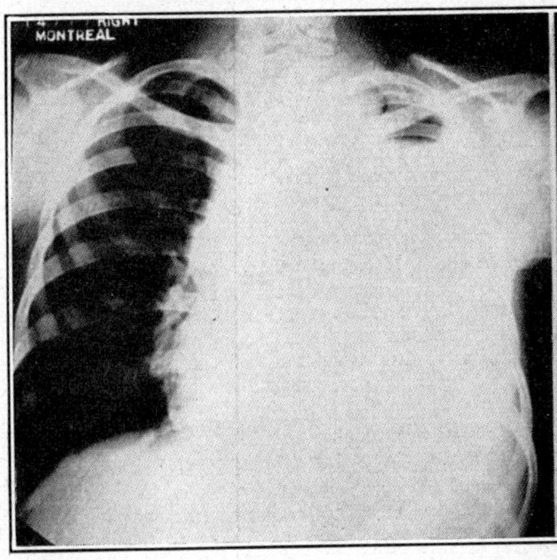

Fig. 9.

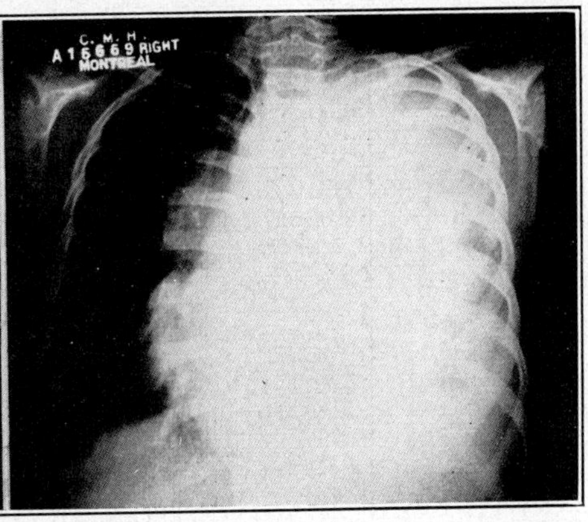

Fig. 10.

Fig. 9.—Case 2. Radiograph of chest following aspiration, showing left-sided fluid and air, a mass in the left upper medial chest, and cardiac displacement.

Fig. 10.—Case 2. Chest seven weeks after admission. The cardiac displacement has increased and air injected on the left side does not rise to the apex.

left of the sternum a diffuse nodular, slightly raised mass could be palpated just beneath the skin. On reflecting the skin of the chest, tumor tissue was encountered. This had reached the body surface by infiltration through the intercostal spaces to invade the muscles and the subcutaneous tissues. Upon opening the chest, the sternum in its upper half was adherent to a large hemorrhagic mass lying behind it.

This mass occupied the superior mediastinum, surrounded the trachea and the adjacent great vessels, had infiltrated and was adherent to the upper medial aspect and apex of the left lung (Fig. 11). Numerous large lymph nodes extended up from the apex of the tumor into the left anterior triangle of the neck. No trace of thymus could be found. The tumor involved the anterior surface and left lateral aspect of the parietal pericardium. A large hemorrhagic mass 3 cm. in thickness extended posteriorly to the pericardium as far down as the diaphragm. As a result of this, the heart was displaced to the right and ventrally. The trachea was displaced to the right of the vertebral column. The esophagus was similarly displaced to the right, but in its lower half it was also displaced anteriorly because of a chain of enlarged lymph glands lying behind it. These extended to the diaphragm. The pericardial sac contained 250 c.c. of thin hemorrhagic fluid. There were smooth, large tumor masses bulging through a grossly intact parietal pericardium. The visceral pericardium and myocardium showed no gross involvement.

The right lung showed nothing of note. A small caseous lymph gland was found at the bifurcation of the trachea. Three-quarters of the left lung resembled a piece of beefsteak, and grossly suggested extensive involvement with tumor. The medial quarter of the lower lobe was atelectatic, but its appearance did not suggest tumor involvement. The left pleura was thickened, and the pleural cavity was filled with a layer of blood clot 3 cm. thick.

The lymph glands of the celiac axis were about four times their normal size, adherent to each other and sarcomatous in appearance. The left adrenal was involved by direct extension from these glands. The involvement of the celiac glands appeared to have taken place by direct extension through the diaphragm. The retroperitoneal and mesenteric lymph glands were grossly normal.

On cross-section, the mediastinal tumor presented a uniformly hemorrhagic appearance with large, white nodules, 3 cm. in diameter, situated posteriorly and

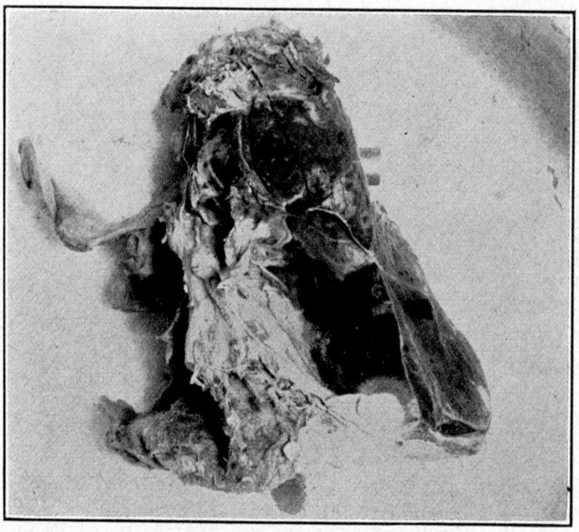

Fig. 11.—Case 2. Gross photograph of autopsy specimen. The mediastinal tumor is at the top of the photograph, part of the left lung can be seen to the right, while the posterior and left lateral aspect of the pericardial sac lies in the lower central portion of the photograph. The heart and anterior portion of the pericardial sac have been removed.

laterally. A few coarse trabeculae could be seen radiating into the tumor from the periphery. After removal of the pleura, masses of hemorrhagic tumor tissue could be seen plastered to the left side of the vertebral column and the posterior ends of the contiguous ribs.

The liver weighed 1,000 gm., as compared with the normal 909 gm. for this age. Its cut surface was yellowish and greasy, suggesting fatty infiltration. There was no evidence of tumor metastases. The spleen weighed 113 gm. as compared with the normal 87 gm. The cut surface was pale, and the pulp was firm to palpation. No nodules could be seen. The kidneys were grossly normal. The right adrenal was normal; the left adrenal was involved by direct extension from the glands of the celiac axis. The pelvic organs were normal.

The metaphysis of the right femur showed a firm white infarct measuring 1.4 cm. in length and 0.8 cm. in width. The metaphysis of the right tibia contained a more recent infarct in that it was soft and deep red in appearance. The surrounding marrow was deeply congested but not unduly soft, and there did not seem to be any decrease in the bony trabeculae. The marrow in the center of the femur was normal.

Microscopic: Tissues were fixed in Zenker and bichromate formol, embedded in paraffin, and stained by differential methods.

The main mass of the tumor and the lymph gland metastases consisted of a fairly uniform cell type. These cells resembled those of the previous case and were of the medium size lymphocytic type (Fig. 12). Most of them appeared to consist wholly of nuclei, but a few had a thin rim of basophilic cytoplasm. The nuclei were vesicular, but less so than reticular cells, and showed some variation in chromatin content. The majority contained one or more nucleoli. They were closely but not densely packed and showed only a few mitotic figures. In addition to the main cell type, there were a few isolated cells which contained more cytoplasm and a vesicular nucleus and which resembled reticular cells. In the connective tissue bands running through the tumor and in the thickened pleura, a few small lymphocytes and neutrophilic and eosinophilic polymorphonuclear cells were present. Numerous sections from the region of the thymus were cut before any trace of thymic

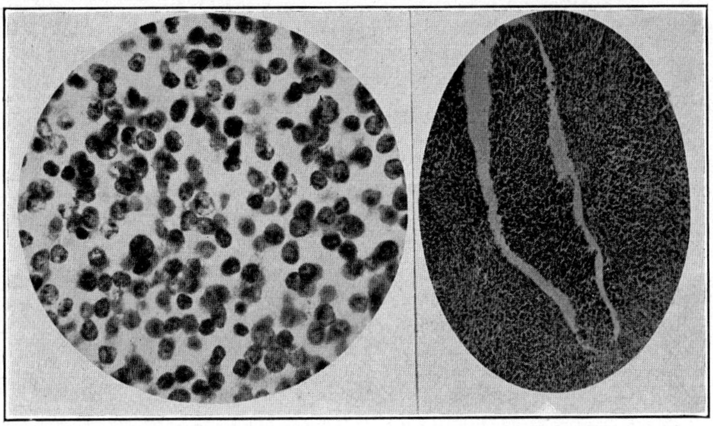

Fig. 12. Fig. 13.

Fig. 12.—Case 2. Oil immersion photomicrograph. The tumor cells are fairly uniform in size but show some variation in chromatin content. This is a more transparent stain than that used in Fig. 6, but the cells are similar. Hematoxylin, eosin azure A stain.

Fig. 13.—Case 2. Low power photomicrograph showing tumor cells in the lumen of a venous channel and attached directly to surrounding tumor by a pedicle passing through a break in the endothelial lining. Red blood cells are present in the lumen.

structure could be seen. In these areas small atrophic thymic corpuscles were present. Their scarcity and the fact that they were not found in the lymph gland metastases demonstrated that they were remnants of the thymus and not newly formed structures. Here, too, there was a rather indefinite suggestion of thymic lobulation.

The white nodules noticed grossly in the main tumor were incorporated lymph glands, with distinct capsules infiltrated by tumor cells. In these glands a few primary and secondary follicles could be seen. These findings would lead one to suppose that these glands were secondarily involved; otherwise it would be difficult to explain why the thymus should so completely lose its characteristic architecture while the lymph glands should maintain theirs. Diffuse hemorrhages were present throughout the tumor, particularly in the thymic region and throughout the connective tissues.

The walls of the arterial trunks were intact, while those of the venous trunks were extensively invaded up to and involving the endothelium. Throughout the whole mass, large venous channels were seen in which the infiltration of the wall had become so extensive that only the endothelial layer separated the tumor cells from the blood stream. In several instances these vascular channels actually contained masses of tumor cells and in a few these masses of tumor cells could actually be seen attached to the surrounding tumor by a pedicle of malignant cells extending through the venous wall (Fig. 13). This finding, and the fact that the lumina of blood vessels with intact walls contained cells closely resembling tumor cells, suggested the possibility of explaining at least in part, if not all, the terminal blood picture in this case. The parietal pericardium, like the veins, was extensively involved.

The left lung presented a most amazing picture which was difficult to interpret at first glance. It appeared to be infarcted in that the lung architecture had been wiped out, and the tissue appeared to have been wholly replaced by red blood cells, the arrangement of which occurred in groups separated by strands of fibrinlike material. With the aid of reticulum and elastic tissue stains, alveoli were indistinctly demonstrated in many places. On the other hand, numerous well-stained nucleated cells arranged either diffusely or in groups could be seen; the red cells were distinct in their outline, and very little fibrin was present. And thus we see that although it had characteristics of both a recent and a late infarct, it could not be classified as either, in that in the former case there would be no loss of lung architecture, while in the latter event there would be extensive necrosis and lack of cell outline.

Throughout the above mentioned lung tissue, groups of tumor cells were present; in some places the infiltration was extensive. In addition, there were numerous cells of different types, consisting of small lymphocytes, neutrophilic and eosinophilic leucocytes, with a scattering of myelocytes and a few plasma cells. The most interesting feature of the lung sections was the presence of giant cells with a large amount of basophilic cytoplasm. The nuclei were polymorphous; the majority were lobulated, stained deeply, and closely resembled megakaryocytes (Fig. 14). The adjoining atelectatic lung tissue contained numerous macrophages in the alveoli whose nuclei and general appearance resembled the above mentioned giant cells. It is possible that these megakaryocyte-like giant cells had risen from the histiocytes of the lung alveoli. There were no giant cells in the tumor. Benzidine stains showed the lung to contain relatively numerous peroxydase-positive cells as compared with the tumor proper, which contained none.

Sections in the region of the intercostal muscles, muscles of the chest wall, and subcutaneous tissues simply showed tumor infiltration between the muscle and collagenous bundles. The cells were of a uniform type.

The parenchymal liver cells showed patchy, fatty degeneration. Many, but not all, of the periportal spaces were infiltrated with cells. Yet the spaces were not enlarged, and there was no cellular invasion of the parenchyma. These cells consisted of small lymphocytes, a few eosinophilic polymorphonuclear cells, and the majority of cells resembled tumor cells. This involvement, although leucemic in type, was not as well developed as one would expect to find in a typical case of leucemia. The architecture of the spleen was not as well outlined as the normal. Malpighian corpuscles could be distinguished, but their boundaries faded indistinctly into the surrounding red pulp. The red pulp was unusually cellular and contained cells not unlike the tumor cells. Many of the cells were in the sinuses, while others appeared to be spreading peripherally from the malpighian corpuscles. Again, as in the liver, these lesions were not as well developed as in typical lymphatic leucemia. The kidneys were normal. The lymph tissue of the intestinal wall showed no deviation from the normal.

The lymph nodes in the region of the celiac axis were almost completely replaced by sarcoma cells, and there was extensive invasion of the surrounding tissues by these cells. The remainder of the retroperitoneal and mesenteric lymph nodes were normal in structure. Unfortunately no sections were made of the superficial lymph nodes. The caseous lymph gland in the mediastinum was histologically tuberculous.

The bone marrow of the sternum, costochondral junctions, ribs, and long bones showed similar neoplastic changes, and with the exception of the long bones, it was replaced completely by neoplastic tissue. The long bones showed extensive focal replacement, but the myeloid elements, while reduced in number, were still present. The megakaryocytes were few, and those that were present showed marked vacuolization. There was no diminution in number of the trabeculae of the bones. The infarcts which had been noted grossly were histologically true infarcts.

Diagnosis.—Primary lymphosarcoma of the thymus with direct metastases to pericardium, left lung, left pleura, left cervical lymph nodes, mediastinal lymph nodes, and the lymph nodes of the celiac axis, with leucemia-like involvement of liver, spleen, and bone marrow.

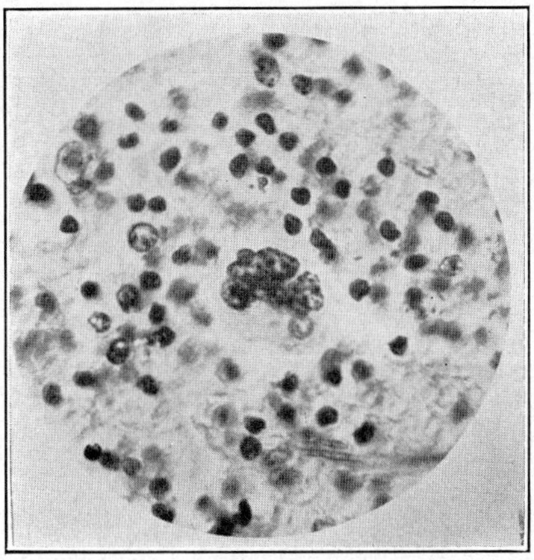

Fig. 14.—Case 2. Oil immersion photomicrograph showing a megakaryocyte-like cell in the infarcted left lung. Hemalum, erythrosin, and saffron stain.

CASE III: CLINICAL AND LABORATORY FINDINGS

T. L. (Case 2112-33), aged six years, was admitted to the Medical Service of the Children's Memorial Hospital on Feb. 9, 1933.

Complaint.—Swelling of the face, trunk, and legs.

Present Illness.—One month prior to admission the child began to lose her appetite, and at that time it was noticed that the eyes became swollen, particularly in the morning. The rest of the face gradually become involved. No other parts of the body were involved at that time, and the condition cleared up in about two weeks. The child returned to school, but two weeks later edema of the face again appeared and since then gradually spread to the trunk and legs. These symptoms closely resemble the so-called superior vena cava syndrome.

Physical Examination.—The child was well nourished. Weight on admission was 49 pounds. The submaxillary, left axillary, and left epitrochlear glands were all moderately enlarged. Otherwise there was no remarkable lymphadenopathy. The left side of the chest was more prominent than the right, but the expansion seemed equal on both sides. No tactile fremitus was present on the left. The percussion note over the entire left chest was flat up to the first rib anteriorly and the second interspace posteriorly. The left border of the heart could not be made out. The right border of the heart was well to the right of the sternal edge. The right lung was resonant throughout. Tubular breathing was audible at the left apex, diminished breathing below. Breath sounds were present on the right side. There were no râles. The heart sounds were very distant, sufficient to suggest a pericardial effusion. There were signs of fluid in the abdomen. The liver was enlarged to the level of the umbilicus. The spleen was just palpable. The diagnosis lay between Pick's disease and a mediastinal tumor.

Laboratory Findings.—White blood cells numbered 17,200; platelets, 321,000; polymorphonuclear leucocytes, 51 per cent; lymphocytes, 38 per cent; monocytes, 6 per cent; eosinophiles, 2 per cent; metamyelocytes, 2 per cent; and basophiles, 1 per cent.

Blood urea nitrogen	17 mg.	Globulin	2.17%
Fibrinogen	0.73%	Total protein	7.56%
Albumin	4.66%		

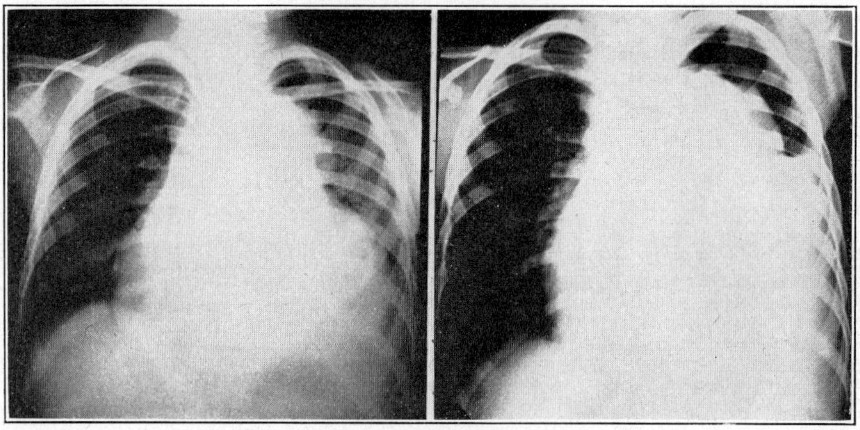

Fig. 15. Fig. 16.

Fig. 15.—Case 3. Film of chest made after aspiration of left-sided pleural fluid. The pericardium is enlarged to the right, and there is a large mass in the left upper medial chest.

Fig. 16.—Case 3. Chest nineteen days later. The pericardium is less markedly enlarged to the right, but the mass in the left upper chest has increased.

The Wassermann reaction was negative.

On aspiration of the chest 25 c.c. of straw-colored fluid was withdrawn. The total cell count was 9,500; specific gravity, 1.008 gm.; total protein, 20 per cent; chlorides, 305 mg.

Several further aspirations were done with rapid reaccumulation after withdrawal. Each successive thoracentesis yielded fluid which was increasingly sanguineous. Dyspnea gradually increased, and the child died April 2, 1933.

Diagnosis.—Lymphosarcoma of mediastinal origin.

Roentgenologic Findings.—The first film made on Feb. 9, 1933, revealed a rather extensive left-sided pleural exudate. A dense mass was present in the left upper medial chest, and the superior mediastinum was broadened to the right. The right border of the pericardial shadow was enlarged to the right, but its left border was obscured. A second film taken the same day following the aspiration of pleural fluid

(Fig. 15) showed the mass in the left upper chest considerably better, but otherwise added little information. The pericardium was still enlarged to the right, and the superior mediastinum was broadened to the right.

Examination during the month of February showed that the pleural fluid accumulated rapidly. A film was made on Feb. 28, 1933, following aspiration of fluid from the left pleural cavity and introduction of air, and also the withdrawal of 500 c.c. of pericardial fluid (Fig. 16). The mass in the left upper chest was seen to be larger and the right border of the pericardium was much closer to the midline. Aspiration of pericardial fluid produced similar changes on March 28, 1933, and by this time the left chest was completely opaque.

Pathologic Findings.—On March 2, 1933, biopsy of the left axillary glands was performed. Grossly and microscopically the glands were normal. Smears and paraffin sections of the pleural fluid were made on two occasions. These showed numerous red blood cells, polymorphonuclears, and discrete masses of atypical lymphocytes. The cells were of uniform size, larger than a small lymphocyte, stained less deeply, and consisted in most instances of an apparently naked nucleus with a nucleolus. Scattered through these were larger cells showing vacuolization, apparently degenerative. A few large cells with vesicular nuclei and basophilic cytoplasm were present. These cells, in view of their appearance and the fact that they formed discrete masses, were undoubtedly malignant lymphocytes.

DISCUSSION

Although the origin of the small lymphocyte-like cell of the thymus is still a moot point, for convenience we shall call them lymphocytes, while not committing ourselves to one or other theory.

It has been stated that in order to make a diagnosis of a primary thymic tumor, one must find typical thymic structures, especially Hassall's corpuscles. As the latter arise from the epithelial reticular cells and not from the lymphocytes, it does not seem logical that when the lymphocytes become neoplastic that they should give rise to Hassall's corpuscles. This appears to be supported by these two cases. In Case 1 the malignant process was obviously arising in the cortex of the thymus, as seen by the numerous areas of primitive cells from which the tumor spreads peripherally. There was an actual invasion of thymic medulla by cortical cells. In the right lobe where the process was more advanced, only a few thymic corpuscles could be found, while in the left lobe where the process was comparatively early, there was only an absolute reduction in the number of corpuscles. On close examination, tumor cells could be seen penetrating Hassall's corpuscles, separating, and peeling their layers off as one would peel an onion. As the process advanced, the corpuscles were destroyed. This also had happened in Case 2, in which only a few atrophic corpuscles could be found after cutting numerous sections. Then again, the direct metastatic infiltrations showed no attempt at formation of these bodies. If these corpuscles were being formed as a part of the tumor process, one would expect the reticular cells to be active, but there was no evidence to support this contention. Although the reticular cells were prominent in the first case, this was due to a degenerative process; in the second case only a few of these cells could be seen. Thus it would seem that, whatever the origin of the lymphocytes, they, and they alone, composed the essential cellular structure of the newgrowth. They reproduced no other cells but themselves, and there was no histologic evidence to show that they were derived from the reticular cells of the tumor.

The first case speaks for itself in indicating that the mediastinal tumor was thymic in origin. There was a large tumor mass lying ventrad to the right lung with its stem attached to the mediastinum. This portion in its periphery showed undoubted thymic lobules, and throughout there were definite traces of thymic architecture and Hassall's corpuscles. This could not have been anything but the right lobe of the thymus. If the process had started in the mediastinal lymph nodes, it does not seem likely that metastases would have so outstripped the mother tumor in growth. Then, too, the lymph gland structure was well retained, and there was only slight infiltration of the tissues surrounding them, while, on the other hand, the tissues surrounding the thymus showed extensive involvement. The early pericardial involvement also points to a tumor of thymic origin.

The fact that the bone marrow may, and one extrathoracic lymph gland did, show early neoplastic changes, does not speak against a thymic tumor if one considers that the process may be a generalized one affecting other lymphoid tissue. That the thymic tumor could not be metastatic from these seems reasonable because the changes in other affected tissues were early—so early in the bone marrow as to make it doubtful that they were present. In addition, these areas did not show the primitive cell islands of the cortex of the thymus.

Ewing[2] states that thymic tumors are characterized by their position in that they surround and compress the trachea, bronchi, pericardium, and adjacent great vessels. The conditions are fulfilled in Cases 1 and 2 and probably in Case 3, as evidenced by the early development of edema of the face, although these conditions were complicated by the metastatic infiltration and the leucemia-like picture in Case 2.

In discussing Case 2, one meets with difficulties because it possessed the characteristics both of lymphosarcoma and leucemia, but, as has already been shown, the lesions have more of the properties of lymphosarcoma than of leucemia. It is becoming more and more apparent that there is no sharp dividing line between these two conditions and that there are undisputed instances which show features of both, but with one of them predominating. The term "leucosarcoma" seems justified for these cases, provided that it is used as a term to classify those cases which as yet, due to insufficient knowledge, cannot be placed definitely either in the group of the lymphosarcomas or the leucemias.

In our second case it seems to us that the thymus is the site of origin of the primary thoracic involvement. In this case Ewing's criteria were fulfilled. The lymph glands in the mediastinum were extensively involved but retained their architecture, while the thymus, except for a rare corpuscle of Hassall, had completely lost its identity. Here again, there was a greater amount of infiltration of the surrounding tissues in the region of the thymus than about the lymph glands. From the tumor in the thymus, the lesion was seen to invade the surrounding structures centrifugally.

Its neoplastic or lymphosarcomatous tendencies were well demonstrated by the infiltrative process which had passed through the thoracic wall to invade the muscles and subcutaneous tissues. The pericardium, the pleura, the left lung, and the lymph glands of the neck and celiac axis were also invaded by direct extension. However, we also found poorly developed lesions of a leucemia-like process in liver and spleen, but, contrary to expectations in a true leucemic process, the kidneys and many lymph glands were completely free of leucemic lesions. The bone marrow changes could be definitely classified as leucemic but were not as extensive as one would expect to find in true leucemia. This is in agreement with Heubner (quoted by Ewing) who says that with thymic tumors the other lesions of leucemia are not always well developed. Here, then, is a case in which were present both lesions of lymphosarcoma and leucemia but with a definite predominance of the characteristics of the former.

A review of the literature reveals that a remarkable feature of leucosarcomas is that the site of greatest involvement is in the mediastinum. Flashman and Leopold,[3] in a survey of the literature, reported that in a series of 107 cases the mediastinum was the probable site of the invasive tumor in 60. The next common site was the skin, the eyes, and eyelids in 22 cases. Ewing[2] states that the existence of a pure lymphocytoma of the thymus, apart from leucemia, does not appear to have been established. This is not in agreement with our first case; moreover cases in recent literature have been reported in which there has been a primary lymphosarcomatous tumor of the thymus without leucemia (Margolis[4]).

In connection with the leucemic changes often seen in association with tumor of the thymus, we would like to draw attention to several facts. In our cases the venous walls appeared unable to resist tumor invasion. This is most marked in the case in which tumor could actually be seen growing in venous channels (Case 2). These tumors were situated in a region where there are numerous and large veins. From these facts it is possible that a terminal leucemic blood picture may result from an outpouring of tumor cells directly into the blood stream. In Case 1 the venous involvement was not sufficiently extensive to permit this to occur. Here, we would like to emphasize again the resemblance between the cells in the circulating blood and those of the tumor.

Whether the lesions apart from the main tumor are metastatic or part of a generalized systemic process affecting lymphoid tissue is a problem which cannot be satisfactorily explained. However, it is a fact that in primary tumors of the thymus distant leucemia-like involvement is common, but in lymphatic leucemia with generalized lymphadenopathy the converse has never been conclusively demonstrated. Margolis,[5] in a series of 32 cases of lymphatic leucemia, found tumor formation in the thymic region in only 4 cases, 3 of which were in children. In the remaining 28 cases, 7 of which were in children, there was no involvement of the thymus. He expressed the opinion that the 4 cases with thymic involvement represented a localized infiltration of the thymus by leucemic cells and that the thymus took no active part in the tumor formation. We are of the opinion that this was not conclusively demonstrated and that these four cases could equally well have been interpreted as being lymphosarcomas of the thymus. In fact, they appeared to resemble our second case. If the origin of the thymic cell is considered to be lymphoid, it is difficult to explain the absence of active involvement in lymphatic leucemia. On the other hand, if these cells are considered to have a different origin, the lesions apart from the main tumor could be interpreted as being metastatic in nature.

Interpretation of the clinical and roentgenologic findings in our cases is easy from the gross pathologic picture. The tumor mass in the superior mediastinum can give rise to symptoms and signs due to pressure on the veins, trachea, and nerves. Involvement of the pleura and the pericardium can be explained by infiltration. This gives rise to pleural and pericardial effusions which are often hemorrhagic. Our third case, from the clinical and roentgenologic standpoint, is identical with the second case, and the findings of typical tumor lymphoid cells in the pleural fluid established the diagnosis of mediastinal lymphosarcoma. In spite of its similarity to the second case, it did not have a leucemic blood picture.

The above signs and symptoms are late manifestations and are easily interpreted. It is unfortunate that the tumors must reach such a relatively large size before they produce symptoms which bring the patient to the physician.

SUMMARY

1. Three cases of mediastinal lymphosarcomas in children are reported. Clinically they were characterized by vague, early symptoms of lassitude, insomnia, and nervousness. Later, they gave rise to a fairly definite train of events, such as edema of the face, dyspnea, a

feeling of suffocation, and, above all, hemorrhagic pericardial and pleural effusions with displacement of heart and trachea. One had a terminal leucemic blood picture.

2. Roentgenologic findings were initially confusing in two of the cases, but in conjunction with the clinical and laboratory examinations, as well as the course, the malignant nature of the condition was soon established. Marked mediastinal enlargement was demonstrated in two cases, but the third case did not present this feature. Here the tumor was mainly situated in the right pleural cavity and simulated an encapsulated effusion.

3. The necropsy findings in two cases were such as to enable the diagnosis of primary lymphosarcoma of the thymus to be made. Both cases were characterized by large mediastinal tumors arising from the thymus, and, whatever the interpretation of the distant lesions may be, the thymic tumors themselves could not have been metastatic. In a large number of cases, a definite dividing line cannot be drawn between the lymphosarcomas and leucemias, and for these cases the term "leucosarcoma" is useful.

We wish to express our thanks to Dr. L. J. Rhea, for his constructive criticism of this paper, and to Dr. A. C. Kallan and Miss J. G. MacLeod, for assistance in preparing it.

REFERENCES

1. Cooke, J. V.: Am. J. Dis. Child. **44**: 1153, 1932.
2. Ewing, J.: Neoplastic Diseases, Philadelphia, 1934, W. B. Saunders Co.
3. Flashman, D. H., and Leopold, S. S.: Am. J. M. Sc. **177**: 651, 1929.
4. Margolis, H. M.: Am. J. Cancer **15**: 2106, 1931.
5. Margolis, H. M.: Arch. Path. **9**: 1015, 1930.

THE EVOLUTION OF THE ADULT TYPE OF TUBERCULOSIS FROM THE CHILDHOOD TYPE: EVIDENCE IN FAVOR OF ENDOGENOUS REINFECTION

A Preliminary Report

J. A. Johnston, M.D.
Detroit, Mich.

TWENTY years ago, Baldwin[1] stated his feeling that "reinfection is mostly autogenous superinfection and due to disease, overstrain, trauma or any cause of lowered vitality, whatever that may mean." Since that time the feeling has grown steadily stronger that this source represents a smaller and smaller fraction of the so-called adult type of cases so that last year at the meeting of the National Tuberculosis Association this statement appears in Pope's communication:[2] "At the present time in this country the weight of scientific opinion leans toward the theory of exogenous reinfection as the determining factor in the etiology of phthisis, but it is doubtful whether the last word has been said upon this subject." Even if it be granted that for practical purposes the exogenous route represents the common source of reinfection, nevertheless completely to discredit the endogenous source, as is implied in Weintraub's report,[3] is going to an extreme not warranted by the facts. Following a group of approximately 500 reactors who were also contacts and 500 who were not, this author reports eleven cases deriving from the contact group and none from the noncontact. The children were followed for varying periods up to five years.

The observations reported here were made on 650 reactors who are wards of the Society of St. Vincent de Paul in Detroit and 150 contacts who were not reactors. On being assigned to this society from the probate court following the rupture of a family group because of disease, economic distress, or legal difficulties, the children are hospitalized and thoroughly checked before being placed in country boarding homes under foster parents. The homes are frequently inspected, and in those instances in which reinfection type disease occurred the foster parents were checked by x-ray when possible.

In seven years there have been detected in this group 23 cases of adult type of tuberculosis. Of these, 7 were discovered on first examination; 16 cases developed under observation. In only 2 of these was

Conducted for the Society of St. Vincent de Paul at the Henry Ford Hospital in cooperation with the Children's Fund of Michigan.
Presented before the American Pediatric Society, Bolton Landing, N. Y., June 13, 1936.

any question raised of reexposure, and in 1 of those 2 the adult lesion did not appear until ten months after the second exposure.

The ages at which the adult lesion appeared coincided with the usual experience; 5 cases appeared between three months and nine years; 15 between ten and seventeen years, and 3 between eighteen and twenty-two years.

One of the several objects of this study was to ascertain, if possible, whether or not we might affect either the incidence of, or the mortality from, the adult type lesion by a system of constant supervision which included preventorium care in a summer camp. Myers and his associates[4] recently stated their feeling that "at the close of fourteen years' observation we are unable to see any difference in the course of the disease regardless of whether the child so treated is a strict bed patient or remains as active as any normal child should be." At the same meeting Hawes[5] pointed to the record of the Prendergast Preventorium to uphold the opposing point of view. Out of 704 children followed, there had developed only 3 adult type of cases with 1 death, while in an identical number of reactors not supervised there had developed 40 cases with 10 deaths. We are unable to show anything like such a low incidence, but our mortality is equally gratifying.

A tabulation of the reports of various groups is interesting in this connection (Table I).

TABLE I

	REACTORS DEVELOPING REINFECTIONS	DEATHS
Pope	38	12
Myers et al.	36	8
McPhedran and Opie[6]	26	5
Hawes (Preventorium group)	3	1
Hawes (No preventorium)	40	10
Detroit group	16	2

This record of a group of children from the lowest economic and nutritional stratum would seem to us, even over so short a period as seven years, to justify the existence of the preventorium plan.

Table II lists reinfection types that have been discovered, together with the time elapsing between the finding of the first infection and the demonstration of the reinfection.

It was our hope to acquire some information on the question of the state of allergy at the time of the reinfection phenomenon, and with this in mind serial dilutions of tuberculin were applied on each examination of the child. The technic involved and the results obtained in another study limiting itself strictly to the first infection were described elsewhere.[7] In that study we found that, quantitatively con-

TABLE II

REINFECTION TYPES OF TUBERCULOSIS DISCOVERED IN SEVEN-YEAR STUDY

NO.	NAME	SEX	AGE REACTIVITY DISCOVERED	X-RAY EVIDENCE CHILDHOOD INFECTION	AGE AT REINFECTION (YR.)	TYPE
1.	J. K.	M	7	Yes	13	Pul.
2.	R. J.	F	13*	No	13	Miliary bone
3.	V. G.	F	14*	No	14	Pul.
4.	I. K.	F	9	Yes	17	Miliary†
5.	G. C.	M	2 mo.	No	3 mo.	Miliary†
6.	E. G.	F	11*	No	11	Pul.
7.	M. C.	F	16*	No	16	Pul. bone
8.	L. DeM.	F	15*	No	15	Pul.
9.	J. DeM.	M	16	No	17	Pul.
10.	D. B.	F	5	Yes	11	Pul.
11.	J. C.	F	4	Yes	6	Pul.
12.	C. K.	F	15	Yes	18	Pul.
13.	R. P.	F	5	Yes	9	Pul.
14.	J. C.	M	10	Yes	12	Pleurisy
15.	M. F.	F	19*	No	19	Pul.
16.	S. F.	M	16	No	17	Pul.
17.	J. F.	F	11	Yes	12	Pul.
18.	M. S.	F	2	Yes	9	Pul.
19.	A. M.	M	10*	Yes	10	Pul.
20.	G. G.	F	9	Yes	15	Pul.
21.	R. C.	F	7	Yes	11	Pul.
22.	G. R.	M	15	Yes	22	Pul.
23.	K. K.	F	7	Yes	14	Pul.

*Reinfection type when first seen.
†Deaths.

sidered, allergy followed a parabolic curve, the rise and fall seeming independent of the immune process, at least so far as that was measurable by the reaction in the peripheral blood, and we concluded that the evidence of that study favored the view that the two phenomena were independent. Observations on this group of children can be similarly interpreted. From Table II it will be seen that in terms of the heights that are commonly seen in first infections, allergy is not particularly high at the onset of the adult type lesion and that instances are found of its occurrence coincidentally with rising, falling, and level thresholds of allergy.

TABLE III

LEVEL OF ALLERGY AT THE ONSET OF THE ADULT TYPE OF LESION

MG. O. T.	NO. CASES	LEVEL IN ADULT TYPE CASES ON 1ST. EXAM.
0.1	7	
0.01	2	4
0.001	4	2
0.0001	2	
0.00001	1	1
Cases showing increase in allergic level on reinfection		7
Cases showing decrease in allergic level on reinfection		5
Cases showing no change in allergic level on reinfection		3

Finally, it was our hope by a study of the individuals showing the transition to learn something of the so-called "lowered vitality," of which Baldwin speaks as a factor influencing the development of the adult lesion.

A comparison of the weights of these children with expected weight yields little information as was pointed out long since in the Philadelphia study, but a study of the individual weight curves over a period of years has been very instructive. There is evident quite regularly a flattening of the curve in the year preceding the development of the lesion which is often the first abnormality to attract attention. With the thought that a study of the metabolism of these children might afford some evidence of subnormality in their nutrition at the onset of their lesion, serial basal metabolism determinations were done and the nitrogen balances were determined. The total metabolic rate in the adult with pulmonary tuberculosis and his nitrogen requirements have been reported by McCann,[8] who found them within normal limits and who reasoned that the elevation which might be expected as a result of infection was offset by the malnutrition that all of his subjects showed. He warned, however, that his conclusions should not be applied to the adolescent. In general, it can be said that our findings do suggest that an element of malnutrition dominates the picture, the total rates being approximately normal, but the basal metabolic mixtures and the retentions of nitrogen suggesting definitely that stores had been depleted. The metabolic mixtures in several instances show a steady rise in the amount of carbohydrate oxidized and the reciprocal fall in fat such as are seen in the recovery from fasting. It can be objected that these findings are impossible to interpret in terms of cause and effect, and that is true, though practically all were obtained before the disease process had advanced far. In any case they disclose elements of depletion often concealed by a deceptively normal weight. The details of this phase of the study will be presented in another communication.

SUMMARY

1. Six hundred and fifty reactors and 150 contacts who were not reactors, from a poor economic stratum, were observed for varying periods up to seven years following removal from their source of infection. There were found 23 adult type of cases, 16 of which developed subsequent to the initial observation.

2. There have been only two deaths, these from miliary tuberculosis, since the study started, a result which is interpreted as favoring the view that something has been accomplished by this system of follow-up and preventorium care.

3. No consistent relationship could be discovered between the onset of the reinfection type of tuberculosis and a quantitative change in allergy.

4. The basal metabolism of this group was found to be approximately normal. The metabolic mixtures and the retentions of nitrogen suggested depletion of metabolic stores.

The x-ray plates were interpreted for the first four years of the study by Dr. Henry D. Chadwick and the author and independently by Dr. H. Doub. In the last three years they have all been reviewed by Dr. Bruce Douglas and the author after an initial reading by Dr. Doub. In the metabolism studies we have had the assistance of Dr. F. W. Hartman, Dr. O. H. Gaebler, and Dr. J. W. Maroney. Dr. F. Janney Smith, of the cardiorespiratory clinic of the Ford Hospital, was in charge of the examinations of all of those patients over fifteen years old.

The tuberculin has been a single lot prepared by Dr. Leroy Gardner, at Saranac Lake.

REFERENCES

1. Baldwin, E. R.: Bull. Johns Hopkins Hosp. **24**: 220, 1913.
2. Pope, A. S.: Nat. Tuberc. A. Tr. **31**: 317, 1935.
3. Weintraub, W. L.: Am. Rev. Tuberc. **33**: 247, 1936.
4. Myers, J. A., Harrington, F. E., Stewart, C. A., and Wulff, M.: Nat. Tuberc. A. Tr. **31**: 300, 1935.
5. Hawes, J. B., Jr.: Nat. Tuberc. A. Tr. **31**: 336, 1935.
6. McPhedran, F. M., and Opie, E. L.: Arch. Int. Med. **52**: 137, 1933.
7. Johnston, J. A., Howard, P. J., and Maroney, J. W.: Amer. Rev. Tuberc. **29**: 652, 1934.
8. McCann, W. S.: Nat. Tuberc. A. Tr. **17**: 422, 1921.

A STUDY OF THE COMPARATIVE VALUE OF COD LIVER OIL, VIOSTEROL, AND VITAMIN D MILKS IN THE PREVENTION OF RICKETS AND OF CERTAIN BASIC FACTORS INFLUENCING THEIR EFFICACY

Martha M. Eliot, M.D., and E. M. Nelson, Ph.D., Washington, D. C., Donald J. Barnes, M.D., and Florence A. Browne, M.D., Detroit, Mich., and Rachel M. Jenss, Sc.D., Washington, D. C.

A SERIES of investigations with the purpose of studying the relative efficacy of cod liver oil, viosterol, and several forms of vitamin D milk given at different dosage levels were carried out in Detroit, Mich., during the winters of 1933-34, 1934-35, and 1935-36. The studies were planned with a view to developing practical methods of testing the value of the various antirachitic substances as administered by physicians and other public health officials to infants living in their own homes.

At the time the investigation was started in the fall of 1933 the belief was current that from 500 to 600 U.S.P. units of cod liver oil and two and one-half to three times as many units of viosterol were necessary to prevent rickets. The work of the first two winters was planned, therefore, to study this supposed relationship between the preventive dose of cod liver oil and of viosterol and to attempt to establish a base line for later comparative studies with vitamin D milks.

During the first winter cod liver oil was prescribed in doses of 540 and 270 units daily and viosterol in doses of 1,350 units daily, or two and one-half times the higher dose of cod liver oil. Due to the high potency of the viosterol (1,350 units in 3 drops) and to the tendency of the mothers to give more rather than less than the number of drops ordered, the amount of viosterol taken by the infants during this first winter was considerably larger than that intended—approximately 2,000 units daily.

The results of the first winter's work showed a complete absence of cases of moderate and marked rickets and a relatively small incidence of slight rickets among infants taking this large amount of viosterol, whereas a few cases of moderate rickets and a somewhat larger percentage of slight rickets occurred among the infants receiving cod liver oil.

From the Children's Bureau, United States Department of Labor, and the Food and Drug Administration, United States Department of Agriculture, with the cooperation and assistance of the Children's Hospital of Michigan, the Detroit Departments of Health and Welfare, the Children's Fund of Michigan, and a number of hospitals that permitted access to their records of newborn infants.

Presented at the Annual Meeting of the American Pediatric Society, Bolton Landing, N. Y., June 11, 1936.

During the second winter, therefore, the dosage level of viosterol was decreased and that of cod liver oil increased. Viosterol was prescribed at dosage levels of 1,350 and 675 units and cod liver oil at 675 and 810 units, with one level, therefore, in common. The dosage levels prescribed for cod liver oil and viosterol during the first two years are shown in Table I.

TABLE I

ANTIRACHITIC SUBSTANCES AND DOSAGE LEVELS IN U.S.P. UNITS PRESCRIBED DURING 1933-34 AND 1934-35

TYPE OF ANTIRACHITIC	AVERAGE NUMBER OF UNITS PRESCRIBED DURING	
	1933-34	1934-35
Cod liver oil	270	675
	540	810
Viosterol	1,350*	675
		1,350

*Dosage prescribed was 1,350 units daily; amount actually taken daily was approximately 2,000 units.

At the end of the second year the findings pointed to the fact that cod liver oil and viosterol administered at the level of 675 units were, to all intents and purposes, equally efficacious or at least that viosterol was no less effective than cod liver oil. It seemed apparent that the differences ascribed to the two forms of vitamin D did not exist in fact and it was believed that the minimum preventive dose (using the absence of moderate or marked rickets as the criterion) was probably in the neighborhood of 675 units. When judged by the presence or absence of slight degrees of rickets, the minimum dose may well be still higher since there is evidence that in the group receiving the higher dosages of viosterol the amount of slight rickets is less than in any other group. The presence of this slight degree of rickets, moreover, among a considerable proportion of infants receiving 675 units made it seem undesirable to repeat the studies of these antirachitic substances at lower dosage levels.

During the third winter attention was turned toward the study of milks. Four forms of evaporated vitamin D milk were used at two quite different dosage levels. Table II shows the types of milks used, the potency desired at the outset, and the potency established on the finished products. The efficacy of the different types of milk as judged by presence or absence of slight rickets will be discussed in detail in another section.

METHOD OF STUDY

Thirteen groups of infants were given an antirachitic substance, either cod liver oil or viosterol (Table I), or some form of vitamin D milk (Table II). The cod liver oil and viosterol were purchased in single lots at the beginning of the study and assayed in the laboratories of the Food and Drug Administration before the actual doses were determined. The milks* were prepared in the late summer of 1935 by reliable firms under expert supervision. All forms of the milk were evaporated and each was prepared from pooled lots to insure uniformity of product. Assays establishing the potency of the finished products were made also by the Food and Drug Administration, but after the milk had been put into use.

TABLE II

ORIGINAL POTENCY DESIRED AND ACTUAL POTENCY ESTABLISHED FOR VITAMIN D MILKS (EVAPORATED)

PRESCRIBED DURING 1935-36

TYPE OF MILK (EVAPORATED)	AVERAGE NUMBER OF UNITS PER RECONSTITUTED QUART	
	POTENCY DESIRED	POTENCY ESTABLISHED
"Yeast" milk		
1	135	170
2	400	400
Cod liver oil concentrate in milk		
1	135	135
2	400	400
Irradiated milk		
1	135	150
Viosterol in milk		
1	400	400

The daily dose of cod liver oil was measured during the first winter in spoons specially furnished to the mothers for this purpose; during the second winter each daily dose was put up in a separate bottle. Droppers calibrated in the laboratory of the Food and Drug Administration were provided with the viosterol so that the correct amount could be measured with a fair degree of accuracy. During the first year the viosterol was used in a concentrated form, 3 drops containing 1,350 U.S.P. units; for the second year's work the viosterol was diluted until 10 drops contained the same number of units. The chance of error in administration was, therefore, greatly reduced the second year.

The general method of procedure used in selecting infants and in organizing the study was that suggested by Powers and Eliot in 1933.[1] The necessity for making careful selection of the infants for the different groups to be studied was pointed out in this preliminary description of method. Analysis of the current material shows this necessity to be even greater than was believed to exist at that time, especially with respect to color, sex, and rate of growth in length.

When first selected, each group was composed of from 45 to 55 infants, of whom approximately two-fifths were colored and three-fifths, white. Efforts were made to select infants who were born at term and were the result of single pregnancies, who were less than eight

*The cooperation of the Evaporated Milk Association in the preparation of the milks is gratefully acknowledged.

weeks of age on admission to the study and were born after the first of September. Only infants who were artificially fed or breast fed with a supplemental formula containing not less than twelve ounces of milk daily were included in the study. Furthermore, no infant was included for final analysis who was known to have received an appreciable amount of any form of vitamin D previous to admission or an additional form of vitamin D during the period under observation other than that prescribed. Infants were accepted during October, November, December, and in a few cases during the early part of January, and were observed no later than the middle of May. Though the final size of the groups was somewhat reduced by necessary exclusions, there remained at the end a total of 567 infants whose records were suitable for analysis. Of these, 59 per cent were white, 41 per cent colored; 52 per cent were males, 48 per cent, females.

TABLE III

NUMBER OF INFANTS RECEIVING VITAMIN D IN THE FORM OF COD LIVER OIL, VIOSTEROL, OR VITAMIN D MILK CLASSIFIED BY SEX, BY COLOR, BY COLOR AND SEX, AND BY AVERAGE NUMBER OF U.S.P. UNITS OF VITAMIN D TAKEN DAILY AS COD LIVER OIL OR VIOSTEROL OR BY NUMBER OF UNITS PER QUART OF RECONSTITUTED MILK

TYPE OF ANTI-RACHITIC	AVERAGE NUMBER OF UNITS ACCORDING TO COLOR OF INFANTS		TOTAL			WHITE			COLORED		
	WHITE	COLORED	TOTAL	MALES	FEMALES	TOTAL	MALES	FEMALES	TOTAL	MALES	FEMALES
Total			567	297	270	335	183	152	232	114	118
Cod liver oil			163	91	72	90	52	38	73	39	34
	273	274	28	10	18	14	4	10	14	6	8
	460	470	34	17	17	19	10	9	15	7	8
	659	652	74	45	29	40	24	16	34	21	13
	821	789	27	19	8	17	14	3	10	5	5
Viosterol			132	57	75	67	29	38	65	28	37
	686	678	47	20	27	22	8	14	25	12	13
	1,392	1,361	50	20	30	24	10	14	26	10	16
	2,185	2,093	35	17	18	21	11	10	14	6	8
Milk (evaporated)			272	149	123	178	102	76	94	47	47
"Yeast"											
170			52	33	19	34	21	13	18	12	6
400			41	18	23	30	16	14	11	2	9
Cod liver oil concentrate											
135			42	22	20	26	17	9	16	5	11
400			40	26	14	30	19	11	10	7	3
Irradiated											
150			47	27	20	29	15	14	18	12	6
Viosterol											
400			50	23	27	29	14	15	21	9	12

The procedure of examination was the same each year. Observations were made by the same two pediatricians and two public health nurses during the first two years of the study and by a third nurse who joined the staff during the last year. An x-ray film of the bones of both forearms and a clinical examination were made at the time of admission and at intervals of approximately one month thereafter. Although x-ray readings were made currently, the complete set of films for each of the 567 infants was reviewed at the end of the investigation. The readings for the three years are, therefore, reasonably consistent. The films were classified as "normal" when there was no evidence of rickets, and as "doubtful" when some change appeared to be present but was not sufficiently clear to make a positive diagnosis. When rickets was present, the diagnosis indicated whether the process was very slight, slight, moderate, or marked and whether active, partially controlled, or with healing far advanced. When evidence of rapidly advancing rickets was found, an increase was made in the amount of the antirachitic factor.

The infants were weighed and the crown-heel length was measured in centimeters at each examination. The average monthly increase in length has been estimated for each infant during the total period he was under observation.

MATERIAL STUDIED

Tables III and IV show the general picture as regards number of children, sex, color, and age at admission and at discharge.

Number of Infants Studied.—The number of infants receiving vitamin D in the form of cod liver oil, viosterol, or vitamin D milk grouped according to color and sex and also according to the daily average number of U.S.P. units* taken in the form of cod liver oil or viosterol or to the number of units per quart of reconstituted milk is shown in Table III. It will be noticed that approximately one-half of the infants received vitamin D milk and that a slightly larger proportion was given cod liver oil than viosterol; also that there is a larger percentage of white than of colored infants, especially in the milk groups, and relatively more male than female infants among the white infants, except for those receiving viosterol. It will also be seen that the number of infants receiving a given number of units of any type of antirachitic is small and that, as a result, there is considerable variability in the sex and color of the infants comprising such a group.

*It should be pointed out that the average dosage levels that are used in the tables which follow are not those prescribed, but the average number of units actually taken daily during the total period of observation or up to the time when the first x-ray evidence of rickets appeared. Dosage was classified in U.S.P. units according to certain broad groups as follows:

TYPE OF ANTIRACHITIC	DOSAGE IN U.S.P. UNITS	
	Range	Theoretical Average
Cod liver oil	150-349	250
	350-549	450
	550-749	650
	750-949	850
Viosterol	500-1,099	800
	1,100-1,699	1,400
	1,700-	----

There were 10 infants who received more than 2,299 units of viosterol. The maximum dosage was 2,990.

TABLE IV

AVERAGE AGE IN DAYS AND RANGE ON ADMISSION AND DISCHARGE FOR 567 INFANTS GIVEN VITAMIN D BY TYPE OF ANTIRACHITIC AGENT AND COLOR

TYPE OF ANTIRACHITIC AND COLOR	MEAN AGE (DAYS)		RANGE (DAYS)	
	ADMISSION	DISCHARGE	ADMISSION	DISCHARGE
Cod liver oil				
White	38	199	17-68	150-258
Colored	34	195	15-69	149-276
Viosterol				
White	39	201	17-64	142-262
Colored	39	199	14-69	153-263
Milk (evap.)				
White	38	188	8-63	126-274
Colored	39	186	10-64	122-258

Age at Admission and at Discharge and Period of Observation.—There is still another factor which tends to complicate the problem: The ages of admission and discharge vary considerably, the age of admission from 8 through 69 days of age, discharge from 122 through 276 days. But, nevertheless, as shown in Table IV, the average age at admission and at discharge in the several antirachitic and color groups was about the same, the age at admission being on the average a little over one month and at discharge, about six and one-half months. It should be noted, however, that the infants in the milk groups were discharged about 10 days earlier than those receiving cod liver oil or viosterol.

It would have been preferable, of course, to have examined all of the infants over exactly the same age interval, but as this was not done, the results presented in the following tables are based on the total period of observation for each child. Since a preliminary analysis of the x-ray findings in a shorter period of observation, but one common to all infants (70-139 days) did not show marked differences* with respect to total incidence of rickets between this short interval and the total period of observation, it was decided for the purposes of the present analysis to use the longer but variable interval. If progression of rickets is to be studied or if one is interested in studying the effect on the healing process of several antirachitic agents and dosage levels, it is obviously necessary to use the longer age period. It should be pointed out, moreover, that the incidence of rickets among the infants admitted prior to 35 days of age tended to be less on the average than for infants who were admitted between 35 and 70 days. Some infants who showed no evidence of rickets during the study might have become rachitic had they been observed over a longer and more comparable time interval.

*A criterion of two standard deviations, taking into account the number of degrees of freedom, has been used as the test of statistical significance.

INCIDENCE OF RICKETS

Incidence of Rickets in Total Group

Of the 567 infants studied, the x-ray films of only 10, or 2 per cent, showed an advance in the rachitic process to a moderate or marked degree. In 164 infants, or 29 per cent, rickets was found but did not develop beyond a maximum* of slight or very slight degree. In 103 infants, or 18 per cent, the diagnosis never progressed beyond the doubtful stage.† Two hundred ninety, or 51 per cent, of the infants showed no evidence of rickets throughout the period of observation. The analysis of the data has been directed chiefly toward a study of the incidence of the slighter degrees of rickets and the evidence of advance or regression of the rachitic process during the period of observation.

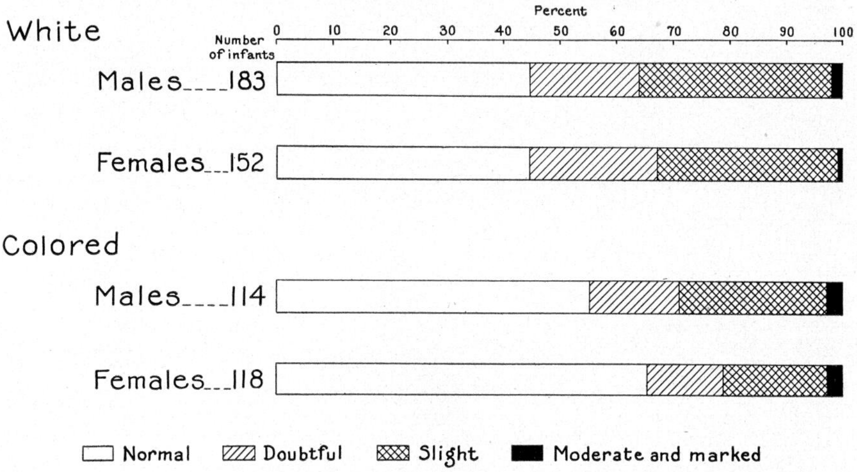

Fig. 1.—Percentage distribution of maximum x-ray findings for 567 infants given vitamin D in the form of cod liver oil, viosterol, or vitamin D milk, by color and sex.

Color and Sex

The incidence of rickets for the males and females in each color group is shown in Fig. 1. A greater percentage of positive cases was found among the white infants than among the colored for both

*The term "maximum diagnosis" will be used to refer to the greatest degree of rickets, whether slight, moderate, or marked, found in an individual infant at any time during the period of observation.

†It is probably of some significance that in 68 per cent of the cases in which a definite diagnosis of rickets was finally made this positive diagnosis was preceded by a "doubtful" diagnosis. This percentage is probably low due to the fact that the interval between x-ray examinations was very variable (anywhere from ten days to two months although the average was approximately one month). In a small group in which the x-ray pictures were taken at intervals of less than a month, all of the first positive diagnoses were preceded by "doubtful" findings. Special study has been made of the x-ray films from which a doubtful diagnosis was made either as a maximum finding in a series or as the finding which preceded a positive diagnosis. It was not possible to find any difference in the appearance of a film classified as doubtful when it preceded a positive or when it occurred alone. The evidence points then to the fact that the so-called "doubtful" diagnoses are in reality the earliest changes to be seen in the x-ray films and their disappearance without further progress of the disease indicates a degree of control that approaches closely that shown by a complete series of normal x-ray films. Further evidence to this effect is found in the fact that the maximum diagnoses of "doubtful" also vary according to the color and sex of the infant as do the maximum diagnoses of "rickets" (Fig. 1 and Table V).

males and females. When the incidence of rickets among colored and white infants is considered, regardless of sex, a significantly larger proportion of positive cases is found among the white infants than among the colored. This picture is the reverse of that which we are accustomed to consider as the usual racial incidence. It should be realized, however, that the well-known difference between white and negro infants is based on the fact that many more negro infants develop rapidly advancing rickets than do white infants. The actual incidence of the earliest stages of the disease might well be the same in the two racial groups or even, as these data demonstrate, reversed. It should be pointed out in this connection, however, that the examinations were all made during the winter when the influence of sunlight was almost negligible, and its absence may be an important factor in the reversal.

There is also a tendency for a larger percentage of cases to occur among the males in a given color group than among the females. But as further analysis indicates that the influence of color is a much more important factor than sex, and since the number of infants in each group would be too small if both sex and color were considered, the detailed tables which follow take only the color of the infants into consideration. In future studies of this type, it would be desirable in the selection of infants to consider sex as well as color, for both factors are fundamental to an understanding of the findings that relate to antirachitic agents and dosage levels.

Antirachitic Substances

With respect to the effect of the different antirachitic substances on the incidence of rickets, analysis of the data has been made first without regard to dosage levels and second taking dosage level into account. Table V shows the incidence of rickets for the total number of white and colored infants given each type of antirachitic substance regardless of dosage level and in addition the incidence in each dosage group.

Efficacy of Antirachitic Substances Regardless of Dosage Level.—Though the findings for the total groups are not based on a large enough number of cases to give throughout results that are statistically significant, nevertheless they do show that the efficacy of the milks (all forms and dosage levels) in preventing rickets is significantly greater than the efficacy of cod liver oil (all dosage levels), in spite of the fact that the average number of units in the milk is considerably lower than that of the cod liver oil. Of the total number of infants receiving vitamin D milks, 53 per cent of the white and 67 per cent of the colored had no rickets as compared with 30 per cent and 45 per cent, respectively, for white and colored receiving cod liver oil. Moreover, comparison of the milks (using again a combination of all types and dosage levels) with viosterol (all dosage levels) shows exactly the same tendency for the white infants, but the number in the viosterol group is too small and the differences between the incidence of either no rickets or rickets in the two groups are too slight to demonstrate significance. Though viosterol appears here to be more effective than cod liver oil, it should be pointed out that the average number of units taken in the form of viosterol by the total group is considerably in excess of that taken in the form of cod liver oil and direct comparisons cannot be made.

No infants receiving viosterol developed moderate or marked rickets, whereas seven who were given cod liver oil and three who were given vitamin D milks developed these more serious degrees.*

Efficacy of Antirachitic Substances by Dosage Levels.—When attempting to study the different antirachitic substances according to dosage levels certain obvious difficulties are encountered, such as the small number of infants in each dosage group and the unequal distribution according to color and sex. The fact that the dosage levels for the different antirachitic substances are the same in only two instances limits the number of direct comparisons that can be made. Furthermore, the dosages of the antirachitic substances used were not at a sufficiently low level to permit moderate or marked rickets to develop in enough infants to allow advanced rickets to be used as one of the criteria for judging success or failure in the prevention of rickets. However, since the investigation was primarily one of prevention, the proportion of infants showing no evidence of rickets throughout the period of observation and the proportion showing a very slight or slight degree are of basic importance. Though in many

*The color and sex of the infants developing moderate or marked rickets, the type of antirachitic substance used and dosage level are as follows:

CASES OF MODERATE AND MARKED RICKETS

AVERAGE NUMBER OF UNITS (DAILY)	TYPE OF ANTIRACHITIC	MAXIMUM DIAGNOSIS OF RICKETS	COLOR	SEX
135	Vitamin D milk, Cod liver oil concentrate added	Moderate	White	Male
135	Vitamin D milk, Cod liver oil concentrate added	Marked	Colored	Female
150	Irradiated milk	Moderate	White	Male
210	Cod liver oil	Moderate	Colored	Male
251	Cod liver oil	Moderate	Colored	Female
325	Cod liver oil	Marked	Colored	Male
340	Cod liver oil	Moderate	Colored	Female
686	Cod liver oil	Marked	Colored	Male
693	Cod liver oil	Moderate	White	Male
735	Cod liver oil	Moderate	White	Female

instances significant conclusions based on statistical analysis cannot be made because of the small number of infants studied, nevertheless certain consistent and repeated tendencies have been found which are worth presenting.

In the upper section of Table V are shown the findings with respect to the incidence of rickets among the infants given viosterol. There can be seen a general tendency for the incidence of rickets to decrease with increase in dosage. It may be seen that the incidence of rickets is

TABLE V

PERCENTAGE DISTRIBUTION OF MAXIMUM X-RAY DIAGNOSES FOR 567 INFANTS GIVEN DIFFERENT AMOUNTS OF VITAMIN D IN THE FORM OF VIOSTEROL, VITAMIN D MILK, OR COD LIVER OIL, BY COLOR

TYPE OF ANTIRACHITIC	COLOR AND AVERAGE NUMBER OF UNITS PER DAY OR PER RECONSTITUTED QUART	PERCENTAGE DISTRIBUTION			NUMBER OF INFANTS
		RICKETS	DOUBTFUL	NORMAL	
Viosterol	White				
	Total	*37*	*21*	*42*	*67*
	686	46	4	50	22
	1392	33	33	33	24
	2185	33	24	43	21
	Colored				
	Total	*12*	*20*	*68*	*65*
	678	24	16	60	25
	1361	4	23	73	26
	2093	7	21	72	14
Vitamin D Milk (evaporated)	White				
	Total	*28*	*19*	*53*	*178*
	"Yeast" milk				
	170	32	21	47	34
	400	30	10	60	30
	Cod liver oil conc. in milk				
	135	38	27	35	26
	400	17	23	60	30
	Irradiated milk, 150	31	10	59	29
	Viosterol in milk, 400	21	21	58	29
	Colored				
	Total	*22*	*11*	*67*	*94*
	"Yeast" milk				
	170	28	0	72	18
	400	27	27	46	11
	Cod liver oil conc. in milk				
	135	19	19	62	16
	400	30	10	60	10
	Irradiated milk, 150	22	11	67	18
	Viosterol in milk, 400	14	5	81	21
Cod Liver Oil	White				
	Total	*45*	*25*	*30*	*90*
	273	36	21	43	14
	460	37	47	16	19
	659	45	20	35	40
	821	65	12	23	17
	Colored				
	Total	*40*	*15*	*45*	*73*
	274	57	7	36	14
	470	27	27	46	15
	652	41	15	44	34
	789	30	10	60	10

no greater among white or colored infants receiving approximately 1,400 units than among those receiving approximately 2,100 units.

The middle section of Table V gives the findings in regard to vitamin D milks. No very definite conclusions can be drawn concerning the relative efficacy of the different types and doses of antirachitic milks though on the whole it would appear that the higher dosage levels are more effective than the lower in preventing rickets. It may be noted that in each of the white groups receiving 400 units in the form of yeast milk or milk with cod liver oil concentrate or viosterol added and in the group receiving 150 units in the form of irradiated milk, approximately 60 per cent of the infants showed no rickets. The evidence is not as consistent for the colored infants, probably because of the fact that there is a much smaller number of colored infants in each group. Among the infants receiving yeast milk, there is apparently no difference in the incidence of rickets among those receiving the higher dosage (400 units) or the lower (170 units).

In the lower section of Table V are given the findings for cod liver oil. With respect to this group it may be pointed out that the general tendency for the incidence of rickets to decrease with the increase of dosage level again appears for the colored group but with certain inconsistencies. There are even more striking exceptions in the white group. For instance, the white infants receiving the lowest number of units (273) show considerably less rickets than those receiving the highest (821). Of course, there is only a small number of cases in the two groups, 14 and 17, respectively, too few to give any stability to the results, but it will be noticed that the sex distribution of the infants in these two groups is quite uneven and in the opposite direction. Thus, there are only 4 males and 10 females in the lower dosage group; in the higher, 14 males and 3 females (Table III). These contradictory findings may be the result of the fact that the lower dosage level is heavily weighted with females, the higher with males, and that, in addition, the infants of a given sex who developed rickets tend on the average to be growing more rapidly in length than those who did not develop the disease. In other words, in the case of these two cod liver oil groups, the reversal of the general tendency for the percentage incidence of rickets to decrease with increasing unitage may well be related to the factors of sex and growth, a subject that will be discussed more fully in the next section.

Comparisons of Antirachitic Substances at Certain Dosage Levels.— It has been pointed out that direct comparisons of different antirachitic substances at the same dosage level can be made in two instances. These are shown in Table VI. First, a group of white infants given approximately 460 U.S.P. units of vitamin D daily in the form of cod liver oil is compared with a group including all white infants given milk containing 400 U.S.P. units to the reconstituted quart. The exact number of units consumed by the latter group is not known, but it is presumably somewhat less than 400 units daily. The incidence of rickets is significantly lower among those taking milk, 23 per cent in comparison with 37 per cent for those receiving cod liver oil. The same tendency was found among the colored infants.

TABLE VI

PERCENTAGE INCIDENCE OF RICKETS FOR WHITE INFANTS RECEIVING CERTAIN FORMS AND CERTAIN DOSAGE LEVELS OF VITAMIN D

TYPE OF ANTIRACHITIC	AVERAGE NUMBER OF UNITS PER DAY OR PER RECONSTITUTED QUART	PERCENTAGE INCIDENCE	NUMBER OF INFANTS
Cod liver oil	460	37	19
*Vitamin D milk (evap.)	400	23	89
Cod liver oil	659	45	40
Viosterol	686	46	22

*Includes "yeast," cod liver oil, and viosterol milks.

The second comparison is for two groups of white infants who received cod liver oil and viosterol at approximately the same dosage level, 659 and 686 units, respectively. There is no significant difference in the incidence of rickets among infants given either cod liver oil or viosterol at these levels.

There is no doubt that in the group of white infants studied the milks at the 400 unit level have been more effective in preventing rickets than cod liver oil at the 460 unit level, and the tendency is the same for the colored infants.

No real difference is found in the efficacy of cod liver oil and viosterol for white infants at the 675 unit level. No real superiority of cod liver oil over viosterol or vice versa has been demonstrated at any dosage level.

GROWTH IN LENGTH

The influence of growth in length on the incidence of rickets and its close association with sex has already been suggested. In order to study this question, the average monthly increase in length has been estimated for each infant included in the study. It should be noted that this method of studying growth* differs from the orthodox cross-sectional approach. A series of measurements on each infant observed for a specified age interval is used to estimate that particular infant's average increase in length for the total period he was under observation. Its advantages over the older method have been clearly defined by Boas,[2]

*The relationship between average percentage increase in weight and incidence of rickets has also been investigated, but up to the present time with negative results.

Palmer and Reed,[3] and others. The exact method of analysis is described in detail in a footnote.*

The mean or average of these individual growth rates is shown by color, sex, and by type of antirachitic substance in Table VII. It will

---

*The method of studying this problem of growth in length consists in estimating the average monthly increase in length for each of the 567 infants. Examination shows that the crown-heel length of an individual infant increases fairly uniformly during early infancy, that is, within the degree of variability of the measurements. Therefore, the straight line, $y = a + bx$, has been taken to describe satisfactory age variations of crown-heel length in the individual infant. The variables, x and y, are respectively age in days, and crown-heel length, measured in centimeters. The b constant is the slope of the line, that is the increase in length per day. The a constant is relatively unimportant, as its value is dependent upon certain arbitrary procedures connected with the solution of the equations. These values have been determined under the least squares criterion. The theory underlying this method is that the observed and theoretical values of y differ by errors which are distributed in accordance with the normal curve.

The b constant multiplied by 30, that is, average increase in crown-heel length measured in centimeters per month, has been used as an index of growth in length. Thus, if 30 b equals 2.38 centimeters, the length of the infant increased on the average 2.4 centimeters per month during the period he was under observation.

The method of determining the constants for the straight line is illustrated for the series of observations given in the following table.

REGRESSION LINE OF CROWN-HEEL LENGTH ON AGE; COLORED FEMALE INFANT (S. C.)

AGE IN DAYS, X	CROWN-HEEL LENGTH IN CM., Y	X²	XY	
23	50.0	529	1,150.0	
51	53.0	2,601	2,703.0	
79	54.5	6,241	4,305.5	n = 6
128	60.0	16,384	7,680.0	S(x) = 621
156	61.0	24,336	9,516.0	S(y) = 341.0
184	62.5	33,856	11,500.0	S(x²) = 83,947.0
S 621	341.0	83,947	36,854.5	S(xy) = 36,854.5

Normal equations:
$$341.0 = 6a + 621\,b$$
$$36{,}854.5 = 621a + 83{,}947\,b$$
Solving:
$$b = 0.07935$$
$$30b = 2.380$$
$$a = 48.62$$
and
$$y = 48.62 + 0.07935x$$

Therefore, during the period of observation, that is from 23 through 184 days of age, the crown-heel length of this infant increased from 50.0 to 62.5 centimeters, or approximately 2.4 centimeters (30b) per month (Fig. 2).

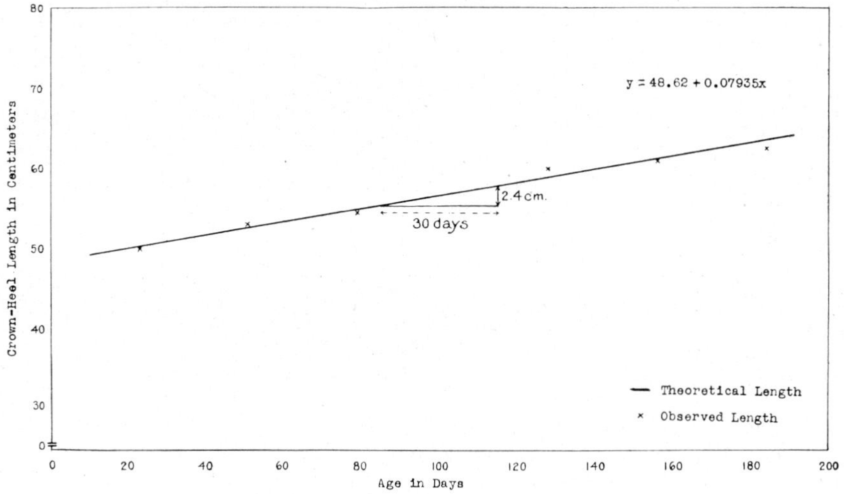

Fig. 2.—Crown-heel length of colored female infant, S. C., measured at irregular intervals from 23 through 184 days of age.

be seen, for example, that the average white male infant grew approximately 2.48 centimeters in length per month during the period he was under observation from one to six and one-half months of age. It should be noted in this connection that these figures are based on observations on a small, highly selected group of Detroit children. It cannot be assumed that the growth rate of infants living in different geographic areas will be the same as those for the Detroit infants included in this study.

TABLE VII

MEAN OF THE AVERAGE INCREASES IN LENGTH (CM.) PER MONTH OF 567 INFANTS GIVEN VITAMIN D IN THE FORM OF COD LIVER OIL, VIOSTEROL OR VITAMIN D MILK (EVAPORATED) BY COLOR AND BY SEX

TYPE OF ANTIRACHITIC AND COLOR	MEAN INCREASE IN LENGTH (CM.) PER MONTH ACCORDING TO SEX	
	MALES	FEMALES
Cod liver oil		
White	2.52 (0.050)*	2.31 (0.086)
Colored	2.54 (0.092)	2.51 (0.106)
Viosterol		
White	2.43 (0.114)	2.26 (0.081)
Colored	2.46 (0.123)	2.34 (0.087)
Vitamin D milk (evaporated)		
White	2.48 (0.047)	2.35 (0.043)
Colored	2.57 (0.089)	2.39 (0.104)
Total		
White	2.48 (0.032)	2.32 (0.029)
Colored	2.54 (0.040)	2.41 (0.045)

*The standard deviation of the mean is shown in parenthesis.

It may be noted that the colored infants tended to grow more rapidly than the white infants of the same sex and that there is a significant difference in the growth in length of the two sexes, the male infants, on the average, growing more rapidly than the female of the same color. As further analysis by type of antirachitic agent shows no real difference between the average increase in length for the infants of a given sex and color who were given any particular type of antirachitic agent and that for the total number of infants of the same sex and color included in the study, only the relation between growth in length and the incidence of rickets according to different dosage levels has been studied.

Growth in Length, Dosage Level and Incidence of Rickets.—The total number of infants was divided, therefore, into two broad, quite distinct dosage groups regardless of type of antirachitic agent. The first group includes those given less than 400 U.S.P. units of vitamin D per day and the second those given 400 units or more. Conservatively stated, the average dosage for the first group was around 275 and for the second, approximately 1,000 U.S.P. units. The lower dosage group includes all those receiving milk and some of the infants receiving cod liver oil; the upper group, all of those receiving viosterol and some of those receiving cod liver oil.

Table VIII shows for these two dosage groups the percentage incidence of rickets for infants whose growth in length was less than and for those whose growth was the same as or more than that of the average infant of the same color and sex. For the infants in the lower dosage group, less than 400 units, there is no consistent difference in the incidence of rickets between those growing slowly and those growing at a faster rate. On the other hand, the infants in the higher dosage group tended to show a consistent difference: In all cases those infants whose growth in length was less than the average* tended to show a smaller percentage of rickets, those who were growing more rapidly, a higher. This evidence indicates that the lower dosage level may not give enough protection to prevent the development of slight rickets in either the infant whose growth in length is below or above the average, but that the higher dosage does tend to protect much more effectively the infant who is growing slowly than it does the more rapidly growing infant. More detailed study of the whole question is needed before definite conclusions concerning the relationship of growth in length to the incidence of rickets can be drawn.

TABLE VIII

PERCENTAGE INCIDENCE OF RICKETS FOR 307 INFANTS RECEIVING LESS THAN 400 U.S.P. UNITS OF ALL FORMS OF VITAMIN D PER DAY AND 260 INFANTS RECEIVING 400 OR MORE UNITS ACCORDING TO COLOR, SEX AND AVERAGE INCREASE IN LENGTH (CM.) PER MONTH

COLOR, SEX AND AVERAGE INCREASE IN LENGTH (CM.) PER MONTH	PERCENTAGE INCIDENCE OF RICKETS FOR INFANTS RECEIVING		NUMBER OF INFANTS RECEIVING	
	LESS THAN 400 UNITS PER DAY	400 UNITS OR MORE PER DAY	LESS THAN 400 UNITS PER DAY	400 UNITS OR MORE PER DAY
White				
Males				
Increase in length				
Less than 2.45 cm.	40	29	58	35
2.45 cm. or more	26	40	51	39
Females				
Increase in length				
Less than 2.30 cm.	23	39	39	36
2.30 cm. or more	25	52	48	29
Colored				
Males				
Increase in length				
Less than 2.55 cm.	30	21	27	29
2.55 cm. or more	36	30	28	30
Females				
Increase in length				
Less than 2.40 cm.	26	17	31	30
2.40 cm. or more	20	22	25	32

*For white females the difference is significant, for males the tendency is the same but cannot be shown to be significant.

PROGRESS AND REGRESSION OF RICKETS

So far only the maximum findings with respect to rickets have been considered. Study of progress of rickets and of regression or healing also brings out some pertinent facts.

Progress of rickets as demonstrated in x-ray films was considered to be present when an initial diagnosis of "very slight" rickets was followed by a diagnosis of "slight," or when a diagnosis of "slight" progressed to a degree classified as "slight-to-moderate." As has been pointed out, in a few cases the process advanced to "moderate" or to "marked." Obviously such changes can be studied most effectively in the group of infants who were observed at reasonably regular intervals from one to six months of age. One hundred twelve infants were so observed. Of them 46 developed rickets and 21 showed evidence by x-ray of progress or advance in the process. Table IX shows the antirachitic substances that were being given and the number of infants in each color group showing x-ray evidence of rickets and progress of the disease.

TABLE IX

NUMBER OF INFANTS OBSERVED BETWEEN 31 AND 179 DAYS OF AGE, NUMBER WHO DEVELOPED RICKETS, AND NUMBER WHO SHOWED PROGRESSION OF THE DISEASE, BY TYPE OF ANTIRACHITIC AGENT AND COLOR

TYPE OF ANTIRACHITIC AND COLOR	NUMBER OF INFANTS		
	TOTAL	DEVELOPING RICKETS	SHOWING PROGRESSION OF THE DISEASE
Cod liver oil			
White	24	11	7
Colored	19	8	7
Vitamin D milk (evap.)			
White	30	12	1
Colored	12	5	2
Viosterol			
White	15	7	4
Colored	12	1	0
Total			
White	69	30	12
Colored	43	14	9

Detailed information with regard to the 21 infants who showed some increase in the degree of rickets is given in Table X. From these data it would appear that progress occurred most often when cod liver oil was given and least often when vitamin D milks were given. The numbers are too few to attempt detailed analysis, but what evidence there is would seem to be in favor of the milks.

Complete regression or healing was considered to be present when the x-ray films showed that all signs of rickets, even the moderately advanced stages of healing, had disappeared and the bones of the forearms again appeared essentially normal.

TABLE X

INFANTS SHOWING PROGRESS OF RICKETS
(OBSERVED FROM 1 TO 6 MONTHS)

CASE	COLOR	SEX	TYPE OF ANTIRACHITIC AND AVERAGE NUMBER OF UNITS PER DAY OR PER RECONSTITUTED QUART	FIRST DIAGNOSIS	AGE AT FIRST DIAGNOSIS (DAYS)	MAXIMUM DIAGNOSIS DURING PERIOD OF OBSERVATION	AGE AT MAXIMUM DIAGNOSIS (DAYS)
			Cod Liver Oil				
J. S.	W	F	206	A_1	97	A_1+	118
R. W.	C	M	210	A_1-	87	A_2+	176
C. S.	C	M	325	A_1	76	B_3	188
J. I.	C	F	340	A_1	84	A_2	126
P. I.	C	M	463	B_1-	90	B_1	118
N. H.	W	M	481	A_1-	70	A_1	112
G. A.	C	M	661	A_1-	117	B_1+	173
C. F.	C	M	686	A_1	115	A_3	178
A. O.	W	M	693	A_1-	108	A_2	170
J. M.	C	F	702	A_1-	44	B_1	98
M. K.	W	M	766	A_1-	65	A_1	100
W. C.	W	M	799	B_1-	104	B_1	132
L. M.	W	M	810	A_1-	52	A_1	80
R. Y.	W	M	926	B_1-	133	B_1	161
			Vitamin D Milk				
C. M.	C	F	CLO conc. in milk 135	A_1-	85	A_1	99
L. W.	W	F	Yeast milk 400	A_1-	79	B_1	170
W. F.	C	M	CLO conc. in milk 400	B_1	132	B_1+	159
			Viosterol				
R. R.	W	F	581	B_1-	124	B_1	159
V. S.	W	F	1459	B_1-	108	B_1	136
J. V.	W	F	2300	A_1-	92	A_1	134
L. S.	W	M	2869	A_1-	86	A_1+	115

Code: A_1-, B_1-, very slight; A_1, B_1, slight; A_1+, B_1+, "slight to moderate"; A_2, B_2, moderate; A_3, B_3, marked. A indicates active rickets; B, under control.

In studying this regression or healing, it became evident that the same factors which enter into the problem of the incidence of slight rickets also influence its disappearance. Dosage level appears to be the most important factor, with sex playing a somewhat more important rôle than it does in the development of the disease. For comparative studies of healing, three distinct, narrowly limited dosage levels were selected: one averaging approximately 150 units, another 400 units, and the third 675. The lower dosage group is composed of infants given the three forms of vitamin D milk at the lower levels, the middle one of infants given vitamin D milk at the higher level, and the third one of infants given viosterol or cod liver oil at the specified level.

TABLE XI

PERCENTAGE INCIDENCE OF HEALING AMONG INFANTS RECEIVING COD LIVER OIL, VIOSTEROL OR VITAMIN D MILKS AT SPECIFIED DOSAGE LEVELS BY COLOR

TYPE OF ANTIRACHITIC AND COLOR	AVERAGE NUMBER OF UNITS PER DAY OR PER RECONSTITUTED QUART	PERCENTAGE OF CHILDREN DEVELOPING RICKETS, WHOSE X-RAY FILMS SHOWED COMPLETE HEALING AT DISCHARGE	PERCENTAGE INCIDENCE OF RICKETS	NUMBER OF INFANTS RECEIVING SPECIFIED TYPE OF ANTIRACHITIC
Cod liver oil				
White	*677	21	42	33
Colored	*662	27	37	30
Viosterol				
White	686	50	46	22
Colored	678	50	24	25
Vitamin D milk (evap.)				
†Lower level				
White	153	27	34	89
Colored	152	17	23	52
‡Higher level				
White	400	50	23	89
Colored	400	33	21	42

*The range of the number of units administered is less than for the group receiving approximately 659 units of cod liver oil, shown in Table V.

†Includes "yeast," cod liver oil concentrate, and irradiated milks.

‡Includes "yeast," cod liver oil concentrate, and viosterol milks.

Table XI shows the type of antirachitic agent, the three major dosage level groups, and the percentage of rachitic infants in whose x-ray pictures complete healing was seen at discharge; it also shows for comparison the total incidence of rickets in each group. The following facts are apparent.

The vitamin D milks at the lower dosage levels (150 units) do not appear to be as effective *in bringing about healing* as the milks at the higher level (400 units) or as viosterol at 675 units. This is of definite interest, since *with respect to the prevention* of rickets the milks, even those of the lower dosage levels, tend (as has been pointed out before) to be at least, if possibly not more, effective than 675 U.S.P. units of viosterol or cod liver oil.

Though the infants in the cod liver oil group were receiving the same number of units as those on viosterol, nevertheless they show a tendency to heal less promptly than did those on viosterol.

The superiority of the milks of the higher dosage level and of viosterol is again brought out.

In Table XII further analysis is made of the effect on healing of the different types of milk at different dosage levels. Milk with added viosterol (400 units) shows a definite superiority over other types of milk containing 400 units ("yeast" and cod liver oil concentrate milk). If these data are compared with those on Table XI, showing the percentage of healing that occurred when viosterol was given alone in doses of approximately 675 units daily, it will be seen that the milk containing 400 units of viosterol appears to be more efficient in bringing about regression of this slight rickets than viosterol when given alone at an even higher level.

TABLE XII

PERCENTAGE INCIDENCE OF HEALING AMONG INFANTS RECEIVING VITAMIN D MILK IN DIFFERENT FORMS AND DOSAGE LEVELS BY COLOR

TYPE OF MILK, NUMBER OF UNITS PER RECONSTITUTED QUART AND COLOR	PERCENTAGE OF CHILDREN DEVELOPING RICKETS, WHOSE X-RAY FILMS SHOWED COMPLETE HEALING AT DISCHARGE	PERCENTAGE INCIDENCE OF RICKETS	NUMBER OF INFANTS RECEIVING SPECIFIED TYPE OF MILK
Vitamin D milk (evaporated)			
"Yeast" milk			
170			
White	36	32	34
Colored	0	28	18
400			
White	44	30	30
Colored	0	27	11
Cod liver oil concentrate in milk			
135			
White	30	38	26
Colored	33	19	16
400			
White	40	17	30
Colored	33	30	10
Irradiated milk, 150			
White	11	31	29
Colored	25	22	18
Viosterol in milk, 400			
White	67	21	29
Colored	67	14	21

COMMENT

In the analysis of the data presented in this study the statistical method has been applied. Though the individual groups of infants at each dosage level were too small to be able to test the reliability of the results in many cases, nevertheless the tendencies shown in the data have been consistent and repeated with but few exceptions. In a fair proportion of cases the data have been adequate to permit tests for statistical significance, and the results so obtained uniformly strengthen the conclusions to be drawn from the general tendencies shown by the data as a whole. The differences that have been shown to exist with respect to the incidence of rickets and healing between white and colored infants, and between the less rapidly and the more rapidly growing infants make it clear that, for each dosage level studied, color and sex should both have been considered in selection of the groups, and enough infants should have been included so that growth in length could have been classified more specifically.

The problem of growth as related to rickets needs to be studied further, as, for instance, the question of whether growth in length during the early months of life is related to length at birth and whether rate of growth may be predicted from measurements at birth. Additional study is needed to determine more satisfactorily whether the several available types of antirachitics are equally effective in the more rapidly growing infants, and whether the basic factors entering into the regression or healing of slight rickets are the same as those influencing the healing of moderate or marked rickets and if so whether their relative importance remains the same.

The conclusions that can be reached as a result of the analysis are included in the following summary.

SUMMARY

1. This paper reports an investigation of the relative efficacy of several different forms of vitamin D at different dosage levels. The study was carried out in Detroit, Mich., during the winter months of 1933-36. Five hundred sixty-seven full-term infants were observed from approximately one through six and one-half months of age. They were given either cod liver oil or viosterol or some form of vitamin D milk at different dosage levels. The dosage administered varied considerably, from approximately 150 through 3,000 U.S.P. units. Diagnosis was based on x-ray films of the bones of both forearms, taken at approximately monthly intervals.

2. The results of this study have demonstrated the necessity of considering such factors as color, sex, rate of growth in length, period of observation, and interval between examinations as basic when attempting to evaluate the efficacy of certain types of antirachitic substances administered at different dosage levels in the prevention of rickets.

3. The evidence presented refers almost exclusively to the incidence of slight rickets as the dosage level was sufficiently high to prevent the development of moderate or marked rickets except in a few infants.

4. The incidence of rickets was significantly less among the colored infants than among the white. The same tendency was found consistently among infants given the different antirachitic agents both when all dosage levels were combined and, with few exceptions, at the different dosage levels.

5. When pertinent basic factors were taken into consideration, it became apparent that, in spite of their lower dosage level, the milks, especially those at the 400 unit level, tended to be more effective in the prevention of rickets than cod liver oil. There is also evidence that viosterol is at least as effective as cod liver oil, and no evidence that cod liver oil is superior to viosterol, unit for unit, in the prevention of rickets.

6. There is no definite evidence from this study that one type of milk at the 400 unit level is superior to another in the prevention of rickets. For the lower dosage levels no clear-cut conclusions with regard to comparative efficacy can be drawn.

7. Within the dosage range used for each type of antirachitic, the higher dosage levels appear to be more effective, provided the basic factors mentioned above are taken into consideration.

8. Advance in the rachitic process occurred most frequently in infants receiving cod liver oil, least frequently in those given vitamin D milk.

9. Regression or healing of the slight degrees of rickets discussed in this paper tended to occur more promptly in infants receiving vitamin D milk of the higher (400 units) dosage level than in those receiving that of the lower level (150 units). Of the different types of vitamin D milk containing 400 units, that to which viosterol was added appeared to be the most efficient. This form also tended to be more efficient than viosterol alone even when the latter was given at a somewhat higher level. When given at a dosage level of approximately 675 units, viosterol tends to bring about regression of slight rickets more promptly than cod liver oil at the same dosage level.

10. The incidence of slight rickets has been shown to be closely and consistently related to growth in length when the dosage of the antirachitic is relatively high, whereas for infants in the lower dosage group there is no consistent difference in the incidence of rickets. These findings indicate that at the higher level the balance between rickets-producing and rickets-preventing factors has been stabilized to such an extent as to allow rate of growth in length to become evident. On the other hand, when a smaller amount is given, the effect of the growth in length is lost in the stronger influence of the inadequate amount of vitamin D.

11. It would appear that if rickets is to be prevented or promptly controlled an amount of vitamin D must be given that will assure

stability in the metabolic processes providing for normal bone growth and allow an adequate margin of safety for the rapidly growing infant. From the data here presented, this amount would appear to be at least as high as that contained in the usual dose of cod liver oil; namely, two to three teaspoonfuls.

Finally in evaluating the results of such a study as this one, it should be borne in mind that from the public health point of view, as well as that of the individual infant, the value of a substance containing vitamin D should be measured first in terms of success in the prevention of rickets under practical conditions and second in terms of economy, and that such economic considerations must include not only the cost of the vitamin but also the need and cost of other nutrients supplied by the vehicle carrying vitamin D.

REFERENCES

1. Eliot, Martha M., and Powers, G. F.: J. A. M. A. **102**: 1823, 1934.
2. Boas, F.: The Growth of Toronto Children. United States Bureau of Education, Report of the Commissioner of Education, 1896-1897, Vol. 2, Government Printing Office, Washington, D. C., pp. 1541-1599.
3. Palmer, C. E., and Reed, L. J.: Human Biology **7**: 319, 1935.

American Academy of Pediatrics

Proceedings

REPORT OF THE COMMITTEE ON HOSPITALS AND DISPENSARIES

Contagious Disease Hospitals

Part II

THE second report concerns contagious hospitals found in Regions II and IV of the American Academy of Pediatrics. Six hospitals are represented from the South and seventeen from the Far West. Sixteen of the total number are contagious divisions of general hospitals. Questionnaires were filled out and returned to the committee by the following hospitals.

HOSPITAL NUMBERS. SECTIONS II AND IV. EXHIBIT A

Section II

NO.	
1	Municipal Hospital, Atlanta, Georgia
2	City Hospital, Louisville, Kentucky
3	Knoxville General Hospital, Isolation Dept., Knoxville, Tennessee
4	Memphis General Hospital, Isolation Dept., Memphis, Tennessee
5	John Sealy Hospital, Contagious, Galveston, Texas
6	Henry A. Wise Hospital, Norfolk, Virginia

Section IV

NO.	
1	San Luis Obispo General Hospital, San Luis Obispo, California
2	Riverside County Hospital, Riverside, California
3	Los Angeles County Hospital, Los Angeles, California
4	No reply
5	San Diego County General Hospital, Contagious Department, San Diego, California
6	San Bernardino County Charity Hospital, San Bernardino, California
7	Santa Barbara General Hospital, Santa Barbara, California
8	Alameda County Hospital, Oakland, California
9	Children's Hospital, Contagious Dept., San Francisco, California
10	City and County Hospital, Contagious Dept., San Francisco, California
11	Santa Clara County Hospital, Isolation Dept., San Jose, California
12	Sacramento County Hospital, Isolation Dept., Sacramento, California
13	Fresno County Hospital, Isolation Dept., Fresno, California
14	Portland Isolation Hospital, Portland, Oregon
15	Salt Lake General Hospital, Salt Lake City, Utah
16	City Contagious Hospital, Tacoma, Washington
17	Isolation Hospital with Firlands Tuberculosis Sanitorium, Seattle, Wash.
18	Rivercrest Hospital, Spokane, Washington

As far as the committee is able to determine, the list represents the only hospitals which may be classified as contagious with the possible exception of one hospital in California and one in Georgia from which no questionnaires were returned.

I. Staff

A. Professional Staff

1. Attending Staff

EXHIBIT B

A. PROFESSIONAL STAFF. I. STAFF. 1. ATTENDING STAFF

HOSP. NO.	ALL PATIENTS UNDER CARE OF PHYS. ON STAFF	ALL PHYSICIANS IN COMMUNITY ALLOWED TO HAVE PATIENTS IN WDS. AND TREAT THEM	QUALIFICATIONS OF OUTSIDE PHYSICIANS	PEDIATRICS				OTOLARYNGOLOGY				ORTHOPEDICS				OPTHALMOLOGY			
				SPECS. ON STAFF	NO. MO. EACH YR.	VISITS AT REG. INTERVALS	ON CALL ONLY	SPECS. ON STAFF	NO. MO. EACH YR.	VISITS AT REG. INTERVALS	ON CALL ONLY	SPECS. ON STAFF	NO. MO. EACH YR.	VISITS AT REG. INTERVALS	ON CALL ONLY	SPECS. ON STAFF	NO. MO. EACH YR.	VISITS AT REG. INTERVALS	ON CALL ONLY
Section II																			
1	Yes	No	Spec. arrangement with hosp. supt.	Yes 19	1 for 12 6 for 3 12 for 1	Yes Yes	Yes	Yes 18	18 for 3 mo.	9 Yes	9 Yes	Yes 8	6 for 12		Yes	Yes 10	3 for 12		Yes
2	Yes	No	None	Yes 6	2 mo.	Pediatrists	Spec.	Yes 6	2 mo.			Yes 6	2			Yes 6	2		
3	No pay pts. have choice	Phys. of pay cases	Good standing	Yes	2-3	Yes		Yes	2-3	Yes		Yes	2-3	Yes		Yes	2-3	Yes	
4	Yes	Yes		Yes	12	1-3 daily		Yes	12	Yes		Yes	12	Yes		Yes	12	Yes	
5	Yes	No	Staff members	Yes 2	Serve continuously			Yes 1	Serve con- continuously			Yes 1	Serve continuously			Yes 1	Serve continuously		
6	No	Yes		No				No				No				No			
Section IV																			
1	Yes	No																	
2	Yes	No			12					Yes					Yes			Yes	

EXHIBIT B—CONT'D

3	Yes	No		Yes 8	6	Yes		Yes 2	12	Yes		Yes			Yes	Yes			Yes
5	Yes Pay	No Private	Cases able to Dr.	Yes 6	2	Yes		Yes			Yes	Yes			Yes	Yes			Yes
6	Yes	Private only in cont.		Yes 2	6	Yes		Yes		Yes		Yes 2	6	Yes		Yes		Yes	
7	Yes	No		Yes 2	6	Yes		Yes 3	4	Yes		Yes 1	12	Yes		Yes 1	12	Yes	
8	Yes	None	None	Yes 5				Yes 8				Yes 9				Yes 4			
9	Yes	No		Yes	12	Yes		Yes			Yes	Yes			Yes	Yes			Yes
10	Yes	Send but not treat					Yes				Yes				Yes				Yes
11	No	No		Yes 3		Yes		Yes 2		Yes		Yes 1		Yes		Yes 1		Yes	
12	Yes	No Only staff mem. allowed		Yes 2	6	Yes		Yes 1	12	Yes		Yes 3	4	Yes		Yes 1	12	Yes	
13	Yes	No		Yes 1	12		Yes	Yes 4	12		Yes	Yes 1	12		Yes	Yes 4	12		Yes
14	No	Yes		Yes	12	Yes													
15	No	Yes		Yes 1	12	Daily	Cont. and T.B.	Yes 4	3		Yes	Yes 6	2		Yes	Yes 4	3		Yes
16	Yes	Yes		County Medical Society gives consultation when needed															
17	Yes	No	May as Con-sultant Mem. King Co. Med. Soc.	Yes 1		Once wk. and call		Yes 1		Once wk. and call		Yes 1		Once wk. and call		Yes 1		Once wk. and call	
18	No Attending Staff—City Health Officer in complete charge																		

EXHIBIT B

A. PROFESSIONAL STAFF. I. STAFF CONTINUED. 1. ATTENDING STAFF

HOSP. NO.	SURGERY				NEUROLOGY				PSYCHIATRY				PSYCHOLOGY				DERMATOLOGY			
	SPECS. ON STAFF	NO. MO. EACH YR.	VISITS AT REGULAR INTERVALS	ON CALL ONLY	SPECS. ON STAFF	NO. MO. EACH YR.	VISITS AT REGULAR INTERVALS	ON CALL ONLY	SPECS. ON STAFF	NO. MO. EACH YR.	VISITS AT REGULAR INTERVALS	ON CALL ONLY	SPECS. ON STAFF	NO. MO. EACH YR.	VISITS AT REGULAR INTERVALS	ON CALL ONLY	SPECS. ON STAFF	NO. MO. EACH YR.	VISITS AT REGULAR INTERVALS	ON CALL ONLY
Section II																				
1	Yes 30	3-12		Yes	Yes 4	6-12		Yes	Yes 1	12		Yes	Yes 1	12		Yes	Yes 2	12		Yes
2	Yes 6	2			Yes 6	2			Yes 6	2			Yes 6	2			Yes 6	2		
3	Yes	2-3	Yes		Yes	2-3	Yes		Yes	2-3	Yes		Yes	2-3	Yes		Yes	2-3	Yes	
4	Yes	12	Yes		Yes	12	Yes		No				No				Yes	12	Yes	
5	Yes 1	Serve continuously			Yes 2	Serve continuously			Yes 1	Serve continuously			No				Yes 2	Serve continuously		
6	No				No				No				No				No			
Section IV																				
1	Yes 4	3	Yes																	
2			Yes					Yes												
3	Yes			Yes	Yes			Yes	Yes			Yes	N.R.				Yes			Yes

EXHIBIT B—CONT'D

5	Yes			Yes	Yes			Yes	Yes			Yes	No				Yes			Yes
6	Yes		Yes																	
7	Yes 3	6	Yes		Yes 1	6	Yes		Same Dr. as Neurology				No							
8	Yes 28				Yes 4				Yes	Same as Neurology			No				Yes 4			
9	Yes			Yes	Yes			Yes	Yes			Yes	Yes			Yes	Yes			Yes
10				Yes				Yes				Yes				Yes				Yes
11	Yes 1			Yes	No				No				No				Yes 1			Yes
12	Yes 12	4	Yes		Yes 1	12	Yes		Yes 1	12	Yes		Same as Psychiatry				Yes 1	12	Yes	
13	Yes 3	12		Yes	Yes 1	12		Yes	Yes 1	12		Yes	Yes 1	12		Yes	Yes 1	12		Yes
14	No reply																			
15	Yes 12	4		Yes	Yes 1	12		Yes	Yes 1	12		Yes	No				Yes 3	4		Yes
16	County Medical Society gives consultation when needed																			
17	Yes 1		Once wk. and call		If necessary			Yes	If necessary			Yes	If necessary			Yes	If necessary			Yes
18	No Attending Staff—City Health Officer in complete charge																			

EXHIBIT B

A. PROFESSIONAL STAFF. I. STAFF CONTINUED. 1. ATTENDING STAFF

HOSP. NO.	DENTISTRY SPECS. ON STAFF	DENTISTRY NO. MO. EACH YR.	DENTISTRY VISITS AT REGULAR INTERVALS	DENTISTRY ON CALL ONLY	ORAL SURGERY SPECS. ON STAFF	ORAL SURGERY NO. MO. EACH YR.	ORAL SURGERY VISITS AT REGULAR INTERVALS	ORAL SURGERY ON CALL ONLY	ORAL HYGIENE SPECS. ON STAFF	ORAL HYGIENE NO. MO. EACH YR.	ORAL HYGIENE VISITS AT REGULAR INTERVALS	ORAL HYGIENE ON CALL ONLY	ROENTGENOLOGY SPECS. ON STAFF	ROENTGENOLOGY NO. MO. EACH YR.	ROENTGENOLOGY VISITS AT REGULAR INTERVALS	ROENTGENOLOGY ON CALL ONLY	PATHOLOGY SPECS. ON STAFF	PATHOLOGY NO. MO. EACH YR.	PATHOLOGY VISITS AT REGULAR INTERVALS	PATHOLOGY ON CALL ONLY
Section II																				
1	Yes 2	12		Yes	Yes 2	12		Yes	Yes 2	12		Yes	Yes 1	12			Yes 1	12		
2	Yes 6	2			Yes 6	2			Yes 6	2			Yes 6	2			Yes 6	2		
3	Yes	2-3	Yes		Yes	2-3	Yes		Yes	2-3	Yes		Yes	2-3	Yes		Yes	2-3	Yes	
4	Yes	12	Yes		Yes	12	Yes		No				Yes	12	Yes		Yes	12	Yes	
5	Yes 1	Serves con-tinu-ously			Yes 1	Serves con-tinu-ously			Yes 1	Serves con-tinu-ously			Yes 1	Serves con-tinu-ously			Yes 1	Serves con-tinu-ously		
6	No				No				No				No				No			
Section IV																				
1													Yes 1	12	Yes					
2			Yes								Yes			12						
3	N.R.				Yes			Yes	N.R.				Yes			Yes	Yes 2	12		

EXHIBIT B—CONT'D

5	Yes			Yes	Yes			Yes	No				Yes			Yes	Yes			Yes
6	Yes 3	On at same time	Yes										Yes 1	12	Yes		Yes 1	12	Yes	
7	Yes 1	12	Yes		Yes 1	12	Yes		Same Dr. as Oral Surgery				Yes 1	12	Yes		Yes 1	12	Yes	
8	Yes 1				Yes 3				Yes 1				Yes 3				Yes 5			
9	Yes			Yes	Yes			Yes	Yes			Yes	Yes			Yes	Yes			Yes
10				Yes				Yes				Yes				Yes				Yes
11	Yes 1		Yes		No				No				Yes 1		Yes		No			
12	Yes 1	12	Yes		Yes 1	12	Yes						Yes 2	6	Yes		Yes 1	12	Yes	
13	Yes 1	12		Yes	Yes 1	12		Yes					Yes 1	12		Yes	Yes 1	12		Yes
14																				
15	Yes 2	6		Yes	No				No				Yes 1	12	3 days wk.		Yes 1	12	Daily	
16	County Medical Society gives consultation when needed																			
17	Yes 1		Daily and call		Yes 1			Yes	Yes 1			Yes	Yes 1		Daily		If necessary			Yes
18	No Attending Staff—City Health Officer in complete charge																			

EXHIBIT B

A. PROFESSIONAL I. STAFF CONTINUED

HOSP. NO.	ALLERGY				TIME		SALARY	
	SPECS. ON STAFF	NO. MO. EACH YR.	VISITS AT REGULAR INTERVALS	ON CALL ONLY	ANY ON FULL?	THOSE ON FULL	ANY ON SALARY?	THOSE ON SALARY
Section III								
1	Yes	12		Yes	Yes	Medical Supt. Prof. Med. & Surg. Pathologist Roentgenologist	Yes	Those on full time
2	Yes 6	2			Yes	1	Yes	2
3	Yes	2-3	Yes		No		No	
4	No				No		No	
5	Yes 1	Serve continuously			Yes	Pathology 1 Surgery 2	Yes	All
6	No				No		Yes	City Physician
Section IV								
1					No		Yes	Roentgenology
2		–			No		No	
3	Yes			Yes	No		N.R.	
5	No				Yes	Chief of Dept. Tuberculosis	Yes	County Psychiatrist

EXHIBIT B—CONT'D

HOSP. NO.	ALLERGY				TIME		SALARY	
	SPECS. ON STAFF	NO. MO. EACH YR.	VISITS AT REGULAR INTERVALS	ON CALL ONLY	ANY ON FULL?	THOSE ON FULL	ANY ON SALARY?	THOSE ON SALARY
Section IV—Cont'd.								
6	Yes 1	12	Yes		No		Yes	Pathologist Roentgenologist
7	N.R.				No		No	
8	No				No		Yes	X-ray Pathology
9	Yes			Yes	No		No	
10				Yes	Yes		Yes	Director $4,200 yearly
11	Yes 2		Yes		N.R.		Yes	Roentgenology $100 per month
12					No		No	
13					No		Yes	$50 per month
14					Yes	City Health Officer	Yes	All City Health Officers
15	Yes 1	12		Yes	No		Yes	2 Med. Drs. part time
16					No		Yes	Director of Health Supt. of Hosp.
17	No				Yes	Infec. Dis. Specialist	Yes	All
18	No Attending Staff—City Health Officer in complete charge							

Among 23 hospitals 17 report that ward patients are under the exclusive care of the attending staff. Only 6 hospitals permit all physicians in the community to send patients to their wards and treat them there. All of the hospitals require that their men be of good standing in their community.

Information concerning physicians on the attending staff in the various specialties is presented in Exhibit B.

None of the hospitals has a full-time staff. Seven report that one or two members of the staff are employed full time. The city health officer is placed in this category in one instance. Fifteen report that one or more members of the staff are paid a salary. This usually applies to individuals in charge of the x-ray department or the laboratories or to a health officer.

Resident Staff.—Eighteen hospitals employ resident physicians. In 6 instances more than one is employed. Women are eligible for this position in 10. All pay the resident a salary. This varies from $50.00 to $200.00 per month; 14 hospitals pay a salary to the resident of more than $50.00 a month. Twelve hospitals require that the resident have at least one year or more of previous hospital experience. Two require more than one year, and the remainder are content with no previous experience except an M.D. degree from a class A school. The length of the service is usually six months or one year, just four services are for one year. The resident has dispensary duties in seven instances. Three hospitals did not reply to this question.

Six hospitals employ assistant residents, women being eligible in four. All pay the assistant resident a salary. Four require previous hospital experience in order for one to qualify for the position. The length of the service is six months in one hospital, one year among the others. Dispensary duties are available in three instances.

Sixteen hospitals employ internes, twelve more than one, and eight more than two. Seven have eight or more. None have more than nineteen. Women are eligible in eight. Fourteen pay a salary to internes. This is usually $25.00 or less per month. Among fifteen hospitals which replied, only one requires previous hospital experience in order to qualify for interneship. All require an M.D. degree from an accredited school. The length of the service varies from 20 days to one year. One-year services are available in eight instances; among the others the service is for three months or less.

Educational Activities.—These are presented in chart form (Exhibit C).

Nine of the 23 hospitals in Regions II and IV are connected with medical schools, 4 among 6 in Region II and 5 among 17 in Region IV. In all but one of these, clinics are available to medical students. Ward rounds are offered for medical students in 7. One did not reply. Eight hospitals have clinics open to practicing physicians, and they may attend ward rounds or walks in 9. Fourteen hospitals hold regular clinical conferences and 16 hold similar pathological conferences, which are usually held weekly. Eleven hospitals have available facilities for research and 8 encourage research in communicable disease.

Special Information.—Presented in Exhibit D with summary following.

Thirteen hospitals report that new cases may be placed in observation wards, cubicles, or one and two bedrooms until the diagnosis is certain. Routine cultures for diphtheria are taken on admission in 14 hospitals, for hemolytic streptococci in 8. Routine vaginal smears are done in 8 hospitals, Von Pirquet or Mantoux tests in 4, Wassermann or Kahn tests in 13, Schick tests in 3, Dick tests in 2. Routine

EXHIBIT C
EDUCATIONAL ACTIVITIES

HOSP. NO.	MEDICAL SCHOOL IN CONNECTION WITH HOSP.	MEDICAL CLINICS GIVEN	STUDENTS WARD ROUNDS WALKS GIVEN	PRACTICING PHYSICIANS: NO. AND CHARACTER CLINICS OPEN TO	PRACTICING PHYSICIANS: NO. AND CHARACTER WARD ROUNDS OPEN TO	POST-GRADUATE COURSES
Section II						
1	Emory Univ.	Yes	Yes	None	None	No
2	Med. Dept., Univ. of Louisville	Frequently	Regularly	Yes—Cont. cases not suitable for gen. clinics	Yes—Daily ward walks. Not often by outside phys.	No
3	None	Yes Internes	Yes	Yes—Out-patient clinic	Yes	No
4	Univ. of Tennessee	Yes	Daily	None	Yes—Any time they desire	No
5	Med. Dept., Univ. of Texas	Yes	Yes	None	None	No
6	None	None				
Section IV						
1	None	None	None			No
2	None					No
3	Univ. of California	Yes	Yes	1 per wk. case demonstration and lectures	N.R.	No
5	None			None	Not in cont. section	No
6	None	N.R.	N.R.	Charity cases for staff men only	N.R.	No
7	None	No	No	Weekly conferences	No	No
8	None	No	No	Surgical medical	Medical and surgical	No
9	Univ. of California	Semimonthly	N.R.	Semimonthly	Daily if desired	No
10	Univ. of California and Standard Med. School	Yes	Yes	None	Yes—No regular schedule	No
11	None			None	None	No
12	None			None	None	No
13	None			None	None	No
14	Univ. of Oregon	Yes	Yes	None	N.R.	No
15	Univ. of Utah Med. School	No	No	Staff-periodic interval	Salt L. Co. Med. Soc. and Utah St. Med. Assn. Mem.	No
16	None	None	None	N.R.	N.R.	No
17	None	None	None	No	Yes—Variable	No
18	None			No	No	No

EXHIBIT C

EDUCATIONAL ACTIVITIES

HOSP. NO.	INTERNES: CLINICAL CONFERENCES HELD AND HOW OFTEN?	INTERNES: PATHOLOGICAL CONFERENCES HELD AND HOW OFTEN?	LIBRARY NO. VOLUMES IN HOSP. MED. LIBRARY	FACILITIES FOR RESEARCH AVAILABLE TO RESIDENT AND HOUSE STAFF	ENCOURAGE RESEARCH COMMUNICABLE DISEASES
Section II					
1	Monthly regular interne Cont.	Weekly entire hosp. staff	550	Use of clinical material and lab. assistance of visiting men and pathologist	No
2	Weekly	As available	Small No.	None	No
3	Monthly	Weekly	? on No.	Yes	Yes
4	Yes—Occasionally	Almost 6 yearly	None	Clinical experiments with serum vaccines and medications	Yes
5	No	Weekly	None	None	No
6					
Section IV					
1			30		
2			300		
3	3 per week	1 per week	Yes	Bacteriological Lab. in Com. Dis. Hosp.	
5	Weekly	Weekly	300	Only on individual effort	No
6	Yes	Yes	325	N.R.	N.R.
7	1 per week	1 per week	50	Limited amount. Study of vascular abnormalities and arteriograms	No
8	Every week	Every week	Co. Med. Soc. Library	To limited extent only	Yes
9	N.R.	N.R.	500	Yes	Yes
10	Daily	Weekly	Being revised	Yes	Yes
11	Semiweekly	At autopsies	100	Nothing special	No
12	No	Weekly	322	None	No
13	Daily ward walks	Weekly	1,000	None	No
14	No	No	No	None	No
15	1 every 2 months	1 every 2 months	No	None	Yes
16	No	No	15	Connected with City Health Dept.	Yes
17	1 per week	Yes	100-125	Well-equipped laboratory with technicians	Not discouraged
18			No	None	Yes

blood counts are taken in 17 hospitals, urinalyses in 18, complete histories are taken and physical examinations are done in 18 hospitals. Five did not reply to this section.

II. Superintendent

This section of the questionnaire concerns the physical set-up of the hospitals. Twenty-two hospitals replied. Among that number only 3 are found in poor residential, tenement and factory districts. The remainder are located in better or moderate, residential, apartment, and shop districts. Only 5 report that their neighborhood is noisy as a result of the presence of factories, trolleys, heavy traffic, or railroads.

Exhibit E presents certain details concerning the physical organization, size, etc., of these hospitals.

Twelve hospitals have one building, 3 have 5, and 2 have 6 buildings. The earliest construction date is 1910, the latest, 1934. First buildings were constructed between 1910 and 1920 for 11 hospitals. First buildings were constructed in 1920 or later among 6. First buildings for 2 after 1930. Nine hospitals have only one or two floors (5-2, 4-1). Six are of fireproof construction. Cost of buildings again shows great variation—from $4,500.00 to $1,000,000, depending on the size and modernity of the plant. Only 11 hospitals supplied the latter information, and among these 6 cost less than $100,000.00.

Bed capacities among 20 hospitals which replied vary from 14 to 456. Only 6 have bed capacities of less than 50. Nine have 100 or more. The three largest report 456, 423, and 350. The three smallest, 14, 18, and 30. Eighteen hospitals report the number of cribs available, which varies from 2 to 26. The three highest report 26, 24, and 22; the lowest, 2, 2, and 2.

Among 19 hospitals which replied, 17 have wards and 8 have cubicles available. These may contain from one to four beds in different hospitals.

Fourteen hospitals exclude no contagious disease; four exclude pertussis, measles and chickenpox; and ten exclude syphilis, one, typhoid fever and the dysenteries.

Seven hospitals did not reply to the question concerning observation wards. Among 15 which replied, 9 do not have them. Three have roms or cubicles which can be used in this capacity.

Contagious Disease Wards (Exhibit F).

Fifteen replies were received to this section of the questionnaire. Fourteen hospitals have contagious disease wards. These vary from one to eight in number. Ten hospitals have 3 or more wards. The total number of beds, of course, varies considerably depending upon the size of the hospital. The lowest number is 3, the highest, 500; but only 3 report a bed capacity of 100 or more. Nine of the 15 hospitals report fewer than 50 beds. Wards for the most part are not large; only one hospital reports 20 or more patients to a ward; the remainder report from 2 to 16. Five hospitals have cubicles and 12 separate rooms. All report that the hospital gets sunlight and 9 have outdoor porches. Adults and children are admitted to the same ward in 10 hospitals.

Admissions.—Admission figures and other relative information for hospitals listed by number for the years 1932, 1933, and 1934 are presented in Exhibit G.

Only three hospitals report admissions of 5,000 or more for any one of the three years considered. Many report fewer than 1,000 admissions. Total admissions for all hospitals is not large when the size of the area involved is considered. Percentages of deaths for all hospitals were 6.2, 6.4 and 7.7 for the years 1932, 1933, and 1934, respectively.

EXHIBIT D

SPECIAL INFORMATION. I. STAFF

HOSP. NO.	OBSERVATION WARDS			PROCEDURES BEFORE ADMISSION TO WARDS										
	WARDS	TIME CASES IN OBSERVATION	TIME CASES MAY BE KEPT	THROAT CULTURE B. DIPH.	THROAT CULTURE HEMOLYTIC STREPT.	VAGINAL SMEARS FOR GON.	VON PIRQUET OR MANTOUX	WASSERMANN OR KAHN	SCHICK TEST	DICK TEST	ROUTINE BLOOD COUNTS	URINALYSIS	HISTORY TAKEN	COMPLETE PHYSICAL MADE
Section II														
1	Yes Rooms	Diag. is certain	Discretion of staff	Yes	No	Yes	As indicated	Taken later	As indicated	No	Yes	Yes	Yes	Yes
2	No to cont. hosp.			Yes	Yes		Man.	Wass.	Yes	Yes	Yes	Yes	Yes	Yes
3	Yes	Attending Drs. judgment		Yes	Yes	Yes	Man.	Kahn	Yes	Yes	Yes	Yes	Yes	Yes
4	Yes		As long as necessary until diag. is made	On all	On all	All formulas	Yes	Wass.	Yes	No	Yes	Yes	Yes	Yes
5	Yes	48 hr.		Yes	Yes	If discharge or inflammation is present	Yes	Wass.	Yes	No	Yes	Yes	Yes	Yes
6														

EXHIBIT D—CONT'D

Section IV

1				No	No	No	No	Kahn	No	No	Yes	Yes	Yes	Yes
2	Yes	As directed by Attending Dr.	As directed by Dr. until diag. is established	Yes	Yes	Not routine	Not routine	Yes	Not routine		Yes	Yes	Yes	Yes
3	Yes			Yes	No	Yes	No	Children no Adults yes	No	No	Yes	Yes	Yes	Yes
5	Cubicles only			Yes	No	If indicated	As ordered	As ordered	As ordered	As ordered	Yes	Yes	Yes	Yes
6	Not admitted for observation													
7	None			As indicated		As indicated		Yes	As indicated		Yes	Yes	Yes	Yes
8	None			Yes	Yes	Yes	Not regular	Yes	Not regular		Yes	Yes	Yes	Yes
9	Yes	24 hr.	Until diag. is made	No	If indicated	No	Routine	Routine			Yes	Yes	Yes	Yes
10	None Cubicle or separate room	10-24 days		2-48 hr. intervals	2-48 hr. intervals	3-5 day intervals	No	Both	Not regular	No	Yes	Yes	Yes	Yes

EXHIBIT D—CONT'D

HOSP. NO.	OBSERVATION WARDS			PROCEDURES BEFORE ADMISSION TO WARDS										
	WARDS	TIME CASES IN OBSERVATION	TIME CASES MAY BE KEPT	THROAT CULTURE B. DIPH.	THROAT CULTURE HEMOLYTIC STREPT.	VAGINAL SMEARS FOR GON.	VON PIRQUET OR MANTOUX	WASSERMANN OR KAHN	SCHICK TEST	DICK TEST	ROUTINE BLOOD COUNTS	URINALYSIS	HISTORY TAKEN	COMPLETE PHYSICAL MADE
Section IV—Continued														
11				Yes	Yes	If indicated	No	Kahn	No	No	Yes	Yes	Yes	Yes
12	None			Yes	No	If indicated			No	No	Yes	Yes	Yes	Yes
13	1 and 2 bedrooms			Yes		Yes		Kahn			Yes	Yes	Yes	Yes
14	None													
15	Yes	3-5 days	As long as necessary			As required			No	No	Yes	Yes	Yes	Yes
16	Yes		Until diag. is established											
17	Yes	Few suspects admitted	Until well at end of quarantine	Yes	Yes	Yes	Occasional	Occasional			Request of staff doctor	3x wk. or daily	Yes	Yes
18	None													

All hospitals in both regions accept both white and negro children. In Region II all are segregated. In Region IV, they are segregated by four hospitals. No hospital in either region limits the number of colored children that may be admitted. Five hospitals have all charity beds. In no hospital are the beds on a strictly paying basis. Five have private rooms for children, 3 have them for adults. Two hospitals have facilities for mothers to stay with the children.

Superintendent.—All of the hospitals derive their funds from either city or county, none from the state. One hospital derives part of its funds from endowment, 2 from private funds, and none receive aid from the community chest. Only 6 hospitals reported their running costs for the last fiscal year. The lowest sum reported was $8,565.31; the highest, $517,631.37. Cost per patient per day varied from $2.22 to $4.68. Average costs for food varied from $0.22 to $1.12 per day. Nursing costs $0.41 to 1.04 per day, and supplies cost from $0.13 to $0.65 per day.

In 12 hospitals the superintendent is a man, a physician in 11, and a lay person in 4. Among 4 women superintendents, 2 are registered nurses, but none are physicians. In one instance, the woman superintendent is also in charge of the nurses' training school.

Nursing.—Among 22 hospitals which replied, 8 are affiliated with other hospitals for the purpose of special training in nursing. Fourteen offer courses in contagious nursing technic. The length of these courses varies from 6 weeks to 3 years. In 6 hospitals only graduate nurses are employed. Immunization of nurses to diphtheria is done in all hospitals of Region II, but is not done in four in Region IV. To immunization of nurses to scarlet fever, in Region II, three replied, "yes" and three, "no"; in Region IV, four, "yes" and twelve, "no." To smallpox immunization in Region II, all replied, "yes"; in Region IV, 13, "yes," and 3, "no." To typhoid fever and other contagious diseases where immunization is possible in Region II, 3 replied, "yes"; in Region IV, 9, "yes." In 1934, one nurse in each of only 2 hospitals in Region II contracted diphtheria, 1 in one hospital, scarlet fever, and none, any other contagious disease. In Region IV, two each in 2 hospitals contracted diphtheria; one, two, three and four, respectively, in 4 hospitals contracted scarlet fever. No other contagious disease was contracted by nurses in any of the 6 hospitals reporting from Region II. In Region IV, 4 hospitals report that nurses contracted rubella, chickenpox, bacillary dysentery, mumps, and one reports that three nurses contracted anterior poliomyelitis. The number of nurses assigned to wards in proportion to the number of patients seems to be adequate in all hospitals. Lengths of assignments vary from 2 weeks to 3 months.

Operating Room.—Fourteen hospitals have at least one special operating room for the contagious division. Only 3 use pupil nurses there. Only 8 hospitals report operations performed in that division in 1934, these varying in number from 7 to 4,070.

Diet Kitchen.—Nine hosiptals have special diet kitchens for infant foods; 6 have them for children.

Supervision Head Nurses

Eight hospitals have head nurses in charge of wards. Fourteen employ one or more graduate nurses for day duty; 11 employ them for night duty.

Supervisors.—Fifteen hospitals employ day supervisors, all of them graduate nurses. Thirteen employ night supervisors, all of them graduate nurses.

Instruction.—Information concerning instruction in contagious nursing was received, but because of the great amount of detailed information we shall not attempt to report it here.

EXHIBIT E

A. GENERAL. II. SUPERINTENDENT

HOSPITAL NUMBER	NUMBER OF BUILDINGS	DATE OF CONSTRUCTION	DATE OF ADDITIONS	NUMBER OF FLOORS IN EACH	FIREPROOF	FIRE STAIRS IN WALLS	OUTSIDE FIRE ESCAPE	COST OF BUILDINGS ONLY
Section II								
1	1	1910 Renovated 1934	None	3	No	No	No	$ 25,000
2	5	1913	None	3 in 3 Bldgs. 1 in 2	Yes	Yes		$1,000,000
3	6	1918 1928 1933		2-4	1		Yes	
4	1	1922		2		Yes		$ 150,000
5	1	1915		2 1 in use	No	No	No	$ 18,000
6								
Section IV								
1	1	1927	None	2	Yes		Yes	
2	Part 2nd floor and a 4-room cottage						Yes	

EXHIBIT E—CONT'D

3	1			4	Yes		Yes	
5	5	New	Not available	3	Partial	Yes	Yes	Not available
6	1	1922	6 beds 1934	1				$ 4,500
7	5 hosp. 12 others	'15-'26 '29-'31 '32-'34	1931 1932	Main—2 Others—1	Main bldg.	No	No	$ 300,000
8		1917 to 1926		3 and basement	Yes			
9								
10	1	1918	0	3	Yes	Yes	Yes	$ 200,000
11	1	1920	1925	1	No			
12					Yes			
13	1	1932						$ 55,000
14	1			2				
15	6	Cont. 1934		5—Main 5—Nurses 1—T.B. 1—Cont.			Yes	$ 400,000
16	1	1912	None	1	No			
17	2	'12-'15		1	No		Yes	$ 30,000
18	1	1910		3	Brick and frame		Porches	$ 85,144

EXHIBIT E

B. BED CAPACITY. II. SUPERINTENDENT

HOSPITAL NUMBER	TOTAL			WARDS	HOW MANY IN CUBICLES	SPECIFY THOSE NOT IN CUBICLES	BEDS IN EACH CUBICLE	CONTAGIOUS CASES EXCLUDED
	BEDS	CRIBS (2 YR. AND UNDER)	BEDS (2 YR. AND OLDER TO 14 YR.)					
Section II								
1	51	15	36	6	All		1	Amebic dysentery, bacillary dysentery, typhoid, Tbc., and syphilis
2	423	22	74	15	1	Isolation—1		None
3	350	24	20	12	Contagious only		1-4	Tbc., syphilis, alcoholism
4	60	10	50	8	None			None
5	14	2	12	3	Movable glass partition used		1	Uncomplicated pertussis, measles, and chickenpox
6								All cases not being handled in homes accepted
Section IV								
1	80	8	6	None				
2	325 25 Communicable	5	10	4	0			None
3	235			7	0			None
5	43	6	37	10	1		1	Whooping cough, measles, chickenpox, unless complicated

EXHIBIT E—CONT'D

6	328	5	As needed	2	8	7 private rooms	1	None
7		10	15	67 rooms	10		1 and 2	None
8	456	26		15	Single rooms to 6 beds			
9	No report							
10	120			4	All		8—3 beds 8—2 beds 1—12 beds 70 single beds	None
11	30	7	23					None
12	18	6	6 adults 6 children	1	All		Varies	None
13	31	6	25			All 1 and 2 beds except 2 rooms in cubicles		None
14	70			4				None
15	228	2		3—Tbc. 2—Cont. 4—Semi-private				None
16	30	2	28	8				Measles, chickenpox, or wh. c. not encouraged
17	60	As needed	As needed	24			16—2 beds 8—3 and 4 beds	None
18	121	5	83 beds 33 cots	8				Accept only diphtheria, smallpox, and scarlet fever

EXHIBIT F

C. DETAILS OF WARD CAPACITY

HOSPITAL NO.	CONTAGIOUS DISEASE WARDS							
	NO. WARDS	TOTAL NO. BEDS	BEDS IN EACH WARD	NO. IN CUBICLES	NO. OF SEPARATE ROOMS	SUNLIGHT	OUTDOOR PORCHES	ADULTS AND CHILDREN IN SAME WARD
Section II								
1	6	51	4-7	All	Only observation rooms	Good except 2 wards	No	No
2	1	79		12	17	Ultra-v. light	Yes	Yes—but not same room
3	4	4-6		24	All cubicles	4 sun parlors	Glass enclosed	No
4	8		4		26	Double doors and large windows	None	According to diagnosis
5	3	10	2-4	Movable partitions		Yes	No	When crowded for space
6					10	Yes	No	Yes
Section IV								
1	2	4	2		None		Yes	Yes
2					Depending on the need	Yes	Yes	No

EXHIBIT F—CONT'D

3	7	235	24 to 39-44	0	59	4	1	Yes
5	10	43	3-7	5	2	East, south and west	Yes	If necessary
6	2	20	5-8	8	7	Outside rooms	No	Yes
7	5	16	3-5	0	When necessary	Yes	1	If necessary
8	2	60	30	None	30	Yes	No	In separate rooms
9	No report							
10	4	120	30			Yes	No	Separate rooms
11	8	30	2-5		1	Yes	No	Occasionally
12	1	18		12		Yes	No	Yes
13	21	31			13 single, 2—3-bed, 6—2-bed	Yes	2	With same disease
14	9	70	6-8		None			Yes
15	3—Tbc. 2—Cont.	17—Cont. 32—Tbc.	3—Cont. 6—Tbc.	0	3 contagious	All	No	No
16	6	28	8 and 4	0	2	Yes	Yes	Yes
17	24	60	2-4	0	24	Indirect	No	Rarely and then if related
18	8		12	0	0	All	9	If necessary

Exhibit G

D. Attendance

HOSP. NO.	PATIENTS		ADMITTED PATIENTS		DISCHARGED		DIED IN HOSPITAL			PATIENTS IN HOSPITAL	
	1932	1933	1934	1932	1933	1934	1932	1933	1934	OPENING LAST YEAR	CLOSE LAST YEAR
Section II											
1	275	Not available	480	Not available	Not available	483	11	Not available	54	21	18
2	11,436	11,852	11,891	11,424	11,873 and died	11,907	966	1,016	1,100	392	373
3	6,268	6,481	7,132	6,236	6,547	7,072				122	144
4	Contagious Tbc.			637 71	920 113	867 75	68 34	83 47	100 26	40	42
5	104	113	July-Jan. 42	104	110	36	0	4	6	1	4
6											
Section IV											
1	1,287	1,260	1,564	1,230	1,394	1,457	52	60	75	45	49
2			84			78			3	0	3
3				4,152	5,095	5,914	415	405	362		

EXHIBIT G—CONT'D

5			561			544			19	36	34
6	3,563	3,673	3,378	3,551	3,678	3,379			326	273	272
7	1,814	2,150	2,191	1,711	2,039	2,050			123	180	166
8	10,405	10,476	10,674				649	699	719	278	278
9											
10	675	742	872	652	675	810	33	53	41	30	51
11	186	211	282	175	201	251	9	9	15	18	23
12		164	166					18	31		
13	192	258	295	190	246	264	19	25	37	12	31
14											
15	101	127	174	116	144	190	30	25	32	29	43
16											
17	275	189		286			1	1			
18	71	56	156	68	57	150	2	0	7	7	13
Totals II	18,083	18,446	19,545	18,472	19,563	20,440	1,080	1,150	1,286	576	581
IV	18,569	19,306	20,397	12,131	13,529	15,087	1,210	1,295	1,790	908	963
	36,652	37,752	39,942	30,603	33,092	35,527	2,290	2,445	3,076	1,484	1,544

EXHIBIT G—CONTINUED

D. ATTENDANCE

HOSPITAL NUMBER	COLORED AND WHITE CHILDREN ACCEPTED	COLORED AND WHITE SEGREGATED	LIMIT TO NO. OF COLORED CHILDREN AT ONE TIME	GENERAL PROPORTION COLORED CHILDREN	STRICTLY CHARITY BEDS	STRICTLY PAY BEDS	NO. PRIVATE ROOMS FOR CHILDREN	PRIVATE ROOMS FOR ADULTS	ANY FACILITIES FOR MOTHERS TO STAY WITH CHILDREN
Section II									
1	Yes	Yes	Only as to space and beds	¼%	51	None	Rare exceptions	Rare exceptions	No
2	Yes	Yes	No	40%	All	None	Emergency Private cases rarely adm.	Emergency Private cases rarely adm.	No
3	Yes	Yes	No		341 and pay				
4	Yes	Yes	No	⅔%	All and private accepted				No
5	Yes	Yes	No	¾%	14	None			No
6	Yes	Yes	No	60%			2	2	No
Section IV									
1	Yes	Yes	No	100:1	Varies	Varies	19	19 for both	Yes
2	Yes	No	No		All	None	2	2	No
3	Yes	No	No						No
5	Yes	No	No	Less than 1%	43 Cont.	None	None	None	No
6	Yes		No	Low	All except for private	As needed			No

EXHIBIT G—CONT'D

7	Yes	As far as possible	No	Very few	225	10 beds part pay	None	1	No
8	Yes	No	No	Not known	All	None	None	None	No
9	Yes	No	No	About 1%					Yes
10	Yes	No	No	2 or 3 a yr.	120	None			No
11	Yes	No	No	Practically more have colored	All	None	None	None	No
12	Yes	No	No	negligible		None			No
13	Yes	As far as possible	No	Small	31				No
14	Yes	No	No	1:10	If unable to pay	All unless unable to pay	None	None	No
15	Yes	No	No	Small	17	None	Not segregated	Not segregated	No
16	Yes	No	No	1:300	30	None	Not segregated	Not segregated	Yes, but not permitted
17	Yes	Not always	No need	1:20	All	None	None	None	If both with same disease
18	Yes		No need		Residents no charge	None	None	None	If absolutely necessary

EXHIBIT H

IV. X-RAY

HOSPITAL NUMBER	DIAGNOSTIC FACILITIES	FULL-TIME TECHNICIANS	AVAILABLE ANY HOUR	AT WHAT HOURS	HIGH-SPEED RADIOGRAPHY	MILLI-AMPERAGE	SUPERFICIAL RADIOGRAPHY	VOLTAGE	DEEP RADIOTHERAPY	VOLTAGE	FLUOROSCOPY	STEREOSCOPIC PLATES
Section II												
1	Yes	2	Yes		Yes	100	Therapy	50-90 Kw	Yes	To 200,000 Kv	Yes 2	Yes
2	Yes	3	Yes		Yes	Ma nax 3,500	Yes	Kv Pk 30 & up	Yes	30-90 Kv	Yes	Yes
3	Yes	1	Yes		Yes		Yes		No		Yes	Yes
4	Yes	1	Yes	All	Moderately high	100	Therapy	All	Yes	185 Peek Kv	Yes	Yes
5	Yes	1	Yes	All	Yes	500	Yes	140 Kv	Yes	200 Kv	Yes	Yes
6	None											

EXHIBIT H—CONT'D

Section IV

1	Yes	No	Yes		Yes	200	No		No		Yes	Yes
2	Yes	1	Yes		Yes		Yes	125 Kv	No		Yes	Yes
3	Yes	1	Yes								Yes	
5	Yes	2	Yes		No		Therapy	100-125	Yes	200 Kvp	Yes	Yes
6	Yes	1	Days	8-5	Yes	100	Yes	30 Kvp up	Yes	200 Kvp	Yes	Yes
7	Yes	1½	Yes		Yes	100 ma	Yes	35 Kvp	No		Yes	Yes
8	Yes	2		7:30 A.M. 4:30 P.M.	No	100	Yes	130 Kvp	Yes	200 Kvp	Yes	Yes
9			Yes						Yes		Yes	Yes
10	Yes	4	Yes	7:30 A.M. 12:00 M.	Yes	200	Yes	20 Ko to 100 Ko	Yes	200 Ko	Yes 2	Yes
11	Yes	3	Yes		Yes	100	Yes		No		Yes	
12	Yes	2	Yes		Yes		No		No		Yes	Yes
13	Yes	1 part time	Yes		Yes		No		No		Yes	Yes
14	None											
15	Yes	2	Yes		Yes	100	Yes	92-102 Kvp	No		Yes	Yes
16	None											
17	Yes	1	No	8-4	Yes	100	Yes		No		Yes	Yes
18	None											

IV. X-Ray

HOSPITAL NUMBER	PORTABLE X-RAY MACHINE	INTERNES X-RAY WORK	IF SPECIAL SPECIFY	EQUIPMENT ADEQUATE	DEPT. SERVE DISPENSARY	OUTSIDE PHYSICIANS	NO. X-RAY PLATES LAST YEAR	NO. SUPERFICIAL TREATMENTS	NO. DEEP THERAPY TREATMENTS
Section II									
1	Yes 2	No		Yes	Yes	No	Unable to ascertain	Included with Grady Hosp.	With Grady Hosp.
2	Yes	No		Yes	Yes	No	50,000	100	200
3	Yes	Some	Special	Yes	Yes	Indigent cases			
4	No	Yes	Attend reading all films and fluoroscopic exams if interested	Old and space not had at present	Yes		Plates not known 8,176 exams.	Total 2,878	
5	Yes	No		Yes	Yes	Yes	4,636	396	793
6	None								
Section IV									
1	No	No		Yes	Yes	Yes	597	0	0
2	No	No		Yes except deep therapy	Yes	No	Communicable diseases not segregated		
3	Yes	No		Yes	No		1,400		

EXHIBIT H—CONTINUED

5	Yes	No		Yes	Yes	No	Communicable diseases not segregated		
6	Yes	No		Yes	Yes	Charity only	2,904 Exam. of film	131	170
7	No	No		For special work insufficient	No	No	3,068 729 dentals	341	0
8	No	No		Yes	No	No	18,440	371	1,580
9	Yes		7 weeks' instruction diagnoses of films	Yes	Yes	Yes			
10	2	No		Business too great for equipment	Yes	City physicians only	N.R.	0	0
11	Yes	Yes	Emergency	Yes	Yes	No		682	0
12	Yes	No		Yes	Yes	No			
13	Yes	No		Yes	Yes	No		0	0
14									
15		Fluoroscopic examinations on fractures		Deep therapy apparatus necessary	Yes	No	Contagious comparatively few	0	0
16									
17	No	No		Yes	No	Through City Health		0	0
18									

Information concerning crossed infections in 1934.

Diphtheria:	14 hospitals—occurred in one
Scarlet fever:	14 hospitals—occurred in five
Measles:	14 hospitals—occurred in one
Pertussis:	13 hospitals—occurred in one
Chickenpox:	13 hospitals—occurred in one
Other diseases:	11 hospitals—occurred in none

X-ray (Exhibit H).

Four hospitals have no x-ray diagnostic facilities. Sixteen have these facilities available at any hour, day or night. Fifteen are equipped for high-speed radiography, 14 for superficial, and 9 for deep radiotherapy. Nineteen are equipped with fluoroscopes, 17 for stereoscopy and 12 have portable machines. Internes do x-ray work in 3 hospitals. Seventeen consider their equipment to be adequate. The x-ray department serves the dispensary in 15 hospitals and outside physicians in 3.

Again our information indicates that these departments in many instances serve an entire general hospital; hence, figures given for number of treatments, plates, etc., are not satisfactory for comparison or estimation of these actually in the contagious department alone.

Laboratories—Pathological—Clinical—Bacteriological—Serological

General.—Thirteen hospitals indicate that a full-time director in charge of laboratories is employed. In 3 the work is done in the city health department, while 7 employ part-time directors.

Pathological.—Twelve hospitals have full-time directors of pathological laboratories. Three have no directors either full or part time. Sixteen employ full-time technicians, 3 have none on full time. Internes do laboratory work in 9 hospitals, routine in 3, special in 6, routine and special in 1. Seventeen of the 19 hospitals that replied consider their laboratory facilities adequate. Only 9 have facilities for research work. Autopsy percentages among 15 hospitals reporting varied from about 30 to a little less than 60 per cent, with a general rough average around 50 per cent.

Clinical.—Fifteen hospitals have full-time directors of the clinical laboratories, 6 have part-time directors, and the others have none or did not reply. Twenty hospitals have full-time technicians, and in 14, the internes do work in the clinical laboratory, routine in 8, and special in 6. Blood chemistry work is available in 20 hospitals; 7 have ''fume hoods''; and 16 have colorimeters. Nineteen possess equipment to do basal metabolic tests. The machines used are usually Sanborn or McKesson's. Seventeen consider their clinical laboratory facilities to be adequate, 2 do not, and 2 do not reply. Twelve afford facilities for research work.

Bacteriological.—Fifteen hospitals have full-time directors of the bacteriological laboratories; four have part-time directors. Nineteen have full-time technicians. Internes do laboratory work in 10, in 5, routine, in 5, special. Nineteen laboratories have electric incubators. Eighteen make all or part of their own media. Nineteen keep animals for experimental purposes. Eighteen have facilities for research work. Eleven consider their bacteriological laboratory facilities adequate.

Serological.—Fifteen hospitals have full-time directors of the serological laboratories and 18 have full-time technicians. Internes do laboratory work in only 2, and this is of a special nature in both instances. Wassermanns are done in their own laboratories in 17, and Kahn tests in 14. Seventeen consider their facilities adequate, and 9 have facilities for research work.

Miscellaneous.—Fourteen hospitals have facilities available for simple photography, 4 for color photography, and 4 for motion pictures. An electrocardiograph is available in 17 hospitals.

Diet Kitchen.—Fourteen hospitals employ trained dietitians. Five employ nurses in this capacity; the remainder did not reply. In 6 hospitals, diets are arranged by both attending physicians and dietitians; in 7, the attending physician alone prescribes the type of diet. One gains the impression that diets are efficiently supervised in most of these hospitals.

Social Service.—Fourteen hospitals maintain a social service department. All but one have a full-time worker in charge, and in most instances these supervisors have had special training for that work.

Fourteen hospitals investigate all patients who are admitted. This is usually done by talking to relatives who bring the patients, but by 9 hospitals home visits are made. Thirteen hospitals take a complete social history in all cases, which is, by 7, filed with the medical history. In 4 an abstract is filed. The social service investigates the patient's ability to pay in 14 hospitals. Convalescent homes are available for patients from 5 of the hospitals, foster homes for 11 hospitals. Only 2 consider their facilities for convalescent care to be adequate.

By 11 hospitals, cases are ''followed'' after discharge. The social service assists in getting patients for recall or ''follow-up'' in 12 hospitals. Volunteers are used for indoor work by 7, for outdoor work by 3. The ward service department is supported by hospital funds in 15, by outside funds in 1; the rest do not reply. Only 2 hospitals have a special ''lay'' committee in charge of the social service department, a physician being on this committee in 1 instance.

General Information (1934).—The following chart reveals the number of cases of the more usual contagious diseases admitted to these hospitals during 1934, together with the total deaths and the percentage death rate in all hospitals for each disease (Exhibit I).

Only 800 cases of diphtheria were admitted to all hospitals in both regions, and of these only 266 were admitted in Region IV. The percentage of deaths was about the same for the 2 regions, but slightly higher for Region II than for Region IV. Scarlet fever deaths show about the same percentage in each region. Measles shows an extremely low rate for Region IV, and both regions had lower percentages of deaths than did Region III. Pertussis has a very high rate in Region II. Both regions are higher than Region III, provided one hospital is omitted which had the remarkable record of only 0.4 per cent deaths among 1,824 cases. There were no deaths from smallpox in either region. This was also true in Region III. There were no deaths from chickenpox in Region IV and only 0.1 per cent in Region II, but here again 1 hospital, the same hospital mentioned in connection with pertussis, reports no deaths among 1,183 cases. Eliminating these figures, the death rate in the rest of the hospitals in Region IV is 3.3 per cent. Percentage of deaths for epidemic spinal meningitis is considerably higher in both regions than in Region III. Typhoid fever percentages are higher in Region II and lower in Region IV than those reported for Region III.

Amebic dysentery occurred with relative infrequency in these two regions considering the area of country involved. The percentage of deaths was about the same, 7.1 per cent and 6.2 per cent respectively. Region III reported more than twice as many cases with no deaths (mortality questionable).

Bacillary dysentery occurred much more frequently in Region II and the percentage of deaths was almost three times as great.

Among other diseases listed under miscellaneous, only 2 cases of poliomyelitis were reported from Region II with no deaths, but Region IV reported 251 cases with 18 deaths, a percentage of 7.1 per cent. Region IV reports 174 cases of erysipelas with a death rate of 10.5 per cent.

As in Region III, other contagious diseases more frequently admitted to the contagious hospitals of Region II and IV are encephalitis, mumps, influenza, strepto-

EXHIBIT I

VIII. GENERAL INFORMATION—1934

HOSPITAL NUMBER	DIPHTHERIA		SCARLET FEVER		MEASLES		WHOOPING COUGH		SMALLPOX		CHICKEN-POX		EPI. CEREBRO-SPINAL MENINGITIS		TYPHOID FEVER	
	CASES	DEATHS	CASES	DEATHS	CASES	DEATHS	CASES	DEATHS	CASES	DEATHS	CASES	DEATHS	CASES	DEATHS	CASES	DEATHS
Section II																
1	273	17	73	1 (pneumonia)	104	7	30	5	0	0	8	0	27	12		
2	127	19	96	2	53	2	40	6	0	0	16	0	5	1	30	4
3	28	1	15	0	11	0	3	0	0	0	8	0	2	2	14	1
4	55	5	50	0	161	7	48	12	4	0	14	0	20	11	69	17
5	35	1	21	0	0	0	32	6	0	0	2	0	3	2	8	0
6	16	4	23	0	23	0	6	0								
Per cent of fatal cases	8.8%		1.08%		4.5%		18.2%		0.0%		0.0%		49.1%		18.1%	
Section IV																
1	4		3													
2	13	3	13	0	2	0	0	0	0	0	4	0	0	0	11	0
3	No report															

Exhibit I—Cont'd

5	67	2	112	2	53	1	4	0	0	0	1	0			51	2
6	30	5	36	1	10	0	0	0	7	0	0	0	0	0	0	0
7	3	0	19	0	15	0	7	0	0	0	2	0	1	1	25	0
8	46	3	69	0	16	0	3	0	0	0	3	0	11	4	9	1
9	No report															
10	33	0	106	6	54	0	35	2	0	0	12	1	5	3	7	0
11	20	0	40	2	24	0	24	2	4	0	6	0	3	3	3	0
12	31	2	40	2	10	0	8	1	0	0	10	0	0	0	25	8
13	11	3	75	1	39	0	27	3	0	0	18	1	3	3	28	8
14*	9	–	578	–	2	–	–	–	32	–	–	–	1	–	–	–
15	0	0	61	3	20	3	18	5	4	0	2	0	2	1	8	2
16	8	0	32	1	2	0	3	0	11		2		1	0	2	0
17	1	0	611	3	275	1	1824	8	135	0	1183	0	2	1	30	0
18	0	0	83	2					4	0						
Per cent of fatal cases	7.0%		1.8%		0.96%		1.07% 10.07% without No. 17				0.1% or 3.3% without No. 17		55.1%		10.5%	

*Does not report deaths. Hence mortality rate is figured without them.

EXHIBIT I—CONT'D

VIII. GENERAL INFORMATION—1934

MISCELLANEOUS DISEASES

HOSPITAL NUMBER	DISEASES	CASES	DEATHS
Section II			
1	Encephalitis	2	0
	Vincent's angina	3	0
	Tetanus	3	2
	Anterior poliomyelitis	2	0
	Mumps	4	0
2			
3	Acute colitis	5	1
	Diarrhea	5	0
4			
5			
6			
Section IV			
1	Influenza	2	
	Poliomyelitis	1	
	Streptococcic throat	2	1
2	Malta fever	5	0
	Influenza	5	0
	Diphtheria carrier	1	0
3			
5	Poliomyelitis	35	0
	Erysipelas	18	2
	Trachoma	19	
	Gc. vaginitis juveniles	5	
	Other Gc. infections	46	
	Other diseases	180	7
6	Erysipelas	10	1
	Lobar pneumonia	23	8
	Poliomyelitis	8	0
	Meningitis	5	5
	Other diseases	8	1
7	Balantidium dysentery	1	0
	Poliomyelitis	2	1
	Trachoma	1	0
	Mumps	1	0
	Leprosy	2	0
8	Erysipelas	27	2
	Encephalitis	5	1
	B. welchii	11	1
	Gc. ophthalmia	5	0
	Other diseases	133	13
9			

EXHIBIT I—CONT'D

10	Erysipelas	55	3
	German measles	11	0
	Gc. vaginitis	32	0
	Gc. ophthalmia	7	0
	Other diseases	269	21
		163	0
11	Gc. vaginitis	10	0
	Impetigo	8	0
	Scabies	16	0
	Vincent's angina	5	0
	Poliomyelitis	17	0
	Other diseases	17	2
12	Anterior poliomyelitis	4	1
13	Poliomyelitis (fiscal year)	17	2
	July-December	9	3
	Impetigo contagiosa	15	1
	Erysipelas	14	3
	Tbc. meningitis	6	4
	Other diseases	4	4

14	Impetigo	1	
	Mumps	3	
	Poliomyelitis	3	
	Erysipelas	41	
15	Influenza	3	0
	Syphilis	64	0
	Tetanus	54	17
	Rheumatic fever	7	0
	Other diseases	179	9
16	Poliomyelitis	6	2
	Tbc. meningitis	1	1
	Other diseases	16	0
17	Erysipelas	9	2
	Poliomyelitis	91	7
	Mumps	2916	0
	German measles	8	0
18	Poliomyelitis	69	5
	Poliomyelitis	253	18
		7.1%	
	Erysipelas	174	133-14
		10.5%	

EXHIBIT I—CONT'D

VIII. GENERAL INFORMATION—1934

HOSPITAL NUMBER	AMEBIC DYSENTERY		BACILLARY DYSENTERY	
	CASES	DEATHS	CASES	DEATHS
Section II				
1				
2	4	0	18	1
3				
4	6	1	65	19
5	4	0	4	1
6				
Per cent of fatal cases	7.1%		24.1%	
Section IV				
1			1	
2	8	0	8	0
3	No report			
5	3	1	3	1
6	3	0	0	0
7	3	0	0	0
8	5	0	0	0
9	No report			
10				
11	0	0	4	0
12	3	0	2	0
13	7	1	1	0
14				
15			1	0
16				
17	N.R.	3	N.R.	1
18				
Per cent of fatal cases	6.2%		8.3%	

coccic throat infections, Vincent's angina, various forms of meningitis and gonorrheal vaginitis in juveniles. None report that syphilitic cases are admitted, but only 2 say that they are barred.

COMMENT

Regions II and IV include the southern states and the Far West. In this entire area, we found only 27 contagious hospitals listed as such. The report is based on replies received from 23 hospitals, representing 9 states, 5 in Region II and 4 in Region IV. No city in either of the 2 regions has more than 1 contagious-disease institution with the exception of San Francisco, California, which lists 2. Among 17 hospitals, of the total number reported from Region IV, 12 are found in California. The figures indicate that there are states in both Regions II and IV which have no contagious-disease hospitals.

There are only three large hospitals in the 2 regions, each of these having more than 300 beds, none more than 475.

Eighteen of the hospitals employ resident physicians and 6 have an active service and employ more than 1 resident physician. Several hospitals unfortunately do not require the resident physician to have had previous hospital experience. The larger hospitals all require at least one year of previous hospital experience before the applicant can be eligible for that position. All hospitals require their internes to have M.D. degrees. Services of one year's duration or more are available in only 8 hospitals.

The contagious hospital is connected with a medical school or affords training to medical students or both in the following cities: Atlanta, Ga., Louisville, Ky., Memphis, Tenn., Galveston, Tex., Los Angeles, Calif., San Francisco, Calif. (2), Portland, Ore., and Salt Lake City, Utah. Facilities for research work are available to the resident and home staff in only the larger hospitals and among these hospitals, as a rule, the organization, particularly as to clinical laboratory and x-ray facilities, appears to be efficient.

Several hospitals apparently do not take routine throat cultures, vaginal smears, or blood counts. We feel that these 3 procedures, at least, should be routine in all contagious hospitals.

Only 8 hospitals have nursing affiliations that afford training in contagious nursing. As in Region III, comparatively few nurses contracted a contagious disease while working in these hospitals.

Several hospitals do not report that they have operating rooms in the contagious divisions, which we feel are very essential parts of contagious hospitals.

Fourteen hospitals reported concerning crossed infections. The record shows that these were comparatively infrequent.

Four hospitals among 23 apparently have no facilities for x-ray work. This is a serious weakness, although these are small tax-supported institutions as in Region III in which the need for x-ray work is probably infrequent. Among the smaller hospitals, again the laboratory services often seem inadequate.

We realize that among small institutions the cost of maintaining a highly organized laboratory, nursing and dietary service would probably be prohibitive, when the relatively small number of cases admitted yearly is considered. However, the patient who is ill of a contagious disease deserves and should have just as efficient care as any other sick person. If an institution for the care of contagious diseases is to be maintained at all, it should be established and run upon that principle. Finally, all of the institutions but two report that their facilities for convalescent care are not adequate.

In general, we might say that most of these institutions seem well equipped and are well run.

Book Review

Allergy of the Nose and Paranasal Sinuses. By FRENCH K. HANSEL, St. Louis, 1936, The C. V. Mosby Company, 820 pages with 58 text illustrations and 3 color plates.

As stated in the Preface, "the object of this monograph is to familiarize the otolaryngologist with the clinical features of allergy as related to the field of otolaryngology, to review the various phases of the subject itself, and to point out the frequent association of the nasal with the other manifestations, particularly asthma, gastrointestinal allergy, allergic skin diseases, and allergic headache." A chapter of twenty-five pages is devoted to allergy and infection of paranasal sinuses in children. This chapter should make the book of considerable interest to all pediatricians.

The subject matter is divided into four general sections. Under the major heading of Fundamental Principles of Paranasal Sinus Diseases, the author discusses the physiology, biochemistry, and bacteriology of the nose and paranasal sinuses. The pharmacologic action of drugs and the cellular reactions of the tissues in allergy and in immunity are described. The second section is devoted to a brief but comprehensive discussion of the theoretical phases of allergy and anaphylaxis and the fundamental clinical characteristics of allergy. In this section, the author presents the conservative, generally accepted ideas which prevail today on this very complex and little understood subject. The third section is devoted to clinical manifestations of allergy as they are expressed in the nasal and paranasal sinus areas of the body. This section of the book probably represents the best efforts of the author, and one will find here excellent discussions of diagnosis of these various conditions. Hay fever is dealt with as a separate section, but may be included for consideration in this section on clinical manifestations. At least as far as children are concerned, it seems difficult to separate nasal pollen reactions from those caused by other foreign substances. The fourth section is devoted to treatment of these various clinical conditions.

The form of the book is entirely satisfactory. The type is large, clear, the style is simple and direct, though inclusive, and the text is easy to read. There are numerous good illustrations which are usually original. There is ample reference to the best work of the most conservative workers, and it would seem that very little of importance in the literature has been missed. Each chapter has an extensive bibliography on that subject. The author has also included to great advantage a résumé, representing his opinion of each phase of the subject. This feature makes the book extremely useful for rapid reference. Numerous case reports in detail are included to illustrate more complex points. These are from the author's own experience in a large otolaryngologic clinic. Part of the pediatric material has been drawn from cooperation with the pediatric allergist.

The work represents a very valuable contribution to this field of medicine. It is recognized that only the beginning of allergy is at present understood and that many factors are mixed with theory and hypothesis, all of which are influenced by personal opinion and experience. These ideas are changing rapidly, and, no doubt, many statements in the book will be questioned in some degree. The general principles, however, are all recognized. It would be difficult to find one person who could combine in his experience all the phases of this very broad subject.

The book should be of value to the otolaryngologist, but it would seem to this reviewer that it would be still more useful to anyone in clinical medical practice, either the internist, the pediatrician, or the general family doctor. The book has considerable reference value and the information is sufficient to be instructive to anyone.

H. McC.

The Journal of Pediatrics

Vol. 9 | October, 1936 | No. 4

Original Communications

PROTAMINE INSULIN IN CHILDREN

Gladys L. Boyd, M.D.
Toronto, Ontario

EVER since insulin was first used, attempts have been made to alter it in such a manner that its absorption would be delayed and its action would be made to resemble more closely that of the normal pancreatic secretion. Efforts during the same time to make the insulin pure have helped to defeat this purpose by reducing the zinc content[1] of the compound and possibly by eliminating split protein products, both of which play a rôle in delaying the absorption of the hormone.

A little over two years ago, Hagedorn and his coworkers[2] at the Steno Memorial Hospital in Copenhagen felt justified in subjecting to clinical trial a mixture of insulin and protamine which they had found after prolonged search to be less soluble in serum and more slowly absorbed than any mixture previously suggested. In the course of some other work these observers discovered that insulin combined with nucleic acid had a more acid isoelectric zone than insulin itself. Accordingly, they sought some basic group with which to combine insulin in order to get its isoelectric zone nearer the pH of tissue fluid than insulin hydrochloride. Such a compound would act as an acid, whereas ordinary insulin acts as a base. Various substances were tried, but protamines alone gave solubility results sufficient to merit trial. Monoprotamines only have been used. The raw material has been the ripe sperm of certain fish. In the past two and a half years these authors have treated eighty-five patients with such a mixture. No ill effects have been seen and much better control has been established in severe cases. These workers used ordinary insulin in the morning and the protamine compound at night.

Presented before The American Pediatric Society, Bolton Landing, June, 1936.

From the Wards and Laboratories of the Hospital for Sick Children, Toronto, and the Department of Paediatrics, University of Toronto, under the direction of Prof. Alan Brown.

Early this year, Root, White, Marble and Stotz[3] reported a series of cases with equally good results. A little later, Kerr, Best, Campbell, and Fletcher[4] reported their results in man and animals, and more recently Sprague and his associates[5] have added further confirmation of the possibilities of this insulin.

The present report is based on the study of twenty-five diabetic children treated with protamine insulin since last December at the Hospital for Sick Children, Toronto. At first the insulin used was made with ordinary insulin mixed with protamine obtained from Hagedorn by Best. Later the protamine was obtained from British Columbia salmon and prepared at the Connaught Laboratories, Toronto. The insulin is prepared for injection by adding to ordinary insulin the right quantity of protamine buffered by sodium phosphate. A flocculent precipitate forms which after shaking is injected in the usual manner. This compound is unstable and should be used within ten days of its preparation. When it is kept in the ice box, a certain amount of shrinkage of the protamine solution occurs, so that it must be warmed to room temperature again before measuring. This instability of the compound is one of the difficulties that must be overcome because it entails too much handling of material by unskilled hands.

The usual procedure has been to observe the patient in the hospital with alternating control periods on insulin hydrochloride with those on protamine insulin. A few of those treated have been well-stabilized cases treated in the out-patient clinic, but in all these close observation of both urine and blood sugar was made.

In none of the children studied was control impossible with ordinary insulin, but in some this was accomplished only with four doses of insulin a day, one before each meal and one at midnight. With protamine insulin alone, or combined with ordinary insulin, equally good, if not better, results were achieved with two doses a day. In both Copenhagen and Boston it was usual to use morning doses of ordinary insulin and evening doses of protamine insulin. In a few this has been found an advantage, but in most cases the "insulin retard" has been used entirely because it is less confusing for the parents to give one kind than to give two kinds. The object of combining the two has been to get the advantage of quick acting insulin to cover the postprandial rise of blood sugar after breakfast. In our experience, the morning glycosuria has been equally well controlled if the protamine insulin was administered by the clock, 8 A.M. and 8 P.M., rather than at mealtimes. Kerr found this adjustment more satisfactory in controlling blood sugar curves in dogs, and it was on his suggestion that we tried it. There is what might be called a refractory period before the best results are obtained. Substitution of equal doses of protamine insulin for ordinary insulin, even if given by the clock, may permit some glycosuria for a couple of days, which completely disappears without any further adjustment by the end of this time. Patients requiring from 80 to 100 units of insulin daily are satisfactorily controlled with two doses of the new insulin or one dose of new and one of old. In milder cases requiring up to as much as 50 to 60 units daily, adequate control is often possible with only one dose in twenty-four hours. The optimum time for its administration is not fixed, but at present an hour before breakfast has seemed a suitable time. It may prove to be better to administer the single dose between eight and nine o'clock at night.

Reactions occur, but they are less severe and less frequent than hypoglycemia. Possibly this is because of the more gradual fall of the blood sugar that occurs. One is amazed how often with a blood sugar content of 40 to 50 mg. per 100 c.c. no symptoms or signs of reaction are apparent, whereas values between 20 and 30 are frequently only accompanied by mild symptoms. Blood sugar estimations appear to be more urgent in the patient who is a glycosuric with insulin retard than with ordinary insulin. Protracted ill feeling, such as tiredness and weakness, due to hypoglycemia is more common and is sometimes sufficiently severe to make the patient desire a return to the old insulin. Such feelings of course may be overcome by the needed reduction of the dose. The well-adjusted patients, on the other hand, speak of increased well-being and particularly about the new restfulness or peacefulness of their sleep. The time of a reaction is, of course, much longer after the insulin is given, usually at least ten hours later, often much longer. Rest is not only more complete for the child, but, as his reactions are more likely to occur in the late afternoon or at breakfast time, the parents rest in greater security. If frequent blood sugar examinations are not made, very severe reactions may develop before symptoms occur. These are not frequent fortunately, but we have seen several patients with blood sugars of 15 to 20 mg. in whom intravenous glucose administration was necessary.

So far, no local reaction has been observed as the result of the administration of protamine insulin, nor has any general protein reaction occurred. There has been no more rapid improvement in carbohydrate tolerance than in those equally well controlled with ordinary insulin. In fact, as Hagedorn himself pointed out, there is no advantage offered by the new insulin to those easily controlled by ordinary insulin, unless this necessitates too frequent needle punctures.

Protamine insulin acts so slowly that it is contraindicated when quick action is desirable, such as in coma, when better results are obtained with ordinary insulin. Likewise in preoperative cases it should not be given, even if the patient is taking it and is being well controlled by it under ordinary circumstances.

SUMMARY

The discovery of protamine insulin is a distinct advance in diabetic therapy. It offers as good or better control of the disease with fewer doses in the day.

Reactions are fewer and, at least for the child, usually occur at more convenient periods when the child is at home, and not during his sleep.

There is a wider margin of safety in errors either in the dose of insulin given or in the food taken.

REFERENCES

1. Scott, D. A., and Fisher, A. M.: J. Pharmacol. & Exper. Therap. **55**: 206, 1935.
2. Hagedorn, H. C., Jensen, B. N., Krarup, N. B., and Wodstrup, I.: J. A. M. A. **106**: 177, 1936.
3. Root, H. F., White, P., Marble, A., and Stotz, E. H.: J. A. M. A. **106**: 180, 1936.
4. Kerr, R. B., Best, C. H., Campbell, W. R., and Fletcher, A. A.: Canad. M. A. J. **34**: 400, 1936.
5. Sprague, R. G., Blum, B. B., Osterberg, A. E., Kepler, E. J., and Wilder, R. M.: J. A. M. A. **106**: 1701, 1936.

A COMPARISON OF THE ANTIRACHITIC EFFECT OF IRRADIATED CHOLESTEROL AND COD LIVER OIL

T. G. H. Drake, M.D., Frederick F. Tisdall, M.D., and Alan Brown, M.D.
Toronto, Ontario

In 1934, Waddell[1] irradiated cholesterol and found that the resultant product had a marked antirachitic effect on rats and chickens. He reported that this product differed from irradiated ergosterol in that it was equally as effective in the cure of rickets in chickens as was cod liver oil, rat unit for rat unit. During the past five winter months we have investigated the antirachitic value in humans of irradiated cholesterol in comparison with that of cod liver oil.

The procedure used was similar to that employed by us in previous investigations on the antirachitic effect of various substances.[2, 3, 4] The observations were made on normal healthy infants varying in age from one to six months at the initial examination (Table I). The infants were practically all of British and Northern European stock.

Table I

Ages of Infants in Months at Time of Initial Examination

Group	Under 1 mo. of age	1 mo. of age	2 mo. of age	3 mo. of age	4 mo. of age	5 mo. of age	6 mo. of age	Total
Irradiated cholesterol	0	15	12	21	17	10	2	77
Cod liver oil	0	13	21	13	17	6	4	74
No vitamin D	1	12	19	18	16	7	2	75

They were attending the infant welfare centers throughout the city and represented a cross-section of the infant population of Toronto. We are indebted to Dr. Gordon P. Jackson, Medical Officer of Health of the City of Toronto, for his cooperation and assistance. Every infant was observed over a period of five winter months. The initial examination was made in October or November, 1935. A second examination was carried out in January, 1936, while the final examination was made in the month of March or April. Each time a physical examination was made and x-ray films were made of both wrists. The infants were all artificially fed on either fresh cow's milk or evaporated milk dilutions. Care was taken to see that none of this milk contained any added vitamin D. Vitamin D free cereals were usually added to the diets at about five months of age. Vegetables

From the Department of Paediatrics, University of Toronto, and the Hospital for Sick Children, Toronto.

were included in the diet at six to eight months of age. Practically none of the infants received egg yolk during the period of observation. Almost all the infants gained in weight either at or above the expected rate.

The infants were divided into two groups. To one group was administered 150 international vitamin D units daily in the form of cod liver oil. This oil was a mixed specimen of cod liver oils obtained from a number of pharmaceutical houses and was of such potency that the daily dose of 20 drops contained exactly 150 international vitamin D units. (One tablespoonful of average good cod liver oil contains 330 international vitamin D units.) The other group received 150 international vitamin D units daily in the form of 10 drops of a solution of irradiated cholesterol in corn oil.* We were also able to observe a third group of infants who received no vitamin D throughout the period of observation.

In order to check thoroughly on the home conditions and to insure that instructions were being carried out, an exceedingly capable public health nurse visited each home every two to four weeks during the period of observation. Occasionally it was found that the instructions were not being accurately observed, and in these instances the infants were discarded from the observation. As previously reported,[2, 3, 4] we found that the usually accepted clinical signs, namely, craniotabes and moderate epiphyseal or costochondral enlargement, were not reliable in the diagnosis of rickets.

We are indebted to Dr. Martha Eliot, Assistant Chief, Children's Bureau, Department of Labor, Washington, D. C., who very kindly interpreted the x-ray findings. The reading of the plates was done without any knowledge as to the antirachitic therapy employed. The degree of rickets was classified by Dr. Eliot as 1–, 1, 2, and 3. In this paper we have called Dr. Eliot's Group 1–, extremely slight rickets (a barely perceptible change which frequently might not be noted); Group 1, mild rickets (a slight but obvious rachitic change); and Groups 2 and 3, moderate and marked rickets (well-defined fringing and cupping at the end of the bone). In addition, the x-ray films were interpreted by Dr. Eliot as to the presence or absence of active advancement of the rachitic process. It should be noted that this last classification indicates only the state of activity of the rachitic process and does not indicate in any way the degree of rickets.

In Table II is given the degree of rickets which was found in the infants of the different groups at the initial examination. It would

---

*We are indebted to Abbott Laboratories, Parke, Davis & Company, and Squibb & Sons for the cod liver oil used in this investigation.

We are indebted to E. I. Du Pont de Nemours & Company for the irradiated cholesterol. The cholesterol (containing the provitamin) was irradiated and after irradiation the unchanged cholesterol was separated from the small fraction which had been activated. This active fraction (containing the vitamin D) was dissolved in corn oil.

Six independent assays were made by different laboratories, including ourselves, in order to check on the vitamin D potency of the products.

seem that the distribution of the cases showing evidences of extremely slight or mild rickets is fairly equally divided among the three groups with the exception that there were slightly more cases with mild rickets in the group receiving irradiated cholesterol.

TABLE II

DEGREE OF RICKETS AT THE INITIAL EXAMINATION IN AUTUMN

GROUP	TOTAL CASES	NO RICKETS (PER CENT)	EXTREMELY SLIGHT RICKETS (PER CENT)	MILD RICKETS (PER CENT)	MODERATE AND MARKED RICKETS (PER CENT)
Irradiated cholesterol	77	84	10	6	0
Cod liver oil	74	91	8	1	0
No vitamin D	75	88	11	1	0

In Table III is shown the maximum degree of rickets observed at any time subsequent to the initial examination.

TABLE III

MAXIMUM DEGREE OF RICKETS OBSERVED AT ANY TIME SUBSEQUENT TO INITIAL EXAMINATION

GROUP	TOTAL CASES	NO RICKETS (PER CENT)	EXTREMELY SLIGHT RICKETS (PER CENT)	MILD RICKETS (PER CENT)	MODERATE AND MARKED RICKETS (PER CENT)
Irradiated cholesterol	77	82	8	10	0
Cod liver oil	74	69	19	12	0
No vitamin D	75	51	16	20	13

In Table IV is given the number of cases in each group showing actively advancing rickets with no evidence of healing at times of observation. As stated before, this classification indicates only the presence of activity in the rachitic process and does not indicate in any way the degree of rickets.

TABLE IV

NUMBER OF CASES SHOWING ACTIVELY ADVANCING RICKETS WITH NO EVIDENCE OF HEALING AT THE TIMES OF OBSERVATION

	TOTAL CASES	AUTUMN (PER CENT)	MIDDLE OF WINTER (PER CENT)	END OF WINTER (PER CENT)
Irradiated cholesterol	77	9	1	1
Cod liver oil	74	7	5	3
No vitamin D	75	9	21	31

In a previous communication[5] we reported that the administration of vitamin D in the form of irradiated cholesterol produced rapid healing of acute rickets during the winter months. Since this report we have observed six additional infants, varying in age from five to ten months, all exhibiting x-ray evidence of moderate or marked rickets. During the winter months we administered to each of these infants 750 inter-

Fig. 1.

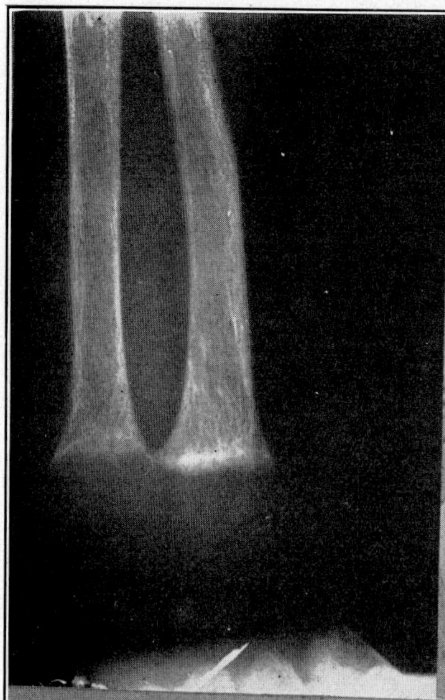

Fig. 2.

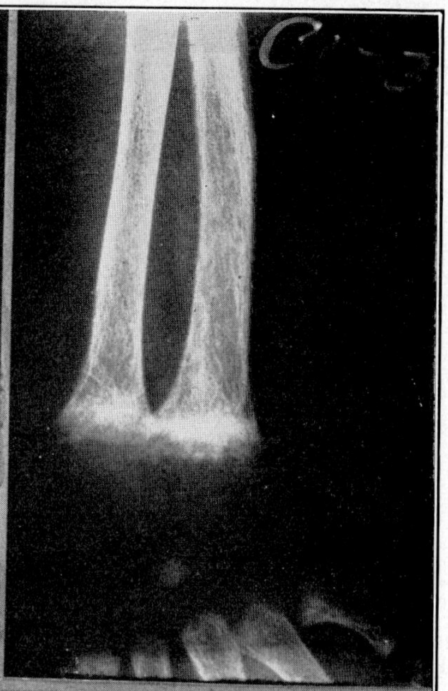

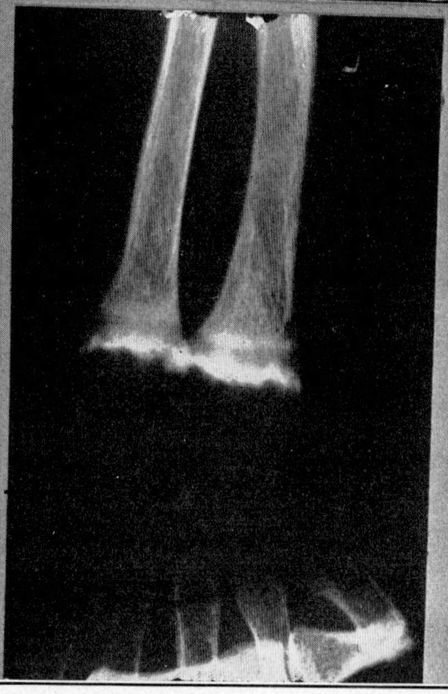

Fig. 3.

Fig. 1.—Case No. 173. X-ray film of wrist of infant aged ten and one-quarter months, showing evidence of marked rickets, April 9, 1935.

Fig. 2.—Case No. 173. X-ray film of wrist of same child after the daily administration for two weeks of 750 international vitamin D units of irradiated cholesterol.

Fig. 3.—Case No. 173. X-ray film of wrist of same child after the daily administration for one month of 750 international vitamin D units of irradiated cholesterol.

national vitamin D units daily in the form of irradiated cholesterol. In every instance marked healing resulted. X-ray pictures taken two weeks and one month after administration was started showed evidences of the healing (Figs. 1, 2, and 3). Also we observed during March and April, 1936, the effect of the daily administration of 300 international vitamin D units of irradiated cholesterol to each of three infants who exhibited moderate or marked rickets. Their ages varied from six to eight months. The weather in Toronto during these two months was so inclement that there was no possibility of the infants receiving any antirachitic effect from exposure to sunshine or skyshine. (The Dominion Meteorological Department reports that in Toronto the month of April, 1936, was the darkest April on record.) Again, in all three cases marked healing resulted (Figs. 4 and 5).

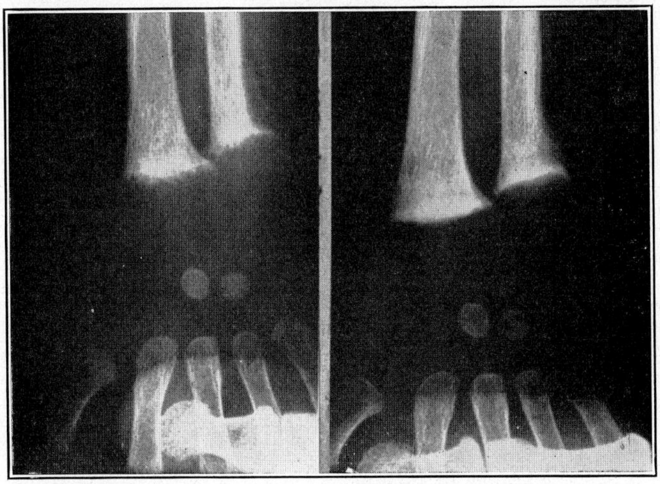

Fig. 4. Fig. 5.

Fig. 4.—Case 102. X-ray film of wrist of infant aged seven and one-half months, showing evidence of marked rickets, March 17, 1936.

Fig. 5.—Case 102. X-ray film of wrist of same child after receiving 300 international vitamin D units of irradiated cholesterol daily for one month.

DISCUSSION

The results reported in Table III show that no infants receiving 150 international vitamin D units of either irradiated cholesterol or cod liver oil daily developed moderate or marked rickets, while 13 per cent of the infants receiving no vitamin D developed rickets of this degree. This is a degree of rickets which is of definite concern to the clinician. The number of infants developing extremely slight rickets and mild rickets is somewhat lower in the group receiving irradiated cholesterol than in the group receiving cod liver oil.

In Table IV we see that 31 per cent of the infants receiving no vitamin D exhibited active rickets at the concluding observation in March or April, while only 3 per cent of the group receiving cod liver oil and 1 per cent of the group receiving irradiated cholesterol showed any evidences of actively advancing rickets.

It is evident from Figs. 1 to 5 that the daily administration of 750 or 300 international vitamin D units in the form of irradiated cholesterol not only prevented the development of rickets but brought about rapid healing of severe rachitic processes.

CONCLUSIONS

1. The antirachitic value of 150 international vitamin D units administered daily to infants in the form of irradiated cholesterol is equally or possibly slightly more effective than 150 international vitamin D units in the form of cod liver oil.

2. The daily administration for five winter months of 150 international vitamin D units in the form of irradiated cholesterol or cod liver oil to 151 normal infants of British or Northern European stock prevented the development in every instance of rickets of a moderate or marked degree.

3. Seven hundred fifty or 300 international vitamin D units administered daily in the form of irradiated cholesterol effectively healed moderate and marked degrees of rickets in infants of British or Northern European stock.

REFERENCES

1. Waddell, J.: J. Biol. Chem. **105**: 711, 1934.
2. Drake, T. G. H., Tisdall, F. F., and Brown, Alan: Canad. M. A. J. **31**: 368, 1934.
3. Drake, T. G. H., Tisdall, F. F., and Brown, Alan: Canad. M. A. J. **34**: 279, 1936.
4. Drake, T. G. H., Tisdall, F. F., and Brown, Alan: J. Pediat. **8**: 161, 1936.
5. Tisdall, F. F., Drake, T. G. H., and Brown, Alan: Canad. M. A. J. **32**: 490, 1935.

ANEMIA OF THE NEWBORN

Report of a Case With Especial Reference to Etiology and Therapy

E. J. Huenekens, M.D.
Minneapolis, Minn.

Ecklin[1] in 1919 was the first to report in detail a case of anemia of the newborn. In 1932 Arthur Abt[2] reviewed fifteen cases reported up to that time, and in 1935 Abbott and Abbott[3] added twenty-six new cases bringing the total number up to forty-one; with the subtraction of seven doubtful cases, this leaves a total of thirty-four unquestioned cases. Since then, a number of other cases have appeared in the literature (Schwartz,[4] Dennett and Ashton,[5] Cohen,[6] Brown, Morrison, and Meyer,[7] Pasachoff and Wilson,[8] Hotz,[9] Dedichen,[10] Noll,[11] and Mannheimer.[12]

The symptoms and signs have been frequently reviewed and need not be reiterated here. Abbott and Abbott[3] report twenty-two cases with a color index of one and above, and six cases below one. The etiology is obscure, so much so that it has been called idiopathic anemia of the newborn. Diamond, Blackfan, and Baty,[13] have shown that erythroblastosis fetalis is associated with universal edema of the fetus, icterus gravis neonatorum, and anemia of the newborn. While erythroblastosis is not present in all cases, there can be no question that there is some relationship between anemia of the newborn and universal edema and icterus gravis. Ecklin[1] and Diamond, Blackfan, and Baty[13] have reported the familial incidence of icterus gravis and anemia of the newborn, and recently Pasachoff and Wilson[14] have done the same for universal edema and anemia of the newborn. Though Pasachoff and Wilson[8] report a mortality of 12 per cent, the prognosis as a rule is good. Some recover without treatment, in others blood transfusions and iron and liver extract have been used either alone or in various combinations.

Baby T. W. was brought to me on Jan. 8, 1936, at the age of twenty-seven days with the following history: He was born on Dec. 12, 1935, in a small Wisconsin town at full term after normal labor and delivery without instrumentation. The birth weight was 7 pounds 5 ounces (3,300 gm.). The father and mother were in good health, and a two-year-old brother was living and well. The mother had vomited at irregular intervals throughout pregnancy, but her blood pressure and urine had remained normal; except for some loss of weight, she felt well. Since the mother was unable to furnish breast milk, the infant was placed at various times on plain milk dilutions, evaporated milk mixture, and S. M. A. Shortly after birth the father (a physician) noticed gradually increasing pallor, but placed no great stress on this.

Read before the American Pediatric Society, June 13, 1936.

At no time was jaundice noted. At the age of three weeks the infant began to vomit regularly (a frequently reported symptom of this disease) and lose weight, and when change of food brought no relief, he was brought to me for examination. Physical examination revealed a well-developed, markedly undernourished infant (weight 3,540 gm.) with marked dehydration as evidenced by poor tissue turgor and depressed fontanel. The pallor of the skin and mucous membranes was very noticeable. The spleen and liver were not palpable, and the examination was otherwise negative. The infant was admitted to Abbott Hospital where a blood examination revealed a hemoglobin content of 42 per cent (Sahli), a red blood count of 1,380,000, and a color index of 1.5. Because of the evident concentration of the blood, the absolute values were undoubtedly still lower. Three hundred cubic centimeters of normal saline solution was injected subcutaneously, and the following morning an intravenous transfusion of 100 c.c. of the father's blood was given.

TABLE I

DATE	HG. (SAHLI)	R.B.C.	W.B.C.	PMNS.	LYMPH.	MONO.	EOS.	BASO.	NORMOBLASTS	PLASMA CELLS	TÜRCK'S IRRITATION CELLS
1/ 8/36	42	1,380,000	30,500	46.0	41.5	8.5	2.0	1.0	9.0	0.5	0.5
1/ 9/36	57	2,870,000	14,950	77.1	19.0	2.6	1.3		9.0		
1/10/36	57	2,720,000	17,750	52.0	40.0	5.0	2.0		1.0	1.0	
1/13/36	58	2,120,000	15,650	40.0	49.0	4.0	6.0		1.0	1.0	
1/14/36	53	2,240,000	14,600	22.0	69.0	5.0	3.0	1.0	5.0		
1/16/36	48	2,040,000									
1/18/36	45	1,840,000									
1/21/36	52	2,510,000	13,800								
1/23/36	58	2,990,000									
1/25/36	56	2,510,000									
1/28/36	58	3,050,000	9,000	25.0	67.0	5.0	2.0	1.0			
1/30/36	60	2,660,000									
2/ 1/36	60	3,050,000									
2/12/36	52	2,550,000	7,500	30.0	56.0	10.0	3.0			1.0	
2/22/36	63	3,190,000	9,700	22.0	62.0	4.0	8.0			3.0	1.0
3/ 6/36	65	3,020,000	7,500	40.0	55.0	2.0	3.0				
3/20/36	75	3,800,000	11,850	40.0	56.0	2.0	2.0				
4/11/36	65	3,340,000	11,550	50.0	47.0	2.0	1.0				
4/24/36	71	3,630,000	13,500	34.0	64.0	1.0	1.0				
5/15/36	80	4,060,000	10,750	42.0	55.0		3.0				
7/ 1/36	82	4,250,000	12,900	52.0	48.0						

1/8/36 Blood Groups (Moss)
Baby Group 2
Father Group 2
Mother Group 2
1/9/36 Fragility Test
Hemolysis begins at 0.46%
and is complete at 0.38%
Control (4-day-old baby from nursery)
Hemolysis begins at 0.44%
and is complete at 0.32%
Wassermann (Kolmer and Kline)
Baby Negative 1/17/36
Father Negative 5/15/36
Mother Negative 5/15/36

1/9/36 Urine
Color—straw
clear
Reaction—acid
Sp. Gr.—1.012
Albumin—very faint trace
Sugar—negative
Pus cells—0-1
Bacteria—few
1/14/36
Platelet count—340,000
Reticulated R.B.C.—4.4%
1/23/36
Reticulated R.B.C.—11.8%
4/25/36
Hemoglobin
Mother—74

2/22/36
straw
cloudy
acid
1.032
negative
faint trace
0-1

5/15/36
Gastric fluid
Free HCl—0
Comb. Ac—54
pH—4.4

There was a rapid rise in hemoglobin and erythrocytes which, however, quickly spent itself (Chart 1). On January 18, ten days after admission, the hemoglobin and red blood cells had sunk close to their levels on admission. On that date, 1 c.c. of liver extract* was injected intramuscularly and repeated at forty-eight-hour intervals for three doses. The effect on the blood was so immediate and so spectacular and the improvement in the infant's general well-being was so marked, that it was very difficult to ascribe it to anything else than the specific effect of the liver. The reticulocytes were 4.4 per cent on January 14, and on January 23 they had risen to 11.8 per cent. After three further injections, the baby was discharged from the hospital. During the twenty-six days of his stay, his feeding consisted of from 720 to 1,000 c.c. of two-thirds lactic acid milk with 5 per cent dextrimaltose No. 1, which produced a gain of weight from 3,540 gm. to 4,520 gm. Viosterol, ten drops, and orange juice were given daily. The infant's temperature was normal throughout

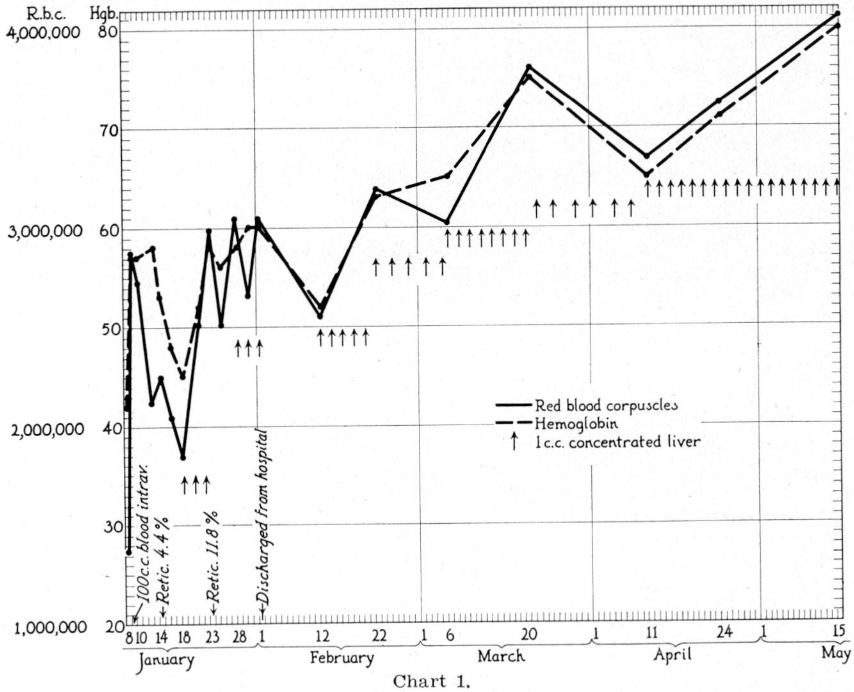

Chart 1.

except for slight temporary elevations due to the blood transfusion and liver injections. The blood Wassermann tests of the infant and both parents were negative. The patient was brought back on February 12 for examination and showed a marked drop in hemoglobin and red blood cells, though it had gained in weight (5,010 gm.). It had received no liver during that time. It was returned home and given 1 c.c. liver intramuscularly every second day. On the next visit, February 21, the blood values had again risen. From February 22 to March 6 liver was given every third day, with a slight drop in red blood cells, though not of hemoglobin. From March 6 to 20 the injections were increased to every two days with a definite increase in the red blood cells and the hemoglobin, to be followed by a decline when the liver was given but twice a week from March 20 to April 11. Thereafter it was given every other day up to May 15, when treatment was discontinued. During the entire time

*Concentrated solution of liver extract (Lederle) 1 c.c. contains active material obtained from 100 gm. liver.

from February 1 to May 15, the infant's diet consisted of equal parts of evaporated milk and water with 5 per cent dextrimaltose, viosterol or oleum percomorphum, ten drops a day, and gradually increasing amounts of orange juice. He received no other food and no medication.

Liver and liver extract have been reported a number of times in the treatment of anemia of the newborn. M'Neil,[15] Gelston and Sappinger,[16] Abbott and Abbott,[3] Dedichen,[10] Hotz,[9] Henry,[17] and Mannheimer[12] have used liver treatment, but in conjunction with iron and multiple blood transfusions, so that it is difficult to judge the specific effect of the liver. When Schwartz[4] gave his patient lextron (containing liver extract, yeast and iron) ½ capsule twice a day, the blood picture remained stationary, but when he increased the dose to one capsule three times a day, the hemoglobin and erythrocyte count immediately improved; his patient recovered without any other treatment. Admittedly, anemia of the newborn is a disease which tends toward spontaneous recovery, and while this fact makes difficult the evaluation of any therapy, our results in this case and those of Schwartz point very definitely toward the specific effect of liver in this condition. If confirmed in future cases, considerable light will be thrown on the hitherto unknown etiology.

The use of liver in anemia is due to the experimental work of Whipple and the clinical observations of Minot and Murphy in pernicious anemia. Castle[18] has shown that the antianemic principle in liver is formed by the interaction of an extrinsic factor derived from beefsteak, yeast, etc., with an intrinsic factor formed by the mucosa of the stomach. The liver stores the substance elaborated by the stomach after it has been acted upon by the extrinsic factor. While Greenspon[19] has attacked the interpretation of the rôle played by the extrinsic factor, there has been no successful challenge of Castle's fundamental work, that pernicious anemia is caused by the permanent absence of the intrinsic factor. There are several diseases besides pernicious anemia, in which the formation or storage of the antianemic principle is interfered with. The one of special interest to us is the so-called pernicious anemia of pregnancy, or, better, macrocytic anemia of pregnancy. In this condition which occurs in the later months of pregnancy, there is a temporary diminution or absence of the antianemic principle; the symptoms are relieved by liver extract and do not recur after the pregnancy has terminated, even though liver is discontinued (Strauss[20]). In anemia of the newborn, we seem to have the same temporary absence of the antianemic principle. The possibility of some relation between macrocytic anemia of pregnancy and anemia of the newborn is suggested by the work of Wintrobe and Shumacker,[21] "Comparison of Hematopoiesis to Macrocytic Anemia of Pregnancy and Anemia in Infants": "It is our impression derived from the study of the changes which take place in the size and number of the red blood corpuscles of the fetus, as well as in the proportion of erythroblasts and reticulocytes, that in many respects the blood of the developing fetus resembles that of cases of pernicious anemia which are being subjected to an effective, continuous and extremely potent stimulus to blood formation. It would also appear from our studies that the macrocytosis of the newborn, frequently considered to be the result of physicochemical changes in the blood, really represents a final stage in the development of the blood in the fetus. In comparison with the blood in pernicious anemia, the blood of the newborn is similar to that of cases in incomplete remission.'' They then suggest that antianemic principle of Castle may be the same substance which causes development of the blood of the fetus and that when a pregnant woman fails to secrete a sufficiency of this substance for both herself and the fetus, one or two things may happen: either the infant receives more than its share, causing macrocytic anemia of pregnancy, or the mother retains the major portion of the antianemic principle, causing anemia of the newborn. They further state that liver therapy has not had a satisfactory trial in primary anemia of the newborn, nor in erythroblastosis of the newborn, the blood picture and findings of which suggest pernicious anemia. This is an interesting working hypothesis and is partially confirmed by our apparent success with liver treatment in anemia of the newborn. Future cases of this disease should be subjected not only to clinical tests of liver therapy, but also to specific tests for the presence of the intrinsic factor. Singer[22] has reported that neutralized normal gastric juice injected into rats produced a definite reticulocyte response, which was absent when the gastric juice of pernicious anemia patients was used, indicating the absence of the intrinsic principle. By the employment of this method or other similar tests, the etiology could be definitely established.

SUMMARY

A case of anemia of the newborn is reported in which improvement followed immediately injection of liver extract. Large doses of liver seem to be necessary. The success of this treatment, if confirmed in future observation, should be of definite aid in clearing up the hitherto unknown etiology of this disease.

I am indebted to Miss Elneita Foscue for technical assistance with the blood examinations.

REFERENCES

1. Ecklin, T.: Monatschr. f. Kinderh. **15**: 245, 1919.
2. Abt, A. F.: Am. J. Dis. Child. **43**: 337, 1932.
3. Abbott, K. H., and Abbott, F. F.: Am. J. Dis. Child. **49**: 724, 1935.
4. Schwartz, A. B.: Wisconsin M. J. **33**: 98, 1934.
5. Dennett, R. H., and Ashton, L. O.: New York State J. Med. **34**: 595, 1934.
6. Cohen, P., J. PEDIAT. **7**: 220, 1935.

7. Brown, S. S., Morrison, M., and Meyer, D. A.: Am. J. Dis. Child. **48**: 335, 1934.
8. Pasachoff, H. D., and Wilson, Leo: Am. J. Obst. & Gynec. **29**: 415, 1935.
9. Hotz, A.: Schweiz. M. Wchnschr. **64**: 1047, 1934.
10. Dedichen, J.: Med. rev., Bergen **52**: 168, 1935.
11. Noll, A.: Ztschr. f. Kinderh. **57**: 21, 1934.
12. Mannheimer, E.: Acta pediat. **18**: 237, 1935.
13. Diamond, L. K., Blackfan, K. D., and Baty, J. M.: J. Pediat. **1**: 269, 1932.
14. Pasachoff, H. D., and Wilson, Leo: Am. J. Dis. Child. **49**: 411, 1935.
15. M'Neil, Charles: Edinburgh M. J. **37**: 175, 1930.
16. Gelston, C. F., and Sappinger, E. E.: Am. J. Dis. Child. **39**: 807, 1930.
17. Henry, W. A.: Canad. M. A. J. **33**: 656, 1935.
18. Castle, W. B.: Science **82**: 159, 1935.
19. Greenspon, E. A.: J. A. M. A. **106**: 266, 1936.
20. Strauss, M. D.: J. A. M. A. **102**: 281, 1934.
21. Wintrobe, M. M., and Shumacker, H. B., Jr.: J. Clin. Investigation **14**: 837, 1935.
22. Singer, K.: Ergebn. d. inn. Med. u. Kinderh. **47**: 421, 1934.

HEMATOLOGY AND PATHOLOGY OF APLASTIC ANEMIA OCCURRING IN A FIVE-YEAR-OLD CHILD

KATSUJI KATO, M.D., AND PAUL E. STEINER, M.D.
CHICAGO, ILL.

IN 1888 Ehrlich,[14] describing a case of a young woman twenty-one years old who developed an extremely severe anemia following incessant uterine bleeding, proposed the name of "aplastic anemia" because of a total absence of regenerative reaction on the part of the bone marrow. From several reviews of the literature made by Cabot,[13] Hirschfeld,[22] Musser,[35] Frank,[16] Smith[41] and Herrman,[20] it may be assumed that over one hundred cases of aplastic anemia are on record, although roughly in about one-third of this number autopsy studies are lacking. It is true that aplastic anemia produces so characteristic a blood picture that no errors in diagnosis are possible; yet such a diagnosis must always be confirmed by the histologic study of the marrow and of other hemopoietic tissues. It must further be emphasized that a typical aplastic blood picture may frequently develop secondary to various other pathologic processes, particularly in acute leucemia and sepsis. For this reason it is preferable, as Bigler and Brennemann[10] have done in reporting their series of cases of "sepsis with granulocytopenia," to avoid the use of the term "aplastic anemia" in describing secondary or symptomatic aplasia.

The occurrence of true aplastic anemia in infancy and childhood must still be regarded as quite a rare occurrence, the greatest majority of reported cases having been encountered in adults. The first pediatric case was probably recorded by Silva[43] (1894) who, however, termed the condition "progressive pernicious anemia." This report was followed by one by Muir[34] (1900), by Acuña[2] (1904), by Babonneix and Paisseau[6] (1910) and by de Elizalde[15] (1913). The first definitely authentic case of aplastic anemia in a child to be recorded in the American literature was that of Smith[41] (1919). The earlier case of Larrabee[27] (1911) reported under the name of "aplastic anemia" showed a lymphatic hyperplasia with evidence of myeloblastic activity. This raises the question whether the condition might not have been one of acute leucemia without leucocytosis. Including both the authentic and probable cases, a total of about thirty instances of aplastic anemia in children are now found in the pediatric literature and are summarized in Table I. The largest series have been published by Morquio and Volpe[33] (1933) from the Children's Clinic of Montevideo. Of the eight cases reported by these authors, the first two had been previously published by Lasnier[28, 29]

From the Department of Pediatrics and Bobs Roberts Memorial Hospital for Children, and the Department of Pathology, the University of Chicago.

(1921 and 1922), and the last is a case of aplastic reaction occurring in the course of acute leucemia.

TABLE I

SUMMARY OF CASES OF APLASTIC ANEMIA IN CHILDREN*

AUTHOR (YEAR)	NO. OF CASES	SEX	AGE (YR.)	DURATION	HB (%)	R.B.C. (MILL.)	W.B.C.	MARROW
Silva (1894)	1	M	12	15 wk.	–	–	–	–
Muir (1900)	1	M	14	2 mo.	12	0.60	7,000	Fatty
Acuña (1904)	1	F	9	1 mo.	–	1.50	4,200	–
Babonneix and Paisseau (1910)	1	F	11	–	25	2.00	–	Fatty
de Elizalde (1913)	1	M	13	–	–	–	–	–
Babonneix and Tixier (1913)	1	F	5	3 mo.	15	0.38	2,000	–
	2	M	11	12 mo.	15	0.55	1,200	Fatty
Heubner (1915)	1	M	2	6 mo.	10	0.98	7,800	Fatty
Kleinschmidt (1915)	1	F	8	6 mo.	10	1.00	3,000	Aplastic
	2	F	4.5	2 yr.	22	0.82	5,800	Fatty
Acuña (1915) Case 2	1	M	3.5	2 mo.	25	1.20	4,500	Fatty
Gorter (1916) Case 1	1	M	6	–	17	0.70	1,600	Yellow
Benecke (1917) Case 1	1	M	3.5	–	18	0.64	2,000	–
Smith (1919)		M	6	8 mo.	10	0.40	4,000	Fatty
Thursfield (1921)	1	F	11.5	7 mo.	30	1.14	5,200	Fatty
Lasnier (1921)	1	F	3	2 mo.	30	1.51	3,500	?
Lasnier (1922)	1	F	11	8 days	–	0.75	–	Fatty
Agnew (1924)	1	F	12	5 mo.	22	1.20	3,500	Fatty
Hurt (1928) Case 1	1	M	13	–	17	0.82	1,800	Fatty
Orrico (1929) Case 2	1	M	2.5	1 mo.	26	1.44	4,600	Fatty
Milhit et al. (1932)	1	F	5	–	8	1.80	6,080	–
Macera et al. (1933)	1	F	10	5 yr.?	20	0.50	6,000	–
Lindquist (1933)	1	M	4.5	acute	25	1.64	200	–
Morquio and Volpe (1933) Case 3	1	M	7	3.0 mo.	10	0.75	2,600	Aplastic
Case 4	2	M	8	1.5 mo.	30	1.00	2,500	Fatty
Case 5	3	M	3	3.0 wk.	52	2.50	5,000	Aplastic
Case 6	4	M	3.5	2.0 mo.	15	1.30	1,000	–
Case 7	5	F	9	1.0 mo.	20	1.00	4,500	Aplastic
Greenwald (1934)	1	F	2	6.0 mo.	10	0.75	2,200	Fatty
Osato et al. (1934) Case 5	1	F	11	7.0 mo.	30	1.14	5,200	Fatty

*A number of cases reported under the name of aplastic anemia in children are purposely excluded from the above list on the grounds that either the clinical or hematological features are atypical, or pathological studies are lacking or contradictory. These omissions refer to the following cases: Benecke (Case 4), Gibson, Gorter (Case 2), Herrman, Hurt (Case 2), Kharina-Marinucci, Larrabee, Morquio and Volpe (Case 8), Orrico (Case 1), Parkinson, and Spak. References to Silva and de Elizalde were not available.

It is clear from the above summary that aplastic anemia in infants and children is still sufficiently rare to warrant an additional report. The present case, of which a fairly adequate hematologic study has been made, followed by a complete histologic examination of all important organs at autopsy, is presented as an addition to the list of authentic cases of aplastic anemia.

CASE REPORT

The patient, a white female child of five and one-half years, was brought to the hospital in a critical condition on Nov. 20, 1935, with a history of recurrent, exsanguinating epistaxis of two months' duration. Bleeding was so severe and persistent as to necessitate cauterization and nasal pack and even then the hemorrhage was controlled only with difficulty. In all, four such hemorrhages had occurred during the two months, and three weeks prior to hospital admission two blood transfusions had been given. The history disclosed the fact that the child was very fond of the odor of gasoline and kerosene and often would saturate her handkerchief with them.

Physical examination upon admission revealed a waxy, pale exsanguinated child, apparently in a comatose condition. Respirations were deep and labored. The nostrils were filled with clotted blood. The lips were pale, and the tongue dry and plastered with dark blood. The tonsils and cervical lymph nodes were not enlarged. Large bubbling râles were heard over both lungs, but no dullness was noted. The heart was greatly enlarged, the left border being in the anterior axillary line and a systolic murmur of functional type, heard at the apex, was transmitted along the sternum and to the axilla. The rate was 160 per minute, the pulse imperceptible. No masses were palpated in the abdomen, and liver, spleen and kidneys could not be felt. No purpuric spots were seen anywhere on the skin. Two incisions, one on the inner aspect of each thigh, about 10 c.m. long (from previous blood transfusions), were noted, and the one on the right was gangrenous for about 2 c.m. at its lower end.

TABLE II

HEMATOLOGICAL CHART OF PATIENT DURING HOSPITALIZATION

(A TOTAL OF 18 TRANSFUSIONS WAS GIVEN DURING THE PERIOD STUDIED)

DATE	R.B.C.	W.B.C.	Hb. (G.M. %)	PLATELETS	L (%)	N (%)	E (%)	B (%)	M (%)	Pl. (%)	Ret. (%)
10/21/35	1.44	2,100	3.6	13,000	75	16	1	0	4	4	0.1
10/22/35	1.52	1,900	3.6	30,000	77	14	0	0	7	2	0.7
10/23/35	2.11	2,050	5.6	40,000	65	24	0	0	8	3	–
10/24/35	2.59	3,500	7.5	75,000	72	12	0	0	10	6	0.3
10/25/35	2.38	2,050	7.7	42,500	78	6	0	0	5	11	0.2
10/26/35	3.50	3,300	9.1	48,000	76	12	0	0	4	8	0.8
10/28/35	3.50	2,600	8.8	20,000	85	4	0	0	8	9	0.2
10/29/35	2.78	2,450	8.4	27,000	89	2	0	0	4	5	0.1
10/31/35	2.71	2,100	6.5	32,500	83	5	0	0	4	5	0.2
11/ 1/35	2.20	1,400	6.0	22,500	85	4	0	0	7	5	–
11/ 2/35	2.39	1,500	6.5	27,500	90	3	0	0	4	3	0.2
11/ 4/35	3.06	1,750	7.0	42,500	81	4	0	0	6	9	0.3
11/ 6/35	3.67	1,600	9.5	32,500	84	6	0	0	2	8	0.1
11/ 8/35	3.83	1,050	9.3	42,500	91	4	0	0	0	5	0
11/10/35	2.97	800	8.8	12,200	85	3	0	0	6	6	0
11/11/35	1.91	660	5.0	63,000	94	1	0	0	2	3	0

Abbreviations: R.B.C., erythrocytes in millions; W.B.C., leucocytes; Hb., hemoglobin concentration in grams per cent (Newcomer); L., lymphocytes; N., neutrophiles; E., eosinophiles; B., basophiles; M., monocytes; Pl., plasma cells; Ret., reticulocytes.

Examination of the blood (tabulated in Table II) disclosed the true nature of the disease. The urine contained a few red cells and hyaline casts and occasional white blood cells; the specific gravity varied from 1.020 to 1.023. The stool gave a negative test to benzidine. Blood cultures were reported to have yielded *B. coli* on one occasion and *Streptococcus viridans* and *B. coli* on another. The first roentgenologic examination (Oct. 23, 1935) revealed a pronounced enlargement of the heart which, however, was found to be slightly decreased in size on the second examination (Nov. 9, 1935). In the last named examination, a mottling about the trunks in the right and upper left lung fields was interpreted to signify the presence of patchy bronchopneumonia. There was also a slight increase in peribronchial markings. (Figs. 1 and 2.) The long bones showed no changes on both examinations (Fig. 2 and 3).

The patient's condition gradually progressed toward fatal termination twenty-six days after admission, the entire course being characterized by a steady, high fever (up to 41° C. at one time) which just before death rose to a height of 42° C. A total of eighteen transfusions were given as listed in Table III.

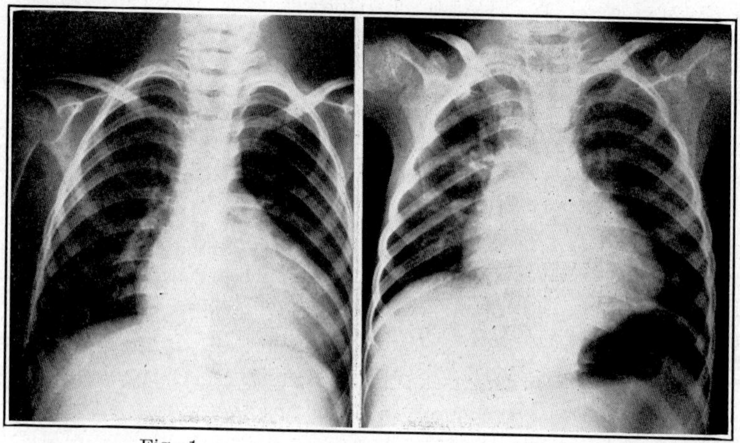

Fig. 1. Fig. 2.

Fig. 1.—Roentgenogram of chest (Oct. 23, 1935) showing an enlargement of cardiac shadow.

Fig. 2.—Roentgenogram of chest (Nov. 9, 1935) showing a decrease in cardiac shadow.

The treatment consisted of iron medication together with cod liver oil and yeast tablets in proper doses. On one occasion a preparation of liver extract was given by injection, but the reticulocyte response, though noticeable, was only transient. Administration of yellow bone marrow extract in large doses had no appreciable effect on the blood picture.

TABLE III

DATE	AMOUNT (C.C.)	DATE	AMOUNT (C.C.)
10/19/35	275	10/30/35	150
10/20/35	200	10/31/35	200
10/21/35	125	11/ 1/35	150
10/22/35	150	11/ 2/35	150
10/23/35	130	11/ 3/35	150
10/24/35	150	11/ 4/35	175
10/25/35	150	11/ 5/35	225
10/27/35	250	11/ 6/35	165
10/30/35	215	11/11/35	200

POSTMORTEM EXAMINATION

The essentials of the anatomic diagnosis at autopsy performed two hours after death were: Marked generalized anemia—aplastic anemia type. Hypoplasia and fatty replacement of bone marrow. Hemorrhages into the skin, pleura, lymph nodes,

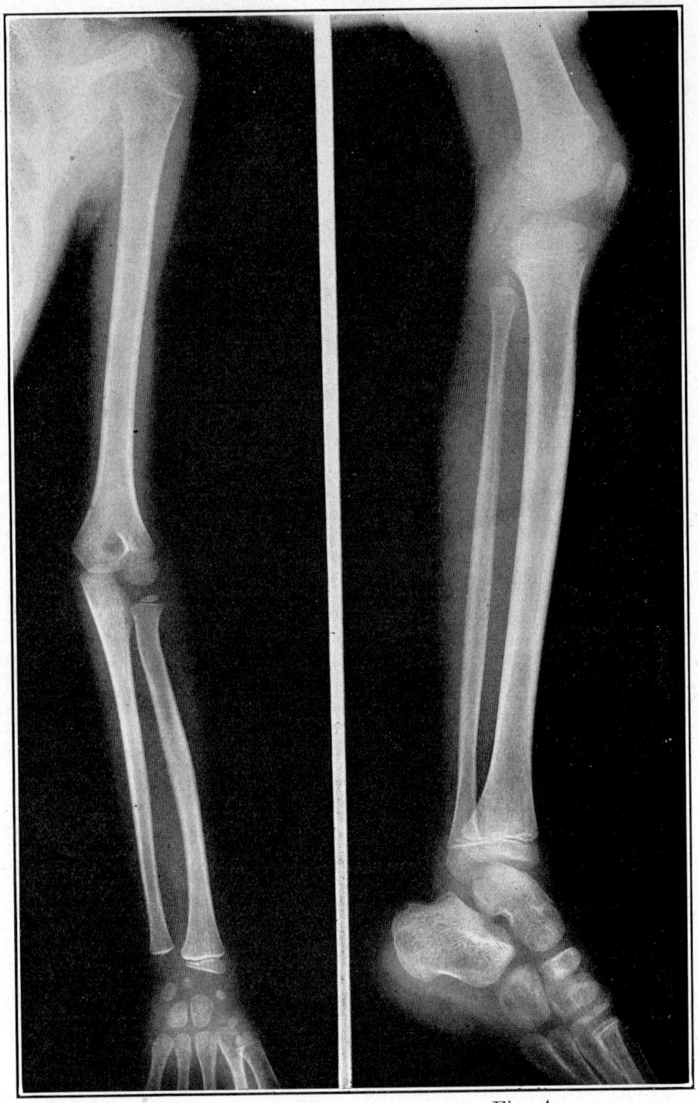

Fig. 3. Fig. 4.

Figs. 3 and 4.—Roentgenograms of the left arm and leg (Nov. 9, 1935).

subserosa of the uterus and cecum, and of the mucosa of the esophagus, stomach, duodenum, rectum, ureters, and urinary bladder. Atrophy of the thymus. Hyperplasia of the spleen and the tracheobronchial lymph nodes. Marked erythrophagia in the liver, spleen, and lymph nodes. Right lobar pulmonary gangrene; disseminated lobular pulmonary gangrene in each lower lobe. Gangrenous necrosis of the gums and rectal mucosa. Acute ulcerations of the jejunum and lower ileum. Hemosiderin staining and fatty degeneration of the liver. Hypertrophy, anemia, and cloudy swelling of the myocardium. Cloudy swelling of the kidneys. Hydropericardium. Focal fibrinous pleuritis. Healing surgical incision over the right upper thigh. Patent foramen ovale.

External Appearance.—The body was that of an emaciated, slender, white, female child, 44.5 inches in length and weighing 32 pounds. The skin was pale, dry and subicteric while the sclerae were icteric. At various places the skin of the trunk and extremities showed petechial and purpuric hemorrhages and an occasional fading ecchymosis. The oral mucous membranes were very pale. The teeth were loosened by marked gangrenous necrosis of the gums. The teeth, buccal mucous membranes, and gums were covered by blackish material, resembling blood, which had apparently oozed from the gums. Over the upper end of each great saphenous vein was a recent surgical incision. That on the left was healed while the one on the right showed some blackish, gangrenous necrosis. The superficial lymph nodes were not enlarged, and there was no edema.

Body Cavities.—The pleural cavities contained no excess fluid, and there were no pleural adhesions. Under the pariental pleura bilaterally were many hemorrhages measuring up to 0.5 cm. in size. The pericardial cavity contained an excess of clear yellow fluid, estimated at 50 c.c. in volume. The heart, the right chambers of which were flabby and overdistended, was greatly enlarged. Its transverse diameter in situ was increased, the apex extending past the midclavicular line. The subcutaneous, subperitoneal and mesenteric fat was pale and small in amount. The mesenteric and retroperitoneal lymph nodes were consequently very conspicuous although not increased in size. A peculiar, irregular blotchy red color also helped render them easily visible. The diaphragm was in normal position. The liver edge was just below the costal margin. There was no excess peritoneal fluid.

Mouth and Pharynx.—As a consequence of the severe necrosis of the gums previously described, the teeth were loosened, and, rigor mortis having set in, the pharynx could not be examined without danger of pushing out the teeth.

Thyroid and Thymus.—The thyroid was not palpably enlarged. Only indefinite traces of thymic tissue remained in the fat at the site of the thymus.

Heart and Blood Vessels.—The enlarged heart, empty but with 1 cm. of aorta, weighed 140 gm. (normal is 90 gm.). The external configuration was slightly altered because of the overdistention of the right chambers. The pericardium was smooth; the epicardial fat, pale and scanty in amount. The myocardium was of an extremely pale, grayish pink color and in it were small focal areas of yellowish fatty change. The wall of the right ventricle measured 2 to 3 mm. while the left ventricular myocarium was 4 mm. thick at the apex and 10 mm. at the base. The chambers contained small, pale postmortem blood clots and pale, watery fluid blood. There were no defects in the valves and no changes in the coronary arteries. The foramen ovale had a defect 4 mm. in diameter which could not be covered by a fold of endocardium. A few small, yellow intimal thickenings were present in the first part of the aorta. The remainder of the aorta, the pulmonary arteries, and the inferior vena cava exhibited no change.

Lungs.—The mucosa of the main bronchi was covered by a tenaceous, slimy exudate, and it was pale. The very pale left lung weighed 110 gm. (normal is 112 gm.). The upper lobe, except for petechial pleural hemorrhages, was normal. The pleura of the lower lobe also had petechial hemorrhages. Throughout this lobe were numerous irregular areas of peribronchial consolidation varying from a few millimeters to several centimeters in diameter. These areas were dark reddish black in color and were extremely conspicuous because of the pronounced paleness and bloodlessness of the surrounding uninvolved portions of the lung.

The right lung was more voluminous and heavier than the left, weighing 200 gm. (normal is 115 gm.). The posterior half of the upper lobe was the site of a sharply demarcated, uniform dark reddish black consolidation. The overlying pleura was roughened by fibrin. The surface made by cutting this peculiar type of consolidation was dry, dark, and not especially friable. The anterior half of this lobe was relatively normal and pale. The middle lobe, except for petechial pleural hemorrhages and hyperemia in its posterior part, was not abnormal. The right lower lobe resembled the left lower lobe.

Liver and Gallbladder.—The liver was enlarged, weighing 865 gm. (normal is 620 gm.). The organ was pale; the capsule, thin and smooth; and the margin, rounded. The surfaces made by cutting bulged markedly. On them the lobular markings were almost indistinguishable on the pale pinkish brown background. There was very little fat and no apparent increase in connective tissue. The gallbladder and the extrahepatic bile ducts were not abnormal.

Spleen.—The spleen was enlarged and weighed 70 gm. (normal is 52 gm.). It was deep purplish red in color, firm, and had a smooth tense capsule. The cut surface of the pulp was moderately firm and the malpighian bodies just discernible.

Pancreas.—There was no recognizable gross abnormality.

Gastrointestinal Tract.—The esophageal mucosa had a few petechial hemorrhages. In the gastric mucosa petechial hemorrhages were very numerous, becoming confluent in a few places. The gastric contents were not blood stained. The duodenal mucosa gave evidence of hyperemia and a few petechial hemorrhages. The tips of the plicae in the lower portion of the duodenum were hyperemic and in a few places were acutely ulcerated in areas measuring several millimeters in diameter. Similar acute ulcerations measuring up to 15 mm. in diameter were present in the mucosa of the ileum. They were not related to Peyer's patches and were most numerous in the terminal part of the ileum. At the base of the appendix and around the tip of the cecum was a subserous hemorrhage. The cecal and rectal mucosa showed a diffuse hyperemia and a few petechiae. The anus was the site of a group of gangrenous ulcers, the largest of which measured 3 mm. They had foul, necrotic bases and reddish black margins.

Adrenals.—The adrenals appeared normal for the age.

Kidneys.—The kidneys were markedly enlarged, together weighing 205 gm. (normal is 131 gm.). The right kidney was very pale and had a yellowish cast on the cut surface. This surface bulged out markedly. The capsule stripped with ease leaving a smooth surface. The cortex was widened, measuring 6 to 7 mm. in thickness. The cortical markings were indistinct. The renal pelvis showed little alteration. The left kidney in all essential respects resembled the right.

Urinary Tract.—An occasional petechial mucosal hemorrhage was present in the urinary bladder and in the ureter.

Generative Organs.—Subserous petechial hemorrhages covered the fundus of the uterus. The ovaries, fallopian tubes, and vagina were normal for the age. There were no ulcers in the latter.

Lymph Nodes.—The superficial lymph nodes were not enlarged. The tracheobronchial nodes were enlarged and on the cut surface showed a dark reddish brown, moist discoloration. The abdominal nodes were not enlarged but were very conspicuous because of the wasting and paleness of the subperitoneal fat and also because of their color. They were irregularly mottled a red or brown color, although parts of some nodes and all of others were normally grayish pink.

Muscular System.—The muscles were very pale and revealed considerable wasting.

Skeleton and Bone Marrow.—The vertebral bone marrow of the midthoracic region was pinkish red in color and that of the lower lumbar region a very pale pinkish gray. The rib marrow was normally red. The extreme upper end of the right femur contained fatty, yellow marrow. In the lower end of the upper third the marrow became pinkish gray mottled with red. This mottling of both the femur and vertebral marrows was not due to foci of hematopoiesis but to hemorrhage as the microscopic examination subsequently revealed.

Brain and Spinal Cord.—No examination was made.

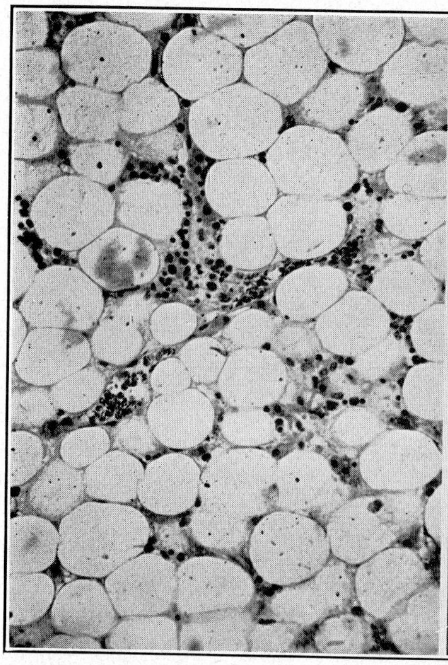

Fig. 5.

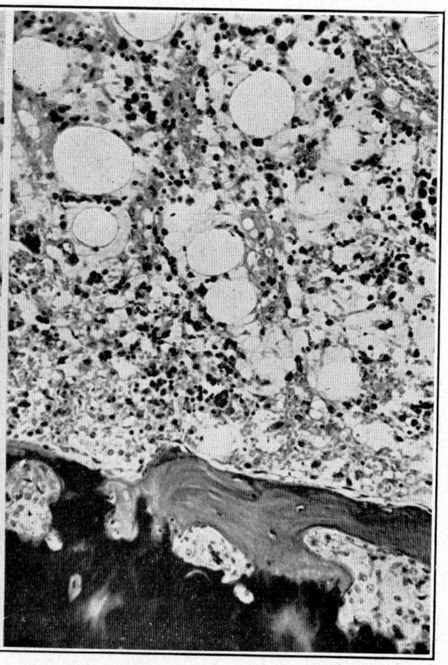

Fig. 6.

Fig. 5.—Photomicrograph of a section of femur marrow showing a hemopoietic focus surrounded by extensive fatty tissue. This focus is the most cellular one of all the foci seen in the section. Hematoxylin eosin, ×285.

Fig. 6.—Photomicrograph of a section of rib marrow showing the most active portion of the myeloid tissue, adjacent to the cartilage. Hematoxylin eosin, ×285.

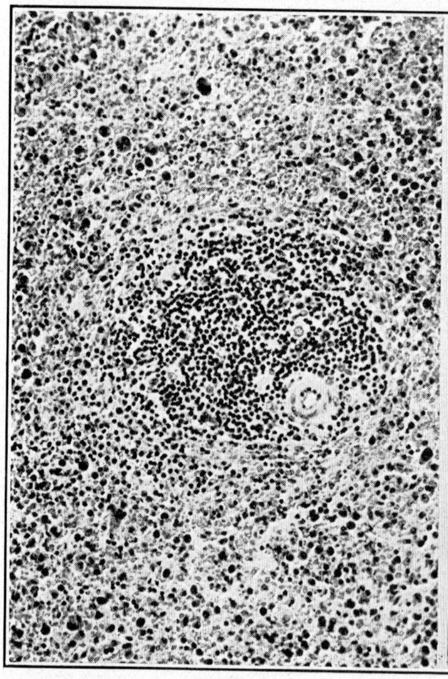

Fig. 7.

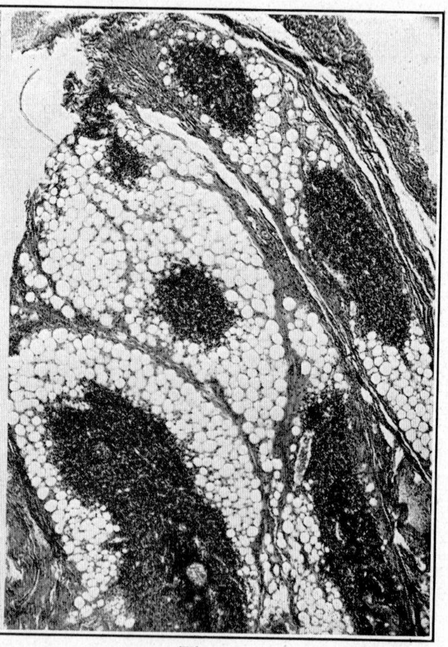

Fig. 8.

Fig. 7.—Photomicrograph of a section of the spleen showing an atrophic condition of malpighian bodies and an increase of reticulum cells. Hematoxylin eosin, ×285.

Fig. 8.—Photomicrograph of a section of the thymus showing a marked atrophy of thymic parenchyma, due to fatty infiltration, the thymic tissue being represented by a few reticulum cells in the connective tissue stroma. Hematoxylin eosin, ×65.

The Journal of Pediatrics, Vol. 9, No. 4, September, 1936

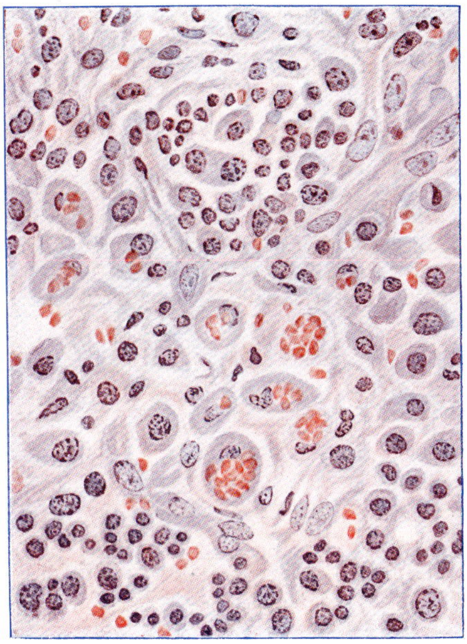

Fig. 9.

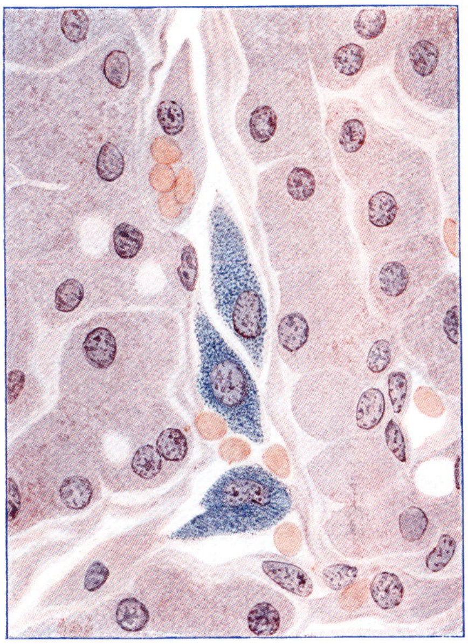

Fig. 10.

Fig. 9.—Camera lucida drawing from a section of the lymph node showing a small follicle surrounded by an accumulation of large reticulum cells with ingested intact erythrocytes. Hematoxylin eosin azur, 4 mm. objective, 10 ocular.

Fig. 10.—Camera lucida drawing from a section of the liver showing several Kupffer cells containing intact erythrocytes and iron pigment in a hepatic sinusoid. Prussian blue stain, counterstained with hematoxylin, oil immersion lens, 10 ocular.

HISTOLOGIC STUDY

The histopathologic study is based on the study of tissues fixed in Zenker's formol and formalin, embedded in celloidin and stained with hematoxylin and eosin, hematoxylin eosin-azur, Scharlach R and by the Prussian blue method for iron

Bone Marrow.—Femur marrow, both pale and red, rib marrow, and upper dorsal and lumbar vertebral marrow were examined. The marrow was found to be fatty with a slight amount of gelatinous edema (Fig. 5). The predominating cells were lipophages, hemophages and plasma cells. Small karyorrhexic lymphocytes and occasional regenerating megakaryocytes were seen between the fat cells. No evidence whatever of erythropoiesis or of granulopoiesis was encountered. One eosinophilic myelocyte was found. In all sections the red color observed grossly was found to have resulted from hemorrhage into the marrow and not from foci of hemopoiesis. Prussian blue stains revealed much iron in the macrophages in addition to the intact red cells shown by other stains. The rib marrow answered to the above description also, but in addition it contained more plasma cells, some of which resembled Maximow's polyblasts (Fig. 6). The vertebral marrow was essentially the same as that of the ribs and femur, but with the addition of an occasional small lymphoid cell nodule and possibly an occasional degenerating myeloblast.

Spleen.—The malpighian bodies were small and were characterized by a reticulum cell increase throughout (Fig. 7). Many of these cells were in mitosis. Lymphorrhexis was pronounced. The outstanding splenic change, however, was a reticulum cell hyperplasia of the pulp and sinuses so extreme as to obscure the latter. Many of these cells were extremely large and actively phagocytic, containing red blood corpuscles and much brown pigment shown by the Prussian blue reaction to be iron.

Thymus.—There was an extreme degree of atrophy, considering the age. Lymphocytes were almost entirely absent, and only a few reticulum cells remained in the connective tissue stroma. Hassall's corpuscles were necrotic (Fig. 8).

Lymph Nodes.—Lymph nodes from three abdominal areas and the tracheobronchial region were examined. They appeared to be normal in size but showed a great decrease in lymphoid tissue. The follicles, small, lymphorrhexic and devoid of reaction centers, were invaded to their centers by large reticulum cells, many of which contained brown pigment resembling iron, while others had ingested one or more intact erythrocytes (Fig. 9). Some of the reticulum cells had several nuclei. The mottled reddish color of the lymph nodes seen at autopsy was found to be caused by a generous invasion of red blood cells in the sinuses. The brown pigment was identified by the Prussian blue reaction as being iron.

Liver.—The liver cells were more or less isolated from one another. In the centers of the lobules they revealed a coarse fatty change and some iron staining (Fig. 11). Here and there were foci of liver cell autolysis apparently due to the great colonies of large bacilli which they contained. The liver sinusoids were unusually wide. The Kupffer cells in them were large and rounded and appeared to be increased in numbers. Many of these cells contained large amounts of iron pigment, while others had engulfed one or more well-preserved erythrocytes (Fig. 10).

Lungs.—The peculiar type of consolidation seen grossly was found to be gangrenous pneumonia. The alveoli in these areas were filled by an exudate which had undergone gangrenous necrosis so advanced that its original cellular nature, except for scattered masses of red blood cells, could not be determined. The alveolar walls were undergoing necrosis, although in a few places stainable nuclei were still evident. Massive bacterial growths of large bacilli had overgrown these areas. The more normal portions of the lungs gave evidence of a slight passive hyperemia and a focal fibrinous exudate. Even in the earliest and most minimal exudates these same large bacilli had caused slight gangrene (Fig. 12).

Kidneys.—The only abnormality noted was a moderate degeneration of the epithelium of the convoluted tubules.

Heart.—The connective tissue showed a mucinous change.

The *adrenal, ovary, pancreas,* and *diaphragm* sections showed no abnormality.

COMMENT

The case here observed presents a typical hematologic and pathologic picture of aplastic anemia. Anemia of this type occurs more frequently in adults than in children for the simple reason that the hemopoietic power of the older individual is more readily exhausted than that of the young. The most distinctive feature of this disease is its unique

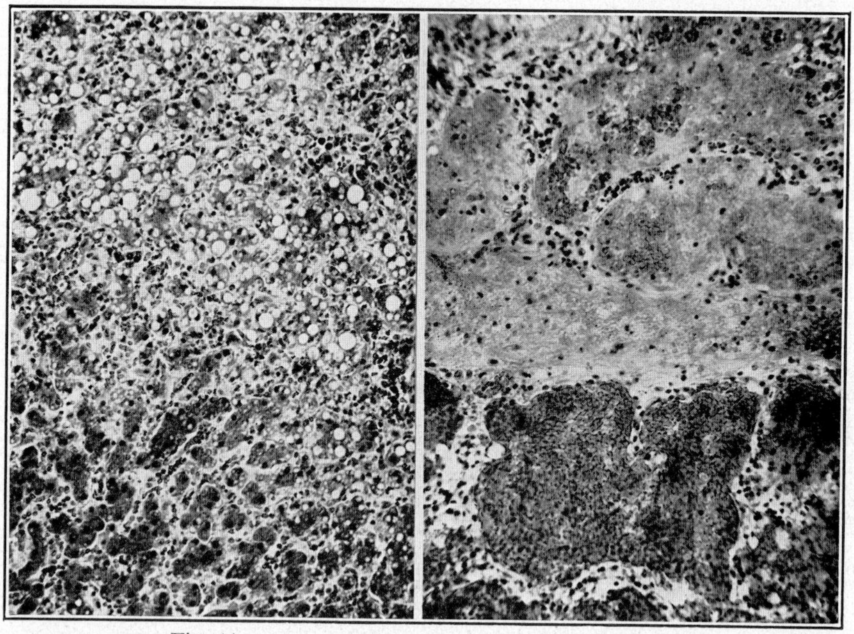

Fig. 11. Fig. 12.

Fig. 11.—Photomicrograph of a section of the liver, showing a central fat necrosis of hepatic lobule, together with an increase in Kupffer cells. Hematoxylin eosin, ×285.

Fig. 12.—Photomicrograph of a section of the lung showing an extensive hemorrhage into the alveoli (lower portion) and an unchecked bacterial growth (upper portion). Hematoxylin eosin, ×300.

blood picture. The decided reduction in the total number of erythrocytes, accompanied by a corresponding diminution in the hemoglobin content, reaches a level seldom seen in any other type of anemia. The lowest figure in children recorded in the literature, namely, 390,000, was observed in a six-year-old female child by Osato and his coworkers, although Ehrlich's original case showed 210,000 in a woman aged twenty-one years. In spite of this great reduction in number, the erythrocytes consistently exhibit no evidence of regeneration. Hypochromia is frequently seen, explaining in part the very low hemoglobin reading; but anisocytosis, poikilocytosis, and polychromatophilia are practically never encountered. Because the regenerative power of the hemopoietic tissue is abolished, nucleated erythrocytes are never present, and reticulocytes are very scarce. The reticulocyte response, if present at all, to liver therapy or to any other type of medication, is usually transient.

Persistent leucopenia is also characteristic of this disease. It, too, may be extreme, the lowest figure (200 per cm.) having been reported by Lindquist[30] in a case of acute aplastic anemia in a four-and-a-half-year-old male child. In the case here reported the lowest level (600) was reached on the day before death. Agranulocytosis is the only other condition in which such a great reduction in the total number of leucocytes is seen; and, as in agranulocytosis, this diminution occurs primarily in the cells of the myeloid series, there being a great decrease in neutrophilic granulocytes. Eosinophiles and basophiles disappear altogether. Unlike agranulocytosis, however, the neutrophilic granulocytes in aplastic anemia never completely disappear, there being an average of approximately 10 per cent present throughout the course of the disease. This relative neutropenia gives rise to a picture of relative lymphocytosis which, however, is not to be confused with absolute lymphocytosis, for the actual number of the lymphocytes is definitely decreased. As a rule, plasma cells are present up to about 10 per cent of the total white cell count. Another constant feature, and one which may constitute the basis for a hemorrhagic tendency, is a conspicuous reduction in platelet count. On stained smears the platelets are to be found only with great difficulty and the direct chamber count shows a low figure ranging between 10,000 and 75,000. Immature forms of leucocytes are never seen in smears made from the peripheral blood, although indirect and amitotic division of leucocytes may be occasionally demonstrated. Even though the bleeding time is usually prolonged and the coagulation time likewise delayed, the fragility of the erythrocyte against hypotonic salt solution reveals no significant deviation from the normal. No evidence of increased hemolysis or of bilirubinemia occurs in aplastic anemia, the plasma generally being water-clear or slightly pale yellow. Serum bilirubin, upon actual estimation, gives a subnormal value. The urobilin reaction in the urine is negative although a urobilinogen test may be positive.

The final and conclusive diagnosis of aplastic anemia is based upon the histologic findings of the hemopoietic tissues. In the present case not only the myeloid tissue, but practically all the lymphoid elements as well, exhibited a pronounced atrophy. Sections of bone marrow taken from the midfemur and from the end of the rib revealed typical changes. The myeloid elements were replaced by excessive amounts of fatty tissue, with consequent reduction in the cellular components. The sinusoidal and capillary spaces were filled with a scant amount of blood-forming tissue consisting mostly of lymphoid elements and a few plasma cells. The most remarkable feature of the bone marrow was the decided diminution in the number of megakaryocytes, only a few of which were seen, these being mostly immature forms (megakaryoblasts).

The lymphoid tissue throughout the body was also found to be atrophic in this case. The thymus was reduced to a thin sheet of atrophic reticular elements. The spleen showed striking reduction in the size of the malpighian bodies and the lymph nodes in general exhibited pronounced atrophy of primary follicles. Macrophages were increased in the lymph sinuses and in the splenic pulp, many of which contained intact erythrocytes in their cytoplasm. Hemosiderosis of these organs, as well as that of the liver cells in the portal triangles, explained to some degree the reduction in circulating erythrocytes. The decided erythrophagia of the macrophages may have resulted from the phagocytosis of foreign erythrocytes introduced into the blood stream by repeated blood transfusions. This phenomenon does not necessarily indicate any incompatibility of the transfused blood, but it does signify that the histiocytic system had been stimulated to acute functional activity by repeated blood transfusions.

In the liver a rather constant finding of central fatty changes of hepatic lobules with hemosiderosis of portal areas was very striking. The free iron granules in the Kupffer cells and in a few hepatic parenchyma cells were definitely demonstrated by Prussian blue reaction, indicating some degree of hemolytic process. This demonstration of free iron in the liver and spleen, however, does not necessarily imply classification of aplastic anemia in the general category of hemolytic anemia, inasmuch as hemosiderosis may occur in conditions other than anemia. The remarkable prolific growths of bacterial masses in various portions of the lungs, together with extensive hemorrhages into the alveoli, are also rather frequently observed in aplastic anemia. This picture closely simulates that found in the lungs of patients dying of agranulocytic angina, as previously reported in a five-year-old female child (Kato and Vorwald[24]).

PATHOGENESIS

Aplastic anemia may develop at any age period, but the occurrence of this condition in children is of extreme interest, for the young individuals are provided with rather reactive hemopoietic tissues, so that such an anemia as seen in this age period is usually of a normoblastic or hyperplastic type. This at once leads us to a consideration of the pathogenesis of aplastic anemia. Originally Ehrlich considered that a severe and chronic hemorrhage may lead to the aplasia of myeloid tissue, but this assumption was controverted by the experiments of Blumenthal and Morawitz,[12] who produced a typical anemia of aplastic type by repeated hemorrhage; but the hematology of their experimental animals differed from that of clinical aplastic anemia in that the marrow showed an increase in lymphocytes. The closest approximation in experimental production of aplastic anemia was achieved by Selling,[39, 40] with chronic intoxication of animals with benzol. His clinical observation of chronic benzol poisoning in industrial medicine corroborated his experimental results. In the case here reported, the history revealed the patient's fondness for the odor of gasoline and kerosene, although it is quite doubtful that such transient inhalation of volatile gas could instigate a fatal anemia of this type. It is to be admitted that the myeloid tissue of this patient may have been so labile as to lead to a state of profound aplasia, following an insignificant degree of intoxication.

As far as our case is concerned, the pathogenesis must be sought in the assumption of a general blood poison acting upon the labile hemopoietic tissue, producing the fatal anemia accompanied by leucopenia and thrombocytopenia. This assumption conforms to the idea of Hirschfeld, who considered aplastic anemia to be undoubtedly erythrotoxic in nature and not a simple aregeneration. Pappenheim regarded aplastic anemia as a form of pernicious anemia, not due to primary myelopathy, but secondary to erythromyelotoxicosis. Both these authors, therefore, use the terms "aregeneratory" or "hyporegenerative" anemia. Frank, on the other hand, characterized the disease as a form of essential thrombopenia (with "aleukia hemorrhagica" and "panmyelophthisis" as synonyms). Our case may with propriety be designated as that of essential erythroleucothrombopenia. Additional synonyms suggested by others are: amyelia (Klemperer); anmyelhemia (Kaznelson); toxic paralytic and anhemopoietic anemia (Schneider); anémie par anhémopoiese (Aubertin); myélose globale aplastique (Morquio and Volpe); and anemia aplastica gravis (Macera and his associates). "Aplastic hemolytic anemia" (Türck) is apparently a misnomer, as there is very little evidence that hemolysis plays any significant part in the causation of the disease. Likewise, the classification of aplastic anemia among the so-called erythronoclastic anemias by Parsons and his associates is erroneous.

SYMPTOMS AND COURSE

Aplastic anemia is a subacute fatal disease with a somewhat insidious onset. In a few instances the patient may show noticeable pallor of the skin for a considerable time before any manifestation of definite symptoms. Most usually, however, the sudden hemorrhage, often very severe and uncontrollable, is the first indication of the disease. Following this initial hemorrhage the disease runs a rather rapid course, usually from a few weeks to a few months at the most. True aplastic anemia is incurable, so far as is known. Cases of recovery following repeated blood transfusions (Herrman) are probably not true cases of aplastic anemia.

The disease is usually accompanied by a moderately high fever and increasing weakness. The patient's resistance is greatly undermined because of the profound leucopenia leading to bacterial invasion of vital organs, particularly of the lungs where resulting abscesses or bronchopneumonia usually cause death. Repeated hemorrhages from the mucous membrane are but one factor of the vicious cycle in the production of anemia.

DIAGNOSIS AND TREATMENT

When the typical blood picture is present, the diagnosis of aplastic anemia is comparatively easy. In cases of a doubtful or ambiguous picture, bone marrow biopsy should be resorted to. This condition can without difficulty be differentiated from thrombocytopenic purpura on the basis of the leucocyte count and the final outcome. In aplastic anemia, leucopenia and thrombocytopenia are the rule; while in hemorrhagic purpura, leucocytosis is most usually present. Aplastic anemia is invariably fatal, whereas Werlhof's purpura is not necessarily so. Another condition liable to be confused with aplastic anemia is acute leucemia during the so-called aleucemic stage; the differentiation here consists mainly in the presence of stem cells in leucemia, while in aplastic anemia immature forms practically never appear. The third condition which may give rise to diagnostic confusion is agranulocytosis, in which leucocytes are greatly reduced, with a total disappearance of granulocytes. In aplastic anemia, however, the neutrophilic granulocytes are always present, even though eosinophiles and basophiles may disappear completely. The greatest difficulty in differentiation seems to arise in distinguishing between aplastic anemia and pernicious anemia, for Ehrlich originally used the term "aplastic pernicious anemia" and Pappenheim and others regarded aplastic anemia not as a primary disease in itself but as a form of pernicious anemia. These two conditions, nevertheless, are totally different clinically as well as hematologically. In pernicious anemia the most significant feature is the occurrence of remissions with or without liver therapy, while in aplastic anemia remissions are never encountered and the disease is progressively fatal. The blood picture in pernicious anemia is macrocytic hyperchromic, characterized by poikilocytosis, anisocytosis, polychromatophilia, and showers of normoblastosis, especially during remissions. In aplastic anemia these morphologic characteristics are totally absent. Aplastic anemia is the extreme type of hypoplastic anemia, while pernicious anemia belongs to the category of hyperplastic anemia, a point which in the latter condition predisposes toward a favorable prognosis.

Treatment of aplastic anemia is unsatisfactory. Iron, arsenic, liver extract, bone marrow extract, high vitamin diet, and light therapy are, in practically all cases, ineffective. Blood transfusions give temporary relief but are never curative. Roentgen ray irradiation, advocated in the treatment of agranulocytosis by Friedmann and Thoma, has also been employed by Osato and his associates[37] in some cases of aplastic anemia. This method, if combined with blood transfusions, is said by them to be the specific curative treatment for aplastic anemia. In fact Osato goes so far as to claim that aplastic anemia is no longer an incurable disease with this combination of treatments. His observations, however, are limited to but two cases of aplastic anemia so treated.

SUMMARY AND CONCLUSIONS

1. A case of idiopathic aplastic anemia occurring in a five-year-old female child, with typical hematology and pathology, is reported.

2. No definite etiologic factor is discernible in this case, although the history of the patient's fondness for the odor of kerosene and gasoline must be noted as playing a possible rôle in causation of the disease in this instance, since these volatile substances may be hemotoxic as is benzol which is regarded as a preeminent leucotoxin.

3. Of the pathologic study the most outstanding finding is the generalized atrophy and aplasia of the hemopoietic organs both of myeloid and lymphoid types.

4. Another interesting finding is the notable erythrophagia of the large phagocytic cells found in the sinuses of the lymph glands and the spleen. The erythrocytes ingested by these macrophages are in all probability the foreign red blood cells introduced into the circulation by blood transfusions, the phagocytic activity of these histiocytes being stimulated by the repeated transfusions. Hemosiderosis in the reticulo-endothelial cells as well as in the hepatic parenchyma cells is notable.

REFERENCES

1. Accolas: L'anémie pernicieuse aplastique, Thèse de Lyon, 1910 (Abstr. Folia Haemat. **12**: 114, 1912).
2. Acuña, M.: Argentina Medica, 1904 (Quoted by Herrman).
3. Idem: Prensa méd. argent. **2**: 49, 1915.
4. Acuña, M., and Casaubon, A.: Arch. latino-am. de pediat. **17**: 1, 1923.
5. Agnew, G. H.: Canad. M. A. J. **14**: 859, 1924.
6. Babonneix, L., and Paisseau, G.: Arch. d. mal. du coeur **3**: 577, 1910.
7. Babonneix, L., and Tixier, L.: Bull. et mém. Soc. méd. d. hôp. de Paris **35**: 227, 1913.
8. Idem: La clin. infant. **11**: 296, 1913.
9. Benecke, E.: Folia Haemat. **21**: 263, 1917.
10. Bigler, J. A., and Brennemann, J.: Am. J. Dis. Child. **40**: 515, 1930.
11. Blumenthal, R.: Deutsches Arch. f. klin. Med. **90**: 132, 1907.
12. Blumenthal, R., und Morawitz, P.: Deutsches Arch. f. klin. Med. **92**: 25, 1908.
13. Cabot, R. C.: Osler's Modern Medicine **4**: 637, 1908, Philadelphia, Lea & Febiger.
14. Ehrlich, P.: Charité-Annalen **13**: 300, 1888.
15. de Elizalde, P.: Arch. latino-am. de pediat. **7**: 234, 1913.
16. Frank, E.: Berlin. klin. Wchnschr. **52**: 961, 1062, 1915.
17. Gibson, A. G.: Lancet **2**: 948, 1926.
18. Gorter, E.: Arch. d. méd. d. Enf. **19**: 525, 1916.
19. Greenwald, H. M.: Am. J. Dis. Child. **47**: 360, 1934.
20. Herrman, C.: Am. J. Dis. Child. **23**: 484, 1922; Arch. Pediat. **39**: 388, 1922.
21. Heubner, O.: Folia Haemat. **19**: 347, 1915.
22. Hirschfeld, H.: Folia Haemat. **12**: 347, 1911.

23. Hurt, A. S., Jr.: Am. J. Dis. Child. **36**: 1080, 1928.
24. Kato, K., and Vorwald, A. J.: Am. J. Dis. Child. **44**: 556, 1932.
25. Kharina-Marinucci, R.: Pediatria **23**: 101, 1915.
26. Kleinschmidt, H.: Jahrb. f. Kinderh. **81**: 1, 1915.
27. Larrabee, R. C.: Am. J. Med. Sc. **142**: 57, 1911.
28. Lasnier, E. P.: Arch. españ. de pediat. **5**: 385, 1921.
29. Idem: Arch. latino-am. de pediat. **16**: 63, 1922.
30. Lindquist, N.: Monatschr. f. Kinderh. **55**: 407, 1933.
31. Macera, J. M., di Firi, M. H., Messina, B., and Vaquer, M.: Arch. argent. de pediat. **4**: 336, 1933.
32. Milhit, J., Levesque, P., and Fouquet, J.: Bull. Soc. de pédiat. de Paris **30**: 553, 1932.
33. Morquio, L., and Volpe, A.: Rev. franç. de pédiat. **9**: 153, 1933.
34. Muir, R.: Brit. M. J. **2**: 909, 1900.
35. Musser, J. H.: Arch. Int. Med. **14**: 275, 1914.
36. Orrico, J.: Arch. latino-am. de pediat. **23**: 125, 1929.
37. Osato, S., Hashimoto, T., and Takigawa, T.: Folia Haemat. **44**: 495, 1931; and **53**: 42, 1934.
38. Parkinson, P.: Proc. Roy. Soc. Med., London, **11**: 15, 1917.
39. Selling, L.: Benzol as a Leucotoxin: Studies on the Degeneration and Regeneration of the Blood and Hematopoietic Organs, Baltimore, 1913, Johns Hopkins Press.
40. Selling, L., and Osgood, E. E.: Internat. Clin. **3** (Ser. 45): 53, 1935.
41. Smith, L. W.: Am. J. Dis. Child. **17**: 174, 1919.
42. Spak, H.: Acta paediat. **1**: 310, 1921.
43. Silva, B.: Riforma med., Napoli **10**: 807, 1894.
44. Thursfield, J. H.: Brit. M. J. **2**: 873, 1921.
45. Türk, W.: Vorlesungen über klinische Haematologie, Part 2, No. 2, 1912, p. 761.

INFLUENZAL MENINGITIS

A Study of Its Clinical Characteristics Based on an Analysis of 54 Cases From the Records of the St. Louis Children's Hospital

Robert W. Huntington, Jr., M.D.,* and
Dorothy Wilkes-Weiss, M.D.,†
St. Louis, Mo.

Although the literature contains many admirable articles on the subject of influenzal meningitis, in most instances the authors' interest was primarily bacteriologic, and there has been but little discussion of the clinical features of this disease. During a study of certain aspects of influenzal meningitis, the results of which are recorded elsewhere,[1, 2, 3] a review was made of the fifty-four case records available at the St. Louis Children's Hospital, and it seemed that the clinical features of this group of cases were of sufficient interest to warrant discussion, although the composite picture was one of diversity rather than uniformity. This paper is based largely upon an analysis of these cases, but occasional references have been made to a series of 500 cases collected by one of us (D. W. W.) from reports in the literature. The latter series was compiled with great care, all doubtful cases being excluded. About fifty more cases could have been added, but it was convenient to keep the number at 500.

The structure of this paper may be outlined as follows:

1. Figures on relative frequency of various kinds of meningitis at this hospital, and on incidence by sex and age, on mortality, etc.
2. Clinical aspects of the disease. Predisposing causes, type of onset, duration of illness, etc.
3. Laboratory findings (blood counts, blood cultures, other cultures), spinal fluid, cytology, and bacteriological study.
4. Problems which may arise in differential diagnosis.

Relative Frequency.—In the experience recorded by Neal,[4] *H. influenzae* ranked forth as a cause of purulent meningitis. The experience at this hospital is similar, as shown by the accompanying table which gives the figures for 1918-35.

Meningococcus meningitis	160 cases
Streptococcus meningitis	74 cases
Pneumococcus meningitis	62 cases
Influenza bacillus meningitis	54 cases
Staphylococcus meningitis	22 cases

From the Department of Pediatrics, Washington University School of Medicine, and the St. Louis Children's Hospital.

*Theron Catlin Fellow in Pediatrics, St. Louis Children's Hospital, 1935.

†Theron Catlin Fellow in Pediatrics, St. Louis Children's Hospital, 1929-32.

Sex and Age.—Only 16 of our 54 patients were females. However, in Neal's group of 111 patients, 59 were females, and it seems likely that our experience in this respect is merely a freak of random sampling. Only 12 of our patients were over two years of age, and here our experience is in accord with the general impression. Of the 500 cases collected from the literature, 127 were in patients more than two years old. The oldest patient in the St. Louis Children's Hospital series was thirteen years old (the hospital admits patients up to the age of fifteen years), and the youngest was two months old.

Mortality.—In our group of fifty-four cases there were three recoveries. Two of these were in patients over two years of age. In the larger series there were thirty-five recoveries, twenty-six of which occurred in patients over two years of age. Clearly the prognosis is not as hopeless in this age period as in infancy.

CLINICAL FEATURES

Onset.—According to the prevailing concept, influenzal meningitis is usually "primary." However, in ten of our cases it seemed clear that the onset of meningitis was preceded by otitis or pneumonia, and in some additional instances there were other features of interest in the recent history. One patient, an eighteen-month-old colored boy, developed osteomyelitis of the tibia following an injury to the ankle and was in the hospital for several days before signs of meningitis appeared. A history of trauma to the skull was obtained in two cases. One of these patients developed meningitis while in the hospital with a fractured skull, while the other, admitted with meningitis, had undergone prolonged manipulation of the middle ear as his physician attempted to remove a foreign body. In the remaining forty cases the meningitis might perhaps be considered "primary," although many of the patients had concomitant otitis and pneumonia. In twenty-five of the forty cases the history was that of an abrupt onset; in the others the onset was more insidious.

Duration of Illness.—In the fifty-one fatal cases the average time elapsing from first symptoms of severe illness to exitus was approximately fourteen days. In the group of cases in which the meningitis was preceded by otitis or pneumonia, the time between the demonstration of meningitis and death averaged slightly less than three days. In the whole series there were two patients who died within two days of the onset of the disease. One of these patients, a white female child sixteen months old, seemed perfectly well the night before admission to the hospital. At 6 A.M. on the day of admission she seemed listless and feverish, at 11 A.M. she vomited, and at 5 P.M. she had a convulsion and was brought to the hospital. On admission she seemed almost moribund, with a temperature of 40.4° C., irregular respiration, and continuous convulsive movements. Lumbar puncture showed 4,500 cells and many influenza bacilli. Death occurred a few hours after admission. This case indicates that influenzal meningitis can kill with great rapidity, but usually the course is more prolonged. The longest duration in any of our fatal cases was thirty-four days, and in this instance serum treatment may have prolonged the course. However, another patient, who received no serum, lived for twenty-two days after the onset of cerebral symptoms, and the average duration in Rivers' series was twenty days.

Miscellaneous Aspects.—In purulent intracranial infection in young children the conventional meningeal signs are often absent, and influenzal meningitis is no exception to this rule. Reference has already been made to the insidious onset which characterized some of these cases. One must be quick to suspect meningitis in any unexplained febrile illness of an infant. A number of our patients looked remarkably well during a considerable portion of their course.

Extrameningeal Lesions.—Concomitant otitis and pneumonia have already been mentioned. One patient with otitis media had a submaxillary abscess. Two patients developed pleural effusions, and in two others necropsy revealed pericarditis. Metastatic lesions were noted during life in six additional patients. One of these, the child with osteomyelitis of the tibia, has already been discussed. Three other children had abscesses of the extremities, and two had cellulitis. An extensive purpuric eruption was observed on one patient.

LABORATORY FINDINGS

Blood Leucocyte Count.—Adequate study of the course of the leucocyte response was not made in any of these cases, and in nine of them there was no count recorded. The remaining 45 cases have been tabulated according to a single leucocyte count. This was the first count recorded except in the cases of patients who developed meningitis in the hospital. In these cases the count selected was the one closest in time to the demonstration of meningitis. The figures are as follows:

Leucocyte count (thousands)	5-10	10-15	15-20	20-30	30-40	over 40
Number of patients	6	9	16	7	4	3

In general the percentage of polymorphonuclears paralleled the total count. It is obvious that patients with influenzal meningitis may have either a leucopenia or a leucocytosis.

Blood Cultures.—Here again our data are fragmentary. Blood cultures were taken in the cases of twenty-four patients, and *H. influenzae* was found on one or more cultures in sixteen of them.

Other Cultures.—In the case of osteomyelitis of the tibia and in those of abscess of the extremities and of pericarditis, pure cultures of *H. influenzae* were obtained from these lesions. No attempt was made to study the antigenic relationship of these strains of *H. influenzae* to those in the meninges. Influenza bacilli were also grown from pleural fluid in one case and from a submaxillary abscess in another. *H. influenzae* was cultured from otitic discharge in two instances, although few ear cultures were made.

Cerebrospinal Fluid.—Dynamics: Definite evidence of block was observed during life in one patient and at necropsy in another. A third patient showed a pressure cone at necropsy.

Cytology: In two cases the first lumbar puncture revealed a normal spinal fluid. In several others the cell count was quite low; in four the pleocytosis was less than 500. In one of these cases a differential count showed 80 per cent lymphocytes. This fluid showed *H. influenzae* on smear and culture. In two of the other three cases the organism was demonstrated on culture though not on smear. In most instances the spinal fluid leucocyte counts were between two and ten thousand with a high percentage of polymorphonuclears. The highest count recorded in this series was 294,000 with 97 per cent polymorphonuclears. In another case the fluid was described as "too thick to count."

Bacteriology: Stained smears of the first spinal fluid sample revealed gram-negative bacilli in all but 12 cases. In 2 of these 12 the first spinal fluid specimen was entirely normal, but the second showed organisms on direct smear. Cultures were made in 53 of the 54 cases, and *H. influenzae* was eventually demonstrated in all of them, although first cultures were negative in 2. No cultures were recorded in 1 case; however, gram-negative bacilli were seen in large numbers in this patient's spinal fluid, and there is a decided probability that they were influenza bacilli. Another case, in which gram-negative bacilli were demonstrated on smear while several cultures were negative, has been excluded, for the failure of the organism to grow on ordinary media suggested that it was not *H. influenzae*. The diagnosis of influenzal meningitis should be confirmed by culture of the spinal fluid in every instance. One cannot assume that gram-negative bacilli in the spinal fluid are always influenza bacilli. One of us has seen a case of meningitis due to a related organism with different growth requirements, and another case in which the gram-negative bacilli readily demonstrated on smear turned out to be aerobic spore-formers. In young infants, of course, *B. coli* meningitis is not uncommon, and differentiation of *B. coli* and *H. influenzae* on morphologic grounds alone is not always easy.

With regard to the interpretation of smears, two points should be stressed: first, the pleomorphism of meningeal *H. influenzae,* and second, technical difficulties in Gram staining a relatively thick film. In several of our cases the house officer who examined the first smear was not certain whether the organisms were gram-positive or gram-negative. This difficulty can be obviated only by familiarity with the Gram stain in use, and each batch of Gram stain has its own peculiarities.

DIFFERENTIAL DIAGNOSIS

The diseases most likely to be confused with influenzal meningitis are meningococcus meningitis, other forms of purulent meningitis, and tuberculous meningitis. In practically all instances bacteriologic examination of the spinal fluid is necessary to settle the diagnosis.

Meningococcus Meningitis.—Since influenzal meningitis is often apparently "primary" and tends to run a prolonged course, the clinical picture in a given instance may strongly suggest meningococcus rather than influenzal infection. While metastatic lesions may be less common in meningococcus meningitis (only one of seventy-four infants with meningococcus meningitis observed at this hospital showed such a lesion), a guess at the diagnosis of influenzal meningitis, whether on this or any other purely clinical ground, would be distinctly hazardous. Moreover, especially to an inexperienced observer, meningeal influenza bacilli may look like diplococci on smear. In cases in which organisms are not relatively abundant in the spinal fluid, an immediate differential diagnosis becomes an impossibility. Sixteen of our fifty-four patients received one or more doses of antimeningococcus serum. This procedure was entirely correct as long as the diagnosis of influenzal meningitis was not established.

Purulent Meningitis, Other Forms.—It would appear that influenzal meningitis occupies an intermediate position between meningococcal and other forms of purulent meningitis. In the case of a patient with a subacute type of meningitis who does not appear particularly toxic, the first guess would be one of meningococcus infection and the second of influenza. Pneumococcus meningitis is likely to be fulminating in character, and a spinal fluid with a low cell count and myriads of organisms is frequently observed. In streptococcus meningitis there is frequently obvious pathology in the mastoid or some other focus of infection. However, the clinical pictures are not sharply differentiated. In particular it should be remembered that pneumococcus meningitis is often apparently "primary"; that, in fact, it may be taken for meningococcus meningitis before the puncture is done; and that influenzal meningitis, as well as epidemic meningitis, may be quite fulminant in character. Here again it is clear that the diagnosis of influenzal meningitis must depend on bacteriologic study of the spinal fluid. Often the diagnosis may be strongly suggested by examination of a direct smear. However, as gram-negative bacilli are not necessarily influenza bacilli, cultures should always be made. If *H. influenzae* is obtained on blood culture, in a case of meningitis it is obviously unlikely that another organism is causing this lesion. However, as will be seen from a case to be discussed later, similar reasoning may not be justified in instances of the isolation of *H. influenzae* from other sources.

Tuberculous Meningitis.—At first sight the possibility of difficulty in differentiating tuberculous and influenzal meningitis might appear remote. That this is not the case is shown by the cases of two patients observed at this hospital.

The first patient, a white boy aged four months, has been listed in our influenzal meningitis series. He was admitted to the hospital on March 24, 1926, with the following story: The illness had begun on March 8, with crying and fever. Retraction of the head was noted on March 11. From March 15 to 21 he seemed slightly better. However, since March 21 the color had been poor. On admission he seemed listless, and there was slight opisthotonos. The left eardrum was bulging and creamy pus was obtained on paracentesis. Physical and x-ray examination of the chest revealed extensive bronchopneumonia, and the roentgenologic diagnosis was disseminated tuberculosis. The white count was 36,000. A lumbar puncture revealed clear fluid with a cell count of 80; 60 per cent of the cells were mononuclears, and smear and culture were negative. Subsequent spinal fluid specimens showed cell counts between 500 and 2,000, with approximately 90 per cent polymorphonuclears. The intradermal tuberculin test was negative to 0.1 mg. On April 5 a culture of the spinal fluid showed *H. influenzae.* The patient died on April 12, and autopsy permission could not be obtained.

The second patient was not included in this series, although the history was filed under a clinical diagnosis of influenzal meningitis. He was a white boy, aged eleven months, who had had many colds during December, 1926, and January, 1927. In February he was admitted to a hospital on account of bronchopneumonia. He improved but developed bilateral otitis. He was discharged February 28. On March 14 his physician found the chest clear although cough continued. During the next week he acquired a ''cold.'' On March 29 a thoracentesis was done, and a few drops of thick pus were obtained. The patient ran a septic temperature. He was admitted to the St. Louis Children's Hospital on April 6. Physical examination revealed a malnourished, poorly developed boy who appeared chronically ill. The fontanel was soft. Both eardrums were bulging, and pus was obtained from each on paracentesis. The respiration was diaphragmatic. Over the right upper lobe the percussion note was flat, and the breath sounds were tubular. X-ray examination suggested the presence of a cavity. Tuberculin test (0.1 mg.) was negative. The patient was put on postural drainage. On April 19 a thoracentesis was done. As the needle entered the chest cavity, air was expelled into the syringe; 2 c.c. of thick green pus was aspirated, and culture showed *H. influenzae.* On operation, April 23, a large cavity was found with a bronchial fistula. On the next day there was rigidity of the neck and back. On April 26 a lumbar puncture showed clear spinal fluid with 17 cells, 9 of which were polymorphonuclears. The Pandy test was one plus, and culture was negative. The following day the patient looked better. On May 1 he again looked very ill. He became spastic with marked opisthotonos and died May 3. A specimen of spinal fluid obtained on the day of death showed 26 polymorphonuclears, 24 mononuclears, and 100 red blood cells. Culture was sterile. Autopsy: Anatomical diagnosis was tuberculous bronchopneumonia, right lung, miliary tuberculosis of spleen and intestines and meninges of brain. There were yellow caseous masses in the right lung, with a few large cavities, and small whitish areas were seen in the subarachnoid space. Histologic examination revealed characteristic tuberculous lesions.

In the second case the influenza bacilli cultured from the thorax were evidently secondary invaders, and a serious diagnostic blunder resulted from another assumption. In the first case it is perhaps not inconceivable that the meningitis may have been primarily tuberculous, and that invasion of the meninges by *H. influenzae* may have been secondary. Since there is no necropsy material there seems no way of settling this point. In any event, these cases indicate that differential diagnosis between tuberculous and influenzal meningitis may constitute a real difficulty.

SUMMARY

On the basis of a group of 54 cases compiled from the records of the St. Louis Children's Hospital, and of a series of 500 cases gathered from reports in the literature, an attempt has been made to discuss influenzal meningitis from the point of view of the clinician rather than of the immunologist. Incidence in hospital practice, incidence by sex and age, and mortality are briefly considered. Data from history and physical examination and from laboratory findings are analyzed, and questions of diagnosis and differential diagnosis are discussed.

REFERENCES

1. Wilkes-Weiss, D.: Studies on Meningeal Strains of H. Influenzae. (To be published.)
2. Wilkes-Weiss, D., and Huntington, R. W.: The Treatment of Influenzal Meningitis With Immune Serum, J. PEDIAT. **9**: 462, 1936.
3. Huntington, R. W., Wilkes-Weiss, D.: Association of Otitis Media and Pneumonia With Onset of Influenzal Meningitis, J. PEDIAT. **9**: 456, 1936.
4. Neal, J. B., Jackson, H. W., and Appelbaum, E.: J. A. M. A. **102**: 573, 1934.

ASSOCIATION OF OTITIS MEDIA AND PNEUMONIA WITH ONSET OF INFLUENZAL MENINGITIS

Robert W. Huntington, Jr., M.D.,* and
Dorothy Wilkes-Weiss, M.D.†
St. Louis, Mo.

CLINICAL observations indicate that in many instances the onset of influenza bacillus meningitis is not associated with noteworthy extrameningeal lesions. The fact that meningeal strains of *H. influenzae* resemble one another and differ from the ordinary respiratory strains in their cultural and serologic characteristics[1, 2, 3] and the uncertainty as to the importance of the species in respiratory infection have led to the belief that this type of meningitis must be "primary" in practically all cases. Nevertheless, recent discussions of influenzal meningitis,[3, 4] while they attribute little significance to preceding or concomitant otitis and pneumonia, indicate that such lesions are relatively common. This paper presents further data on their frequency, and the question of their significance is discussed.

In the cases of patients with meningitis, it is often difficult to decide whether other lesions are present. For example, in very toxic or comatose patients, especially infants without striking meningeal symptoms, shifting atelectasis and transmitted rhonchi may lead to a tentative diagnosis of bronchopneumonia, not justified by later examination. However, in the cases of pneumonia cited in this paper, the diagnosis was confirmed by persisting signs, and in many instances by x-ray or autopsy. Cases of doubtful or terminal pneumonia were not included. Similarly, in the case of a very sick child, especially of one with purulent meningitis, the examiner is sometimes too easily convinced that the ears look abnormal. The diagnosis of catarrhal otitis media, based only on some redness of the drum, has not seemed definite enough to warrant discussion here. The term otitis media has been applied only to cases with definite middle ear suppuration.

In a series of influenzal meningitis cases from the St. Louis Children's Hospital, preceding and concomitant otitis and pneumonia were much more frequent in infants than in older children. Of fifty-four patients, twelve were over two years of age. Only one of these showed pus in the middle ear on admission, and none had signs of pneumonia. Of the forty-two patients under two years of age, more than half had otitis or pneumonia on admission to the hospital. Although in general such lesions are common in this latter age group, this incidence seems suggestively high.

From the Department of Pediatrics, Washington University School of Medicine, and the St. Louis Children's Hospital.

*Theron Catlin Fellow in Pediatrics, St. Louis Children's Hospital.

†Theron Catlin Fellow in Pediatrics, 1929-1932.

An analysis of the cases of the forty-two infants with influenzal meningitis reveals certain features of interest. In ten of the cases signs of meningitis developed in the hospital and were preceded by pneumonia or otitis (Table I). From a critical study of the duration of

TABLE I

10 CASES IN WHICH OTITIS OR PNEUMONIA PRECEDED MENINGITIS

PATIENT	LESION PRECEDING MENINGITIS		DURATION OF ILLNESS		FROM DEMONSTRATION OF MENINGITIS	COMMENT
	PURULENT OTITIS	PNEUMONIA	FROM BEGINNING DAYS	FROM ADMISSION DAYS	DAYS	
1	+	Broncho	7	2	1	First CSF negative
2	–	Lobar	15	8	1	Culture of pleural fluid *H. Influenzae* and pneumococcus
3	+	Lobar	9	5	1	Seemed "improved" second day in hospital Twitching began on fourth day
4	+	Broncho (post-pertussis)	?	4	1	CSF culture *H. influenzae* and streptococcus
5	+	Lobar	20	13	3	Vomiting and prostration first noted tenth day in hospital
6	+	Broncho	19	12	2	Mastoidectomy third day in hospital Bronchopneumonia found 3 days after operation, stiff neck 8 days after
7	+	Broncho	20	13	1	First CSF clear. Discharging ear 1 week before admission. Fever for 3 days
8	–	Broncho	16	14	3	Autopsy showed marked peribronchial thickening. Seemed quite well on fifth day in hospital
9	+	Broncho	Recovered			Sterile pleural effusion present on admission
10	+	–		49	4	Admitted to hospital for repair of spina bifida. Pus from left ear twenty-fourth day in hospital. CSF culture negative same day, later became positive

symptoms in each instance, it seems clear that in this group the other infections actually preceded the meningitis; in two the first lumbar punctures, done because of suspicious symptoms, revealed clear sterile spinal fluid, and in these there can be no doubt of the time relation of the meningitis and the extrameningeal lesion. In twelve cases the patients admitted with meningitis showed otitis or pneumonia on admission, and in two others (Nos. 23 and 24) the children admitted with signs of bronchopneumonia may well have had meningitis at the time, although lumbar punctures were not done until later (Table II). Of these 14 patients, five were admitted before the third day of their disease and four more before the end of the first week. In the cases of patients seen early in the disease, it is unlikely that an otitis or pneu-

TABLE II

OTHER PATIENTS SHOWING OTITIS OR PNEUMONIA ON ADMISSION

PATIENT	DURATION OF ILLNESS TO ADMISSION DAYS	ADMISSION FINDINGS		TOTAL DURATION OF ILLNESS DAYS	COMMENT
		OTITIS (PURULENT)	PNEUMONIA		
11	2	–	Broncho	2	Autopsy showed extensive purulent pneumonia
12	4	+	–	14	Mastoid tenderness on admission
13	10	+	–	11	
14	16	+	Broncho	34	
15	1	+	–	2	Bilateral labyrinthitis at autopsy
16	6	+	–	7	
17	14	+	–	16	
18	2	+	–	6	
19	17	+	–	31	
20	19	+	–	22	
21	5	+	–	6	
22	5	+	–	13	
23	2	–	Broncho	19	Lumbar puncture not done until tenth day
24	2	–	Broncho	14	Lumbar puncture not done until fourteenth day

monia could be classed as secondary to the meningitis. In patients seen late in the disease, of course, this point is difficult to decide. However, for purposes of comparison, it seems safe to summarize this series with the statement that the onset of meningitis was definitely preceded by pneumonia or otitis in ten cases, and may have been concomitant with such lesions in fourteen other cases. Thus out of forty-two cases there were twenty-four in which it seemed likely that the beginning of meningitis was associated with ear or pulmonary infection.

A comparison of this series with a series of cases of meningococcus infection indicated that evidence of preceding or concomitant pneumonia and otitis was significantly less common in the latter group. A series of seventy-four cases of epidemic meningitis in children under two years of age was compiled from the St. Louis Children's Hospital records. In two of these cases the meningitis was preceded by bronchopneumonia and in one case by mastoiditis. Eight other patients had otitis media on admission to the hospital with meningitis, and two of these also had bronchopneumonia. From elementary statistical considerations it appears unlikely that the higher incidence of such lesions in the influenzal meningitis series could be attributed to coincidence.[5, 6]

Although the cases of influenzal meningitis with otitis media were carefully studied in an attempt to determine whether the ear was the source of intracranial infection, data on this point were meager. Postmortem examination of seven patients who had shown purulent otitis on admission and of three others who had anatomic evidence of temporal bone involvement although there was no aural discharge during life, revealed no instance in which the meningitis could confidently be classed as otogenic. In one case there was a pachymeningitis of undetermined duration, while in the others the dura was uninvolved. Osteomyelitis of the skull, localized temporal abscesses, and sigmoid sinus thrombosis were not found, and their absence was sometimes of considerable interest. Patient No. 1 (Table I), for example, admitted two days before death, was found to have pus in both ears and a negative spinal fluid. At necropsy a very recent influenzal meningitis was found; yet even in this case there was no evidence of temporal localization. The fact that no definite indication of an otitic source of the meningitis was found in any of these cases does not exclude such an origin. According to Alexander,[7] diffuse meningitis is the common intracranial complication of ear infection in infancy, localized processes being rarely encountered. It is possible that the ear might be the source of the meningitis in these cases, and the labyrinthitis found in two of the three instances in which serial sections of the temporal bone were made could perhaps be construed as evidence for this view. It is also possible, however, that the inner ear infection was secondary to the meningitis. Clinical histories in the cases with preceding or concomitant otitis add nothing of value to these inconclusive anatomic findings. Definite mastoid tenderness was noted in one case only, and in this case the mastoiditis could not have been much older than the meningitis.

While association between respiratory disease and the onset of influenzal meningitis is apparently more than a coincidence, present knowledge is inadequate to explain the nature of the relationship. It would be interesting to know whether influenzal organisms related to those in the meninges played any part in the development of the pneumonic or otitic lesion. Since it is generally agreed that meningeal *H. influenzae* invade the body by way of the respiratory tract and since these organisms exhibit diversified pathogenic potentialities, there is nothing inherently improbable in this hypothesis. Meningeal *H. influenzae* differ from ordinary respiratory strains in their invasiveness upon inoculation into laboratory animals, as well as in their cultural and serologic characteristics. In laboratory animals meningococci are definitely less invasive. Metastatic lesions are apparently quite common in influenzal meningitis since they were observed during life in six of our fifty-four cases. One of these patients had an osteomyelitis of the tibia, and three had abscesses of the extremities. *H. influenzae* was recovered in pure culture from all of these lesions. No cultures were made from the cellulitis which occurred in the two remaining cases. Bacteriologic study of pericarditis found at necropsy in two additional cases of influenzal meningitis revealed pure cultures of *H. influenzae.* In another instance influenza bacilli with pneumococci were recovered during life from a pleural effusion. For comparison, among the group of 74 cases of meningococcus meningitis cited in this paper, there was but one instance in which a metastatic lesion was found during life, while in another endocarditis was discovered at necropsy. This difference between the two groups is suggestive, though not quite enough to be statistically significant, and is in accord with the impression gained from animal experiments that the meningeal influenza bacillus is a more versatile pathogen than the meningococcus. Hence the observation that the latter organism seldom damages the respiratory mucosa does not indicate that meningeal *H. influenzae* must also be harmless to this tissue. Using a strain of *H. influenzae* which may not have been related to the meningeal type, but which clearly differed from the usual strains in its invasive properties, Blake and Cecil were able to produce an experimental bronchopneumonia in monkeys.

On the basis of the hypothesis that meningeal *H. influenzae* can produce respiratory pathology, it would be interesting to look for this organism in the respiratory tracts of patients with influenzal meningitis. The recovery of ordinary *H. influenzae* would be of little significance, for it is frequently found in the respiratory tract, and its relation to meningeal strains is as dubious as its pathogenicity. Meningeal strains, however, are not often met with in the absence of meningitis, and their isolation from the respiratory tracts of two patients with influenzal meningitis is perhaps of some interest. No other reports of this sort have come to the author's attention, and little work has been done along this line since convenient technics for identification of meningeal strains have only recently been developed. In the two cases cited, the cultures may merely indicate that the organisms passed through the nasopharynx on their way to the meninges. In a case recently observed at the St. Louis Children's Hospital, the nose culture showed large numbers of influenza bacilli which proved to be serologically identical with those in the meninges. The child had an otitis media, but satisfactory ear cultures were not obtained. Meningeal *H. influenzae* has also been isolated from the nasopharynx in one case reported by Pittman. These cultures, while they show the feasibility of isolation of meningeal *H. influenzae* from the respiratory tract, offer no evidence of its importance as a respiratory pathogen. Evidence on this question would be difficult to obtain, for influenza bacilli may spread within the respiratory tract in infections due to other agents. Even the recovery of invasive influenza bacilli in pure culture from an area of pneumonic consolidation would not establish their pathogenic rôle in this lesion with certainty. However, an intensive search for meningeal *H. influenzae* in otitic and pneumonic lesions of patients with and without influenzal meningitis might lead to results of interest. Such a study might possibly help to clarify our general concepts of the pathogenic activity of influenza bacilli.

Since in the cases cited, there is no proof that influenza bacilli took part in the induction of the respiratory lesions, two other hypotheses suggest themselves, both of which assume that these lesions are caused by other agents. According to the first hypothesis, changes in the respiratory mucosa may facilitate the passage of influenza bacilli across this membrane into the blood and meninges. A spread of influenza bacilli within the respiratory tract, such as is seen in a variety of infections, might, if the influenza bacilli were potentially virulent, contribute to the development of generalized *H. influenzae* infection. The second hypothesis disregards local tissue changes, and assumes that a constitutional susceptibility to *H. influenzae* infection might be induced by respiratory disease. However, at the present time discussion of these or other hypotheses would be purely speculative.

To conclude, association between respiratory disease and the onset of influenzal meningitis is more than a coincidence, since analysis of the experience at this institution showed preceding and concomitant otitis and pneumonia to be significantly more common in a group of infants with influenzal meningitis than in a similar group with meningococcus meningitis. However, the nature of the relationship between respiratory infection and influenzal meningitis cannot be determined at present since there are no cogent data available.

REFERENCES

1. Pittman, M.: J. Exper. Med. **53**: 471, 1931.
2. Idem: Ibid. **58**: 683, 1933.
3. Rivers, T. M.: Am. J. Dis. Child. **24**: 102, 1932.
4. Neal, J. B., Jackson, H. W., and Appelbaum, E.: J. A. M. A. **102**: 513, 1933.
5. In contrasting the two series, it will be noted that the difference between the proportion of cases in which the meningitis was preceded by pneumonia or otitis is more than three times the calculated standard deviation. So is the difference in the proportion of cases in which the patient, admitted with meningitis, showed pneumonia or otitis on admission.
6. Yule, G. Udney: An Introduction to the Theory of Statistics, ed. 9, London, 1929, C. Griffin Co.
7. Alexander, Gustav: Die Ohrenkrankheiten im Kindesalter, Bd. VII, Pfaundler and Schlossman Handbuch der Kinderheilkunde, ed. 3, Leipzig, 1927, F. C. W. Vogel.
8. Huntington, R. W., Jr.: J. Clin. Investigation **14**: 459, 1935.
9. Ward, H. K., and Wright, J.: J. Exper. Med. **55**: 223, 1932.
10. Blake, F. G., and Cecil, R. L.: J. Exper. Med. **32**: 691, 1920.

THE TREATMENT OF INFLUENZAL MENINGITIS WITH IMMUNE SERUM

DOROTHY WILKES-WEISS, M.D.,* AND
ROBERT W. HUNTINGTON, JR., M.D.†
ST. LOUIS, MO.

INFLUENZA bacillus meningitis is one of the commoner infections of the central nervous system. In the experience of Neal[1] *H. influenzae* ranked fourth as a cause of purulent meningitis. The figures for the St. Louis Children's Hospital from 1918 to 1935, as shown in the accompanying tabulation, give a similar impression.

Meningococcus meningitis	160 cases
Streptococcus meningitis	74 cases
Pneumococcus meningitis	62 cases
Influenza bacillus meningitis	54 cases
Staphylococcus meningitis	24 cases

Since influenzal meningitis is relatively common and since the mortality is high, it was logical to investigate the possibility of treatment with immune serum. Ordinary respiratory strains of *H. influenzae* exhibit a marked antigenic heterogenicity, i.e., a serum made from one strain will probably show little or no reaction with the next strain tested, but the close antigenic relationship exhibited by meningeal strains[2, 3] might encourage hopes for the development of an immune serum which would be therapeutically effective in infections due to those strains.

In interpreting the reports of cases of influenzal meningitis in which recovery was associated with the use of serum, it is important to remember that recovery was not unknown before the introduction of serum. Moreover, while the prognosis is always poor, recovery is more frequent in patients over two years of age than in infants. Our own experience includes 39 cases in which no serum was used. Nine of these cases were in children over two years of age, and in this group there were two recoveries, while of the 30 infants only one recovered. A critical survey of the individual reports of 500 cases of influenzal meningitis from the literature was made by one of us (D.W.W.), including only those in which the diagnosis seemed certain. Although this series included 10 patients treated with serum with 1 recovery, it can be considered as a satisfactory control group. There were 373 infants under two

From the Department of Pediatrics, Washington University School of Medicine, and the St. Louis Children's Hospital.
*Theron Catlin Fellow in Pediatrics, 1929-1932.
†Theron Catlin Fellow in Pediatrics, 1935.

years of age with 9 recoveries, giving a mortality of 97.6 per cent, while 26 of the 127 patients over two recovered, or a mortality of 79.5 per cent. This series of unselected cases illustrates the higher incidence of the disease as well as the higher mortality in infancy.

The literature contains but few papers on serum treatment of influenzal meningitis. From the very paucity of such reports, one might assume that the results had been as disappointing as the few available data would indicate. Ward and Wright[4] have reported on eight cases with one recovery. Recovery occurred in one of Pittman's 18 cases. Our own material includes 15 patients treated at this hospital and 4 treated elsewhere. One of these patients recovered, a boy aged seven years, under the care of Dr. John A. Kolmer. Kuttner's patient (reported by Ward and Wright) was also more than two years old. One would have been more inclined to attach significance to these recoveries if the individuals had been infants. If these patients had been the only ones in the older age group who had received serum, a stubborn optimist, while conceding that the serum was perhaps useless in infants, might have continued to hope that it would be useful in older patients. However, 6 of our 16 treated patients were more than two years old. The age is given in but 10 of the other recorded cases, and in 6 of these it was more than two years. Evidently the ultimate results are discouraging in both age groups.

A temporary sterilization of the spinal fluid was noted in 5 of Ward and Wright's cases, in 3 of Pittman's, and in 2 of our own. Before the introduction of serum treatment, little attention was paid to the spinal fluid after the diagnosis had been made, and our material does not enable us to determine whether such a temporary sterilization may occur spontaneously. Since the course of the disease often tends to be somewhat prolonged and since recovery from influenzal meningitis was not unknown before the introduction of immune serum, it may well be that such sterilization occurs spontaneously.

The possibility that the poor results cited here may be attributable in part to the age of the patients and to delay in the institution of treatment immediately suggests itself and cannot be excluded. However, among 74 children with meningococcus meningitis observed in this hospital whose ages were under two years, there were only 31 deaths, and many of the patients who recovered were not treated until late in the disease. Hence it does not seem that either of these factors can altogether account for the apparent failure of serum treatment in influenzal meningitis.

Neal[1] has mentioned the possibility of the development of a more effective serum. However, an exhaustive analysis of the antigenic structure of *H. influenzae* has already been made by Pittman and by Ward and his coworkers, and the serums used by them seem theoretically adequate from our present knowledge. Serum of the same type was used in six of our cases. Although we do not feel hopeful about the improvement of serum therapy in influenzal meningitis, we believe that any further work along this line must take account of the experimental studies just mentioned, and it seems desirable to accord them a brief review.

Freshly isolated strains of meningeal *H. influenzae* exhibit many salient characteristics by which they differ from most strains from other sources. A capsular structure is present; growth on suitable media is mucoid in character; and the organisms are invasive upon inoculation into laboratory animals. Supranatant fluid from a centrifuged culture will produce a precipitin reaction in suitable serum, thereby demonstrating the presence of a soluble antigen. A close correlation exists among all these properties, and all may be rapidly lost on subculture unless due precautions are taken. Pittman has shown that nearly all strains of meningeal *H. influenzae* possess the same type of soluble antigen. This specific soluble substance, or S-substance, is apparently not the entire explanation of the serologic homogenicity of this group of organisms since serum prepared from old cultures which have lost this component may agglutinate both old and fresh strains. However, there is considerable evidence to suggest the importance of this S-substance in influenza bacillus infections.

The observations of Ward and Wright[4] indicate that this S-substance possesses the property of protecting influenza bacilli from the bactericidal action of serum of normal animals and that, if a test strain is well endowed with S-antigen, significant bactericidal activity is shown only by immune serum containing S-antibody and is closely correlated with the concentration of this antibody. Serum prepared from old strains which had lost the S-antigen agglutinated freshly isolated strains but had little or no bactericidal power against them. Similar observations are recorded by Weiss.[7]

Data on pneumococcal structure and immunity provide a close analogy to the observations recorded for meningeal *H. influenzae*. In pneumococcus infections, it appears that an S-antigen-antibody reaction is of considerable importance in determining the course of the disease, while antibody for another antigenic component of the pneumococcus may cause agglutination of the organisms in vitro, while conferring little if any benefit on an infected host.[5, 6] Some of Weiss'[7] observations on experimental infection of rabbits with virulent *H. influenzae* might suggest that serums with relatively little S-substance showed some tendency to retard the progress of the infection. There is, however, little theoretical justification for the clinical use of such serums. Nine of our patients were treated with a serum of this sort, and no evidence of beneficial effect was noted. In four of our case histories the nature of the serum used was not recorded, so that in six cases only can one be certain that the serum used contained S-antibody. The one recovery occurred in this group. However, in all the cases reported by Pittman and by Ward and Wright, the serum used contained S-antibody, and such serum apparently offers little hope for improvement in the ultimate prognosis.

On the basis of experimental data, Ward and his colleagues believe that fresh human serum should be added to immune serum in the treatment of influenzal meningitis. This procedure, based on the demonstrated absence of complement in the spinal fluid of influenzal meningitis and the apparent necessity for complement in bacteriolysis, was carried out in all their cases and in all of ours. However, in the case of recovery reported by Pittman, the spinal fluid became sterile after two treatments with immune serum alone, and two of the three patients who showed temporary sterilization of the spinal fluid received no fresh complement added to the serum. Nevertheless, theoretically the addition of active serum seems indicated.

Although in the reported cases the treatment has not been as uniform as might be desired for an optimum clinical experiment, the published data indicate quite clearly that despite much study of the rationale and mechanics of the procedure, treatment with immune serum offers little hope for the patient with influenzal meningitis. These discouraging results are not altogether surprising, for although a variety of clinical infections have been treated with *antibacterial* serums, in general the results have been disappointing. Antimeningococcus serum and Type I pneumococcus serum are perhaps the only well-established exceptions to this statement. The usefulness of the latter is restricted within sharp if ill-understood limits since it seems to be quite ineffective in the treatment of purulent processes and specifically of meningitis, due to pneumococcus Type I. It is remarkable that so far no serum with a clinical effect remotely resembling that of antimeningococcus serum has been discovered. The analogies between influenzal and meningococcus meningeal infections would make it appear possible to produce an effective antiserum for influenzal meningitis. However, anti-influenzal serum is not a success despite the brilliant and arduous work which lies back of some of the clinical experiments which we have discussed. Clearly there is some unknown factor which makes the dislodgment of the meningococcus relatively easy, while meningeal *H. influenzae* is not readily evicted.

In conclusion, it may be stated that the results of serum treatment of influenzal meningitis have been discouraging, and that there is no obvious justification for optimism as to the possibilities of future work. The use of such serum is purely experimental, and its commercial exploitation seems quite unjustified. If investigation of serum treatment is to be continued, the serum should contain anti-S-substance, since there is little theoretical justification for the use of serum devoid of this component. Active human serum should probably be added to the immune serum, though one can only guess at the optimum proportions. Furthermore, the organism should be typed in every case. There seems no justification whatever for continuing this mode of therapy unless such stipulations are fulfilled.

REFERENCES

1. Neal, J. B., Jackson, H. W., and Appelbaum, E.: J. A. M. A. **102**: 573, 1934.
2. Rivers, T. M.: Am. J. Dis. Child. **24**: 102, 1932.
3. Pittman, M.: J. Exper. Med. **58**: 683, 1933.
4. Ward, Hugh K., and Wright, Joyce: J. Exper. Med. **55**: 223, 1932.
5. Avery, O. T., and Neill, J. M.: J. Exper. Med. **41**: 355, 1925.
6. Topley, W. W. C.: An Outline of Immunity, Baltimore, 1933, William Wood and Company.
7. Wilkes-Weiss, D.: Studies on Meningeal Strains of H. Influenzae (to be published).

A FOLLOW-UP STUDY OF AMBULATORY CHILDREN WITH TUBERCULOSIS INFECTION

Ernst Wolff, M.D., and Samuel Hurwitz, M.D.
San Francisco, Calif.

THIS study was undertaken to determine the course of tuberculous infections in ambulatory children. The majority of follow-up reports deals with sanitarium cases of childhood tuberculosis and offers no comparison for this group. Many statistical studies of school surveys have disclosed the incidence of tuberculous infection in apparently healthy children. However, these individuals have not been observed for a sufficient length of time to know their ultimate fate. An attempt is made to answer this last question from an analysis of the subsequent data.

Our material originally consisted of 639 children who attended the out-patient children's chest clinic at the University of California Hospital. They were referred from the general pediatric clinic because of exposure to tuberculosis or as tuberculous suspects. Only 162 patients returned for the final recheck. All cases were tested by the Mantoux method with 0.1 mg. of old tuberculin. Complete physical and x-ray examinations were performed at the initial visit and at intervals thereafter. At the initial examination two children had negative tuberculin tests but were included here because of definite roentgen evidence of tuberculous infection. A brief summary of the records of these two patients is as follows:

Case 1.—H. B., a male eleven years of age, had had no history of contact but was brought to the clinic because of cough and night sweats for three months. There were no abnormal physical findings, but the x-ray plates showed calcified hilar glands. At reexamination, eight years later, the patient was perfectly well. The tuberculin test was still negative; there were no physical signs, and the roentgen picture was unchanged.

Case 2.—H. A., a six and one-half-year-old female child, was brought in because of malnutrition. There was no definite history of exposure. Physical examination was essentially negative, but x-ray pictures revealed hilar gland calcification. Ten years later the patient was perfectly well with no physical evidence of tuberculosis. The tuberculin test was again negative, and the x-ray picture unchanged.

The division into age groups and the number of years these cases have been followed is shown in Table I. Sixty-four per cent were observed for more than six years.

The sources of infection are illustrated in Table II. Over two-thirds gave a definite history of exposure, and of these patients 89 per cent were exposed to members in the same household.

From the Pediatric Department of the University of California Medical School.

TABLE I

UNIVERSITY OF CALIFORNIA CHILDREN'S CHEST CLINIC FOLLOW-UP RECORD

INITIAL AGE (YEARS)	NUMBER OF CASES	NUMBER OF YEARS FOLLOWED				
		(3-5)	(6-8)	(9-11)	(12 AND OVER)	AVERAGE
0- 4	54	22	18	11	3	6.6
5- 9	73	26	21	20	6	7.2
10-15	35	10	13	10	2	7.0
Total = 162 Males = 88 Females = 74		58	52	41	11	

TABLE II

SOURCE OF INFECTION

AGE YEARS	INTRA-FAMILIAL	INTRADOM-ICILIARY	EXTRADOM-ICILIARY	MILK	NEGATIVE
0- 4	30	6	3	1	14
5- 9	37	3	6	0	27
10-15	20	3	1	1	10
Total	87	12	10	2	51

Exposed = 68%
No History of Exposure = 32%

A comparison of the clinical and roentgenologic findings at the onset with those after the follow-up period is given in Table III. It is quite evident that the incidence of symptoms and physical signs is materially decreased at the final examination.

TABLE III

COMPARISON OF CLINICAL AND ROENTGEN FINDINGS

	ONSET		RECHECK	
	NO. OF CASES	PERCENTAGE	NO. OF CASES	PERCENTAGE
SYMPTOMS	67	41	8	5
Physical signs	68	42	32	20
Roentgen findings				
Negative	68	42	68	42
Doubtful	50	31	12	8
Latent	25	15	79	49
Active	19	12	3 (1 death)	2

The chest roentgenograms have been classified as follows:

a. Negative—no evidence of tuberculous infection.

b. Doubtful—enlarged hilar shadows but no other tuberculous manifestations.

c. Latent—including focal calcification of the lung, parenchymal fibrosis, hilar gland calcification, and pleural calcification.

d. Active—infiltration and cavitation of the lung tissue.

Seventy-three per cent of the initial x-ray examinations were either negative or doubtful. The percentage of latent cases increased from

15 per cent initially to 49 per cent at the final recheck. This increase was due to the change of the doubtful and active groups to a latent stage. Only 2 per cent were active, whereas originally 12 per cent had been so.

The x-ray changes for the different age groups are analyzed in Chart 1. The doubtful cases are grouped with the negative ones. In all age divisions the initial negative cases remained so or finally showed evidence of a latent process but did not develop changes of active tuberculosis with the exception of one individual in the 0-4 year group. Those patients showing latent tuberculosis at the initial examination were found to be latent at the final recheck in all age sections. The group with active tuberculosis initially became latent with the exception of four cases. Two of the latter became negative while two remained active. In our 10-14 year age division no activation of the pulmonary

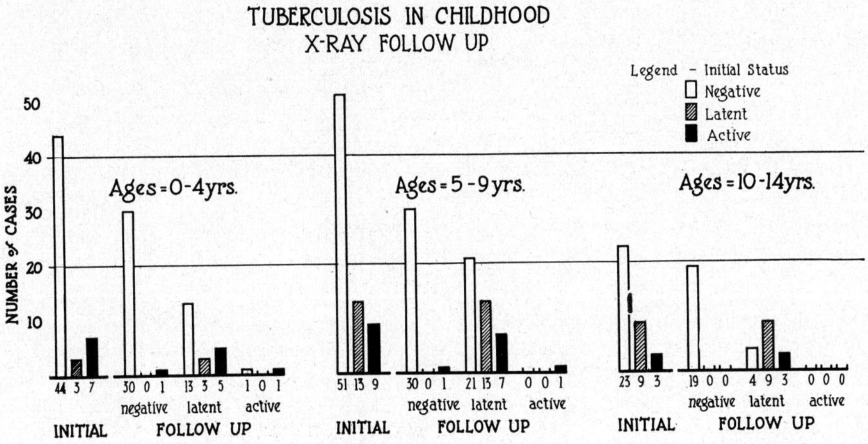

Chart 1.

tuberculous infection was shown by roentgenogram. One patient who initially had had infiltration of the right apex at the age of thirteen years now, after four years of observation, showed parenchymal fibrosis and hilar gland calcification. However, there was an active tuberculous process in the lumbar vertebrae.

The interval history reveals that 30 patients (18.5 per cent) required sanitarium care; 10 were in the 0-4 age limit, 15 in the 5-9 year group, and 5 in the oldest age group. One patient in the youngest division died of tuberculous meningitis, the only death in this series. Examination of the death certificates of San Francisco for the whole period of this study revealed only one death from tuberculosis in the remaining 477 cases of the original group of 639 children. This is strong supportive evidence that our assumption that the mortality rate from primary tuberculous infection in ambulatory children is extremely low is correct. Only two patients at present have active pulmonary lesions.

Austrian,[1] who observed dispensary children for a period of eight to twelve years, concluded that the number of young individuals exposed to tuberculous infection who develop tuberculous disease is relatively small provided contact with the infecting source is abolished when its existence has been established and provided ordinarily good hygienic and dietetic regimens are maintained. In only eight patients of the whole group was the exposure continued, and the active and fatal cases described previously were all in this group. This study again illustrates the well-known fact that reinfection from continued exposure is responsible for the activation of tuberculous processes in childhood.[2]

One of the striking features in this study was the loss or diminution of skin sensitivity to tuberculin manifested by four patients. Initially positive to 0.1 mg. of old tuberculin, three were negative on recheck to dilutions up to 10 mg., while one did not react to 0.1 mg. but was not tested with stronger solutions. A varying sensitization to tuberculin has been previously recorded.[1, 2] A brief résumé of the preceding cases is appended:

CASE 1.—A. E., a white female, six years of age, was first seen because of cough and lassitude. She had had no known exposure. Physical examination revealed râles at the left apex and the roentgenogram showed enlarged bronchial glands and increased parenchymal markings in the left upper lobe. At recheck, eleven years later, she was well except for intermittent asthmatic attacks. The roentgen ray examination showed calcified nodes at the tracheal bifurcation. The tuberculin test was negative to 0.1 mg. of old tuberculin.

CASE 2.—A. T., an eleven-year-old white female, had no history of exposure. Her symptoms were anorexia, failure to gain, and fatigability. Physically there were no positive findings and x-ray examination showed only increased bronchial markings. Reexamination at twenty-one years of age, two years after marriage, showed a well-developed individual with no abnormal physical signs or x-ray changes. Her tuberculin test proved to be negative with a dilution of 10 mg. of old tuberculin intradermally.

CASE 3.—B. B., a female child of five years, had been exposed over a four months' period to the grandfather who had active pulmonary tuberculosis. She had no complaints, and physical and x-ray examinations were negative. Five years later the patient was still perfectly well, and the status was unchanged clinically and roentgenologically. Exposure had been discontinued. The Mantoux reaction was negative up to 10 mg. of old tuberculin.

CASE 4.—J. O., a female child, was first seen at the age of seven years with symptoms of anorexia, fatigability, and listlessness. Physical examination was negative. The roentgenogram revealed enlarged bronchial glands. In the interval between the initial and final visit at seventeen years of age the patient had been in a sanitarium for eight months. At the last check-up she was symptom-free and without physical signs or positive x-ray findings. Her skin test was negative with 10 mg. of old tuberculin intracutaneously.

SUMMARY

One hundred and sixty-two ambulatory children with pulmonary tuberculous infection were followed over an average period of approximately seven years. Initial and subsequent studies included tuberculin testing and complete physical and roentgenologic examinations.

Clinically all patients, with four exceptions, are now perfectly healthy. These latter cases belong in the group of eight, in which exposure continued. In the whole series there was but one death; this caused by tuberculous meningitis occurred in the 0-4 year division.

The roentgen ray findings became negative or latent in 98 per cent of all cases. The 12 per cent initially active lesions diminished to 2 per cent at the last recheck. The majority of patients with doubtful x-ray shadows at the commencement later revealed evidence of latent tuberculous processes.

Four patients initially positive to 0.1 mg. of old tuberculin intradermally showed altered skin sensitivity on follow-up. Three were negative to old tuberculin in dilution up to 10 mg. and have always had negative chest plates. One individual did not react to 0.1 mg. of tuberculin but could not be tested with stronger dilutions. Her roentgenogram revealed calcification at the tracheal bifurcation.

CONCLUSION

The subsequent course of ambulatory children with pulmonary tuberculous infection is extremely favorable provided that they are adequately supervised and are not exposed to reinfection.

We appreciate gratefully the thoughtful cooperation of Miss Dorothy Keane and Mrs. Hazel Leseque of the Children's Out-Patient Department of the University of California in the preparation of the material for this paper.

REFERENCES

1. Austrian, C. R.: Am. Rev. Tuberc. **16:** 501, 1927.
2. Opie, E. L., McPhedran, F. M., and Putnam, P.: Am. J. Hyg. **22:** 644, 1935.

450 SUTTER STREET

HYPERPYREXIA OF SIXTEEN MONTHS' DURATION OF UNKNOWN ETIOLOGY

HARRY M. GREENWALD, M.D., AND JACOB KOOTA, M.D.
BROOKLYN, N. Y.

IN THIS communication we report the case of a boy eight years old who has had a continuous elevation of temperature of unknown origin for over sixteen months.

S. R., male, eight years old, was admitted to the Israel Zion Hospital of Brooklyn, N. Y., on Nov. 4, 1934, because of fever and pain in the right leg of six days' duration. The onset occurred with hyperesthesia which increased to such a degree that even the bed sheet could not be endured, and, in addition, there was severe pain in the right leg, prohibiting all motion. For six days before admission the temperature ranged from 101° to 102° F. Because of the hyperesthesia, the elevation of temperature, and the inability to move the right limb, a diagnosis of poliomyelitis was made by the family physician, and a lumbar puncture was done before the child was admitted to the hospital. Examination of the fluid showed ten cells—all lymphocytes.

We saw the child for the first time on the day he was admitted to the hospital. Examination at that time revealed the following: the temperature was elevated to 104.2° F.; the patient, however, did not appear particularly ill; marked diffuse tenderness was present in both lower extremities and the boy seemed to be unable to move his right leg; the knee jerks were absent; there was no rigidity of the neck; but rigidity of the back was present; the cremasteric and abdominal reflexes were normal, and the Babinski sign was absent; there was no swelling or tenderness about the joints. The remainder of the physical examination was negative. On admission the white blood count was 24,900, of which 87 per cent were polymorphonuclear leucocytes, 12 per cent lymphocytes, and 1 per cent eosinophiles; the red blood count was 4,728,000; the hemoglobin (Sahli) was 73 per cent. The urinalysis was negative. Lumbar puncture was done and 10 c.c. of clear fluid was removed for examination; there were 100 cells, practically all lymphocytes, in 1 c.mm. of fluid. All the subsequent laboratory data are given in Tables I and II.

Because of the absent knee jerks and the pleocytosis in the spinal fluid, a diagnosis of acute poliomyelitis with an involvement of both lower extremities was entertained and a transfusion of 400 c.c. of whole blood from an immune donor was given intravenously. The temperature, however, continued to remain elevated and fluctuated daily between 100° and 106° F. Two days later, because of the septic temperature and because of an almost immediate and complete return of motion in the

From the pediatric service of the Israel Zion Hospital.

right leg, the diagnosis of poliomyelitis was discarded. It is difficult to explain the pleocytosis in the spinal fluid on the second puncture, but we believe that the increase in the number of cells may have been due to an irritation of the meninges caused by the first lumbar puncture done at home. The knee jerks became active again six days after admission. We have no explanation for their absence early in the disease.

TABLE I

LABORATORY DATA—BLOOD STUDY

Hemoglobin and Cell Count

DATE	HEMOGLOBIN (SAHLI)	R.B.C.	W.B.C.	P.	L.	E.	B.	M.	SMEAR
11/ 3/34	73%	4,728,000	24,900	87	12	1			Neg.
11/ 7/34	85%	5,000,000	15,900	87	11	2			Neg.
11/16/34	75%	3,700,000	16,200	75	22			3	Neg.
11/23/34	91%	4,800,000	22,100	92	4	1	1	2	Neg.
11/29/34	75%	4,792,000	23,800	95	5				Neg.
12/17/34	90%	5,250,000	41,200	91	7			2	Neg.
2/ 7/35	78%	4,250,000	22,400	87	12			1	Neg.
3/ 7/35	65%	3,400,000	18,600	83	10	3		4	Neg.
5/22/35	76%	4,200,000	15,700	82	14			4	Neg.

Blood Culture

DATE	RESULT
11/ 6/34	Positive culture (*Streptococcus hemolyticus*)
11/ 6/34	No growth
11/16/34	No growth
12/ 3/34	No growth
1/ 3/35	No growth
1/25/35	No growth
2/ 6/35	No growth
2/12/35	No growth (Aerobic and anaerobic cultures)
5/21/35	No growth

Serology

DATE	TEST	RESULT
11/23/34	Wassermann and Rosenthal	Negative
11/23/34	Widal for typhoid and paratyphoid	Negative
12/17/34	Agglutination for melitensis abortus	Negative
2/15/35	Agglutination for melitensis abortus	Negative
3/ 1/35	Mouse test for *Spirocheta morsus muris*	Negative
3/15/35	Mouse test for *Spirocheta morsus muris*	Negative

Chemistry

DATE	GLUCOSE	UREA NITROGEN	CREATININE	URIC ACID
11/23/34	94.8 mg. %	16.8 mg. %	1.49 mg. %	4.06 mg. %

Sedimentation Rate

DATE	WESTERGREN INDEX
5/21/35	64.6 (normal 12-15)

A blood culture taken on November 6 at 11:45 A.M. revealed the presence of hemolytic streptococci, but, unfortunately, no report of the number of colonies was made. A second culture taken on the same day at 9 P.M., after the child's temperature had fallen precipitately to 96° F., showed no growth, and every subsequent culture taken over a period of nine months, anaerobic as well as aerobic, was consistently negative (Table II). For a time, however, the case was considered one of septicemia because of the single positive blood culture, but every effort to find a focus of infection was futile. Finally, on Feb. 15, 1935, the diagnosis of sepsis, too, was discarded because of the repeated negative blood cultures. During this time nine transfusions of 200 to 250 c.c. of whole blood each were given intravenously at irregular intervals.

TABLE II

ADDITIONAL LABORATORY DATA

Spinal Fluid

DATE	APPEARANCE	PRESSURE	CELLS	ALBUMIN	GLOBULIN	GLUCOSE
11/3/34	Clear	Normal	10	--	--	--
11/4/34	Hazy	Normal	100 (lymphocytes)	2 plus	Absent	Present

N.B. First tap was done at patient's home on day before admission.

Urine

Examinations were made every 3-5 days during entire hospital stay. Only findings were those of a febrile urine (e.g., an occasional pus cell and hyaline cast).

Tuberculin Tests

DATE	TEST	CONCENTRATION	RESULT
11/ 6/34	Mantoux	0.1 c.c. 1-1,000 O.T.	Negative
11/13/34	Mantoux	0.1 c.c. 1- 100 O.T.	Negative
11/20/34	Mantoux	0.1 c.c. 1- 10 O.T.	Negative

Electrocardiographic Studies

DATE	RESULT
1/10/35	Normal tracing
4/16/35	Normal tracing
3/ 7/36	Normal tracing

Roentgenographic Studies

DATE	AREA EXAMINED	FINDINGS
11/ 9/34	Dorsolumbar spine	Normal
11/ 9/34	Pelvis	Normal
11/12/34	Pelvis	Normal
11/18/34	Sinuses	Normal
11/19/34	Pelvis	Normal
11/23/34	Chest	Normal
11/30/34	Mastoids	Normal
2/26/35	Pelvis	Normal
3/ 6/35	Dorsolumbar spine	Normal

N.B. Since discharge from hospital repeated fluoroscopic examinations of the heart and lungs failed to reveal any abnormal findings.

On Nov. 9, 1934, tenderness was present over the upper and outer aspect of the right thigh; rectal examination also revealed an area of tenderness about the left pubic bone near the ischium, but subsequent observation and repeated roentgen ray examinations of the pelvis and of both femurs failed to show the presence of any osseous pathologic changes. Similarly, repeated roentgen ray studies of the lumbodorsal spine and pelvis at intervals of several weeks failed to disclose any evidence of skeletal infection. The generalized hyperesthesia gradually subsided, but the elevation of temperature continued with a fluctuation of six to eight degrees in twenty-four hours.

From Nov. 4, 1934, the day of admission, until March 25, 1935, there was a daily fluctuation of temperature from 99° to 106° F., a difference of 7°. On March 25 and 27 there was no elevation of temperature for the first time. On March 28 the temperature again began to rise but did not reach the previous levels daily although on many occasions the temperature rose to 105° F. This continued until June 2, approximately seven months after the onset of the disease, when the temperature curve became irregular and, although many days followed in which fluctuations of five degrees still occurred, there were days when only a slight rise was observed. As time went on, the number of days when little or no elevation of temperature occurred increased until fever-free intervals of three and four days were quite common. During the last week of the child's stay in the hospital (July 17 to 23) the highest temperature was 101° F. (Chart 1). Elevations to 103° F. and even 104.5° F., however, occurred for a few hours every four to five days during August. During September the highest temperature noted was 103° F. and the longest fever-free interval was six days; and thus the tendency to subsidence continued so that the elevations became fewer and lower until finally, in January, 1936, the highest temperature observed was 101° F. and the longest fever-free interval was two weeks. The child had only two distinct chills; one on November 16 and the other on December 9. In both instances the chill ushered in a sharp rise in temperature.

On November 10, six days after admission to the hospital, a maculopapular eruption appeared on the posterior aspects of the left thigh and left buttock. It resembled the rash seen in serum sickness, but it was nonpruritic. After a few days it began to fade, and in two weeks it disappeared completely. The rash reappeared in two to three weeks, however, and continued to come and go for approximately fourteen months. At times the distribution resembled that of the erythema annulare encountered in rheumatic fever, that is, it appeared over the buttocks, on the extensive surfaces of the arms and legs, and occasionally on the chest; at other times it was more generalized and also involved the trunk; often it was a bright red and then again a pale pink. Several times the rash resembled measles so closely in its appearance and distribution that, were it not for the absence of Koplik spots and catarrhal symptoms, the rash could easily have been mistaken for that of measles. On April 14 the eruption was present on the abdomen and thighs and looked like urticaria.

Interestingly enough, in spite of the marked elevation of temperature over a long period of time, the child never looked dangerously ill; indeed, he was at all times bright, alert, cheerful, and cooperative.

As already stated, after Feb. 15, 1935, the diagnosis of septicemia was discarded, and a renewed search for the cause of the fever was made. The child was carefully studied for tuberculosis, malaria, sinus and

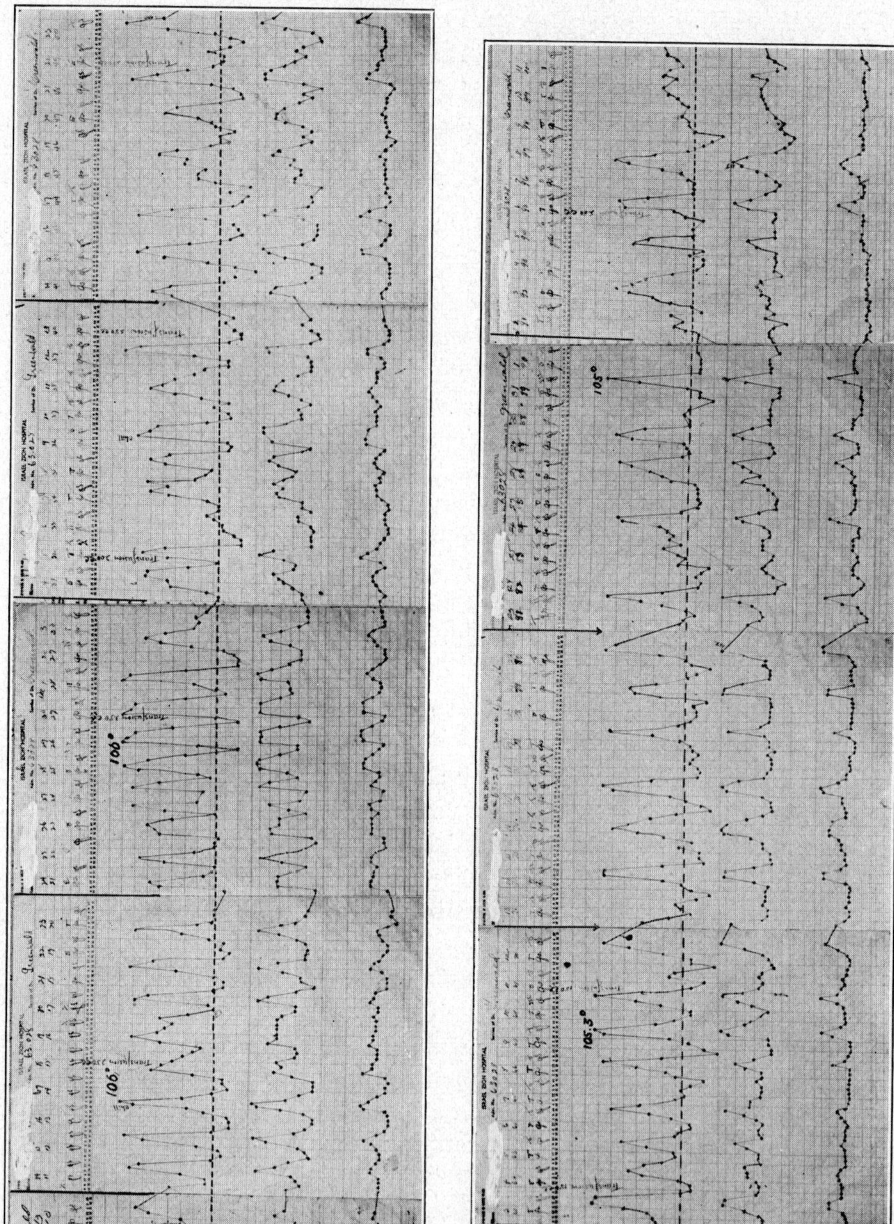

Chart 1.—The temperature curve during the patient's stay in the hospital. The heavy lines at the top of the chart indicate the weekly periods.

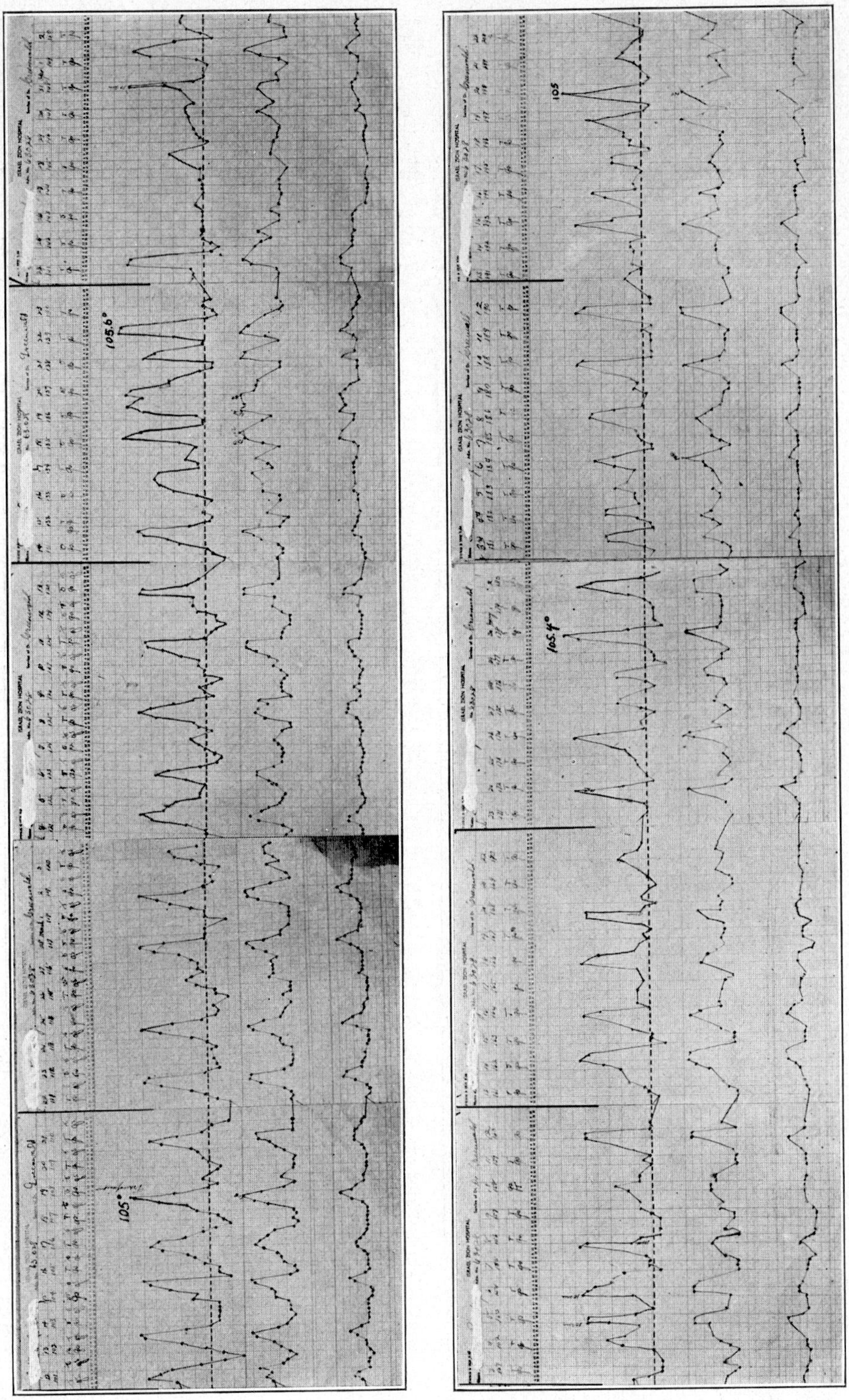

Chart 1 (Cont'd).

mastoid infection, ratbite fever, leucemia, Hodgkin's disease, rheumatic fever, syphilis, disease of the genitourinary tract, and subacute bacterial endocarditis (Tables I and II). The reasons for excluding these conditions as a cause of the fever will be discussed later.

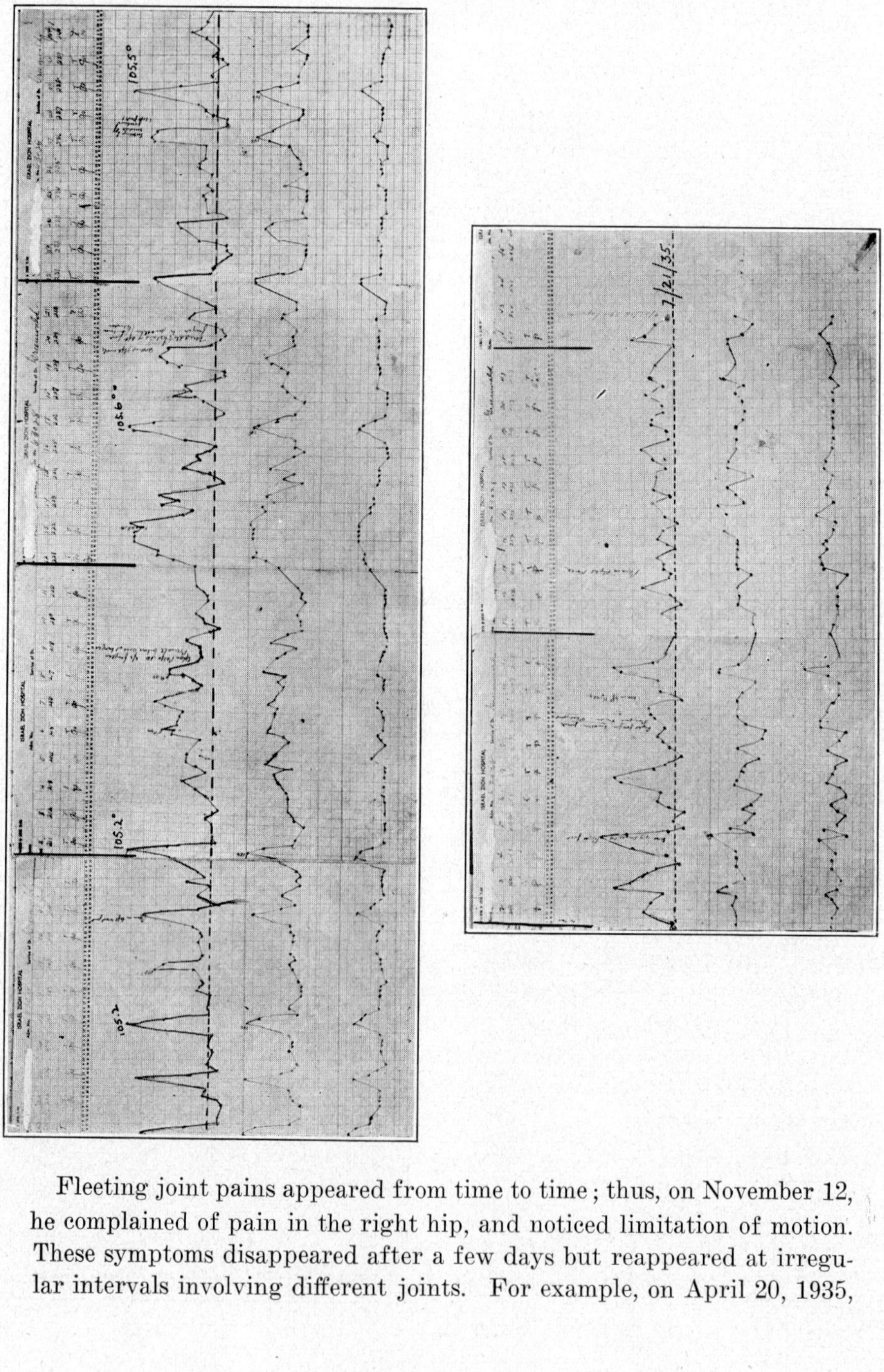

Chart 1 (Cont'd).

Fleeting joint pains appeared from time to time; thus, on November 12, he complained of pain in the right hip, and noticed limitation of motion. These symptoms disappeared after a few days but reappeared at irregular intervals involving different joints. For example, on April 20, 1935, pain and tenderness in the interphalangeal joints of the right thumb were present for four days; on May 20 the left wrist was involved; on June 20 the left ankle, as well as the interphalangeal joints of the left forefinger, became swollen and painful; on July 9 there was pain and swelling of the interphalangeal joints of the right second finger; on July 10 the left knee and on July 14 the right knee became tender and painful. In August the cervical vertebral joints became affected with the development of torticollis which lasted about twelve weeks. Apparently, as time went on, the joint manifestations became more pronounced and seemed to reach a peak about September, 1935. The increase in the joint manifestations seemed to coincide with the subsidence of the fever. In other words, it appeared that, as the fever-free intervals increased, the joint involvements simultaneously became more frequent and prominent. Limitation of motion in the involved joints persisted long after the swelling and tenderness had disappeared. We have described the joint manifestations in some detail because the course of this patient's illness so closely resembled that of Bilderback's patient. In the description of his patient's illness, Bilderback[3] stated "after eighteen months of almost continuous fever, marked with wide fluctuations, sometimes with a variation of nine degrees in twelve hours, the patient began to show unmistakable evidence of chronic infectious arthritis."

In our case rheumatic fever was considered but ruled out because of the prolonged course without clinical evidence of cardiac involvement and because repeated teleroentgenograms of the heart failed to show any enlargement or change in configuration. At no time did repeated electrocardiographic studies show any evidence of myocardial damage. The sedimentation rate was high (Table I), but we feel that, while this is of definite prognostic value, it is of little diagnostic value in rheumatic fever.

After nine months, July, 1935, no diagnosis could be made, in spite of all efforts. As may be seen from the temperature chart, however, the fever showed a tendency to subside although fluctuations of five and six degrees in one day still occasionally occurred. On July 23 the child was discharged from the hospital and was kept under observation at home. His fever gradually disappeared. The temperature-free intervals increased from one or two days to four and five days, then to a week and finally to two weeks until, in February, 1936, a period of one month went by with only a single elevation of temperature to 102° F. The joint manifestations are still present (April, 1936) although not as severe as six months before.

Early during his stay in the hospital the patient was given frequent transfusions; later these were discontinued and amidopyrin and sodium salicylate in fairly large doses were given. These drugs were apparently without influence on the temperature or joint involvement. From the onset of the disease the child was given a full diet; special efforts were made to see that a sufficient amount of the accessory food substances was ingested. His weight on discharge from the hospital was almost exactly what it was on admission, 73 pounds. During his stay at home the child gained weight rapidly and at the last examination on April 20, 1936, he weighed 95 pounds.

COMMENT

In the last few years several papers on fever of unknown origin have been published.[1] These papers dealt with the cases of children who had an obscure fever for periods varying from one to several weeks. In practically every case careful clinical laboratory studies revealed the diagnosis, and it was found that tuberculosis, rheumatic fever, undulant fever, syphilis, Hodgkin's disease, leucemia, sinus infection, typhoid fever, infection of the genitourinary tract including perinephric abscess, subdiaphragmatic abscess, septicemia, or subacute bacterial endocarditis was responsible for the elevation of temperature. On the other hand, reports in which fever was of more than one year's duration and in which the diagnosis remained in doubt, in spite of careful clinical and laboratory investigation, are extremely rare. As far as we know, only three cases that can be placed in this category have been thus far reported. Two of these cases were of adults who eventually developed pericarditis with cardiac enlargement, polyserositis, and glomerulonephritis with fatal termination. The diagnosis in these cases was established by necropsy studies.[2] The third case was that of Bilderback[3] who reported the case of a boy six and a half years old who had an almost continuous elevation of temperature since the age of four years. In many respects Bilderback's case closely resembles our case. For example, the age and sex of Bilderback's patient correspond with those of our patient; the duration of the temperature with the wide fluctuations; and the final development of arthritic manifestations also correspond to the signs and symptoms observed by us. It is interesting, too, that Bilderback's patient showed general hyperesthesia, a sign so prominent in our case that it led us to entertain a diagnosis of poliomyelitis.

In the differential diagnosis, rheumatic fever, tuberculosis, malaria, ratbite fever, syphilis, infection of the genitourinary tract, Hodgkin's disease, leucemia, sinus and mastoid infection, and subacute bacterial endocarditis were considered. Although the disease more closely resembled rheumatic fever than any other condition, we feel that rheumatic fever can be definitely excluded for the following reasons: First, the prolonged course of the disease was entirely unlike that of rheumatic fever; second, there was no evidence of enlargement of the heart or myocardial changes as determined by clinical, roentgen ray, and electrocardiographic studies; at no time were the cardiac sounds abnormal; third, although the joint involvement was fleeting in character, the residual stiffness and impairment of motion observed in our case after the acute phase had subsided certainly were unlike the usual joint manifestations seen in rheumatic fever; and fourth, the marked leucocytosis in our patient was further evidence against rheumatic fever.

Tuberculosis was excluded because of the three negative Mantoux tests with increasing doses of old tuberculin. While we are aware that in rare instances active tuberculosis may be present in spite of repeated negative Mantoux tests with large doses of old tuberculin,[4] we eliminated this disease as an etiologic factor because careful clinical and roentgen ray studies of the lungs and the osseous system of our patient failed to show any evidence of tuberculosis.

Malaria was ruled out because of repeated negative blood smears and the failure to respond to quinine in large doses.

Ratbite fever was considered and discarded because of the absence of a characteristic lesion about the finger and because of the absence of the spirochete in the blood. In order to rule out this condition definitely, however, 10 c.c. of blood from the patient was injected into mice on two different occasions; examination of the blood of the mice failed to reveal the presence of the *Spirocheta morsus muris.*

Subacute bacterial endocarditis was eliminated because of the persistent negative blood cultures, the absence of cardiac murmurs, and the absence of clinical signs, e.g., substernal pain, café au lait color, embolic phenomena, and enlargement of the spleen. (The spleen became palpable one-half fingerbreadth below the costal margin on June 9, 1935, but could not be palpated again a few days later.)

Roentgenographic studies of the accessory nasal sinuses and mastoid processes were made to rule out the presence of an infectious process in these regions. At no time did the films show any abnormalities.

Typhoid and paratyphoid were eliminated as a possible cause almost immediately because of the high leucocyte count; in addition, a Widal test made on Nov. 23, 1934, was negative.

Undulant fever was considered, but two agglutination tests done on Dec. 17, 1934, and Feb. 15, 1935, were negative.

Still's disease, or chronic polyarthritis, was considered a likely etiologic factor in our case because cutaneous manifestations, such as erythema, erythema multiforme, and urticaria, as well as protracted fever, occur in this disease. Cases of Still's disease have been reported in which the patient had an elevation of temperature for three months or longer before joint involvement occurred.[5] In our case, too, the temperature was elevated for at least three months before the joint manifestations became marked. Against the diagnosis of Still's disease, however, are the absence of symmetrical joint involvement, the absence of wasting and marked limitation of motion, and the absence of enlargement of the liver and superficial lymph nodes. Roentgenologic examination of the elbow, wrist, hip, knee, and ankle joints of our patient on April 20, 1936, failed to show thickening of the periarticular structures, osteoporosis, or distention of the joints—changes characteristic of Still's disease. The lower pole of the spleen could be felt one-half fingerbreadth below the costal margin for the first time on June 9, 1935, and for several days after. Later it could not be felt. While it is true that enlargement of the spleen in Still's disease may not be marked, it is Poynton's opinion that it can be felt at least one or two inches below the costal margin in practically every case.[6] Another dissimilarity is the moderate leucocytosis found in Still's disease. Our patient had a marked increase in the number of white cells; indeed, the count reached 41,000 on one occasion. Eosinophilia is observed occasionally in Still's disease; it was absent in our case. Our patient, however, did have a definite increase in the sedimentation rate (Table I). We mention this because Dawson and Boots[7] stressed the increased rate in Still's disease.*

We have mentioned the fact in favor of and against the diagnosis of Still's disease because we feel that it is impossible at this stage of the patient's illness to make a definite diagnosis of Still's disease or to rule it out.

*We have since learned that the case reported by Bilderback in 1930 as a case of fever of unknown etiology of one year's duration is now considered to be definitely one of Still's disease.

REFERENCES

1. a. Berkman, John M.: Wisconsin M. J. **32**: 809, 1933.
   b. McMullen, Edwin C.: Tri-State M. J. **7**: 1433, 1935.
   c. Schott, Charles: Illinois M. J. **64**: 485, 1933.
   d. Schlesinger, Bernard: Clin. Journal **63**: 191, 1934.
   e. Dreyfus-Sée, G.: Presse méd. **41**: 307, 1933.
2. Christian, Henry C.: M. Clin. North America **18**: 1023, 1935.
3. Bilderback, J. B.: Am. J. Dis. Child. **14**: 686, 1930.
4. Jacobsen, A. Wilmot: J. Pediat. **8**: 292, 1930.
5. Holt, Jr., L. Emmett and McIntosh, Rustin: Holt's Diseases of Infancy and Childhood, New York, 1933, D. Appleton-Century Co., p. 634.
6. Poynton, F. J.: Quoted by Garrod, Archibald E., Batten, Frederick E., Thursfield, Hugh, and Paterson, Donald: Diseases of Children, New York, 1919, William Wood & Co., p. 901.
7. Dawson, M. H., and Boots, R. H.: J. A. M. A. **95**: 1894, 1930.

ISOLATED PERIPHERAL RADIAL NERVE PARALYSIS IN THE NEWBORN

SOL M. ABELSON, M.D., AND JOSEPH GREENGARD, M.D.
CHICAGO, ILL.

ISOLATED peripheral radial nerve palsy in the newborn has received very little attention in this country. The only reports in the American literature were made by Smith.[1, 2] There are a number of reports in the German literature, and among them two rather comprehensive accounts which contain reviews and comments on all reported cases.[3, 4] We wish to report a case which we believe merits recording, first, because such instances have received little attention in American writings and, second, because other factors than those recognized by writers on this subject may have operated in this infant.

REPORT OF CASE

Maternal and Birth History.—The last menstrual period occurred Sept. 28, 1932, or Oct. 30, 1932. Pregnancy was uneventful except for slight edema of legs and occasionally of face, and with albumin 1+ at times. The measurements were as follows: intercristal 27 cm., intertrochanteric 30 cm., interspinous 23 cm., and Baudelocque 16.5 cm. An unsuccessful attempt at induction of labor with castor oil and an enema was made July 16. The patient was admitted to Mount Sinai Hospital, service of Dr. A. F. Lash, on August 14. At 10 A.M. castor oil, 1½ ounces, was given, followed by quinine sulphate, 5 gr., at 9:45, 10:15, and 10:45 A.M., and an enema at 1 P.M. Irregular pains resulted, which were only slightly influenced by intranasal pituitrin. At 5:35 P.M. pituitrin, minims 3, was given hypodermically and the bag of waters ruptured at 6:50 P.M. At 7:25 nembutal (sodium pentobarbital), 3 gr., was given by mouth and repeated at 7:45 P.M. when dilatation of the cervix was practically complete. Progress was satisfactory until the resistant perineum was encountered, where the head remained one hour with very little advance. At 10:40 P.M. delivery was easily effected by low forceps and episiotomy under ether-nitrous oxide anesthesia. The position of the occiput was left posterior, but rotation anteriorly occurred spontaneously.

Infant History.—The child was a baby girl weighing 6 pounds and 12 ounces (3030 grams) in good condition and with a vigorous cry. The following morning examination revealed a flaccid paralysis of the extensors of the right wrist with resulting wrist drop and slight adduction of the thumb. The circumferences of both forearms and arms were alike. There were no pressure marks or other external or palpable evidences of injury in either the shoulder, arm, forearm, or wrist. Movements at the right shoulder and elbow were normal. The triceps muscle was not involved.

A diagnosis of isolated peripheral radial nerve paralysis was made and the hand placed in a cock-up splint. Massage was done daily. Improvement was rapid, and after ten days the splint was discarded. Recovery was complete in two weeks, and no abnormality was noted after that time. At present, at the age of two years, the child is well and normal in every respect.

From the Department of Pediatrics, University of Illinois College of Medicine.

COMMENT

Trauma is considered the essential causative factor in the production of isolated peripheral radial nerve palsy. The radial nerve is most exposed to injury at the lateral surface of the lower one-third of the arm. Compression does occur here at times since hematomas are described at this point in several case reports. Ottow[5] observed a case in which a hematoma was present without radial nerve paralysis. Langen[3] has interpreted these hematoma-like swellings and pressure grooves which occur occasionally in these paralyses of the newborn as due to amniotic bands which are subsequently absorbed. Ottow, however, thinks that the grooves are more likely due to pressure by the umbilical cord and the hematoma-like swellings to compression by the pelvis, since amniotic bands appear very early in gestation and result in more severe deformities and malformations. In our case the absence of involvement of the triceps indicates that the radial nerve was affected below the axilla. The absence of muscular atrophy and the rapid recovery would argue against constriction of the arm by amniotic bands and would indicate pressure recently applied as a more likely etiologic factor. Absence of pressure marks would not necessarily militate against pressure as a possible cause, since none were noted in several reported cases due to compression.[2, 5, 6, 7, 8] In our case arrest of the head at the resistant pelvic floor occurred for about one hour after satisfactory progress. Ottow explains the mechanism of paralysis as due to the compression of the humeri between the promontory and the symphysis at the level of the entrance to the true pelvis, when the head is arrested by the resistant pelvic floor. That compression of both humeri takes place seems likely since Smith's recently reported case and one of Ottow's showed bilateral radial nerve paralysis. Krafft[9] stresses uterine wall pressure and reports a case associated with subcutaneous adiponecrosis reaching to the lateral aspect of the lower third of the forearm (radial point).

Another factor which has hitherto escaped attention and may be of importance is the rôle of maternal medication in the production of this condition. In our case castor oil, pituitrin, quinine, and sodium pentobarbital were administered. The first two may readily be excluded as possible etiologic agents. Quinine and barbiturates, however, may be suspected. No reports could be found in the literature where either of these drugs taken orally by the mother produced peripheral neuritis in the fetus, except perhaps Taylor's case[10] of deafness of the newborn in which the inner ear was involved because of quinine. Nevertheless, cases are recorded in which the intramuscular injections of quinine and urea[11] and barbituric acid derivatives[12] in the upper arm caused radial nerve paralysis. In his explanation, von Uhlenbruck considers a generalized intoxication with localization of the drug in the radial nerve. From this standpoint our case might possibly be included in the group of Saturday night palsies in which pressure on the arm in addition to an intoxication (alcoholic) causes the paralysis. In only one other of the twenty-nine cases reported, however, was quinine given to the mother. Barbiturates were not given in any of these. In some ten cases of the group, fractures of the humerus were associated with the nerve paralysis.

SUMMARY

1. A case of isolated peripheral radial nerve palsy in the newborn is reported.

2. Compression of the upper arm by the pelvis appears to be the major causative factor in these cases.

3. In our case it is possible that fetal intoxication from a barbiturate and quinine was a contributory causative factor.

REFERENCES

1. Smith, L. Howard: Am. J. Dis. Child. **11**: 333, 1916.
2. Idem: Am. J. Obst. & Gynec. **30**: 283, 1935.
3. Langen, P.: Arch. f. Gynäk. **139**: 560, 1930.
4. Kehrer, Erwin: Die Armlähmungen bei Neugeborenen. Suppl. to Ztschr. f. Geburtsh. u. Gynäk. **107**: 1934.
5. Ottow, B.: Zentralbl. f. Gynäk. **56**: 2714, 1932.
6. De Tone, G. (Cited by Langen): Arch. de méd. d. enf. **30**: 406, 1927.
7. Petersen, E.: Gynéc. et Obstét. **12**: 68, 1925.
8. Hasslinger, J.: (Abst.) Zentralbl. f. Gynäk. **23**: 3173, 1899.
9. Krafft, H.: Zentralbl. f. Gynäk. **59**: 2773, 1935.
10. Taylor, A. M.: South. M. J. **28**: 125, 1935.
11. Babcock, W.: Surg. Clin. North America **8**: 813, 1928.
12. Von Uhlenbruck, P.: München. med. Wchnschr. **78**: 1256, 1931.

3201 West Sixty-Third Street
185 North Wabash Avenue

INTESTINAL OBSTRUCTION DUE TO MECONIUM ILEUS IN A NEWBORN INFANT

Case Report

Katharine Dodd, M.D.
Nashville, Tenn.

INTESTINAL obstruction due to stenosis and atresia of various parts of the gut or to constricting bands is not uncommon in newborn infants. From time to time there have appeared in the literature reports of obstruction due apparently to no tumor or congenital malformation of the gastrointestinal tract but to an accumulation of mucilaginous meconium in the tract itself. The term "meconium ileus" has been adopted by most writers to describe this condition. Even in the more complete textbooks of pediatrics there is usually no mention of such a condition. Pfaundler and Schlossman refer to it briefly in their 1935 English edition, quoting a case report from the literature. Finkelstein in his German textbook of diseases of infants says, "Sometimes with the first portion of meconium a gelatinous gray or yellow mucoid mass is passed, 'the meconium plug.' In occasional cases symptoms of intestinal obstruction are caused by mucous plugs rather than malformation; sausage-like, gelatinous or hard masses which consist of mucus, epithelial cells, calcium concretions and sometimes fibrin. They are perhaps related to meconium plugs or may be an evidence of membranous enteritis."

As this form of obstruction is apparently rare, the diagnosis usually difficult and the cause obscure, it seems of interest to report the following case:

Baby C. was born on the outside obstetric service of the Vanderbilt Hospital on Sept. 5, 1934. The child was the result of a full-term normal pregnancy and was born after a normal labor. The mother's blood Wassermann was negative. From birth he refused to take fluids well and vomited what he did take. On the second day after birth it was noticed that he was becoming dehydrated. He was admitted to the hospital the next day, Sept. 7, 1934. He was said to have had one small meconium stool. Nothing abnormal was noted on admission, except marked dehydration. The baby weighed 6 pounds and 10 ounces. The temperature was normal. The hemoglobin was 21 grams; the urine, normal. The Wassermann test was negative. No obstruction was met on rectal examination, but, when the finger was removed from the anus, it was found covered with a thick, dark, gelatinous material which did not resemble ordinary meconium. The child was given subcutaneous saline and placed on a formula of diluted whole milk with sugar. He nursed badly and continued to vomit everything taken. The stools were large grayish green to yellow and resembled

From the Department of Pediatrics, Vanderbilt University Medical School.

thick gelatin. The abdomen became markedly distended. A diagnosis of congenital atresia of some part of the intestine was considered, but the passage of such large amounts of material by rectum seemed to make the diagnosis unlikely. As the vomiting and distention increased steadily, it was decided to institute duodenal suction, with attempts at feeding through the duodenal tube later if the vomiting ceased. Meanwhile parenteral fluids were continued. The child's condition improved temporarily, but the vomiting and distention recurred when feeding was started. On the third day after admission the temperature rose sharply; the respirations became rapid; and signs of bronchial pneumonia developed. Ten days after admission the child died.

At postmortem examination the stomach and small intestines were distended and the colon relatively contracted. There was no evidence of volvulus, constricting bands or other external obstruction to the intestine. On examination of the interior of the gastrointestinal tract nothing abnormal was found until the ileum was

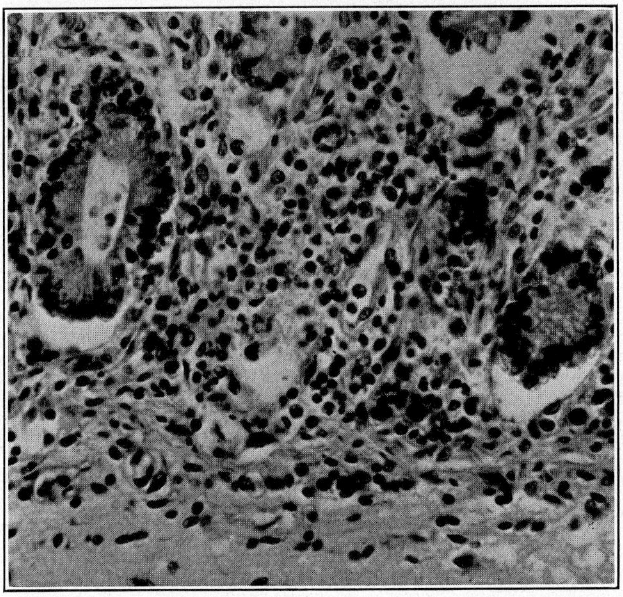

Fig. 1.—Section from ileum showing focus of inflammation in base of mucosa. Note inflammatory cells invading intestinal gland at left. The exudate is composed principally of mononuclear cells; however, a few polymorphonuclear leucocytes are present. (×550.)

reached. Here the intestinal lumen was filled with tenacious, gray mucoid material similar to the material found in the stools during life. When this was removed, the mucosa appeared normal and free from congestion, hemorrhage or ulcers. No obstruction was found in the intestine. The colon was filled with the same tenacious, gray mucoid material. It was described as being of the consistency of stiff jelly and seemed to contain little true fecal matter. The liver appeared normal, and bile was easily expressed from the gallbladder into the duodenum. The spleen was not enlarged. The only abnormality grossly was a small amount of yellow exudate along the notched border. All the organs were normal except the lungs. Here a moderate amount of bronchopneumonia was found. The bones showed no evidence of congenital syphilis.

When microscopic sections of the organs were made, most of the tissues were found to be normal. There was a slight inflammatory reaction of the small intestine with an increased number of mononuclear cells in the mucosa and even below the muscularis mucosa in the submucosa. A few polymorphonuclear leucocytes were present in the mucosa and submucosa of the duodenum. There was no necrosis or ulceration of the intestine. The muscularis was prominent but not hypertrophied. The serosa was normal. There was partial desquamation of the epithelium of the mucosa. The goblet cells showed no evidence of hypersecretion. A microscopic section of intestine is shown in Fig. 1. A small area of bronchopneumonia was found in the lungs. The liver was normal on microscopic section.

The only organ showing marked changes was the pancreas. Here there was an interstitial pancreatitis characterized by increased fibrosis and a slight degree of inflammation. The fibrosis was marked and was both interlobular and intralobular in distribution. The inflammation was composed principally of mononuclear cells,

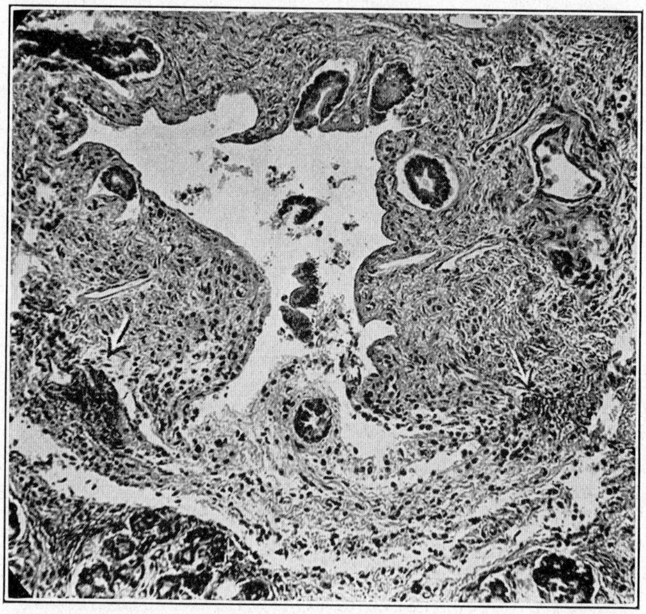

Fig. 2.—Section showing slightly dilated pancreatic duct with desquamation of epithelium and acute inflammation of the wall. Arrows point to fibrinous exudate. (×190.)

lymphocytes, and large mononuclear phagocytes; however, occasional polymorphonuclear leucocytes were present. The inflammation was most prominent in the walls of the ducts and the surrounding fibrinous tissue. There were hemorrhage and fibrin with many polymorphonuclear leucocytes in the wall of two or three of the ducts. A striking feature was the dilatation of the ducts and some of the acini. Many of the ducts and the acini contained a loose pink finely granular precipitate, while some were empty. A few had desquamated epithelium. In no instance was there demonstrable occlusion of the ducts. The islands of Langerhans were normal, and the acini were normal except for dilatation. Microscopic sections of the pancreas are shown in Figs. 2 and 3. From the appearance of the pancreas it seems possible that there may have been a stenosis of the main pancreatic duct. This possibility was not thought of at the time of the postmortem examination, and the sections of the pancreas which were preserved did not permit of settling this point.

In a review of the literature twenty-one reported instances of an apparently similar condition were found. In five cases[1-5] the child after showing symptoms of intestinal obstruction for several days passed one or more large plugs of puttylike meconium and then was well. In the majority of the other cases[6-19] the child had no bowel movements, and the condition was thought to be a congenital developmental obstruction of the gastrointestinal tract. The true cause, obstruction due to thickened intestinal contents, was first revealed either at operation or at postmortem examination. The gastrointestinal tract was always patent, and no external causes of obstruction were found. In most cases the intestine was enormously dilated above the

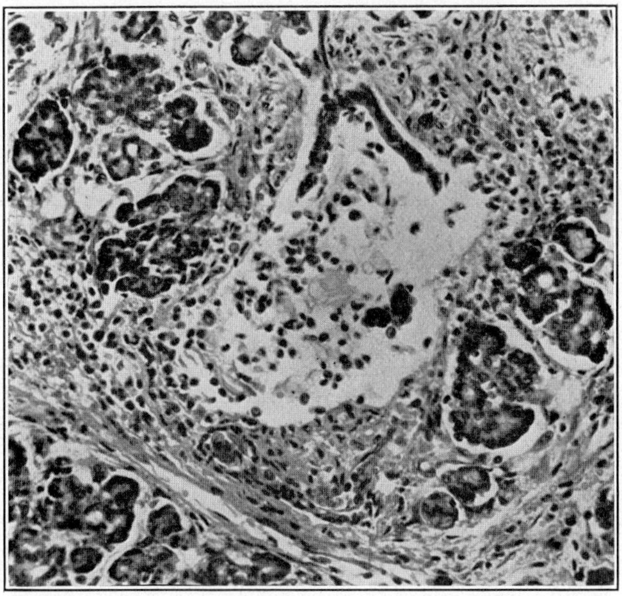

Fig. 3.—Section of dilated pancreatic duct and surrounding acinic tissue. Note the desquamated epithelium and acute inflammation in the duct wall and adjacent tissue.

obstruction, which was usually in the ileum, and was completely collapsed below. In several cases the intestinal musculature was hypertrophied at the point of obstruction. In a few cases there had been rupture of the intestines, and fluid was found in the peritoneum. Many different terms were used to describe the intestinal contents, but the favorite one was that they were of the consistency of thick putty. In the majority of instances only the peritoneal cavity and the gastrointestinal tract were examined, or if other organs were examined only a description of the gross appearance was given. Various theories were then advanced as to the cause of the gummy, puttylike meconium. The favorite theory was that the intestinal contents were thickened because of lack of secretion or too late secretion of bile or pancreatic juice, or perhaps of the glands of the gastrointestinal tract itself.

In five cases in which the other organs were examined, an abnormality of either the liver or the pancreas was found. Kornblitt, Borris, and Otani[7] describe a typical case in a four-day-old child. No meconium had passed from birth. Vomiting and distention appeared on the third day. At operation the child had gas in the peritoneal cavity. There were markedly distended loops of small intestine covered with a pasty brown material. The operation was discontinued because of the poor condition of the child. Death occurred the next day. At postmortem examination a diagnosis of meconium ileus with perforation and generalized meconium peritonitis was made. Microscopic sections of the pancreas showed findings very similar to those reported in the present case. There was a marked increase in the stroma of the pancreas; the acini were atrophic; and in many areas replaced by connective tissue. The main pancreatic duct was extremely widened, and the dilatation of the ducts extended even into the terminal portions involving the acini with the result that the acinic cells were flattened, occasionally resembling small ducts. A small amount of lymphocytic infiltration was the only evidence of reaction about the ducts. Serial sections were made through the head of the pancreas, and the main pancreatic duct was found to be stenotic. It was suggested that the changes in the pancreas corresponded almost exactly to those brought about experimentally after ligation of the pancreatic duct, and that absence of pancreatic juice had caused inspissation of meconium with subsequent intestinal obstruction. Landsteiner[12] describes an almost exactly similar case with operation and death. Here again on postmortem examination marked changes were found in the pancreas. There were an increase in the interlobular and intralobular connective tissue and an infiltration of this tissue with round cells. The ducts were markedly dilated, and the acini and the islands of Langerhans, normal. The pancreatic duct near its lumen was tortuous and folded and without contents. Further on in the pancreas it was wider and filled with exfoliated, mostly unstained, epithelial cells. Landsteiner believes that it was lack of pancreatic secretion that caused the thickening of the meconium. At the end of his article he mentions another case of obstruction due to thickened meconium. The pancreas was normal, but there was no secretion of bile. He says that it looks, therefore, as if both bile and pancreatic juice might be necessary for the formation of meconium of normal consistency. Fanconi[13] also reported a case in which the pancreas was normal. There was bile in the gastrointestinal tract, and yet the liver showed the typical picture of jaundice due to obstruction. The liver cells were bile stained, and the smallest capillary bile ducts were plugged with bile. There is one more case with a cystic liver described by von Meyenburg,[16] in which the meconium was said to be of a puttylike consistency.

Lesions in the pancreas in infants without symptoms of meconium ileus are not uncommon. In cases in which we have seen interstitial pancreatitis in infants dying from other causes, the lesion was, however, not as severe as it was in our case of meconium ileus. Lack of biliary secretion is also not rare without symptoms of intestinal obstruction. In few of such children seen after the neonatal period is the character of the first stools known.

In the six cases of meconium ileus, including our case, in which complete postmortem examination was done, abnormalities were found in either the liver or the pancreas in every case. It seems probable, therefore, that failure of pancreatic secretion or bile to reach the gastrointestinal tract during fetal and neonatal life is at least part of the cause of meconium ileus.

REFERENCES

1. Ullman: Deutsche med. Wchnschr. **20:** 37, 1894.
2. Longuet: Quoted by Ullman.[1]
3. Soldin, Max: Jahrb. f. Kinderh. **77:** 453, 1913.
4. Berti: Quoted in Centralbl. f. inn. Med. **19:** 276, 1898.
5. Frick, P.: Indian J. Pediat. **1:** 223, 1934.
6. Monnier: Schweiz. med. Wchnschr. **65:** 94, 1935.
7. Kornblith, Borris A., and Otani, Sadao: Am. J. Path. **5:** 249, 1929.
8. Bullowa, J. G. M., and Brennan, R. E.: J. A. M. A. **73:** 1882, 1919.
9. Hughes, E. E.: Brit. J. Child. Dis. **19:** 32, 1922.
10. Torkel, K.: Deutsche med. Wchnschr. **31:** 344, 1905.
11. Rothman: Discussion of Torkel's paper.[10]
12. Landsteiner, K.: Centralbl. f. allg. Path. u. path. Anat. **16:** 903, 1905.
13. Fanconi, Guido: Virchows Arch. f. path. Anat. **229:** 207, 1920.
14. Gidionsen: Inaug. Diss., Freiburg, 1898, quoted by Fanconi.[13]
15. Farrer: Inaug. Diss., Straussburg, 1895, quoted by Fanconi.[13]
16. Von Meyenburg: Habilitationsschrift, Zurich, 1918, quoted by Fanconi.[13]
17. Trumpp: Jahrb. f. Kinderh. **76:** 678, 1912.
18. Exalto: Deutsche Ztschr. f. Chir. **189:** 52, 1924-25.
19. Boikan, W. S.: Arch. Path. **9:** 1164, 1930.

A COMPARATIVE STUDY OF AGGLUTININ RESPONSE AFTER PERTUSSIS VACCINATION WITH THE SAUER VACCINE AND WITH A TOXIN VACCINE AND IN UNTREATED CLINICAL PERTUSSIS

LUCY MISHULOW
ASSISTED BY ISABELLE MOWRY AND RUTH ORANGE
NEW YORK, N. Y.

PERTUSSIS vaccination has been the subject of study for many years, but until fairly recently the results reported by various investigators differed so widely that it was hard to judge whether pertussis vaccine was of any value. Recent reports, however, have been rather encouraging. Madsen[1] found in a carefully controlled investigation on the Faroe Islands that there were a definite reduction in incidence and a marked decrease in mortality due to pertussis among the vaccinated children as compared with the unvaccinated controls. Sauer[2] reported very favorable results when he used large doses of pertussis vaccine.

There is at present, however, considerable difference of opinion as to the optimum method of preparing pertussis vaccines and the total dosage that is to be used. The dosage formerly employed was comparatively small, seldom exceeding 10 to 15 billion bacteria. Madsen found that a total of 22 to 30 billion bacteria gave very favorable results. Sauer has tripled this dose. He recommends a dosage of 80 to 90 billion, which is by far the largest ever employed.

The chief points of controversy with regard to the preparation of pertussis vaccines are: (1) whether stock cultures of pertussis are as antigenic as freshly isolated cultures; (2) whether the Bordet-Gengou medium is the only medium suitable for maintaining pertussis cultures and for the preparation of the vaccine; (3) whether human, goat, or sheep blood should be used to enrich the medium.[3]

In considering the above points it is well to bear in mind that the antigenicity of bacteria depends to a large extent upon the conditions under which they are maintained in the laboratory. Some cultures alter rapidly, whereas others retain their original characteristics for a period of years when they are kept under optimum conditions. In preparing typhoid and paratyphoid vaccines, for instance, stock strains of proved antigenicity may be kept for many years, whereas newly isolated strains may be entirely unsuitable.[4] Stock diphtheria bacilli of proved toxigenicity, such as P.W. No. 8, are used for pre-

From the Research Laboratories, New York City Department of Health, Director of Bureau of Laboratories, Dr. William H. Park.

paring toxins in preference to newly isolated virulent cultures. Other examples may be given to show that the date of isolation of a culture is by far less important than the condition of the culture at the time that it is used in preparing the vaccine.

With regard to pertussis bacilli, Leslie and Gardner[5] found that the bacilli could be divided into four groups on the basis of their virulence for guinea pigs and the differences in their serologic characteristics; the authors considered these groups as phases of the same type. They found that freshly isolated cultures were virulent for guinea pigs and they placed these in Phase I. Stock cultures that were nonvirulent were placed into Phases III and IV, and a small group of stock bacilli that were slightly virulent, they designated as Phase II. All of the above phases differed serologically. They succeeded in changing pertussis cultures of Phase I to Phases III and IV by special methods of cultivation; thus showing that cultures in Phases III and IV are degeneration stages of Phase I. These changes, however, were slow to appear, and it required special methods of cultivation to induce them. In one instance it took twenty-five months to change Phase I to Phase IV; and that only after the culture was grown on mediums that were not optimal for pertussis bacilli, and by fishing out certain individual colonies. In other instances the change of phase was induced by growing the culture on an Antiphase I Serum and again selecting individual colonies. These artificially induced changes are not comparable to the changes that take place under ordinary conditions in the laboratory. Toomey, Ranta, and Takacs[6] found that pertussis bacilli retain their virulence and antigenicity for a long time when the cultures are maintained on blood medium. Similarly Shibley and Hoelscher[7] found that stock cultures maintain their "S" or virulent form for a period of years when they are maintained on a suitable medium. We found in a study extending over a period of years that pertussis bacilli retain their original morphologic, cultural, and serologic characteristics for a long time (in some instances for a number of years) when the cultures are maintained on an infusion medium that has 25 to 30 per cent of normal blood and that the percentage of blood in the medium determines the loss or retention of its original characteristics. When the amount of blood is decreased below 20 per cent, or when the organisms are grown on blood-free mediums, the growth becomes atypical; the ability to lyze blood is decreased or entirely lost; and the cultures agglutinate poorly in specific serum. On the other hand, cultures that are maintained on Bordet-Gengou medium, or infusion agar plus 25 to 30 per cent of normal animal blood, are characteristically coccoid in form, produce hemolysis on both the above mediums and are agglutinated by specific serums. It therefore appears that pertussis cultures can be maintained in stock without loss of their original characteristics if they are grown under suitable conditions, and there seems to be no adequate reason for discarding them in favor of newly isolated strains.

The question of the kind of blood that should be incorporated in the medium for growing the cultures should be considered first for its growth-accessory substances and second for the possibility of sensitizing the vaccinated children to the corresponding serum if there should be any need subsequently to use a therapeutic serum.

As far as the growth-accessory substances are concerned, there is no evidence at present that human blood has better growth-promoting substances than animal blood. On the other hand, adult human blood may contain antipertussis antibodies which may cause dissociation and possibly alteration in type, and for that reason it may be undesirable to use human blood.

The possible sensitization to subsequent use of therapeutic serums through the injection of vaccines that are grown on horse's or sheep's blood has probably been the main reason for advocating the use of human blood. In view of the work of Mackenzie,[8] however, there seems to be little danger of sensitizing by the minute amount of serum that may be present in vaccines that are grown on solid blood mediums. Mackenzie found that it was necessary to give a minimum of 100 c.c. of undiluted horse serum to sensitize humans to horse serum and also to some extent to sheep, rabbit, and chicken serums. But the degree of sensitization to the heterologous was very much less than to the homologous serum. In calculating the maximum amount of sheep serum that may be present in pertussis vaccines that are prepared by our method, we find that they contain approximately 0.00041 c.c. of sheep serum per cubic centimeter of vaccine or 0.00328 c.c. of serum in the total dose of 8 c.c. of vaccine, which is the dosage recommended by Sauer. It therefore seems most unlikely that there is any danger of sensitizing to either horse or sheep serum by the minute amount of serum that is present in the vaccine.

Because of the differences of opinion with regard to optimum dosage and methods of preparing the vaccine, we began an investigation about three years ago to determine, if possible, the following points:

1. The comparative antigenicity of vaccines prepared of newly isolated cultures and of stock cultures.

2. The optimum dosage and the optimum intervals between injections for antibody stimulation. The intervals used by different investigators at present vary from two to seven days.

3. A comparative study of agglutinin response after intracutaneous, intramuscular, and subcutaneous vaccination. Tuft, Yagle, and Rogers[9] found in a study of different methods of antityphoid vaccination that small intracutaneous doses of vaccine stimulated agglutinins to the

same or slightly higher degree than much larger subcutaneous doses. We were able to confirm their results with regard to antityphoid vaccinations,[10] and it occurred to us that the intracutaneous method may prove equally satisfactory in pertussis vaccination.

The clinical tests to determine the above points were carried out by Dr. T. E. Waldie, of the New York Foundling Hospital, and it was through his cooperation that we were able to obtain bleedings from the vaccinated children as well as from corresponding unvaccinated controls. We hoped that by studying the agglutinin response after vaccination we may get some information as to the adequacy of the dosage employed, the comparative value of the intramuscular and the intracutaneous methods of injection, and the antigenicity of vaccines that were made of freshly isolated and of stock cultures. Although the presence of agglutinins may not be a direct index of immunity it might help to evaluate the immediate response to vaccination.

We have also studied agglutinin response in clinical pertussis in order to see whether there was any similarity between the time of appearance, the height of the titer attained, and the length of time that agglutinins persist after infection and after vaccination. With these problems in mind we carried through the following experiments:

EXPERIMENT 1: AGGLUTININ RESPONSE AFTER INTRAMUSCULAR AND INTRACUTANEOUS VACCINATION WITH PERTUSSIS TOXIN VACCINE GIVEN AT TWO- AND SEVEN-DAY INTERVALS

This experiment was in the nature of a preliminary test. The vaccine employed in this test was prepared in such a manner that it contained a toxic substance in addition to the pertussis bacilli. We found in a previous investigation[11] that pertussis bacilli are capable of producing a toxic substance and that vaccines containing this toxic substance stimulate agglutinins to a greater degree than those which lack this substance. We therefore prepared our vaccines in such a manner that they contained this toxic substance in addition to the pertussis bacilli. The toxin vaccine was prepared as follows:

Preparation of Pertussis Toxin Vaccines.—Stock cultures were maintained on beef infusion agar, pH 7.2 to 7.4, to which 30 per cent blood was added. Before the vaccine was prepared the cultures were plated on infusion blood agar and on Bordet-Gengou medium, and each culture was examined for characteristic morphology, for hemolysis, and from time to time for agglutination with specific serum. Only those cultures were used in the vaccine that were characteristic morphologically, culturally, and serologically.

Preliminary transplants were made on 1-inch tubes of sheep blood –beef heart agar and incubated for forty-eight hours at 37° C. The growth from each tube was emulsified in 12 c.c. of 1 per cent sheep serum–beef heart broth of pH 7.2 to 7.4, and 4 c.c. of this broth suspension was inoculated on 30 per cent sheep blood–beef heart agar in Blake bottles. The bottles were incubated for twenty-four hours at 37° C. and were then tilted back and forth to cover the entire surface of the bottle with the liquid inoculum. After an additional twenty-four hours' incubation the growth was washed off with 10 to 15 c.c. of sterile physiologic saline which contained 1 per cent phenol. The vaccine was tested for purity by inoculating blood agar with a sample of the vaccine, and the vaccine was then incubated at 37° C. for twenty-four hours, which is usually sufficient to sterilize it. It was tested for sterility and stored in the ice box at 8 to 10° C. The vaccine was standardized by Wright's method and diluted to contain 10,000 million bacteria per cubic centimeter, also the phenol content was diluted to 0.5 per cent. Each lot of vaccine was tested for the toxic substance, by Shwartzman's method[12] as follows:

A portion of the vaccine was centrifuged to sediment the bacteria, and the supernatant fluid was passed through a W Berkefeld filter. The bacteria-free filtrate was used for the test. Rabbits were given an intracutaneous injection of 0.25 c.c. of the filtrate, and from eighteen to twenty-four hours later they were given an intravenous injection of the filtrate using 1.0 to 1.5 c.c. per kilogram weight of the rabbit. An inflammatory reaction appeared at the point of intracutaneous injection in about four to eight hours after the intravenous injection; this reaction deepened in color until it was dark purple. Some of the rabbits died within one-half hour to three hours after the intravenous injection when the filtrate was very toxic. There was, however, a fairly large percentage of rabbits that were not susceptible to this toxin, and therefore three or four rabbits were used in each test. Either the skin reaction or death was taken as an index of toxicity.

The agglutination studies were carried out as follows:

A group of 190 children was subdivided into eight groups. The children in Group 1 were given intramuscular injections at two-day intervals, and in Group 2 at seven-day intervals. The total dosage in this group was 39 billion bacteria. The third and fourth groups were given a total of 8.5 billion bacteria intracutaneously at two- and seven-day intervals, respectively. Groups 5, 6, 7, and 8 were injected with corresponding amounts of sterile milk instead of vaccine. The milk was diluted to the same opacity as the vaccine, and the injections were given in the same way as the vaccine. So that for each group of children that received the vaccine, there was a corresponding group of controls who received milk.

Bleedings were obtained from the children before the injections and at intervals beginning one week after the last injection was given.

Each case was designated by a number so that the person who read the test did not know whether it was a vaccinated or a control child. The same person made all the readings of the test in order to eliminate individual variations.

The agglutination antigen used in these tests was a suspension of the bacteria in physiologic saline containing 0.1 per cent formalin. This suspension was diluted to the desired concentration and standardized with a known pertussis serum. A control of the antigen with this serum was used in every test in order to control the sensitivity of the antigen. Every new antigen that was prepared was standardized in this manner.

The serums were diluted with saline beginning with a 1:5 dilution and doubling each succeeding dilution. Then equal amounts of serum dilution and antigen were mixed in small tubes and incubated at 55° C. overnight. The titer of the serum was determined by taking the highest dilution of the serum that showed definite clumps.

With very few exceptions the normal preinjection bleedings were either negative or agglutinated in a low titer, usually below a 1:20 dilution of the serum. In two instances the normal bleedings showed a titer of 1:60 and 1:80, respectively, but on investigation it was found that one of these children was recently transferred from the Misericordia Hospital and that he had just recovered from pertussis and that the other was intimately exposed to pertussis and may have had an abortive attack. Both of these children were excluded when the results were charted.

In charting our results we considered agglutination not above 1:20 as within the normal range and 1:20 or above as positive. The results of the first experiment are given in Table I.

TABLE I

AGGLUTININ RESPONSE AFTER INTRAMUSCULAR INJECTIONS OF PERTUSSIS TOXIN VACCINE AND OF STERILE MILK

VACCINE	METHOD OF INJECTION	INTERVAL BETWEEN INJECTIONS	TOTAL PERTUSSIS BACTERIA	NUMBER OF CASES	AGGLUTININ INCREASE*	PER CENT POSITIVE
Toxin vaccine, 10 billion per c.c.	Intramuscular	2 days	39.0 bil.	23	8 cases	34.7
		7 days	39.0 bil.	19	2 cases	10.5
	Intracutaneous	2 days	8.5 bil.	25	9 cases	36.0
		7 days	8.5 bil.	25	2 cases	8.0
Control, sterile milk	Intramuscular	2 days	0	28	5 cases	17.8
		7 days	0	24	5 cases	20.8
	Intracutaneous	2 days	0	20	0 cases	0
		7 days	0	26	2 cases	7.6

*Agglutination titer varied between 1:20 and 1:960—average 1:70.
Total vaccinated, 92.
Total controls, 98.

The agglutination response in this test was rather low. Most of the children showed no increase in agglutinins above the normal range. But of those that did show some increase, the response was better in the two-day than in the seven-day interval group and was somewhat better in the intracutaneously vaccinated group than in the intramuscular, although the total dosage given intracutaneously was one-fourth of the intramuscular dose.

The results in the control group were somewhat disconcerting. As shown in Table I there was an increase of agglutinins in some of the children who were injected with milk instead of vaccine—17 per cent and 20 per cent, respectively, in the two- and the seven-day intramuscularly injected children, and 7 per cent in the seven-day interval intracutaneously injected children. None of the children in the two-day interval intracutaneously injected group showed any increase in agglutinins. It seems difficult to explain why milk should stimulate agglutinins for pertussis, except on the basis of nonspecific stimulation of latent agglutinins due to a possible previous infection, as some of these children must have had ample opportunity of exposure before they were brought to the hospital.

From the results obtained in this test, it would seem that intracutaneous injections at short intervals might be the method of choice. However, since the groups studied in this experiment were rather small, no definite conclusions can be drawn at this time until further comparative tests are made.

EXPERIMENT 2: AGGLUTININ RESPONSE AFTER VACCINATION WITH LARGE DOSES OF PERTUSSIS VACCINES MADE OF NEWLY ISOLATED AND OF STOCK CULTURES

This experiment was planned to determine whether large doses of vaccine would give a corresponding increase in agglutinins, also to compare the antigenicity of vaccines made of stock cultures that have retained their original morphologic, cultural, and serologic characteristics and of freshly isolated cultures. A group of 60 children was used in this test. These children were divided into two groups. One group of 30 children was given a vaccine prepared according to Sauer's method, i.e., newly isolated cultures grown on human blood–Bordet-Gengou medium*; and a similar group was given our toxin vaccine which was made of stock cultures that have retained their original characteristics. The cultures used in our vaccine were grown on sheep blood infusion agar, and the vaccine contained a toxic substance in addition to the bacteria. The concentration of bacteria was the same in both vaccines—10 billion bacteria per cubic centimeter. The injections were made intramuscularly at seven-day intervals giving 1, 1.5,

*This vaccine was obtained through the courtesy of Dr. Sauer from Eli Lilly & Co.

and 1.5 c.c. into each arm, a total of 80 billion bacteria. This method was chosen in order to make the test comparable with the method employed by Sauer.

Bleedings were taken from the children before the vaccines were injected and again one, two, three, and four weeks after the last injection of the vaccine. These bleedings were tested in the same manner as in the first experiment. Due to various unforeseen conditions, the immunization was not completed in eight children of the Sauer vaccine group, and in 5 of our vaccine group; they were therefore excluded when the results were charted. This left a group of 22 chil-

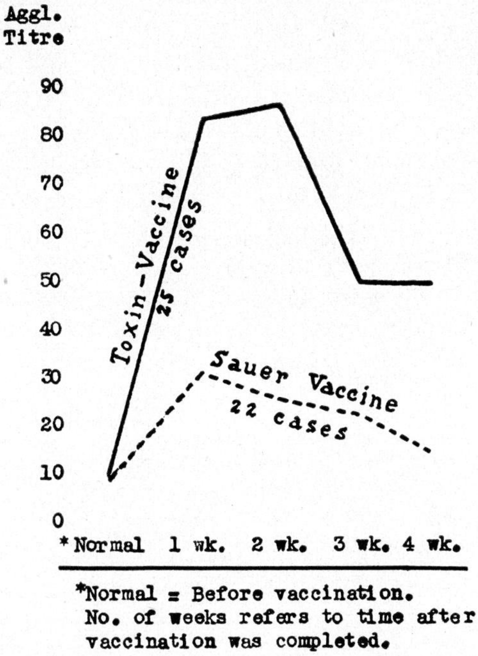

Chart I.—Average agglutinin titers of children injected prophylactically with 80 billion bacteria of the Sauer and of the toxin vaccine.

dren who received 80 billion bacteria of the Sauer vaccine and 25 children who received a similar dose of our toxin vaccine.

The agglutinin response in both these groups was very much better than in those who received a much smaller dosage as shown in Experiment 1 although there were still a considerable number of children among them who showed no increase in agglutinins.

In the Sauer vaccine group of 22 children, 12, or 55 per cent, showed an increase of agglutinins, and 10 remained within the normal range. In the group of 25 children who received our toxin vaccine, 21, or 84 per cent, showed an increase, and 4 remained in the normal range.

There was considerable variation in the individual agglutinin titers in both groups. In charting the results we used the average response of the group as a whole, including those that showed no increase in agglutinins. The results are given in Chart I.

As shown in this chart, the average agglutinin response of the toxin vaccine group was very much higher than that of the Sauer vaccine group. This may have been due to the additional stimulation of the toxic substance in the vaccine and confirms our previous findings in rabbits.[11]

The maximum titer in both groups was attained between one and two weeks after the last injection of the vaccine, and then it dropped rapidly although it was still above normal at the end of four weeks. We did not make any examinations later than four weeks and, therefore, do not know how long they remained above normal. This corresponds with the results obtained by Kristensen and Ahrend Larsen[13] in complement fixation studies of vaccinated children. They found that the highest complement fixation titers were obtained in the first two weeks and that they decreased rapidly after that.

From the results obtained in this experiment two things stand out clearly: (1) That the agglutinin response to vaccination was largely proportional to the dosage employed. In cases in which the dose did not exceed 8.5 billions given intracutaneously or 39 billions given intramuscularly (Experiment 1) only a small percentage of the children showed an increase in agglutinins. When the dose was 80 billion bacteria, 55 to 84 per cent of the children had an increase of agglutinins. (2) That a vaccine prepared of stock cultures compared very favorably with the one prepared of newly isolated cultures in that it stimulated agglutinins to a higher degree.

EXPERIMENT 3: A STUDY OF AGGLUTININS IN UNTREATED PERTUSSIS CASES AND IN NONPERTUSSIS RESPIRATORY INFECTIONS

Our next problem was to study agglutinins in pertussis cases in order to determine whether there is any similarity between the time of appearance, the height of the titer attained, and the length of time that agglutinins persist after infection and after vaccination. Through the courtesy of Dr. I. Herbert Scheffer, of the Willard Parker Hospital, we were able to obtain sequent bleedings from 65 definite and suspected pertussis cases, and also from 12 patients with nonpertussis respiratory infections. The bleedings were taken as soon as the patients were admitted to the hospital, and in most cases weekly bleedings were obtained until early convalescence. The bleedings were tested for agglutinins in the same manner and with the same antigens as in the previous experiments.

There was a marked variation in the agglutinin titers of the individual pertussis cases which apparently did not correspond to the severity of the infection. In 9 cases there was no increase above the normal range; in 8 cases it was approximately the same as in the vaccinated; and in 40 cases it was high. In every case in which there was an increase in agglutinins, they increased rather rapidly until the maximum was reached and after that there was a more or less rapid decrease.

Chart II shows the highest and lowest titers that were obtained in individual cases of clinical pertussis, and these are compared with those of the children who were vaccinated with the Sauer vaccine, and with

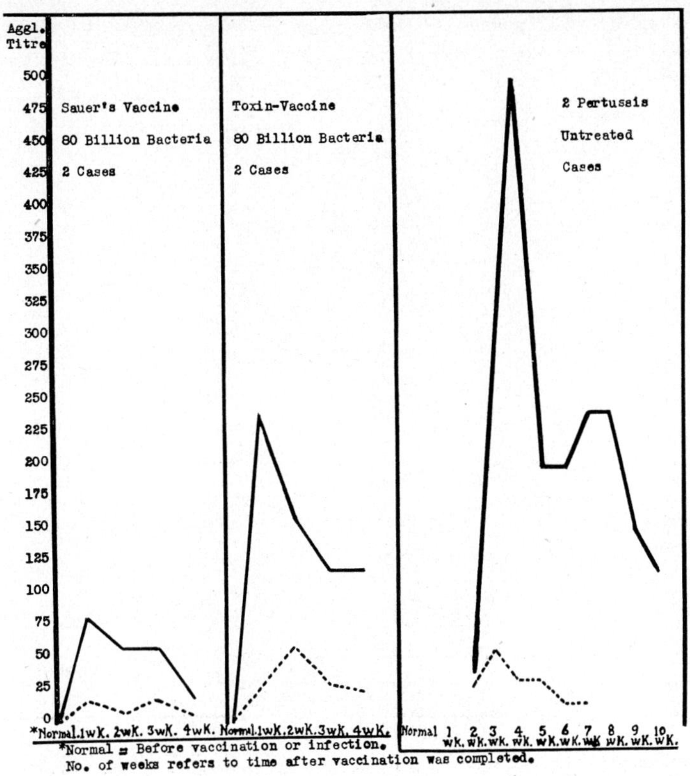

Chart II.—The highest and lowest agglutinin responses that were obtained in the groups of children who were injected with the Sauer vaccine and with toxin vaccine and in the untreated cases of pertussis.

the toxin vaccine. In none of the vaccinated children did the agglutinin titer attain the height of the infected children. Among the vaccinated children, however, the highest titer was obtained in the group that received the toxin vaccine.

In Chart III are summarized the results obtained in Experiments 2 and 3. The average agglutinin response in the group of 65 pertussis cases is compared with those of the normal children who were vaccinated with the Sauer and the toxin vaccines. The initial time given in the graph of the pertussis cases is only approximate, as we had to rely on the histories in each case, and they were dated from the time symptoms were first noted.

The average agglutinin titer in the pertussis cases differs markedly from that of the vaccinated children in the length of time at which the maximum was obtained and in the height of its curve, but it resembles it, in that having reached the maximum, it dropped very rapidly. Dr. Scheffer[14] observed that in most of the pertussis cases in this group there was a marked clinical improvement at about the time that the maximum agglutination titer was obtained. It appears therefore that agglutinins decreased almost as soon as active infection stopped and convalescence began. This corresponds closely to the decrease in

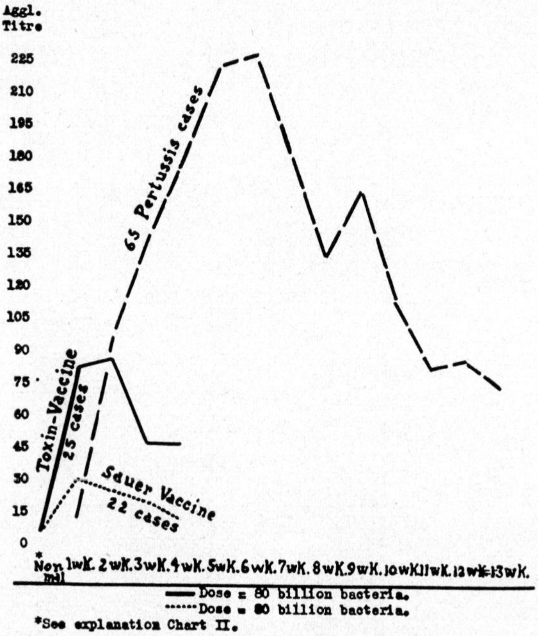

Chart III.—Average agglutinin titers of children injected prophylactically with Sauer's vaccine and with toxin vaccine and of untreated cases of pertussis during the infection and early convalescence.

agglutinins in the vaccinated children soon after the stimulation by the vaccine is discontinued.

The results obtained in the agglutinin studies of the 12 cases of nonpertussis respiratory infection were as follows:

Ten children had normal titers, i.e., negative or not over 1:20 dilution; 1 child had a titer of 1:60, and another of 1:200. These last two children, however, had a history of definite exposure and may have had a mild infection which would account for the high agglutinin titers.

SUMMARY

Agglutination studies were made on several different groups of children who were given injections of pertussis vaccines, in untreated clinical pertussis and in nonpertussis respiratory infections. The object of these studies was to determine the following points:

1. The optimum dosage for vaccination.

2. The comparative antigenicity of vaccines that are made of freshly isolated and of stock pertussis bacilli.

3. The comparative value of the intramuscular and the intracutaneous methods of administering the vaccine when given after short or long intervals.

4. The agglutinin response after vaccination and during infection and early convalescence. The results obtained were as follows:

a. The average agglutinin response in the vaccinated children was, on the whole, proportional to the dosage given. In those in whom the maximum dose did not exceed 8.5 billion bacteria given intracutaneously or 39 billion bacteria given intramuscularly, only a few of the children showed an increase in agglutinins; although the titer of some of those that did show an increase was fairly high. On the other hand, a dose of 80 billion bacteria stimulated agglutinins in a large percentage of the children (55 per cent in the group that received Sauer's vaccine and 84 per cent in the group that received our toxin vaccine).

b. The intracutaneous method compared favorably with the intramuscular method in stimulating agglutinins although the dose used intracutaneously was very much smaller than the intramuscular dose.

c. The agglutinin response was better in the groups that were given the injections at two-day than at seven-day intervals. However, the groups studied were very small, and therefore definite conclusions cannot be drawn at present.

d. The agglutinin response was better in the group of children who were injected with a vaccine that was made of stock cultures that were grown on sheep blood infusion agar (toxin vaccine) than in those who were injected with a vaccine that was made of freshly isolated cultures that were grown on human blood–Bordet-Gengou medium (Sauer).

e. The agglutinin response in pertussis cases differed markedly from that of the vaccinated children, in the length of time at which the maximum was attained and in the height of its curve (Chart 3). But having attained the maximum (the maximum titer differed widely in different cases) it dropped rapidly. It corresponded closely in this respect with the drop in the agglutinin titer of the vaccinated children. It seems therefore that there was a decrease in agglutinins almost as soon as infection ceased and convalescence began. This again corresponds with the decrease in agglutinins in the vaccinated children soon after the active stimulation of the vaccine was discontinued.

f. The agglutinin content of the serums of all but 2 of 12 children who had nonpertussis respiratory infections was in the normal range. These 2 children were definitely exposed to pertussis and may have had a mild infection which would account for their high agglutinin titers.

CONCLUSION

1. As far as it can be judged from the agglutinin studies, a dosage of 50 to 80 billion bacteria seems indicated in pertussis vaccination when given intramuscularly or subcutaneously.

2. The intracutaneous method of administering the vaccine has given very promising results and may prove to be the method of choice if further tests will confirm our present findings.

3. Potent vaccines may be prepared of stock cultures provided they retain their original morphologic, cultural, and serologic characteristics. The potency of the vaccine may be increased by preparing the vaccine in such a manner that it contains a toxic substance in addition to the bacteria. Sheep blood infusion agar of pH 7.2 to 7.4 was found suitable for preparing pertussis vaccines.

REFERENCES

1. Madsen, T.: (a) Whooping Cough, Boston M. & S. J. **192**: 50, 1925. (b) Vaccination Against Whooping Cough, J. A. M. A. **101**: 187, 1933.
2. Sauer, L. W.: J. Pediat. **2**: 740, 1933.
3. Sauer, L. W.: Am. J. Pub. Health **25**: 1226, 1935.
4. Perry, Marrian H., Findley, H. T., and Bensted, H. J.: J. Roy. Army M. Corps **63**: 1, 1934.
5. Leslie, P. H., and Gardner, A. D.: J. Hyg. **31**: 423, 1931.
6. Toomey, J. A., Ranta, K., and Takacs, W. S.: J. Infect. Dis. **57**: 286, 1935.
7. Shibley, G. S., and Hoelscher, H.: J. Exper. Med. **60**: 403, 1934.
8. Mackenzie, G. M.: J. Immunol. **9**: 333, 1924.
9. Tuft, L., Yagle, E. M., and Rogers, S.: J. Infect. Dis. **50**: 98, 1932.
10. Mishulow, L., Mowry, I. W., and Stocker, A. K.: To be published.
11. Mishulow, L., Mowry, I. W., and Scott, E. B.: J. Immunol. **19**: 227, 1930.
12. Shwartzman, G.: J. Exper. Med. **48**: 247, 1928.
13. Kristensen, M., and Ahrend Larsen, S.: Compt. rend. Soc. de biol. **95**: 1110, 1926.
14. Scheffer, I. H.: Personal communication.

RHEUMATIC HEART DISEASE IN CHILDHOOD

A Clinical and Postmortem Study of Seventy-Three Cases

Stanley Gibson, M.D., and E. J. Denenholz, M.D.
Chicago, Ill.

THE outlook for the rheumatic child both as to morbidity and mortality has been studied in the mass in many cardiac clinics. The average wastage over periods of years has been computed in large groups of cases. Less attention has been given to the factors which influence the prognosis in the individual case. What determines an early fatal issue? Does the manner of onset, whether with chorea, polyarthritis, or carditis play a significant rôle? Is the child overwhelmed by a single virulent rheumatic attack, or does he succumb to repeated bouts of infection? To what extent do rheumatic nodules, or pericarditis, or multivalvular involvement influence the prognosis? Is the age of the child at the onset of the rheumatic infection of importance in determining the outlook?

In the effort to gain information on these and other points concerning the life history of the rheumatic infection, we have made a critical study of the clinical and postmortem findings in seventy-three cases of rheumatic heart disease observed at the Children's Memorial Hospital. Inasmuch as the hospital does not retain patients who have attained the age of thirteen years, the present material includes only those patients whose illness terminated below this age limit.

Because of the fact that the work has been chiefly statistical in nature, we shall first set out our findings in tabular form, followed by a discussion of those features which seem to us to be worthy of comment.

Total number of cases, 73
Males—30
Females—43

A. History	
1. Incidence of predisposing causes	
a. Sore throats	
Frequent	18
Infrequent	21
b. Tonsils	
In	55
Out	18
Before first rheumatic attack	11
After first rheumatic attack	4
Questionable	3
c. Growing pains	5
d. Scarlet fever	4
e. Family history	
Rheumatism in other member of family	13

From the Cardiac Service of the Children's Memorial Hospital, Chicago. Dr. Joseph Brennemann, Physician-in-Chief.

2. Incidence of rheumatic phenomena
   a. Chorea
      - One attack 15
      - Two attacks 4
   b. Joint pains
      - One attack 33
      - Two attacks 10
      - Three attacks 3
      - Many attacks 4
   c. Carditis
      - One attack 29
      - Two attacks 22
      - Three attacks 8
      - Four attacks 6
      - Five attacks or more 4
      - Questionable 3

B. Physical Examination

1. Valvular involvement
   - Mitral 49
   - Mitral and aortic 19
   - Functional murmur 2
   - No murmur 3
2. Pericardial friction 35
   - Complaint of pain 26
   - Absence of pain 9
3. Arrhythmia
   - Fibrillation 7
4. Nodules
   - Present 27

C. Postmortem Examination

1. Valvular involvement
   - Mitral 16
   - Mitral and tricuspid 9
   - Mitral and aortic 14
   - Mitral, aortic, and pulmonary 1
   - Mitral, tricuspid and pulmonary 1
   - All valves 6
   - No valvular involvement 1
2. Pericarditis 62
3. Amount of pericardial fluid in cases of pericarditis
   - No fluid 39
   - Less than 100 c.c. (5 to 75 c.c.) 16
   - 100 c.c. 3
   - 125 c.c. 2
   - 150 c.c. 1
   - 200 c.c. 1
   - Over 200 c.c. 0
4. Cause of death
   - Rheumatic heart disease 67
   - Bacterial endocarditis 2
   - Staphylococcic septicemia 2
   - Renal insufficiency 1
   - Pneumonia 1

D. Observations Relative to Duration of Rheumatic Infection (First rheumatic manifestation to death)

1. Average age at onset 6.3 yr.
   Average duration 1.4 yr.

2. Age at onset

Age at onset	No. of cases	Average duration
3 yr.	5	0.4 yr.
4 yr.	12	1.5 yr.
5 yr.	14	1.5 yr.
6 yr.	9	1.5 yr.
7 yr.	9	1.1 yr.
8 yr.	6	1.8 yr.
9 yr.	9	1.7 yr.
10 yr.	7	1.1 yr.
12 yr.	1	0.5 yr.
Questionable	1	

3. Mode of onset

	Average duration
Of 6 cases beginning with chorea	1.7 yr.
1 died within 3 months of onset	
2 died within 2 years of onset	
6 died within 3 years of onset	
Of 41 cases beginning with joint pains	1.5 yr.
11 died within 3 months of onset	
16 died within 6 months of onset	
20 died within 1 year of onset	
30 died within 2 years of onset	
34 died within 3 years of onset	
37 died within 4 years of onset	
41 died within 5 years of onset	
Of 25 cases beginning with carditis	1.1 yr.
8 died within 3 months of onset	
14 died within 6 months of onset	
16 died within 1 year of onset	
20 died within 2 years of onset	
22 died within 3 years of onset	
24 died within 4 years of onset	
25 died within 5 years of onset	

4. Combinations of rheumatic manifestations

Chorea, joint pains, and nodules	5 cases	2.5 yr.
Chorea	5 cases	1.8 yr.
Joint pains and nodules	19 cases	1.7 yr.
Chorea and joint pains	9 cases	1.4 yr.
Joint pains	17 cases	1.1 yr.
Carditis alone	15 cases	0.8 yr.
Nodules	3 cases	0.4 yr.
Chorea and nodules	0 cases	

DISCUSSION

An analysis of our figures relative to what are usually regarded as predisposing causes of rheumatism shows that these predisposing causes were absent in a large percentage of the cases. That the rheumatic infection occurs more frequently in regions where respiratory infections are prevalent is a well-recognized fact. A cold or sore throat often occurs a few days or weeks before the onset of definitely rheumatic phenomena. These observations have naturally raised the question of the etiologic significance of upper respiratory infections in the rheumatic process. In our group of cases, only one-fourth gave a history of frequent sore throats; about one-fourth were subject to infrequent attacks; and almost one-half gave a negative history. It is doubtful whether these figures differ significantly from those which would obtain from a group living under similar conditions without any rheumatic manifestations.

Not only has the occurrence of sore throats been emphasized as a probable etiologic factor in the rheumatic infection, but chronic tonsillar infection has also been considered an important predisposing cause. Indeed the tonsil has been viewed with so great suspicion that in many clinics the appearance of any rheumatic manifestation is considered an indication for tonsillectomy as soon as the patient's condition will permit, and this regardless of evidence of tonsillar infection. In this connection it is of interest that eleven children, or 15 per cent of the group, had been subjected to tonsillectomy prior to the first rheumatic attack.

"Growing pains" were encountered in only five of the histories. The fact that this complaint was so rarely obtained in this group of cases would seem to indicate that the indefinite aches which the laity usually interpret as growing pains are of minor importance in the rheumatic infection.

In only four instances was there a history of scarlet fever. In all four of these cases joint pains occurred within a few weeks or months following the scarlet fever. This would suggest that the scarlet fever acted as a predisposing cause, just as other respiratory infections seem to do in an appreciable percentage of cases.

When we come to a consideration of the admittedly rheumatic phenomena, we find that chorea was present in one-fourth of the patients. This figure is surprisingly high in view of the fact that chorea is considered the rheumatic manifestation least likely to be accompanied by cardiac involvement and that, when carditis does occur, it is usually of milder type than when the invasion of the heart is ushered in by an acute polyarthritis.

The involvement of the joints is the "most rheumatic" of all the rheumatic phenomena, being the most frequent mode of onset, and the symptom-complex which calls attention to the danger which threatens the heart. Yet in almost one-third of the cases, there was a complete absence of joint pains. Of those who gave a history of joint pains, the majority had but a single attack, and only 10 per cent had more than two attacks.

One of the most interesting findings concerned the number of attacks of carditis. In 40 per cent the first attack proved fatal. This is so strikingly at variance with the usual teaching that it is deserving of emphasis. Sir Thomas Lewis,[1] in writing on rheumatic carditis, says, "Death may occur in acute and very severe cases, but these are rare. A first attack is rarely fatal." White,[2] discussing the course and prognosis of rheumatic heart disease, says, "It is usual for the child to survive the first rheumatic infection whether it is frank rheumatic fever, chorea, ill-defined sickness, or rheumatic heart infection alone." Other authorities make similar statements. We are frank to confess that we had held the same view, even though we had observed the course of the majority of the children whose case histories comprise this report. Only when we were confronted by the statistics did we appreciate how large a percentage of the children succumbed to the initial bout of carditis. Perhaps our own erroneous impression, and that of others, may be explained by the fact that the patient with chronic heart disease who has been followed in the out-patient department, and who has been repeatedly in the hospital, is naturally more familiar to the clinician and is better remembered than the patient who has not been in attendance at the out-patient clinic, and whose first hospital stay closes the picture.

Turning to a discussion of the physical findings, we find pericardial friction was heard at some time during the course of the illness in practically half of the cases. This is a significantly high percentage when one considers that the early stages of the infection were rarely followed in the hospital, that a transient friction rub might easily escape notice, and that pericarditis might occur in the absence of a friction rub. The importance of precordial or upper abdominal pain in pointing to pericardial involvement is revealed by the fact that pain was complained of in twenty-six of the thirty-five cases in which pericardial friction was heard.

Auricular fibrillation occurred in seven instances. Once established it persisted until death in all except one. In this case fibrillation continued over a three-week period seven months before the fatal termination and recurred during the last week of life. Our findings were in accord with other observations to the effect that auricular fibrillation is an ominous sign in the rheumatic heart disease of children and may usually be looked upon as a terminal event. Of the seven children who exhibited fibrillation, two were nine years old, and the remaining five were ten years old when the fibrillation began.

Rheumatic nodules were found in twenty-seven of the seventy-three cases. Here again the figures doubtless fail to give the full incidence of this important rheumatic manifestation. We do believe, however, that they represent very nearly the percentage occurring during the period of hospitalization. Not only were the children inspected repeatedly by members of the attending staff, but our nurse in charge was very zealous in her search for nodules and was deeply chagrined if she failed to be the first to detect them. All writers on rheumatism emphasize the importance of the rheumatic nodule as indicating a heavy degree of saturation with the rheumatic virus and a consequent bad prognosis. The significance of their absence has not been so fully considered. Indeed the failure to discover rheumatic nodules in over 60 per cent of the cases implies that their absence is by no means a necessarily good omen. In fact, it was in the children whose courses ran rapidly downhill that nodules were least often found. In other words, rheumatic nodules are seldom found in children who are lightly infected by rheumatism and are often absent in those who are overwhelmed by it. Nodules appear in the children who are seriously infected, but who show some degree of resistance to its ravages.

The postmortem studies revealed the presence of mitral involvement in every case except one. This verified the usual teaching that the mitral valve is practically always invaded in the rheumatic heart disease of childhood. The aortic valve was involved in 46 cases, the tricuspid in 41, and the pulmonary in 8. The most frequent combination of valvular involvement was mitral, aortic, and tricuspid, occurring in 25 instances.

Only eleven patients in the series failed to show the presence of pericarditis. Four of these eleven died a noncardiac death. The high incidence of pericarditis found postmortem emphasizes its importance in the severe carditis of childhood. It also emphasizes the fact that even though the presence of pericarditis cannot be proved by the detection of a friction rub, one has a right to suspect pericardial invasion in the child who shows the signs of serious rheumatic heart disease.

One of the perplexing problems presented by the child with rheumatic heart disease who reveals on physical and roentgenographic examinations a markedly increased cardiac outline is whether the enlargement is due to cardiac hypertrophy and dilatation or to pericardial effusion. We feel that the postmortem observations offer convincing evidence on this point. In no case was there more than 200 c.c. of fluid in the pericardial sac. Only one contained this amount, and six others contained between 100 and 200 c.c. of fluid. Certainly amounts so small would in no way embarrass the heart, nor would they be easy of detection either by physical or roentgenographic examination. White[2] says, in speaking of pericardial effusion, "An amount less than 150 c.c. is probably not discoverable by any method of examination since it produces no definite signs."

Numerous writers have emphasized the rarity of massive effusion in rheumatic heart disease. Carey Coombs[3] said, "The diagnosis of pericardial effusion in rheumatic heart disease is still a field for much erroneous thinking, in spite of the work of Lees, Poynton, and others, who have shown by correlation of clinical with postmortem data that effusion rarely attains a bulk sufficient to cause physical signs and that the signs commonly supposed to be due to effusion are in reality caused by acute dilatation of the heart. Skiagraphy is rarely practicable, the patient being too ill to be moved; and it is only in the presence of large effusions, such as do not occur in cardiac rheumatism, that skiagraphy is of any value. Exploratory puncture should be resorted to with the utmost caution: no case in which subsequent events have shown that it would have been justifiable has come under my notice." Yet this view has not gone unchallenged. Sutton[4] has advocated paracentesis of the pericardium as a therapeutic measure in rheumatic pericarditis. Using the posterior site, she did pericardial taps on eleven children, removing varying amounts of fluid up to 400 c.c. In most instances 200 to 300 c.c. of fluid were obtained. Sutton admits that it is doubtful whether the ultimate result in rheumatic pericarditis is altered, but she is convinced that the symptoms of marked dyspnea, orthopnea, cyanosis, and a sense of pressure and suffocation may be ameliorated by the removal of part or all of the pericardial fluid. We are unable to explain the large amounts of fluid in the cases reported by Sutton compared with the absence or minimal amounts of fluid which were obtained in our cases unless it be a difference in climate and environment influencing the behavior of the rheumatic infection. Certainly there was no indication for paracentesis of the pericardium in the group here reported, either to increase the patient's comfort or as a lifesaving procedure.

The mode of onset of the rheumatic infection has been considered an important factor in determining the prognosis. Findlay[5] says, "Of 80 cases of cardiac disease following chorea, 22.5 per cent ended fatally; whereas of 313 examples following arthritis, 27.7 per cent ended fatally during the same period of time. The prognosis is, however, most serious when carditis is the first or only manifestation of the disease. The mortality incidence in the examples which commenced with carditis, but which were afterwards followed by rheumatism (chorea, arthritis, or nodules) was 42.8 per cent, and in those in which carditis was the sole manifestation of the disease, 66.6 per cent." In the estimation of the seriousness of the prognosis by the duration of the infection in fatal cases rather than the percentage mortality in a given period of time, our figures are in complete agreement with those of Findlay. Of six cases beginning with chorea, the average duration was 1.7 years. In the forty-one instances in which arthritis was the first manifestation, the average duration was 1.5 years. When the carditis itself was the first manifestation, the period of survival averaged only 1.1 years; and when carditis was the sole rheumatic episode, the average time from onset to death was only 0.8 year.

The above statistics do not convey an adequate notion of the behavior of the rheumatic infection in this group. A closer scrutiny of the figures reveals the fact that whereas a relatively small percentage survived for several years, a surprisingly large number survived for only a few months. Twenty children died within three months of the first rheumatic manifestation, and within the succeeding three months eleven others had succumbed. The second half year accounted for the death of six others. Thus it is seen that 27 per cent had died within three months, 42 per cent had died within six months, and 50 per cent had died within one year of the onset. We have already called attention to the fact that the initial bout of carditis resulted fatally in 40 per cent of the cases. The figures just quoted show that the course of the fatal attack was relatively rapid. Any disease which claims an appreciable percentage of its victims within three months of onset can scarcely be said to be an essentially chronic disease. While numerous writers have called attention to the occasional fulminant case of rheumatic carditis, we do not believe that the frequence of this type has been sufficiently appreciated. Yet we are convinced that our findings are not exceptional, if comparison be made where climatic conditions are similar to those obtaining in Chicago. In a study of the development of mitral stenosis in young people, Bland, White, and Jones[6] reported the duration of rheumatic infection in one hundred patients living in the vicinity of Boston who died at or before the age of twenty-one years. Of their group, twenty died within six months of the onset. This percentage, while lower than in our series, is high, especially when it is recalled that their material included individuals through the age of twenty-one years while our own series was comprised wholly of children under thirteen years of age.

SUMMARY

A clinical and postmortem study of seventy-three children with rheumatic heart disease has revealed the following:

1. Predisposing causes of the rheumatic infection, such as sore throats, chronic tonsillar infection, growing pains, and scarlet fever, were encountered with less frequence than was anticipated.
2. Chorea occurred in 26 per cent and joint pains in 68 per cent.
3. The first bout of carditis proved fatal in 40 per cent.
4. Pericardial friction was heard in 48 per cent.
5. Pericarditis was found on postmortem examination in 85 per cent. In no instance was a large amount of fluid present in the pericardial sac.
6. Auricular fibrillation was infrequent, occurred in the older patients, and was usually a terminal event.
7. Nodules were found in 37 per cent.
8. Average duration of life was longest when the attack began with chorea, less prolonged when joint pains initiated the infection, and shortest when the invasion of the heart itself was the only evidence of rheumatism.
9. The total duration of the rheumatic infection was less than three months in 27 per cent.

We are indebted to Dr. William G. Hibbs, attending pathologist, for the privilege of reviewing the postmortem records.

REFERENCES

1. Lewis, Sir Thomas: Diseases of the Heart, New York, 1933, The Macmillan Company.
2. White, P. D.: Heart Disease, New York, 1931, The Macmillan Company.
3. Coombs, Carey: Rheumatic Heart Disease, New York, 1924, William Wood & Co.
4. Sutton, Lucy Porter: Am. J. Dis. Child. 48: 1934.
5. Findlay, Leonard: The Rheumatic Infection in Childhood, New York, 1932, William Wood & Co.
6. Bland, Edward F., White, Paul D., and Jones, T. Duckett: The Development of Mitral Stenosis in Young People, Am. Heart J. 10: 995, 1935.

Critical Review

SURGICAL PEDIATRICS

HERBERT E. COE, M.D.
SEATTLE, WASH.

TO THOSE who for many years have been keenly cognizant of the definite and distinct differences between the surgery of adults and that of infants and children, it is most gratifying to note the recent trend toward a more general recognition of these differences and of the fundamental conditions upon which they depend. Among the several excellent articles in the medical literature of the past year those by Penberthy,[1] Burton,[2] and Brunkow[3] are particularly worthy of mention. They point out clearly the differences in structure, proportions, reactions, growth factors, psychology, physiologic requirements and pathologic processes between the rapidly growing infant or child and the adult. The child is an organism in a relatively unstable state of rapid evolution while the adult is in a comparatively stable condition with a gradual progression toward the major involution so well described by Warthin.[4] These differences have resulted in the development of the specialty of pediatrics which requires a constant appreciation and evaluation of these various factors and has given rise to such terms as the "pediatric attitude" or the "pediatric approach." The knowledge of these fundamental differences forms a subconscious screen or filter through which one dealing with children must pass all observations if he is to see conditions in true perspective and arrive at correct conclusions.

Broad experience and keen surgical judgment are evident in the articles mentioned, attention being directed particularly to conditions peculiar to infancy and childhood, the necessity of conservation of body heat, adequate fluid and food supply, skill and delicacy in handling tissues, hemostasis, anesthesia, and especially to the necessity and value of close cooperation between the surgeon and pediatrician. The last point is particularly to be heeded by the occasional surgeon who considers it an unwarranted invasion of his domain for the pediatrician to make suggestions or recommendations regarding the condition of the patient or the choice of time for operation.

Until the rather exclusive specialty of surgical pediatrics develops further, there should be in every community some surgeon particularly adept at handling children[5] who will devote his attention to a study of the essential differences between children and adults and develop ability in this branch of surgery. The differences are not only physical but mental, and he should take into account the effect of illness, therapeutic procedures and hospitalization upon the emotional development of the child,[6] recognizing that many of the psychologic maladjustments of adult life have their origin in childhood, and being particularly careful to minimize the psychic shock which is too frequently associated with illness and the child's contact with the medical profession.

ANESTHESIA

With the great variety of anesthetic agents at present available, individualization of anesthesia is particularly important and relatively easy to accomplish.[7] It seems superfluous to say that the anesthetist should know the condition of the child, but too frequently there is a lack of cooperation between the surgeon and the anesthetist with the result that the anesthetist has little time to determine the type of anesthetic best suited to the patient and no time to gain the child's confidence. Conservation of the surgeon's time is given preference over the present physical and future psychic condition of the patient. This situation is no doubt due to the safety and widespread use of ether, which is so well suited to the average case that its disadvantages as compared to the newer anesthetic agents are overlooked. Especially to be mentioned in this connection are avertin, the barbiturates, cyclopropane, and the use of preanesthetic medication. The statement that these agents are contraindicated in the extremes of life should be revised. Such a generalization is unwarranted as regards children and would appear to indicate unfamiliarity with this age group rather than the result of careful observation and study. Due care and judgment must be exercised in the administration of anesthetics as well as of any other potent drug regardless of the age of the patient, and unwillingness to study the requirements of infants and children and to make the necessary adjustments in suitable cases is a type of mental inertia which should not be tolerated as an excuse for the use of inferior methods.

Cyclopropane is steadily gaining in favor. It is emphasized, however, that it must be used by a skilled anesthetist[8] and requires special apparatus. In one series of 1,108 cases the youngest patient was ten days of age,[9] and in older children, when combined with avertin as a basal anesthetic, it has proved to be as near the ideal as any anesthetic yet employed. There is less postoperative nausea, vomiting, distention, and general discomfort than with any other type of anesthesia. It is best administered by the endotracheal method using the carbon dioxide absorption technic. The cost is still rather high, averaging $1.14 in a large number of cases, which figure, however, includes all accessory supplies. The advantages, however, outweigh this adverse item as it can be used in nearly all types of cases including many bad risks, and it almost entirely avoids the unpleasantness of ether. At the Mayo Clinic it is rapidly displacing ethylene,[10] which for several years has been rather extensively used. On the other hand, vinethene, which at first seemed to promise much as an inhalation anesthetic, has not maintained its popularity. While it is excellent for short anesthesia such as for the reduction of fractures or the extraction of teeth, being followed by prompt and complete recovery,[11] the reflexes are not easily controlled during the longer operations, and in addition the cost is rather high and the material relatively unstable. It is excellent as an induction agent preceding ether.

It is most gratifying to note the rapidly increasing use of basal anesthesia or narcosis; children present the ideal field for this type of premedication. They usually come to the surgery without their consent and often with their active opposition, frightened by strange surroundings and persons, mentally too immature to understand why they should be subjected to a painful or at best a disagreeable procedure, and although in some instances outwardly calm, inwardly so disturbed as to upset the endocrine balance completely. Gwathmey[12] very wisely states that the ideal condition of a child previous to operation is deep sleep and that the usual anesthetic methods, especially in tonsil and adenoid operations, are unsafe and inhumane. Children tolerate the barbiturates well in doses adjusted to age and size. Nembutal in over 1,200 cases has given highly satisfactory results. It should be given thirty to forty minutes before operation either by mouth or rectum, the patient moved with gentleness, supplemental ether induced by ethylene and oxygen and followed by carbogen until the throat reflex and respiration return to normal. Such a sequence and combination for tonsil operations is superior to the use of any one anesthetic agent alone as it results in a minimum amount of secretions, frequently no nausea or vomiting, a wider margin of safety between the therapeutic and toxic dose, and a postoperative period of quiet rest lasting from thirty to sixty minutes. It requires modern anesthetic equipment and should be under the supervision of a skilled anesthetist. This method may differ radically from the usual ones, but it carries the sanction of authority and is based upon an analysis of over 488,000 anesthetic records throughout the United States.

The barbiturates are of two classes, heavy and light, nembutal and sodium amytal being examples of the former, and evipal and pentothal sodium of the latter. The former objection to intravenous and rectal anesthesia that it is not controllable has been met by the light barbiturates.[13] They are used in dilute solution and are broken down and excreted with extreme rapidity. While the end products of the heavy barbiturates may be present in the excretions for seventy-two hours, those of the light type disappear so rapidly that only a bare trace remains in twelve hours, and for all practical purposes the effect has passed off in from three to thirty minutes, depending upon the dose. This characteristic places them definitely in the class of controllable anesthetics and hypnotics. Since the effect is upon the respiratory and not the cardiac centers, respiratory stimulants and artificial respiration can easily be used until the effect has completely disappeared, if there should be an instance of idiosyncrasy to the drug. They are usually administered intravenously and induction is smooth, pleasant, and rapid, unconsciousness being complete within one minute. Too rapid administration causes respiratory depression which is easily counteracted by coramine or picrotoxin. The dose for children is in proportion to the weight, based upon an average adult weight of 150 pounds. In a series of over 1,000 cases pentothal sodium was held to be slightly superior to evipal, the induction being smoother with less twitching, less fall in blood pressure, and no postoperative restlessness. It is from 30 to 50 per cent more potent than evipal and hence is more depressant to the respiratory center,[10] a characteristic which makes careful supervision particularly necessary in children. As a rule, however, children tolerate well the dosage appropriate to their weight.

The most recent development in basal anesthesia is the rectal use of the quick-acting barbiturates. Experimental investigation of evipal as a preanesthetic agent has shown that less supplemental anesthetic is required to produce anesthesia, more to produce respiratory failure and that the animals survive toxic amounts twice as long and have fewer lung lesions than animals which do not receive this preanesthetic medication. Following these observations this method was used in 150 cases with most satisfactory results,[14] there being quiet sleep in over 80 per cent, an induction period of about five minutes, good relaxation, and little tendency to obstruction of the airway. It was much more satisfactory in abolishing psychic influences than morphine, which when used alone as a preanesthetic medication does not destroy them. The unfavorable comments were a rather slow postoperative reaction and a considerable amount of postoperative restlessness.

The intravenous use of evipal has been so extensively and favorably reported that further comment seems superfluous. In one series of 120 cases,[15] many children were included, one of whom was an infant eight months old in whom 140 mg. were used for a ten-minute anesthetic.

Until further reports upon the rectal use of the barbiturates are available avertin will continue to be the most popular and widely used drug for basal anesthesia by this route. The 100 mg. table is generally considered best for children[16] although less in tonsil cases is advocated by some observers. While it has been combined with morphine, atropine, and novocaine as total anesthesia in children,[17] its outstanding field is as a basal anesthetic.[18] The amount should be adapted to the condition of the patient, higher dosage being necessary in those patients who are nervous or frightened and in vigorous children or athletic individuals. Second doses for any reason should be used with extreme caution on account of cumulative effects upon respiration. Since the action on the liver is similar to that of chloroform, protection of liver function by preoperative intravenous glucose is advisable.

In all types of preanesthetic medication sufficient time should be permitted to elapse for the full physiologic effect to be obtained before the supplemental anesthetic is administered, as otherwise a combined action may occur with a rather alarming respiratory depression. Such depression yields readily to coramine by the intramuscular or intravenous route, depending upon the urgency of the condition. An experimental study of this action of coramine[19] has shown that it is a true physiologic antidote for the barbiturates, being distinctly superior to ephedrine or adrenalin,[20] which frequently have a rather serious secondary depressing effect. It is usually given intramuscularly but in urgent cases may be used intravenously in doses from 2 to 5 c.c. repeated every ten minutes until effective. In these large doses it occasionally causes hiccoughs, flushing and projectile vomiting, but these untoward symptoms are of short duration and leave no aftereffects.

The demand for preanesthetic medication and basal anesthesia has originated for the most part with the pediatricians and pediatric nurses rather than with the surgeons and anesthetists,[21] and the increasing use of these humane procedures will probably depend upon their tactful and persistent insistence.

For infants ether will perhaps continue to be the anesthetic of choice[22] although basal anesthesia may be used when indicated and nitrous oxide is valuable. Conservation of body heat is an important factor in this class of patients. The vague fear of thymus still persists, but the continued insistence of Waldbott that the so-called thymic syndrome has an allergic basis seems gradually to be placing consideration of this troublesome condition on a more scientific foundation.[23] In the presence of an allergic family history skin tests with the proposed anesthetic agent or the administration of a small amount of it followed by a blood count for eosinophilia are of more diagnostic value than a roentgenogram.

Convulsions under ether anesthesia have been mentioned more frequently in the British than in American literature.[24] They begin with facial twitchings and dilated pupils, extend to the rest of the body, and if allowed to continue terminate fatally in over 30 per cent of the cases. They occur in toxic patients in whom there has not been opportunity for adequate preoperative preparation. The treatment consists in elevation of the head and the administration of 20 to 40 c.c. of 50 per cent glucose intravenously followed by 5 per cent glucose in saline.[25]

BURNS

An analytical study of the symptom-complex of burns shows that there is a rather constant sequence of events.[26] Pain and fright first induce reflex shock; loss of fluid from the circulation into the tissues begins at once and reaches a peak in about twenty-four hours, after which it gradually returns; bacterial contamination, which also occurs early, progresses to active infection and gives systemic evidence of toxic absorption in thirty-six to forty-eight hours. When this sequence is recognized, the rationale of treatment becomes apparent. Opiates and heat combat reflex shock; protection of the affected area from bacterial invasion if seen sufficiently early, and from absorption if later; maintenance of adequate fluid in the circulatory system. Fluid may be supplied by intravenous administration of normal saline solution even up to the amount of the normal blood volume, checking the amount by estimation of hemoglobin rather than the blood pressure[27] and the appearance of tissue edema. A hemoglobin of 125 per cent is not unusual, but, if it reaches 140 per cent, it indicates a concentration of the blood which is often fatal.[28] There is usually depletion of the blood chlorides but not of blood sugar, so glucose solutions are not indicated. Serum albumin, however, is lost and must be replaced by liberal blood transfusions if the administered fluid is to be kept in the blood vessels. In the absence of suitable donors gum acacia solution may be used, but blood is preferable. The large quantities of fluid necessary to maintain normal blood concentration are easily excreted when adjustment between tissue fluids and circulation takes place, and a reassuring sign is a transient polyuria. If edema develops, it usually indicates retention of chlorides, and the intravenous saline may be replaced by water if there is still blood concentration. An amount of sodium chloride equal to 0.5 to 0.8 gm. per kilogram of body weight in twenty-four hours is a reasonably safe standard.[29]

Protection of the burned surface by adherence to the principles of the tannic acid treatment is still fundamentally sound although many minor modifications are advocated by various writers. The addition of silver nitrate[30] as described by Bettman increases the speed of tanning, simplifies nursing, and reduces shock; mercurochrome forms a thin, transparent film through which any accumulation of pus easily penetrates[31]; gentian violet is particularly effective against the streptococcus and is distinctly analgesic[32]; ferric chloride is stable in solution and forms a rather transparent coagulum which is elastic enough to permit early motion of joints, but the application is so painful that it should be preceded by liberal morphine or barbiturate analgesia.[33] The prime essential of the local treatment is protection from irritation, whether the irritation be from contraction of the surface due to air drying, from bacterial products, from frequent treatments, or from disturbing changes of dressings. The age-old principle of healing by rest applies as well to burns as to wounds.

A rather radical and novel departure in the treatment of the shock and pain incident to burns is the cold water treatment.[34] The pathologic changes in tissues injured by burning and by freezing are practically identical, and reasoning by analogy the initial treatment by application of cold should be as effective in one as the other. This is accomplished by immersion of the burned part, or the entire body, in cool water or by the application of cool wet dressings to burns of the face or small areas. Tap water at a temperature of 60° to 70° F. is used, the temperature being gradually increased to 80° F. during the first hour, to approximately 92° F. during the second hour, and to 98° F. during the third hour. The rate of increase is dependent upon the sensation of pain. The treatment is applicable to patients in the initial stage of shock soon after the accident. No attempt is made at extensive removal of clothing or devitalized tissue until after recovery from shock, when morphine is usually given and the area cleaned thoroughly, rinsed with sterile water, dried with a current of warm air and the usual protective measures instituted. The relief from pain and shock is spectacular. In a series of 52 cases the results were markedly superior to those in a preceding series of 130 cases treated by the usual antishock methods. There is no variation from the usual treatment of the various secondary local and general conditions, such as fluid administration, tannic acid, protection from contractures, skin grafting, etc.

The more recent studies of the circulation and the water metabolism associated with burns have changed the former concept that suppression of urine is due to toxic irritation of the kidneys. The anuria is known now to be due to lack of circulating fluid, and death occurs from that cause rather than from uremia. The absolute necessity of maintaining an adequate circulation is increasingly apparent.

INTRACRANIAL CONDITIONS

The fact that many cases of brain tumor progress steadily to a fatal termination has been responsible for the development of a rather fatalistic attitude, not only on the part of the laity, but also on the part of a considerable proportion of the medical profession. This is unfortunate, for the prognosis in some instances is good, and this attitude may in such cases prevent the early diagnosis and treatment which are so necessary to recovery. There is a fairly constant group of symptoms which to the alert medical attendant should suggest intracranial tumor, and a thorough neurologic analysis or a prompt reference to a neurologic surgeon will permit the institution of treatment which in many cases will be lifesaving. Suggestive symptoms[35] are vomiting, particularly of the projectile type which does not yield to usual medical measures, persistent headaches, disturbances of vision, a tendency to clumsiness in play, falling or variations in gait, and disturbances of smell, hearing, or speech.

Children differ essentially from adults in the relative frequency of certain types of brain tumor; especially to be noted are the astrocytomas, the meduloblastomas and the adamantinomas. Astrocytomas may become cystic and in many instances be successfully removed. Meduloblastomas are often markedly relieved by operation or by roentgen therapy, but the relief is usually only temporary. Adamantinomas arise from the ducts of the hypophysis and cause disturbances of vision and pituitary dysfunction. They often respond satisfactorily to treatment. Lumbar puncture in cases of suspected brain tumor may be extremely dangerous. If there is clinical evidence of increased intracranial pressure, rest in bed, restriction of fluids, and dehydration by rectal administration of magnesium sulphate is a safe method of relief. The two symptoms to be kept constantly in mind by those who are in frequent contact with children are vomiting and persistent severe headache, as they occur in over 70 per cent of cases.

A condition which may closely simulate intracranial tumor is lead poisoning.[36] All of the usual symptoms may be present and to confuse the diagnosis further there may be absence of lead lines on the gums and of stippling of the red cells. However, roentgenography will usually show lines of increased density near the epiphyseal lines of the long bones and the blood, urine, and cerebrospinal fluid may show a positive lead test. Careful search will often reveal a source of supply of lead, such as paint from toys or water from the old type of lead pipes. Reduction of the intracranial pressure by dehydration methods or by surgical decompression relieves the symptoms and usually results in recovery.

An unusual and serious postoperative complication in infants and small children is intracranial thrombosis.[37] It occurs in clean as well as septic cases usually in the superior longitudinal sinus, and the onset varies from a few hours to two weeks after operation. Symptoms are convulsions, vomiting and delirium, or in some cases milder toxic symptoms. The cases reported occurred following operations for cleft palate, pyloric stenosis, and hernia. A report of eight cases of so unusual a condition is interesting and merits further study and analysis. It suggests the possibility that a careful search of the intracranial vessels might reveal this condition in some of those autopsies which have noted the cause of death rather vaguely as toxemia from postoperative infection, or postoperative shock. Convulsions of the jacksonian type with other localizing signs of an intracranial lesion may be due to an intracranial hemangioma.[38] The diagnosis is suggested by the presence of a nevus on the face or scalp on the same side. Such lesions are usually amenable to radium treatment. While multiple nevi of the skin are not uncommon, the suggestion that they may be associated with similar lesions within the body is logical and deserves careful consideration in the interpretation of an unusual symptom-complex.

CHEST AND LUNGS

In the treatment of empyema in infants and children certain concepts are generally accepted. These are that the mortality is highest in infants; that closed drainage is particularly adapted to infants;

that before the mediastinum has become stabilized or before the subsistence of the pneumonia, aspiration alone is permissible; that the variety of the infecting organism is a factor in determining the type of treatment; and that some form of open drainage either intercostal or by rib resection will be necessary in a large proportion of older children. A controversial point seems to be regarding the length of time aspiration should be used before resorting to open drainage. It is contended on the one hand[39, 40, 41] that open drainage at the appropriate stage of the process shortens the period of treatment, permits more efficient evacuation of purulent material, and relieves toxemia; and, on the other,[42, 43] that aspiration should be continued as long as the patient shows improvement, that complete evacuation of the pus is unnecessary, that fibrinous coagulums will undergo autolysis and disappear, and that open drainage should be delayed until there is insufficient response to repeated aspirations. It is difficult to reconcile these two views which seem to be in the nature of personal opinions. A comparison of mortality and morbidity is most unsatisfactory on account of the well-recognized fact that the severity of cases varies greatly in different localities and in different years in the same locality and by the fact that empyema is a localized collection of pus, the significance of which may be affected by diverse etiologic factors. Mortality and morbidity will be increased by a rigid adherence to any one method of treatment, and the highest degree of success will be attained only when there is the ability to evaluate the signs and symptoms and the judgment to use the method of treatment which is adapted to the type and stage of the pathologic process. In other words, the best mortality statistics over a long period of years will be obtained by those who have a thorough knowledge of the fundamental pathology of the condition and of the various methods of treatment. Such a statement is so self-evident that it would seem almost puerile, but repeated emphasis on fundamental principles would seem indicated when one considers the great numbers of articles which are continually appearing stressing some one method of treatment as responsible for good or bad results and failing to evaluate or to correlate other important factors which have equal or greater significance in an analysis of end-results.

Bronchoscopy and esophagoscopy require special training and teamwork, and the symptoms indicating the use of these procedures should be widely known.[44] A foreign body in the trachea or bronchus causes one or more of the following symptoms: choking, gagging, coughing, wheezing heard more distinctly at the mouth than over the chest wall, hoarseness, and cyanosis. These symptoms appear at varying periods after the foreign body has entered the air passages: nonobstructive metal objects may give few signs for several weeks, whereas vegetable substances usually set up violent reactions at once with cough, toxemia, and irregular fever. When the foreign body has been lodged in the lungs for some time, it may cause bronchiectasis, lung abscess, massive collapse of the lung, unexplained dyspnea, or symptoms suggesting tuberculosis with persistent absence of tubercle bacilli. In the presence of such findings a bronchoscopic study is indicated. Roentgenography may fail to show the foreign body, but its presence may be suspected if there is a constant area of increased density, often lobular in its shape and distribution.[45] A movable object in the trachea may produce a snapping sound by being alternately drawn down to the bifurcation and blown up against the larynx.[46] If such an object is in one of the bronchi, it may act as a valve permitting the entrance but not the exit of air, and producing an obstructive emphysema with a high pitched percussion note and hyperresonance. Fluid secretions due to the irritation of a foreign body follow the laws of gravity, and this fact should be remembered for the purpose of postural drainage and in the endeavor to prevent fluid from entering the unaffected lung.

Foreign bodies in the esophagus often lodge behind the cricoid cartilage causing pain on swallowing and a sensation of pressure which may be referred to some point at a distance from the lesion.

Bronchoscopy permits accurate differential diagnosis instead of "inferential diagnosis"[47] in many conditions affecting the air passages in infants and children; among which may be mentioned especially asphyxia neonatorum, congenital atelectasis, congenital anomalies of the larynx, thymic compression of the trachea, and acute and chronic suppurative diseases of the respiratory system. The personnel of the modern obstetric hospital should include a bronchoscopist and every obstetric department should have available the services of some one sufficiently expert to examine the larynx and upper trachea of infants.

Diaphragmatic hernia in infants and children is being reported with increasing frequency, and the operative treatment shows a good percentage of satisfactory results. The operation should be performed early because the diaphragm is a muscular structure and its development is dependent upon function.[48] When its activity is diminished or prevented by a hernia, normal development during the period of growth is impossible, resulting in disturbances of digestion, respiration, and circulation which give the typical picture of malnutrition and lowered resistance. Following successful operation, there is a rapid return to a normal state of nutrition, rate of growth, and physical activities. The condition in some instances causes few symptoms, and the diagnosis may be made only as a result of a careful general examination including roentgenography of the chest to determine the cause of slow gain in weight and vague respiratory symptoms. In other instances feeding difficulties, dyspnea, small abdomen, and full tympanitic chest indicate the diagnosis so definitely that the roentgenogram is merely confirmatory.[49] The operation presents certain technical difficulties which places it clearly in the domain of major surgery. It is best done under positive pressure anesthesia. The replacement of the ectopic viscera may be difficult on account of size, number, or adhesions; the line of closure of the diaphragmatic opening may stretch or open postoperatively; or there may be associated congenital anomalies.[50] A condition which may be confused with diaphragmatic hernia is congenital elevation of the diaphragm sometimes mistakenly called eventration.[51] In this condition there is no enlargement of the normal diaphragmatic openings, the diaphragm being intact and thinned out into a translucent fibrous sheet, and the abdominal viscera do not pass into the true thoracic cavity. A careful roentgenographic study will show that while the viscera are above the normal position of the diaphragm, their relations are more constant than in hernia; they do not pass through a diaphragmatic opening; and the shadow of the diaphragm cannot be seen, or is much less distinct than in the case of hernia. The differential diagnosis is important as surgery is not indicated, and if the infant survives the first few months the condition is not incompatible with long life.

Atresia of the esophagus with the usual accompaniment of tracheoesophageal fistula is so uniformly fatal that a suggested procedure for treatment is interesting.[52] The diagnosis is not difficult but is sometimes delayed until aspiration pneumonia has occurred. There is excessive mucus in the mouth from accumulation in the blind esophageal pouch. The lower segment is the one which usually communicates with the trachea and the gastric secretions, the production of which is stimulated by attempts at feeding, regurgitate into the lungs causing cyanosis and dyspnea with the coughing up of quantities of frothy fluid. This causes marked prostration, and the infant appears almost lifeless but gradually recovers only to repeat the same performance at the next feeding. Death is due to starvation and dehydration if it does not occur earlier from accumulation of fluid in the lungs. When the condition is suspected, a catheter may be passed very gently into the throat until it meets the obstruction, and the mucous contents of the pouch withdrawn to prevent aspiration. When the obstruction is well below the level of the larynx, lipiodol may be injected and the condition visualized by roentgenography. Barium should never be used as it is irritating. Immediate surgery is indicated and consists of tying off the cardiac end of the esophagus with tape to prevent regurgitation of stomach contents, followed by gastrostomy to permit feeding. The esophageal pouch must be kept clear by aspiration. Later the pouch may be brought out to a subcutaneous position and a skin tube prepared to construct an anterior thoracic esophagus. The many technical difficulties of this series of steps are so apparent that for the present it will have mainly an academic interest and should be attempted only in an institution having extensive equipment and the services of a highly skilled staff.

GASTROINTESTINAL TRACT

The medical literature on appendicitis continues to be voluminous, and there is little to distinguish that of the past year from that which has been previously reviewed in this department. Occasional articles stress the value of cooperation between the pediatrician and the surgeon, the necessity for a careful, unhurried examination, the evaluation of the reactions of the individual child, and appreciation of the anatomic and physiologic differences between children and adults.[53-57] Much information may be gained by a quiet inspection after the abdomen is uncovered, noting posture, activity, respiration, and facial expression. The child with an acutely inflamed appendix protects the tender organ by lying quietly and avoiding changes of intraabdominal pressure or tension, such as are caused by unnecessary movements of the legs or trunk or the abdominal type of respiration. His expression is apprehensive if he anticipates an attempt to touch the abdomen. Quiet inspection while obtaining the history also gives the child time to inspect the examiner and gain confidence so that palpation of the abdomen beginning on the side which is not tender seems only a continuation of the conversation. Time is necessary also to obtain the child's confidence after a thoroughly bad psychologic attitude has been quite effectively produced by repeated assurances on the part of the family that the doctor will not hurt him. It is regrettable that statements occasionally appear to the effect that rectal examinations are of doubtful value. While it is, of course, true that rectal examination is not to be considered a fixed and unvariable part of the diagnostic procedures, its value should not be minimized. It may be unnecessary or merely confirmatory for the keen, trained pediatrician and definitely contraindicated for the examiner whose finger is large and whose methods are brutal, but there still remains a great proportion of cases in which definite and valuable information may be obtained in this way, and especially is this true in infants and small children.

The position of the appendix in children is variable and often quite different from the usual adult location, a fact to be remembered when the point of maximum tenderness is on the left side, in the midline, at the edge of the liver, or in the lumbar region. A retrocecal appendicitis may be indicated by frequent loose or mucous stools and may give none of the usual signs of peritoneal irritation. In certain parts of the country symptoms suggestive of appendicitis but accompanied by bloody or mucous stools may indicate amebic or bacillary dysentery,[58, 59] and operation is definitely contraindicated. There may be the usual pain, tenderness, and temperature of appendicitis, but there is usually little or no rigidity or leucocytosis, and there are often eosinophilia, spasticity of the colon, palpable mesenteric lymph nodes, and a positive stool culture. When the differential diagnosis is difficult and there is the possibility that the symptoms may be due to an extraabdominal condition, the fact that the blood sedimentation time in acute appendicitis is usually normal may be of distinct assistance.

In definitely doubtful cases it is better to perform an occasional unnecessary operation than to lose a life on account of delay.[60] This advice, however, is not to be confused with the recommendation still too frequently seen that appendicitis should be operated upon as soon as the diagnosis is made, regardless of the stage of the pathologic process. Such practice results in unnecessary mortality when the operation is performed during the danger period between the second and the seventh day, the period of dehydration, carbohydrate depletion, toxemia, and negative phase of bacterial resistance. If adhesions have not formed and there is evidence of peritonitis, it is difficult to comprehend the conception that the protective activities of the peritoneum can be aided by operative trauma. The first ten hours is a relatively safe period, but after this time the postoperative mortality rises steadily to a peak on the fourth and fifth days[61]; analysis of the mortality statistics cited by those who advise immediate operation regardless of the stage of the pathologic process will usually show this well-defined danger period. The conviction is steadily growing that children seen after the second day of symptoms show a definitely lower mortality rate under the nonoperative treatment than following immediate operation. If there is evidence of abscess formation, it is better to allow time for a definite wall to form rather than to attempt early drainage.[62] During the two or three days required for this process, the general condition of the patient may be markedly improved by appropriate measures.

Conditions which are often impossible to differentiate from acute appendicitis are acute regional ileitis and mesenteric lymphadenitis,[63, 64, 65] the diagnosis in most instances being made only after the abdomen is opened. Ileitis usually occurs in older children and adolescents and is characterized by marked, hyperemic thickening of the terminal portion of the ileum involving the wall of the bowel rather than the mucosa and accompanied by extensive lymphadenitis of the mesenteric glands. The glands may suppurate, and there may be local gangrene of the bowel wall with perforation and peritonitis. The appendix often shows little or no involvement, and the temptation to remove it should be resisted unless it is acutely inflamed. If, however, the process appears to be chronic, the appendix may be removed but it is unwise to invert the stump, and, in general, surgical procedures should be reduced to a minimum. Both conditions seem to be secondary to infections of the upper respiratory tract, and if tonsillar infection is present, a subsequent tonsillectomy is advisable. When the mesenteric adenitis is the predominating condition, the enlarged glands may in some instances be palpable during periods of relaxation in abdominal rigidity. There is usually a history of repeated attacks of mild abdominal pain, and vomiting is not as constant a symptom as in appendicitis. In general it may be said that mild symptoms, general rather than sharply defined local tenderness, cervical adenitis and an upper respiratory infection are more suggestive of mesenteric lymphadenitis than of appendicitis, but it is safer to operate and find only an adenitis than to miss the diagnosis in acute appendicitis.

However subject to criticism the term chronic appendicitis may be, a condition characterized by irregularly occurring abdominal pain, digestive disturbances, changed disposition, and interference with nutrition is occasionally encountered which is completely relieved by the removal of the appendix. Appendices removed under these circumstances and occasionally those removed during abdominal operations for other conditions will often show under careful special methods of staining definite nerve lesions consisting of hyperplasia of the nerve tissue in the mucosa or localized neuromas,[66] which may well cause reflex disturbances of digestion and pain referred to other parts of the abdomen.

It has been frequently emphasized that early diagnosis of intussusception is a prime factor in successful operative treatment and that early diagnosis depends upon both the profession's and the laity's becoming intussusception conscious. The most suggestive symptom is severe, intermittent, colicky pain in a strong, previously well baby. The infant shows pallor and the appearance of shock during the attacks but at first appears normal and happy between attacks. The severity of symptoms increases, and the characteristic sausage-shaped mass appears in the upper abdomen together with scanty mucous stools tinged with blood. When the diagnosis is made early, reduction can be accomplished in about 50 per cent of the cases by rectal injection of normal saline solution. In a series of 210 cases the average duration of symptoms in cases which yielded to this treatment was sixteen hours[67] while the average duration of those which could not be so reduced was thirty-one hours. All preparations for operation should be made and the infant anesthetized. With the container at a height of three and a half feet the solution is allowed to run in-slowly for three or four minutes, then is expelled, and the injection is repeated a second and third time. The appearance of flatus is a reasonably sure indication that reduction has taken place. Another indication of reduction is an increase of 1½ to 2 inches in the circumference of the abdomen which does not disappear with the return of the solution. This increase is dependent upon the passage of some of the solution through the ileocecal valve and is determined by measuring the abdomen before and after reduction. If there is doubt as to whether reduction has been accomplished, a small incision should be made and the abdomen should be explored. In cases where a confirmatory operation is not done, satisfactory evidence of reduction may be obtained by administering a teaspoonful of powdered charcoal before the child leaves the table. The charcoal may be recovered by enema about four hours later. Hipsley has not found the use of barium under fluoroscopic observation of any advantage over saline. When barium is used, reduction can be observed and its progress assisted by kneading and massage during the introduction of the enema.[68] This procedure is probably safer in recurrent intussusception than in the usual acute type on account of the temptation to be too vigorous when progress becomes slow and the eye is not able to determine the condition of the bowel wall.

Irreducible intussusception is encountered more frequently in older children and in the ileac type, in whom the symptoms are more likely to be indefinite and the diagnosis delayed. There is usually vomiting without fever, abdominal rigidity or distention and a somewhat tender abdominal mass can be felt.[69] In four such cases the bowel was gangrenous, all patients recovering after resection or lateral anastomosis. The intussusception passed in one instance and was apparently absorbed in two. There is no tendency to peritonitis or hemorrhage when the bowel is left in place following lateral anastomosis; therefore procedures such as splitting the bowel with removal of the intussusception, enterostomy, or exteriorization are not favored. A record of four consecutive recoveries from this very serious condition is unusual to say the least, a factor being perhaps the age of the children, two and one-half to twelve years.

Intussusception may be initiated in later life by a Meckel's diverticulum which has caused intestinal hemorrhage and pain in childhood suggesting gastric or duodenal ulcer.[70] If a careful roentgenographic study fails to reveal a gastric or duodenal ulcer or no other cause can be found for gross or occult blood in the stool a Meckel's diverticulum should be considered present. It may not be visualized following ingestion of barium because the entrance is so directed that intestinal contents rarely enter. The diverticulum should be removed at a time of choice because of the ever present danger of perforation, hemorrhage, or intestinal obstruction.

Persistent vomiting during the first few days of life usually indicates atresia rather than pyloric stenosis. When the atresia occurs in the duodenum the vomitus may contain bile and after the first few hours usually contains blood. The blood is thought to come from mucosal vessels ruptured by the extreme gastric distention and peristalsis. The diagnosis is easily corroborated by the roentgenogram which shows a dilated stomach and duodenum with absence of gas in the intestine. The defect is often associated with other anomalies, such as malrotation of the intestine, fetal type of mesentery, multiple atresias, and fetal position of the cecum.[71, 72] Early operation has not given as good results as when it is delayed for one or two weeks, nutrition being maintained by intravenous or rectal injections.

Early jaundice which grows progressively deeper is usually due to a congenital obstruction of the bile ducts[73] either by a plug of mucus or bile or from atresia. The presence of bile in the stools or urine is no evidence of patency of the ducts as it may be excreted from the blood in sufficient quantity to give positive tests. Other conditions which cause early jaundice are icterus neonatorum, erythroblastosis, and hemolytic icterus, in all of which the diagnosis becomes apparent within a few days, whereas the jaundice due to a congenital obstruction is not associated with other symptoms or signs but continues to increase gradually. There is no harm in waiting for a month or two if necessary to rule out other conditions, and to improve the nutrition of the infant. The operation may be performed at the age of three or four months, although one child in a series of forty-five cases lived for a year before operation. At operation the obstructing plug may be dislodged by distending the duct with saline solution, or in cases of atresia an anastomosis with the duodenum may be possible. When there is atresia of the hepatic duct, the results are not as satisfactory as when the common duct is involved. In only about one-third of the cases was the condition suitable for surgery, and of these, 60 per cent recovered. If the ducts are patent, a complete absence of the gallbladder and cystic duct may cause no symptoms and be discovered accidentally.[74]

An interesting observation with a possible bearing upon Hirschsprung's disease has been recorded in the case of a young adult having a stricture of the anus due to a burn in infancy.[75] Typical symptoms of the disease gradually developed, and operation at the age of seven and one-half years to relieve the stricture failed to affect them. Several years later a sympathectomy was completely successful. The interesting point is the possible effect of long-continued irritation of the anal nerve endings upon the neuromuscular mechanism of the large bowel and whether it may suggest a possible cause of Hirschsprung's disease. Treatment by section of the sympathetic nerves is more satisfactory than bowel resection because it is productive of less shock, permits shorter hospitalization, and is physiologically more rational. It is preferably done during childhood before faulty bowel function has become too thoroughly established.[76]

In the diagnosis of intestinal obstruction or of ileus, roentgenography gives valuable assistance, permitting recognition of the condition before clinical symptoms have advanced to a point where surgical relief is difficult.[77] Gas and liquid levels can be seen in the upright or side positions and give an indication of the location of the obstruction. They are more marked in strangulation obstruction than in the simple type. Moderate general distention is seen normally in children under the age of two years and is rather common after any abdominal operation.

Chronic duodenal ileus is a condition in which the attempt to obtain relief by surgery is usually unsatisfactory.[78] It is characterized by marked gastric and duodenal distention, vomiting, gastric retention, anorexia and malnutrition and may persist for several years. It is usually due to compression of the duodenum by a peritoneal band or by the root of the mesentery containing the superior mesenteric artery, in which case surgery can accomplish nothing. In the newborn it is to be differentiated from duodenal atresia by the fact that a thin trickle of barium will be seen to pass gradually through the obstructed region, and the same method in older infants will rule out pyloric stenosis, the opaque medium passing readily into the duodenum. Treatment by gastric lavage with 1 per cent sodium chloride at twelve-hour intervals for several days usually gives marked relief. The interval may then be lengthened to two or three days for about three months, but if distention and vomiting recur the more frequent washings must be resumed. Most cases improve under this treatment and the improvement tends to become permanent at about the age of eight years.

The possibility of duodenal ulcer should be considered if an infant or small child has a history of digestive disturbances and chronic, vague, recurrent pain in the abdomen.[79] There may be occasional vomiting and the passage of blood by bowel. Perforation may occur, giving symptoms of shock, with marked epigastric rigidity and tenderness without distention, and operation should be performed at once. When perforation occurs in the newborn the diagnosis is difficult and is rarely made except at autopsy.

Perforation of the jejunum may occur as a result of trauma.[80] Suggestive symptoms are steadily rising pulse rate, vomiting, local or general rigidity, and severe persistent abdominal pain, although in some instances pain is absent in the early stages. There is not usually a great escape of intestinal contents on account of the reduced peristalsis and the eversion of the mucosa, and the presence of shifting dullness is much more indicative of massive hemorrhage from torn mesenteric vessels than of intestinal contents. No operative procedures should be instituted until the initial shock has been relieved.

While it is well known by the profession that most swallowed foreign bodies pass spontaneously, it will no doubt be a relief to many a distracted mother to know that in an observed series of 849 cases this occurred 818 times and that the mere presence of a foreign body in the stomach is not an indication for removal.[81] Among the few objects which may require surgery may be mentioned radium, bodies so long that they cannot pass the angles of the duodenum, and a matted mass of several articles. The progress of any ordinary object can be checked by roentgenography, and gastrotomy should be performed only if the object cannot be removed by gastroscopy or if it seems unsafe or otherwise inadvisable to allow it to remain.

OTHER ABDOMINAL CONDITIONS

In early suspected peritonitis or when it is desirable to obtain definite information regarding the causative organism or probable source of the infection diagnostic aspiration of the abdomen is a valuable aid.[82] There is little danger of injuring the intestine if the puncture is made below the level of the umbilicus using an ordinary spinal needle with an obtuse bevel and if the point of the needle is turned to lie parallel with the parietal peritoneum as soon as it is felt to enter the abdomen. When the amount of peritoneal exudate is small, it is usually more easily found against the parietal peritoneum, and often only a drop or two is obtainable. A smear and culture should be made, of which the former is more essential for immediate diagnosis,

The failure to obtain fluid should not be considered as evidence against the presence of peritonitis or permitted to outweigh other clinical evidence, but a positive result gives a definite basis upon which to outline treatment. "One may dispute about symptoms, but one cannot take issue with a drop of pus containing great numbers of cocci." It is particularly to be emphasized that a positive finding is rarely, if ever, to be used as an indication for laparotomy for the surgical treatment of peritonitis is productive of higher mortality than the nonsurgical. The value of the procedure lies in the information which it gives as to the causative organism and the consequent ability to institute appropriate specific measures. Particularly is this so in the early diagnosis of pneumococcal peritonitis.

When peritonitis is found upon opening the abdomen, stimulation of the reticuloendothelial system by peptone broth has resulted in a high percentage of good results.[83] In a series of 43 cases including several children, there was but one death. This occurred in a ten-year-old child who developed an acute perforating appendicitis during the early stages of an attack of influenza and died on the fourth postoperative day from a generalized infection. Of the 42 cases with recovery one was complicated by bronchopneumonia, and two were complicated by mild symptoms of ileus which cleared up easily. Any treatment of peritonitis which results in uneventful recovery in 39 out of 43 cases and a mortality of only 2.3 per cent deserves careful consideration, even though the series of cases is comparatively small. The solution is made by diluting commercial peptone broth with normal saline, and it is freely introduced into the peritoneal cavity at the time of operation.

Inguinal hernia in infants is not particularly uncommon, but in premature infants it may be serious. In a study of forty-four such cases there were six instances of strangulation or incarceration.[84] Such an occurrence is an indication for immediate surgery regardless of age. It is especially important that when a hernia exists any cause of increased intraabdominal pressure should be relieved. Among these may be mentioned excessive crying, vomiting, straining at stool, and phimosis. In seven infants early circumcision so reduced the straining that the hernia disappeared. Truss treatment is likely to be ineffective if the causes of straining are not first relieved.

With the exception of diabetes, pancreatic lesions are rare in children. That they may occur, however, is evidenced by a report of a primary carcinoma of the pancreas in a fourteen-year-old boy.[85] The usual cachexia of malignancy gradually developed, but there was nothing else to suggest the diagnosis, and the case is mentioned here simply on account of its extreme rarity. Acute pancreatitis, however, is occasionally encountered,[86] giving symptoms of acute onset with severe abdominal pain, persistent vomiting, general abdominal tenderness often without rigidity, and systemic symptoms of shock. The urinary diastatic index is usually high. The condition may follow a septic process elsewhere in the body, and surgery is suggested for the drainage of pancreatic ferments and blood-stained fluid. It would seem wise to refrain from surgical intervention except on very definite indications of abscess formation or peritoneal irritation under which circumstances the preliminary preparation of a drainage tract walled off from the peritoneal cavity is a valuable procedure. Children recover slowly from such upper abdominal surgery and, wherever possible, conservative treatment results in a shorter period of convalescence.

Multiple hemangiomas of the liver causing fatal pulmonary edema are reported in a three-month-old infant.[87] The enlargement of the liver and abdomen was accompanied by vomiting and constipation, and there was a small elevated hemangioma on the right side of the chest. Earlier in this review[38] reference has been made to the possible association of hemangiomas in the underlying organs with similar superficial lesions, and in this case such an association was suggestive in explaining the symptoms.

Abdominal cysts arising from various structures usually cause symptoms by pressure upon adjacent viscera after a gradual painless enlargement of the abdomen. The more common forms are omental, ovarian, mesenteric and enteric, or enterogenous cysts.[88, 89, 90] Diagnosis is often difficult and requires a most careful study including such aids as gastrointestinal and renal studies and aspiration, the final step usually being exploratory laparotomy. A suggestive symptom in cases of enterogenous cysts is pain associated with the taking of food. Mesenteric cysts attached near the intestine occasionally cause intestinal obstruction.

Splenectomy is of proved value for certain conditions which are encountered in childhood, and the indications are reasonably clear.[91] They are, first, to stop a perverted activity of the spleen; second, to check the progress of some obscure pathologic process; third, to relieve the body of an organ grossly enlarged and useless; and fourth, to remove a focus of infection. The best results are obtained in hemolytic icterus and purpura hemorrhagica. In splenic anemia and splenomegaly with gastric hemorrhages results are good when the anemia is associated with leucopenia but not when there is leucocytosis. In sickle-cell anemia there is usually an improvement in symptoms but not in the blood picture. The large size of the spleen in erythroblastic anemia causes so much discomfort that splenectomy often gives welcome relief, but the progress of the disease is not affected. Erythroblastosis of the newborn which does not yield to transfusions has apparently been cured in some instances by splenectomy. In hemolytic icterus it is unwise to undertake splenectomy during a crisis. The operation should be deferred until the red cells and hemoglobin have returned to a reasonably good level.

ORTHOPEDICS

Osteomyelitis causes as great a degree of disability, crippling, and invalidism as tuberculous joints or infantile paralysis, and on account of its serious nature should be equally feared. Early diagnosis is as essential for adequate treatment as in appendicitis, a fact which should be constantly in the minds of the profession and of the laity. The importance and significance of the usual symptoms of appendicitis have been so emphasized by leading surgeons that the general public is becoming appendix-conscious and a similar condition must be brought about if the serious secondary results of osteomyelitis are to be avoided. To this end the dictum should be: Any child under thirteen years of age with pain in an extremity, loss of function, fever, and leucocytosis has acute osteomyelitis until proved otherwise.[92] It is essentially and, in the hematogenous form, almost exclusively a disease of infancy and childhood, and the responsibility for early diagnosis rests upon the general practitioner or pediatrician who first sees the child. Too often the orthopedic surgeon is called to treat the sequelae of neglect: bone necrosis, multiple metastases, fracture, deformity, secondary contractures, and interference with bone growth, with the associated anemia and parenchymatous and cardiac lesions. The visible and palpable signs of inflammation are usually absent at first, with the exception of local tenderness, and there is often a history of previous otitis media or boils. The joints are rarely involved except in older children where the epiphyseal cartilage is thinner and the infection penetrates more easily, making the disease progressively a more urgent and serious problem with the increasing age of the child. In differentiating osteomyelitis from arthritis, it is to be remembered that an infected joint cannot be moved without pain, whereas, when the process is near a joint, painless motion is possible if due care is exercised.

The osteomyelitis of infants differs distinctly from that of older children.[93] The bones are softer, with larger cancellous spaces, and the periosteum is more closely attached. This permits infection to pass more readily through the cortex to the subperiosteal space with more frequent formation of a subperiosteal or soft tissue abscess. In such instances it is often unnecessary to make an opening through the cortex. There is more rapid formation of bone than in older children and with reasonably early drainage there is rapid healing with rare formation of sequestrums. Care must be exercised in choosing the time for drainage as the general condition of the infant is of first importance and a delay of two or three days especially in streptococcic infection may be required to develop an extremely necessary resistance. Such a delay does not necessarily mean a bad result in an infant, whereas too early operation is dangerous. Drainage should be thorough, the wound packed with vaseline gauze, the part immobilized and the local condition left strictly alone for at least one or two weeks. The more infrequent the dressings, the more rapid the recovery in the average case. In older children it is to be remembered that the bone infection is usually a local manifestation of a general process, and operation before the development of general resistance may add the shock of operative trauma to a defense mechanism which is struggling to overcome a septicemia.

The highest mortality occurs in those patients operated upon during the first week of the disease, but nice judgment is necessary as to the time of election for operation, because too much delay favors the formation of multiple foci.[94] As is true with appendicitis, treatment should be based on a knowledge of the pathologic process and an inflexible rule as regards time of operation may usually be considered evidence of a lack of that knowledge. Early operation regardless of positive blood culture or number of areas involved is at times advised in older children, but this may be followed by secondary hemorrhage seven to ten days later. This is a serious complication requiring blood transfusions.[95] In older children when the disease has become firmly established, recurrences are not uncommon, and it has been suggested that in reporting series of cases a terminology similar to that used in analyses of cancer would be desirable, listing cases as five-, ten- or fifteen-year cures.

During the operation it is necessary to keep constantly in mind the characteristics of septicemia, such as the formation of bacterial emboli or of septic thrombi and the effect of toxemia on other organs and on the child as a whole. The location of an embolus or thrombus in a terminal capillary or in a large vessel will determine the amount of bone destruction; rough operative manipulation such as curetting the medulla, the indiscriminate use of chiseling instead of motor-driven instruments, too vigorous gauze sponging, etc., tends to dislodge infected material and favor the formation of multiple secondary lesions especially when general resistance has not yet developed,[97] and the same result may be produced in a lesser degree by too frequent postoperative dressings and lack of immobilization. The value of the Orr treatment may be due in some measure to the formation of a bacteriophage. This suggests the use of stock bacteriophage and excellent results are reported in traumatic primary osteomyelitis of the phalanges following such treatment, frequent injections being used.[98] Staphylococcus antitoxin is recommended if the blood culture is positive, as free circulating toxin has been demonstrated and is a cause of hemolysis.[99] The blood serum of normal adults usually has a high titer, and a transfusion from a person who has recovered from a staphylococcic process supplies a serum of particularly high titer. Such treatment is, of course, not necessary after the blood stream has become sterile and the process has become definitely localized in the bone. Stimulation of the reticuloendothelial system by the use of peptone broth packs, as referred to earlier in this review under the treatment of peritonitis, has been found effective and has interesting possibilities. The use of maggot therapy, although still rather frequently reported,[100] is apparently being supplanted by less discomforting forms of treatment and is being restricted to those conditions requiring removal of necrotic tissue or stimulation of healthy granulation,[101] and again the necessity of judgment and the application of measures based upon a knowledge of the pathologic stage or individual condition rather than the use of routine treatment are emphasized.

In the consideration of postural defects a careful distinction is necessary between the accentuation of normal physiologic curves seen in the earlier years of life and pathologic conditions which are precursors of later deformities.[102] As examples of the former may be mentioned early bowlegs, knock knee and lordosis which should be kept under observation but usually become normal under a proper dietary and hygienic regimen. Flat feet, round shoulders, winged scapulae, and scoliosis, however, belong in a different category and may develop into serious deformities unless recognized and subjected to vigorous and well-supervised treatment, such as corrective shoes, exercises, muscle training, braces, casts, or operative procedures. It is not sufficient to advise parents that children need more out-of-door exercise or should be encouraged to play more. Definite instructions must be given, specific exercises detailed, and periodic supervision required over a sufficiently long period to be sure that the desired results are obtained, a period of observation of two to four years often being necessary.

The effect of ultraviolet radiation upon the healing of bone has been the subject of so much diverse comment, and so much loose information has been disseminated by commercial firms to both the profession and the laity, that a course of animal experimentation was undertaken to clarify the situation.[103] Treatment by means of carbon arc radiation was used in a carefully controlled series of fractures. The period of bone healing was slightly improved, averaging between 5 and 10 per cent less in the treated cases than in the untreated controls; no correlation could be determined between the healing of fractures and the calcium-phosphorus ratio in the blood serum; and healing was definitely retarded by the type of radiation which produced vasodilation, confirming the results following vasodilation produced by sympathectomy.

Fractures about the elbow are rather common in children, and good ultimate function is more dependent upon careful reduction than in fracture of the shaft of long bones, where growth tends to compensate for shortening or moderate deformity.[104] Complete anesthesia and early reduction are essential, and open reduction may be necessary, particularly in fracture of the lateral condyle of the humerus.[105] This fracture is often unrecognized and if unreduced goes on to deformity from irregular growth which may not become apparent until later years. Careful physiotherapy gives excellent results, it being particularly important to avoid forced or vigorous passive motion, to use massage and heat as early as possible, and to encourage active motion as soon as it is safe.[106]

The adolescent period is characterized by a rapid increase in weight and muscle power, which often outstrips the ossification of the epiphyseal lines and results in a number of rather characteristic lesions. Participation in athletics involves falls and sudden muscular exertion which put such strain upon these regions that epiphyseal separation frequently occurs. When the medial epicondyle of the humerus is torn away, it may be drawn downward into the elbow joint by the flexor pronator group of muscles, causing limitation of motion and tenderness at the point of fracture.[107] Open operation is necessary in practically all instances and gives excellent results, whereas disability, limitation of motion, and possible injury to the ulnar nerve occur if the fragment is not replaced. Avulsion of the epiphysis of the lesser trochanter is also caused by direct muscle pull, giving symptoms of generalized pain throughout the entire thigh, local tenderness, and rather marked muscle spasm, which limits all motions of the hip except adduction.[108] The remaining insertion of the muscle prevents any distinct degree of displacement, and fixation in a short spica gives good results, walking with crutches or cane being permitted in one week and the plaster being removed in four weeks.

Slipping of the capital epiphysis of the femur, which also occurs most frequently at this period, is apparently due to trauma and muscle tension, possibly combined with rapid increase in weight.[109] Microscopic study has shown that this condition is not associated with rickets or osteomalacia but that the lesion consists of a fracture through the epiphyseal plate including a small portion of the adjoining osseous tissue. As noted in this review last year, the degree of disability varies with the degree of displacement; bed treatment is always necessary; open operation may be required; and results are not particularly satisfactory, shortening and limitation of motion being not uncommon sequelae.

Avulsion or displacement of the tibial tubercle with occasional fragmentation—Osgood-Schlatter's disease—gives symptoms of local pain, tenderness, and swelling with limitation of motion[110] and requires immobilization with application of heat until the acute symptoms subside. This should be followed by elastic pressure for several weeks and complete healing may require two or three years. Recovery is more rapid if immobilization by splint or plaster is continued four to six weeks.

A sacroiliac syndrome occurring during adolescence is thought to be due to changes in the sacroiliac region resembling those seen in Osgood-Schlatter's disease or in Legg-Perthes' disease.[111] Roentgenographic studies of normal individuals show that the sacroiliac space is wider in children than in adults and that epiphyses develop about the fifteenth or sixteenth year. Symptoms of low back strain appear in children who engage in vigorous activities, the initial injury often being so slight as to escape notice. Forward bending and lateral bending to one side are limited; straight leg raising from a lying position is much restricted and causes severe sciatic pain; there is localized tenderness over the affected sacroiliac region; and there is a limp characterized by a short-stepping gait on the side involved. Without treatment the condition tends to improve gradually but recurs on very slight strain. The best results are obtained by support and protection with restriction from athletics for at least one year.

Congenital dislocation of the hip in infants is successfully reduced in about 80 per cent of cases by fixation in a position of extreme abduction.[112] This places infants in a special class as regards this condition and imposes upon the obstetrician and pediatrician the obligation of early diagnosis. On account of the rounded contour and usual position of flexion of an infant's thighs the usual signs of shortening, absence of the head of the femur from the acetabulum upon palpation, and limitation of abduction from a position of right-angle flexion may easily be overlooked. For that reason special attention should be paid to the hips in the examination of all infants. When facilities are available and in all cases of doubt, a measurement of the acetabular angle is valuable. This is shown on the roentgenogram by drawing a base line through the lowest points of the iliac bones in the acetabular fossae and a line from the upper outer pole of each acetabulum through this lowest point of the iliac bone of the same side. It is essential in taking the roentgenogram that the tube be centered exactly over the middle point of the upper border of the pubis. The angle formed between this oblique line and the base line has been called the acetabular index,[113] but as it is read in degrees it is not a true index and should more properly be called the acetabular angle. In the normal newborn infant this angle averages 27.5 degrees. If it is greater than 30 degrees, there is either an actual or potential dislocation of the hip, and the thigh should be maintained in marked abduction until the acetabulum and head of the femur have become adjusted to each other, and there is clinical evidence of stability. The average acetabular angle as determined by a study of normal children three years of age was 20 degrees, and in children two years of age with congenital dislocation of the hip it was 37.5 degrees.

In older children conditions vary so widely that treatment must be individualized. In general, manipulative reduction is not successful after the fourth year, but it should be attempted in all favorable and even in doubtful cases. When open reduction is necessary, plastic reconstruction of the acetabulum commonly called the shelf operation gives a high percentage of good results, as shown by the absence of pain or limitation of motion within ordinary ranges, and the ability to engage in milder forms of athletics.[114] There are usually a slight limp and a variable amount of shortening. If the structures surrounding the hip are so short that the head is placed in the acetabulum with difficulty or under tension the final results are not good.

Acute purulent infection of the hip joint may follow or complicate a pyogenic process elsewhere in the body, such as otitis media.[115] In addition to the usual signs and symptoms of sepsis, the thigh is flexed, abducted, externally rotated, and all motions are restricted by muscle spasm. There is usually a tender mass, which may be fluctuant, below Poupart's ligament, and the inguinal glands may be palpable and tender. If there is fullness above Poupart's ligament, it may indicate a pelvic extension of the process from the joint. Every means should be employed to improve the general condition and more than one incision may be necessary for adequate drainage. If the arthritis has been of long duration, osteomyelitis of the ilium may occur with the formation of an involucrum so large that it may displace the bladder, or there may be actual perforation by the sharp point of a sequestrum.[116] In any case of osteomyelitis of the ilium, especially if there is pyuria, a cystogram should be made. The shadow of the involucrum may be obscured or confused in the usual roentgenogram by the shadows of the pelvic bones, but the cystogram will show a marked displacement or distortion of the bladder. Even though there is no pyuria in cases showing such displacement, the possibility of perforation should be considered; the involucrum should be opened, the sequestrum removed, and the osteomyelitic lesion drained through an extraperitoneal incision above the pubis. This will prevent perforation, clear up the osteomyelitis and improve the general condition of the child more rapidly than if drainage is done by the usual route over the joint or through the adductor region.

The treatment of tuberculosis of the spine by operative fusion is superior in the final analysis to the nonoperative treatment since cure depends upon ankylosis, and ankylosis cannot take place in the presence of constant motion.[117] Plaster jackets and braces cannot be effective on account of the uncontrollable mechanical influences of respiration and muscle spasm, and exacerbations or progress of the disease are almost certain to occur. Another adverse effect of nonoperative treatment is interference with respiration which prevents proper oxygenation of the blood and tends to lower resistance. Operation in early childhood is apparently not contraindicated, an adequate preoperative period of rest on a frame or in a plaster shell of some two to three years being the controlling factor in determining the time for operation. During the preoperative period the general condition should be brought to the best possible state by thorough antituberculosis measures. The actual technic of the fusion varies with different surgeons, some preferring the Hibbs method supported by an osteoperiosteal graft,[118] and others relying upon a short rigid graft fusing the fewest possible number of vertebrae and allowing the development of compensatory curves above and below the fused area.[119] The length of treatment by operative methods is not materially less than by nonoperative ones as prolonged postoperative rest is essential for cure, but the permanence of results is much more secure and satisfactory.

There is a marked tendency to recurrence in a certain type of clubfoot. In this type the heel is often represented by a dimple rather than a prominence, and there is such an imbalance of muscle groups that normal development is impossible, and the forces of growth are constantly working against the corrective measures.[120] Relapses will occur in spite of good early correction, and later operation will become necessary. This is the type in which muscular growth of the lower leg is much slower than normal and in which prolonged cast treatment usually causes bone atrophy. In the more usual type there are three problems, adduction, inversion, and equinus, each of which should be treated in turn beginning with the adduction.[121] Gentle correction by means of casts and wedging, with frequent changes, produces excellent results in about 90 per cent of these cases. Forcible manipulation under anesthetic causes damage which tends to produce rigidity, and a rigid foot in partial correction is less serviceable than a completely untreated one. In the milder type or in cases seen very early, the method of treatment by elastic traction is often effective.[122] This consists of the use of a sole plate with a projection at the outer side from which an elastic band passes upward to be attached above the knee. Traction is maintained continuously and causes rapid correction and overcorrection. After full correction is obtained, the traction may be discontinued during the day in children who are walking; later a plaster night boot should be prepared and its use continued for several years.

One of the effects of lumbar sympathectomy is to increase the circulation to the legs. This has been found useful in relieving the cold, blue extremities of poliomyelitis. A study has been made to determine whether it will not also cause an increase in the rate of growth of the bones of such legs and thus make the difference in length between the sound and the affected side less noticeable.[123] Varying degrees of improvement occurred: in some the rate of shortening was diminished; in others the rate of growth was normal so that there was no change in the relative length of the two legs; and in a few the growth was more rapid than on the opposite side so that the difference in length was diminished. In one group the shortening progressed in spite of the operation. The factors favorable to good results were considered to be paralysis limited to one lower extremity, a mild or moderate degree of involvement, and operation at the age of six or eight years during the period of rapid growth. Growth depends upon normal muscular activity as well as circulation, and in extreme paralysis there is not enough such activity to permit growth even though the circulation is increased by sympathectomy. Since muscles partially paralyzed respond better when thoroughly warm, whether the heat is applied externally or internally, it would be interesting to compare the effect of external heat and muscle reeducation on a similar series of cases. Comparisons, however, are particularly difficult in this disease because of the variation in severity in different localities and different epidemics, the lack of standards for accurate measurement, the marked influence of psychic factors and the variations in personality and methods of different physiotherapists. With such a diversity of factors influencing the choice of patients and the evaluation of end-results, it is possible to say only that sympathectomy has apparently been a stimulus to growth in some cases, that in others it has done no harm, and that it is impossible to predict for the individual case whether or not it will be of value.

Slipping patella is a condition in which the patella dislocates to the outer side when the knee is flexed. It may cause definite disability. Congenital dislocation or displacement of the patella also occurs and is a somewhat similar condition. There is usually a tight adhesion or band connecting the patella with the intermuscular septum of the external hamstring or with the fascia lata, or both. Operative correction is usually quite satisfactory.[124]

The fate of the average spastic child is deplorable. He is usually dismissed by the examining physician with the statement that this is another case of Little's disease, that very little can be done aside from ordinary care, that he may live a long time or be carried off by some intercurrent disease, and that it would probably be well to send him to an institution. Because the child cannot express himself easily or cannot control the flow of saliva, a diagnosis of mental defect is made, and he is condemned to association with mental defectives or is given about the same intellectual training that is bestowed upon an animal. The parents wander from one medical consultant to another and finally in desperation try anything that attracts easy money by rosy promises. One of the main reasons for the shunning of the spastic child by so many of the members of our profession is that proper treatment calls for so comprehensive a knowledge in such varied fields of medicine and surgery that no one mind is capable of encompassing it all,[125] and the failure to obtain good results is often due to one-sided treatment. There should be a well-rounded team in charge of all such cases, including the orthopedic surgeon, neurosurgeon, medical consultant, dentist, psychologist, and physiotherapist. Endocrine dysfunction and foci of infection require attention; nutrition is partially dependent upon good teeth; knowledge of the intelligence quotient and mental capacity will influence the amount and type of exercise to be recommended; intracranial adhesions or a cyst may require surgery. Only after a thorough study of the individual case is rational and well-planned treatment possible. When normal or fair intelligence is present, physiotherapy and muscle training teach relaxation and control; speech training is necessary in some 15 per cent of cases; occupational therapy is valuable; rest periods or stretching in plaster casts or molds, tenotomies, tenoplasties, and joint stabilization are to be used when indicated. Operations on nerves are of limited usefulness, sympathectomy is unsatisfactory, and transplantation of spastic muscles is disappointing. There are of course occasional cases where there is so great a degree of intracranial damage that little hope can be held out, but the great majority of these unfortunate children can be markedly benefited, and no one should be denied a most thorough examination and careful estimation of the possibilities of improvement. Many of these children have normal or even brilliant minds and what could be more cruel than to condemn casually such an intellect to constant misunderstanding and association with mental defectives?

GENITOURINARY TRACT

Persistent pyuria is the most constant symptom in anomalies of the upper urinary tract and is an indication for a thorough urologic study in any child who does not respond to medical treatment within four weeks.[126] If operation is too long delayed nephrectomy may be necessary when earlier diagnosis might have resulted in saving a functioning portion of the kidney. The prognosis of polycystic kidney is poor, and, in general, it may be said that the less surgery performed the longer the patient will live. A solitary renal cyst may be excised unless it involves the entire organ thus placing it in the class of large fluid tumors of the kidney which should be treated by initial drainage with secondary nephrectomy. An ectopic kidney held down in the pelvis by an anomalous blood vessel must be removed. Incontinence may be due to an ectopic ureteral opening below the vesical sphincter, the ureter being an accessory one and usually draining the upper portion of the kidney. When this portion of the kidney is infected, it may be resected. A ureter ending blindly may give rise to a large abdominal tumor, the correct diagnosis being difficult and being usually made after the abdomen is opened. Strictures, congenital kinks, and aberrant blood vessels occasionally occur and can be relieved by appropriate surgical treatment.

Perinephric abscess causes pain, fever, leucocytosis, and tenderness in the costoiliac region. History of a previous pyogenic process elsewhere in the body is suggestive, and the roentgenogram usually shows a deviation of the spine away from the affected side, elevation of the diaphragm, and the shadow of a mass. There is, however, no definite, pathognomonic sign; abscesses have been found which failed to show typical signs, and abscesses have not been found when supposedly typical signs were present.[127] A fourteen-year-old patient had osteomyelitis of the twelfth rib; a thirteen-year-old one had an infected, ruptured hydronephrosis; and a six-year-old child operated upon after study and repeated consultation showed no local pathologic process.

Tuberculosis of the kidney is not uncommonly associated with surgical tuberculosis elsewhere in the body.[128] The onset is insidious and usually painless, the first sign often being a slight intermittent hematuria. After a variable period frequency and pyuria appear, with perhaps slight loss of weight and gradual impairment of health. The frequency is more noticeable during the day. Incontinence indicates a progressive involvement of the bladder. The diagnosis is confirmed by careful urologic examination and the finding of tubercle bacilli. The condition is often bilateral and always serious, but in suitable cases nephrectomy is advisable and gives good results.

Wilms' tumor is the most common malignant growth in childhood.[129] The onset is painless, and the first sign is usually enlargement of the abdomen by a mass which is firm and not tender. There is usually a mild degree of anemia, but the urinalysis is often normal. By excretory urography the ureter is seen displaced toward the midline, and there is deformity of the kidney pelvis. These tumors are very susceptible to roentgenotherapy, radiation causing a marked and rapid reduction in size. Nephrectomy should be performed during the period of recession as there is always a secondary increase in growth. Two or three postoperative series of radiation should be given at intervals of one month, but recurrence is the rule. An occasional cure is reported, however, and every possible means of eradication should be employed.

About 60 per cent of all valvular obstructions in the posterior urethra or neck of the bladder occur in infants and children under the age of ten years. Such children are usually anemic and undernourished, and give a history of gastrointestinal upsets, dribbling, enuresis, straining on urination, and pyuria.[130, 131] Diagnosis is made by a thorough urologic study. Careful preliminary treatment is necessary, and operation is contraindicated until the general health is excellent and the local condition has been improved as much as possible; flushings, urinary antiseptics, and continuous drainage by indwelling catheter often being necessary. Transurethral operation, using the cautery punch and small instruments adapted to the size of the child, is most satisfactory, and recovery with complete restoration of health is often spectacular.

Infection of the urinary tract by colon bacilli is frequently resistant to the usual urinary antiseptics. Clinical investigation of the use of mandelic acid for this purpose is showing encouraging results.[132] A girl, aged three years, who had urinary stasis with pyelitis, megaloureters, hydronephrosis on one side, uretheral stenosis on the other and a heavy infection with colon bacilli, showed little improvement under treatment by ketogenic diet, methenamine, and ammonium chloride. The urine became completely sterile following the maintenance of a concentration varying between 0.25 and 0.43 per cent of mandelic acid in the twenty-four-hour specimen over a period of ten days. The treatment must be carried out with close attention to detail, it being essential that a high degree of acidity of the urine be maintained and that the fluid intake be not greater than 1,200 c.c. daily. A few patients have had nausea, vomiting, and diarrhea, but under close observation and careful management a high percentage of excellent results have been obtained.

Diverticula of the urethra are rare. A case is reported in a six-month-old infant in whom suppression of the urine was caused by the pressure of the infected diverticulum on the urethra.[133] There was a history of dysuria and dribbling with sudden onset of septic symptoms when the diverticulum became infected, and a tender, rounded, bulging mass in the course of the urethra at the base of the penis, which could be emptied by pressure. Before infection it was not tender. Suprapubic cystotomy was necessary for temporary drainage and diversion of urine while the local condition was being improved, the diverticulum removed, and the urethra repaired. Roentgenography following the injection of an opaque medium is suggested as a diagnostic measure, and removal of the diverticulum before infection has occurred is recommended.

Extensive study and clinical observation have demonstrated that spermatogenesis is absent or at best abnormal in the undescended testis. In experimental animals it has been found to return to normal after the testis is placed in the scrotum, variation in local temperature being a determining factor. Clinical observation suggests that after orchidopexy the human testis becomes fertile, but not to a normal degree,[134] and the obvious difficulty of accurate statistics in unilateral orchidopexy is pointed out. The presence of the testis in the scrotum is not alone an index of fertility, and a clinical study has been made in a series of 336 cases after standards of fertility were established by carefully controlled estimations in normal individuals.[135] Fertility was definitely proved to be far below normal in a high percentage of all cryptorchids, being rated at 10 per cent before orchidopexy. After orchidopexy 82 per cent of individuals were determined to be fertile.

In the hormone treatment of undescended testis there is some tendency to confusion in the standardization of dosage between the gonadotropic pituitary extract and that obtained from pregnancy urine. Both appear to be equally effective in suitable cases, but the former is administered in doses containing 10 rat units[136] as contrasted to the latter which is recommended in doses of 250 to 1,000 rat units.[137, 138] This treatment should be used near the age of puberty, as excessive development and precocious sexual activity may result in younger children from frequent or large doses. The testes increase to the size which is normal for the age, but the increase of the genitals is greater. The diversity of detail in the many reports on the hormone treatment of undescended testis indicates clearly that, since the last word has not yet been said, a clear, accurate statement of indications and technic cannot be made. In general, it is agreed that this form of treatment has distinct value in most cases where there is not a physical impediment to descent; that it is indicated in those cases which show an associated endocrine dysfunction as with Fröhlich's syndrome; that it is not indicated in young children; and that after the age of eleven or twelve years it should be pushed vigorously using frequent and large doses for nine to twelve months before deciding upon surgical treatment. It may be necessary to discontinue treatment for a period of three months after a course of six to nine months to avoid a loss of sensitivity to the stimulus and possibly to prevent gonadic atrophy which has been observed in experimental animals after prolonged treatment. In some instances orchidopexy has seemed indicated after the testis has descended in response to the hormone treatment to prevent a secondary retraction when treatment is discontinued. There is usually a distinct improvement in the general condition with decrease of weight when there has been obesity, increase when there has been underweight, and improved mental reaction; the latter, however, may well be entirely psychologic in older patients.

When surgery is necessary, the Torek technic is generally considered best for the great majority of cases. The transplantation operation, however, has been advocated,[139] the contention being that the scrotal septum exercises elastic traction. In this operation the testicle is passed through an opening in the septum and fixed by suturing the tunica albuginea to that of the normal testis, thus placing both testes in one side of the scrotum. When the Bevan operation is chosen, it is particularly necessary to cut the lower margin of the internal ring and separate very thoroughly the fibers, which will be found just within the abdomen beneath the peritoneum attached to the cord, preventing the descent of the testis.[140]

The question of malignancy in the undescended testis has been thoroughly discussed at great length. A particularly careful and unbiased analysis of approximately 40,000 hospital admissions of male patients shows that tumors of the testis occur twenty times as frequently in undescended as in normally located testes.[141] Two per cent of patients with undescended testes developed testicular tumors, and only 0.01 per cent of testicular tumors occurred in persons with normally descended testes. Other factors are concerned, however, and it was not determined whether all undescended testes are potentially malignant or whether the factor of nondescent is the determining factor in the development of malignancy.

The treatment of hypospadias requires many operative stages, and it is well to be certain that the parents of a child so afflicted understand this fact distinctly. If there is contraction of the ventral side of the penis, this deformity should be corrected before the age of two years after which three or four years should be allowed for development of the parts before plastic reconstruction of the urethra is begun.[142, 143] Several methods are available, and the choice for the individual case will depend upon the type and degree of the defect and the experience of the surgeon. The technic is difficult and requires special skill and careful observation of the principles of plastic surgery, but reasonably satisfactory results can be obtained. To be classed as satisfactory, the urethra should be of full length and adequate caliber, and the meatus should be at or near the normal position of the frenum. The attempt to bring the urethra through the glans so that the meatus shall be in the normal position involves the danger of hemorrhage and hence is inadvisable in most instances. The parents are usually concerned regarding ultimate function, and they may be assured that with the physical result mentioned function will be normal.

Cysts or canals of the genitoperineal raphe may be found in young children.[144] They occur at any point along the midline of the perineum, scrotum, or ventral surface of the penis and are usually symptomless unless infected. They are lined with dermoid or mucous cells, depending upon their origin. They do not communicate with the urethra and hence do not cause pyuria even when infected, but they sometimes cause pressure upon the urethra. If infected, they should be laid open widely; but, if uninfected or if the infection is subsiding or chronic, excision is advisable and is followed by rapid healing.

Malignant tumors other than those of the kidney are rare in infancy. Myosarcoma of the prostate in an infant eight months old caused suddenly developing suppression of urine with pain, straining, and edema of the perineum.[145] The rapidly growing mass caused death in about three weeks in spite of suprapubic and perineal incisions. Carcinoma of the uterus in an infant fourteen months of age caused vaginal bleeding, discharge of varying amount and foul odor, and a palpable mass on rectal examination.[146] Deep roentgenotherapy was of little effect, and after one year metastases and a rapid increase in growth took place with death at the age of thirty-two months. The possibility of hysterectomy was not mentioned.

The sex-linked characteristic of hemophilia has stimulated study of the treatment of this condition with female sex hormones and placental extracts.[147, 148] Theelin has been found to be the most potent ovarian extract. The oil solution is the preparation of choice, as the aqueous solution has little effect. It is available in 1 c.c. ampules containing 1,000 international units each. Marked improvement or complete control of bleeding in hemophiliacs and nonhemophiliacs usually follows the injection of one ampule every two hours for three or four doses. If the condition is urgent, two ampules may be given at the first dose. Severe stinging pains at the site of the injection may be prevented by drawing 4 or 5 drops of novocaine into the syringe after the theelin, injecting it first, and waiting some thirty seconds before injecting the theelin. A blood coagulant extract of human placenta has proved effective in eleven of fifteen cases of hemophilia.[148] Oral administration is effective in fifteen or twenty minutes, whereas the effect of intramuscular injection may not be apparent for several hours. Extreme care is necessary to avoid entering a vein as this has proved fatal in experimental animals. The good effect remains for two to nine days, and the treatment may be repeated, children having been able to live normal, active lives for a period of several months under the continued administration of this material.

The treatment of hemangiomas depends upon the size and type of the growth.[149] An experience extending over four and one-half years and including 697 cases indicates that 80 per cent of port-wine marks are cured or markedly improved by treatment with the Kromayer light; over 50 per cent of the spongy, capillary type are cured by carbon-dioxide snow; and endothermy under anesthesia is effective in the large, lobulated ones or those having raised purplish bases. Excision is advisable when the location and size are favorable. The results from treatment by radiation and fulguration have not been as satisfactory as by these other methods, as the sequel is often rather marked scarring. The treatment by the Kromayer light and carbon-dioxide snow requires many stages over a long period of time but usually results in a skin slightly smoother than normal without scar contraction.

TREATMENT

In determining the prognosis and treatment of many conditions, the blood sedimentation rate is of great value and should be more generally used.[150] The cause of this reaction has not been definitely determined, but sufficiently extensive observations have been made to bring out a number of facts regarding it. The test should be done with exactness and interpreted with the knowledge that minor variations are usual and are not significant. In the newborn, sedimentation is normally slow, but for children and adolescents the normal values are the same as for adults. Changes in the sedimentation rate occur more slowly than changes in the leucocyte count and temperature, and the return to normal is slower. Complications developing in the course of an acute infection cause a rapid increase in the sedimentation rate. In simple catarrhal inflammation or in the early stages of acute inflammation of the appendix, it is normal. In joint tuberculosis it is increased, providing a valuable differential point between this condition and Kohler's or Legg-Perthes' disease. It is especially useful in indicating the presence of occult organic disease and in estimating the progress of chronic infections, such as tuberculosis or rheumatic fever. Its value is increased when it is used in conjunction with the Schilling blood count, and these two tests should be considered as supplementary. A series of tests is better than isolated ones.

In the treatment of chronic staphylococcic infections of the skin, staphylococcus toxoid has given good results.[151] It is recommended in gradually increasing weekly doses beginning with 0.05 c.c., controlling the dose by the patient's response and general condition. The toxoid gradually deteriorates and will lose 40 per cent of its antigenic power in six months even when kept in the ice box.

A study of the treatment of wounds by hypertonic solutions of sodium chloride or magnesium sulphate applied as wet dressings indicates that they are of little value.[152] With the lower concentrations the layers of gauze in contact with the wound soon become isotonic, and even with high concentrations the strength of the solution in the innermost layers is markedly reduced. The amount of water which can be withdrawn from a fresh wound is 1.2 to 1.5 c.c. per square inch of surface per hour, regardless of the degree of hypertonicity, and with granulating surfaces there is great variation. As water leaves the tissues, the concentration of serum becomes greater, and there is soon a return flow of a weak solution of salts, according to the laws of osmosis, and the tissues become boggy and edematous. The effect on phagocytosis could not be determined, but the action of the hypertonic solution does not extend into the deeper tissues where active infection is often located.

Contused, lacerated wounds, and recent burns which are contaminated may be treated effectively by cod liver oil dressings.[153] Gauze saturated with oil is applied directly to the wound and on a burn where a minimum of manipulation is desirable it may be applied without preliminary removal of the greasy detritus which is often the result of first-aid treatment. At the end of twenty-four hours the superficial dressings are removed, and the lower layers of gauze are resaturated with oil. Changing of dressings once in forty-eight hours is usually sufficient. Cod liver oil is bacteriostatic and stimulates the formation of healthy granulations. Epithelialization proceeds rapidly with formation of a smooth scar without pigmentation even in third-degree burns. Granulations may become exuberant at the end of a week, and some other type of dressing may become necessary to inhibit them. It seems possible that the action of cod liver oil may be similar to that of peptone broth in stimulating activity of the reticuloendothelial system.

Of especial value in children is the novocaine pack as applied to minor wounds requiring suture.[154] After oozing has been controlled by pressure or adrenalin, gauze soaked in novocaine is applied directly to the wound. Any available solution from 1 to 5 per cent may be used, effective anesthesia for a distance of nearly 1 cm. from the edges of the wound being obtained in from five to eight minutes, depending upon the strength of the solution. It may be used before cleansing, making that procedure less painful, and since distortion of the tissues by infiltration is avoided it is possible to obtain better cosmetic results.

The treatment of surgical shock is directed primarily toward the restoration and maintenance of blood volume which is accomplished satisfactorily in most instances by the intravenous administration of saline and dextrose solutions.[155] Blood transfusions and the use of acacia solutions are of great value, but caution is necessary in the case of the latter that it be not used in too large amounts. The use of sodium bicarbonate solutions intravenously is not advisable, but 10 per cent alcohol in a solution of 10 per cent dextrose is recommended. The administration of alcohol in this manner is rather unusual, and it is doubtful whether it possesses any advantage over dextrose combined with insulin, as whatever value it may have is no doubt due to its being a quickly available, diffusible carbohydrate.

In surgical shock, fluid does not usually leave the body, and the problem consists in returning it to circulation. In dehydration from other causes, however, it is often necessary to supply salts as well as fluid. This is particularly true in children, in whom the necessity of fluid for the maintenance of normal function is even greater than in adults. The loss of fluid from discharging wounds and vomiting should be estimated and careful attention paid to blood concentration and urinary output when there is the least possibility of dehydration. A loss of fluid amounting to 6 per cent of the body weight produces a serious dehydration and is often accompanied by albumin, blood, and casts in the urine, indicating that there is insufficient fluid to maintain normal kidney function.[156] In the presence of these signs water must be supplied in plentiful amounts in as short a time as possible. If vomiting has been a factor in the dehydration, sodium chloride should be supplied until the blood chemistry is normal but not in greater amounts on account of the danger of causing edema. If more fluid is necessary, glucose solution may be used as the glucose will be oxidized leaving the water to supply the body tissues. The necessary amount can be determined by the urinary output, as the kidney excretes only what is left after the tissue requirements are satisfied, a daily excretion of about 1,500 c.c. being a reasonable standard. When the necessity for fluid is acute, 5 per cent glucose in saline intravenously is widely used.[157] Ten per cent glucose in saline is used to supply carbohydrate and for the treatment of acidosis or insulin shock. Dextrose in Ringer's solution or Hartmann's solution is used when other salts are needed. Opinions regarding the speed of large volume injections vary, 500 c.c. per hour being an average rate for adults. A safe rule is that dextrose solutions should not be injected at a more rapid rate than ⅓ gm. per hour per pound of body weight. Hypertonic solutions should be given more slowly than isotonic ones. In shock, fluids may be injected at the rate of 20 to 40 c.c. per minute until the pulse reacts, then more slowly. The temperature of the solution is not important when it is given slowly.

Fluids may be given by continuous intravenous infusion for periods of several days, but this method should be used only with judgment and under careful observation as it is not without danger.[158] There should be no cessation of flow through the needle since this favors backflow of blood and clot formation. General edema or edema of the lungs may occur from an overburdened circulation or improper proportion of salts. Kidney irritation as indicated by hematuria may follow a too prolonged intravenous administration of 5 or 10 per cent glucose, and embolism has been reported. In general, it is better to use intermittent rather than continuous intravenous infusion, the indication for the latter usually being a paucity of suitable veins and the probability that the treatment will be required for a long period.

The value of blood transfusions is unquestioned, particularly in the treatment of shock and hemorrhage, and transfusion may be used to good advantage in many of the infectious and nutritional disturbances in children. The indirect gravity citrate method is perhaps the most suitable for general use as it is less expensive and requires less apparatus and less teamwork.[159] Cross-matching should be done even though donor and recipient are in the same group, as occasionally there is incompatibility due to difference in subgroups. Even with this precaution, nonspecific reactions may occur consisting of rise of temperature from 0.5 to 2 degrees and lasting from a few minutes to an hour. In a series of 207 transfusions such reactions seemed to be beneficial rather than otherwise, and there were no hemolytic reactions. The blood must be kept warm; special care is recommended in preparing and cleansing the apparatus. At variance with the experience in this series in which the value of transfusions in septicemia is questioned is a report that multiple small transfusions every forty-eight hours until the blood culture is negative produce excellent results in septicemia.[160] Transfusions should be begun early before resistance has broken down and metastatic lesions have developed. Immunotransfusions are best. Septicemia, particularly that due to the staphylococcus, is always a serious condition, and the factors influencing individual resistance are so diverse that differences of opinion based on different series of cases are inevitable. Any method of treatment which has produced good results should be reported so that it may be available to others in case of need.

Interesting observations have been made in Russia upon the use of cadaver blood for transfusions.[161] The blood is obtained from persons dying from accidents and may be preserved in the ice box for a period of four weeks. Such blood does not clot and hence does not require citration. There is ample time for Wassermann tests and tests for sterility, and the therapeutic effects are the same as when blood from living donors is used. It may be possible that if regimentation becomes more general in this country or perhaps in cases of extreme emergency cadaver blood will be used, but for the present a certain psychic factor will probably limit the popularity of this procedure.

REFERENCES

1. Penberthy, G. C.: Surgery of Childhood, J. Michigan M. Soc. **35**: 293, 1936.
2. Burton, J. F.: Principles Involved in Surgical Diseases of Newborn, J. Oklahoma M. A. **28**: 406, 1935.
3. Brunkow, C. W.: Contrast Between General Surgery of Infants and Children and That of Adults, Northwest Med. **35**: 259, 1936.
4. Warthin, A. S.: Old Age: The Major Involution, New York, 1929, Paul B. Hoeber.
5. Boland, F. K.: Surgical Diseases of the Gastro-Intestinal Tract in Children, Internat. Clin. **2**: 26, 1936.
6. Beverly, B. I.: Effect of Illness Upon Emotional Development, J. Pediat. **8**: 533, 1936.
7. Maurits, R.: Individualized Anesthesia, J. Michigan M. Soc. **34**: 463, 1935.
8. Sise, L. F., Woodbridge, P. D., and Eversole, U. H.: Cyclopropane; New and Valuable Gas Anesthetic, New England J. Med. **213**: 303, 1935.
9. Griffith, H. R.: Cyclopropane Anesthesia, Anesth. & Analg. **14**: 253, 1935.
10. Lundy, J. S., Tovell, R. M., and Tuohy, E. B.: Annual Report for 1935 of the Section on Anesthesia; Including Data on Blood Transfusion, Proc. Staff Meet., Mayo Clin. **11**: 421, 1936.
11. Marvin, F. W.: Clinical Use of Vinethene, Anesth. & Analg. **14**: 257, 1935.
12. Gwathmey, J. T.: Premedication and Inhalation Anesthesia for Tonsil and Adenoid Operations in Young Children: Humane and Safe Method, Am. J. Surg. **31**: 272, 1936.
13. Jarman, R., and Abel, A. L.: Intravenous Anaesthesia With Pentothal Sodium, Lancet **1**: 422, 1936.
14. Gwathmey, J. T.: Rectal Administration of Evipal Soluble, Am. J. Surg. **32**: 411, 1936.
15. Garrey, W. E. (Boston), and Cohn, R. B.: Use of Sodium Evipal as Anesthetic for Short Surgical Procedures, New England J. Med. **213**: 301, 1935.
16. Mueller, L. B.: Report of 3,000 Cases of Avertin Anesthesia, J. Indiana M. A. **29**: 175, 1936.
17. Boyd, J.: Avertin as Complete Anaesthetic in Children: Survey of 700 Cases, Brit. M. J. **1**: 1120, 1935.
18. Shipway, F. E.: Avertin: Analysis of 1,600 Administrations, Canad. M. A. J. **34**: 2, 1936.
19. Schube, P. G.: Study of Use of Coramine in Dealing With Effects of Barbituric Acid Derivatives, New England J. Med. **214**: 926, 1936.
20. Wood, P. M.: Denarcotization or Resuscitation of Anesthetized Patients, Anesth. & Analg. **14**: 234, 1935.
21. Leech, B. C.: Preanesthetic Medication in Children, Anesth. & Analg. **14**: 283, 1935.

22. Botsford, M. E.: Anesthesia in Infant Surgery, California & West. Med. **43**: 271, 1935.
23. Waldbott, G. L.: Allergic Shock From Local and General Anesthetics, Anesth. & Analg. **14**: 199, 1935.
24. King, H. J.: Convulsions Under Ether Anesthesia, Am. J. Surg. **30**: 182, 1935.
25. Wilson, W. S.: Convulsions Under Ether Anesthesia, Anesth. & Analg. **14**: 281, 1935.
26. Gunn, J., and Hillsman, J. A.: Thermal Burns, Ann. Surg. **102**: 429, 1935.
27. Harkins, H. N.: Bleeding Volume in Severe Burns, Ann. Surg. **102**: 444, 1935.
28. Walsh, J. N.: Treatment of Severe Cutaneous Burns, J. South Carolina M. A. **31**: 189, 1935.
29. Seeger, S. J.: Treatment of Burns, Texas State J. Med. **31**: 488, 1935.
30. Cotter, A. P., and Kimbell, N. K. B.: Tannic Acid-Silver Nitrate Treatment of Burns, New Zealand M. J. **34**: 384, 1935.
31. Turner, A. C.: Contribution to Treatment of Burns, Brit. M. J. **2**: 995, 1935.
32. DeHart, R. M.: Treatment of Burns With Gentian Violet, Virginia M. Monthly **62**: 594, 1936.
33. Coan, G. L.: Ferric Chloride Coagulation in Treatment of Burns, With Résumé of Tannic Acid Treatment, Surg. Gynec. Obst. **61**: 687, 1935.
34. Rose, H. W.: Initial Cold Water Treatment of Burns, Northwest Med. **35**: 267, 1936.
35. Frazier, C. H.: Brain Tumors in Children, Arch. Pediat. **53**: 295, 1936.
36. Bucy, P. C., and Buchanan, D. N.: Simulation of Intracranial Tumor by Lead Encephalopathy in Children, With Remarks Concerning Surgical Treatment of the Latter, J. A. M. A. **105**: 244, 1935.
37. Evans, P. R.: Post-Operative Intracranial Thrombosis in Childhood, Lancet **2**: 12, 1935.
38. Greenwald, H. M., and Koota, J.: Associated Facial and Intracranial Hemangiomas, Am. J. Dis. Child. **51**: 868, 1936.
39. Mason, J. M.: Acute Empyema in Children, J. A. M. A. **105**: 1114, 1935.
40. Maes, U., Veal, J. R., and McFetridge, E. M.: Mortality of Empyema; Analysis of 100 Consecutive Deaths From Records of Charity Hospital in New Orleans, J. Thoracic Surg. **4**: 615, 1935.
41. Bodley, J. W.: Empyema in Children, South. Surgeon **5**: 1, 1936.
42. Strong, R. A.: Aspiration Treatment of Empyema in Children, J. Iowa M. Soc. **25**: 334, 1935.
43. Burpee, C. M.: Treatment of Empyema in Children by Aspiration, J. M. A. Georgia **24**: 326, 1935.
44. Coyle, J. A., and Sycamore, L. K.: Foreign Bodies in the Air and Food Passages, New England J. Med. **214**: 677, 1936.
45. Butler, E. F.: Recognition of Radioparent Foreign Bodies at Periphery of Lung, Am. J. Surg. **29**: 285, 1935.
46. Lewis, C. K.: Diagnosis and Removal of Foreign Bodies From Lower Air Passages, J. Tennessee M. A. **29**: 48, 1936.
47. Jackson, C.: Recent Advances in Bronchoscopy of Children, Pennsylvania M. J. **39**: 685, 1936.
48. Truesdale, P. E.: Diaphragmatic Hernia in Children With Report of 13 Operative Cases, New England J. Med. **213**: 1159, 1935.
49. Weinberg, J., and Hamilton, H.: Congenital Diaphragmatic Hernia in Infant, With Successful Operation, Nebraska M. J. **20**: 241, 1935.
50. Stephens, H. D.: Diaphragmatic Hernia in Children, Australian & New Zealand J. Surg. **5**: 161, 1935.
51. Landon, J. F.: Eventration of Diaphragm, J. Pediat. **8**: 593, 1936.
52. Gage, M., and Ochsner, A.: Surgical Treatment of Congenital Tracheo-Esophageal Fistula in New-Born, Ann. Surg. **103**: 725, 1936.
53. Rosamond, E.: Appendicitis in Childhood, J. Arkansas M. Soc. **32**: 35, 1935.
54. Risser, A. S.: Acute Appendicitis in Infants and Children, J. Oklahoma M. A. **28**: 254, 1935.
55. Bauer, E. L.: Appendix Vermiformis in Infancy and Childhood, Pennsylvania M. J. **38**: 787, 1935.
56. Heyl, J. H.: Acute Appendicitis in Infants and Children Under 5 Years of Age, New York State J. Med. **36**: 332, 1936.
57. Helmholz, H. F.: Diagnosis of Acute Appendicitis in Children, Journal-Lancet **55**: 681, 1935.
58. Barbour, P. F.: Acute Appendicitis in Children, South. M. J. **29**: 500, 1936.

59. Felsen, J.: Appendicular Form of Bacillary Dysentery, With Notes on Mesenteric Adenitis and Inflammation of Distal Portion of Ileum, Am. J. Dis. Child. **50**: 661, 1935.
60. Skrentny, S. H.: Acute Appendicitis in Childhood, J. Indiana M. A. **29**: 122, 1936.
61. Leonard, E. D., and Derow, S.: Mortality Factors in Acute Appendicitis: Study of 1,000 Cases, New England J. Med. **214**: 52, 1936.
62. Pattison, A. C.: Factors in Mortality of Acute Appendicitis, Ann. Surg. **103**: 362, 1936.
63. Collins, D. C.: Mesenteric Lymphadenitis in Adolescents Simulating Appendicitis, Canad. M. A. J. **34**: 402, 1936.
64. Coleman, E. P.: Diagnosis of Mesenteric Lymphadenitis, Illinois M. J. **68**: 408, 1935.
65. Probstein, J. G., and Gruenfeld, G. E.: Acute Regional Ileitis, Ann. Surg. **103**: 273, 1936.
66. Simard, L. C.: On Frequency of Nervous Lesions of Vermiform Appendix: "Neuro-Appendicopathy," Canad. M. A. J. **33**: 518, 1935.
67. Hipsley, P. L.: Intussusception, Brit. M. J. **2**: 717, 1935.
68. Miller, M. M., and Beatty, C. L.: Recurrent Acute Intussusception: Treatment With Barium Enemas and Massage Under Fluoroscopic Control, Ohio State M. J. **31**: 759, 1935.
69. Elliot-Smith, A.: Irreducible Intussusception: Report of 4 Cases, Lancet **2**: 992, 1935.
70. Greenblatt, R. B., Pund, E. R., and Chaney, R. H.: Meckel's Diverticulum: Analysis of 18 Cases With Report of One Tumor, Am. J. Surg. **31**: 285, 1936.
71. Kellogg, E. L., and Collins, J. T.: Congenital Duodenal Obstruction, Am. J. Surg. **30**: 369, 1935.
72. Donovan, E. J.: Congenital Atresia of Duodenum in New-Born: Duodenojejunostomy, Ann. Surg. **103**: 455, 1936.
73. Ladd, W. E.: Congenital Obstruction of Bile Ducts, Ann. Surg. **102**: 742, 1935.
74. Danzis, M.: Congenital Absence of Gall Bladder, Am. J. Surg. **29**: 202, 1935.
75. Fowler, L. H., and Hanson, W. A.: Megacolon, With Report of Traumatic Case Treated by Left Lumbar Sympathectomy, Minnesota Med. **18**: 646, 1935.
76. Rankin, F. W.: Treatment of Hirschsprung's Disease, Kentucky M. J. **33**: 474, 1935.
77. Schneider, H. H.: Use of Roentgen Ray in Diagnosis of Ileus, J. Kansas M. Soc. **37**: 148, 1936.
78. Miller, R., and Gage, H. C.: Chronic Duodenal Ileus in Infancy and Childhood, Lancet **2**: 115, 1935.
79. Tashiro, K., and Kobayashi, N.: Duodenal Ulcer in Infancy and Childhood: Case of Perforated Duodenal Ulcer in Child of 7, Am. J. Surg. **29**: 379, 1935.
80. Counseller, V. S., and McCormack, C. J.: Subcutaneous Perforation of Jejunum, Ann. Surg. **102**: 365, 1935.
81. Clerf, L. H.: Foreign Bodies in Stomach: Removal by Peroral Endoscopy, Surg. Gynec. Obst. **61**: 210, 1935.
82. Denzer, B. S.: Abdominal Puncture in Diagnosis of Peritonitis in Childhood, J. PEDIAT. **8**: 741, 1936.
83. Feagles, H., and Bain, C. G.: Peptone Broth in Peritonitis, Northwest Med. **35**: 62, 1936.
84. Goldberg, S. L., and Rambar, A. C.: Strangulated Inguinal Hernias in Premature Infants, Am. J. Surg. **32**: 478, 1936.
85. Smith, W. R.: Primary Carcinoma of Pancreas in Children: Report of Case in Boy 14½ Years of Age, With Generalized Metastases, Am. J. Dis. Child. **50**: 1482, 1935.
86. Dobbs, R. H.: Acute Pancreatitis in Childhood: Report of Case, Lancet **2**: 989, 1935.
87. Howard, W. A.: Multiple Hemangio-Endotheliomas of the Liver, J. PEDIAT. **8**: 588, 1936.
88. Horgan, J.: Cysts of Omentum: Review and Report of Case, Am. J. Surg. **29**: 343, 1935.
89. Livingston, L. G.: Mesenteric Cyst: Case Report, South. M. J. **28**: 1028, 1935.
90. Mayer, O. B.: Enteric Cysts, Ann. Int. Med. **9**: 797, 1935.
91. Penberthy, G. C., and Cooley, T. B.: Results of Splenectomy in Childhood, Ann. Surg. **102**: 645, 1935.

92. Dillehunt, R. B.: Osteomyelitis in Infants, Surg. Gynec. Obst. **61**: 96, 1935.
93. Green, W. T., and Shannon, J. G.: Osteomyelitis of Infants: Disease Different From Osteomyelitis of Older Children, Arch. Surg. **32**: 462, 1936.
94. Wilson, J. C., and McKeever, F. M.: Hematogenous Acute Osteomyelitis in Children, J. Bone & Joint Surg. **18**: 328, 1936.
95. Buzby, B. F.: Acute Hematogenous Osteomyelitis, J. M. Soc. New Jersey **33**: 193, 1936.
96. Weaver, J. B.: Statistical Study of Osteomyelitis at University of Kansas Hospital, J. Kansas M. Soc. **36**: 402, 1935.
97. Owen, W. B.: Diagnosis and Treatment of Osteomyelitis, Ann. Surg. **103**: 1007, 1936.
98. Kirschenmann, J. J.: Osteomyelitis, Am. J. Surg. **29**: 465, 1935.
99. Stookey, P. F., Scarpellino, L. A., and Weaver, J. B.: Immunology of Osteomyelitis, Arch. Surg. **32**: 494, 1936.
100. Robinson, W.: Progress of Maggot Therapy in United States and Canada in Treatment of Suppurative Diseases, Am. J. Surg. **29**: 67, 1935.
101. Ferguson, L. K., and McLaughlin, C. W., Jr.: Maggot Therapy; Rapid Method of Removing Necrotic Tissues, Am. J. Surg. **29**: 72, 1935.
102. Badgley, C. E.: Physiological Postural Deformities in Contrast to Pathologic Postural Deformities, J. Michigan M. Soc. **34**: 469, 1935.
103. Sweeney, H. M., and Laurens, H.: Effect of Carbon Arc Radiation on Healing of Bone, Arch. Surg. **31**: 395, 1935.
104. Goldblatt, D., and Jewett, E.: Injured Child, With Review of 312 Cases, Am. J. Surg. **29**: 11, 1935.
105. Wilson, P. D.: Fracture of the Lateral Condyle of Humerus in Childhood, J. Bone & Joint Surg. **18**: 301, 1936.
106. Ritter, H. H.: Physical Therapy in Surgical Practice, Arch. Phys. Therapy **16**: 715, 1935.
107. Dunlop, J.: Traumatic Separation of Medial Epicondyle of Humerus in Adolescence, J. Bone & Joint Surg. **17**: 577, 1935.
108. Fitchet, S. M.: Fracture of Epiphysis of Lesser Trochanter of Femur, New England J. Med. **213**: 164, 1935.
109. Sutro, C. J.: Slipping of Capital Epiphysis of Femur in Adolescence, Arch. Surg. **31**: 345, 1935.
110. Elward, J. F.: Bilateral Osgood-Schlatter's Disease, Radiol. **26**: 630, 1936.
111. Rogers, M. H., and Cleaves, E. N.: Adolescent Sacroiliac Joint Syndrome, J. Bone & Joint Surg. **17**: 759, 1935.
112. Gill, A. B.: Evaluation of Present-Day Methods of Dealing With Congenital Dislocation of Hip, J. Bone & Joint Surg. **18**: 487, 1936.
113. Kleinberg, S., and Lieberman, H. S.: Acetabular Index in Infants in Relation to Congenital Dislocation of Hip, Arch. Surg. **32**: 1049, 1936.
114. Howorth, M. B.: Shelf Stabilization of Hip: Report of 53 Cases With Particular Emphasis on Congenital Dislocation, J. Bone & Joint Surg. **17**: 945, 1935.
115. Freiberg, J. A., and Perlman, R.: Pelvic Abscesses Associated With Acute Purulent Infection of Hip Joint, J. Bone & Joint Surg. **18**: 417, 1936.
116. Hepler, A. B.: Bladder Displacement Secondary to Suppurative Arthritis of Hip and Osteomyelitis of Pelvic Bones in Children: Operation for Impending Perforation, J. Urol. **35**: 32, 1936.
117. Albee, F. H.: Spinal Tuberculosis: Climatic and Operative Treatment, Am. J. Surg. **30**: 60, 1935.
118. Compere, E. L., and Jerome, J. T.: Treatment of Tuberculosis of Spine in Young Children, Ann. Surg. **102**: 286, 1935.
119. Calvé, J., and Galland, M.: Osteosynthesis in Spinal Tuberculosis, J. Bone & Joint Surg. **18**: 46, 1936.
120. Forrester-Brown, M.: Treatment of Congenital Equinovarus (Club-Foot), J. Bone & Joint Surg. **17**: 661, 1935.
121. Kite, J. H.: Treatment of Congenital Club-Feet, Surg. Gynec. Obst. **61**: 190, 1935.
122. Brown, L. T.: Treatment of Club Feet, J. Bone & Joint Surg. **18**: 173, 1936.
123. Harris, R. I., and McDonald, J. L.: Effect of Lumbar Sympathectomy Upon Growth of Legs Paralyzed by Anterior Poliomyelitis, J. Bone & Joint Surg. **18**: 35, 1936.
124. Ober, F. R.: Slipping Patella or Recurrent Dislocation of Patella, J. Bone & Joint Surg. **17**: 774, 1935.
125. Brockway, A.: Problem of the Spastic Child, J. A. M. A. **106**: 1635, 1936.
126. Campbell, M. F.: Surgical Treatment of Anomalies of Upper Urinary Tract in Children, J. A. M. A. **106**: 193, 1936.

127. Rusche, C. F., and Bacon, S. K.: Unusual Conditions Simulating Perinephric Abscess: With Report of 10 Cases, J. Urol. **34**: 504, 1935.
128. Addison, O. L.: Tuberculosis of Kidney in Childhood, Brit. M. J. **2**: 565, 1935.
129. Priestley, J. T., and Broders, A. C.: Wilms' Tumor: Most Common Malignant Growth Affecting Children, Proc. Staff Meet., Mayo Clin. **10**: 81, 1935.
130. Counseller, V. S., and Menville, J. G.: Congenital Valves of Posterior Urethra, J. Urol. **34**: 268, 1935.
131. Caulk, J. R.: Obstruction at Bladder Neck in Infants and Children, South. M. J. **29**: 142, 1936.
132. Helmholz, H. F.: Successful Treatment by Means of Mandelic Acid of Child With Urinary Stasis and Infection, Proc. Staff Meet., Mayo Clin. **11**: 231, 1936.
133. Kretschmer, H. L.: Diverticula in Anterior Urethra in Male Children, Surg. Gynec. Obst. **62**: 634, 1936.
134. Wangensteen, O. H.: Undescended Testis: Its Fate After Satisfactory Scrotal Anchorage, Ann. Surg. **102**: 875, 1935.
135. MacCollum, D. W.: Clinical Study of Spermatogenesis of Undescended Testicles, Arch. Surg. **31**: 290, 1935.
136. Werner, A. A., et al.: Effect of Gonadotropic Extract of Pituitary in Cryptorchidism, J. A. M. A. **106**: 1541, 1936.
137. Dorff, G. B.: Maldevelopment and Maldescent of Testes: Further Observations on Treatment With Anterior Pituitary-Like Gonadotropic Hormone, Am. J. Dis. Child. **50**: 1429, 1935.
138. Spence, A. W., and Scowen, E. F.: Use of Gonadotropic Hormones in Treatment of Imperfectly Migrated Testes, Lancet **2**: 1335, 1935.
139. McCrea, E. D'A.: Treatment of Undescended Testis, Lancet **2**: 753, 1935.
140. Eisenstaedt, J. S.: Technic of Orchidopexy, Illinois M. J. **69**: 161, 1936.
141. Hinman, F., and Benteen, F. H.: Relationship of Cryptorchidism to Tumor of Testis, J. Urol. **35**: 378, 1936.
142. Cabot, H.: Treatment of Hypospadias in Theory and Practice, New England J. Med. **214**: 871, 1936.
143. Walters, W.: Successful Operations for Hypospadias, Ann. Surg. **103**: 949, 1936.
144. Neff, J. H.: Congenital Canals and Cysts of Genito-Perineal Raphe, Am. J. Surg. **31**: 308, 1936.
145. Ray, E. H.: Sarcoma of Prostate in Infants: Case Report and Brief Review of Literature, J. Urol. **34**: 686, 1935.
146. Lockhart, H. A.: Cancer of Uterus in Childhood, Am. J. Obst. & Gynec. **30**: 76, 1935.
147. De Silva, E. B.: Treatment of Hemorrhage in Hemophiliacs and Nonhemophiliacs With Theelin in Oil: Preliminary Report, Illinois M. J. **69**: 81, 1936.
148. Eley, R. E., Green, A. A., and McKhann, C. F.: Use of Blood Coagulant Extract From Human Placenta in Treatment of Hemophilia, J. PEDIAT. **8**: 135, 1936.
149. MacCollum, D. W.: Treatment of Hemangiomas, Am. J. Surg. **29**: 32, 1935.
150. Wintrobe, M. M.: Erythrocyte Sedimentation Test, Internat. Clin. **2**: 34, 1936.
151. Connor, J. I.: Staphylococcal Infections of Skin and Their Treatment, Brit. M. J. **2**: 1195, 1935.
152. Taylor, F. W.: Hypertonic Wet Dressing: Experimental Study, Surg. Gynec. Obst. **61**: 623, 1935.
153. Steel, J. P.: Cod-Liver Oil Treatment of Wounds, Lancet **2**: 290, 1935.
154. Fritz, M., and Tanner, E. K.: Novocain Pack; Contribution to Therapy of Fresh Accidental Wounds, New York State J. Med. **35**: 1217, 1935.
155. Frazier, C. H.: Modern Treatment of Surgical Shock, J. A. M. A. **105**: 1731, 1935.
156. Coller, F. A., and Maddock, W. G.: Study of Dehydration in Humans, Ann. Surg. **102**: 947, 1935.
157. Cutter, R. K.: Use of Large Volume Intravenous Injections, J. A. M. A. **106**: 1250, 1936.
158. Orr, T. G.: Continuous Intravenous Infusion; Consideration of Its Possible Dangers, Minnesota Med. **18**: 778, 1935.
159. Jones, R. H.: Report of Blood Transfusion Service at University of Colorado School of Medicine and Hospitals, Colorado Med. **32**: 714, 1935.
160. Stenn, F.: Merits of Blood Transfusion in Septicemia, Illinois M. J. **69**: 65, 1936.
161. Yudin, T. I.: Transfusion of Cadaver Blood, J. A. M. A. **106**: 997, 1936.

American Academy of Pediatrics

Proceedings

SIXTH ANNUAL MEETING OF THE AMERICAN ACADEMY OF PEDIATRICS

KANSAS CITY, MO., MAY 11 AND 12, 1936

Round Table Discussion on Childhood Psychiatry

Chairman: Dr. Franklin G. Ebaugh, Denver, Colo.
Assistants: Dr. Leo Kanner, Baltimore, Md., and Dr. James S. Plant, Newark, N. J.

CHAIRMAN EBAUGH.—I want (1) to present briefly the psychobiologic point of view as applied to the handling of children's problems, (2) to outline what is now being done by the departments of pediatrics and psychiatry to prepare students to deal with the behavior problems of children, and (3) to offer some suggestions as to the fundamentals of a psychiatric training program.

Everyone accepts the pediatrician as the general practitioner of childhood. Pediatrics has been defined by Veeder as "that branch of the medical sciences which has to do with factors influencing the growth and development of individuals from birth to maturity," but pediatricians have, in the past, limited their attention principally to the child's physical development—to heart, lungs, kidneys, weight, and body fluids—and have ignored the interesting problems of the child as a behaving or misbehaving personality. They have avoided, in teaching schedules and in clinical practice, the emotional and personality problems of childhood. Yet we all agree that this phase of modern pediatrics is now assuming great significance, since educators, psychologists, and psychiatrists have been accused of taking it over. Furthermore, parents who have always taken their children to the pediatrician for physical care frequently decide to go elsewhere with problems relating to behavior.

The pediatrician has several methods of dealing with this situation: he may be on the defensive, scoff at and belittle the achievements in the field of behavior studies, or he may decide to meet his difficult situation by acquiring an understanding of the principles that underlie the development of the personality, its emotional disorders and their adequate management. But the physician who adopts the second course is often bewildered and antagonized by what Dr. Brennemann has aptly designated as a "confusion of theory and authority." Wishing to enter the field of behavior study, he notices that there are many psychologic schools, each with biased emphasis on one factor or another. He does not know which way to turn and usually loses his interest in a feeling of resignation, deciding to get along as best he can without psychiatric assistance.

For these physicians, who are lost in a confusion of doctrines of focal infection, endocrinology, theoretical brain localization, behaviorism, or the cultural-mythological theories of the various psychoanalytic schools, it seems to me that the present-day emphasis on the psychobiologic point of view in dealing with problems of behavior offers a practical solution. The psychobiologic point of view avoids one-sided approaches and offers no ready-made formulas that can be immediately applied to all children. It deals with demonstrable actualities rather than hypothetical claims and is willing to accept from any worker or any school of thought that which has been satisfactorily proved to be a factual contribution. It adapts its methods to the need of the individual child instead of adapting the child to the rigid postulates of a theory.

In recognizing the importance of psychobiology, I have no intention of belittling the part played by anatomy, histology, or physiology in adding to our understanding of the human organism. What I wish to point out is that they, in themselves, present only single aspects of this highly complex and integrated unit, while psychobiology takes into consideration this unit as a whole, inclusive of all the ''ologies.'' It deals with mentally integrated behavior in its human totality, that totality of the behaving organism to which Meyer refers as ''he,'' ''she,'' ''you,'' or ''I''—in other words the individual or person; and it deals with this individual in his relationships to other behaving individuals. We cannot approach, therapeutically, a mysterious brain center, the location or even existence of which is uncertain, but we can work with a child as a person and with his parents or teachers, as well as with the situation to which the child is reacting in the home, the school, and the community. In the mental development of the child, there are critical periods and successive levels of mental integration or personality formation. In the study of the child at any given moment, we are dealing with every experience the child has had previously, in a genetic-dynamic relationship. In the words of Tennyson's Ulysses, it is literally true that ''we are a part of all that we have met.''

Psychobiologic Methods as Applied to Children's Problems

In the care of the child, how are psychobiologic methods applied? How practicable are these methods for the use of the general practitioner? The psychiatrist has no short cut and but few instruments of precision at his disposal in dealing with behavior problems. From the very nature of the subject matter, the understanding of childhood behavior is a complicated and often laborious business. I do not like the term ''psychiatric technic''; I doubt if such a technic actually exists. The child is brought to the physician's attention with a complaint, which varies from an exanthematous condition, otitis media, whooping cough, lesion of the skin, to constant blinking of the eyes. The means of investigative pursuit do not smack of the metaphysical, nor do they imply special procedures known only to a select few. On the contrary, they embrace the common-sense approach which any physician utilizes in sizing up a problem with which he is confronted. The patient's complaint forms a nucleus about which the study proceeds. We overlook a great deal that is important when we do not give the child and the parent an opportunity to talk. Psychiatrists, therefore, pay particular attention to the complaint, and complaints should always be obtained from several sources. This has been especially emphasized in a recent paper by Kanner.

The significance of the data secured by this method can perhaps best be illustrated by a clinical example:

> Complaint from teacher: ''John is failing in everything. He can't do mental arithmetic.''
>
> Complaint from mother: ''John is slow, just like his dad. It must be hereditary.''
>
> Complaint from John: ''They don't like me in school. I have a hit-and-run teacher. I won't go to school.''
>
> The ''hit-and-run'' teacher, he later explained, before assigning problems in mental arithmetic would point or lunge at him, stating that he was so slow she didn't expect him to answer the problem, and she would never repeat the problem given. John admits that he responded by doing nothing,

although occasionally he spent his time carving initials on the school desk. It is of interest to know that the complete examination in this case indicated that we were dealing with a child of superior intelligence and that the mother of the boy was enmeshed in a most turbulent and unsatisfying marital situation, along with the stress and strain of bringing up a family of four children, of whom John was the youngest and the result of the most undesired pregnancy.

The clinical advantage of the complaint in psychopediatric work is the clue that it gives to the attitude of those dealing with the children—its general educational and self-educational significance to the physician. It lends itself to a systematic grouping of the many items and difficulties commonly met with in psychopediatrics, at the same time serving as an indicator in the reformation or diagnosis and as a check on one's therapeutic success or lack of it.

Having obtained the complaint, we proceed to develop the story, reconstructing the setting in which the difficulty arose, tracing its development from its outset to the present time, and particularly noting its effect upon the individual and his environment. In short, we approach the problem as we would any that challenges us in the scientific world, by ascertaining the conditions under which it develops, the predisposing factors, their work or course, and the results to which they have given rise.

In addition, a personal history is taken, with emphasis on the personality make-up of the child, his characteristic performance, parent-child relationships, school and group behavior, and the like, as well as the physical factors. The family history completes the indirect examination.

The direct examinations of the child consist of the usual routine, complete physical studies including indicated contributory examinations, that is, laboratory, x-ray, etc., mental measurements, and the so-called psychiatric examination, in which special emphasis is placed on the child's emotional life and habits, as well as on the various features of his environment and their possible direct or indirect connection with the difficulty to be treated. Here we are dealing to a large extent with interpersonal relationships between parents, teachers, and the child. The mental health of the child may be determined by his maximum ability to get along with people in a manner that will contribute mutual satisfaction on a constant give-and-take basis, without the interference of inner conflict or external friction. The child is not only a biologic, but also a highly differentiated sociobiologic, unit. A study of the child's environment demands no unusual theoretical preparation, but simply an elaboration of the complaint in the light of the actual manner in which the child gets along at home, in school, and in the community. The physician becomes increasingly aware of certain home situations centering around parent-child relationships and poor personal relations, such as domination by one member of the family, interfering by relatives, favoritism, maladjustment due to the fact that the child was unwanted, clash of authority, dissension between parents either overt or otherwise, oversolicitude, overseverity, neglect, jealousy, difficulties with a step-parent, ineffectuality of parent, important physical and mental disabilities in parents, as well as significant social, economic, and moral maladjustments in the home.

Also contributing are school situations which influence behavior, such as (1) personal relationships based on antagonism between pupil and teacher, conflicts between home and school, and the like; or (2) disabilities of the teacher which influence a child's behavior; such as neuroticism or poor physical health, insecurity, and lack or inadequacy of training. In the same way, a rigidity or poorly organized school curriculum often influences the behavior of the child, as do community situations, especially lack of public interest in school and health problems; inadequate provision of recreational outlets for children; community attitudes toward delinquency; isolation of groups differing in language, customs, and race; and congestion of population.

To summarize, therefore, the psychobiologic approach to the study of childhood behavior problems is based on a pluralistic attitude in which we single out some happening or group of happenings, either pathologic or normal, in the transit of a person through life and study it for what it does and is in relation to the whole situation of that individual. In the consideration of a child, we wish to ascertain (1) the conditions that gave rise to the complaint, (2) the predisposing factors, (3) their working or course, (4) their results, and (5) the modifiability of the whole.

In dealing with children, the diagnosis is expressed in terms of the individual problems with which we are confronted. This tells us more than general terms such as "nervousness," "neurosis," "neurasthenia," "behavior disorder," and the like. It is always the child, as a person, that we wish to treat, not merely his tics, enuresis, temper tantrums, or fears, as diseases or symptoms. The therapeutic program depends on the completeness of the direct, indirect, and contributory examinations, with the conclusions we have drawn from them and what we have recognized to be the child's personality assets and liabilities.

Psychiatric treatment is, therefore, the total of efforts made in behalf of the adjustment of an individual with personality difficulties. Its first aim is to set up in the patient a condition of comfort and well-being and, in general, a feeling of security. This means the utilization, by the physician, of a psychotherapeutic approach. Psychotherapy is essential in the therapeutic armamentarium of any physician. I define psychotherapy as "an effort to influence in the right direction the attitude of the patient toward himself, toward his mental and physical processes, toward his environment. It is an effort to teach him to understand himself, his illness, and the cause or causes of his illness, whether this cause or these causes lie in the body, in his environment, or in the superficial or deeper layers of his mental life." Psychotherapy, as it deals with the child, rests on an aeration or ventilation of the conflict material presented by the child, by means of direct interviews in which the child is given an opportunity to discharge and bring out into the open all the life experiences that have been causing him serious concern. Psychotherapy includes also desensitization, whereby the patient is required to face frankly the traumatic experience of the past. Suggestion, persuasion, reassurance, and reeducation are necessary psychotherapeutic adjuncts in dealing with the child. Reeducation especially leads to the establishment of new habits of response and the development of social, recreational, and activity programs to insure future stabilization. In psychotherapy, there is always a need to desensitize the patient's family to his illness and to influence them in new habits of response to the child. This is of great significance in the type of behavior manifestation so often encountered in the "overprotected child," who frequently develops temper tantrums, hypochondriasis, loss of initiative, and continued dependence.

Other types of treatment center around the fundamentals of general medical treatment, especially as it pertains to the physical well-being of the child. Environmental shifts, such as placement of the child in a foster home, may be an essential phase of the treatment occasionally, although as a general principle it is best to further the adjustment of the child directly in the home. For this purpose, the social worker's aid will be more and more solicited and utilized to the fullest extent possible. I need not emphasize the importance, in the social-therapeutic regime, of establishing general recreational facilities in the community.

I have briefly reviewed the psychobiologic viewpoint as applied to children's personality difficulties. I hope that it does not appear mysterious and that the terminology, aside from the use of the word psychobiologic, has not confused you. Because of its emphasis upon the person rather than upon the disease, psychobiology is fundamental for all of us if we accept our full obligations in dealing with the child. In our medical training, we are apt to be preoccupied with organs and systems, or with physiologic segments and part-functions, instead of with the more sweeping and total functionings of the individual, in which he must be viewed, as described by Adolf Meyer, as a mentally integrated behavior. I feel that the pediatrician who is responsible for the care of children should adopt this pluralistic attitude in meeting the interesting problems of childhood, instead of becoming confused by the various schools of thought and involved in controversy among ourselves. Psychiatrist, pediatrician, and general practitioner should adopt a conjunct approach based upon thorough and practical medical training, which should include both undergraduate and postgraduate studies. This seems to me the real solution of what Dr. Brennemann has signated as a ''confusion of theory and authority.'' For practical purposes, it is to be expected and accepted that the pediatrician and the general practitioner dealing with children should assume their shares of responsibility for the personality difficulties of childhood. This means that they should take care of the majority of such problems. The psychiatrist may be utilized, like any other consultant, to deal with the more complex and involved behavior problems. It is anticipated that we will have fewer of these problems if the pediatricians adopt an attitude in dealing with the mental phenomena of childhood similar to the attitude they have so successfully utilized in dealing with the physical care of the child. It may be accepted that psychiatry must assume the responsibility for court work and many other special phases pertaining to childhood delinquency and the relation of these problems to future mental conditions, especially the minor psychoses (the psychoneuroses) and the more sweeping mental reactions of the adult.

Present Status of Training in Child Psychiatry in Relation to Pediatrics

A review of a recent study of the situation in our medical schools is most pertinent to our discussion. The teaching content of the departments of pediatrics during the current year indicated that only brief formal instruction in the field of child psychiatry and mental hygiene was given in fourteen of the sixty-eight four-year medical schools visited. In the remaining schools many professors of pediatrics volunteered the information that no attempt was being made to present the psychiatric viewpoint throughout the instruction in pediatrics, or that, owing to lack of time, there was a complete omission of teaching in this field. In fact, at the time of this study, only four schools gave evidence of formal organization for such teaching within the department of pediatrics, although several other schools had made arrangements for staff participation in seminars or an occasional lecture in child psychiatry and mental hygiene. Liaison work between the departments of psychiatry and pediatrics, in some degree or other, existed in nine schools. Opportunities for such elective work in pediatrics were also meager. Child guidance facilities of some kind were available in twenty of the schools visited. In several localities adequate child guidance clinics were available but were not utilized in the teaching schedule, because of isolation, lack of interest on the part of the university departments, or lack of desire to participate in teaching on the part of the director of the clinic. It was most striking to note this lack of utilization for pediatric teaching of the facilities available. In the schools that have a psychopathic hospital or institute, facilities for child psychiatry have usually been established as a part of the regular out-patient activities and more extensive individual instruction is given, frequently at the request of the pediatric department. However, these facilities are not utilized in the general interne training. The outstanding work at Cornell University Medical School under Dr. La Mar, at Johns Hopkins University School of Medicine under Dr. Kanner, at Washington University Medical School under Dr. Kubitschek is well known to you.

The groundwork, therefore, for the complete care of the child, utilizing the experience of both fields, has been established and much good work is now being done which promises further progress in the near future. This again will lead back to the objectives of the general medical curriculum. If we accept psychiatry as that phase of medicine which deals with the pathology and therapy of the person, we must aim to produce a practitioner who, on graduation from a Class A medical school, has acquired a sound attitude toward professional duties and responsibilities and an ability to deal reasonably well in the early days of practice with the rank and file of patients and conditions that will confront him. The medical curriculum, likewise, throughout each year in the medical course should be directed primarily toward health, its preservation, perfection, or restoration, and not toward disease. From this point of view, we are compelled to accept a psychobiologic approach to problems of health and disease, in that we are always dealing with a person and not a walking test tube containing some fascinating disease process. Likewise, the medical curriculum should not continue to be divided into separate blocks of study, but all departments should be to some extent interdependent. In this connection, I believe again that psychobiology is an excellent connecting link, correlating the preliminary medical sciences with the clinical sciences. It is to be anticipated that the medical curriculum of the future will not prescribe or standardize any strict uniformity of method in the teaching schedule. There will be a wide liberty of choice in the different schools, each of which should provide broad general foundations and requirements for the basic medical training. When the general practitioner and the pediatrician get their grounding in psychiatry in the medical school, "the confusion of theory and authority" will no longer exist. If this comes about in the undergraduate teaching schedule, we may anticipate a similar development in the field of graduate education, with specialization based on thorough experience and fundamental training as elected by the individual physician.

Fundamentals of a Psychiatric Training Program for Pediatricians

I have often been asked the difficult question: What constitutes the irreducible minimum in the way of a foundation for the orientation of the general medical man or the pediatrician who assumes responsibility for the emotional and personality problems common in childhood? It would be impossible to formulate such minimum instructions. Too much depends upon the individual who is doing the teaching, the content of the course, and the special interest and initiative of the person receiving instruction. Such instruction should be very flexible, but I would consider the following as fundamental:

The physician or pediatrician should know how to administer the Binet-Simon test and be sufficiently aware of its limitations to interpret it wisely. He should develop insight into the individual aspect of behavior problems. When intensive individual study is required, the case may be one appropriate for psychiatric consultation, but the pediatrician must be capable of caring for the less complex cases and of appreciating the length of time necessary in psychiatric study, where formulas of "do this" and "don't do that" are of no value. The pediatrician who desires such training should spend at least one year in preparation (preferably two), having contact with the important phases of social and clinical psychiatry. Special elastic training programs and requirements should be established in various centers to meet these needs and to give the pediatrician some understanding of such fundamentals as these:

Mental growth and development of the child.

Behavior as an interaction between the child and his environment (motivation of behavior, symptomatic and genetic-dynamic aspects).

Common home, school, and community situations that influence child behavior.

Factors that enter into the development and training of habits (eating, sleeping, elimination, sex, etc.).

Etiologic classification of the common behavior problems of childhood.

Methods of behavior study (social, physical, psychometric, psychiatric).

Methods of management and treatment (direct, indirect, social-manipulative, psychotherapeutic; in general, clarification and interpretation in contrast to direct corrective measures).

Origin, development, aims, and application of mental hygiene.

Individual discussions concerning the hospital care of behavior disorders and borderline states in childhood indicate clearly that the consensus of opinion in both the pediatric and the psychiatric groups is that these problems should be handled in a children's hospital and that adequate facilities should be developed there. This certainly is preferable to the tendency in some psychiatric hospitals to add wards for children and consider these problems in relation to the major adult problems.

Conclusion

In conclusion, I should like to reemphasize the following points:

First, psychiatry in the care of a child has a clear-cut contribution to make to general medicine and pediatrics in its psychobiological attitude; that is, the attitude that deals with the total child by the general principles of clinical history and examination, with special emphasis on the complaint factor. Psychobiology gives us a pluralistic attitude toward behavior problems and is based on demonstrable facts and not on any theory or system or special school of psychology.

Second, it is evident that the general practitioner and pediatrician must stand as the first line of defense in dealing with the personality and emotional problems of childhood and that, in actual practice, the responsibility will fall on them for handling such problems in their incipiency.

Third, medical education and practice cannot be separated. We, therefore, should bring about throughout the whole medical curriculum greater correlation between the preclinical and the clinical sciences, along with psychobiologic concepts, emphasis upon prevention, and greater recognition of medicine as a social agency. Interdepartmental and liaison activities between the departments of medicine, pediatrics, and psychiatry are now demonstrating the practical applicability of a conjoint approach to personality problems in childhood which promises much for future clinical and therapeutic endeavors, as well as for the training of a personnel in the field of general medicine and pediatrics that will be competent to deal with the rank and file of childhood behavior manifestations.

But either way it goes, it's interesting. Either way it goes, it leads us to fields of adjustment that are richly carpeted with strange and exciting flowers. Either way it goes, we meet sickness and health just as truly as in the matters of organ function.

For many of you—as for many psychiatrists—I have said nothing that is new. For the rest, psychiatrists as well as pediatricians, if you care for rare adventure, if you can stand failure and foolish error, if you don't become too disturbed over exotic theories and practices that burst into flower overnight in a new field—you will enjoy practice in a community more than you ever enjoyed practice in a person.

The Practice of Psychiatry in a Community Clinic*

James S. Plant, M.D., Newark, N. J.

The position of the psychiatrist in community work is much the same as is that of many of your leading pediatricians. We in psychiatry have just as many in our field who are preoccupied with the symptoms of mental disorder as you have who

*The author apologizes that this material rather closely parallels his longer article, "The Promise of Psychiatry" (Am. J. Dis. Child. **44**: 1308, 1932). It is less interesting but a bit more honest to recognize how slowly one develops.

are interested in the diseases of children rather than in children. If you point with some apprehension to the glittering blandishments of psychoanalysis, are you not really equally disturbed by such as your own vitamin "racket"? If you are struggling to adjust yourself to a new level of integration and to questions and problems which have not come to you before, so are we.

In other words, I see pediatrics and psychiatry moving shoulder to shoulder out of the realm of weight charts and hallucinations, out of the realm of disease entities and syndromes, into the field of the adjustment of the individual in a complex world. In the light of these common interests and problems let us review simply what it is which we face.

First, with a marked and rather sudden decrease in the time and energy occupied in the mechanics of living, many bewildered people have turned to bridge, golf, and mad rushing about in speeding automobiles. The significant change, however, has been that of a marked increase in the interest in the relationships of living. The harassed parent of a large family who for centuries has asked "What can I do for others?" is now querying "What do I mean to others?" Problems of food were earlier few because for the busy mother Johnny could jolly well eat his spinach or do without. (Notice that the tasks of life managed to produce something of that same detachment which in various ways we labor for now.) Today the same difficulty principally raises the questions, "What does this *mean?*" "Who's going to win?"—questions which soon completely supersede all problems of the food itself.

Posterity will look upon this rapid shift of interest from the mechanics to the relationships of living as the most dramatic and, in the end, most worthwhile development of our generation. And let us not fool ourselves—psychiatry is little, if any, ahead of pediatrics in meeting the issues that have been raised.

Second, and this is probably rather closely related to the above, there is a widespread and discomfiting question as to *why* things are happening. Parents earlier satisfied if the youngster ceased sucking his thumb now ask why he has been persisting in the habit; families earlier happy over the clearing of a conduct disorder now seem more interested in the reasons for the change than in the change itself.

Here again we progress. "Why" will lead us much farther than "what." But for the present this means serious trouble for both of our groups. We have, to date, moved farther than you in this sector. Psychoanalysis, for all you may wish to say against it, is at least an attempted answer to a question which most of us are only trying to run away from. We shall not still these queries by making fun of them. If you do not like such answers as we have made as to "why" people behave as they do, build some answers of your own; do not just stick your heads in the sand.

Third, while every generation has had to consider itself "critical," has had to feel that its problems surpass those of other times, it seems fair to say that our times have been presented with problems of social adjustment rather more complex and pressing than those of any other time since the Renaissance. Urbanization, staggering problems in facility of communication, and rapidly changing types of machinery have tumbled upon us in dismaying rapidity. And for various reasons a bewildered populace seeks an answer from the physician. The overanxious mother and the questioning young wife are no less "sick" than are those with some organic disturbance. True, the illness is less sure of diagnosis, the "history" lacks clean-cut points, the therapy is a long, hard struggle through a maze quite as baffling to the doctor as to the patient. Are you and I blind that we would try to pretend that these are not real illnesses just because we cannot circumscribe them with our usual diagnostic terminology? Are we quitters, that we would turn away because the problems seem too complex?

Most of my colleagues feel that at this point psychiatry has gone much farther than has pediatrics. With this I personally cannot agree. I feel that the psychiatrists in general have been quite as blind to the problems raised by the social pressures as have your group been. The psychiatrist is still satisfied to bring the patient for treatment many miles from his accustomed milieu—is still willing to study the lion at the zoo, quite oblivious to the fact that what he sees there is no real lion.

Such are the problems which face us, and, right or wrong, some assay of the effectiveness of our various approaches. Just because I can use social workers I think that certain avenues of information and therapy are open to me—avenues I think you know very little about. Just because I sit in various classrooms or know the recreation leaders or policemen in my area better than I know the parents, I think that I have certain insights into the problems the child has to solve—insights which are beyond the view of the practicing pediatrician. Just because I like to think of myself as a sociologist rather than a psychologist, I think that I came upon my problems with a point of view different from yours. Yet I would have failed utterly today to make myself clear if I gave you any other impression than that the problems and perplexities that are yours are really also mine and are those, too, of my colleagues.

The platform upon which I work is a very simple one. It has only two important planks. One bolsters and patches, repairs, and makes fancy additions, but the practice of pediatrics or psychiatry in the community can comfortably operate on two very homely principles.

The first is to recognize that in every sort of conduct disorder the child is trying to solve a problem. There are times when we adults can see that no problem really exists, but it exists for the child. There are times, aplenty, when we feel that the child's method of solution is faulty. I can assure you, gentlemen, that when a child sucks his thumb, or plays hookey, or springs a temper tantrum, he is trying in his own way to solve what he sees as some sort of a problem, and I can assure you that until we find what problem the child was trying to solve, we can do nothing to help him. Virchow taught us not so long ago that physical disease is nothing but this same effort on the part of the normal body to solve a problem. He revolutionized the practice of medicine. To preoccupy yourselves with the disappearance of lying, truancy, nail biting, or masturbation is about as sensible as to persuade yourself that your pneumonia patient has no fever or your fracture case, no pain.

The second is to rigidly follow the rules of Dr. Anna Freud as to the practice of psychiatry in children. There are three of these rules. They come from an analyst, but they are good ones. They will carry you farther than all the trick technics of a technic-crazy culture.

The first is easy. Have unending patience.

The second is hard. Have faith in the child. With most of the enuritic patients I see, I soon become convinced that it must be the pediatrician rather than the child who is wetting the bed. The doctor is making all the plans, deciding on the medicine, assaying the results. Over and over again in the whole field of conduct disorders, I find myself the first one to ask the child what *he* thinks to be the matter and what *he* wants to do about it. See your children *alone*. See them at other times than you see the parents. Give them, through your every action, the feeling that you have faith in their ability to solve the difficulty if they care to. And drive for the same thing with the parents—that it is for us adults to stand by the child's efforts, not to stand in place of them.

The third is hard. See the problem as the child sees it. This does not mean "solve the problem as the child has solved it." This does not mean to excuse the child; it means to understand him. It does not mean to let the child do as he will and to hell with the rest of the world; it means that you cannot change a course of action effectively unless you understand why it was undertaken. This third rule of Anna Freud's is the most difficult and most interesting of all your ventures. Often the child, in wide-eyed amazement at the first person who has tried to see what he is trying to do, will tell you the whole problem in ten minutes. Often our myopic adult eyes and our set adult ways mean (at least in my own practice) that we never really can find out what the child is *trying to do*.

The Contribution of a Psychiatrist as a Member of the Pediatric Hospital Staff

Leo Kanner, M.D., Baltimore, Md.

Pediatricians are in agreement that a considerable number of children's problems with which they are confronted are concerned not so much with the patients' organs as with the patients themselves. They are also in agreement that their early medical training has considered largely, if not exclusively, the pathology and treatment of organs, organ systems, and more diffuse somatic diseases, but has usually neglected to include the pathology and treatment of unhealthy performances of the whole person, of the maladjusted, misbehaving, mismanaged, suffering human being. Children are brought to them daily with complaints of food capriciousness, sleep disturbances, school failures, excessive shyness or aggressiveness, anxiety, temper tantrums, breath-holding spells, restlessness, tics, nail biting, thumb-sucking, speech disorders, masturbation, and what people refer to as general nervousness. The days when all these problems were handled with the prescription pad only are fortunately over. No one realizes this more than the conscientious pediatrician himself, who is eager to learn how to deal with his patients and their parents in an informed and really helpful manner. The demand for an inclusion of psychiatric understanding in the diagnostic and therapeutic armamentarium of the pediatrician has come and grown in recent years as a spontaneous expression of this realization.

To supply this need at the Johns Hopkins Hospital, a close full-time working relationship was established in 1930 between the psychiatrist privileged to undertake this task and the staff of the Harriet Lane Home, the pediatric department of the hospital. The psychiatrist entered upon this assignment with the clear awareness of the fact that he came to learn at least as much as to teach. He considered his functions not as a chance to descend upon his pediatric collaborators with a rigid set of rules to be imposed upon them *ex cathedra,* but as a challenge to demonstrate his usefulness through practical work with the patients in whose behalf he was consulted. He did not come to create needs artifically, but to study the really existing and felt needs and help to satisfy them to the best of his ability.

For this reason, the first step was of necessity one of orientation. What were the complaints and situations that made the members of the pediatric staff feel that psychiatric assistance might contribute something to their amelioration—something which at that time was not available to themselves? The proverbial courtesy of the pediatricians led them to come to the psychiatrist with the question: What kind of cases do you want us to refer to you? However, no specifications were handed out. It was suggested that any child, regardless of the nature of his difficulty, be referred if the pediatrician felt that a consultation might be of benefit to his own understanding of the case or to the child himself. It is interesting to note what happened under the circumstances. Among the first one thousand cases selected by the pediatricians for psychiatry consultation, the leading complaints or reasons for referral were as follows (often there were two or more leading complaints in the same case):

Poor progress or conduct at school	315
Enuresis	256
Food capriciousness and pica	222
Temper tantrums	217
Nail biting	163
Restlessness	154
Fear reactions	153

Problems of epileptic children	142
Spoiled child reaction	126
Speech difficulties	124
Tics	75
Hypochondriac trends	72
Psychogenic headaches	68
Sleep disturbances	65
Sex problems	63
Psychogenic vomiting	54
Thumb-sucking	36
Crying spells	34
Stealing	29
Encopresis	26
Psychogenic constipation	24
Disobedience	22
Breath-holding spells	22
Destructiveness	21
Lying	21

A number of things were learned from this list of complaints in one thousand cases, covering a period of a little over two years. They represented a cross-section of the problems which the pediatrician meets in his daily practice. They amounted to approximately 10 per cent of all children examined and treated during that period in the Harriet Lane dispensaries, wards, special clinics, and private consultation service. The list does not include reference to the not infrequent requests for advice in the handling of delirious or stuporous children in the wards or dealing with unreasonable, belligerent, or otherwise difficult parents. Nor does it include requests for the intelligence testing of blind, deaf, orthopedically and neurologically handicapped children or those considered for adoption and for boarding home or institutional placement.

The psychiatrist regarded his functions as twofold. Aside from an unparalleled opportunity for satisfying investigative curiosities, he envisioned his task as one of helping the patients who were sent to him and at the same time imparting to the pediatricians the insight and skill necessary for the adequate handling of the common behavior disorders of children. These two functions cannot be separated. Lectures and reading assignments alone are of relatively little help. It is mainly through actual work with concrete issues that psychiatric as well as any other practical medical efficiency can be acquired. In our own setting, the amalgamation of clinical case work and clinical instruction has shaped itself in the following manner:

The referring pediatrician, when he sends a child for psychiatric consultation, is expected to formulate the problem briefly and concisely. He learns to express the facts of the complaint and his own findings and impressions lucidly in plain English, steering clear of terminologic confusions and generalizations. He thus has a chance to become aware of factors which he may have heretofore neglected, factors concerning the individual and his relations to the world in which he lives. Much is gained if the physician, in dealing with human behavior, is satisfied with the recognition and formulation of essential facts and happenings, instead of trying to translate into questionable diagnostic labels or fantastic interpretations something which he has not taken the trouble to investigate. Only those who do not appreciate the importance of clear statements of fact will be surprised to find that these simple formulations, occupying less than half a page, have been of great educational value, replacing bewildering abstractions by concrete data in everyday language.

After the child has been examined, the pediatrician receives a report which becomes an integral part of the pediatric case history and in which every step of the examination is recorded. A summary, refraining from nosologic terms, tells him: The child was brought to us with such and such a complaint. It proceeds to inform him of the patient's, his family's, teacher's, or other people's attitudes about the child and his difficulties, of the nature and development of the problem, the patient's intelligence, his emotional responses, the domestic and social implications, complicating features of his physical health, life experiences that have a bearing on the problem, and difficulties of interpersonal relationships. Recommendations are made on the basis of the findings, giving reasons for each step of the therapeutic plan and at the same time pointing out the obstacles which may lie in the way of ideal adjustment.

In addition to this, the members of the hospital staff are given an opportunity for more direct contact with the psychiatrist. The older members of the group have a standing invitation, of which they often make use, to sit in during the examination and therapeutic interviews and observe the work while it is in progress. The internes spend routinely three days a week for a period of two months at the psychiatric establishment at Harriet Lane. They see what is being done with the children and eventually learn to make themselves responsible for the taking of histories, psychiatric examinations including psychometric tests, and the working out of therapeutic programs. When they go back to the wards and dispensary, they do so with a broadened horizon, with a far better knowledge of the facts concerning children and standards of behavior. They have become less dependent on the psychiatrist in the understanding and treatment of the common personality and adjustment difficulties of their patients. They have gained a knowledge of the facilities existing in the community in behalf of maladjusted children, recreational, boarding, correctional, and custodial opportunities, and the existing possibilities of cooperation with the schools.

This arrangement is supplemented by still another mode of collaboration. The psychiatrist and his assistants are on daily call to the wards and dispensary. The pediatricians thus receive psychiatric advice not only after children had been referred, but also at the time of first contact with the patient. This takes care, among other things, of psychiatric emergencies and immediate problems in the wards, such as delirium, acute excitements, violent resentment of hospitalization, psychogenic vomiting, or excessive masturbation, at the clinic. On occasions, advice is sought and given in cases, for instance, when the parents fail to give their consent to the performance of an imperative operation or do not permit certain necessary tests to be done. In other words, the hospital physicians are aware of the presence of a psychiatrist in their midst and make use of his functions in a large variety of situations.

A similarly close relationship is maintained with the so-called special clinics of the children's hospital, the cardiac, epilepsy, endocrine, syphilis, and tuberculosis clinics. Epileptic children are referred routinely and repeatedly for assistance in home and school adjustment, intelligence rating in reasonable intervals, and vocational guidance. The pediatricians turn to us for help when a child on an antidiabetic or ketogenic diet steals prohibited food, when a rheumatic child would not stay in bed as prescribed, when a patient with severe cardiac ailment further endangers his health by fierce temper outbursts, when the sensitiveness and irritability of a choreic child become too bothersome, or when repeated psychometric tests are expected to throw light on the development of thyroid-treated cretins.

All these arrangements are governed by a spirit of mutual give-and-take collaboration. The psychiatrist has an opportunity to obtain first-hand information about many things which the average child guidance clinic, removed from a pediatric hospital, has little opportunity to learn. Being placed in the main stream of a busy pediatric center, he sees in a constant flow the everyday problems of the everyday child as they come to the practicing pediatrician. He learns of the difficulties that may arise from hospitalization, acute illness, chronic ailments, and convalescence. He observes the problems that face the ward nurses and the social workers of the hospital. He has a chance to study the nature and extent of behavior disorders of children suffering from asthma, eczema, and spastic colon. He has a chance to follow for years the personality development of premature, rachitic, malnourished infants, of early ruminators and nystagmoid head shakers, of children with encephalitis, meningitis, epilepsy, or lead poisoning. And, above all, he has the great advantage that all his patients have had a thorough physical examination prior to being referred to him.

Just as the child psychiatrist in this manner has an opportunity to become a better child psychiatrist, so, I venture to say, does the pediatrician emerge from this arrangement as a better pediatrician. He soon learns to slough off some of the current misunderstandings about psychiatry. Some pediatricians came with the notion that psychiatry is concerned merely with extremes and end-products of mental aberrations and therefore did not see how it could possibly apply to their work with children. Some thought that it is interested merely in classifications. Some felt that it is a weird and mysterious hunt for mythologic complexes. Some thought of it in terms of hypnotism and peculiar forms of suggestion. Others believed that it was synonymous with a search for the intelligence quotient. A few had at first to overcome a definite fear of the psychiatrist whom they expected to be endowed with some supernatural powers. And some came prepared to be initiated in the use of a few quick tricks, similar to the miracles of Lourdes or the notorious chiropractic snap: You take a child, turn the magic key, and, presto, you have turned him into a perfect specimen.

The internes and other members of the staff are helped to cure themselves of these notions. They learn to humanize their patients. They learn to make themselves responsible for human beings, instead of dealing merely with collections of organs of specimens of a supposedly homogeneous species. They learn to consider the fact that some things are problems of one or another organ, others are problems of the child, still others are problems of the family and the environment, and most of them are combinations of several of these. Having learned sets of facts about tissue structures, organ functions and dysfunctions, and biochemistry, they get acquainted with new, similarly objective and concrete sets of facts about behavior, performance, the functions and dysfunctions of the individual child and his reactions to people and to life situations. They are helped to develop a curiosity for the whence and why of children's behavior disorders and are taught to satisfy this curiosity in a scientific and factual manner. They perceive that the psychiatrist who works with concrete facts can well afford and really manages to refrain from glib toying with hypothetical assumptions of unproved mechanisms and complexes. They are saved from being embarrassed by modern parents who refuse to accept at its face value the assertion that stuttering or nightmares are merely the result of bad tonsils or mild anemia. Their knowledge of pathology, limited hitherto to body structures, is broadened by the inclusion of the pathology of the acting, feeling, and reasoning person. Their knowledge of therapy is broadened by the inclusion of psychotherapy, that is, informed and understanding treatment of whole dysfunctions, of the person, the mentally integrated functioning of the individual and the group. In doing so, they are no longer likely to keep behavior problems out of their domain with an impatient shrugging of their shoulders, the prescription of tonics and sedatives, and a self-commiserating sigh which indicates: "Just another nervous, neurotic, neurasthenic, or neuropathic child!" As a matter of fact, they no longer need any of these terms if they know the child well enough and are acquainted with his problems and the proper therapeutic procedure. And they no longer look for quick tricks but soberly and in orderly fashion use the knowledge which they have obtained in their patient work with the child, his family, his teachers, and, whenever necessary, the social agencies of the community.

Thus, the contribution of a psychiatrist as a member of a pediatric hospital staff may be summarized as follows:

1. Service to the children who are referred to him because of behavior and personality disorder.

2. Demonstration of objective, common sense methods of examination and treatment which the pediatrician can learn to use in his own practical work when dealing with common, everyday behavior difficulties of children.

3. Helping the pediatrician to assume full responsibility for the child as an individual, regardless as to whether the child does or does not present behavior difficulties.

One observation has impressed me so strongly during the six years of collaboration with the pediatric group at Harriet Lane that I cannot refrain from mentioning it briefly. Some people are in the habit of agitating themselves with the question: Who should be responsible for the handling of behavior problems of children? The psychiatrist? The pediatrician? The educator? The social worker? The psychologist? I must say that in the actual work at Harriet Lane the question of competency has not arisen even once. Its very formulation, as a matter of fact, seems to me to be based on false premises. The question should not be: Who should do this and who should do that? but: What am I prepared to do competently and what am I not prepared to do competently? I cannot see how the field of psychopathology can possibly be relegated to medically untrained people. Unless we wish to return to the medieval dualistic separation of body and mind, we must concede to the physician the right and obligation to treat sick people, whether their sickness lie in the domain of organ pathology or the pathology of the person. The psychiatrist is not competently prepared to deal with the complexities of pediatric organ pathology. Nor is the pediatrician competently prepared to deal with the complexities of psychopathology. But, without being an ophthalmologist, he has learned how to take care of uncomplicated conjunctivitis and how to use the ophthalmoscope to advantage. Without having specialized in immunology, he contributes a lion's share to the treatment and prevention of contagious diseases. And without specializing in psychiatry, he can obtain sufficient information and skill to concern himself with the everyday psychopathology and psychotherapy of childhood. This does by no means eliminate the psychiatrist, just as it does not eliminate the ophthalmologist or the immunologist. As a matter of fact, it definitely creates for him a place as an adviser and teacher of the pediatrician, who is then helped and encouraged to assume hitherto neglected responsibilities.

How do the pediatricians themselves feel about the kind of collaboration described in this presentation? The appetite for it has grown considerably in recent years. Four medical schools, those of Columbia, Western Reserve, Iowa State, and Tennessee State Universities, have made definite arrangements for a one year's training of capable and interested young pediatricians at the Harriet Lane psychiatric establishment, so that they may return to their pediatric hospitals with a knowledge of child psychiatry. The organization of this round table conference is in itself eloquent proof of this trend. Dr. Edwards A. Park, director of Johns Hopkins pediatric department, made this statement before the 1935 Conference on Psychiatric Education: "It is difficult to give an estimate of the value of the Psychiatric Clinic in the Harriet Lane Home. I feel tempted merely to say, 'We could not possibly get along without it!' On analysis, its value lies chiefly in three particulars: the care of individual children, the education of physicians and students, and the investigation of abnormal behavior in the human being. . . As a result of his instructions, Dr. Kanner has supplied the pediatric staff with the tools for psychiatric work and has given them an ability to use those tools, for he has taught a systematic method for the examination of a child with a behavior disturbance and has made clear the principles of understanding and management.''

DISCUSSION

Dr. Ebaugh asked Dr. Veeder to open the discussion.

DR. BORDEN S. VEEDER (ST. LOUIS) pointed out the great field of child psychiatry in pediatrics. He stressed the changes in the attitude of the pediatrist toward the problem during the past thirteen years. The pediatrist formerly looked upon the entire field as one of mystery shrouded in a nomenclature beyond the comprehension of the rank and file. There was a demand that the problems of child psychiatry be presented in a simpler language with a saner understanding. Dr. Veeder feels that this has been and is the job of the pediatrist as evidenced by the deeper insight displayed in attacking our everyday problems. He stressed the point that success in this field is utterly impossible without a complete understanding of the problem at hand—further, that probably no greater service can be rendered by the pediatrist in the field of child psychiatry than that of prevention. His unique position in the family, his intimate association with the child from birth, his clear understanding (as a rule) of the social, cultural and economic status of the family, his cognizance (often) of marital discord, and indeed his knowledge of most of the intimate family relationships—all these place him in a most favorable position to detect impending psychiatric problems. The alert pediatrist in his routine visits to the home, occasioned by the usual illnesses of childhood, senses the attitude of the parents and the atmosphere of the home, and he may well be in a position to predict, in his patient, the psychiatric disturbances of the future and institute even in the early months of life those measures of prevention which seem indicated. Dr. Veeder cited here in illustration the too often encountered psychogenic constipation, having for its background the overanxious mother obsessed with the necessity that her baby have a daily evacuation of the bowels at a stated time. The child finally ''feels'' the worry of the mother and becomes equally concerned with the problem. Such disturbances can and should be anticipated by the pediatrist and prevented. His close observation of the attitude and atmosphere of the baby's environment will enable him to be successful in meeting these situations. To do this he must develop an analytical attitude.

Dr. Veeder contrasted the position of the pediatrist in the home of the patient with that of the psychiatrist who meets the patient only in his office; he stated that he felt the former had certain distinct advantages. He further stated that, although he appreciated the value of the social worker in child psychiatry, her importance had been definitely overemphasized. His own contacts with the family in the home provided ample opportunity for study of environment and relations from which study he finds no trouble in estimating his ability to handle the problem.

DR. C. ANDERSON ALDRICH (WINNETKA, ILL.) stressed the importance of attitude in the field of child psychiatry. He emphasized the point that attitude, not knowledge, was the all-important feature in dealing with these problems, and finally raised the question ''Is attitude contagious?''

CHAIRMAN EBAUGH stated that attitude must be considered in all problems, especially in school where he believes attitude is undoubtedly transmitted from teacher to child. As an example, he cited the instance of thyrotoxicosis in the teacher, with its resulting effect upon the students.

DR. HENRY F. HELMHOLZ (ROCHESTER, MINN.) feels that the pediatrist is probably responsible for the ''worry attitude'' so frequently encountered in the mother. The importance placed upon the child's routine as to habits of food, stool, rest, etc., has been carried to extreme. He believes that the pediatrist appreciates this situation and is getting away from its overemphasis. Dr. Helmholz drew attention to the absolute necessity, in dealing with psychiatric disturbances, of getting at the *child's* problem as in contrast to the mother's problem.

CHAIRMAN EBAUGH asked how and under what circumstances do pediatrists refer their cases to psychiatrists. He discouraged the "last resort" attitude which so frequently is assumed by both pediatrist and parent toward the psychiatrist. He rather took the pediatrist to task for the superficial manner in which the referred case is studied before reaching the psychiatrist.

DR. VEEDER took exception to a statement made by Dr. Ebaugh in his leading discussion that the pediatrist should do his own Binet-Simon tests. He feels that the trained psychiatric worker should actually carry out the technic of the test, after which the pediatrist should interpret the findings.

CHAIRMAN EBAUGH stated that, not only is the technic of the test of value, but the attitude of the child toward the test is of great importance and therefore well worth the time consumed in its doing.

DR. GUSTAVE F. WEINFELD (RAVINIA, ILL.) stated that he feels it is extremely difficult for the pediatrist to get at the root of these psychiatric disturbances. The time-consuming investigations necessary to arrive at a proper understanding of the hereditary and environmental phases of the problem and the proper evaluation of the social and family relations are well-nigh impossible for the pediatrist.

CHAIRMAN EBAUGH feels that the situation is not so hopeless as depicted. Often the problem is found in the parent's attitude. Oversolicitude probably is encountered most often, resulting in the overprotected child, the dependent child devoid of initiative. At times the solution is found in some very obvious occurrence in the family life, such as illness or death; at other times, in the more obscure family relationships, such as marital difficulties, etc. Finally, Dr. Ebaugh suggested that the pediatrist might enlist the service of a trained psychiatric worker.

DR. KANNER stressed the importance of working with the child himself. Get the problem from the child; the parent sees it intellectually, not emotionally.

DR. CARROLL M. POUNDERS (OKLAHOMA CITY, OKLA.) asked Dr. Kanner whether he believes that allergic children have inherent nervous make-up.

DR. KANNER stated that the allergic child is not essentially neurotic. Much depends on attitude of parent toward allergic condition. He feels that all such terms as neuropathic, neurotic, congenital neuropath, be discarded and that only the particular problem in the particular child be considered.

DR. VEEDER emphasized the importance of inherent characteristics as opposed to environment in any consideration of growth and development. He asked if it is not logical to assume the existence of a congenital emotional type.

DR. PLANT disliked the term "congenital emotional type." He prefers to speak of the vulnerability of the individual. It is important to determine the load which a child can stand. It is found remarkably consistent and can be fairly accurately predicted throughout childhood.

He feels that attitudes are most certainly contagious. Attitudes are communicated through psychomotor tensions. It is the *way* things are said, not *what* is said. It is impossible to explain attitudes—one shows faith in them. Finally, Dr. Plant took issue with Dr. Veeder in regard to the pediatrist's knowledge of family relations. He feels that the pediatrist is unable to learn much of the environment and interrelationships as he encounters the family in the home. The parents are dressed up mentally and physically for the physician's visit; only the trained psychiatric social worker and nurse see the family undressed.

DR. ALDRICH.—In what does inability to bear load consist? Might the violent reaction of certain newborn infants to their environment mean that in later infancy and childhood such children would be unable to bear the expected load?

DR. PLANT.—Yes.

DR. STANLEY D. GIFFEN (TOLEDO. OHIO).—What are the commoner problems the child is attempting to meet when enuresis is established?

DR. PLANT.—1. Desire to regain the preeminence of babyhood, as when the new baby arrives.

2. Responding to the family's interest in enuresis. The parent is interested in the wrong thing instead of the right. The child appreciates this—only by concentration on wrong things does he get attention.

3. Playing with older child—carrying the load of an eight-year-old by a six-year-old may produce enuresis. Sometimes in school the child is carrying a load too heavy for his mental and physical make-up.

Finally, Dr. Plant advised: Do not concentrate on enuresis; concentrate on the child's problem.

DR. LEROY A. WILKES (TRENTON, N. J.).—Who knows the family? Granted the pediatrist in his contact is unable to learn the true situation while the visiting nurse does get at the root of the problem, does her success depend upon technic or is it simply a matter of her continued presence breaking down resistance?

DR. PLANT.—Her success does not depend upon any technic which is not available to the pediatrist. She is more one of the family. The mother gets off her dignity. The time element probably plays a less important rôle than the intimacy of the relationship.

CHAIRMAN EBAUGH criticized the pediatrist for the manner in which cases are referred to the psychiatrist. Typical of the pediatrist's so-called diagnosis on these cases might be mentioned such terms as "neurotic child," "hyperactive child," "terrible delinquency," etc. Most of the children present very definite problems. The diagnoses or labels as applied by pediatrists mean nothing. He asked the question: What is the pediatric technic in average personality and emotional problems?

DR. VEEDER.—The technic employed by the pediatrist is much the same as that of the psychiatrist when and if the case is investigated at all. Dr. Veeder reiterated that he feels the pediatrist *does* know the family by his visits to the home. He anticipates impending problems and institutes measures of prevention in the early years.

DR. PLANT warned against the possibility of producing fear of what may come by adopting Dr. Veeder's idea of prevention.

DR. KANNER, discussing further technic, emphasized the importance of an intelligent story of the family, its environment and problems, rather than the stereotyped history so frequently obtained. He was particularly bitter against the "Father L & W, Mother L & W" type of history. He urged that the mother be given full range to tell her own story as she chooses. She should be taken seriously.

DR. JOHN A. BIGLER (HIGHLAND PARK, ILL.).—How does one get information from the child? How does one find out why the child is doing what he is doing?

DR. KANNER.—Obtain information first from parent, school, physician, social worker, nurse, and then from child. The interview with the child should not be a third degree. The questions should be simple, the answers taken seriously; get his reason for his behavior.

DR. PLANT stated that his technic is different from Dr. Kanner's. He interviews the child first and knows absolutely nothing about him at the first conference. He allows the child to tell his own story, beginning with his first memories. The child should not be asked why he commits his digression; this immediately places him on the defensive; rather he should be guided in telling his own story of himself, and in the nature of things he finally works into the problem itself. Above all else, keep faith with the child. Do not be jockeyed into the position of a whip for the family.

DR. H. K. TENNEY, JR. (MADISON, WIS.).—What can we do toward the prevention of difficulties? How can we educate the parents to anticipate the problems?

DR. KANNER.—Prevention is difficult, but by solving one problem the parent gains confidence and comes with the new ones before they are too advanced. Give the parent confidence in dealing with problems. Do not frighten him by anticipating the problems too much. Have the parents steer clear of confusion.

DR. PLANT: Dr. Tenney's question has always been of great interest to me. Teachers can do things with other children that they cannot do with their own. The love factor complicates matters. It removes objectivity and blinds parents so they cannot see the important facts.

DR. LANDY.—Are not the factors in the problem so many as to defy solution?

DR. KANNER.—Parents come to us with a definite problem. We must examine the physical and environmental factors and try to help as much as possible. Often the outstanding difficulty cannot be removed, but we do the best we can to help the situation.

DR. P. J. ZENTAY (ST. LOUIS).—How can we discover the problem of parent-child relationship early? Most of the problems can be traced to the first few months of life. Overanxiety of the mother over the possible difficulties that may arise should be handled by the pediatrician. We are dealing with a complexity of personalities, and, if we cannot influence the parents, nothing can be done. Our entire work is premised on the fact that we can influence the parents.

DR. KANNER.—I thought I was in for a fight, but I see you agree with me. I feel that genus homo will improve. I see children at four to five months. It is a challenge to pediatricians to start work with the parents when the children are at that age, to keep them from getting false anxieties, which do so much harm. Psychiatry in the last thirty years has rediscovered common sense.

CHAIRMAN EBAUGH.—An analysis of 500 cases has shown that oversolicitude, and overprotection have been the chief causes of temper tantrums, daydreaming, and hypochondriasis. In adolescence those children remain overdependent on their parents and are emotionally retarded. Parents should be made aware of this condition so they can correct it.

DR. MITCHELL.—Parents have an idea that all their children can reach the higher grades. Are not graded schools bad?

DR. PLANT.—We must go into the schools and teach them what to do. In our county we have done away with the Binet classes. We must carry the child along according to his chronologic age. Special classes are garbage heaps and should be done away with. We are realizing that school is life, not just a preparation for life. The child should live to the fullest each year of his life. This idea is gaining hold. The fullness of a child's adult life depends on the fullness of his child life. With regard to attitudes, they cannot be taught by words, but only by example.

DR. BUFFORD.—Do you think that the school report cards cause conflicts in a child?

DR. PLANT.—Yes. We are trying out a card without grades. It is general, showing the strengths and weaknesses of the child without resorting to figures. The usual grade report cards do much damage.

DR. MITCHELL.—How long are you going to keep the children in school?

DR. PLANT.—An enormous number of children who would otherwise be working are forced to remain in school, due to the economic depression. The schools are facing unusual and unprecedented problems, but I believe it is a good thing for them. They will solve them by getting away from their academic tradition and so will prepare the child for life.

CHAIRMAN EBAUGH.—I am concerned with two things now:

1. Why the doctors are not using psychiatric social service workers to deal with behavior problems in private practice.

2. The lack of information accompanying the case when the child is referred to a psychiatrist. Labels like nervousness, incorrigibility, etc., are meaningless. Formulate the complaints in chronologic order. Give the complete history as it is told to you and all the pertinent facts.

DR. TENNEY.—This sort of conference lets us see what we are expected to do. To most of us the expense of a psychiatric social worker is prohibitive.

DR. ZENTAY.—The pediatrician cannot use this method because of the small fee he commands. The problem child requires long consultations with the parents for which they are willing to pay only the general charge for an office call.

DR. KANNER.—The time factor is very important. I am aware of it. But how little time it takes to do harm. Parents can easily be frightened by having them anticipate illnesses and by exaggerating symptoms. By learning the technic, the time required in handling these cases can be shortened. Listen to the complaint. Find out the situation. By educating the parents, they will be willing to pay for the extra time.

M. HINES ROBERTS, Recorder.

News and Notes

The following physicians have been certified by the **American Board of Pediatrics** since the last report. Twenty-three of these men were examined.

John A. Bigler, Highland Park, Ill.
Arthur Proctor Black, Peiping, China
Frederick B. Burke, Detroit, Mich.
Garabed A. Z. Garabedian, Tulsa, Okla.
Flora K. Rubinstein, Brooklyn, N. Y.
Harry Apfel, Brooklyn, N. Y.
Samuel Sheppard Brown, Brooklyn, N. Y.
John B. Burns, Binghamton, N. Y.
John Walker Canaday, Glens Falls, N. Y.
Fred T. Cavanaugh, Troy, N. Y.
John Frank Coppolino, Philadelphia, Pa.
Louis Klein Diamond, Boston, Mass.
Katherine Jean Edgar, Rochester, N. Y.
H. Louis George, Jr., Watertown, N. Y.
George Courtenay Glass, Jr., Hartford, Conn.
Edward Scott Goodwin, Albany, N. Y.
Milton J. H. Grand, New York, N. Y.
John Bolter Griggs, Hartford, Conn.
Irving LeBell, New York, N. Y.
Walter Levy, New York, N. Y.
Charles H. O'Regan, New York, N. Y.
William Panitch, Newark, N. J.
Henry Nickerson Pratt, Boston, Mass.
Hugh Currie Thompson, Jr., Albany, N. Y.
Henry Woodruff Titus, New Rochelle, N. Y.
J. Alfred Trackman, New York, N. Y.
Mark J. Wallfield, Brooklyn, N. Y.
Henry Washeim, Jr., Utica, N. Y.

Comments

Nearly fifteen years ago the Section on Pediatrics of the American Medical Association voted to establish the Abraham Jacobi Memorial Fund. Each subscriber to the fund receives a copy of the current *Transactions of the Section on Pediatrics,* and the balance of the money is used by the fund to pay the expenses of guest speakers, special publications, special committee expenses, and the like. As a balance gradually accumulated, it was voted several years later to accumulate an endowment fund of $10,000. Approximately $6,000 was accumulated and invested in this way, to which $2,000 was added by a gift from the Central States Pediatric Society. When the latter was disbanded to form Section III and part of Section II of the American Academy of Pediatrics, it was voted to turn over the funds remaining in the treasury to the Jacobi Memorial Fund. The endowment fund thus stands at approximately $8,000 at the present time. When the endowment fund was founded, it was with the idea that an endowment of $10,000 would produce an annual income of $500, and no further annual subscriptions would be necessary.

In the early days of the fund the usual subscription was $5 although many contributed more to get the endowment fund under way. There has been a steady decline in the number of subscribers in the past four years. The Fund Committee, consisting of the last four Section chairmen, with the secretary, Dr. Frank Neff, of Kansas City, whose individual work and interest over these years has to a large extent been responsible for the success of the fund, has recently circularized the friends of the Section in regard to the fund and transactions. The American Medical Association must be guaranteed a minimum distribution of 350 copies if the Transactions are to be continued. The Fund Committee is reducing the amount asked from each subscriber to $3. It is hoped by this means to increase the number of subscribers to the fund. The fund has served a useful purpose and has aided materially in the work of the Section and in furthering worthwhile pediatric projects. It has been carefully managed, and the committee deserves our support as well as our thanks. The question is raised as to whether the *Transactions of the Section on Pediatrics* should be continued. While from a sentimental standpoint the older members would dislike to see the Transactions discontinued, the value of publishing together a group of articles on unrelated subjects, all of which are published elsewhere, is questionable.

The Journal of Pediatrics

Vol. 9 November, 1936 No. 5

Original Communications

CONGENITAL SYPHILIS

In the Light of Thirty Years' Investigation of the Spirochete and Twenty-Five Years' Experience With Salvarsan*

Erich Hoffmann,† Bonn, Germany

Translated by H. A. Haynes, Jr., M.D., Ann Arbor, Mich.

FOREWORD

IT WAS for three reasons that I decided to publish my lectures given in Santander on the problem of congenital syphilis. First, much confusion and misunderstanding remained in spite of Matzenauer's advances (1903) and the definite results of etiologic investigations in Germany since 1905. Newly acquired facts made a new presentation desirable, especially as they can be vouched for from personal experience.

Second, I wished to present the results of German research in other countries for the information of physicians and to clear up misunderstandings which are still hindering the battle against this world epidemic.

And third, I am convinced that today this subject demands closer cooperation between pediatricians, syphilologists, gynecologists, pathologists, and those engaged in other branches of medicine. However, in the successful struggle for the freeing of humanity from the scourge of syphilis, it is especially important to prevent the transmission of the disease, falsely called hereditary syphilis, and thereby free innocent children from the curse of a generalized infection with which they become afflicted even before birth. May this goal soon be reached by every friend of humanity, and may further useful contributions follow this unified presentation. Then, indeed, the elimination of syphilis will no longer be pointed to as Utopian.

Bonn, December 31, 1935.

Erich Hoffmann.

*Die Angeborene Syphilis im Lichte 30 jähriger Spirochäten—un 25 jähriger Salvarsanforschung: Abhandlungen aus der Kinderheilkunde un ihren Grenzgebieten, Heft 40, 1936, Berlin, S. Karger.

Lectures given in Spanish (August 12-17, 1935) at the International University at Santander, Spain, in the amphitheater of the Casa de Salud de Valdecilla.

†Professor of Dermatology.

I. INTRODUCTION

THE advances which have been made during the past thirty years in the etiology and experimental investigation of acquired syphilis have become very important in the presentation of the theory of congenital syphilis. In spite of these advances, widespread fallacies exist which have not yet been clarified. As in the field of tuberculosis, famous clinicians and pathologists, such as P. Ricord, R. Virchow, A. Fournier, A. Neisser, endeavored to determine the limits and nature of syphilis before the discovery of its etiologic agent and before satisfactory experimental animals were available. In spite of clinical experience, they reached false conclusions which have persisted and which even today influence some physicians. In both of these chronic and polymorphous diseases, whose differentiation from diseases clinically resembling them was once so difficult, a well-grounded study could begin only after discovery of their etiologic agents. By the introduction of exact methods of investigation Robert Koch, who died twenty-five years ago, first lightened the gloom of tuberculosis with the flame of his genius more than fifty years ago (1882), while only thirty years have passed since the discovery of the spirochete of syphilis (Schaudinn and Hoffmann[1]). By the introduction of experimental syphilis (Metschnikoff-Roux[2]), the serologic reaction (A.v. Wassermann[3]), and spinal fluid diagnosis,[4] valuable supplements were found which, together with the discovery of Fritz Schaudinn, placed us for the first time on a definite basis regarding the recognition of the pathogenesis of congenital syphilis. In connection with proof of the curative and preventive action of atoxyl (P. Uhlenhuth, E. Hoffmann, Salmon, and others), Paul Ehrlich created modern chemical therapy, which, following the introduction of arsenobenzol (1910),[5] has laid the foundation for the prevention of and for an efficient battle against congenital syphilis.

If I review, in four lectures, the greatest advances in a field which is covered by a voluminous literature, it seems to me better to consider more fully the new discoveries of worth rather than the older pathology and symptomatology. These new discoveries have altered our position in regard to this problem and have made us more optimistic, in spite of some erroneous views which have persisted. The time has come to draw

[1]First discovery March 3, following joint research at the Berliner Hautklinik (Charité), first publication April 25, 1905, in the publication of the Kaiserlichen Gesundheitsamt (see Wien. klin. Wchnschr. 1935, No. 32 and Vorträge und Urkunden, etc., Verlag S. Karger, 1930). Here there is an exact description of the discovery of the etiologic agent of syphilis (Appendix 122-124) as well as a reprint of the first four original articles.

[2]In apes in 1903; in rabbits; Bertarelli and Volpino in the eye in 1906. Parodi in the testicle in 1907, and E. Hoffmann, Löhe and Mulzer in the skin of the testicle in 1908 first found the virus (primary syphiloma).

[3]In 1906, on the basis of the complement fixation reaction of Bordet, in conjunction with A. Neisser and C. Bruck.

[4]After Quincke's discovery of the lumbar puncture, Ravaut. Sicard, and others introduced its use, and Wassermann and Plaut supplemented it by the specific reaction.

[5]Salvarsan in rabbits in 1909 (in collaboration with Bertheim and Hata); in man in 1910; neosalvarsan in 1912.

conclusions, clearly and emphatically, from these advances and to make our goal the elimination of this once dreaded scourge, laying stress on familial and social problems. Many details are to be found in the new Handbuch, in articles by Rietschel, E. Müller, Péhu, Kerl, and others,[6] while as yet the fourth volume of the French work "Traité de la Syphilis"[7] (Jeanselme) has not been published. As the literature is voluminous and many publications are of doubtful value, I believe it better to limit myself to the accepted facts and views which are of practical import for the elimination of congenital syphilis.

Owing to the frequency of transmission of syphilis to the fetus, syphilis has always assumed a special position among the chronic infectious diseases. Premature interruption of pregnancy and expulsion of a macerated fetus are consequences of this disease which have been ascribed to a very early infection, explained by "germinative transmission" and even blastophthoria. This assumption was made by Paracelsus, who wrote in 1529, "Fit morbus hereditarius, et transit a patre ad filium." In a noteworthy manner, Ambroise Paré in 1633 said, "Souvent on voit sortir les petits enfants hors le ventre de leurs mères ayant cette maladie, et tôt après, avoir plusieurs pustules sur leurs corps; lesquels estant ainsi infestés, baillent la vérole à autant de nourrices qui les allaitent."[8]

Such strictly clinical observations explain the choice of the term "hereditary," which was formerly so generally accepted that its exclusion from the terminology of many countries appears to be difficult. Nevertheless, this term should be avoided, because the transmission of the spirochete of syphilis has nothing to do with heredity, the laws of which are now known. Instead, the present term "congenital syphilis" has become fairly generally accepted. Objection has at times been raised to this designation because it suggests infection through conception, and the terms "syphilis innata" and "connatalis" have been suggested to replace "congenital syphilis." I support this change in terminology and E. Müller, Péhu and Kerl have cited the latter names in their new Handbuch articles. Thus I may designate as "syphilis innata" the severe fetal forms now called congenital syphilis in the French literature, and as "syphilis connatalis and postnatalis" the milder forms which first appear after birth. From these diaplacental infections, those infections occurring during and after birth must be distinguished as acquired infant syphilis, "syphilis acquisita infantum," and, as we shall see later, the rarer mixed infection, "syphilis binaria."

[6]In Arzt-Zieler, Haut- und Geschlechtskrankheiten, Urban und Schwarzenberg, 4,541 (bibliography here given).

[7]Now being completed by Sézary (Masson et Cie., Paris, publishers).

[8]Quoted from C. F. Marshall, Syphilology, etc. (London, 1906, p. 317). As Rietschal stated, Fallopia, the personal physician of Popes Alexander I and Julius II, had already recognized the syphilitic fetus and infection of wet nurses (Jadassohn's Handbuch, 19, 1).

II. PATHOGENESIS (METHOD OF TRANSMISSION)

Whether a germinative transmission is possible or whether in syphilis, as in all other infectious diseases, infection becomes established later in the course of pregnancy through the placenta and umbilical cord, is a question of decisive importance in regard to further problems, especially that of prevention. As will be seen below, the course of infection is explained in the latter sense by our investigations. The opposing views of certain physicians, who cannot renounce old familiar and beloved theories, similar to the opposition of Rudolf Virchow to Robert Koch's discovery, cannot seriously oppose the newly won facts.

A. *Theory of Germinative (Paternal) Syphilis.*—The studies of the late Rudolf Matzenauer in 1903, shortly before the discovery of the spirochete, had shaken the theory of paternal syphilis so strongly that many experienced clinicians were already turning from it. Although my teacher, Edmund Lesser, as well as E. Finger and others, strongly supported this theory of paternal transmission, which was contrary to sound reasoning and which confused rather than helped the young physician, I had known it to be incorrect even before Matzenauer's famous publication in Vienna. However, at that time, I refrained from opposing this theory out of consideration for my teacher. Since the discovery of the spirochete, this theory[9] has become entirely untenable.

Because syphilis is usually introduced into the family by the father, the older physicians suspected that a "purely paternal transmission" could occur, thus sparing the mother from the disease, and that the "guilt" of the procreator would be visited on the children (and children's children). This supposition, which was indeed incompatible with the known contagious nature of the virus of syphilis, became strengthened in the minds of clinicians. Before the discovery of the Wassermann reaction, mothers of syphilitic children were at times found to exhibit no symptoms or clinical manifestations of syphilis, even after most thorough examinations. It was already known at that time that the tendency of syphilis was prolonged latency in the early as well as in the late stages. But the entirely asymptomatic course, the "silent infection," was only admitted later after animal experimentation (rabbits) by Kolle and others. Certainly Matzenauer had already referred to it and to the fact that in a series of mothers of definitely syphilitic children, suggestive and even positive signs (adenopathy, leucoderma, essential alopecia, etc.) could be demonstrated by a very thorough clinical examination. This idea of an asymptomatic syphilis later became confirmed by numerous serologic examinations and has given rise to the idea that every mother of a syphilitic child has either a latent or active infection,

[9] E. Hoffmann, Aetiologie der Syphilis, Springer, 1906, p. 42. The importance of spirochetes in the mother and fetus as well as in the fetal membranes is emphasized here.

and that she is the carrier of the infection. Statistics which support this are so frequently published and cited in texts that I need not discuss them here.

In support of the theory of paternal syphilis, which formerly Kassowitz, A. Fournier, etc., and even today Finger, Hochsinger,[10] Fischl, Almkvist, Mutzer, and others would not renounce, are a few observations which are regarded by critical clinicians only as rare accidents. Thus, families are described in which a syphilitic husband has been the father of a syphilitic child by a supposedly healthy wife, while she has later given birth to a normal child by a healthy husband, and all serologic examinations of the mother and child (spinal fluid, roentgen ray evidence?) have remained consistently negative. One such observation was published in 1929 by J. Almkvist, the well-known Swedish syphilographer. This was translated into French by Péhu.

Nov. 4, 1914, a mother gave birth to an infant weighing 2,950 gm. who had a syphilitic papular eruption and positive Wassermann reaction. Examination of the mother did not reveal any reason for supposing the existence of syphilis, either clinically or serologically. This woman has been serologically examined 36 times in the past 14 years, always with negative results. June 29, 1935, about 10½ years after the birth of the syphilitic child, she married another husband and was delivered of a child weighing 3,920 gm., completely healthy and showing no symptoms of syphilis. This infant and his mother have been followed by Almkvist; neither has presented clinically or serologically any evidence of syphilis. Thus this physician concludes that the syphilis of the first infant was of paternal origin.

The above case shows more than ten years' interval between the births of the syphilitic and the healthy infant. During such a long period the transmissibility of syphilis usually disappears spontaneously, thus making possible the formulation of the "laws of marriage" of the older clinicians. The birth of a healthy infant is easily explained by the long lapse of time and the fact that the mother probably had a previous latent or manifest syphilis, perhaps healing later spontaneously. Negative serologic reactions do at times occur in syphilis of long duration. Significant conclusion can obviously not be made on the basis of one or two rare cases.

This is still more true in cases in which treatment of the father alone has led to the birth of a normal child after or between the birth of other syphilitic children. Today, such observations must be regarded as coincidences, because formerly treatment consisted only of mercurials, which could influence the transmission of syphilis but slightly, as compared with salvarsan.

Through similar clinical observations, the opinion became established that the sperm of syphilitic men commonly contained and transmitted the germ of the disease. However, since the size of the spirochete in comparison with the sperm head has become known, this theory has had

[10]In Abhandlungen aus der Kinderheilkunde und ihren Grenzgebieten, No. 15, the old doctrine is presented by one well versed in this theory.

to be abandoned. The partisans of paternal transmission now consider a "granular virus form" to account for the infection of the ovum. That is also not justifiable, in spite of the intercession of Levaditi, Hochsinger, Meirowsky, and others.[11]

Further, through experiments on apes and rabbits, the "infectiousness of the sperm" of syphilitic men has been proved, and it cannot be denied that, in contrast to reported negative results (A. Neisser, E. Hoffmann and others), at times positive results ensue (Finger and Landsteiner, Uhlenhuth and Mülzer and others). These experiments cannot be of great value because, if the sperm flow contains many spirochetes, the mother will be infected by such a contagious disease before the ovum, which in early development is protected so well by Nature by virtue of its membranes and living metabolic processes.

All clinical observations support the fact that syphilis is usually transmitted by spirochetes occurring in erosions, etc., of the skin or mucous membranes, while it has not been proved that the sperm alone is infectious in men free from such lesions. During the secondary stage, men infect their wives by means of spirochetes transmitted from erosions, papules, and mucous membranes. Spirochetes frequently occur in the urethra, and I believe them responsible for the occasional infectious nature of the sperm flow.[12] Nothing is definitely known about the spirochete content of spermatic fluid in late syphilis. However, I know of one significant fact bearing on this matter. Physicians who have acquired syphilis in the course of their professional duties (usually primary lesions of the fingers) and, in spite of a roseola, have remained free of genital lesions, do not often infect their wives, even when continuing marital relations during the course of the secondary period, when their infection was still undiagnosed. This observation, which I have occasionally made in physicians and also in nurses and laymen, is evidence against the virus content of the spermatic fluid, even during late primary and early secondary stages; this fact is important because of many repeated negative findings. So far as I know, infection of rabbits by repeated injections of naturally obtained spermatic fluid of an infected buck has not been successful.

Finally, the so-called exceptions of Colle's law formerly played an important rôle. They occurred very rarely, and not once were they described by reputable clinicians of wide experience. The appearance of an apparent primary (pseudoprimary lesion) on the nipple of the mother of a syphilitic child was considered a new infection, while today

[11]On the basis of implantation experiments using the method described by Schaudinn, v. Prowazek, and E. Hoffmann, the rolled-up forms (formes en boucle et en pelote) were recently described by Levaditi, Schoen, and Vaisman as a stage of development of the *Spirocheta pallida* (Zentralbl. f. Haut- u. Geschlechtskr: 52, 249).

[12]Czerny and other pediatricians emphasize the fact that in foundling asylums (e.g., Prague) the contagiousness of congenital syphilis is not great and transmission is rare. As the virulence of protozoa is enhanced by characteristic passage of insects, a similar augmentation of the virulence of *Spirocheta pallida* may be possible in weeping papules, erosions, etc. (under anaerobic conditions) which would be of importance in contact infection and may explain the greater frequency of genital lesions compared with extragenital infections.

we know that only a reinduration (superinfection) can occur on a latent syphilitic.[13] Such exceptions to Colle's law are no longer heard. Our greater knowledge of symptom-free reinfection and superinfection, obtained from experimental syphilis, has aided much in the explanation of this fact.

The theory of paternal transmission had progressed far, as shown by the theory of "choc en retour," formulated by the great Ricord. Péhu interpreted this as an indirect infection of the mother by the sperm-infected child, as well as infection by the father, and regarded this theory with scepticism. To us, this theory must appear exaggerated and erroneous; today it is considered only a curiosity.

Here may also be mentioned the theory of syphilis by conception (syphilis conceptionelle précoce), which assumes an especially malignant form of the disease when conception and infection occur simultaneously. Even in a definite postconceptional infection of a mother who was previously healthy at the time of conception, adherents of the theory of paternal transmission have regarded the infection as being carried from the sperm to the ovum, with subsequent infection of the mother through "choc en retour."

As well-known clinicians still cling to these erroneous views, the facts which contradict "paternal transmission of congenital syphilis" will be clearly presented once again. First of all, the records of very rare, doubtful cases are no longer tenable in the face of modern knowledge, even though occasionally they appear significant. We know today that syphilis is so contagious that were a syphilitic man to transmit spirochetes by his sperm to a woman, he would first infect her and not the ovum alone. Spirochetal infection of the ovum and not the more accessible mother is therefore to be regarded as improbable, if not impossible. Also it is hardly conceivable that a holoblastic ovum,[14] such as the human, would continue to develop if it were syphilized, because even later, in the fetus, immunity is lacking or is so slight that with early diaplacental infection spirochetes overwhelm it and can cause its death. A matter of decisive importance is the fact that spirochetes have never been found in the fetus of syphilitic mothers nor in the fetal portion of the membrances before the fifth month of pregnancy. Rare exceptions toward the end of the fourth month, such as the fetus described by Gräfenberg and others, are not definite, while others carefully described by Oluf Thomson, Paul Schneider, etc., showed nothing. If a germinative infection occurred, spirochetes would be expected to develop in such numbers in the fetus during the first half of pregnancy, that they could be demonstrated without difficulty in the first months of pregnancy.

---

[13] E. Hoffmann, Dermat. Ztschr. 12: 491, 1905.

[14] As interesting as they may be, the observations made by Levaditi on mereoblastic ova (spirochete of chickens) have no importance for human pathology; similarly, the experiments with pébrine (a disease of silkworms) have no bearing on the question.

How enormously spirochetes can multiply in very young animals, e.g., chickens, is shown by the inoculation of *Spirocheta gallinarum* into newly hatched chicks; the research done in my laboratory by Kroó[15] is also significant in regard to this question. The germinative—that is, the oogenic as well as the spermatogenic—transmission of syphilis may therefore be regarded today as entirely unproved. Attempts to preserve this doctrine by older and even by more recent clinical observations are of minor importance when opposed by the great mass of available research.

B. *Diaplacental Infection.*—As has been emphasized by G. Herxheimer in his excellent article (Wiesbaden, 1928) and in my papers (Hamburg, 1928, and Koenigsberg, 1929), only the diaplacental route of infection remains, and Matzenauer's statement, "Without a syphilitic mother there can be no syphilitic child," may today be considered entirely valid. Matzenauer's theory, which Rietschel and I have long supported (Handb. d. Hautkr. 19), that transmission first occurs by way of the placenta and umbilical cord during the second half of pregnancy, most frequently in the sixth and seventh months, can be amplified on the basis of new research, confirmed by Klaften in conjunction with O. Thomson, P. Schneider, and others. Thus, the earlier view that syphilis was the result of a germinative infection has lost favor, this chronic infection following the rule of transmission of the etiologic agents from the mother to the child.

The transmission of *Spirocheta pallida* occurs regularly from the infected mother to the fetus; in general, it occurs more intensively and more frequently if the mother's infection is fresh and severe. In cases of severe, untreated infection, this results in the early expulsion of a diseased and dead fetus. In the course of time, the intensity of the syphilis gradually diminishes, even without specific treatment, and children are born at term, manifestly infected or apparently uninfected, the latter sooner or later showing signs of syphilis. The birth of a completely healthy infant can occur between stillbirths or infected children. The "spontaneous gradual diminution of the intensity of syphilitic transmission," according to Kasowitz' rule, which in general holds good, is thereby broken. The cause of this lapse lies, first, in the fluctuation of intensity of the mother's infection and the number of virulent organisms which enter the blood stream, and, further, in the extent of localized infection within the mother's placenta, conditioned by the organisms in the blood. This irregularity of fetal infection is well illustrated by the fact that twins are not necessarily equally severely infected; indeed, one may be healthy and the other syphilitic. One such occurrence was reported in uniovular twins and, I believe, can be explained by the localization of foci of infection in the placenta and umbilical cord.

[15]The chicks do not react clinically to the immense multiplication of spirochetes. Hoffmann, Aetologie der Syphilis, Springer, 1906, 42.

It has recently become recognized that habitual abortion during the first months of pregnancy is not always due to syphilis but to the same causes as in nonsyphilitic women, while stillbirths and premature births occurring during the second half of pregnancy (fifth and sixth months on) are suggestive of syphilis. However, in spite of this, in actual practice, abortions should always be investigated for the presence of syphilis.

The participation of the obstetrician in the investigation of and battle against congenital syphilis has become very important. In addition to the course of the pregnancy, the pathologic-anatomic changes which are found in the placenta and umbilical cord are of great significance and can frequently be shown to be specific by the presence of spirochetes. The placentas of syphilitic fetuses and of syphilitic children are usually abnormally large and heavy in proportion to the body weight of the child. I have termed this proportion of placental to infant or fetal weight the placental quotient. At the end of gravidity, it is usually 1:6 for the normal, 1:5 for the syphilitic, and even 1:4 and more in premature births, thus at least arousing suspicion of syphilis.[16] The placenta also shows pathologic changes which consist of proliferation of capillary endothelium and stroma cells, diminution of intervillous spaces, the so-called abscesses in the villae, and vascular changes which are manifested as an obliterating endovasculitis, which Kaufmann found in 16 per cent of cases. Anemic infarcts, which Virchow first thought to be gummas, and infiltrates containing giant cells occur especially in the maternal portion of the placenta. Frequently the umbilical cord likewise shows perivasculitis, mesovasculitis, and endovasculitis with small cell infiltration, which is more pronounced in the adventitia and media at both ends of the cord. The focal arrangement stands out in a characteristic manner in and around the umbilical vein, which is frequently involved.

All these changes, in themselves not characteristic of syphilis, demand consideration, and further studies, such as dark-field examination and silver stains of sections, should be carried out in establishing proof of the etiologic agent. Spirochetes are frequently present in the walls of the umbilical vessels and can be found at times in scrapings of the intima and media of the umbilical vein which is generally involved severely. In the placenta, spirochetes are often as numerous in the fetal as in the maternal portion, although they invade primarily from the latter portion; this may be due to the influence of immunity developed in the maternal organism, as well as to its high oxygen content.[17] The transmission of the anaerobic spirochetes into the fetal portion does not occur before the fifth month of gestation. Probably an occasional spirochete suffices to infect the fetus owing to an almost complete absence of immunity in

[16]E. Hoffmann: Dermat. Ztschr. 54, 369 and 57, 145.

[17]The small number of *Spirocheta pallida* in the oxygen-rich placenta and in the blood, as well as their situation in the tissue, led me in 1905 to infer that the spirochete was anaerobic, a fact which Schaudinn at first doubted.

the latter, the severity of the infection being proportional to the invading masses of microbes (involvement of the vessel walls). This invasion can enter directly into the blood stream or, in addition, can occur through the lymphatic passages,[18] in which case, as I stated in 1928, a sort of primary complex can develop in the fetal placenta and in the umbilical cord up to the liver vessels. Thus, occasionally, a specific phlebitis can appear in the infected liver (Beitske). By animal experimentation (rabbits), healthy placentas have been penetrated by the *Spirocheta pallida* and similar spirochetes (Philipp and others); this is not true for the larger parasites, such as trypanosomes. These tedious experiments, however, do not have any great significance when applied to human pathology. My hope that animals with longer periods of gestation (e.g., llamas) could be used in these experiments has thus far remained unfulfilled.

Transmission of *Spirocheta pallida* can occur until the end of pregnancy. The number of transmitted germs may depend on the age and intensity of the maternal infection and on the number of spirochetes still motile and present in the blood stream, as well as on the extent of localized infection in the maternal placenta. Thus, the protecting barriers to the fetal portion of the placenta may break down in the case of a maternal infection acquired shortly before or during pregnancy, with an ensuing high spirochetal content of the maternal blood resulting in numerous placental foci. The earlier this fetal invasion occurs (fifth to sixth months) with consequent greater invasion of the fetal blood, lymphatic and tissue routes, the more intense will be the infection of the fetus which is not yet protected by any immunity. Because of the absence of immune processes, an unchecked increase of parasites may occur in the fetus and thereby cause its death. Involvement of vessels with narrowing of their lumen, as observed in the syphilitic placenta, results in deficient nourishment. Transmission of spirochetes may occur long after the original maternal infection, due to the fact that acquired syphilis may run a course of exacerbations and, when untreated, recurrences are possible during many years.

On the other hand, even with a fresh syphilis of the mother which has not been specifically treated, transmission may occur late or, more rarely, not at all. Thus may apparently normal or really normal children be born. The fact that the former frequently show evidences of syphilis four to eight weeks or within the first four years after birth has given rise to the opinion that transmission of spirochetes first occurs shortly before birth or—what may be rare—during it, due to loosening of the placenta (H. Rietschel).[19] This type of congenital syphilis, becoming

[18]H. Rietschel first suggested this possibility in 1913.

[19]Late transmissions are frequently reported, as for example, I. Levin considered an infection as occurring fourteen days before birth on the basis of the appearance of a primary lesion on the mother ten days later (ten days postcoitus and four days prepartum!) and the infant having Coryza syphilitica twenty-five days after birth, and an exanthema and weakly positive serologic reaction forty-four days after birth. (Zentralbl. f. Haut- u, Geschlechtskr. 51, 589).

recognizable some weeks or months after birth, could be designated as syphilis postnatalis, or as syphilis congenita, innata, and connatalis.

All degrees of severity of infection are evident, ranging from a macerated fetus and severe visceral and bone syphilis of affected children (syphilis innata) to the apparently healthy infant (syphilis connatalis or postnatalis asymptomatica). These types are explained by the manner and severity and, above all, by the time of invasion and numbers of spirochetes invading through the maternal placenta whose protective function eventually fails to a greater or lesser degree. It is not clear as to the extent to which antigenic substances traversing the placenta play a part in mitigating the infant infection.

It should be further emphasized here that the severity as well as the frequency of fetal syphilis has significantly become reduced during the last decades. This fact is cited in the new Handbuch and in many individual articles and is ascribed to salvarsan therapy during pregnancy, a therapy which has also aided in a reduction of syphilis in general. Before I discuss this further, some questions of acquired infant syphilis must be considered.

C. *Binary and Acquired Syphilis.*—Pasini questioned whether there was a sharp distinction between congenital and acquired syphilis of the newborn, and I explained the possibility of mixed infections, i.e., a binary congenital syphilis.

All infections occurring by hematogenous or lymphogenous routes and not exogenous (with or without a primary lesion) are considered as syphilis congenita; infection takes place through the umbilical cord, which may present a phlebitis. Rare cases of deep or superficial, chancrelike, umbilical ulcers, which, according to Hutinel, L. F. Meyer and others, appear about three weeks after birth, have been regarded as lymphatic infections occurring through the umbilical cord. Similar forms of infection, rarely noted, approach acquired infant syphilis in appearance and are difficult to differentiate from an exogenous infection of the umbilicus occurring during or shortly after birth.

As I have pointed out in previous articles, a double infection is possible, giving rise to syphilis congenita binaria, only one case of which, reported by Schilling and V. Hoffmann,[20] was I able to accept as definite. This mixed form can occur when a child, infected before birth by diaplacental transmission of spirochetes from the mother, receives a second or superinfection of spirochetes through the skin during the passage through a birth canal containing infectious papules or erosions. This superinfection can be manifested by a primary on the head, or more rarely elsewhere, but may occur asymptomatically. The spirochetes, derived from the same source, namely, the still infectious mother, reach the child by two different routes: most important, before birth through the umbilical cord, and then later through the skin at time of delivery.

[20]Jadassohn's Handb. d. Haut- u. Geschlechtskr. 17/3, 168.

Naturally there remains the possibility that an exogenous infection after birth can originate from the same or from another source of infection (wet nurses, nurses, etc.).

Such infections "en passage" are very rare, A. Fournier stating that he had never seen one. In my article on binary syphilis of nursing infants,[21] I referred to ten cases of proved primaries on the heads of nursing infants and believe that these are frequently overlooked because they are often insignificant and the regional lymphadenitis may be minimal. Consequently, the question whether there is a sharp borderline between acquired and congenital syphilis in infants deserves more consideration, and our best efforts must be given to the study of the possibility of superinfection and to careful investigation of binary syphilis of the newborn. Thus might be explained the appearance of keratitis profunda, etc., following what would appear to be an acquired syphilis in infancy.

Tarnowsky described binary syphilis of older individuals with signs of late congenital syphilis, which should be differentiated from binary syphilis of nursing infants and should be considered as a reinfection or superinfection of an older congenital syphilitic, in whom the skin immunity, with or without specific therapy, has decreased to such an extent as to permit a true primary or a pseudoprimary lesion. The possibility of a symptom-free superinfection should always be considered; also, reinfection without an obvious primary lesion may prove to be more important than was formerly thought in doubtful cases, causing late recurrences after an apparently successful cure of adults and of children.

Most pediatricians regard acquired infant syphilis as rare and proportionately unimportant; as Czerny emphasizes, it usually runs a less severe course than in adults.[22] Unfortunately erroneous views prevail which have been represented by illustrations and descriptions in well-known textbooks and thereby have been uncritically disseminated. Pictures of older children of six years or more with alopecia microareolaris, which is a typical early manifestation of an acquired syphilis and is encountered in adults only in the first year, are presented as "late recurrences of congenital syphilis" (Ledermann in Jadassohn's Handbuch,[23] E. Müller in Pfaundler's Handbuch, Feer,[24] etc.). Also, leucoderma and vegetating condylomas occurring in well-nourished infants and older children are indicative of an acquired (or binary) and not a congenital infection.[25] The primary lesion may frequently be concealed, for example, on the tonsil, and is easily overlooked.

---

[21]Deutsche med. Wchnschr. 1929, 1289; Schweiz. med. Wchnschr. 1929, 1213; and Dermat Ztschr. 54 (1928), 369 and 57 (1930), 150.

[22]Other authors, such as Rietschel, do not share this view.

[23]Jadassohn's Handbuch, 19, 73.

[24]Lehrb., 9, Edition 1926, 723 (Condyloma).

[25]Experienced pediatricians, such as H. Rietschel, believe that such condylomata are never observed as an original lesion, but rather as a recurrent lesion after the first year of life, and then only rarely.

D. *Frequency of Congenital Syphilis.*—The occurrence of congenital syphilis has been significantly reduced. E. Müller, Klaften, Péhu, Lomholt, and others have made statistical studies and have attributed this reduction to successful treatment with salvarsan preparations, which has also caused a decrease in the formerly marked polymorphism and severity of congenital syphilis. The statistics presented by authors in different countries vary considerably.

In many countries (e.g., Brazil, Russia, etc.) they are higher than in Germany. Years ago Buschke estimated the number of stillbirths in Germany as 20 per 25,000, and Baisch as 20 per 10,000. According to the German census of 1927, there were about 7,500 living children with congenital syphilis. In the children's clinics, from 2 to 4 per cent of infants were found to be syphilitic. In England and France these figures are higher and reach 10 per cent, and in France and its colonies even 20 per cent and more. To be sure, doubtful cases (hereditary distrophies, etc.) have been included. The number of premature and stillbirths due to syphilis was given as 50 to 90 per cent by Weber and Reischig; Reischig found 81.1 per cent and Gräfenberg found 92 per cent of the stillborn to be macerated. The mortality of the infants born alive was high; Noeggerath showed that it was from 50 to 67 per cent in hospitals, from 24 to 35 per cent in nursing homes, and from 15 to 19 per cent in out-patients (those less severely involved). The greatest number of these infants died in the first year, especially during the first four months. The devastating effect which syphilis exercises on progeny is shown by Hochsinger's great work; he followed 266 pregnancies in 67 families and found that 46.6 per cent of the pregnancies resulted in premature stillbirths, 28.6 per cent in infant mortality within the first year, while only 24.8 per cent of the infants remained alive. Gammeltoft found only 7 (3.5 per cent) healthy children among 201 children of untreated syphilitic mothers. Hata could prove only 5 healthy children over five years of age in 100 syphilitic marriages.

These few but startling figures suffice to show the devastating effect of syphilis on progeny before the introduction of modern therapeutic methods.

Another arresting fact is the percentage of pregnant women who have syphilis. This was investigated by Blumenthal and myself in 1908[26] and also by others since then.

The figures obtained ranged from 8 to 10 per cent, and in Halle, reached even up to 20 per cent; they fell to 5 to 6 per cent and are now still lower (4 per cent). On the basis of compilation, Klaften estimated the average frequency of syphilis among pregnant women in Europe as about 4.5 per cent to 5.5 per cent; in America, 6.8 per cent. These figures have been greatly reduced wherever there is satisfactory treatment. In 1926-27 Philipp and Richter[27] found 65 syphilitic children among 5,028 births in the Berliner Frauenklinik, which is scarcely 1.3 per cent. In 1931-32, there were only 22 syphilitic children among 4,073 births, or only 0.5 per cent. The number of macerated syphilitic stillborn decreased during this period from 42 in 1926-27 to 7 in 1931-32, which fact is still more striking.

In Denmark, where the statistics are exceptionally accurate, due to an excellent central card index system, the yearly census of congenital syph-

[26]Dermat. Ztschr. 15, 23 and 17, 1 and 82.
[27]München. med. Wchnschr. 1933, 1540.

ilis has dropped from 280 in 1920 to 29 in 1931 (Lomholt[28]). I understand that in Vienna, in spite of weak doses of salvarsan (only 0.3 gm. of neosalvarsan per week) used in the treatment of pregnant syphilitic women, there is a disappearance of the macerated fetus, as well as a significant reduction of congenital syphilis, a fact noted by different authors. The statistics of the northern countries are similar to the Danish, thus demonstrating the success of treatment.

There is much in the literature about the transmission of syphilis to the second generation (termed by many, the third generation).

That an insufficiently treated or an untreated woman with congenital syphilis can exceptionally transmit syphilis to her child is admitted by clinicians, and a compilation made by Feige under my direction and newer studies show that a few cases may meet the rigid requirements of Fournier, Finger, and others. That transmission is also possible to the third generation (also termed the fourth) is asserted but has not been ascertained. These questions cannot be further discussed here because they have no bearing on the problem which interests us and, due to our modern therapeutic knowledge, are no longer as important as formerly.[29]

E. *Doubtful Infections (Malformations, Hereditary Dystrophies, and Syphilis Larvée).*—Finally there is another question, much discussed in the French literature, as to whether syphilis can engender monstrosities, malformations and dystrophies. This question has been exhaustively treated and criticized by Péhu. There is also the question as to whether a syphilitic toxin is capable of impairing the germ plasm, thus producing a blastophthoria. In my articles (1928-29), I opposed the idea that injury to the germ plasm can result without a diaplacental transmission of *Spirocheta pallida*. It also appears to me that this stand, already supported by Husler and others, is justified and I believe that it is worthy of being reemphasized. Whoever considers such a vague theory[30] must admit that syphilis by its influence on the germ plasm would have greatly damaged the human race during the last hundred years in the countries in which it is widespread. We know, however, that children of otherwise healthy syphilitic parents who are no longer infectious can be entirely normal. Indeed it is remarkable that extremely good-looking and healthy children have been born into otherwise unblemished families of old syphilitics and paralytics, when marriage occurred after loss of transmissibility of the syphilis. The regularity with which healthy children are born, after intensive prenatal therapy with modern preparations (neosalvarsan, bismuth), supports this view.

The statements about the occurrence of monstrosities, malformations, and dystrophies are likewise derived from the experience and imagination of older clinicians and are vague and far-reaching and in need of

---

[28]Dermat. Wchnschr. 100, 173.

[29]Schönfeld: Dermat. Ztschr. 72: 119.

[30]Fr. v. Müller formerly supported this theory on the basis of several observations in syphilitic families, which, however, can be explained otherwise.

revision. When syphilis was still more rife, and in regions where it was widespread (Paris, Morocco, etc.), even great clinicians ascribed unrelated conditions to syphilis. Thus Lewin once believed that maculae caeruleae, which are due to pediculosis, were a special type of syphilitic exanthemas, while in France, vitiligo, alopecia areata, the tubercle of Carabelli, and many other conditions were ascribed to syphilis. The famous A. Fournier, who first included tabes, general paralysis and aneurysms as syphilitic manifestations, also ascribed numerous dystrophies of the teeth and other organs to syphilis, thus making, in addition to his observations of lasting value, unfortunate statements which have proved to be completely fallacious. It is still held that tuberculosis, rachitis, and other ills can occur on the basis of a congenital syphilis; a lamentable interpretation which, similar to the error of the great Hunter, has resulted in serious consequences. Recently French authors, such as Hutinel and others, considered such disturbances as residues of persisting infections of the infant and due to a specific involvement of the endocrine glands. Schneider, in his article in 1928, collected and reviewed the pathologic changes and spirochetal findings in these glands; also E. Müller, Péhu, and Kerl mentioned them. Interesting as this problem may be, I cannot discuss it further because of my limited personal experience. J. Darier in his excellent text (1928) included, in addition to "hérédosyphilis virulente," the "hérédodistrophies"; he characterized them as "troubles of physical development, a disposition to malformations such as an alcoholic or tuberculous father might cause," and said that these hereditary dystrophies can occur with or without a congenital syphilitic infection.

It is a recognized fact that certain severe dystrophic manifestations, such as the cicatrices of Parrot and other stigmas of the teeth, bones, sensory organs, etc., are evidence of congenital syphilis. These are explained by a lower degree of spirochetogenic involvement. If monstrosities, malformations, and dystrophies in syphilitic families occur without diaplacental transmission of spirochetes, they cannot be ascribed to syphilis. In this respect, it seems to me that the viewpoint accepted in Germany (Rietschel, E. Hoffmann, and others) is critical and correct. Whoever maintains a relation between syphilis and dystrophies must demonstrate the cause and prove the presence of the etiologic agent itself or its acknowledged consequences (inoculation, spinal fluid, serologic reactions, etc.). Because syphilis is extremely polymorphic in its manifestations and because of the possibility of simulation of other diseases (it has been termed the "great imitator"), the opinions of the French school should not be shared when it comes to diagnosis and delimitation. Instead, the rule, "Consider syphilis," should always be followed. If such vague and insufficiently proved theories, which still persist in France, of the "dystrophic sequences of syphilitic toxins" and the influence of hereditary factors were seriously admitted, the progress made by the research of the last three decades would be lost. The theory of "syphilis larvée" and Péhu's fourteen subdivisions,[31] which include all the dystrophies and malformations as well as monstrosities in the various organs, would permit the possibility of a syphilitic origin for all human pathology, as Péhu himself admitted.

Rietschel devoted an article (Med. Klinik, 1931) to a critical résumé of these questionable doctrines and cited reasons why such a position is uncritical and untenable from a clinical standpoint.

Today it is a requisite of medical science to establish more stringent diagnostic criteria for the hereditary dystrophies and to eradicate exaggerated and uncritical theories. Only where the *Spirocheta pallida* can be found, or definite manifestations of it can be proved, are dystrophic processes to be considered as specific. All other dystrophies and malformations should be investigated on the basis of familial inferiority (mental or otherwise) or of true toxic causes (alcohol?) and, even if they are present in the same patient along with congenital syphilis, they should not necessarily be ascribed to the syphilis.

Before a syphilitic toxic influence from the mother to the ovum or fetus can be established, experimental proof on pregnant animals (rabbits) must be obtained. This could be done by repeated injections, before and after coitus, of macerated organs rich in spirochetes—after heating to the death point of the spirochetes. Similar experiments could be carried out with alcohol and other substances having a possible influence on heredity. The assertion made by prominent clinicians—I mention here only R. Sabouraud, the world famous mycologist—that the abnormal tubercle of Carabelli be regarded as a sign of congenital syphilis shows how misleading purely clinical observations and statistics can be. In countries where syphilis was, or still is, widespread, it is often present along with other diseases, as well as tuberculosis, and may be so masked by them that false conclusions are understandable. The difficulty of correcting such errors is repeatedly shown in the history of medicine, and not infrequently even the most outstanding clinicians and pathologists (A. Fournier, E. Finger, R. Virchow) have at times held on to opinions in the realm of the chronic infectious diseases (syphilis, tuberculosis), which were later proved erroneous. In the French literature the opinion is held that tuberculosis can be considered only when it can be proved to be the result of infection with Koch's bacillus. When the same requirements are accepted for the *Spirocheta pallida*, a lengthy and violent controversy will end abruptly.

---

[31]According to Péhu. hérédosyphilis larvée can be manifested by : (1) developmental disturbances, (2) nutritional disturbances, (3) endocrine disturbances, (4) osteoarticular manifestations, (5) nervous involvement, (6) digestive syndromes, (7) hepatic syndromes, (8) respiratory syndromes, (9) cardiovascular affections, (10) renal syndromes, (11) cutaneous manifestations, (12) blood changes, (13) involvement of the lymphatic system, (14) congenital malformations.

III. PATHOLOGIC ANATOMY

Only a few important points of general pathology will be presented here, the subject having been thoroughly discussed by G. Herxheimer and P. Schneider in their Wiesbaden publications.

A. *General Considerations.*—Shortly after their transmission to the fetus, during the fifth month of pregnancy or later, the spirochetes multiply in the fetal organism without producing a reaction and disseminate through the fetus in immense numbers. To a much less degree, this is also true for acquired syphilis, where a severe, occult proliferation is present, not only in the early incubation period before the appearance of the primary lesion, but also in the secondary period in the roseolas and papules, etc., which are hematogenous in origin. As I have emphasized for thirty years, tissue reactions, not only the inflammations that are recognizable microscopically, but also the clinical manifestations, occur considerably after the invasion of the spirochetes. We know today that an asymptomatic infection[32] may persist which merits attention in connection with gravid and congenital syphilis. As I have explained, the limited numbers of *Spirocheta pallida* in the blood and in the maternal placenta are due to the high oxygen content which destroys the anaerobic spirochetes; but under anaerobic conditions in the macerated fetus, an unlimited multiplication of spirochetes can take place. The opinion that this unchecked proliferation occurs after death has only been partially ascertained; as soon as there is a lack of oxygen due to edema and constriction of the lumena of the placental vessels, favorable cultural conditions prevail in the fetus, and, owing to lack of immunity, an unlimited increase of the microbes takes place. Expulsion of the fetus occurs several weeks after its death, thus affording in its oxygen-free tissue a great opportunity for unlimited multiplication of spirochetes. This finally results in partial decomposition of the fetus as a consequence of maceration following fermentative processes. G. Herxheimer has justly emphasized the anergy present in the young fetus of this type; and transmission of protecting immunity from the mother through the diseased placenta cannot really be considered when such severe endovasculitis is present.

The histological pathology of congenital syphilis is similar to that of acquired and experimental animal syphilis. It is distinguished by an inflammation of the blood vessels which may involve the walls of the veins, arteries and lymph vessels, even the capillaries and lymph spaces. The *Spirocheta pallida,* as I have emphasized since 1905, is a lymphatic and connective tissue parasite which behaves differently than the blood spirochetes. In spite of my repeated references to this fact, this difference is underestimated, as is the importance of the anaerobic tendencies of the *Spirocheta pallida.*

[32]Experimentally proved by Kolle and others in mice and rabbits.

It does not seem, therefore, justifiable to speak of a septicemia in congenital or even acquired syphilis (septicémie syphilitique primo-secondaire[33]). Proof of the presence of *Spirocheta pallida* in the oxygenated blood stream is very difficult in the living child, even in the most severe forms of congenital syphilis.[34] Anaerobic *Spirocheta pallida* do not thrive in the blood but escape from the blood stream as quickly as possible, and are much more frequently found in the endothelium and perithelium of the blood capillaries and lymph spaces, and in the vessel walls, often surrounding the vasa vasorum. The endothelium becomes irritated, with resultant edema, proliferation, and hypertrophy; this has been determined experimentally in my laboratory during the primary incubation period of syphilis in rabbits, by G. Armuzzi, a student of mine for many years, who carried out my suggestions carefully. In the perivascular lymph spaces and in blood and venous thrombi, which have a low oxygen content, occasional or numerous *Spirocheta pallida* can be found, and also a few in regional lymph glands as early as twenty-four hours after infection, while they have been found in the spleen forty-two hours after infection by silver staining of sections (my student, Emil Zurhelle).

The true cytotropic reaction, which appears in addition to the endovasculitis, mesovasculitis, and perivasculitis, follows as a more or less allergic reaction, is related to vascular endothelium, and is considered by Aschoff as a defense mechanism of the reticuloendothelial system. This reaction is not uniform but appears in isolated islands, so that free zones always remain between the foci of perivascular infiltration. This focal distribution is also characteristic of the nests of spirochetes and is reflected in the histologic picture. In addition, there appears a unmistakable sclerotic change of the collagenous tissue, which in rabbits is accompanied by a myxomatous exudation, and in man by lymphedema and a less noticeable degeneration of the connective tissue.

The characteristic cell picture of syphilis does not consist of a pure plasmoma, as Unna assumed. Cell counts of tissue from chancres and later syphilomas, which have been made by various French authors (Nanta, Laurentier, and others), show from 35 to 63 per cent small lymphocytes, about 10 per cent large lymphocytes, and 10 per cent each of mononuclears and plasma cells; however the number of plasma cells is usually considerably greater, according to my experience and that of other German pathologists and syphilologists. In congenital syphilis, plasma cells are at first absent and later are more rarely found than in acquired syphilis.

French authors further assume a proliferation and even a wandering of the endothelium. They emphasize that giant cells, which are more

[33]Sézary; Traité de la Syphilis (Jeanselme) III, 65.

[34]I sometimes found them in dark-field examination in severely involved nursing infants (Berl. klin. Wchnschr., 351, 1907).

frequent in the many lupoid forms of syphilis and even involve vessel walls, are of endothelial origin. I frequently have seen convincing examples of this in small vessels (veins) which are being destroyed by endovasculitis.

B. *Bone Involvement.*—In the dearth of other symptoms, the bony involvements have become very important in the detection of fetal and early forms of congenital syphilis, not only because of their spirochetal content, but because they are recognizable roentgenologically. The most important form is the classical Wegnerian involvement of the epiphyseal borders of the long bones (femur, tibia, etc.) which is also manifested in the cartilaginous borders of the ribs and elsewhere. These changes can occur from the fifth fetal month onward. The great frequency of bone involvement and its significance in Parrot's disease (a pseudoparalysis due to epiphyseal separation) give it a special value for syphilologists, pediatricians, obstetricians, and pathologists. Next in importance to osteochondritis is periostitis syphilitica; this form may begin in fetal life but usually appears somewhat later. In addition, German authors mention the osteomyelitis fibrosa rareficans of Pick, and Péhu also cites a productive hyperplastic form. A type characterized by transverse shadow bands (Klaften) has recently been reported which can be recognized roentgenologically and which occurs following prenatal specific therapy in Wegner's disease.

On the basis of thorough researches by O. Thomsen, P. Schneider, L. Pick, M. Péhu, and others, it may be said that spirochetes are present in their classical form in the growth centers of the bones, but not before the fifth month of pregnancy. In the absence of any reaction the spirochete is the only certain indication of a progressive but otherwise latent infection; the stratum of cartilaginous development is its site of predilection, while this form of involvement does not occur in the membranous bones. Osteochondritis regularly occurs symmetrically, is often recognizable by roentgenographic examination before and at birth, and is easily differentiated from rachitis up to the third month. In the course of the first three or four months, the osteochondritis recedes spontaneously and disappears as a generalized symmetrical involvement, while other forms become more pronounced (periostitis, localized lesions, etc.).

Thus, osteochrondritis syphilitica is not, as its name signifies, an inflammatory process from the beginning, but is a characteristic alteration at the border of the developmental zone between the diaphysis and epiphysis of the long bones, ribs, etc., the ossification of which is disturbed in the cartilaginous stratum. The normal epiphyseal borders, which ordinarily appear as a regular narrow white line, become an irregular, zigzagged, yellowish white streak seldom more than 4 mm. in width. At a further stage in development, a striking zone of yellowish tissue arises which projects in tonguelike forms of different lengths into the epiphysis. Under the influence of the *Spirocheta pallida*, which causes little or no reaction in the fetal organism, bone formation is disturbed and greatly delayed, while the cartilaginous columns develop in the usual manner. Gratelike arrangements of calcified cartilage appear in the widened zones of calcification, the so-called "Kalkgitter" or calcified grate, between which normal cartilage remains. With severe degrees of involvement, in the course of time, a band of granulation tissue, which arises from the connective tissue of the young bone marrow, is interpolated between the bones and the zone of calcification. This results in a spongy connection between the bony diaphysis and the cartilaginous epiphysis, and at times in a complete epiphyseal separation due to a fracture in the region of the "Kalkgitter" or at the border between the zone of calcification and uncalcified cartilage, thus producing the clinical picture of Parrot's pseudoparalysis. This anatomic process is usually more frequently and more marked in the lower extremities at the distal ends of the femur and tibia, while the hip and proximal ends of the tibia and humerus, as well as the radius and ulna, are less frequently and less severely involved. The ribs and smaller round bones are also more or less altered, as can be demonstrated roentgenologically (L. Pick and others). Parrot's pseudoparalysis shows a preference for the upper arm, which is easily traumatized. These sequences, which do not always occur in a regular order (Wimberger), demonstrate that primarily the lower extremities and wrists of the newborn merit roentgenographic study (Péhu and others[35]).

The degree of involvement recognizable anatomically as well as roentgenologically has been divided into three stages. In the first stage, the provisional zone of calcification is somewhat broadened. In the second stage, it is 3 or 4 cm. wide and is visibly serrated with granulation tissue projecting into the region of the "Kalkgitter" zone. In the third stage, in addition to the other disturbances named, this granulation tissue has so increased that it results in sponginess and even in epiphyseal separation (pseudoparalysis).

This gradual process, which is very marked in the premature and the newborn, is demonstrable to a less extent by roentgenograms of the fetus in utero. Péhu and Policard believe that at first a clear zone, broader than normal, and near the diaphysis is characteristic of the roentgenogram, and that longitudinal serrations in the "Kalkgitter" zone become visible as dark lines resembling pencil marks. This roentgen evidence is often still more striking because of the presence of double-contoured dark stripes.

Periostitis syphilitica can likewise begin in intrauterine life but occurs less commonly in the first months, becoming marked usually after the third month of life, and assuming more importance in later childhood. This condition is manifested in the long bones and elsewhere and is

[35]Good illustrations are found in L. Pick's article, "Angeborene Knochensyphilis," in the Handb. d. pathol. Anat. (9/1), and in other textbooks, and are therefore not included here.

recognizable roentgenographically, in consequence of its ossification, as a cup-shaped dark line. Periostitis ossificans also appears in the phalanges and skull bones during childhood. Also periostial hyperostoses can be present on the skull in early life; they later produce characteristic stigmas, especially of the tibia (saber shin).

Schneider has called attention to two types of osteochondritis which are not strictly delimited; namely, the passive type with marked spirochetal infiltration of the fetal tissue, and the later active type, in which more and more reactive processes slowly appear with formation of granulation tissue.

C. *Active and Passive Process (Miliary Syphiloma).*—Schneider's division into passive and active processes is basically important for the changes in other organs. Thus, many organs are infiltrated by immense masses of spirochetes without evidence at first of a perivascular or an interstitial inflammation, while later, if the defense mechanism in the last fetal months or at the time of birth develops slowly and thereafter becomes stronger, these reactive processes stand out more prominently. A dense spirochetal infiltration is found, for example, in the suprarenal gland, where the microbes are ordinarily found between the cells. Here, as French authors have pointed out, a marked opposition exists to the ultravirus, which lies within the parenchymal cells or within the nuclei. The difference between an early anergic reaction, then a hypoallergic reaction, and rarely an allergic reaction, is decreased about the time of birth and later becomes still less; then the so-called miliary syphilomas and nodular pseudogummas can occur in addition to an interstitial proliferative inflammation. These pseudogummas were formerly considered to be veritable gummas (R. Virchow and others), but can be differentiated from gummas by their extraordinarily rich spirochetal content. Indeed, the first case of congenital syphilis in which I found *Spirocheta pallida* in the liver, lymph glands, etc. (spring of 1905), was distinguished by such pseudogummas.[36]

Miliary syphilomas, which I have produced experimentally in rabbits,[37] occur as small nodules most frequently in the liver, but also in other organs (bones, etc.) and consist of polymorphic, degenerated, occasionally necrotic cells, and usually contain spirochetal colonies which can be stained by silver methods. Similar in structure are the larger nodules, which resemble gummas more closely; whether a hyperallergic inflammation has played a part in these as in the true gummas appears doubtful in view of their rich spirochetal content. The so-called thymus abscesses of Dubois, as well as the characteristic pneumonia alba, contain large numbers of spirochetes.

---

[36]Berl. klin. Wchnschr. 1905, 728 and 1022-5.

[37]I found miliary nodules containing giant-cells in the tumorlike, older primaries in the rabbit cornea. (Dermat. Ztschr. 41, 236, Plate II, Fig. 3).

Unfortunately, it is not possible for me to enter further into these interesting pathological changes and their significance. I may, however, refer to articles by G. Herxheimer, P. Schneider[38] and to the new Handbuch.

IV. CLINICAL MANIFESTATIONS

In connection with this general presentation of the pathogenesis and frequency of congenital syphilis, its symptomatology, which is easily found in textbooks, will only be mentioned briefly before I discuss the early diagnosis and treatment. As has already been stated, the severe symptoms, which previously were so frequently encountered by clinicians in their classical forms, have become rarer, and the picture of congenital syphilis has changed much more than that of acquired syphilis, in that it has become essentially more uniform and presents fewer symptoms.

Pathologic changes present in the dead fetus, placenta, and umbilical cord are of interest primarily to the obstetrician and pathologist. Because they have already been discussed, I will only mention that they result in the expulsion of the macerated fetus, or in the premature birth of syphilitic children, who are retarded in their development. A macerated fetus occurs rarely in the fifth, usually in the sixth to seventh, month of pregnancy; the living infants are delivered at this period. As already mentioned, with a young macerated fetus, there is a complete absence of reaction on the part of the tissue in spite of the immense numbers of spirochetes. Foci of spirochetes are present in the cartilaginous borders of the long bones, as well as changes indicative of the osteochondritis of Wegner. The resultant widening and irregularity of the cartilaginous border is diagnostically the most important sign of fetal syphilis. The chemistry of the developmental processes has been considered as an explanation for the fact that the spirochetes settle in these locations, after having previously flooded the liver from the blood stream. According to Schneider and others, the spirochetes occur here in large numbers and also at times, as Bertarelli found, in the osteoplastic centers.[39] Similar residual or inactive foci—also in the periostium, etc.—are of significance in the explanation of persistent positive serologic reactions, or reactions becoming positive upon provocative treatment; if the foci are small and walled off, a continuing negative serologic reaction can occur, though this is rare.

A. *Severe Forms of Involvement.*—Osteochondritis is often accompanied by a severe nutritional disturbance, which is evidenced by the senile, atrophic appearance of the fetus and of the child. The color of the skin is a peculiar brownish yellow with gray undertones; in addition, there exists a striking pallor and emaciation. In very severe infections, there is a simultaneous involvement of the palms and soles by a pem-

[38]This author presents numerous excellent illustrations.

[39]E. Hoffmann: Atlas der ätiologischen und experimentellen Syphilisforschung, J. Springer, 1908. Plate 24, Fig. 2; here many other illustrations of congenital syphilis are found.

phigoid syphilide, which in typical cases consists of pea-sized vesicles, first clear, then cloudy, and rarely containing blood or pus—the "pemphigus syphiliticus" of the older syphilologists. The vesicles are surrounded by a ham-red to copper-colored zone of infiltration; in contrast to the pyogenic pemphigus of the newborn (impetigo neonatorum) which involves the trunk, the base of the syphilitic vesicles is compactly infiltrated and numerous spirochetes can be easily found in scrapings of the floor of the vesicles.

The coexistence of osteochondritis and pemphigoid syphilides, which at one time was much more frequent, is characteristic of the severe and early diaplacental infections. In such cases in which the pemphigoid eruption extends further and may even involve the entire cutaneous surface, at times a papulocrustaceous syphilide develops, and a visceral syphilis is also present in the liver, spleen, adrenals and in many other organs. The visceral involvements are usually more severe than the cutaneous manifestations; however there is an exception in the case of the pemphigoid syphilide which is a manifestation of syphilis congenita gravis. Between this severe form and the other specific exanthemas, there is a gradual transition, resulting in less severe visceral as well as external symptoms.

The cutaneous manifestations can be very polymorphic, as in acquired syphilis; but their regular sequence and typical morphology may be altered. In children with marked visceral syphilis whose severe fetal infection extends into the nursing age, as Huebner aptly stated, in addition to an irregular, coppery, atypical roseola and palmar and plantar papules, the diffuse, superficial, infiltrated syphilides are an especial indication of recent and severe infantile syphilis. These infiltrations, which may be as large as the palm of the hand, frequently occur on the face, especially around the mouth, and there result in rhagades of varying depth, which later leave characteristic cicatrices (Parrot) as stigmas. Also similar diffuse infiltrations are frequently noticed on the palms and soles and are characterized by their hamlike color. They are less common elsewhere (anus, buttocks). In addition to the coppery, irregular, and frequently atypical roseola, they characterize a severe to medium-severe infection. Macules, maculopapules, and crusting syphilides, which first appear in the less intense infections some weeks and months after birth (syphilis congenita postnatalis), will not be discussed further; they deviate from the appearance of acquired syphilis more or less by their atypical appearance and the absence of the more regular sequences of acquired syphilis. Even ulcerating ecthyma-like syphilides can occur early, and psoriasiform lesions and an infiltrated eruption similar to erythema multiforme[40] (hyperallergy) are also occasionally described, as well as the appearance of infiltrated early gummas.

[40]Stroscher, Dermat. Ztschr. 1910, 17, Plate 3.

Another manifestation is the rare but symmetrical perinychia or paronychia on several or all the fingers, from which spirochetes can easily be demonstrated. These lesions, characterized by a brown to ham-red infiltration, can appear early or late and even become ulcerated; they are pathognomonic of congenital syphilis. With the involvement of one nail and a regional lymphadenitis, a primary lesion of acquired syphilis (A. Fournier's chancre panaris) should be considered; the importance of this is often undervalued.

B. *Other and Late Forms.*—In addition to the cutaneous manifestations, the mucous membranes play an important rôle. Coryza syphilitica is exceptionally important as an early symptom and not infrequently yields proof of spirochetes on dark-field examination. The characteristic "snuffles" of such infants are due to an edema with decreased secretion of the nasal mucous membranes, on which bloody and purulent scabs are also formed; these changes lay the foundation for deeper processes and later malformations of the nasal structure. Other mucous membranes, such as the conjunctivae, are less commonly involved, and sometimes contain spirochetes. Erosions and plaques appear at times in the buccal mucous membrane and can recur later. Rhagades at the angles of the mouth and on the tonsils, which at times are eroded and frequently contain spirochetes, should always be investigated. Experienced syphilologists, such as Hochsinger and others, emphasize the value of a hard enlargement of the cubital and thoracic (paramammillary) lymph glands.[41] In addition to the hutchinsonian triad, Hochsinger considers a somewhat equivalent early triad of congenital syphilis, consisting of skull deformities (caput natiforme, saddle nose, etc.), radiating scars around the mouth (Parrot), and palpable cubital adenopathy. Gland puncture, which is so frequently practiced with acquired syphilis, seldom yields spirochetes in congenital syphilis. However, this practice should not be overlooked in case of doubt.

Alopecia appears diffusely or in small patches, and the involvement of the eyebrows and cilia, as well as the scalp, is particularly characteristic; in older nursing infants and in small children it may be suggestive of syphilis acquisita infantum.

Especially after prenatal salvarsan therapy, superficial manifestations are frequently only minimal or may be absent. Because of this, syphilis congenita tarda may occur in which, after a more or less asymptomatic course, characteristic stigmas and involvements develop later. Besides the hutchinsonian triad of keratitis profunda,[42] nerve deafness, and typical alterations of the upper and middle incisors, as well as of the first molars, there are characteristic or suggestive signs (signs of certainty and probability of the French school), such as

[41] I also advise examination of the lymph nodes in the axillae, etc.

[42] For newer presentation, see Yokota (Zentralbl. f. Haut- u. Geschlechtskr. 51, 589).

widened knee joints, saber tibia (periostitis ossificans), changes of the ocular fundus (frequent, usually chorioretinitis), saddle nose, testicular atrophy, dwarfism or giantism, etc. The various tooth changes, which the young Fournier described in a very exaggerated manner as being produced by the syphilitic virus (microdontia, diastasis, hypoplasia of enamel, irregularity of form), have become much disputed since then. While definite signs are not known for the milk teeth, the real hutchinsonian tooth is typical of the permanent teeth, and is characterized by crescentic identation of the cutting edge, barrel or pear-shaped, screwdriver-like form, and frequently deviation of the converging axis. The collarlike atrophy of the first upper (six-year) molars is, to a certain extent, also characteristic, as well as the so-called Moon's tooth (better described by Pflüger). Other tooth changes should suggest a thorough examination for syphilis; they occur, however, in other morbid disturbances (idiocy, convulsions, etc.). Furthermore, the high arched palate may be mentioned here as a suggestive sign although this condition is more frequently a result of rachitis.

Besides megalosplenia and occasional enlargement of the liver, there are other symptoms in infants which are more or less suggestive: undernourishment, a peculiar pallor, no gain in weight or even a loss in spite of rich food, hydrocephalus, frequent vomiting and crying at night, nervous disturbances and convulsions (with striking venous dilatation, especially on the head). Nephrosis (albumin, edema) seldom occurs.

The manifestations of the so-called period of recurrences (second to fourth year of life), consisting of exuberant condylomas on the genitals and anus, alopecia microareolaris, erosions of the mucous membranes, etc., in vigorous infants, should be considered as syphilis acquisita infantum. Some communications in the literature (chancres in ano and otherwise located extragenitally on the head and face, single or multiple) indicate how difficult the demonstration of chancres can be and how often they are not even considered. Acquired syphilis in infants usually does not run a severe course and, according to the opinions of experienced pediatricians, is rare compared with congenital (and binary) syphilis. This undervaluation of acquired forms of syphilis (condyloma, alopecia, etc.) is in need of revision, as I have often emphasized. It is known that children frequently run a lighter course with otherwise severe infections (e.g. typhus), and the same may commonly be true with syphilis.

C. *Central Nervous System Disturbances (Spinal Fluid Changes) and Other Sequences.*—Important as they may be for the physical and mental development of the child, endocrine dysfunctions and nervous system disturbances can only be mentioned briefly. Many cases of dystrophia adiposogenitalis, infantilism, dwarfism or gigantism, myxedema, eunuchoidism, contraction of the visual fields, diabetes, etc., have been explained on this basis, and in this case their treatment may become important.

With regard to the central nervous system, I may say that spinal fluid changes are common in early infancy, but are less frequently encountered later. This difference between early and late infancy may at times be explained by an early death of the severely infected infants, and by a spontaneous or therapeutically conditioned retrogression of spinal fluid syphilis as in acquired syphilis. A special form of spastic involvement is described by Marfan and is manifested in syphilis. In addition to syphilitic meningitis, which can cause hydrocephalus, convulsions, and other signs (paresis, lameness, hemiplegia), there are other more or less obvious defects of the nervous system and disturbances of the intelligence, even to the point of idiocy. Late manifestations occur in the form of juvenile tabes and paresis[43] and become recognizable at the earliest in the fourth year of life; perhaps earlier spinal fluid examination would facilitate its diagnosis and treatment. Involvement of the vessels (arteritis or phlebitis in the brain and elsewhere) is also observed.

Gummas have been observed in all organs. Severe deep tertiary ulcerations often simulate lupus, etc., and can occur on the face, mouth, palate, nose (perforations), and other sites, causing deep ulceration and leaving as stigmas severe mutilating scars, often with bony involvement.

So much for the clinical manifestations, the polymorphism of which has not been completely discussed. When rachitis, tuberculosis, etc., develop along with congenital syphilis in infants, clinical pictures are observed which have given rise to the French theories of syphilis larvée. Here, however, there is the question of a combination of factors whereby in children, weakened through diaplacental infection, other diseases can occur more severely and in peculiar clinical forms. In these cases, specific therapy is often of striking benefit.

V. RECOGNITION AND EARLY DIAGNOSIS

Diagnosis, prognosis, therapy, and, finally, the social problem and prevention of congenital syphilis will now be briefly considered.

Of real help in the recognition of congenital syphilis are:

1. Carefully taken family history.
2. All methods of clinical investigation (inclusive of roentgenograms).
3. Investigation for the presence of spirochetes.
4. Serologic examinations.
5. Spinal fluid examinations.
6. Other methods (luetin reaction, blood sedimentation rate, etc.).

[43]A large number of cases of juvenile neurosyphilis were recently reported by Menninger (Zentralbl. f. Haut- u. Geschlechtskr, 51, 680).

The importance of a thorough history, including that of the parents, siblings and nearer relatives, is universally admitted. It should include all suggestive symptoms (also stigmas) and the investigation of all suspects. French authors emphasize this especially; they have included investigation of all diseases which could be confused with syphilis, and properly so. Further, the history of births (abortion, premature, stillbirth) is very significant, as has already been noted. The placenta, umbilical cord, and macerated fetus should always be thoroughly examined, because they can offer proof or arouse suspicion of congenital syphilis.

A. *Obstetric Aspects.*—An early obstetric diagnosis is extremely important. All pregnant women should be thoroughly investigated clinically after taking their history; but syphilis may be present in spite of negative findings. In addition, it is essential to make a serologic examination of all pregnant women, as far as possible in the fourth month (at the latest at the beginning of the fifth month), always using the standard methods (Wassermann reaction, Kahn test, Müller, Meinicke reaction, and also the sensitive Schreus-Wassermann reaction), which should be repeated in case of inconclusive results. Thus, patients with syphilis can be diagnosed in time for effective treatment to be instituted.

In addition to examination of the retroplacental blood, which seldom shows nonspecific reactions, the placenta and umbilical cord should be thoroughly examined (weight, placental quotient, macroscopic, and microscopic appearance). In all suggestive cases, a thorough search for spirochetes should be made by careful dark-field examinations (tissue scrapings from the vein walls of the fetal and placental ends of the umbilical cord); at times the silver staining of formalin-fixed sections will quickly reveal spirochetes (Armuzzi and others). For this purpose, the preservation of a 5 cm. length of the end of the umbilical cord is advisable, as I pointed out in 1928, for later demonstration of spirochetes by staining of sections. Employing silver stains, my students, Edm. Hofmann, Klaften, Philipp, and others, have frequently demonstrated spirochetes in the fetus and in newborn babies. When negative results are obtained from all of these methods, the investigation of the father and siblings at times may help the physician.

Many suggestions as to the clinical diagnosis have already been given. The differentiation of the simple pemphigus neonatorum (more superficial, noninfiltrated, paler lesions) from the syphiloid pyodermia on the buttocks, etc., is often possible by observation of the lesions, and can be proved by the finding of spirochetes. Although the serologic reactions are extremely important, they should be interpreted with caution during the first ten to fourteen days after birth. Instead of provocative reactions in infants, I advise multiple tests and observations of the serologic curve, which does not decrease as rapidly in the presence of syphilis as it does in the case of false positive reactions.

B. *Examination for Spirochetes.*—Examination for spirochetes is still altogether too infrequent. India ink preparations (E. Müller and others), which pediatricians still use, are inadequate, being much too uncertain. Repeated dark-field preparations of scrapings or tissue serum,[44] which I have employed since 1905 with success, are always advisable since the demonstration of spirochetes on the first trial can be expected only when they are present in large numbers (Jahnel). In addition to vesicles and their floors, papules, erosions, rhagades, etc., the nasal and conjunctival mucous membranes are productive sites for scrapings. For the demonstration of spirochetes in adolescents and in children, I advise scrapings of the palatine tonsils, which frequently harbor spirochetes. In the newborn during the first nine months, no spirochetes can be found in the mouth (Erika Schneider, Eva Löb[45]). Scrapings and small pieces excised from portions of the skin (soles and heels) rich in spirochetes are often easier than obtaining preparations from the base of artificially produced vesicles (cantharides, carbon dioxide snow). For the early diagnosis of asymptomatic syphilis, the nasal mucosae and tonsils should always be thoroughly examined for *Spirocheta pallida* by repeated dark-field preparations. I have already stressed that by this method the diagnosis can be made immediately, while serologic examination requires one or more days. Therefore, the repetition of dark-field examinations is very important.

The luetin reaction is of little significance, and increased blood sedimentation rate is often suggestive but is not decisive.

C. *Roentgen Ray Procedures.*—Roentgen ray examination of the epiphyses of the lower and upper extremities is very important for early diagnosis due to the frequent presence of Wegner's disease. Up to the third month it is pathognomonic; later, confusion may arise with rachitis, Möller-Barlow disease, etc. The essentials of Wegner's disease and of other forms (periostitis, etc.) have been stated previously. Many pediatricians consider roentgen ray examination very important, and this has been confirmed in Germany (Moro, etc.), as well as in France (Péhu).[46] It should always be employed, as well as spirochetal and serologic investigation, especially for the differentiation of congenital from acquired syphilis. At times, hutchinsonian teeth can be recognized in roentgen ray films before erupting through the alveolar ridges. (Stokes, Meyer-Buley[47]). Spinal fluid examination is also important

[44]This alone made it possible for Schaudinn and myself to find *Spirocheta pallida* in 100 per cent of the cases, even in the serum obtained from lymph glands, in March and April, 1905.

[45]Dissertation, Bonn, 1934. In collaboration with my student, Erika Schneider, Löb never found spirochetes in the tonsils or in the mouth before the ninth month.

[46]Cervini and Bogani: Zentralbl. f. Haut- u. Geschlechtskr. 52, 330.

[47]Dissertation, Bonn, 1929, and Dermat. Ztschr. 58: 313.

and to be recommended in cases in which the diagnosis is in doubt. Transient or permanent spinal fluid changes occurring in infants suffice for the definite diagnosis of syphilis. The lumbar puncture is to be preferred to cisternal puncture in small children, the latter needing great skill.

D. *Miscellaneous Facts.*—In consequence of prenatal salvarsan therapy of most pregnant syphilitics, the early recognition of congenital syphilis has become more difficult than formerly. It cannot be doubted that this sovereign therapy, as well as bismuth, is transmitted to the fetus through the placenta in efficacious form, and thus controls or produces a latency of the infection in the fetus. Whether a complete cure or an asymptomatic congenital syphilis results is very difficult to say. Symptoms, or positive serologic (and spinal fluid) reactions, can be absent up to the third or, at times, even to the fifth or sixth month. An examination three months after birth, which many believe to be sufficient, does not suffice for the exclusion of a congenital infection; it is much more practical to demand a follow-up of six months. Infants with normal placental quotients and negative spirochetal findings, who are entirely normal clinically, also should have this supervision if they are born of mothers who have had syphilis or are still syphilitic, even when a sufficient guarantee of cure seems certain due to intensive treatment before or during pregnancy.

Consideration of all of the above mentioned clinical symptoms (lymphadenopathy, splenomegaly, etc.) is again advised. The significance of the stigmas (Hutchinson, Fournier) has already been stressed. Spinal fluid examination is necessary in all nervous disturbances of childhood.

VI. PREVENTION AND TREATMENT

Preventive measures and treatment, as already stated, have produced striking results. In order to reduce the incidence of congenital syphilis, there are two means at our disposal: specific therapy, which has long been well developed and has recently been simplified, and a far-sighted prophylaxis of syphilis in general. This may necessitate making exception to the otherwise valid rule: "Never institute specific therapy without a definite diagnosis."

A. *Preventive Measures of Familial Syphilis.*—The pregnant woman is the sole carrier of the causal agent of congenital syphilis and then only after the fifth month of pregnancy. This is the basis upon which we can and must work for the elimination of congenital syphilis. Because of confused and groundless theories of congenital syphilis ("germinative transmission" and "influence on the germ plasm, i.e., heredity"), the progress made has not been sufficiently great for an effective battle against it. When I presented my above mentioned articles in 1928-29, I tried to show the value of this fact.

The pregnant woman is also the starting point for our measures to reduce syphilis as a generalized affliction. She calls on the physician for other conditions and often for prenatal care. The axiom is then valid: "Always consider syphilis, as well as tuberculosis and cancer." There are social and charitable facilities for the care of pregnant women. Would it not be possible to examine every gravid patient for syphilis before the fifth month of pregnancy, without arousing suspicion? The family physicians of those who do not attend social clinics could also make a fundamental advance, for the sake of healthy future generations, by discreetly conducting a clinical and serologic examination. Thus, all syphilitic women—or almost all—could be reached at the opportune time and the birth of healthy children could be assured.

However, our efforts must extend still further, namely, to the prevention of infection of the mother by the syphilitic father, thus avoiding the introduction of infection into the family, with consequent prevention of familial syphilis in general. Today the attainment of this goal is not so difficult, because salvarsan in sufficient dosage quickly and efficiently checks the spirochetes which migrate to the surface and are thus capable of transmitting the disease. This rapid reduction of the danger of inoculation is also important for the reduction of familial syphilis, because infected men, with recently acquired syphilis, who allow themselves to be treated immediately, usually do not transmit their infection, even during treatment. I advise immediate treatment for women who have been exposed and probably infected by husbands whose syphilis is still infectious, even if proof of the spirochete is not found either in a cervical smear or elsewhere (urethra, tonsils, etc.). For these possible, indeed probable, infections of short duration, the preventive treatment of one or two courses with short rest periods will suffice, provided that the serologic reaction remains negative on repeated examinations. Thus, the danger of familial syphilis is banished, and the possibility of congenitally syphilitic offspring is eliminated.

However, if that is not feasible, there remains the possibility of accomplishing not only the healing of the gravid mother, but also the birth of a healthy child by means of treatment during pregnancy. Our three-course system (Bonn) suffices for a final cure of early syphilis if it is not too old and unusually stubborn, which, however, our experience seldom shows to be the case. I emphasize again, along with experienced obstetricians, that this treatment, instituted early enough in the second half of pregnancy, should continue until parturition, in order to avoid danger of premature termination. A new course of treatment is not necessary in later pregnancy in women who have been treated intensively and systematically and whose cure may be assumed with sufficient probability. In my article, "Is Syphilis Curable?"[48]

[48]"Ist Syphilis heilbar?" Dermat. Ztschr. 59: 279, 1930.

I have explained the signs which are to be considered as indicating cure and a sufficiency of treatment; the publications of Zieler[49] may also be referred to in this connection.

A further simple measure for the prevention of familial and congenital syphilis is to advise the use of accepted methods of venereal prophylaxis by husbands who indulge in extramarital relations. Also, anticonceptional prophylaxis is to be recommended, that is, the conscious avoidance of impregnating syphilitic women until they have been sufficiently treated. If, in spite of this, pregnancy ensues before complete cure appears to have been accomplished, the prenatal treatment advocated under all circumstances by so many obstetricians must be carried out through the period of pregnancy, in order to ensure the birth of a healthy child.

B. *Prenatal and Preventive Treatment.*—It has been our experience in general that two combined courses with a four-week rest period suffice for the prenatal treatment of the fetus, even in the presence of obvious syphilis. The assumption that gravid women after an initial dose of 0.3 gm. cannot tolerate individual doses of 0.45 gm. of neoarsphenamine twice a week (thus 0.9 gm. weekly doses) is not in accordance with our long years of experience.[50] Ten or, better still, twelve injections combined with bismuth constitute a course. Even larger doses of neosalvarsan (0.52 and 0.6) have been given to vigorous pregnant women in my clinic without any disturbance. The normal dose of 0.45 gm. twice weekly ordinarily suffices to safeguard the fetus.

Frequently the mother as well as the child cannot receive this complete course during pregnancy, and are thus undertreated. These partially treated mothers and newborn babies must receive further therapy until the entire course has been given.

That leads us to the question which I brought up years ago, as to whether a preventive treatment of the newborn is advisable before the syphilitic infection can be definitely demonstrated. I have affirmed this for a long time and have found much support. Today, since the prenatal treatment has been further extended, a preventive treatment, representing only a continuation of that instituted prenatally, may be required. After the delivery, the mother and child are in the hands of the physician and, with sufficient explanations, should be amenable to proposals for therapy; later, it is more difficult to persuade the mother to continue treatment. Valuable time is lost and the chance of an early cure is decreased[51] with expectant observation. The damage which can occur from too intensive treatment is slight; much greater is the danger of further involvement which requires difficult and pro-

[49]International Derm. Congress, Budapest 1935.

[50]In many countries (Japan, Java) the tolerance seems to be less (German preparations?).

[51]The publications of the Spiethoff clinic do not alter this standpoint; the customary treatment of salvarsan alternating with other preparations is the basis of the Bonn system, which has also been accepted in Denmark, Austria, Spain, etc.

tracted treatment, and which can have further sequelae, while the prognosis becomes poorer the longer one waits. A six-month observation period, therefore, is necessary in order to ascertain freedom from syphilitic involvement.[52]

That is basis enough to justify the preventive treatment of all newborn children of mothers who are still infectious or in whom infection is suspected. This should begin immediately after birth, if they have received inadequate, or no prenatal therapy. This standpoint is well grounded, because it offers the most for individuals and family, as well as for social-hygienic indications, and would contribute efficiently to the limitation of syphilis. Much care and expense is saved by such a procedure. Finally, babies, in whom the presence of syphilis is not definitely established, withstand antisyphilitic treatment very well, according to our experience. Against the advantages enumerated, a few really healthy infants will be treated. Their number will weigh slightly with most experienced physicians; furthermore, simple stovarsol therapy is regarded as sufficient by many clinicians.

C. *Postnatal Therapy.*—While I have seen good results from combined neosalvarsan-bismuth (or mercury) therapy with medium dosage (.01 gm. neosalvarsan per kilogram), recently stovarsal[53] treatment has been preferred by most pediatricians, gynecologists, and dermatologists and has been regarded as sufficiently efficacious. An intensive ninety-four-day course has been advocated by E. Müller, after he had previously—like myself—interceded for a very intensive combined calomel-neosalvarsan therapy. Also, I have employed the stovarsol therapy occasionally usually, however, with bismuth injections (0.002 to 0.003 gm. metallic bismuth per kilogram) or mercury inunctions. Details are given in my textbook of dermatology.[54]

E. Müller advises stovarsol therapy alone with large doses for ten days with four-day rest periods between (first dose, ½ tablet of 0.25 gm.; with vigorous infants, 1 tablet, and then a rapid increase to 2, 3, or 4 tablets daily). With a course of 7 x 10 = 70 treatment days and 6 x 4 = 24 rest days between, he tries to give 40-60 gm. of stovarsol and thus conclude the treatment in ninety-four days. With this treatment, the children become and remain healthy and serologically negative.

Other noted pediatricians advise beginning with small doses, then increasing slowly from ¼ to ½, ¾, and 1 tablet of 0.25 gm. in order to employ larger doses, according to tolerance, after the second or

---

[52]Recently, Coppolino advanced the opposite view, that children, who presented no clinical, serological and roentgen findings one month after birth, did not require treatment. (Zentr. Bl. Hautkr. 52, 63).

[53]No. 594 of Ehrlich's series is called spirozid in Germany, stovarsol in France, and acetarsone by the American Medical Association's "New and Non-Official Remedies." The tablet is 0.25 gm. by weight (translator's note).

[54]E. Hoffmann: Behandlung der Haut- und Geschlechtskrankheiten, ed. 5, 1930, new edition in preparation.

third weeks; many combine this with mercury inunctions (0.1 gm. of 33 per cent ointment per kilogram) or bismuth injections. The total of the stovarsol—with or without short rest periods—amounts to from 24 to 30 gm.; by repetition of this course during the first half-year twice, and in later months even three times, this total can be reached.

Tolerance is usually high with good care and nourishment (as far as possible with mother's milk) and dosage suitable to the individual case; complications, such as vomiting, diarrhea, and exanthemas, are rare and can be controlled by suitable means (sodium thiosulphate). Severely involved newborn and infants occasionally die sooner, due to too intensive specific therapy (spirochetal toxicity), which deaths are no great misfortune since the infants would probably be backward physically and mentally. Preliminary small doses of mercury protiodide or several mercury inunctions and cautious stovarsol doses are suggested. Heavily infected infants, and preferably all, should at first be treated in hospitals. After retrogression of symptoms, and provided there is good tolerance, the simple stovarsol therapy can be continued as an out-patient treatment.

Stovarsol is not sufficiently efficacious for the prenatal treatment of pregnant women and is, therefore, no more permissible than malaria therapy during gravidity (transmission of plasmodia).

According to most experienced syphilologists, intensive stovarsol therapy, with dosage and duration adapted to the severity of the congenital syphilis, is very effective and so efficacious that neither recurrences nor nervous involvements ensue. Mental deficiency due to severe fetal infection cannot always be prevented,[55] but sufficient prenatal neosalvarsan and bismuth therapy must be given in order to make this prevention possible. Older infants and small children, as well as adults, should be treated by neosalvarsan (0.01 per kilogram) and bismuth as outlined in my book. In cases in which stovarsol is not sufficient, this treatment is to be advised and may be repeated once or twice, according to indications. The saturation therapy of Schreus or, better still, malaria followed by the Bonn method of therapy, should be considered.

Minor late involvements of other types do not always require intensive salvarsan-bismuth therapy; here, iodine and bismuth therapy suffice, especially if it is a quiescent noninfectious process or a benign-appearing latent process (positive serologic reaction).

One more word about the intensity of the treatment. We have already mentioned that congenital syphilis shows a characteristic tendency toward spontaneous healing; thus, spinal fluid changes and visceral processes, with the exception of the bony involvement of Wegner, often disappear entirely, or to a large extent. It remains undecided whether, as a consequence of the growth process, infants and small children

[55]Recently, Kis and Rajka advised stovarsol therapy immediately after birth for all children of syphilitic parents, especially as a means of preventing defective intelligence.

possess a particular resistance to agents of infection, such as the *Spirocheta pallida,* but syphilis acquisita seldom runs a serious course. At all events, an excessively large dosage of stovarsol and neosalvarsan does not appear necessary because here the aid of *vis medicatrix naturae* can perhaps be relied upon. Therefore, in spite of my inclination for the maximal dosage, I have usually avoided dosages of more than 0.01 gm. neosalvarsan per kilogram and have usually had success with these small doses. Large doses, approaching the limit of tolerance, are not necessary with stovarsol; indeed, the goal at which maximal therapy aims, namely, a complete cure in a limited time, need not be considered.

VII. CONCLUSIONS

Great advances, which justify further hopes, have undoubtedly been attained during thirty years of etiologic and twenty-five years of therapeutic investigation. The specter of "hereditary syphilis" and "hereditary dystrophies," as well as "hereditary corruption" has been banished.[56] The pregnant woman has been recognized as the sole intermediary for the transmission of congenital syphilis. The danger of transmission of spirochetes to the fetus is first present during the fifth month of pregnancy. This is the definite basis upon which we can lead an effective battle. Through suitable medical and social care, we must succeed more and more in getting in contact with all syphilitic pregnant women before the fifth month. With two prenatal courses of treatment extending from the middle to the end of pregnancy, healthy children can be produced, who are, and remain, free from signs of mental and physical inferiority.[57] Postnatal preventive therapy administered to apparently healthy children, born of infected or infectious mothers, is justifiable and later avoids much affliction and expense. Postnatal therapy of infected children has been simplified by stovarsol therapy which, according to the opinion of experienced clinicians, is efficacious; I have had good and lasting results with it, when combined with bismuth (or mercury) and neosalvarsan therapy.

The introduction of syphilis into the home can best be precluded by the preventive treatment of women who have been exposed to it. Measures have been suggested for the treatment of the infected man before marriage, in order to avoid the misfortune of familial syphilis. After getting in touch with the syphilitic pregnant woman, by means of her history and family investigation, further infectious cases can be traced and treated. By this procedure, which has been supplemented

[56]Husler has discussed, but leaves open, Lenz's question of whether treatment of the parents by iodides, mercury, and arsenicals could influence, by heredity, the progeny: such an apprehension is as groundless as the presumption that syphilitic toxins could influence heredity.

[57]Husler (Ztschr. f. Kinderh., 43: 555, 1927) has never found syphilis in the third generation. I allowed Feige to discuss this subject in his dissertation (Bonn, 1917): a syphilitic blastophthoria was never evident, nor even surmised. The physical and mental condition of forty-two congenital syphilitic adults was found by Husler to be above the average.

in most civilized countries by the formation of regulatory laws for the control of venereal diseases, and by the sympathetic cooperation of gynecologists, dermatologists, and pediatricians, a further diminution must result in the incidence of congenital syphilis and of acquired syphilis.

The definite reduction of congenital syphilis, as shown by yearly census in Denmark,[58] to about one-tenth the former number in twelve years, with elimination of stillbirths and severe forms of the disease, must be an inspiration to us to continue the eradication of this disease which was once so greatly feared. The Danish and German results have been attained with German salvarsan preparations, the efficacy of which has been proved in the Ehrlich Institute at Frankfort;[59] I have no experience with other arsenobenzine products. As the elimination of leprosy was accomplished in civilized lands in the Middle Ages without a specific therapy, we may hope for a still greater success in the battle against syphilis, with the aid of our modern knowledge of early diagnosis and treatment. The marked decrease of congenital syphilis and the elimination of its severe forms give us great confidence that we are on the right path and will be victorious. This goal would be reached still more quickly if the intensive combined treatments with short rest periods, shown by statistics to be most effective, were universally[60] employed and if preventive therapy were more accepted.

[58]Lenstrup (Copenhagen) stated on the basis of 250 congenital syphilitic children that syphilis is not the cause of imbecility; instead, it is due to hereditary inferiorities of other types. Therefore, he proposed the sterilization of such individuals (Sixth Northern Congress of Pediatrics, August, 1934).

[59]E. Hoffmann, Über die zweckmäszigste Behandlung der Syphilis (Wien. klin. Wchnschr. 1935, 1010). It remains to be decided whether the recently recommended solusalvarsan is as good as the standard neosalvarsan.

[60]Particulars are given in the article mentioned in the preceding footnote (59).

EDEMA ASSOCIATED WITH HYPOGENESIS OF SERUM PROTEINS AND ATROPHIC CHANGES IN THE LIVER

With Studies of the Water and Mineral Exchanges

W. H. Thompson, M.D., Irvine McQuarrie, M.D., and E. T. Bell, M.D.
Minneapolis, Minn.

RECENT advances in our knowledge concerning the physiologic mechanisms involved in the exchange of body fluids have greatly heightened our interest in cases of so-called "idiopathic edema." It is obvious from an examination of published case reports that a variety of etiologically unrelated clinical entities have inadvertently been grouped together under this general designation merely because the origin of the edema in each instance has been undetermined. As a tentative diagnosis, therefore, "idiopathic edema" simply signifies that all known causative factors, such as nephritis, nephrosis, circulatory insufficiency, inflammatory and allergic disorders, severe anemia, protein starvation and the excessive ingestion of sodium chloride and water, have been excluded.

The present report deals with a case falling into this general category, which was the first of its particular kind to be recorded, so far as we are aware. As indicated in the above title, the underlying pathogenesis of the edema in this instance involved a marked degree of hypoproteinemia believed to be due to a deficiency in the physiologic mechanism for fabricating serum proteins. The postmortem discovery of a peculiar zonal atrophy in the liver lobules suggests the likelihood that this was the responsible pathologic lesion. Since our preliminary presentation of this case,[1] Myers and Taylor[2] have reported interesting clinical studies on a man fifty-one years of age, who was likewise suffering from chronic hypoproteinemic edema apparently due to an inability to produce serum proteins at a normal rate. During the past few months we have had the opportunity to observe an additional child presenting a somewhat similar clinical picture. It is not unreasonable, therefore, to believe that this entity will be recognized with increasing frequency, if searched for among the assortment of cases ordinarily classified under the designation, "idiopathic edema."

CLINICAL FEATURES OF CASE

The patient, E. N., was a girl two years of age, who was admitted to the Pediatric Service of the University of Minnesota Hospital on Oct. 5, 1931, because of intractable, generalized edema. According to her past history, she was delivered

---

From the Departments of Pediatrics and Pathology, University of Minnesota.

Presented in preliminary form before the American Pediatric Society at Rochester, Minnesota, May 26, 1932.

Aided by a grant from the Medical Graduate Research Fund of the University of Minnesota.

at term, weighing 9 pounds. Labor was "dry" and was prolonged to thirty-six hours. The face was observed to be swollen at the time of birth. This did not persist, however, and so was in all probability merely a result of difficult labor. Her early infancy was not remarkable except for frequent attacks of coryza. She was fed at the breast for nine months but was given cow's milk in addition after the first month. Cod liver oil and orange juice were given regularly after the first few weeks of life, and cereals and vegetables were added after the fifth month. After she was weaned from the breast, standard diets appropriate for the age were given. It is worthy of special note that her feeding and general care were under the supervision of a competent pediatrician throughout her entire life before she was

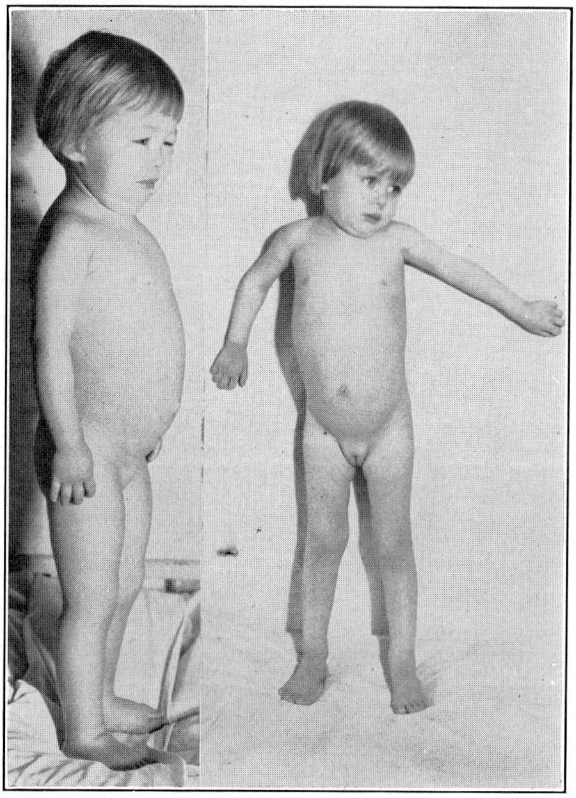

Fig. 1. Fig. 2.

Fig. 1.—Showing persistence of edema nearly five months after admission to the hospital in spite of high-protein, "salt-free" diet.

Fig. 2.—Appearance of patient after loss of edema and ascites as a result of blood transfusion.

referred to us for special study and treatment. Her development and growth were essentially normal. She walked at fourteen months and learned to talk shortly thereafter. She perspired unusually freely and always tended to be somewhat constipated. In all other respects she seemed to be essentially normal up to time of the present illness. The family history was not remarkable. Her parents, who were of Bohemian extraction, were both fairly healthy. She had no brothers or sisters.

Present Illness.—Edema of the face and extremities sufficiently marked to attract the attention of her parents first appeared in January, 1931, following a "cold." This edema persisted without much change until March, when it apparently subsided partially during an attack of whooping cough. Soon thereafter, however, it recurred and by July had become fairly marked. In September it was observed that the abdomen had enlarged considerably and the edema of the face and extremities had become still more conspicuous. Because of increasing irritability and abdominal discomfort, the patient was admitted to the University Hospital for more intensive study and treatment.

It is worthy of special emphasis that her diet had always been adequate as regards its protein and vitamin content. At no time was there any demonstrable evidence of cardiac, renal, or hepatic disease. Shortly after the first appearance of edema, when the patient was but fourteen months of age, the urine was examined carefully for albumin, casts and blood cells, but no abnormalities were found. Repeated examinations thereafter likewise yielded negative results.

On admission the patient appeared very much as she did when the photograph shown in Fig. 1 was taken. The general physical examination was essentially negative except for the obvious edema and abdominal enlargement. The edema was generalized but was more in evidence over the face and extremities than elsewhere. Protrusion of the abdomen was clearly due to the presence of freely shifting fluid. The texture and color of the skin and mucous membranes were essentially normal. The tongue was not enlarged. The hair was normal in amount, texture, and distribution. Except for fairly marked edema of the eyelids and slight hypertrophy of the tonsils, the eye, ear, nose, and mouth examinations were negative. Temperature was normal. *Heart:* Size, action, sounds and response to effort were entirely normal. Systolic blood pressure was 106 and diastolic, 72. Eyegrounds appeared normal. Lungs were clear. Nervous reflexes were all normal. *X-ray* examinations of the wrists, arms and legs showed her bone development to be normal. The urinary tract showed no abnormality by x-ray. The *urine* was negative for albumin, casts, blood cells, and glucose. Specific gravity ranged between 1.010 and 1.030. Phenolsulphonephthalein test showed 50 per cent excretion in two hours on one occasion and 60 per cent on another. *Blood Findings:* The Wassermann test was negative; nonprotein nitrogen 22.5 mg. per 100 c.c. The serum proteins were: albumin 1.9 per cent, globulin 1.5 per cent, total protein 3.4 per cent; plasma cholesterol 226 mg. per 100 c.c.; plasma chloride 357 mg. per 100 c.c.; serum calcium 11.25 and inorganic phosphorus 5.58 mg. per 100 c.c. Unfortunately fibrinogen was not determined, but the coagulation of the blood appeared to be entirely normal. Blood counts were as follows: erythrocytes, 4,480,000 per c.mm.; hemoglobin, 87 per cent; total leucocytes, 8,300 per c.mm. with 78 per cent polymorphonuclears, 17 per cent lymphocytes, 4 per cent eosinophiles and 1 per cent large mononuclears. Platelet counts were not made.

Clinical Course.—Because of the intractable nature of the edema and because her home lacked facilities adequate for her care, the patient was kept in the hospital for a period of 201 days, during which the special studies reported here were carried out. The urine remained albumin-free throughout this entire period except for a trace found in a single sample at the height of her terminal infection. Except for a brief period following blood transfusion, the edema persisted in spite of a high-protein, low-salt, vitamin-rich diet and a constantly positive nitrogen balance. During the greater part of this period, she consumed daily between 2.5 and 3.5 gm. of protein per kilogram of body weight. Variations in the degree of edema occurred as a result of special procedures being tested, but none of the latter appeared to stimulate regeneration of the serum proteins. That the edema was due to a reduction in the colloidal osmotic pressure of the blood incident to marked hypoproteinemia was proved by its complete disappearance following blood transfusion, which raised the serum proteins above the critical level. Figure 2 shows the patient several days after the transfusion, when no edema was demonstrable. After a remission of a few weeks' duration, she again showed a

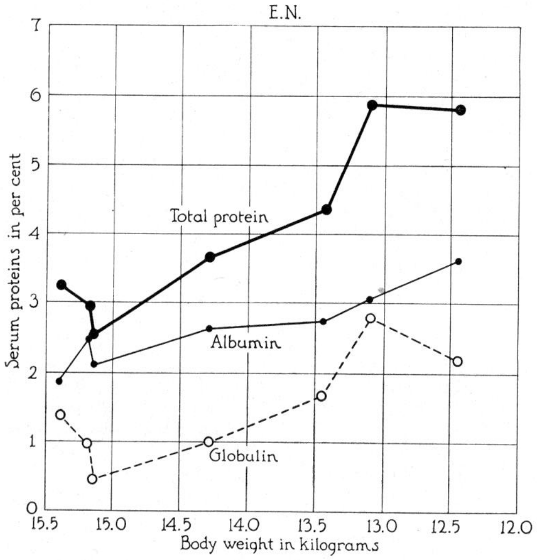

Fig. 3.—Showing inverse relationship between concentration of serum proteins and degree of edema, as indicated by changes in body weight.

gradual gain in weight due to retention of fluid. After the edema had become apparent at the end of seven weeks, it was discovered that the serum proteins had again declined toward the original low level. At no time did the serum globulin fraction exceed the albumin in amount. The close relationship between the serum proteins and the degree of edema, as indicated by changes in body weight, is shown in Fig. 3.

WATER AND MINERAL EXCHANGES

Obscurity regarding the underlying pathogenesis of this unusual form of hypoproteinemic edema suggested the desirability of measuring the water and mineral exchanges under a variety of conditions. The individual effects of parathyroid extract, of posterior pituitary extract, and of blood transfusion are shown in the accompanying charts, which are largely self-explanatory.

The methods used for measuring the water balance were those which we have employed in previously reported studies.[3] In brief they were as follows: The patient was kept in a special metabolism room in which the temperature was maintained between 67 and 74° F. and the relative humidity between 40 and 60 per cent at all times. A specially trained nurse supervised the administration of all food, drink, and medication, collected excreta, checked the room conditions and weighed the patient on a Troemner balance. During periods of special study the daily diet, which was given in four equal meals at six-hour intervals, was made up of powdered whole milk, egg yolk, egg white, cane sugar, clear lemon juice, and water. At other times the patient was given in addition meats, vegetables, fruits, yeast, and cod liver oil. Stools were separated by means of carmine given at the beginning of each period. They were dried to determine the water content. The

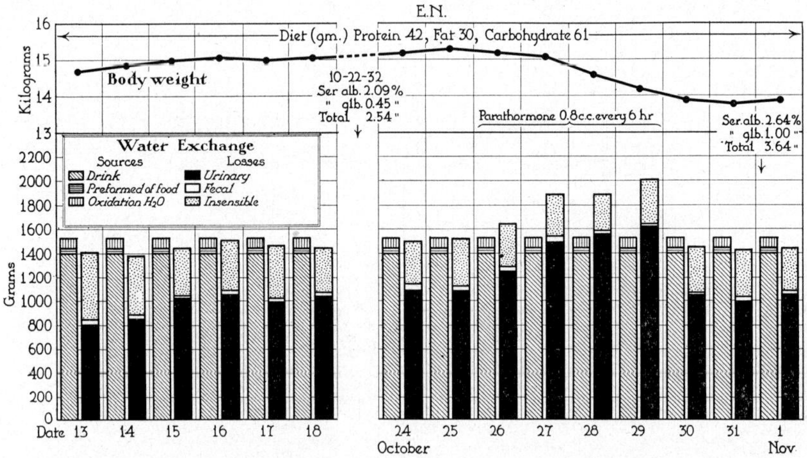

Fig. 4.—Partition of water exchange before and during administration of parathyroid extract. The latter is seen to cause a moderate reduction in edema in spite of low serum protein concentration.

insensible water loss of the body was calculated from body weight changes and a rough estimate of the metabolic mixture according to the method of Newburgh, Johnston, and Falcon-Lesses.[4] Serum proteins were determined according to the procedure of Howe as modified by Hawk and Bergeim.[5] The methods used for determination of the various minerals of the urine and stools were as follows: Sodium, Butler and Tuthill[6]; potassium, Shohl and Bennett[7]; chloride, Volhardt, as modified by Harvey[8]; phosphorus, Fiske and Subbarow[9]; calcium, Tisdall and Kramer[10]; and nitrogen, Kjeldahl.[11]

The data presented in the first part of the chart shown in Fig. 4 are typical of the water balance throughout the greater part of the patient's sojourn in the hospital. The measurements recorded are presented merely as a sample to illustrate the fact that edema persisted in spite of a "salt-free," relatively high-protein diet. It will be observed that the total serum protein was barely half the value usually cited as approximating the critical level below which edema develops. In contrast to the reversal of the albumin-globulin ratio, which is characteristic of nephrosis, the globulin fraction was reduced to a greater degree than the albumin in this instance.

The effect of parathyroid extract (parathormone), as shown on the right half of the chart, was fairly effective in producing a negative water balance during the period of its administration. It is apparent that the negative balance was due exclusively to an increase in the urine volume. While the concentrations of both the albumin and the globulin of the serum were found to be somewhat increased following the period

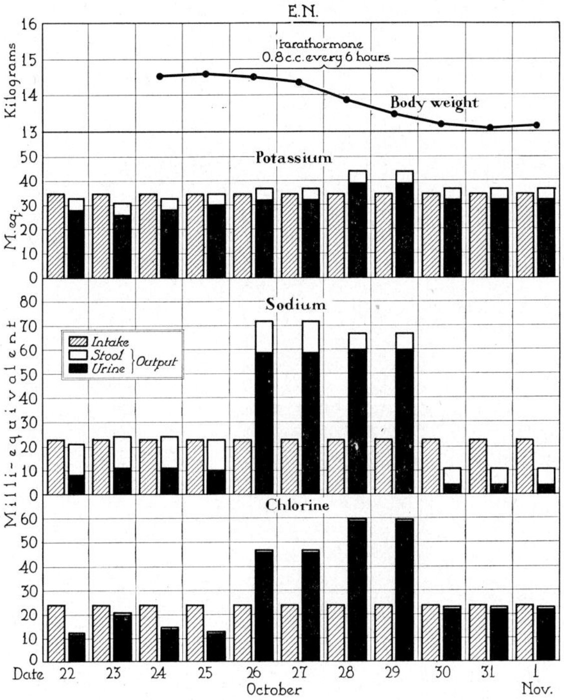

Fig. 5.—Effect of parathyroid extract on potassium, sodium and chlorine excretion.

of diuresis, they were not elevated above the "critical level" for edema formation. In fact, the extra water lost as a result of the administration of parathyroid extract was regained within a few days after withdrawal of the hormone.

In Fig. 5 are charted the intake and output of potassium, sodium, and chloride before, during, and after the period of parathyroid extract administration. That most of the edema fluid lost during the diuresis period was extracellular in origin is indicated by the excessive loss of sodium and chlorine. The slight negative balance of potassium during the third and fourth days may indicate a small loss of intracellular water during that portion of the period, but the amount is comparatively insignificant. Following omission of the parathyroid extract, sodium began at once to show a positive balance, whereas the intake of chloride and potassium was equalled by the output. These observations merely indicate that the composition of the edema fluid in this case is essentially the same as that found in other forms of edema.

The effects of parathyroid extract on the calcium, the phosphorus, and the nitrogen balances are shown in Fig. 6. It will be seen that the nitrogen output remained unchanged. It is especially notable that the patient remained in positive nitrogen balance during the succeeding five months also, but failed to maintain her serum proteins at a level sufficiently high to prevent edema. The output of calcium and phosphorus by way of the kidneys and the intestines was significantly in-

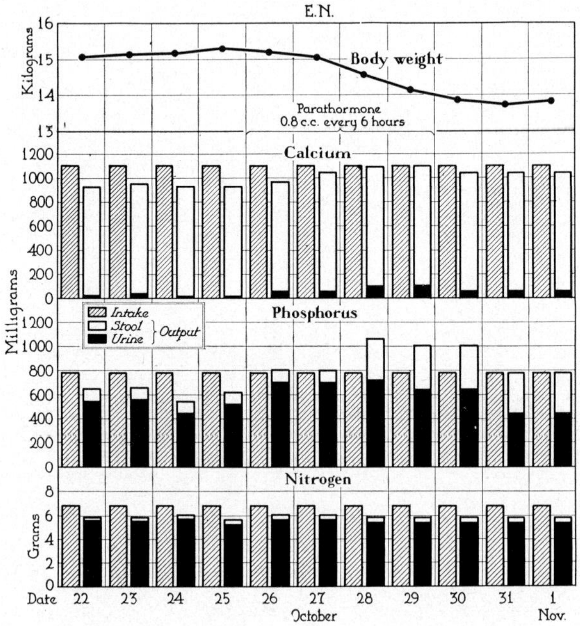

Fig. 6.—Effect of parathyroid extract on calcium, phosphorus and nitrogen balances.

creased by the hormone. Whereas the total calcium excretion had been definitely below the intake previously, the two were essentially equal during the parathormone period. The positive balance of phosphorus noted in the foreperiod was superceded by a definitely negative balance when the extract was administered. Unfortunately serum calcium and protein determinations were not made at the height of the period of diuresis and so it is impossible to say whether or not the degree of blood concentration was sufficient to explain the parathormone diuresis alone on an osmotic pressure basis. The nitrogen, the calcium, and the phosphorus excretion studies throw no light on this phase of the subject, but merely indicate that the patient's response to the extract was entirely normal as regards the calcium and phosphorus metabolism.

Because it had previously been found possible to cause loss of edema in certain cases of nephrosis by the administration and withdrawal of pitressin, the antidiuretic principle from the pituitary gland,[3] the procedure was carried out in the case of this patient. While she responded

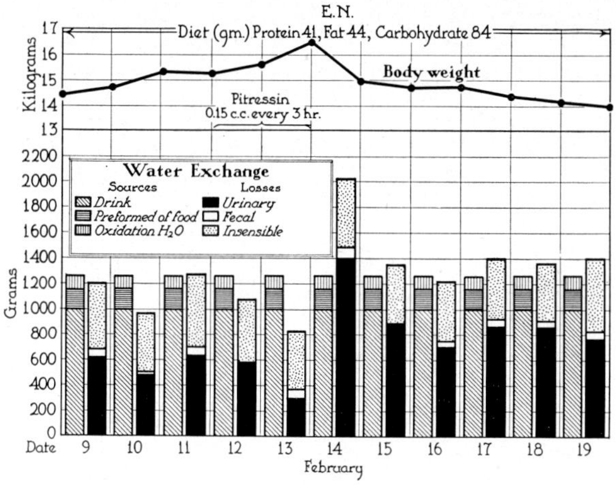

Fig. 7.—Effect of sustained pituitary antidiuresis and withdrawal on the water exchange.

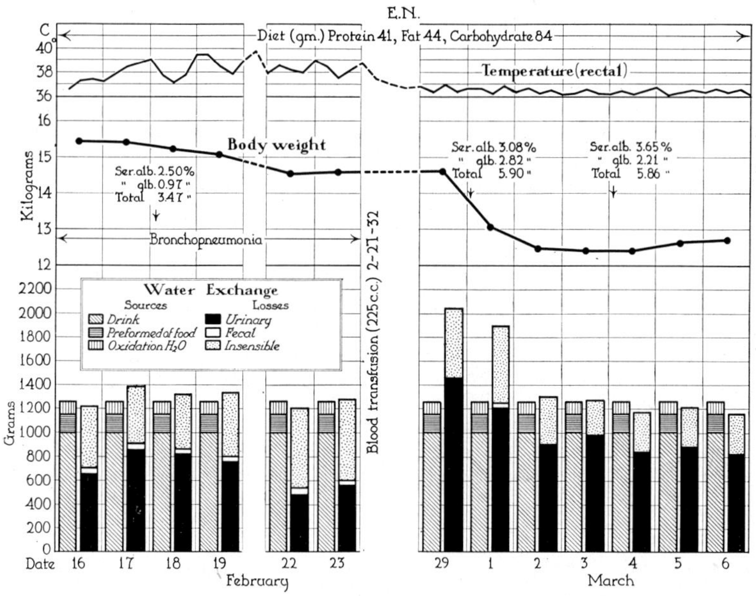

Fig. 8.—Effect of blood transfusion on the serum proteins and the water exchange. Rapid loss of edema fluid.

to the sustained pituitary antidiuresis like other edematous subjects do, that is by a gain in body weight and an obvious increase in the degree of edema, her response to withdrawal of the hormone differed from that of the other patients mentioned in that the period of active diuresis was not sufficiently prolonged to result in a significant net loss in body water. This failure was probably due to the fact that her serum proteins totalled less than 3.0 per cent at the time of the test.

The causative relationship between the depressed level of the serum proteins and the occurrence of edema is strikingly shown in Fig. 8. During the course of a mild attack of bronchopneumonia, the patient was given a fairly large transfusion of blood. Following a latent period of nearly two days, active diuresis set in. This resulted in a net loss of 2.3 kilograms of edema fluid within forty-eight hours. The total serum

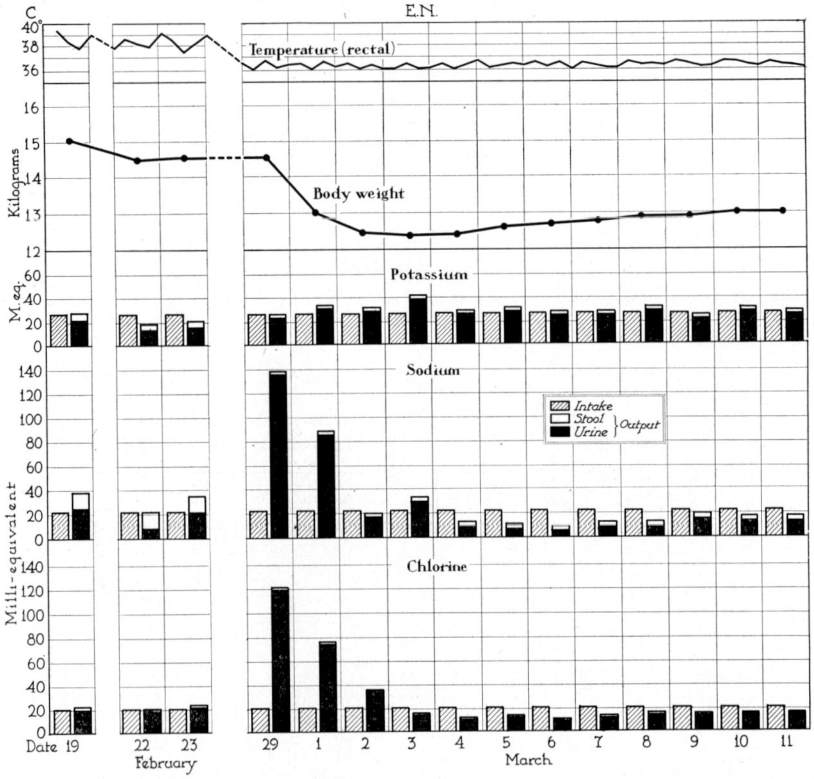

Fig. 9.—Potassium, sodium, and chlorine losses accompanying excretion of edema fluid after blood transfusion.

proteins were increased from approximately 3.5 to 5.9 per cent as a result of the transfusion. Since the serum protein value, 5.25 per cent ± 0.25, may be regarded as the critical level below which edema develops, it is reasonable to assume that the elevation in serum protein level is alone sufficient to account for the result obtained. No adequate reason can be offered at the present time for the delay in appearance of diuresis following the transfusion.

It is obvious from the chart that practically all of the extra water lost was excreted by the kidneys. It will be observed that the amount of water lost as insensible perspiration was significantly greater when the patient was edematous than it was after the edema had disappeared. Since the insensible water loss has been shown by Gilman and Barbour[12] to be inversely proportional to the osmotic pressure of the blood plasma, this observation might be interpreted as indicating a decrease in the value of the latter during the edema period, when the patient was on a low sodium chloride intake. The subject should be further investigated in patients with edema receiving various amounts of salt in the diet.

The mineral exchange data presented in Fig. 9 show that the water lost during the period of diuresis was derived from the extracellular fluid compartments of the body because the balances of sodium and chloride were strongly negative. In contrast the potassium balance

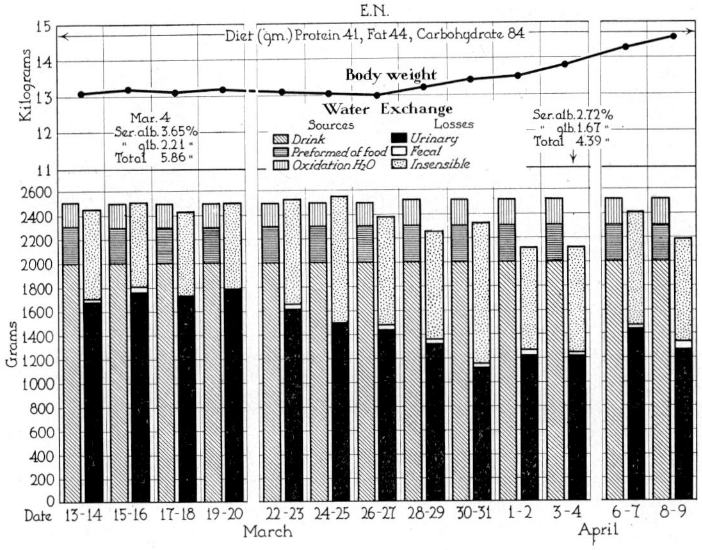

Fig. 10.—Water exchanges in posttransfusion period in two-day periods. Occurrences of edema associated with lowering of serum proteins in spite of high-protein diet.

was but slightly altered. There was, nevertheless, a definite, though slight, increase in the excretion of potassium, which persisted well beyond the period of active diuresis. This might be interpreted as indicating a small outward shift of intracellular water.

Following a slight increase within a few days after cessation of diuresis, the body weight remained essentially stationary for approximately three weeks, as shown in Fig. 10. Thereafter, it rose gradually because of the recurrence of edema. Determination of the serum proteins after reappearance of edema showed their total value to have fallen somewhat below the accepted critical level for edema formation. The rather long period of freedom from edema following a single transfusion and the apparent gradualness of serum protein decrease suggest a slow loss of the circulating serum proteins by ordinary "wear and tear" rather than by an active destructive process. Since the ascitic fluid present had but a low protein content and the urine contained no protein, it appears almost certain that the underlying defect lay in the patient's inability to form new serum protein molecules at a normal rate.

During her long period of hospitalization the general clinical picture remained essentially unchanged except for one mild attack of pneumonia, which she survived, and a later acute attack of unilateral otitis media with complicating mastoiditis. Following operation for the latter, the patient again developed bronchopneumonia from which she died on April 23, 1932. The total period covered by this latter episode was but a few days.

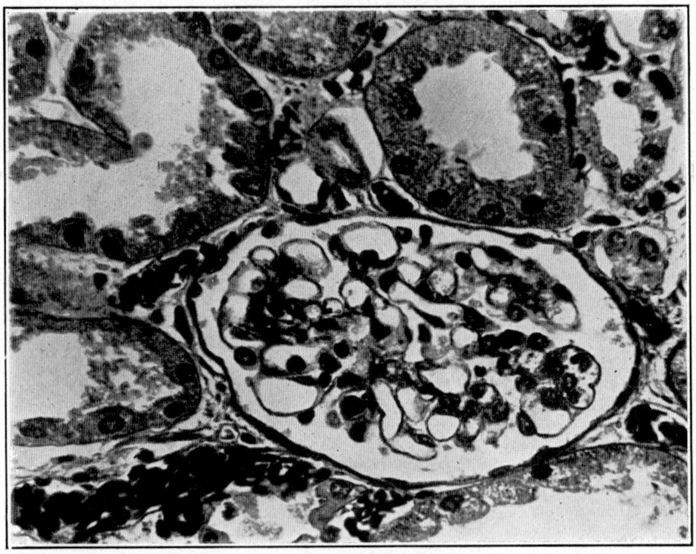

Fig. 11.—Section of the kidney. Note that the glomerulus and the tubules are entirely normal. Photomicrograph.

POSTMORTEM EXAMINATION

Grossly the postmortem examination was negative, except for purulent exudate draining from the mastoid wound, early bronchopneumonia, and the presence of a moderate degree of generalized edema with excess of translucent fluid in the serous cavities. The *heart* was of normal size and development and appeared to be entirely free from acute and chronic disease. The *kidneys* were normal in size. The capsule was stripped from the cortex with ease, leaving a normal appearing surface. Microscopic sections (Fig. 11) showed that both tubules and glomeruli were entirely normal. The endothelial cells were small and inconspicuous, as they are normally in a child, and there was no thickening of the capillary basement membrane. The tubules contained no precipitated protein, and the tubular cells were entirely normal in every respect. There was no evidence of disease in the interstitial structures.

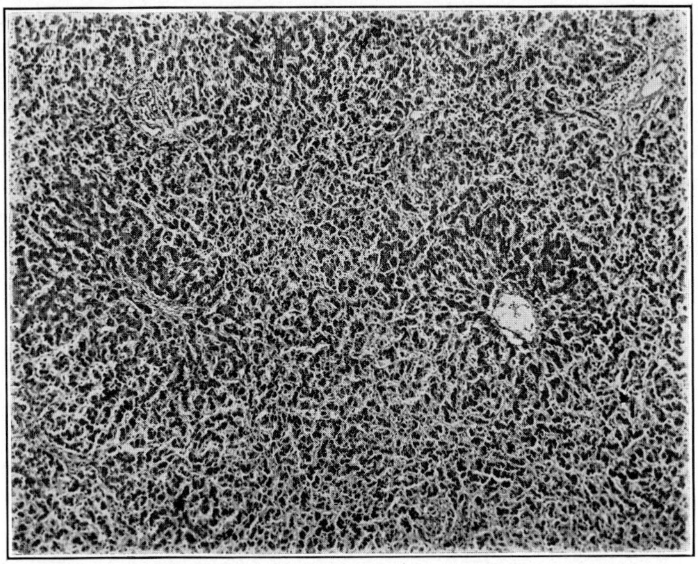

Fig. 12.—Section of the liver under low magnification. Note the persistence of the hepatic cords about the central veins and the extensive atrophy in other parts of the lobules. Photomicrograph.

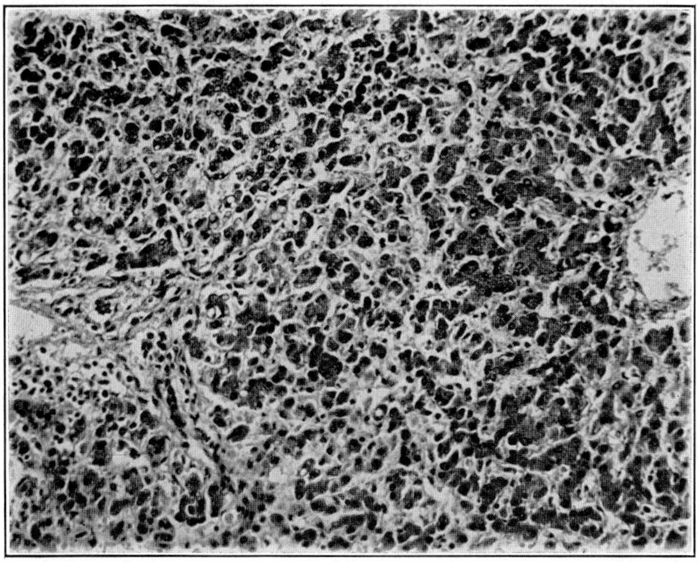

Fig. 13.—An area from Fig. 12 under moderate magnification. Note the preservation of the hepatic cords adjacent to the central vein (on the right side of the illustration) and the atrophy of the intermediate and peripheral zones of the lobule. Photomicrograph.

While the *liver* appeared normal macroscopically, a microscopic study revealed striking changes. Under low magnification (Fig. 12) a marked atrophy of the hepatic cords, especially in the intermediate and peripheral zones of the lobules, could be seen. The hepatic cells about the central veins were usually intact. In Fig. 13 a part of a lobule is shown under higher magnification. The central vein is shown on the extreme right of the photomicrograph. The hepatic cords around the central vein were practically normal in appearance, while the cords in the intermediate and peripheral zones were broken and discontinuous. A portion of the atrophic zone of a lobule is shown in Fig. 14. It will be noted that the hepatic cords did not form a continuous network, an appearance evidently due to the complete degeneration and disappearance of adjacent cells. Fragments of necrotic cells could be seen, but there was no evidence of a diffuse necrosis of cells such as is seen in acute atrophy

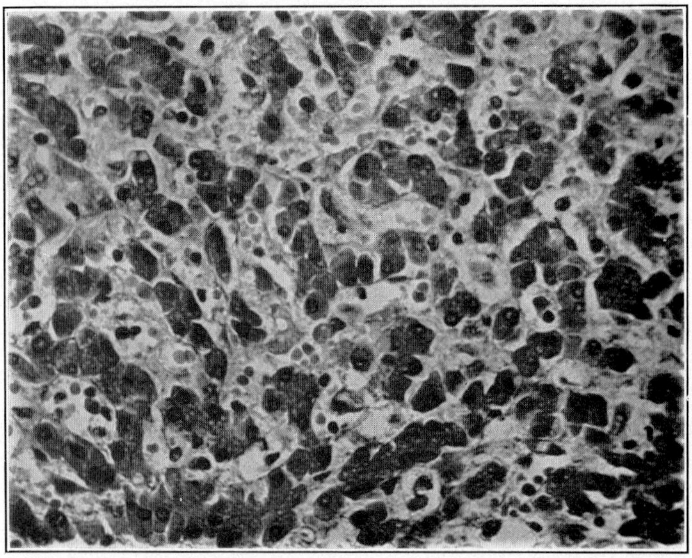

Fig. 14.—An area from the intermediate zone of a lobule under high magnification. Note the discontinuity of the hepatic cords due to the disappearance of a great many liver cells. Many cells are decreased in size and their surfaces are rounded because of absence of adjacent cells. Photomicrograph.

of the liver. The microscopic appearances were rather those of a chronic progressive atrophy of the hepatic cords. In some sections of the liver, lobules were found which showed instead of atrophy occasional small necrotic foci. The atrophy described above was, therefore, not uniform in degree throughout the liver. No explanation for the unusual lesion was found. It differed from the common forms of acute atrophy in the absence of extensive areas of nercosis. It was unlike subacute and chronic atrophy in that there was no cirrhosis. In states of prolonged severe malnutrition appearances similar to those in this case may occur. However, it is perhaps best to classify this disease as *primary atrophy of the liver,* i.e., one of undetermined etiology.

DISCUSSION

The features of special interest in the foregoing report are two: (1) that pertaining to the nature of the hypoproteinemia which was responsible for the edema and (2) that concerning the unusual pathologic lesions in the liver. Two unusual points regarding the serum proteins should be emphasized. The more important is that this patient manifested an unmistakable deficiency in her mechanism for fabricating these important blood constituents. This appears to us to be definitely proved by the fact that marked hypoproteinemia persisted over a period of many months in spite of a high-protein diet with constant maintenance of a strongly positive nitrogen balance. The proteins included in the diet were of good quality for serum protein regeneration, according to the recent work of Whipple and his coworkers[13] on the comparative efficiency of different dietary proteins. It was satisfactorily determined that extra protein was not lost by way of the urine, feces, or ascitic and edema fluids. Abnormal destruction of serum proteins appears to have been ruled out by the fact that the descent of their levels following blood transfusion was extremely slow. The second unusual point is the symmetrical reduction in the serum albumin and globulin fractions. At no time was the albumin-globulin ratio reversed. In fact, the regeneration of globulin appears to have been slightly more impaired than that of the albumin.

The characteristic lesion in the liver lobules was unique in that no true cirrhosis, no infiltration of wandering cells, and no necrotic cellular débris were apparent. Since the morphologic blood picture remained essentially normal and no other parenchymatous lesion than that in the liver was found, this observation appears to us to substantiate the theory of Whipple and coworkers[14a and b] that the liver is the chief site of formation of the serum proteins. The peculiar distribution of the lesions further suggests that this process may be a more or less specialized function of those cells situated in the intermediate and peripheral zones of the hepatic lobules.

The direct cause of the liver lesions is unknown. The early age of the patient at the onset of edema, the lack of any clear-cut history of preceding infection or intoxication and the small size of the hepatic cells might be interpreted as suggestive evidence of a congenital defect in the development of these structures, but no further proof of this somewhat fantastic explanation is available. It is of passing interest, however, that three years after the death of this patient, her parents brought a second child, eighteen months of age, to us with the complaint that she seemed at times to show slight edema similar to that shown by E. N. at the onset of her illness. No pitting edema could be demonstrated at the time of our examination, but her serum proteins as well as those of the parents were determined. From the point of view of heredity it may or may not be significant that this sister's total serum protein was found to be but 6 per cent, and her father's but 6.12 per cent, while the mother's was 7.4 per cent. The parents were to report to us in case edema became apparent in this child. An additional year has passed, but no report has been received.

Various observers[15, 16, 17, 18] have reported a decrease in serum or plasma proteins in liver disease, particularly in cases of cirrhosis with ascites and edema. This has usually been attributed to underfeeding of protein in such cases, and the edema has often been referred to as being a result of cardiac insufficiency and venous obstruction. Myers and Keefer[18] found, however, that certain patients with severe cirrhosis lost significant amounts of protein into the ascitic fluid. They concluded that such patients probably suffer also from decreased ability to produce serum proteins, particularly albumin. They, like other contributors to the subject, found the albumin-globulin ratio of the serum to be reversed in the majority of instances. The case reported here and that reported by Myers and Taylor[2] differ from cases of ordinary cirrhosis in that there was never any tendency to a reversal. These two patients showed a marked deficiency in their capacity to fabricate globulin as well as albumin. This deficiency was the primary factor in their abnormal retention of water. The ascites was a feature of the generalized edema, just as it is in the case of lipoid nephrosis. There was no evidence of venous obstruction or of cardiac or renal insufficiency.

SUMMARY AND CONCLUSIONS

1. Clinical and metabolic studies were carried out over a period of many months in the case of a patient suffering from "idiopathic" hypoproteinemic edema.

2. No evidence of cardiac or renal disease was obtained during her lifetime. The formed elements of the blood were repeatedly found to be entirely normal.

3. The low levels of the serum albumin and globulin were uninfluenced by high protein feeding, although a strongly positive nitrogen balance was known to be maintained thereby over a period of more than six months.

4. Since no other cause for the symmetrical lowering of the serum proteins could be found, it was assumed that the body's mechanism for their regeneration was defective.

5. Studies on the water and mineral exchanges showed the edema per se to differ in no essential way from that due to the hypoproteinemia of protein starvation or that due to excessive protein loss.

6. Elevation of the serum proteins by means of blood transfusion resulted in complete disappearance of the edema, demonstrating a direct relationship between the low serum proteins and edema formation.

7. Postmortem examination revealed a comparatively widespread atrophy of hepatic cells, which was confined chiefly to the intermediate

and peripheral areas of the liver lobules, the central zone being spared. No lesions were present in the kidneys, heart, or other parenchymatous organs.

8. In the light of these data the tentative conclusion has been drawn that this unusual liver lesion was responsible for hypogenesis of the serum proteins and consequently for the development of edema and ascites.

9. Hypoproteinemia in the absence of albuminuria and protein starvation should be regarded as at least presumptive evidence of one form of hepatic insufficiency.

REFERENCES

1. Thompson, W. H., Ziegler, M., and McQuarrie, Irvine: Am. J. Dis. Child. **44**: 650, 1932.
2. Myers, W. K., and Taylor, F. H. L.: J. A. M. A. **101**: 198, 1933.
3. McQuarrie, Irvine, Thompson, W. H., and Ziegler, M.: J. PEDIAT. 8: 277, 1936.
4. Newburgh, L. H., Johnston, M. W., and Falcon-Lesses, M.: J. Clin. Investigation **8**: 161, 1930.
5. Hawk, P. B., and Bergeim, O.: Practical Physiological Chemistry, ed. 10, Philadelphia, 1931, P. Blakiston's Son & Co., p. 449.
6. Butler, A. M., and Tuthill, Elizabeth: J. Biol. Chem. **93**: 171, 1931.
7. Shohl, A. F., and Bennett, H. B.: J. Biol. Chem. **78**: 643, 1928.
8. Harvey, S. C.: Arch. Int. Med. **6**: 12, 1910.
9. Fiske, C. H., and Subbarow, Y.: J. Biol. Chem. **66**: 375, 1925.
10. Tisdall, F. F., and Kramer, B.: J. Biol. Chem. **48**: 1, 1921.
11. Kjeldahl, J.: Ztschr. f. anal. Chem., Wiesb. **22**: 366, 1883.
12. Gilman, A., and Barbour, H. G.: Am. J. Physiol. **104**: 392, 1933.
13. Pommerenke, W. T., Slavin, H. B., Kauber, C. H., and Whipple, G. H.: J. Exper. Med. **61**: 261, 1935.
14. a. Kerr, W. J., Hurivitz, S. H., and Whipple, G. H.: Am. J. Physiol. **47**: 379, 1918.
    b. Whipple, G. H., Belt, A. E., and Smith, H. P.: Am. J. Physiol. **52**: 54, 1920.
15. Gilbert, A., and Cheray, M.: Mém. Soc. de biol. **63**: 487, 1907.
16. Salvesen, H. A.: Acta med. Scandinav. **72**: 113, 1929.
17. Peters, J. P., and Eisenman, A. J.: Am. J. M. Sc. **186**: 808, 1933.
18. Myers, W. K., and Keefer, C. S.: Arch. Int. Med. **55**: 349, 1935.

TRAUMATIC PNEUMOTHORAX IN THE NEWBORN

Jerome S. Leopold, M.D., and Frederick Castrovinci, M.D.
New York, N. Y.

PNEUMOTHORAX is of uncommon occurrence in children. Scott[1] in 1928 collected 177 cases in children of various ages. In reporting his own case of pneumothorax, Davies[2] reviewed twenty-seven previously reported. In 1931 Coccheri and Rossi[3] reported 300 cases from the literature dating from 1844 to 1930, including sixteen cases of their own.

Stoloff[4] is of the opinion that tuberculosis is probably the most frequent single cause of pneumothorax in children. On the other hand, according to Anderson and Cathcart[5] tuberculosis as an etiologic factor is rare as compared to the 3 per cent occurrence in pulmonary tuberculosis in adults. However, in considering the nontuberculous causes of pneumothorax in infants and children, Lereboulet and his associates[6] and Royer de Véricourt[7] list pneumonia, empyema, lung abscess, and pertussis as the most frequent. Cases of spontaneous pneumothorax either accompanying or following pneumonia have been reported by Bashinski,[8] Lacchia,[9] Acuna and his coworkers[10] and others.[11, 12, 13] In reporting a case of pyopneumothorax from our service, Rogatz and Rosenberg[14] found only twelve similar cases in the literature occurring during the first year of life. Direct trauma to the chest (Macera and Perissé[15]) or prolonged difficult deliveries (Donahoe[16]) may also cause pneumothorax. Pissavy and Zimmer[17] report a case of pneumothorax following puncture of the pleura in a fifteen-year-old child. Ruge[18] in 1878 described the first case of pneumothorax in the newborn. In 1930 Stein,[19] in a report with a review of the literature, described four cases and added one of his own. Gasul and Singer[20] brought the series up to eight cases. In an excellent monograph, Glaser and Landau[21] reported seventeen cases, including one of their own, with a mortality of 47 per cent in pneumothorax in the newborn. Flipse[22] is the only author to report a case of pneumothorax following hypodermic medication. The following report of a case of pneumothorax in the newborn is of interest because we were unable to find in the literature a report of a similar case caused by attempted cardiac puncture.

From the Abraham Jacobi Division for Children of the Lenox Hill Hospital, New York, Service of Dr. Jerome S. Leopold.

CASE REPORT

(Courtesy of Dr. Arthur Stein)

H. P. H., male, newborn infant, was born by a precipitous delivery on Dec. 2, 1935, ten hours after the onset of labor. The birth weight was 5 pounds 8½ ounces.

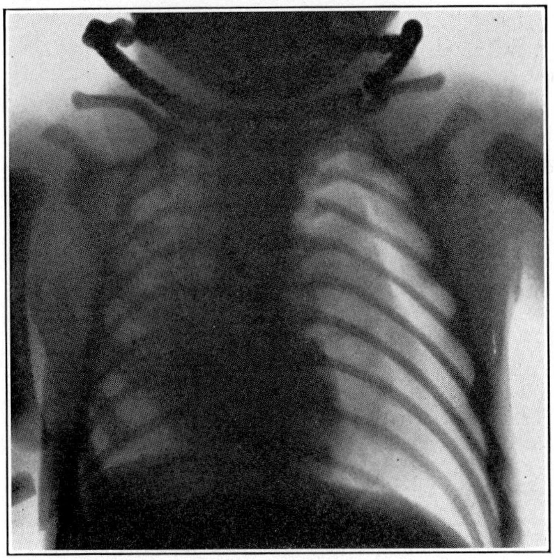

Fig. 1.—Showing a 50 per cent pneumothorax, partial collapse of the left lung, and shifting of the mediastinum to the right.

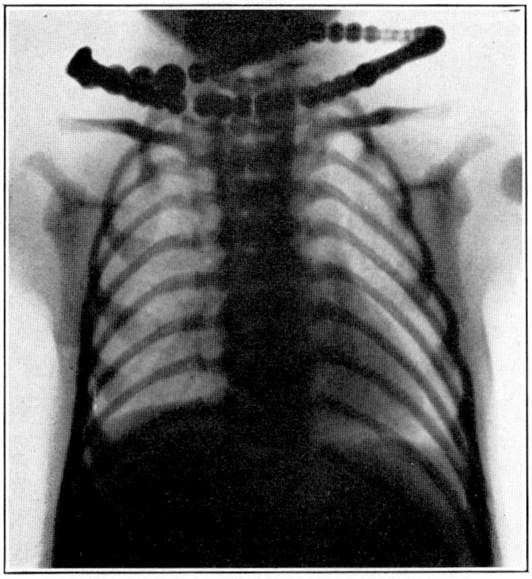

Fig. 2.—Showing complete absorption of the air, with the mediastinum normally located.

At birth the infant appeared very pale, listless, and did not breathe. In attempts at resuscitation, besides immersion in hot and cold water tubs, alternately, and dilatation of the rectum, one ampule of medication was injected supposedly into the heart by means of a 24 gauge, ¾ inch needle. When a weak cry was heard, the infant was at once placed in an incubator and oxygen was administered continuously. Complete physical examination several hours later revealed the following findings:

The infant appeared apathetic and somewhat cyanosed. Stimulation produced a very weak cry. The respirations were rapid and shallow. The skin was pale and dry. The mucous membranes and the extremities were slightly cyanotic. The anterior fontanel was patent, of normal fullness, and admitted two fingers. The neck was normal. On the chest wall, a needle puncture wound was present in the third intercostal space, just to the left of the sternum. On the left side the thorax appeared fuller than on the right. The respiratory excursions were markedly diminished; tactile fremitus was practically absent; percussion produced a tympanitic note. The breath sounds were exaggerated over the entire right side, and were markedly diminished over the left chest. No râles were heard. The heart sounds were heard best to the right of the sternum. The abdomen was soft. The liver edge was easily palpated just below the right costal margin. The spleen was not felt. The genitals and extremities were negative. A diagnosis of left-sided pneumothorax was made and was confirmed by roentgen ray examination (Fig. 1). During the first thirty-six hours of life, the infant had four stools consisting of meconium and mucus streaked with fresh blood. The blood was explained on the basis of the trauma to the anus produced secondary to the dilatation procedure instituted as a stimulating measure at birth. The infant was kept in the incubator, and oxygen was administered continuously. The physical findings improved daily. It was noted that the point of maximum intensity of the heart sounds was steadily shifting from the right of the sternum to the left. The breath sounds on the left side gradually became normal.

On Dec. 9, 1935 (7 days after birth), the physical examination of the chest was entirely normal. Roentgen ray examination (Fig. 2) revealed complete disappearance of the pneumothorax. The oxygen was discontinued. The stools had become free of blood, and the infant was taking breast milk with a complementary formula satisfactorily. When discharged from the hospital on Dec. 11, 1935, the infant weighed 5 pounds 6½ ounces. When seen at the age of five months, he weighed 14½ pounds, was 25¾ inches long, and had two teeth. The infant was of normal development and well nourished.

DISCUSSION

In reviewing the literature on pneumothorax in the newborn, the explanation most frequently advanced for the mechanism of production is the rupture of an alveolus during resuscitation causing a bronchopleural fistula. Flipse[22] feels that forceful respiratory movements at the onset of respiration in his case were caused by an aplasia of the epiglottic cartilage with subsequent collapse obstructing the glottis. In Stein's[19] case there was apparently a permanent bronchial communication with the pleural cavity because at the end of two years no expansion of the right lung had occurred. In the case presented by Gasul and Singer,[20] the pathogenesis was described on the basis of aspiration of infected material at birth with the production of a localized pneumonitis. This process, going on to abscess formation, ruptured at the age of three weeks, causing pyopneumothorax and leading to death in three days. In the case reported by us, it is felt that air entered the pleural cavity through the needle puncture wound during the first few respiratory efforts. With the onset of the respiratory movements and the subsequent production of a negative pressure in the pleural cavity, air was most likely sucked in through the puncture wound. This readily explains the rapid clearing up of the pneumothorax within seven days.

SUMMARY

A case of a newborn infant is presented in whom pneumothorax developed apparently secondary to puncture of the left chest. The air was spontaneously absorbed within seven days. Complete recovery resulted.

REFERENCES

1. Scott, A. J.: Tr. Sect. Dis. Child. A. M. A., p. 58, 1928.
2. Davies, Willard J.: M. Times & Long Island M. J. **62**: 237, 1934.
3. Coccheri, Pietro; and Rossi, Vittorio: Arch. di. pat. e clin. med. **11**: 46, 1931.
4. Stoloff, E. Gordon: Am. J. Med. Sc. **176**: 657, 1928.
5. Anderson, William Willis, and Cathcart, Don F.: J. M. A. Georgia **23**: 456, 1934.
6. Lereboulet, P., Lelong, Marcel, and Even, R.: Nourisson **17**: 257, 1929.
7. Royer de Véricourt, E.: Gaz. méd. de France, pp. 879, Oct. 15, 1934.
8. Bashinski, Benjamin: South. M. J. **22**: 525, 1929.
9. Lacchia, Paolo: Pediatria **37**: 901, 1929.
10. Acuna, M., Bettinotti, S. I., and Vallino, M. T.: Arch. argent. de pediat. **2**: 349, 1931.
11. Geyman, Milton J., and Clark, Daniel M.: Radiology **23**: 622, 1934.
12. McClendon, S. J.: Arch. Pediat. **48**: 511, 1931.
13. Reitter, George S.: Am. J. Roentgenol. **31**: 770, 1934.
14. Rogatz, J., and Rosenberg, A.: Am. J. Dis. Child. **41**: 1104, 1931.
15. Macera, Jose M., and Perissé, Juan M.: Semano med. **39**: 2B:1450, 1932.
16. Donahoe, Will E.: Journal-Lancet **52**: 699, 1932.
17. Pissavy, A. and Zimmer: J. de méd. et chir. prat. **98**: 443, 1927.
18. Ruge, C.: Ztschr. f. Geburtsh. u. Gynäk. **2**: 31, 1878.
19. Stein, Jacob: Am. J. Dis. Child. **40**: 89, 1930.
20. Gasul, Benjamin, and Singer, Harry A.: Am. J. Dis. Child. **45**: 1050, 1933.
21. Glaser, Jerome, and Landau, Daniel B.: Am. J. Dis. Child. **50**: 986, 1935.
22. Flipse, M. Jay: J. Florida M. A. **14**: 403, 1928.

26 East 63rd Street

2 East 54th Street

THE BACTERIAL FLORA OF MECONIUM SPECIMENS COLLECTED FROM SIXTY-FOUR INFANTS WITHIN FOUR HOURS AFTER DELIVERY

MARSHALL L. SNYDER, PH.D.
DENVER, COLO.

IN HIS dissertation of 1886 Escherich[1] stated that the meconium of the infant was sterile and bacteria did not appear until four hours after birth in the summer and seventeen hours in the winter. Subsequent workers, Schild,[2] Szego,[3] Sittler,[4] Tissier,[5] Cruickshank and Cruickshank,[6] and Passini,[7] furnished data supporting Escherich. Statements to this effect may be found in the texts of Ford,[8] Topley and Wilson,[9] Zinsser and Bayne-Jones,[10] Park and Williams,[11] and Kendall.[12]

Exceptions to these findings, however, have been recorded which suggest strongly that bacteria may occasionally be present in the meconium at birth. Hymanson and Hertz[13] found bacteria in nine of thirty-nine meconium specimens collected by rectal swab shortly after birth and streaked out on serum glucose agar. Burrage[14] in 1927 reported the cultivation on solid media of bacteria from thirty-eight of one hundred first passage specimens of meconium, the first of which was collected at delivery and was found to contain many bacteria. A similar series of fifty first passage specimens was recorded in 1934 by Hall and O'Toole[15] who obtained the same percentage of positive results as Burrage. They used both solid and liquid media. In the last two instances most of the specimens were obtained from sterile diapers brought to the laboratory from the nursery. No attempt was made to collect the specimens regularly at or within a short time of delivery.

The present investigation undertook to determine the presence of bacteria in the intestinal contents at birth, as well as in the four-hour period following delivery. The mode of invasion was also considered.

METHODS OF COLLECTION AND EXAMINATION

The time of collection ranged from four minutes to three hours and ten minutes after delivery. A swab on a fairly stiff copper or iron wire which was placed in a short length of glass tubing was used to collect the specimens. This combination, with a small amount of castor oil for lubrication, was placed in a test tube and sterilized in the autoclave at fifteen pounds' pressure for one-half hour. Several tests showed the oil to be sterile. The anal region of each of the first few infants was sponged with Sharpe and Dohme S. T. 37, but this was

From the Department of Bacteriology and Public Health and the Child Research Council, University of Colorado School of Medicine and Hospitals.

discontinued because of its slow evaporation and 95 per cent alcohol was used for the remaining cases. A control test of this area was made by rubbing it with an ordinary swab which was placed in glucose broth. These control cultures showed that this method of sterilizing the anus and buttocks was not entirely efficacious, but no other satisfactory method was found. The meconium was collected by inserting the tube well past the anal sphincter, pushing the swab still farther into the rectum, and withdrawing the swab, which brought meconium into the tube.

The following technic was employed for examining the meconium. When the meconium was present in sufficient quantity, it was examined microscopically by cover slip as well as Gram's stain. The results of these examinations were invariably negative. A small amount of meconium was streaked across eosin methylene blue and blood agar plates to determine the presence of gram-negative and gram-positive aerobic organisms, respectively. An additional amount was placed in freshly boiled and cooled brain medium for the enrichment of what few bacteria might be present whether aerobic or anaerobic. In a few cases when brain broth was not available glucose broth was used. Occasionally the meconium was streaked out on blood agar slants which were made anaerobic under alkaline pyrogallol; these were all sterile.

RESULTS

To date, the meconium collected by this method within four hours after delivery was examined from sixty-four infants, including two of cesarean birth. These cases were divided in respect to time as follows: twenty-nine were collected within thirty minutes after delivery; ten between thirty minutes and one hour; sixteen between one and two hours; and nine between two hours and three hours and ten minutes.

The thirty-minute period was selected arbitrarily to cover as many cases as possible within a short time after the arrival of the baby. The babies who came within this limit, the organisms isolated, and the control cultures of the skin surface of the anal area are listed in Table I.

Table I shows that three out of twenty-nine specimens of meconium obtained within thirty minutes after delivery showed positive bacterial growth on streaked plates. That these organisms must have been present at birth in Case 6 seems indisputable, for the specimen was collected nine minutes after delivery, and there were numerous colonies along the streak on the blood agar plate. The failure of the *L. acidophilus* to grow in enrichment media cannot be explained. In Case 29, colonies appeared in large numbers along the streak on the blood agar plates. Among these were hemolytic colonies of *Streptococcus pyogenes* whose presence in a meconium specimen collected within a half-hour after delivery caused some concern for the mother, but nothing abnormal was recorded for the postpartum period of ten days in the hospital.

Str. mitis was also isolated from the plate, and both species of streptococcus and *B. coli* were recovered from the enrichment culture. In Case 27 there were only three colonies of *B. coli* at the beginning of

TABLE I

BACTERIAL FLORA OF SPECIMENS OF MECONIUM COLLECTED WITHIN THIRTY MINUTES AFTER DELIVERY

NO.	TIME*	RESULTS		
		PLATE	ENRICHMENT	SKIN CULTURES
1	4	Sterile	Sterile	Sterile
2	8	Sterile	Sterile	Sterile
3	8	Sterile	Sterile	Sterile
4	8	Sterile	Sterile	*B. coli*
5	9	Sterile	Sterile	*M. epidermidis*
6	9	*L. acidophilus*	Sterile	Sterile
7	10	Sterile	Sterile	Sterile
8	10	Sterile	Sterile	Sterile
9	10	Sterile	Sterile	Sterile
10	10	Sterile	Sterile	Sterile
11	10	Sterile	Sterile	Sterile
12	11	Sterile	Sterile	Sterile
13	11	Sterile	Sterile	Sterile
14	13	Sterile	*B. coli*	*B. coli*
15	13	Sterile	Bacteroides species	*M. epidermidis*
16	14	Sterile	Sterile	Sterile
17	14	Sterile	Sterile	Sterile
18	15	Sterile	Sterile	Sterile
19	15	Sterile	Bacteroides species	Sterile
20	16	Sterile	Sterile	Sterile
21	16	Sterile	*M. aurantiacus*	*M. epidermidis*
22	17	Sterile	Sterile	Sterile
23	18	Sterile	Sterile	Sterile
24	19	Sterile	Sterile	*Str. mitis*
25	20	Sterile	Sterile	Sterile
26	20	Sterile	Anaerobic coccus	Sterile
27	20	*B. coli*	*B. coli* *Str. fecalis*	*B. coli* *Str. fecalis*
28	26	Sterile	Sterile	Sterile
29	30	*Str. pyogenes* *Str. mitis*	*Str. pyogenes* *Str. mitis* *B. coli*	Not taken

*Time in minutes from birth to collection of specimen.

TABLE II

SPECIMENS OF MECONIUM COLLECTED BETWEEN THIRTY AND SIXTY MINUTES AFTER DELIVERY

NO.	TIME BETWEEN DELIVERY AND COLLECTION	RESULTS		
		PLATE	ENRICHMENT	SKIN CULTURES
1	31*	Sterile	Sterile	Sterile
2	34	Sterile	Sterile	Sterile
3	35	Sterile	*L. acidophilus*	*M. epidermidis*
4	39*	Sterile	Sterile	Sterile
5	52	Sterile	Sterile	Sterile
6	55	Sterile	Sterile	Sterile
7	57	Sterile	Sterile	Sterile
8	59	Sterile	*B. coli*	Sterile
9	59	Sterile	*M. epidermidis*	Sterile
10	59	Sterile	*B. coli* *C. hofmanni*	Sterile

*Cesarean birth.

the streak, but *B. coli* and *Str. fecalis* were isolated from the enrichment cultures as well as the skin area. Bacteria were demonstrated in five more of the specimens by enrichment procedures. The isolation of the unidentified species of the genus Bacteroides and the anaerobic coccus indicates the necessity for anaerobic methods in this type of study. The relation of the organisms isolated from the meconium and skin areas by enrichment is discussed later.

Specimens of meconium were collected from ten babies between thirty and sixty minutes after delivery; the results are summarized in Table II.

In the small series listed in Table II no bacteria were isolated directly, but in four of the ten specimens bacteria were shown to be present by enrichment methods. Only one control culture from the skin was positive for bacterial growth, and no duplication occurred with the corresponding culture of meconium in enrichment medium.

Sixteen specimens of meconium were collected between one and two hours after delivery; the results are recorded in Table III.

TABLE III

SPECIMENS OF MECONIUM COLLECTED BETWEEN ONE AND TWO HOURS AFTER DELIVERY

NO.	TIME BETWEEN BIRTH AND COLLECTION	RESULTS		
		PLATE	ENRICHMENT	SKIN CULTURES
1	1:00	Sterile	*C. hofmanni*	Sterile
2	1:00	Sterile	*M. albus*	*M. epidermidis*
3	1:03	Sterile	*M. candidus* *D. catarrhalis*	Sterile
4	1:04	Sterile	*L. acidophilus*	Not taken
5	1:05	Sterile	*B. coli*	Sterile
6	1:10	Sterile	Sterile	Sterile
7	1:15	Sterile	*B. welchii* *C. hofmanni* *M. epidermidis*	Sterile
8	1:15	Sterile	Sterile	Hay bacillus
9	1:15	Sterile	Sterile	Not taken
10	1:16	Sterile	Sterile	Sterile
11	1:21	Sterile	*M. epidermidis* *S. salivarius*	*M. epidermidis*
12	1:30	Sterile	*B. coli* *M. epidermidis*	Sterile
13	1:43	Sterile	Sterile	*M. epidermidis* *Str. salivarius*
14	1:46	Sterile	Sterile	Sterile
15	1:53*	Sterile	*Str. fecalis* *B. coli*	Sterile
16	1:56*	Sterile	*Str. fecalis* *B. coli*	Sterile

*Twins.

No bacteria were demonstrated by direct plating in any of the sixteen meconium specimens recorded in Table III. With enrichment media, however, ten of the sixteen specimens yielded positive results. This is a distinct increase in the positive results over those obtained in the preceding time periods. The isolation of *B. welchii,* the one species of sporulating anaerobe encountered, indicates again the necessity of anaerobic methods.

Nine specimens were obtained between two hours and three hours and ten minutes after delivery. These are shown in Table IV.

TABLE IV

BACTERIAL FLORA OF SPECIMENS OF MECONIUM COLLECTED BETWEEN TWO HOURS AND THREE HOURS AND TEN MINUTES AFTER DELIVERY

NO.	TIME BETWEEN BIRTH AND COLLECTION	RESULTS		
		PLATE	ENRICHMENT	SKIN CULTURES
1	2:00	Sterile	*M. aurantiacus*	Sterile
2	2:05	Sterile	Sterile	Sterile
3	2:17	Sterile	*Str. salivarius*	Not taken
4	2:25	Sterile	*M. epidermidis*	Sterile
5	2:35	Sterile	*M. albus*	*M. albus*
6	2:46	Sterile	*M. epidermidis*	Not taken
7	3:00	*L. acidophilus*	*M. candidus* *L. acidophilus*	Not taken
8	3:03	Sterile	*M. candidus*	Sterile
9	3:10	Sterile	Sterile	Sterile

Table IV shows that in only one case were bacteria numerous enough to be demonstrated by direct plating, but nine of the ten specimens gave positive results with enrichment methods. Only one of seven control cultures from the skin was positive for bacterial growth; the same species, *M. albus,* was also isolated by enrichment from the corresponding meconium specimen.

The species isolated from the specimens of meconium from sixty-four newborn infants within four hours after delivery are summarized in Table V in respect to frequence, time intervals, and methods of isolation. The cultures from the skin tests are included for comparison.

Table V shows that only four species of bacteria were isolated by direct plating methods. These species included two strains of *L. acidophilus* and one each of *B. coli, Str. pyogenes,* and *Str. mitis.* Thirteen known species, two unidentified species of the genus Bacteroides, and one unidentified anaerobic coccus were isolated by enrichment methods. Their frequence is given: *B. coli,* nine times; *M. epidermidis,* six; *L. acidophilus,* four; *C. hofmanni, Str. fecalis,* and *M. candidus,* three; *M. albus, M. aurantiacus, Str. salivarius, D. catarrhalis,* and Bacteroides species, two; and *Str. pyogenes, Str. mitis, B. welchii,* and an unidentified anaerobic coccus, once each.

The bacteria recovered from the skin cultures were six strains of *M. epidermidis,* three of *B. coli,* and one each of *Str. mitis,* hay bacillus, *Str. fecalis,* and *M. albus.*

DISCUSSION

Although specimens of meconium were obtained up to three hours and ten minutes after delivery, it was obvious that those collected as soon

TABLE V

FREQUENCY OF BACTERIAL SPECIES IN SPECIMENS OF MECONIUM COLLECTED WITHIN FOUR HOURS AFTER DELIVERY

	METHODS														
	DIRECT PLATING					ENRICHMENT					SKIN CULTURES				
	0-30 MIN.	30 MIN.-1 HR.	1-2 HR.	2-4 HR.	TOTAL	0-30 MIN.	30 MIN.-1 HR.	1-2 HR.	2-4 HR.	TOTAL	0-30 MIN.	30 MIN.-1 HR.	1-2 HR.	2-4 HR.	TOTAL
B. coli	1				1	2	3	4		9	3				3
M. epidermidis							1	3	2	6	2	1	3		6
C. hofmanni							1	2		3					
L. acidophilus	1			1	2		1	1	1	3					
M. candidus								1	2	3					
M. albus								1	1	2				1	1
Str. salivarius								1	1	2			1		1
Str. fecalis						1		2		3	1				1
M. aurantiacus						1			1	2					
D. catarrhalis								1	1	2					
Bacteroides species						2				2					
Str. pyogenes	1				1	1				1					
Str. mitis	1				1	1				1	1				1
B. welchii								1		1					
Anaerobic coccus							1			1					
Hay bacillus													1		1
Specimens	29	10	16	9	64	29	10	16	9	64	26	9	14	6	55
Negative	26	10	16	8	60	22	6	6	2	36	19	8	10	5	42
Positive	3	0	0	1	4	7	4	10	7	28	7	1	4	1	13
% Positive	10.4			11.1	6.3	24.1	40.0	62.5	78.0	48.3	24.6	12.5	28.0	16.7	23.6

as possible were of more value in answering the question whether bacteria are present in the meconium at birth. The most striking proof was the specific case where the collection was made nine minutes after delivery. Nothing had been done to the infant, such as washing or taking the rectal temperature. No organisms were isolated from the skin of the anal region by enrichment, but numerous delicate colonies appeared in from forty-eight to seventy-two hours along the streak on the blood agar plate inoculated with the meconium. These organisms were tentatively classified as Doederlein's bacillus or *L. acidophilus,* the identity of which was pointed out by Thomas[16] in 1928. The presence of such numbers of bacteria, even if not seen microscopically, would seem to be proof of their multiplication in the meconium before birth.

The relation of the bacteria isolated from the skin surface of the anal areas to those recovered from the meconium by enrichment methods warrants some consideration because it would seem that the isolation of organisms from the anal area might limit the value of the positive results obtained by enrichment of the respective meconium specimens. Three possibilities exist: First, when bacteria are isolated from the meconium and not from the anal area, it would indicate the presence of a few organisms in the meconium and either that cleansing of the skin of the anal region was satisfactory or that the surface was sterile at birth. Second, the culturing of bacteria from the skin and not the meconium suggests that although the cleansing was not completely efficient, organisms had not invaded the meconium. Third, isolation of the organisms from both skin and meconium may be interpreted in two ways. The isolation of a species from the anal area unlike the species recovered from the meconium would not necessarily interfere with the assumption of bacterial growth from a few cells in the meconium. The isolation of the same species from both skin area and meconium, however, suggests either the occurrence of per anum invasion with natural duplication of results from these two sources or direct exterior contamination of the meconium specimen from the skin.

If the thirteen cases of positive skin cultures are analyzed in light of these possibilities, it is found that in five cases bacteria were recovered from the anal areas only, in four cases different species were isolated from anal areas and the corresponding meconium specimens, and in only four cases were the species from the two sources identical. Therefore, it would appear that only the last four cases should be eliminated on the ground of exterior contamination. In addition, there were six cases in which no skin cultures were made. One was sterile, one had hemolytic streptococci in the meconium as demonstrated by direct plating, and the other four were positive for bacteria by enriching methods. If the four cases of duplication and the four positive cases with no skin cultures be eliminated from the series, there remain fifty-six specimens of meconium from the series, in twenty of which bacteria were demonstrated by enrichment methods. These results indicate the presence of only a few bacterial cells, except possibly the cases from which anaerobes were isolated, in the meconium.

In this series the percentage of positive results with solid media was only 6.3 per cent, which is much lower than the 23 per cent reported by Hymanson and Hertz,[13] the 38 per cent by Burrage,[14] and the 30 per cent by Hall and O'Toole.[15] Enrichment results gave 35.7 per cent, a figure which is not significantly different from the 38 per cent obtained by Hall and O'Toole with both solid and enrichment media. It is possible that some of the discrepancies may be explained by the failure of Hymanson and Hertz to cleanse the skin of the anal area before the specimen was collected, and that Burrage, Hall and O'Toole limited their studies to first passage specimens. Hall and O'Toole reported specimens microscopically positive which were collected thirteen, twenty-six, and seventeen hours, respectively, after birth which findings led Hall (personal communication) to believe that postnatal bacterial invasion accounted for many of the positive results in the study of first passage meconium specimens. The present investigation was designed to cover these points and to get the specimens within a short period after delivery under aseptic precautions, and it would seem that the positive cases reported furnish reliable evidence that bacteria are present in the meconium at birth in a small percentage of cases. Thus the essential point in this investigation is not that the solid media results are so greatly different or that the enrichment results approximate the figures given previously, but that the meconium is not always sterile at birth.

To explain the presence of bacteria in the meconium of newborn infants in numbers to be demonstrated by plating or enrichment media, if contamination can be ruled out, three routes of infection may be considered. First, it is possible that bacteria invade the meconium during passage of the fetus through the birth canal, but the natural process of delivery prevents any serious investigation. Second, the bacteria may have been deposited in the intestine from the blood stream. In this study no attempt was made to run control tests on the blood of the mother and child. Third and most plausible, the amniotic fluid may have been infected by the organisms of the vaginal flora. Since the fetus is surrounded by amniotic fluid, which enters the intestinal tract, as evidenced by the presence of lanugo hair, epidermal cells, and vernix caseosa in the meconium,[17] it would not be unreasonable to expect bacterial invasion of the meconium if the fluid became infected. Therefore, a relation should exist between the time of rupture of the fetal membranes and birth with the appearance of bacteria in the meconium; that is, the longer the time between fetal membrane rupture and delivery, the greater should be the chance of finding bacteria in the intestinal tract. A similar relation of time between rupture and inflammation of the fetal membranes and congenital pneumonia in stillborn and newborn infants dying in the first three days was pointed out by Johnson and Meyer.[18] Hall and O'Toole,[15] however, could not show that time elapsing from rupture of the fetal membranes to birth influenced the presence of bacteria in fifty first passage meconium specimens. Similarly, in the present study little or no relation could be established between the time from fetal membrane rupture to delivery, inflammation in the membranes, and the presence of bacteria in the meconium of fifty of the sixty-four cases studied.

SUMMARY

In three of twenty-nine specimens of meconium collected within thirty minutes after delivery, bacteria were demonstrated by plating methods. These three positive cases indicate that prenatal bacterial invasion of the intestinal tract does occur in a small percentage of cases.

Some of the positive results obtained by enrichment might be invalidated by the failure to sterilize thoroughly the skin surrounding the anus, but a large number with corresponding sterile skin cultures, or skin cultures showing other bacterial species than in the meconium, indicated that a few organisms were present in the meconium at birth in about 36 per cent of this series of sixty-four specimens.

REFERENCES

1. Escherich, T.: Die Darmbakterien des Sauglings, 1886, Stuttgart, F. Enke.
2. Schild, W.: Ztschr. f. Hyg. **19**: 113, 1895.
3. Szego, K.: Arch. f. Kinderh. **23**: 25, 1897.
4. Sittler, P.: Centralbl. f. Bakt., Orig. **47**: 145, 1908.
5. Tissier, H.: Recherches sur la flore intestinale des nourrissons, Thèse de Paris, 1900.
6. Cruickshank, J., and Cruickshank, R.: System of Bacteriology, Medical Research Council, London **8**: 344, 1931.
7. Passini, F.: Ztschr. f. Kinderh. **53**: 175, 1932.
8. Ford, W. W.: Textbook of Bacteriology, Philadelphia, 1927, W. B. Saunders Co., p. 795.
9. Topley, W. W. C., and Wilson, G. S.: The Principles of Bacteriology and Immunity, Baltimore, 1931, William Wood and Co., Vol. 2, p. 1256.
10. Zinsser, H., and Bayne-Jones, S.: A Textbook of Bacteriology, New York, 1934, D. Appleton-Century Co., p. 137.
11. Park, W. H., and Williams, A. W.: Pathogenic Microorganisms, Philadelphia, 1933, Lea and Febiger, p. 418.
12. Kendall, A. I.: Bacteriology, General, Pathological, and Intestinal, Philadelphia, 1928, Lea and Febiger, p. 663.
13. Hymanson, A., and Hertz, J. J.: Am. J. Obst. **75**: 662, 1917.
14. Burrage, S.: J. Bact. **13**: 47, 1927.
15. Hall, I. C., and O'Toole, E.: Am. J. Dis. Child. **47**: 1279, 1934.
16. Thomas, S.: J. Infect. Dis. **43**: 216, 1928.
17. Williams, J. W.: Obstetrics, New York, 1930, D. Appleton-Century Co., p. 181.
18. Johnson, W. C., and Meyer, J.: Am. J. Obst. & Gynec. **9**: 3, 1925.

THE BACTERIAL FLORA OF THE INTESTINAL CONTENTS OF TWENTY-SEVEN STILLBORN INFANTS

MARSHALL L. SNYDER, PH.D.
DENVER, COLO.

IT WAS shown in a preceding study of newborn infants that bacteria could be demonstrated by plating methods in three of twenty-nine specimens of meconium collected within thirty minutes after delivery.[1] These findings indicated that bacteria were present in the intestinal tracts of infants at birth in a small percentage of cases. In order to study further the occurrence of bacteria in the intestinal tract at birth, segments of the intestines of twenty-seven stillborn* babies were examined.

Despite the large amount of work recorded on the sterility of the meconium at birth and the bacterial invasion of normal living infants, only two references dealing directly with intestinal examinations of stillborn material were found in the available literature. Both Escherich,[2] who examined three stillborn infants, and Popoff,[3] who killed newborn kittens and puppies, were unable to demonstrate bacteria in any of these and concluded that the fetal meconium was sterile at birth.

METHODS OF COLLECTION AND EXAMINATION

In the first fifteen cases only one segment was taken from the intestinal tract. This was from the ascending colon as close as possible to the cecum, and was selected because it was thought to be least exposed to either oral or anal bacterial invasion. Therefore, if bacteria were found, it would seem indisputable evidence that bacteria were present in the intestinal tract at birth. In the remaining twelve cases segments were taken from the descending colon, ascending colon, ileum, and duodenum. The segments were tied off, cut, and placed in sterile Petri dishes, and in the first fifteen cases they were dipped momentarily in boiling water. Those from the other twelve were seared with a hot spatula. The sections were opened with instruments that had been boiled or flamed. Smears of the contents were stained by Gram's method and were negative except in one case where large gram-positive rods were observed. The contents were also streaked across eosin methylene blue and blood agar plates and were placed in freshly boiled and cooled deep brain medium.

From the Department of Bacteriology and Public Health and the Child Research Council, University of Colorado School of Medicine and Hospitals.

*No distinction is made between the terms "stillborn" and "deadborn."

RESULTS

The fifteen infants from whom only one section of the intestine was taken are recorded in Table I in the order of the time elapsing between death and autopsy.

Table I shows there is apparently little relationship between the time of delivery and autopsy and the presence of bacteria in the intestines

TABLE I

BACTERIAL FLORA OF THE INTESTINAL CONTENTS AT THE ASCENDING COLON OF 15 STILLBORN INFANTS

NO.	HOURS*	SECTION	RESULTS	
			PLATES	ENRICHMENT
1	3	Ascending colon	Sterile	Sterile
2	14	Ascending colon	Sterile	Sterile
3	18½	Ascending colon	Sterile	Sterile
4	27	Ascending colon	Sterile	Sterile
5	30	Ascending colon	Sterile	Sterile
6	30	Ascending colon	Sterile	Sterile
7	57	Ascending colon	Sterile	Sterile
8	63	Ascending colon	Sterile	Sterile
9	66	Ascending colon	Sterile	Sterile
10	66	Ascending colon	Sterile	Sterile
11	72	Ascending colon	Sterile	*M. aureus*
12	73	Ascending colon	Sterile	Sterile
13	109	Ascending colon	Sterile	*M. epidermidis*
14	?	Ascending colon	Sterile	Sterile
15	?	Ascending colon	Sterile	Sterile

*Time in hours between delivery and autopsy.

of stillborn infants. In only two of the fifteen cases were bacteria demonstrated, and in both of these only after enrichment. These cases are discussed in detail as follows:

CASE 11.—No clinical history was available for this premature infant, who weighed about 5 pounds. Autopsy revealed extensive subarachnoidal hemorrhage. Other sites of hemorrhage were in the pleurae, epicardium, scalp, tentorium cerebelli, and falx cerebri. The heart's blood was sterile. *M. aureus* was isolated by enrichment from the ascending colon. Time of the rupture of the fetal membranes and the condition of the membranes and placenta were unknown.

CASE 13.—This premature infant of about six months' gestation was apparently dead from the nephritic toxemia of the mother. Autopsy showed slight maceration, petechial hemorrhages in the thymus, parietal pericardium, epicardium, scalp, and epicranium, and slight congestion of the cerebrum. The membranes ruptured eighteen and one-half hours before delivery and were acutely inflamed. The heart's blood was sterile. *M. epidermidis* was isolated from the ascending colon by enrichment. The mother made an uneventful recovery.

The significance of the positive enrichment cultures will be considered in the discussion.

The bacteriologic study of the sections taken from various portions of the intestinal tract of twelve stillborn infants is given in Table II.

In contrast to the first series, the data presented in Table II show that the intestinal contents of only one of twelve stillborns to be sterile in

TABLE II

BACTERIAL FLORA OF THE CONTENTS OF VARIOUS PORTIONS OF THE INTESTINAL TRACT OF STILLBORN INFANTS

NO.	TIME HOURS*	DUODENUM	ILEUM	ASCENDING COLON	DESCENDING COLON
16	14	Sterile	Sterile	Sterile	*M. epidermidis* *Str. fecalis*
17	16¾	*B. welchii*†	*B. welchii*†	*B. welchii*†	*B. welchii*†
18	22	Sterile	Sterile	Sterile	*M. citreus* *Str. nonhemolyticus II*
19	23	Sterile	Sterile	Sterile	Sterile
20	24	Sterile	Sterile	Sterile	*B. alkaligenes*‡ *M. flavus*‡ *Str. ignavus*‡
21	24	*B. alkaligenes*‡	Sterile	Sterile	*M. citreus* *B. coli*
22	24	Sterile	Sterile	*M. aurantiacus*	*B. coli*
23	28½	*B. tertius*	Sterile	Sterile	Sterile
24	30	Sterile	Sterile	Sterile	*B. coli* *Sarcina lutea*
25	30	Sterile	*M. luteus*‡	*M. luteus*‡	*M. luteus*‡
26	50	*C. hofmanni*‡	Sterile	Sterile	Sterile
27	53	Sterile	Sterile	Sterile	*M. varians*‡

*Time in hours between delivery and autopsy.
†Observed microscopically in contents.
‡Isolated by direct plating.

sections taken from the duodenum, ileum, ascending colon, and descending colon. Bacteria were isolated by direct plating and enrichment methods in the other eleven cases. These cases are reported as follows:

CASE 16.—This was a full-term infant, weighing about 9 pounds, anatomically normal. The heart's blood was sterile. *M. epidermidis* and *Str. fecalis* were isolated by enrichment from the descending colon.

The mother had a massive hemorrhage from a duodenal ulcer before she was brought to the hospital on the evening before delivery. Fetal movements could not be discerned at the time of entrance. Death of the baby was believed to be due to the anemia of the placenta which resulted from the hemorrhage; the placenta and membranes were free from inflammation.

CASE 17.—The body was that of a full-term child who weighed about 8 pounds. The delivery was a breech presentation, and apparently the head was retained in the cervix until death occurred. The placenta, the membranes, and the cord were acutely inflamed. Autopsy showed atelectasis, slight bilateral tentorial tears with no hemorrhage, and aspiration of amniotic fluid. Large gram-positive rods were observed microscopically in the duodenum, the ileum, the ascending colon and the descending colon. These were isolated and identified as *B. welchii.* Since the child was born in this hospital and remained most of the sixteen and three-fourth hours from birth to autopsy in the ice box, it would seem that the presence of organisms in sufficient number to be demonstrated microscopically would be clear-cut evidence that the bacteria invaded and multiplied in the meconium before birth.

CASE 18.—This full-term, 8-pound infant was delivered by version and extraction after a shoulder presentation was determined. The cord was not pulsating before the patient was taken to the delivery room. The placenta was normal; no information was available about the rupture of the membranes. Autopsy revealed a broken neck and atelectasis. The heart's blood was sterile. The inoculated plates were negative, but *M. citreus* and *Str. nonhemolyticus II* were isolated by enrichment from the descending colon.

CASE 20.—The clinical history furnished no definite reason for the death of this 6½-pound full-term infant. The doctor who delivered this case in an outside institution reported a velamentous insertion of the cord with rupture of the membranes adjacent to the site of insertion, but there was no record of hemorrhage. The gross pathology was limited to atelectasis. *B. alkaligenes, M. flavus,* and *Str. ignavus* were isolated by both plating and enrichment from the descending colon.

CASE 21.—This was a premature infant of about the seventh lunar month of gestation, weighing about 3 pounds. It was brought in from another hospital, and no information was secured about the clinical history. Autopsy showed pneumothorax. *B. alkaligenes* was isolated by both plating and enrichment methods from the duodenum; *M. citreus* and *B. coli* were isolated by enrichment from the descending colon.

CASE 22.—This was a full-term infant who was delivered in another hospital. The mother's labor was prolonged. Forceps were applied unsuccessfully and with heavy laceration which apparently caused the death of the baby. The body had already been opened. No heart's blood was taken, but *M. aurantiacus* was isolated from the ascending colon by enrichment, and *B. coli* was recovered from the descending colon after enriching of the contents.

CASE 23.—This infant was about one month premature, and weighed about 5 pounds. The heart was beating at birth, but no respirations were made. The delivery was a footling presentation, and great difficulty was encountered in removing the head. Membranes ruptured about one and a quarter hours before delivery; the placenta was normal. The heart's blood was sterile. Tentorial tears with resultant hemorrhage were found at autopsy. *B. tertius* was recovered by enrichment from the duodenum. All other cultures were sterile.

CASE 24.—The body was that of a full-term infant weighing 8½ pounds. It was born in an outside institution, and no clinical history was available. Autopsy showed tentorial tears with hemorrhage. The heart's blood was sterile. *Sarcina lutea* and *B. coli* were isolated by enrichment from the descending colon.

CASE 25.—This was a full-term infant whose heart was beating up to twelve hours before delivery but was not beating at birth. There was no apparent clinical cause for death. Autopsy showed moderate congestion of the lungs and some "congenital pneumonia." The heart's blood was sterile. The membranes were moderately inflamed, having ruptured thirty hours before delivery. *M. luteus* was isolated directly by plating methods from the ileum, the ascending colon and the descending colon.

CASE 26.—This full-term infant was delivered after a breech presentation. The heart was beating, but the infant made no attempt to breathe. Resuscitation was abandoned after forty-five minutes. Autopsy showed fetal atelectasis and tentorial tears. The membranes ruptured two hours before delivery; neither placenta, membranes, nor cord was inflamed. The heart's blood was sterile. From the white mucoid material of the jejunum, which was microscopically negative, *C. hofmanni* was isolated by direct plating. The other sections were sterile.

CASE 27.—This infant was slightly premature and was delivered dead after a breech presentation. Autopsy showed fetal atelectasis and a patent intraventricular septum. The heart's blood was sterile. Three colonies of *M. varians* were found at the beginning of the streak on blood agar, and this species was also isolated by enrichment. All positive cultures were obtained from the descending colon.

If the study is analyzed in respect to the intestinal segments studied rather than according to the case, it is noted that four of the twelve duodenal specimens yielded bacteria, and in three of the four cases organisms were demonstrated by plating methods or microscopically. Only two ileal segments were positive but one showed bacterial cells when examined microscopically. Bacteria were demonstrated three times by plating and enrichment in the ascending colon sections and once microscopically. Nine of the twelve descending colon segments showed bacteria to be present by plating or enrichment methods, and one, microscopically. This might indicate a more frequent per anum bacterial invasion of the intestine than per os.

Sixteen species were isolated from the intestinal contents of the twenty-seven stillborn infants. Their frequence is given as follows: *B. coli, B. alkaligenes,* and *M. citreus,* three times; *M. epidermidis,* two times; and *M. flavus, M. luteus, M. varians, M. aureus, M. aurantiacus, Str. ignavus, Str. fecalis, Str. nonhemolyticus II, C. hofmanni, B. welchii, B. tertius,* and *Sarcina lutea,* once each.

DISCUSSION

Proof for prenatal bacterial invasion of the intestinal tract in stillborn as with newborn infants depends entirely upon microscopic and cultural examination of the intestinal contents. The presence of organisms in the intestinal contents of a stillborn child as demonstrated by the microscope soon after birth would seem to furnish absolute proof that bacteria may be present at or before birth. The observation of gram-positive rods similar to *B. welchii,* which was subsequently isolated, in Case 17, is offered as the most suggestive evidence in this series. Next in value to microscopic proof is the culturing of organisms directly on solid media so that the position and number of the resultant colonies cannot be mistaken for contamination. This condition occurred in Cases 20, 21, 25, and 26. Positive enrichment cultures are least valuable because growth in liquid media may result from either too few organisms to be demonstrated by plating methods or from exterior contamination. Although there was no skin sterilizing factor in this study, the surfaces of the segments had to be cleansed. This was accomplished by either dipping momentarily into boiling water or searing with a spatula. The segments were opened with either freshly boiled or flamed scissors and forceps. Despite these precautions the isolation of such organisms as *Sarcina lutea* would lead one to doubt the validity of positive enrichment results in all cases. This leaves the obvious conclusion that reliable data are best obtained with solid media and positive microscopic evidence.

Three possible methods for prenatal invasion of the intestinal tracts of stillborn infants are to be considered: (1) neonatal septicemia, (2) infection of the amniotic fluid, and (3) during passage of the fetus through the birth canal.

A possible relation exists between the septicemias of the stillborn and the organisms found in the intestinal tracts of these cases. Some cases of neonatal septicemias have been described in detail by Slemons,[4] DeLee,[5] and Serbin.[6] In the present series only two of twenty-one cases gave positive blood cultures at autopsy, and the organisms isolated, *M. tetragenus* and *Bact. pyocyaneum*, respectively, were not recovered from the intestine in any case studied. Therefore, it may be said that there was no correlation between the organisms isolated from the heart's blood and those isolated from the intestinal tract in this group of stillborn infants.

The early rupture of the fetal membranes with subsequent infection of the amniotic fluid by the vaginal organisms and invasion of the intestinal tract of the fetus either per os or per anum or both offers the most plausible method of infection. The somewhat analogous rôle between early rupture of the fetal membranes and congenital pneumonias in the newborn and stillborn was pointed out by Johnson and Meyer.[7] However, Hall and O'Toole[8] could not establish any relation between the time elapsing between the rupture of the fetal membranes and the presence of bacteria in the first passage of meconium. In the preceding study of a series of sixty-four specimens of meconium from newborn infants collected within four hours after delivery,[1] this relationship could not be determined. It seemed important, nevertheless, to compare the stillborn with the normal newborn in this respect. It was difficult to secure accurate information about the rupture of the fetal membranes; the available data, however, are listed in order of increasing time from rupture to delivery, and the histologic examination of the placentas in these and other cases is also included in Table III.

Too few cases are included in Table III to establish any definite relation between the time elapsing between rupture of the fetal membranes and delivery, the condition of the membranes, and bacteria in the intestinal contents of stillborn infants. It does seem significant, however, that in four of the five cases showing moderate to acute inflammation of the fetal membranes, bacteria were isolated from the intestinal contents. On the other hand, *C. hofmanni* was isolated directly in large numbers from Case 5 in which the membranes ruptured allegedly forty-five minutes before delivery and the fetal membranes showed no sign of inflammation, and in Case 13 the fetal membranes were acutely inflamed, but no bacteria were isolated from the intestinal contents.

This problem is confused by the inability to collect accurate information about the rupture of the membranes because so-called "high" ruptures may pass unnoticed but permit invasion of the amniotic fluid by

TABLE III

RELATION BETWEEN THE TIME OF RUPTURE OF THE FETAL MEMBRANES TO DELIVERY, INFLAMMATION OF THE MEMBRANES, AND THE PRESENCE OF BACTERIA IN THE INTESTINAL CONTENTS OF STILLBORN INFANTS

NO.	TIME IN HOURS*	CONDITION OF FETAL MEMBRANES	BACTERIAL FLORA OF THE INTESTINAL CONTENT
1	At birth	Normal	Sterile
2	At birth	Normal	Sterile
3	At birth	Normal	Sterile
4	At birth	Normal	Sterile
5	0:45	Normal	*C. hofmannii*†
6	4:45	Normal	Sterile
7	14:30	Normal	Sterile
8	15:45	Normal	Sterile
9	17:00	Acute inflammation	*B. welchii*‡
10	18:45	Acute inflammation	*M. epidermidis*
11	30:00	Moderate inflammation	*M. luteus*†
12	?	Acute inflammation	*M. aureus*
13	?	Acute inflammation	Sterile
14	?	Normal	Sterile
15	?	Normal	Sterile
16	?	Normal	Sterile
17	?	Normal	*M. citreus* *Str. nonhemolyticus II*

*Time in hours from rupture to delivery.
†Isolated by plating.
‡Observed microscopically.

the vaginal flora. After membrane rupture some time must elapse before bacteria can multiply in the amniotic fluid, and then the fetus may or may not swallow the infected fluid. The same possibility exists for the invasion by bacteria per anum. The fetus may be delivered before inflammation of the membranes occurs and still have bacteria in the intestinal tract. Finally, the hygiene of the individual mother frequently determines the number and type of organisms in the vaginal tract[9]; that is, the flora ranges from a homogenous but scanty flora of gram-positive rods, Doederlein's bacillus or *L. acidophilus*,[10] with a highly acid secretion (Grade I) to a mixed flora with a more alkaline secretion (Grade III). Thus it is probable that the type of vaginal flora determines the amount of infection of the amniotic fluid and in turn the organism isolated from the intestine of the newborn and the stillborn infant.

The remaining possible route of prenatal infection of the intestinal tract is during the passage of the fetus through the birth canal. As in the newborn series this mode of invasion could not be studied seriously.

SUMMARY

The presence of *B. welchii* microscopically and culturally in the duodenum, the ileum, the ascending colon and the descending colon of a stillborn infant is considered as reliable evidence that bacteria may invade the intestinal tract of the infant before or during birth. Additional evidence of slightly less value was obtained by finding numerous colonies along the streaks on plates inoculated from the intestinal contents of four stillborn infants. The results obtained by enrichment were regarded as of doubtful significance because of the possibility of accidental contamination, except in the one case where *B. welchii* was isolated after being observed microscopically.

REFERENCES

1. Snyder, M. L.: J. PEDIAT. **9**: 624, 1936.
2. Escherich, T.: Die Darmbakterien des Säuglings, 1886, Stuttgart, F. Enke.
3. Popoff, D.: Centralbl. f. Bakt., Orig. I, **11**: 214, 1891.
4. Slemons, J. M.: J. A. M. A. **65**: 1265, 1915.
5. DeLee, J. B.: J. A. M. A. **67**: 344, 1916.
6. Serbin, W. B.: Am. J. Obst. & Gynec. **15**: 682, 1928.
7. Johnson, W. C., and Meyer, J.: Am. J. Obst. & Gynec. **9**: 3, 1925.
8. Hall, I. C., and O'Toole, E.: Am. J. Dis. Child. **47**: 1279, 1934.
9. Cruickshank, R., and Sharman, A.: J. Obst. & Gynec. Brit. Emp. **41**: 190 and 369, 1934.
10. Thomas, S.: J. Infect. Dis. **43**: 216, 1928.

ACTIVE ARTIFICIAL IMMUNIZATION IN DIPHTHERIA

The Relative Effectiveness of Various Antigens and the Duration of Immunity

Jean V. Cooke, M.D.
St. Louis, Mo.

ALTHOUGH the value of diphtheria immunization is unquestioned, there is still some uncertainty about the best method of producing it; i.e., the method which will result regularly in the maximum percentage of immune subjects with a minimum of injections and unpleasant reactions. Certainly, effectiveness and simplification are the two primary requisites for any method of immunization advised on a large scale. The high incidence of susceptibility in children, especially those in the preschool age, has led to the general acceptance of the view that preliminary Schick tests in children should be omitted and that every child should be immunized. Another advance in simplification of the general procedure will be made when a method of immunization can be shown to result regularly in such a high percentage of immunes that subsequent Schick testing may be safely omitted.

This report summarizes the results of immunization against diphtheria in more than 500 young adult student nurses during an eighteen-year period, with the use of several types of antigens and with a variance in the number and spacing of the injections. A number of subjects immunized from six to sixteen years previously were retested to determine the duration of the immunity.

Methods.—All student nurses of the Washington University Nurses' Training School were given Schick tests in groups of 15 to 50 early in their probation period during the years 1918-1935. Those with positive tests were immunized and were retested from four to six months later. This interval of several months before a retest seems important since in several instances Schick tests which were negative four to six weeks after immunization had again become positive three to four months later. Any who remained Schick-positive were given a second immunization identical with the first, usually from six to ten months after the initial injections. Previous to 1925 the Schick test toxin and immunizing antigens were obtained from the New York City Board of Health, and since then all material has been furnished by Eli Lilly and Company. Controls of the identical toxin preparation used for the Schick test heated for five minutes to 75° C. were always included, and readings of the tests and controls were made on the fourth day. All tests, readings, and im-

From the Department of Pediatrics, Washington University School of Medicine.

munizations were done by the author to guarantee uniformity in interpretation and procedure. Some pupils who left training before immunization was finished are omitted from the tabulations, only those being included upon whom complete observations were made.

Results.—Susceptibility: Of 1,054 nurses tested, 664, or 63 per cent, gave positive Schick tests. A large proportion of these girls came from rural or suburban communities and a rather high percentage of susceptibility seems to be the rule in persons not reared in larger cities where diphtheria is endemic.

TABLE I

RESULTS OF DIPTHERIA IMMUNIZATION BY VARIOUS PROCEDURES

ANTIGEN USED	DOSES	INTERVAL	NUMBER VACCINATED	PER CENT NEGATIVE
1. T.A.T. (3L+)	3	1 wk. + 1 wk.	62	79.0
T.A.T. (2nd set)	3	1 wk. + 1 wk.	8	38.0
2. T.A.T. (0.1L+)	3	1 wk. + 1 wk.	274	59.3
T.A.T. (2nd set)	3	1 wk. + 1 wk.	96	92.6
T.A.T. (3rd set)	3	1 wk. + 1 wk.	5	100.0
3. Toxoid	2	3 wk.	53	75.5
Toxoid (2nd set)	2	3 wk.	13	92.4
Toxoid (3rd set)	2	3 wk.	1	100.0
4. Toxoid	2	5 wk.	46	78.2
Toxoid (2nd set)	2	5 wk.	10	100.0
5. Toxoid	3	3 wk. + 2 wk.	37	100.0
6. A.P. Toxoid	1	–	64	80.0
A.P. Toxoid (2nd set)	1	4-5 mo.	13	100.0

Immunization: The results of the immunizations with the various antigens have been summarized in Table I. In the two groups (1 and 2) with toxin-antitoxin (T.A.T.), it will be noted that a single series of three injections at weekly intervals did not regularly produce as high a percentage of immunes as might be expected. This was especially true of the 0.1L+ antigen which produced about 59 per cent of immunes. A second series of three injections resulted in the immunization of a very large proportion of the remainder, and the small number not immunized by the preceding injections became Schick-negative after a third set. The results with two doses of toxoid (Groups 3 and 4, Table I) given at an interval of three weeks or five weeks were quite similar to those from toxin-antitoxin. When three doses of toxoid (Group 5, Table I) were given at intervals of two and three weeks, the results were much better. A single dose of alum-precipitated toxoid resulted in only 80 per cent immunes, but a second dose immunized all the remainder. Although a few required a third set of injections with toxin-antitoxin and with toxoid, all became Schick-negative eventually.

In the immunization of infants and young children, it has been our experience, as well as that of others, that a rather high proportion of those inoculated with two doses of toxoid or a single dose of alum-precipitated toxoid develop negative Schick tests. There is a very definite impression, however, among certain health officers in rural communities that the response to diphtheria immunization is less satisfactory in rural children than that reported in cities. It may be that the relatively lower percentage of immunes obtained among the young adults here reported after their first series of injections is related to the fact that a large proportion of them were reared in suburban communities or that adults are more difficult to immunize with the same doses used in children. At any rate, the fact that, as a group, these nurses responded only moderately well to the initial vaccination gave a somewhat better opportunity to observe the relative effectiveness of the various procedures used.

Certain features of the results may be summarized briefly. Toxoid and especially alum-precipitated toxoid were relatively more effective than toxin-antitoxin. Two doses of toxoid or a single injection of alum toxoid immunized only 75 to 80 per cent. By far the best results were obtained by two doses of alum-precipitated toxoid, the second after a considerable interval, and by three doses of plain toxoid separated by intervals of several weeks. This tends to confirm the well-known experimental observations that the immunity following the first or "primary" response to the diphtheria antigen is slow, feeble and transient, but the "secondary" response following a later antigen stimulus results in rapid, pronounced and persistent antitoxin formation. It would appear, therefore, that those who become immune following a single injection or series of injections have already responded previously to the diphtheria antigenic stimulus such as occurs in the development of "natural immunity," and develop the permanent immunity characteristic of a "secondary" stimulus. On the other hand, those who have not reacted previously to the diphtheria antigen and consequently do not become immune following a single injection or series of injections will require a second immunization. It was hoped that alum toxoid, being insoluble and, therefore, slowly absorbed, would serve as both the primary and secondary stimuli and that a single antigenic injection would be adequate. The results in the series reported here, however, do not confirm this, since 20 per cent of those receiving a single dose remained Schick-positive.

The results obtained by the several methods used indicate that the maximum percentage will be immunized by two doses of alum toxoid with an interval of one to several months between them. While a considerable number may be immunized by a single injection, the percentage remaining Schick-positive is sufficient to warrant the advisability of giving a second later dose whenever possible. The larger number of injections of toxin-antitoxin and plain toxoid make them less desirable for routine use, although the latter seems quite effective when given in three doses at intervals of about three weeks.

Reactions following toxoid injections are rare in infants and young children although often a somewhat tender nodule persists for some days after alum-precipitated toxoid. The occasional occurrence of moderately severe local pain and swelling accompanied by a febrile general reaction in older children and more frequently in adults has tended to limit the use of toxoid and alum toxoid. During the past six years several hundred young adults (nurses and medical students) have been given toxoid and alum toxoid. Most of them have had a slight local reaction only, while a few have had headache, mild fever, and malaise for the day following. Alum-precipitated toxoid seemed somewhat more likely to produce such an effect than plain toxoid. Rarely a very severe local reaction with general febrile toxic symptoms has occurred and persisted for several days.

In general, such reactions have been only slightly more severe than those following toxin-antitoxin and there has been no suggestion of discontinuing the use of toxoid because of them. It must be emphasized, however, that the foregoing applies only to the products of one manufacturer used routinely. In the few instances in which two other commercial toxoid antigens were tried, the number and the severity of the reactions were so great that they were considered unsuitable for use in adults.

Clinical Results.—All student nurses of the group tested spent from four to six weeks on duty in the contagious wards of the St. Louis Children's Hospital where they attended patients with clinical diphtheria as part of their training. During the three years immediately preceding the adoption of immunization in 1918, seventy student nurses were on duty in the contagious wards and twenty of them developed clinical diphtheria. Since 1918 only two cases of diphtheria have occurred among almost 1,000 students, both in known nonimmunes, accidentally exposed to the disease before immunization. This contrast in incidence before and after immunization is striking proof of the clinical effectiveness of the procedure in persons intimately exposed.

Duration of Immunity After Active Artificial Immunization.—The immunity which develops after diphtheria vaccination has generally been assumed to be lasting, although it is the general belief that in many instances the artificial immunity produced by injections merely protects the child over a certain limited period of susceptibility to diphtheria, and that during this time many develop an additional "natural immunity" which is solid and permanent. This belief is fostered by the frequent observation that even without artificial immunization there is a considerable tendency for older children and adults to have negative

Schick tests. That this tendency is apparently not constant, however, is shown by the fact that, in the adult nurses reported in this paper, 63 per cent were still susceptible. While in occasional instances diphtheria has occurred in vaccinated children, it has been extremely rare in those known to have been Schick-negative after vaccination. The published observations, however, on the duration of immunity based on Schick tests done some years after vaccination have been few because of the difficulty of collecting groups of immunized persons some years afterward. Such as I have been able to find are given in Table II. The first two show the results after toxin-antitoxin while the others report results with Ramon's anatoxin. The largest series, that of the Mosers (often mistakenly attributed to Ramon in the literature), gives somewhat misleading percentages, since no previous Schick tests had been made and many children may have been immune even before the anatoxin injections. In general, the results reported, however, indicate that the immunity

TABLE II

DURATION OF IMMUNITY AFTER ACTIVE IMMUNIZATION

OBSERVER		INTERVAL AFTER IMMUNIZATION—YEARS	NUMBER TESTED	PER CENT SCHICK-POSITIVE
Schroeder	T.A.T.	5	28	10.7
Parish and Okell	T.A.T.	1 to 4	440	5.0
Moser, M., and Moser, G.	Ana.	2	498	5.0
		3	162	4.3
		4	250	3.6
Cerruti	Ana.	2½	29	17.2
Calisti	Ana.	1	54 (adults?)	0.0
Bosco	Ana.	4	10	40.0
Ronchi	Ana.	5	27	14.8

persists in a large proportion of those vaccinated. Many of those found to have positive Schick tests later were observed to become reimmunized quickly after another vaccination.

In the groups of young adult nurses considered in this report, 102 were retested six to sixteen years after immunization by toxin-antitoxin and subsequent negative Schick tests. Of these, 12 had been done fourteen to sixteen years previously, and three of these, all after sixteen years, again gave positive Schick tests, one of them only weakly positive. Ninety who had received the injections six to twelve years previously included only two with positive tests, one of these (after nine years) being strongly positive and the other (after eight years) being only faintly positive. The fact that more than 95 per cent of this group of 102 were immune from six to sixteen years after vaccination is striking proof of the degree of effectiveness and persistence of the protection afforded by active artificial diphtheria immunization.

SUMMARY

In more than 1,000 young adult student nurses, 63 per cent were found susceptible to diphtheria by the Schick test.

Groups were immunized by toxin-antitoxin, toxoid, and alum-precipitated toxoid over a period of eighteen years. Of the methods tried, the most effective procedures were found to be (1) two injections of alum toxoid with an interval of several months between or (2) three injections of plain toxoid with intervals of several weeks between the doses.

As a result of immunization, the clinical incidence of diphtheria among these nurses has been reduced from 28.6 per cent to 0.2 per cent.

In a group of 102 nurses, immunized by toxin-antitoxin and retested six to sixteen years later, more than 95 per cent were still immune.

REFERENCES

Schroeder, M. C.: Arch. Pediat. 38: 368, 1921.
Parish, H. J., and Okell, C. C.: Lancet 2: 322, 1928.
Moser, M., and Moser, G.: Presse méd. 37: 1543, 1929.
Cerruti, C. F.: Bol. soc. d. internaz. d. microbiol., sez. ital. 3: 423, 1931.
Calisti, E.: Bol. d. soc. internaz. d. microbiol., sez. ital. 5: 36, 1933.
Bosco: Quoted by Cerruti.
Ronchi: Quoted by Cerruti.

MECHANICAL LESIONS OF THE APPENDIX IN CHILDREN AS A BASIS FOR APPENDICITIS

Percival Nicholson, M.D.
Ardmore, Pa.

THIS is an investigation based on the study of 127 consecutive cases of mechanical lesions affecting the appendix in children exhibiting symptoms not generally attributed to a disturbance of this organ, but clearly distinguishable by clinical and laboratory investigation. These findings were confirmed in all cases by careful study of the gross anatomical changes at operation, as well as by microscopic examination. In these lesions was found a basis for an explanation of a large number of cases of appendicitis in both childhood and adult life generally considered as acute primary forms. A diagnosis of mechanical lesions of the appendix was possible at such an early stage that by surgical removal of the causative factor the mortality rate was kept at a minimum. In this series it was zero.

It is also proposed to show that by early surgical intervention, not only is mortality reduced, but the nutritional development of the children, by its return to the normal, produces ideal weight and development.

This work on mechanical conditions in and around the appendix was suggested by the failure of some cases of bad posture in children to improve when abdominal supports were applied, or if they did improve they failed to maintain their improvement. In a certain number there were associated mild attacks of abdominal pain; a diagnosis of chronic appendicitis was made; and appendectomy was performed. At operation distinct mechanical lesions in and around the appendix were found and removed together with the appendix. The symptomatic relief and the nutritional improvement were so marked and rapid that they led to a very careful survey of similar cases; these after appendectomy had equally good results. This work clearly demonstrates the value of accurate laboratory work, the importance of very careful and detailed histories, and a diagnosis largely by exclusion.

Mechanical conditions involving the appendix have been described by numerous authors under the headings of "chronic appendicitis," and "appendical syndrome." The subject, "chronic appendicitis," has been a controversial one in surgical circles for years. Myers[1] quotes Watkins as reviewing 662 papers up to 1932 and reviews the literature to September, 1934. In his summary he states: "The more

From the Pediatric Service of the Bryn Mawr Hospital.

recent literature, especially that of the last five years, on chronic appendicitis indicates a growing opinion that there is such a malady, that it is more prevalent, more dangerous, and more frequently overlooked than has been previously taught. Indications are that failures of the past have been largely due to a lack of diagnostic thoroughness. Certain medical centers have published statistics showing from 60 to 90 per cent of the patients who had operations for chronic appendicitis were completely relieved by appendectomy alone. Muller recently (1932) has said that a campaign of instruction of the public regarding appendicitis is more important than a campaign against cancer. It seems fair to say that such a campaign should be directed to the laity regarding acute appendicitis, but a like campaign is needed for the profession regarding chronic appendicitis."

Freed[2] states, "In the United States and Canada twenty-five thousand die yearly from acute appendicitis, that is one death every twenty-five minutes, or seventy deaths every day, Sundays and holidays included, and the mortality is on the increase." In childhood there is an average mortality of about 14.5 per cent.

Farr[3] states, "I also believe that there is such an entity as chronic appendicitis and that it applies to children fully as often as to adults." Tenny[4] is convinced of the importance of a mechanical obstructive condition in and around the appendix as a producer of appendicitis, and he emphasizes reflex constipation and pylorospasm. Wilkie,[5, 6] one of the first to describe acute obstructive appendicitis, lays emphasis on constriction of the appendical lumen, with associated fecal concretions, and describes both an acute and a chronic form.

In making a diagnosis of mechanical conditions in and around the appendix, it is first necessary to know the normal anatomy. The appendix hangs down freely from the cecum and has a uniform and patulous lumen, and a terminal and limited arterial blood supply. Any kinking, twisting or constriction of the wall of the appendix, whether produced by Lane's bands, Jackson's membrane, short mesentery, or constriction of the lumen due to contracting fibrous tissue from a previous inflammatory reaction, will cause fecal retention, and this in turn will produce chronic irritation of the appendix. Through the sympathetic and vagus nerves, there is an intercommunication with the stomach, often producing pylorospasm with nausea or vomiting, or with the colon, producing spastic constipation.

When the lumen of the appendix is constricted, fecal material may be forced in from the cecum. But since the weaker contraction of the appendical wall is not able to evacuate completely the contents, a portion remains, and its moisture is absorbed through the appendical wall and produces a beginning inspissation which may lead to concretion. If this change is not severe enough to obstruct the lumen completely, there are chronic symptoms, such as pain, spastic constipation, "bilious attacks," vomiting, etc. If the concretion completely obstructs the lumen, more severe changes may follow, often ending in gangrene. These cases produce, according to Wilkie,[5, 6] 90 per cent of the mortality of acute appendicitis. On the other hand, a constriction of the blood supply from a twist, short mesentery, membrane, or bands, causes edema of the wall and predisposes to an inflammatory process.

A typical history is that of a child who has had short attacks of recurrent abdominal pain for a considerable period, either daily or at longer intervals. The pain varies from a dull ache, a burning sensation, or sense of fullness to one of a sharp stabbing character. The attacks may be very fleeting but they have a marked tendency to recur, and at times there is associated nausea or actual vomiting. The *recurrence* of attacks, in spite of a well-regulated simple diet and good hygiene, is of great significance. Children often stop in their play, turn a little white, have a slight generalized abdominal pain, over in an instant. These cases are commonly diagnosed as indigestion. The pain is very likely to come on during or from one-half to two hours after a meal, or pains may have no relation to food intake. Pain frequently is increased by exercise, its location is umbilical or epigastrical at first, but later may become localized in the right iliac fossa. A bowel movement, passage of gas, or vomiting usually gives prompt relief. There are associated poor color, poor muscle tone, poor nutrition, and poor posture. Abdominal supports will often relieve the symptoms for a time, but there is frequently a recurrence. This failure to produce a permanent cure with abdominal supports is very suggestive. There is poor appetite, and constipation is the rule. The temperature, pulse, respiration, and blood count at this time are normal. A careful abdominal examination at the time of the attack will reveal in most cases slight deep right iliac tenderness with but little if any muscular rigidity. If a review of the family history reveals appendicitis in the near relatives, it is very suggestive, as heredity seems to play an important part; in this series the rate was 63 per cent. The physician should inquire as to any pylorospasm in infancy and any causeless attack of vomiting or cyclic vomiting, as in our 127 cases 66 per cent had vomiting and 6 per cent cyclic vomiting.

Later pain may move over to the lower right quadrant. A white blood count with careful study of the neutrophiles, including a nuclear shift, then shows slight irritative changes but not much elevation of the total count. As the case becomes more acute, there may be a slight temperature elevation during the attacks. At operation bands, adhesions, Jackson's membrane, a short mesentery, or stricture of the appendix with fecal concretions is found. The appendical lumen usually shows cystic dilatation and some atrophy of the mucous membrane with a possible old fibrosis of the walls from a previously healed acute attack. If operation is performed very early in the course of the infection, no appendical lesion may be found.

Another frequent type is that found in a child who has been in apparently good health, but usually whose nutrition is poor, as shown by a searching history. He goes to bed to awake several hours later with sharp abdominal pain which causes him to double up. The pain is soon relieved, and he sleeps again only to awaken a second time with a return of colic, and he frequently vomits. At first the pain is in the umbilical region, acute and spasmodic; later it becomes less acute but more continuous, and becomes localized in the right lower quadrant. The temperature, the pulse, and the respiration are normal, but there is always a slightly anxious expression. These attacks of appendical colic may have numerous remissions. Examination during attacks shows deep right iliac tenderness. A prompt operation is indicated; at operation the appendix presents some form of constriction and contains inspissated fecal material or a concretion and often gangrene.

There is also a type of mild acute appendicitis, probably embolic, secondary to an infection from sinusitis, tonsillitis, etc. The patient has malaise and nausea, a furred tongue, loss of appetite, and constipation with a very slight temperature. There is vague abdominal pain at the umbilicus which later becomes more or less localized in the right side. The patient may be in bed a day or two, at the end of which time the symptoms gradually clear up. Deep iliac tenderness can be obtained, and if an operation is performed, edema of the appendical wall is found. It is often these overlooked attacks which cause inflammatory reaction with subsequent fibrotic stricture of the appendix.

There are numerous other combinations of symptoms neither so definite nor so suggestive of chronic appendicitis, but equally important to the child. A child who on automobile trips has nausea or actively vomits, or who has had periodic attacks of vomiting, either repeated mild attacks often in the morning before breakfast or severe ones with associated acidosis, probably has chronic appendicitis. He may, however, never have had any abdominal pain. A white blood count with a nuclear shift may show slight irritative changes, as increase in rod nuclears, in addition to changes suggesting a more chronic inflammation, as lymphocytosis and monocytosis. An examination of the abdomen at the time of a vomiting attack frequently discovers deep iliac tenderness and less often right rectus rigidity. These patients are treated as a rule for an imbalance of the sympathetic nervous system causing reflex vomiting and spasticity of the colon, resulting in colicky pains and constipation. A roentgen ray study of the gastrointestinal tract may occasionally disclose a partially filling appendix which does not empty in the normal time (only one case in this series), but, as a rule, roentgen rays are not conclusive except as evidence of spasticity of the colon. Roentgen ray examinations were not used in this series on account of the expense and the fact that the diagnosis could be made without their aid. It was also felt that the barium and bismuth retained would complicate convalescence following operation. It is necessary to proceed with extreme

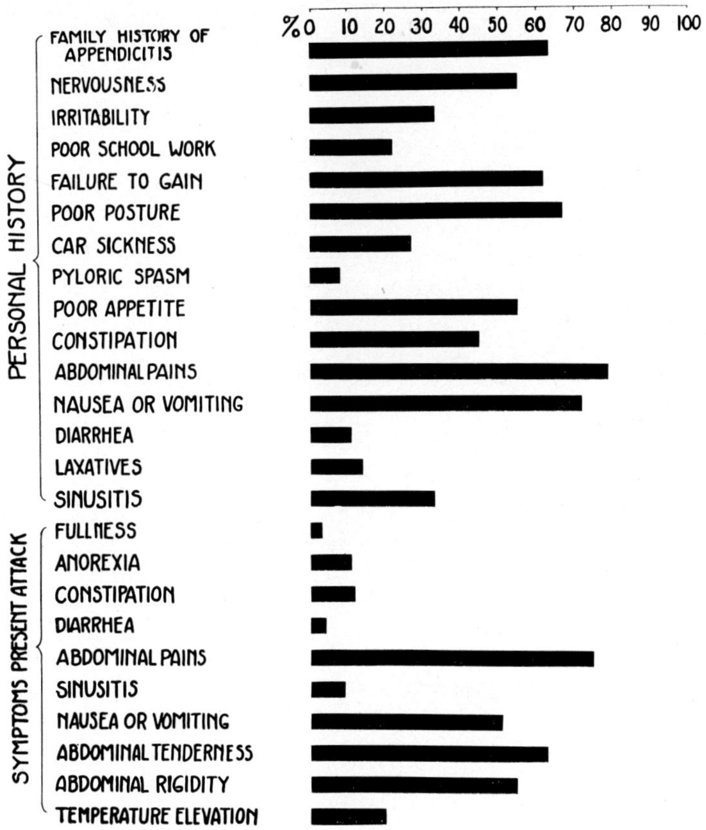

Chart 1.—Symptomatology.

caution and observe these patients for some time and to rule out any involvement of the genitourinary tract, by urinalysis and roentgenograms if necessary, but when by a process of elimination focal infections are excluded, one is justified in making a diagnosis of mechanical lesions in or around the appendix. Diagnoses are largely based on a history of long-continued symptoms and by elimination rather than by physical findings.

There is another group of children with definite symptoms of chronic appendicitis; in these the blood count usually shows an eosinophilia, with an average of 4 per cent. Most of these patients in our series had seatworms in the appendix and were completely relieved by appendectomy. This condition was first recognized in 1899 by Still[7] and has been lately reviewed by Margaret Warwick.[8]

Once a diagnosis is established, an immediate appendectomy is undoubtedly the only treatment. In cases in which a diagnosis of chronic or mild acute appendicitis is associated with a sinusitis or other upper respiratory infection, one should operate at once. It used

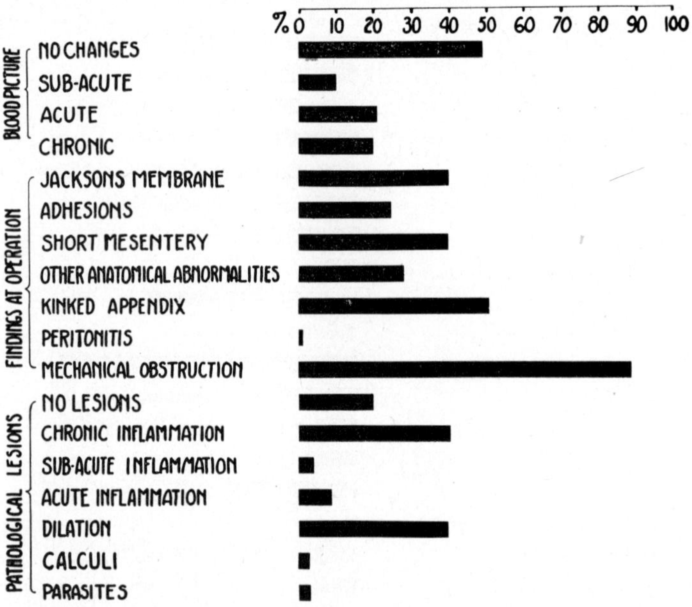

APPENDIX:		NO LESIONS	CHRONIC	SUB-ACUTE	ACUTE	DILATION
BLOOD PICTURE	NO CHANGE	70	52			53
	CHRONIC	13	20	34		27
	SUB-ACUTE		14	33	11	13
	ACUTE	17	14	33	89	7

Chart 2.—Blood picture and pathologic findings.

to be our custom to delay operation until the infection cleared up, but we found that severity of the appendical condition is greatly increased, and there is grave danger of a gangrenous appendix and peritonitis if operation is delayed. By use of tribrom-ethanol (avertin) and the postoperative use of 10 per cent carbon dioxide and 90 per cent oxygen we have had uniformly good results.

In only one of our series of 127 cases was it necessary to use drainage. That patient was first seen two days after the onset of acute symptoms. Recovery was complete in thirty-nine days.

The most constant symptoms in our cases were attacks of abdominal pain, generalized at first, later sometimes localized with associated nausea or vomiting. The most common physical finding was deep tenderness in the right iliac fossa.

Charts 1, 2, and 3 give the frequency of occurrence of the various symptoms, findings at operation, pathologic conditions, and the results.

The pathologist in cases of chronic appendicitis must examine the appendix not only for signs of chronic fibrosis and acute inflammatory changes but also for evidence of cystic dilatation as is shown in microscopic section by flattening out of the rugae and also by atrophic changes in the mucosa.

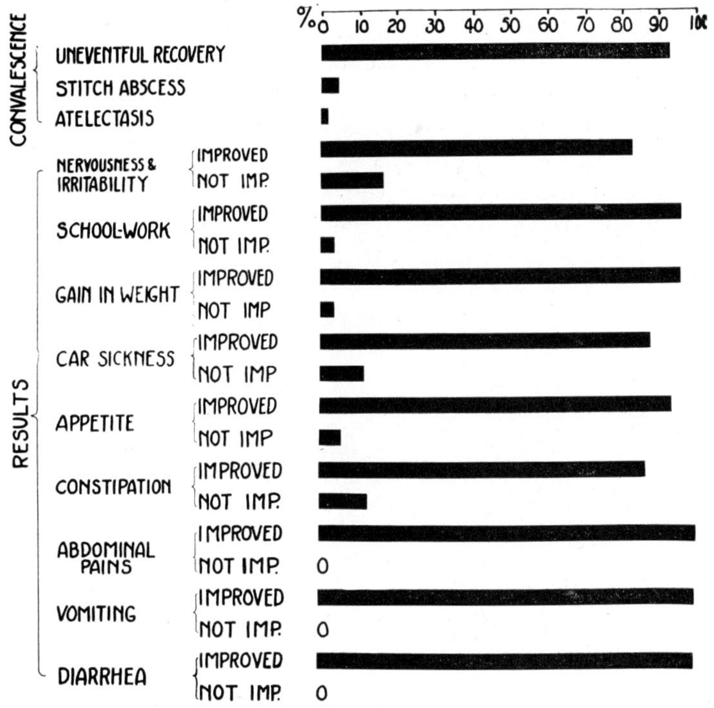

Chart 3.—Postoperative course and results.

In an analysis of the Bryn Mawr Hospital pathologic records of acute appendicitis in adults, approximately 95 per cent showed evidences of preceding fecal retention and cystic dilatation.

CONCLUSIONS

1. In 127 consecutive cases of mechanical lesions affecting the appendix in childhood, the symptoms usually began at an early age in mild form and recurred over a long period, the most constant being recurring abdominal pain, frequently associated with vomiting and deep right iliac tenderness.

2. In addition to complete recovery and relief from symptoms in all cases following appendectomy, the children showed a very notable increase in weight.

3. The extrinsic causes of obstruction of the appendix predominated, often leading to obliteration of the lumen and retention of fecal material.

4. Approximately 95 per cent of adult appendices removed at the Bryn Mawr Hospital showed evidence of obliteration of the lumen with fecal retention preceding the terminal inflammatory attack.

5. By a careful diagnosis in childhood and early operation, nutrition and development could be made normal at this age period, and mortality could be minimized at all ages.

REFERENCES

1. Myers, B. L.: J. Missouri M. A. 31: 363, 1934.
2. Freed, C. E.: Pennsylvania M. J. 39: 5, 1935.
3. Farr, C. E.: Surg. Clin. North America (April), 1935.
4. Tenny, Charles F.: New York State J. Med. 35: 977, 1935.
5. Wilkie, D. P. D.: Brit. M. J. 1: 253, 1931.
6. Wilkie, D. P. D.: Canad. M. A. J. 22: 314, 1930.
7. Still, George F.: Common Disorders and Diseases of Childhood, ed. 4, Oxford University Press, page 322.
8. Warwick, Margaret: Am. J. Clin. Path. 5: 238, 1935.

A STUDY OF THE BIRCH-HIRSCHFELD PHOTOMETRIC TEST FOR VITAMIN A DEFICIENCY

CHARLES E. SNELLING, M.B.
TORONTO, ONTARIO

VITAMIN A is one of the thirty-seven food substances essential for normal nutrition. A lack of this vitamin results in pathologic changes in many parts of the body. The most obvious changes are in the epithelial cells which tend to lose their columnar shape and become stratified. The occurrence of these changes in the conjunctiva and lacrymal glands results in the development of the eye condition known as xerophthalmia. This condition, however, develops only after an almost complete deprivation of vitamin A for many months.

Xerophthalmia is rarely encountered in the United States and Canada. During the past ten years at the Hospital for Sick Children in Toronto, we have seen only one case of xerophthalmia out of 802,000 attendances at the hospital. Similar figures indicating the rarity of this condition have been obtained from Harriet Lane Home, Johns Hopkins Hospital, Baltimore; the Children's Hospital, St. Louis; Minnesota General Hospital, Minneapolis; the Children's Memorial Hospital, Chicago; the Massachusetts General Hospital, Massachusetts Eye and Ear Infirmary, and the Children's Hospital, Boston; and the Montreal General Hospital, Montreal.[1] These findings are what one would expect when one considers the distribution of vitamin A in the foods ordinarily consumed. It is found in large amounts in the fats of dairy products, animal fats, liver, and egg yolk. Carotene, the precursor of vitamin A, is found in large amounts in spinach, chard, carrots, and many other vegetables and fruits. Vitamin A is probably the most widely and abundantly distributed of all the vitamins.

In harmony with this widespread and abundant distribution of vitamin A in foods is the absence of evidence of vitamin A deficiency at postmortem examination. At Boston, in the Children's Hospital, in 1,756 autopsies, keratinizing epithelial cells were demonstrated in only 15 patients.[2]

It is well recognized that night blindness may be caused by a lack of vitamin A. When this condition is present, the individual is unable to adjust his vision to decreasing amounts of light. The defect may be produced by a lesser deficiency of vitamin A than that necessary to cause

From the wards and laboratories of the Hospital for Sick Children and the Department of Paediatrics, University of Toronto, under the direction of Alan Brown, M.D., F.R.C.P.(C).

xerophthalmia. Demonstration of this defect, which can be present without any other obvious changes, might therefore indicate that the individual was suffering from a lack of vitamin A.

Reports have recently appeared in some European countries on the prevalence of night blindness.[3] Of much more interest and importance to us, however, are the reports of Jeans and Zentmire of Iowa City. These investigators found defective dark adaptation in 21 per cent of a group of children just admitted to the hospital.[4] In their more recent report of a survey of Iowa school children,[5] they found definitely subnormal dark adaptation in 26 per cent of the children from the rural districts, 53 per cent of the children from the villages, and no less than 56 to 79 per cent of the urban children, depending on their economic level. Furthermore, on the administration of vitamin A to 87 of these children with subnormal dark adaptation, they found either improvement or a return to the normal level in 84, or over 95 per cent.

These are most unexpected results. Although no details of the diets are given, it can be assumed that the diets are of the same standards as those used throughout most of the United States and Canada. Thus the work of Jeans and Zentmire would indicate that the average diet today does not contain an adequate amount of vitamin A.

The question of the adequacy of the supply of vitamin A is of such importance that we undertook an investigation using the instrument and technic as described by Jeans and Zentmire.[4]

The instrument used in making the test was a Birch-Hirschfeld No. 329 photometer obtained from Carl Zeiss, Inc. The photometer consisted of a metal tube 18 mm. in diameter with an electric light bulb in the end. At the other end of the cylinder there were in respective order, an opal glass, an iris diaphragm, and a second opal glass 40 mm. in diameter. The diaphragm was opened and closed by a lever with a scale marked with the diameter of the opening in millimeters. A metal disk, with five circles punched out, slid in a groove distal to the second opal glass. The holes were circular, 4 mm. in diameter. Four of the holes were situated in the form of a 2 cm. square. The fifth hole was in the center equidistant from all the others. In front of this was a Goldberg wedge, which is a glass slide with a uniformly increasing depth of opacity from one end to the other and marked off with a scale from 1 to 13, the numbers varying directly with the opaqueness.

The bulb in the metal cylinder was illuminated by a transformer connected to 110 volt circuit. The transformer stepped the voltage down to 3.5 in the light circuit. The source of light thus did not vary. The subject was placed in front of the photometer and observed the light from the bulb coming in the following order through opal glass, the iris diaphragm, opal glass, the fivepoint disk and the Goldberg wedge. The amount of light coming through varied directly with the size of the opening or scale reading of the diaphragm and inversely with the reading of the Goldberg wedge. Also because the wedge is graded from clearness to near opacity, the five points were not all equally visible. The end-point of the test was taken when the subject could definitely distinguish only three of the five points.

The examinations were carried out in a completely darkened room. The subject was placed with the head on a chin rest 24 inches from the photometer. The subject faced a six-foot square-white screen placed at a distance of 40 inches from his eyes. Immediately behind the subject was a 150 watt electric light with a metal reflector which illuminated the white screen.

The subject, seated in the position described above, was directed to observe the middle of the screen for five minutes, estimated by the use of an interval timer. At the expiration of the time, the timer was again set for ten minutes. The lights were put out and the subject was directed to look at the photometer. He was asked to tell the number of points of light he could see. The Goldberg wedge was adjusted and the diaphragm opened or closed until the minimum amount of light was found at which the subject perceived constantly three of the five points of light. The instrument was covered for a few seconds with the hand to make sure that the subject was answering correctly. This is in accord with the technic described by Jeans and Zentmire.[4] They state, "The operator always confirmed the accuracy of an end-point by covering the wedge with the palm of the hand for a few seconds in order to rest the patient's eyes and then by having the subject again report on the number of points of light constantly visible."

Jeans and Zentmire[4] found that normal persons gave readings with the wedge set at 7 and the diaphragm at 14 to 20 at the first test, i.e., immediately after the eyes have been exposed to the bright light. It would appear that our light source before being reduced by a wedge and the diaphragm was of lesser intensity than that used by Jeans and Zentmire, as very few of the individuals we tested gave an initial reading with the wedge set higher than 5 and the diaphragm at 14 to 20 mm.

The subject will require more light for the first reading if it is taken immediately rather than a moment or two later. Thus it is impossible to make duplicate determinations of the end-point of the first reading because during the first few seconds after the room is made dark the recovery or adaptation is extremely rapid to a certain point and then slowly approaches the level that it reaches at the end of the ten-minute period in the dark. The latter level is the one which Jeans and Zentmire used to determine whether the adaptation was normal or not. They state that with their instrument the normal eye recovers to readings with the wedge set at 7 and the diaphragm at 3 to 6 mm., inclusive. In individual tests we confirmed that the second reading was constant by using different combinations of wedge and diaphragm settings which gave the same light values. At the end of the ten-minute interval the subject's ability to perceive does not vary as it does at the first test. Thus in considering the readings the one taken at the end of the ten-minute period is the important one. The smallest amount of light required by the subject after the period in the dark gives the greatest adaptation.

In the winter and spring of 1935, 163 subjects were tested for dark adaptation as outlined above. Eighteen of these were adults (laboratory staff and nurses), and 145 were ambulatory patients in hospital or attending the out-patient clinic. At this time we were interpreting our results in terms of the position of the Goldberg wedge and the size of the diaphragm opening. Because, as mentioned above, the instrumental readings obtained by us were in a different range from those of Jeans and Zentmire, we had to set our own normal level. We took the readings of 15 of the normal adults (laboratory workers and nurses) who were on a good dietary regime and used them as a standard. We decided that any reading with the wedge set at 7 or higher was normal. Using this standard, 53 of the subjects tested, or 32 per cent, showed poor dark adaptation. Twenty-eight of the group with poor adaptation to the dark were given 2 teaspoonfuls of cod liver oil daily, and 18 of these, or 64 per cent, showed what we considered was improvement after a period of from two to six weeks' therapy. We believed that the above group were suffering from vitamin A deficiency and that we had confirmed the findings of Jeans and Zentmire.[4]

Later while carrying out further tests it seemed to us that there was an overlapping of the light values with different wedge settings and size of opening of the diaphragm. The physics department of the University of Toronto very kindly measured with a photoelectric cell the amount of light that was being transmitted to the subject at all the positions of the wedge and diaphragm. The measurements were made using the center light spot. The calibrations are given arbitrarily, allowing 1,000 for the wedge setting of 1 and the diaphragm wide open. Thus in terms of this apparatus, with a wedge setting of 1, diaphragm 20 mm. (wide open) the light value was 1,000 and with a wedge setting of 13 and the diaphragm of 2 mm. the value was 0.9. (Table I.) Any amount of light between can be obtained by suitable settings of the wedge and the diaphragm. The constancy of the light source was further checked by testing the transformer circuit with a sensitive voltmeter. The fact that the variations in potential were negligible indicated that the amount of light emitted by the lamp in the photometer did not vary.

We applied this table to the findings made in the winter and spring of 1935. It was observed that our arbitrary normal range obtained from the fifteen adults varied from 37 to 136. These adults were all taking what had been considered to be adequate diets, and, if we use this spread of readings for normality, then very few of our original group had poor adaptation.

In order to determine the optimum light adaptation we decided to test a group of children who were receiving more than adequate amounts

TABLE I

Light values for the photometer with the various positions of the wedge and diaphragm. This table was estimated for us by the Department of Physics of the University of Toronto. They measured with a photoelectric cell the amount of light transmitted to the subject through the center hole of the 5 points of light.

W† / D*	1	2	3	4	5	6	7	8	9	10	11	12	13
20	1000.0	722.0	513.0	364.0	258.0	187.0	136.0	100.0	77.0	57.0	45.0	33.0	24.0
18	994.0	717.0	510.0	362.0	256.0	186.0	135.0	99.4	76.5	56.6	44.7	32.8	23.9
16	986.0	712.0	506.0	359.0	254.0	184.0	134.0	98.6	75.9	56.2	44.4	32.5	23.6
14	956.0	690.0	490.0	348.0	247.0	179.0	130.0	95.6	73.6	54.5	43.0	31.6	23.0
12	807.0	583.0	414.0	294.0	208.0	151.0	110.0	80.7	62.2	46.0	36.3	26.6	19.4
10	628.0	453.0	322.0	228.0	163.0	117.0	85.4	62.8	48.3	35.8	28.2	20.7	15.1
8	450.0	325.0	231.0	164.0	116.0	84.1	61.2	45.0	34.6	25.6	20.3	14.8	10.8
6	272.0	196.0	139.0	99.0	70.2	50.8	37.0	27.2	20.9	15.5	12.2	9.0	6.5
4	141.0	102.0	72.2	51.4	36.4	26.4	19.2	14.1	10.0	8.0	6.3	4.7	3.4
2	38.5	27.8	19.7	14.0	9.9	7.2	5.2	3.8	3.0	2.2	1.7	1.3	0.9

*D refers to setting of diaphragm.
†W refers to setting of wedge.

of vitamin A. To do this we tested 64 normal children from six to sixteen years of age, receiving in their daily diet 30 to 35 ounces of milk, butter, meat, fruit, two vegetables other than potato, cereal and bread. This diet supplies large amounts of vitamin A. In addition, they were given daily, 21,000 units of vitamin A* for a period of six weeks. It was found that this group required light values ranging from 19 to 258 for the test. The same children had been tested prior to the administration of the additional vitamin A and the spread of readings likewise was from 19 to 258. No difference was observed in the range of readings before or after the administration of the additional vitamin A. This is shown in Chart 1.

During the six-week period in which the additional vitamin A was being administered, the children were tested at biweekly intervals. In

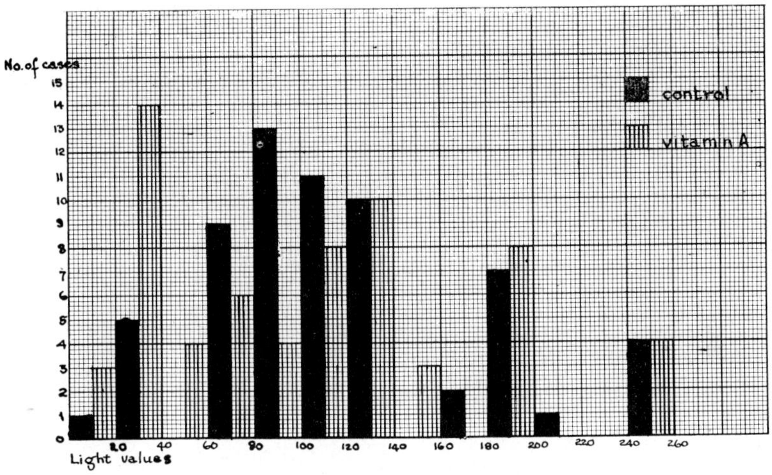

Chart 1.—Number of cases for the various readings for the test, before and after the administration of additional vitamin A.

Light value means the least amount of light necessary for the constant perception of the 3 points at the end of the ten-minute period in the dark. The cases are grouped with light values ranging from 0 to 20, 20 to 40, etc.

most cases the results obtained showed marked variations in the four tests on the same individual. A group of these selected at random are shown in Table II.

Because of the variability of the results we became concerned about the accuracy of the test. Dr. Walter W. Wright, chief of the ophthalmologic service of the Hospital for Sick Children, after examining the instrument and observing the technic of the test, stated that from his experience with other subjective eye tests with children he questioned the probability of obtaining reliable results.

In carrying out the test, the operator is entirely dependent on the veracity and personal reaction of the subject. If the subject reports

*Ten drops of viosterol in halibut liver oil. Kindly supplied by Mead Johnson and Company.

seeing three points of light, unless the light is turned out or covered so as to be hidden, the operator must accept that as what the subject sees. We found it absolutely impossible to test children under six years of age because of this, as their imaginations took them into realms away above the number of points of light on the instrument.

In order to rule out as far as possible factors which are difficult to control in children, such as imagination and personal reaction of the subject, twelve adults, physicians and technicians, working in the labora-

TABLE II

READINGS OBTAINED DURING THE ADMINISTRATION OF ADDITIONAL VITAMIN A*

SUBJECT	PERIOD OF ADDITIONAL VITAMIN A			
	0	2 WEEKS	4 WEEKS	6 WEEKS
I	19	85	45	37
II	134	85	130	45
III	208	117	45	130
IV	85	134	84	258
V	61	179	130	110
VI	37	37	130	110
VII	130	85	85	130
VIII	110	135	85	37
IX	247	151	110	184
X	85	136	179	26

*The lower the reading, the better the dark adaptation.

TABLE III

RECORDS OBTAINED FROM TESTS OF LABORATORY WORKERS AT APPROXIMATELY DAILY INTERVALS*

SUBJECT	TEST 1	2	3	4	5	6	7	8	9	10	11	12	13	14
A	116	163	116	208	116	179	163	179	50	85	84	85	84	50
B	70	70	116	36	186	151	84	151	179	179	179	151		
C	116	50	36	151	50	84	26	50	50	26	50			
D	26	84	37	85	26	50	50	26	37	50	26			
E	84	163	184	70	116	187	117	208	50					
F	37	50	26	50	26	50	26							
G	254	208	228	208	116	179	151							
H	208	208	163	116	163									
I	84	247	50	50	247									
J	184	70	184	84	117									
K	186	151	117	151										
L	116	151												

*The lower the reading, the better the dark adaptation.

tory were tested daily for varying periods. There was no change made in the routine of these individuals. The record of the tests from these subjects is given in Table III. Two consistently required a small amount of light to perceive the points; 3 consistently required a large quantity; 4 varied from day to day; 2 improved and 1 became less adapted to the dark as time went on. Also the subjects would observe when the light was near the limit of perception, that they saw 3, 2, 0, 5, etc., points when the source was not varied in any respect. The statement was also made that the lights were being moved. Our tests with adults showed wide variation for individual subjects, similar to the results obtained with the children.

It was pointed out to us that adaptation to the dark may be somewhat a matter of experience. Persons living in rural districts have little difficulty going about in the dark because they have good adaptation. However, the same individuals residing in urban centers for a period lose that ability and then will regain it when on a vacation in the country after a week or so.

CONCLUSIONS

In our hands the Birch-Hirschfeld photometer has been unsatisfactory for the estimation of small variations in dark adaptation, such as might be produced by vitamin A deficiency.

REFERENCES

1. Personal communications received by Dr. F. F. Tisdall, Hospital for Sick Children.
2. Personal communication received from Professor K. D. Blackfan, Harvard Medical School, Children's Hospital, Boston, Mass.
3. Frandsen, Helga: Hemeralopia as an Early Criterion of A-avitaminosis, Copenhagen, 1935, Nyt Nordisk Forlag: Arnold Brusck.
4. Jeans, P. C., and Zentmire, Zelma: J. A. M. A. **102**: 892, 1933.
5. Jeans, P. C., and Zentmire, Zelma: J. A. M. A. **106**: 996, 1936.

CARBON TETRACHLORIDE POISONING

Henry L. Heyl, M.D.
Boston, Mass.

INSTANCES of carbon tetrachloride poisoning have been frequently described.[1-4] Without attempting a comprehensive review, we are reporting an additional case, partly because the drug was contained in a common household material, but principally because clinical discussions of the treatment of this intoxication have been rare.

USES FOR CARBON TETRACHLORIDE

Most instances of poisoning from this drug occur because of its use in certain fire extinguishers, in various cleansing solutions, and in the treatment of hookworm disease. The fact that its vapor is heavier than air makes it valuable to the fire fighter, but dangerous to the recipient of a "dry" shampoo who breathes the intoxicating fumes that settle around her face,[5] or to one using the chemical as a grease remover inside a closed automobile. Poisoning due to absorption through the gastrointestinal tract has occurred chiefly in the treatment of hookworm disease.

PROPHYLAXIS

The Egyptian Board of Health in its wholesale treatment of villages for hookworm disease has found carbon tetrachloride intoxication occurring often enough with the therapeutic dose of 4 c.c. to warrant a routine set of precautions enforced within the temporary compounds where all treatments are given. The routine may be briefly outlined as follows: All persons who have recently taken alcohol are refused treatment. Ascaris infection also is considered a contraindication to the use of carbon tetrachloride because of the possibility of obstruction to its rapid excretion. All persons to be treated are placed on a high carbohydrate, low fat diet by advance agents. Immediately before the therapeutic dose of carbon tetrachloride, sugar in the form of molasses is given each patient. Following the administration of the carbon tetrachloride, each patient receives a saline cathartic. Patients may not leave the compound until the purge has proved effective. Those showing toxic symptoms are treated immediately with calcium and glucose.

From the Department of Pediatrics, Harvard Medical School, and the Infants' and Children's Hospitals.

PHARMACOLOGY

The drug is absorbed through the gastrointestinal tract, the lungs, or injured skin.[7] Overdosage may cause hemorrhages in the gastrointestinal mucosa, albuminous infiltration of the glomeruli of the kidneys, and central necrosis with cirrhosis or terminal acute yellow atrophy of the liver.[8, 4] Lipemia has been a frequent finding.[3, 4] Toxic symptoms progress through vomiting, stupor, temporary recovery, jaundice, fever, amblyopia, edema, anuria, hematuria, albuminuria, convulsions and coma, to death. Alcohol, fat, or protein in the diet increases the drug's toxicity.[7, 9] High carbohydrate and calcium intake reduces intoxication and frequently is associated with recovery.[7, 10]

Minot and Cutler[11] have pointed out a guanidinemia in carbon tetrachloride poisoning which they believe is responsible for interruption of carbohydrate metabolism. They believe that glucose is not resynthesized from lactic acid and that this results in both a hypoglycemia and an accumulation of lactic acid in the blood and its excretion in the urine. Finding that guanidine and calcium are antagonistic[11] and believing that calcium is necessary for activating the adrenal mechanism that normally compensates for a low blood sugar,[10, 12] Minot and Cutler feel that intravenous glucose becomes permanently effective in compensating for the hypoglycemia only when given with calcium.

CASE REPORT

The two-year-old boy (weight 25 pounds) who stimulated our interest in this type of poisoning was brought in on April 9, 1935, two hours after swallowing 1 to 25 c.c. of the noninflammable cleaning fluid Energine (90 per cent carbon tetrachloride, 10 per cent hydrocarbon with petroleum base).[13]* He had vomited immediately and become drowsy. Physical examination on admission showed no abnormalities except stupor and the odor of carbon tetrachloride about his mouth. The essential feature of his treatment, which started immediately, was the intensive administration of glucose and calcium with a minimal fat and protein intake. Milk and fruit juices were the only foods allowed. Parenteral fluids were given on each of the first six days of the intoxication. The details of treatment are given in Table I.

Within twelve hours he was up playing around the crib, seemingly normal. The second day he refused to eat, had a temperature of 104° F., and a urine containing a trace of albumin, 2 red blood cells, 2 white blood cells, and occasional granular casts in each high dry field of an uncentrifuged, voided specimen. The blood at this time contained 80 per cent hemoglobin (Tallqvist), with 4,500,000 normal red cells and 25,000 white cells per cubic millimeter; 95 per cent of the latter were polymorphonuclear. On each of the first three days he vomited twice and had 5 stools which, though watery yellow, contained no blood, and grew no typhoid or dysentery organisms when cultured.

On the third day he refused to eat and was irritable. The temperature rose again to 103° F. (pulse 160), and at 6:00 P.M., following a few generalized twitchings, he

*This particular product carried no announcement on the label to indicate either its chemical or toxic nature.

TABLE I

CHEMISTRY OF THE BLOOD							CLINICAL STATE	THERAPY (IN C.C.)										
								INTRAVENOUS					S.C.	INTRAMUSC.		ORAL		
DAY OF DISEASE	CO_2 VOL. %	N.P.N. MG. %	SERUM PROT. GM. %	CALCIUM MG. %	CHLORIDE M. EQ./L.	ICTERIC INDEX		10% GLUCOSE	20% GLUCOSE	50% GLUCOSE	10% Ca GLUC.	PLASMA	NORMAL SALINE	10% Ca GLUC.	LIVER EXTRACT	SKIM MILK	FRUIT JUICE	CALCIUM LACTATE
1	57	27	6.8	10.2			Stupor in A.M. Lively in P.M.	200 200			15 10					800	800	
2							Anorexia	200			10		300				1,100	5 gr. 5 gr. 5 gr.
3				7.0			Listless in A.M. Convulsions and unconscious in P.M.	200	120	25	10 20		300				500	5 gr. 5 gr.
4	30	45	3.5	10.0	90		Semicomatose Liver 1.5 cm. Slight jaundice		130 130 130		10 10 10	140	350				250	
5	38	60	4.5		90	15	Semicomatose Liver 3 cm. Slight edema		100 100		10 10			10 10	5	1,200 gav.		
6		64	4.5	11.0	90	15	Interested in surroundings Edema, ascites, anuria		200	25	10			10		700 gav.		
7	50	68	4.5		90	15	Brighter Anuria, edema								5	780	600	15 gr.
8							Playing; voiding Liver at umbilicus									780	600	15 gr.
9	50	88	4.5			10	Playing Edema and ascites less Liver 3 cm.								5	Soft solid diet with whole milk from this point on.		15 gr.
10							Sitting up											15 gr.
11																		15 gr.
12		80	5.8				Liver 2 cm.											15 gr.
13																		15 gr.
14		40		11.8			Liver 1.5 cm.											15 gr.

suddenly became rigid, cyanotic, pulseless, and unconscious, breathing irregularly. Intravenous sodium luminal (1 gr.) was ineffective. Ether relaxed the rigidity and clonic twitchings slightly; after receiving 25 c.c. of 50 per cent glucose intravenously at 7:30 P.M., the extreme rigidity of his early attack relaxed; moderate opisthotonus and mild twitchings still remained at 11:30, when he received 120 c.c. of 20 per cent glucose with 20 c.c. of 10 per cent calcium gluconate intravenously. At this time the blood pressure was 100/78; there was no papilledema. Spinal fluid collected at this time was normal. After midnight he was completely relaxed.

During the fourth and fifth days he was semicomatose and was fed chiefly by gavage. The liver for the first time became palpable, increasing in size so rapidly that by the seventh day it was at the level of the umbilicus. There was never real jaundice. Peripheral edema, ascites, and anuria were the prominent clinical findings from the fifth to the eighth day. The urine continued to show cells, casts, and appreciable albumin until the ninth day; it was normal thereafter. By the end of the second week edema and ascites were gone; the boy was sitting up playing in bed and eating a soft solid diet enthusiastically. The liver receded slowly and at the time of discharge, three weeks after admission, was still 1 cm. below the costal margin.

Three months after discharge he was reexamined. His appetite was poor. He had not gained weight. The liver edge was not palpable. When given 25 gm. of galactose by mouth, he showed no reducing substance in the urine collected for the next six hours. Phthalein excretion was within normal limits and the nonprotein nitrogen at this time was 23 mg. per cent.

COMMENT

It would be presumptuous to attach much significance to the limited data represented by this case. Yet certain points are of interest.

In the presence of the low chlorides, a constant hematocrit (4,500,000 red cells per cubic millimeter on the fourth day), and a rising nonprotein nitrogen level, it could be assumed, according to the theories of Minot and Cutler, that the low CO_2 was related to the accumulation of lactic acid in the blood. Whether the severe convulsive episode on the third day was due to hypoglycemia must remain uncertain, inasmuch as studies of the blood sugar were not made during the acute phase; the blood calcium just an hour before the attack was low enough to make it conceivable that tetany may have played a part. We could not help but be impressed by the possible significance of calcium and glucose in the treatment of this intoxication. In the presence of adequate hydration we felt that the urinary findings, anuria, and the nonprotein nitrogen represented definite renal injury. We wondered whether the abrupt fall in serum protein was due to liver damage or to starvation. Liver extract was given because of certain evidence that it has a substitution value in instances of acute hepatic damage.[14] Plasma was used in transfusion because of the low serum protein and adequate hematocrit.

Because there have been so few clinical reports of recovery from a severe poisoning by this drug and because the therapy or theories involved are not well known, we are including in our report the following outline for the study and treatment of similar cases:

a. Emergency gastric lavage; catharsis.

b. Low fat, low protein, high carbohydrate diet.

c. Calcium intake maintained at 0.5 gram intravenously, or 2.0 grams by mouth, daily.*

d. If vomiting is predominant, continuous intravenous drip (calcium gluconate, 5 per cent glucose, normal saline).

e. Parenteral fluids and transfusion as indicated.

f. Studies of blood sugar, CO_2, nonprotein nitrogen, calcium, serum protein, fat, guanidine, and lactic acid.

SUMMARY

We have reported an instance of severe poisoning from carbon tetrachloride contained in a common household cleaning fluid and have emphasized certain forms of available therapy, notably the intensive use of calcium and glucose.

REFERENCES

1. Davis, P. A.: J. A. M. A. **103**: 962, 1934.
2. McGuire, L. W.: J. A. M. A. **99**: 988, 1932.
3. McMahon, H., and Weis, S.: Am. J. Path. **5**: 623, 1929.
4. Butsch, W. L.: J. A. M. A. **99**: 728, 1932.
5. Moller, K. O.: J. Indust. Hyg. **15**: 418, 1933.
6. Tomb, J. W.: J. Trop. Med. **36**: 265, 334.
7. Lamson, P. D.: J. Pharmacol. & Exper. Therap. **22**: 215, 1923.
8. Gardner, G. H., et al.: Bull. Johns Hopkins Hosp. **36**: 107, 1925.
9. Cutler, J.: J. Pharmacol. & Exper. Therap. **45**: 209, 1932.
10. Minot, A. S.: J. Pharmacol. & Exper. Therap. **43**: 295, 1931.
11. Minot, A. S., and Cutler, J.: J. Clin. Investigation **6**: 369, 1928.
12. Underhill, F. P.: J. Biol. Chem. **25**: 447, 1916.
13. Cummer Products Co., Bedford, Ohio: Personal communication.
14. Castle, W. B., Boston, Massachusetts: Personal communication.

*One gram of calcium is contained in 1,000 c.c. milk, 10 gm. of calcium gluconate, 4 gm. of calcium lactate, or 3 gm. of calcium chloride.

Correspondence

The Relation of Tuberculosis to Generalized Atypical ''Tuberculosis'' Adenitis—A Manifestation of Lymphogranulomatosis Benigna (Schaumann)

Dr. Torben K. With, Copenhagen, Denmark

In a recent number of THE JOURNAL OF PEDIATRICS, A. Wilmot Jacobsen in a paper, ''Generalized Tuberculosis of the Lymph Nodes and Multiple Cystic Tuberculosis of the Bones,'' has reported what he claims to be a case of proved tuberculous disease in a child in good general condition, who failed repeatedly to react to large doses of tuberculin.

To his statement, ''With the Mantoux test, except the false negative reactions during the acute stage of some of the febrile diseases and in moribund patients, and those with overwhelming infections . . ., we have never seen another case of proved tuberculosis in a child who persistently gave a negative tuberculin test,'' can be added that the same rule holds true for the adult as shown by Hart[1] and Lichtenstein.[2] This rule is founded on a vast material of clinical and pathologic studies and is of the greatest value to the clinician and to the pediatrist. As Jacobsen claims to have described a case which is an exception to this rule, his statement is of the greatest interest from the standpoint of the biology of tuberculosis. If his case is studied in the light of recent investigations, however, doubt arises that his case is a proved exception to the above mentioned rule. The reasons for this are the following. The type of lymph gland enlargement in his two cases, as he states, are of the same characteristic type, both clinically and histologically, as seen in Boeck's sarcoid. The disease of skin and mucous membranes ''sarcoid Boeck-Besnier,'' the osseous condition of ''osteitis multiplex cystoides'' of Jungling, the lymph gland swelling of the type mentioned above, together with certain forms of pulmonary disease and splenomegaly have been grouped together by Schaumann[3] under the term ''lymphogranulomatosis benigna'' as manifestations of a general systemic disease with many points in common with Hodgkin's disease. The recent communications of Mylius and Schürmann,[4] Pautrier,[5] Salvesen,[6] Kissmeyer,[7] Chevallier and Führer,[13] and Nielsen[14] may be referred to for the details of interpreting these conditions as manifestations of the same systemic disease. The etiology and pathogenesis of benign lymphogranulomatosis, as well as of Hodgkin's disease, are obscure. Some hold that it is a disease *sui generis* with its own etiology—an unknown infectious agent (Kissmeyer[7]); others hold that it is merely a syndrome—a mode of reaction to different agents as tuberculosis, leprosy, or lues (Darier[8]); while a large group of clinicians hold that the disease is a special form of tuberculosis with a very low allergic reaction (''positive anergie,'' Martenstein and Noll,[9] of the Breslau Dermatological School).

Whatever may be the etiology, it is far from being proved as tuberculous in nature. Jacobsen states (p. 305), ''It is reported that the tuberculin test may be negative in lupus pernio, Boeck's sarcoid, and osteitis multiplex cystoides, as for example in Jüngling's Cases 2, 3, 7 and 9. These, however, and most of the other similar cases in the literature, were tested by the relatively insensitive Pirquet method, and it is by no means assured that the intradermal tests with the stronger dilutions would likewise have failed to produce positive tests in these individuals.''

The following data show that a complete lack of reaction is seen in about one-third of the cases. Martenstein and Noll[9] found 5 of 16 cases of lupus pernio and Boeck sarcoid negative to 0.1 mg. of tuberculin intracutaneously. Danbolt[10] found 7 of 11 cases of Boeck's sarcoid negative with 5 to 50 mg. Bonnevie and With[11] found 7 of 23 cases negative to 1 mg., and of these 4 also were negative when tested with 10 mg. In light of the extensive work of Hart[1] this should be considered as a strong argument against the tuberculous nature of the disease.

If the cases of Jacobsen are reviewed in light of their findings, the following points may be considered.

1. The two children suffer from a typical benign lymphogranulomatosis. Case 1 of the glands, bones and lungs, Case 2 of the glands and lungs only.

2. Both children have been exposed to infection with the tubercle bacillus by the father who was at home with open pulmonary tuberculosis from July, 1930, to January, 1934.

3. With these facts in view, the following explanation is at hand:

The first child with the strongly positive tuberculin reaction has besides her benign lymphogranulomatosis a tuberculosis which has nothing to do with her primary disease. The fact that she died after a couple of years from generalized tuberculosis has no influence on this statement. Tuberculosis has been reported several times as a complication which has been the cause of death in both benign and malignant lymphogranulomatosis.

It is to be noted in Case 2, with the negative tuberculin reaction, that the reactions were not performed after January, 1933, and the child did not die until May 31, 1934. In the interval, January, 1933, to May, 1934, she was at home at the same time as the father and had opportunity to be infected with tuberculosis. Moreover, the fact that she was infected with tuberculosis and died from tuberculous meningitis within this interval is in agreement with the findings of Wallgren and Nilson[12] that meningitis follows as a rule a few months after primary infection. The question remains as to why she was infected so late, as she had been living with, and exposed to, the father previously. It may be answered that in an exposed family some children are infected early while others avoid infection for a long time (Hart[1]).

4. As this child, provided that the interpretation is correct, was not infected with tuberculosis at the time of the negative tuberculin reaction, the case is not contradictory to the doctrine of the absolute value of the negative tuberculin reaction.

REFERENCES

1. Hart, P. D'A.: Med. Research Council, Special Report, Series No. 164, London, 1932.
2. Lichtenstein: Am. Rev. Tuberc. **29**: 190, 1934.
3. Schaumann: Brit. J. Dermat. **36**: 315, 1924.
4. Mylius and Schürmann: Beitr. z. Klin. d. Tuberk. **73**: 166, 1929.
5. Pautrier: Bull. Soc. franç. de dermat. et syph. **41**: 1012 and 1054, 1934.
6. Salvesen: Acta med. Scandinav. **86**: 127, 1935.
7. Kissmeyer: La maladie de Boeck, Copenhagen, 1932.
8. Darier: Bull. Soc. franç. de dermat. et syph. **41**: 999, 1934.
9. Martenstein and Noll: Arch. f. Dermat. u. Syph. **168**: 409, 1929.
10. Danbolt: Nord. med. Tidskr. **10**: 1398, 1935.
11. Bonnevie and With: Arch. f. Dermat. u. Syph., in press (a part of the material is found in the reports of the Ninth International Dermatological Congress at Budapest: Sv. Lomholt zu Ramel "Quantitative intracutane Tuberculin-untersuchungen—").
12. Wallgren and Nilson: Rev. franç. de pédiat. **11**: 37, 1935.
13. Chevallier and Führer: Bull. Soc. franç. de dermat. et syph. **41**: 1144, 1934.
14. Nielsen, Jens: Ibid., pp. 1187-1218.

Remarks to the Foregoing Paper of Torben K. With, "The Relation of Tuberculosis to Generalized Tuberculous Adenitis—A Manifestation of Benign Lymphogranulomatosis"

Kornel L. Terplan and A. Wilmot Jacobsen, Buffalo, N. Y.

The histologic diagnosis of the lymph nodes in both of the cases published by one of us (A. W. J.) and the postmortem examination in Case 1 were made by the other (K. L. T.). Therefore, we feel that we ought to comment jointly on the foregoing paper of Dr. Torben K. With, which is based solely on citations from the literature of cases more or less similar to ours. We feel that more emphasis should be placed upon the pathohistologic features than was done by Doctor With. First, however, we wish to note a distinct disagreement as to the nomenclature. There is a most unfortunate tendency in present-day medicine to create new names for combinations of pathologic lesions which heretofore have been known under less misleading simple descriptive terms. One of these new names is "benign lymphogranulomatosis." It was introduced by Schaumann[1] to designate tuberculoid granulomas in lymph nodes, skin, bone marrow, lungs, and sometimes in tonsils, and probably also in the spleen and liver. The characteristic histologic feature in all these organs is typical epithelioid cell tubercle formation, usually with absence of caseation, although slight central necrosis may be present, especially in the lymph nodes. This name has not been adopted by pathologists. Mylius and Schürmann[2] speak of the same lesions in lymph nodes as "universal tuberculous large cellular hyperplasia." They call attention to the later stages with hyaline sclerosis instead of caseation and calcification. They consider these lesions as a peculiar form of atypical tuberculosis, identical with the systemic large cellular hyperplasia described long ago by Ziegler. This hyperplastic type of lymph node tuberculosis is well known to all pathologists. Some of them prefer the term "fungoid," designating tuberculous granulation tissue without caseation.

In discussing the etiology of "benign lymphogranulomatosis," Doctor With fails to mention that Schaumann,[1, 3] who originated this term, and also Schürmann and Mylius, interpret these lesions as atypical tuberculosis in an etiologic sense. The causative agent in their opinion is a tuberculous virus. Schaumann tried to explain the absence of the tuberculin reaction by a state of anergy or a sensibility to tuberculin. We wish to call attention to the discussion of Schürmann and Mylius of their own cases, one of which showed a combination of tuberculous lymph node hyperplasia and ordinary progressive tuberculosis of the lungs. They state that "the negative reaction to tuberculin in pure cases of tuberculous lymph node hyperplasia should not impress us as being so strange when we consider the entire histologic picture, especially the absence of caseation. However, behind this symptom (i.e., the negative reaction) there are more problems hidden, which at the present time cannot be answered." These authors discuss further the different possible combinations of the noncaseating tuberculous hyperplasia with the ordinary tuberculosis. These two varieties may appear simultaneously, or a more caseating type may complicate a mere hyperplastic tuberculosis at a certain time which at postmortem examination may be estimated from the anatomic findings. This latter type possibly could be produced by two different tuberculous viruses. In most cases, however, it is, according to Schürmann and Mylius, impossible to learn anything certain about the time at which caseating tuberculous processes may appear in a patient suffering from tuberculous lymph node hyperplasia. On the other hand, in their opinion, this combination of the caseating and noncaseating types especially suggests the tuberculous etiology of the epithelioid cell hyperplasia in lymph nodes (so-called "benign lymphogranulomatosis").

If as careful an observer as Schürmann admits the difficulty inherent in any attempt to analyze these cases of combined atypical and ordinary caseating tuberculosis in exact pathogenetic and etiologic terms, it is rather surprising to see the readiness of Doctor With to explain either the presence or the absence of the tuberculin reaction in our two cases. Doctor With bases his discussion on the assumption that the noncaseating or fungoid type of lymph node tuberculosis is not tuberculosis at all in an etiologic sense and that in both of our cases there were two different diseases which had nothing to do with each other. The literature which Doctor With himself quoted, especially the papers of Schaumann, and Schürmann and Mylius, suggests strongly that his interpretation is not necessarily correct. How can he feel sure that the benign lymphogranulomatosis was the "primary disease" and that only later as indicated by the positive tuberculin reaction a real tuberculous infection occurred? How did this "primary disease" enter the body? There was ample opportunity for tuberculous infection in the home of this negro family through all the years in which the two children were seen. The term "benign lymphogranulomatosis" was not used in our paper for reasons mentioned herein, just as Schürmann and Mylius, like many other pathologists, prefer the term "atypical lymph node tuberculosis." As to the etiology, in addition to Schaumann, and Schürmann and Mylius, Beintema[4] and Jadassohn[5] speak of tuberculoids. There are, of course, other dermatologists, especially of the French school, who do not feel that epithelioid cell granulomas in the skin and lymph nodes are tuberculous in nature, among these especially Pautrier.[6] However, to introduce still another designation for this syndrome, as Pautrier does in speaking of "reticulo-endotheliose," seems to us inappropriate inasmuch as the term is already markedly overburdened and used for entirely unrelated diseases.

We strongly recommend discarding the term "benign lymphogranulomatosis," as it has proved to be confusing, especially when used to suggest a relationship to tuberculosis similar to that borne by Hodgkin's disease. Indeed it inevitably implies such a similarity, as in many European countries the term "lymphogranulomatosis" is used synonymously with Hodgkin's disease, which condition in a high percentage of cases is entirely unassociated with tuberculosis. With regard to this question, we might refer to the paper by one of us[7] dealing with the nature, pathogenesis and etiology of Hodgkin's disease.

From the postmortem findings in our first case it is clear that the tuberculous infection occurred several years previous to death. Several calcified foci were found in the parenchyma of the lungs. When and why at a later time the picture of tuberculous peritonitis and caseating bronchogenic spread in the lungs was brought about is just as difficult to explain as in so many other cases of chronic tuberculosis in children and adults. The entire complex question of exogenous reinfection or endogenous exacerbation should be carefully examined in all cases of this type. Inasmuch as in our second case a complete postmortem examination was not performed, we would prefer not to comment on the relation of the progressive tuberculous lesion terminating in tuberculous meningitis to the tuberculous lymph node hyperplasia. There is, however, no reason to assume, as Doctor With does, that we are dealing with a recent tuberculous infection, which resulted in tuberculous meningitis. The first infection with tubercle bacilli may have occurred several years previous to death in this case just as well as in the first one. To the statement of Doctor With, based on a quotation of Wallgren and Nilson that tuberculous meningitis follows as a rule a few months after the primary infection, which he uses to prove the recent nature of the tuberculous infection in Case 2, there is a large number of exceptions in children and adults. We could cite from our own material several postmortem protocols proving that tuberculous meningitis is found in children and adults with entirely stony tuberculous complexes.

The fact that we do not understand the tuberculin reaction in the individually different types of tuberculous tissue processes, especially in the purely hyperplastic type, should make us very careful not to arbitrarily dismiss the possibility of tuberculosis on the evidence of a negative tuberculin test alone. All the environmental factors, the family history, signs of tuberculous infection in all children, linked with the anatomic histologic findings in both of our cases speak strongly for a common tuberculous etiology. The histologic picture is that of atypical epithelioid cell hyperplasia. There is so far no other etiologic agent known which can bring about a universal tuberculous lymph node hyperplasia with epithelioid cells and Langhans' giant cells, with or without slight central necrosis, except the tubercle bacillus or a tuberculous virus in a wider sense.

REFERENCES

1. Schaumann, J.: Brit. J. Dermat. **36:** 515, 1924.
2. Mylius, K., and Schürmann, P.: Beitr. z. Klin. d. Tuberk. **73:** 166, 1929.
3. Schaumann, J.: Bull. Soc. franç. de dermat. et syph. (Reunion dermat., Strasbourg) **41:** 1296, 1934.
4. Beintema, K.: Bull. Soc. franç. de dermat. et syph. **41:** 112, 1934.
5. Jadassohn, W.: Bull. Soc. franç. de dermat. et syph. **41:** 1344, 1934.
6. Pautrier, L. M.: Bull. Soc. franç. de dermat. et syph. (Reunion dermat., Strasbourg) **41:** 1054, 1934.
7. Terplan, K.: Zentralbl. f. d. ges. Tuberk.-Forsch. **39:** 561, 1933.

Critical Review

TUBERCULOSIS IN CHILDREN

Lee Forrest Hill, M.D.
Des Moines, Iowa

The most comprehensive survey ever undertaken of the facilities for caring for tuberculous patients in the United States has been completed by the Council on Medical Education and Hospitals of the American Medical Association and was fully reported in the December 7, 1935, issue of the *Journal of the American Medical Association;*[1] 471 sanatoriums, 740 tuberculosis departments of hospitals, and 29 preventoriums provided the statistical data upon which the report is based. The total capacity for tuberculosis is 95,198 beds: 64,997 in the sanatoriums, 28,534 in the tuberculosis departments, and 1,667 in the preventorium group. The total replacement value of the tuberculosis institutions is estimated at approximately $328,937,777.36, or a general average of $3,455.30 per bed. The annual cost of the tuberculosis hospitalization in the United States exceeds $70,000,000. The average cost of maintaining a tuberculous patient in the sanatoriums is $2.37 a day; in the tuberculosis department, $2.95; and in the preventoriums, $1.39.

More pertinent for the purposes of this review is that part of the report which deals with children. A total of 11,647 beds are available for this group of patients in all the tuberculosis institutions. Of these the sanatoriums provide 9,036; the tuberculosis departments of hospitals, 944; and the preventoriums, 1,667. All together, 230 sanatoriums admit children. Over half of the sanatoriums admitting childhood tuberculosis also admit children with pulmonary tuberculosis of the adult type. The figures given for admissions to the tuberculosis sanatoriums show that of a total of 12,629 children, 1,191 had adult type tuberculosis; 6,659, the childhood type; 824 had extrapulmonary lesions; 3,236 were nontuberculous; and 701 were unclassified. Sixteen of the twenty-nine preventoriums reported 2,479 patients admitted, of whom 12 had the adult type tuberculosis; 424, the childhood type; 24 had extrapulmonary lesions; 1,326 were nontuberculous; and 693 were unclassified. The report further states that many of the sanatoriums admitting children have a waiting list for adults and properly questions the wisdom of such a procedure, pointing out that the prime objective in tuberculosis control is the isolation of tuberculous patients who give off tubercle bacilli. For the most part, the report indicates that the children in tuberculosis institutions received adequate protection from "open" cases of tuberculosis, but that in some there were opportunities for contact between adult patients and children, and in a few sanatoriums it was observed that children with pulmonary tuberculosis were hospitalized together with other children in the preventorium unit.

It is rather surprising to learn that over 37,000 tuberculous patients were admitted to general hospitals in a one-year period (1934). Undoubtedly the majority of these institutions provide adequate segregation facilities, but it is a fair surmise that there are many thousand other unrecognized tuberculous patients admitted to hospitals in general who are a source of contagion for other patients, nurses, doctors, and attendants. That such a surmise is correct is attested by observations on nurses and medical students among whom the percentage of positive reactors to tuberculin is relatively low at the beginning of training, but approaches 100 per cent by the time the training period has been completed. The medical profession as a whole still pays too little attention to the communicability of tuberculosis. The time is not far distant when the same contagious technic will be applied to the care of tuberculosis as is now applied to diphtheria and scarlet fever. In fact it is not improbable that within a few years it will have become the custom in many of our hospitals to require satisfactory evidence of the absence of tuberculosis in a communicable form before the admission of the patient to the general wards. This could be accomplished at slight expense by means of routine fluoroscopy for all patients over ten years of age. Such a procedure should be but little more troublesome than the requirement of throat cultures and vaginal smears enforced in many pediatric departments and should reduce the hazard to doctors and nurses, as well as benefit the patient. If it were carried out in obstetrical departments, loss of life among infants due to fatal forms of tuberculosis could be materially reduced.

Another point worth dwelling on briefly and which the report brings up is the matter of institutional care of children who are in contact with tuberculosis in their homes or who have only the first infection type of tuberculosis. From the report it will be seen that there were many such admitted to sanatoriums and preventoriums. Obviously a considerable sum of money was involved in the care of these children. Was it worth it, or could this money have been spent to better purpose in other ways?

Myers[2, 3] believes that knowledge gained from years of observation of large numbers of children with primary tuberculosis has amply demonstrated that these children do not need treatment in sanatoriums, preventoriums, special schools, fresh air classrooms, or summer camps, to heal their tuberculous foci. Treatment in such institutions neither hastens the healing process nor makes it more complete than that which occurs in the child's own or a foster home. If the child remains in his own home, it is of course desirable that the infecting source be removed. He cites as substantiating evidence of his opinion the results of treatment in 155 children who were observed from the time the disease was in the acute inflammatory stage until lime or fibrous strands were deposited in sufficient quantity so that they could be visualized in the x-ray film. Nineteen were treated in sanatoriums; 50 in the Lymanhurst school; and 86 in their homes. Among 136 whom it was possible to trace, no difference could be seen in the course of the disease, whether the children were treated as strict bed patients, sent to a special school, or remained as active as any normal child is in the home. Consequently, Lymanhurst has discontinued its treatment division and has diverted its funds into other channels of tuberculosis control.

Nor "have we been able," states Myers,[2] "to obtain any evidence to show that hospitalization, special schools, summer camps, or any other form of treatment except breaking contact with tubercle bacilli has any influence upon the later development of reinfection type of disease." Again the point should be made that the admission of a child to a tuberculosis institution does not insure that contact with tubercle bacilli will be prevented. On the contrary, the opportunities may actually be increased.

In addition to the argument that institutional treatment of first infection tuberculosis is unnecessary, the proponents of this line of reasoning draw attention to its futility. For instance, Myers[2] speaks of the situation at Lymanhurst in Minneapolis, where there were estimated to be 20,000 children infected with tuberculosis and 70,000 others who needed protection from infection. The capacity for treatment at Lymanhurst was 175. Certainly the expenditure of funds for the care of this small number in view of the much larger problem accomplished very little.

Consequently, the money formerly used to maintain these children in the preventorium unit is now employed to do tuberculin testing on large groups of children; to search out and segregate the source of contamination of the positive reactors, thus making not only the child in his own home safe, but also giving protection to the rest of the community; and finally to follow up the adolescent positive reactors by frequent x-ray examinations in order to detect the reinfection form of tuberculosis sufficiently early to institute therapeutic measures aimed at arrest of the process and prevention of the victim's in turn becoming a spreader of bacilli. Such a program would seem to yield far greater returns, in terms of tuberculosis control, for the financial outlay involved, than the preventorium method. According to Stewart,[4] similar changes to those going on at Lymanhurst are now in process of development elsewhere.

Pastor,[5] in discussing the fight against tuberculosis in Puerto Rico, advances further arguments against the value of the preventorium in his locality. He found it cost as much to maintain a well child in a preventorium as to support a tuberculous patient in a sanatorium. Taking the child away from the home to protect him from contagion is an expensive and impractical procedure. It is far easier, more effective, and less costly to send away the focus of contagion, leaving the rest of the family at home. Beds in sanatoriums should be for sick persons who are potential sources of contamination. He suggests that tuberculosis workers adopt the slogan, "Make every home a preventorium."

Moreover, if protection of the infected child is to be effective, it must not be limited to a few months of institutional care, where the child merely gains a few pounds of weight only to lose it when he returns to his poor home, but it must extend over a period of years into adult life, since most childhood infections that do light up do not become activated until the age of puberty or thereafter. "By keeping the home free from foci of contagion, raising its standards, educating parents, and affording facilities for systematic clinical supervision of contacts, we could probably achieve more in the prevention of tuberculosis than has been achieved by all the preventoria of the past and of the present," says Pastor.

Hawes,[6] on the other hand, is convinced that properly run preventoriums and summer camps are decidedly worth while in the campaign against tuberculosis. On the basis of fifteen years' experience with the Prendergast preventorium in Boston, he states that he knows "of no more effective way in which our present knowledge of tuberculosis may be extended than by means of the preventorium and the summer camp, providing that active and practical measures are used to educate not only the children themselves in the principles of health and hygiene, but also their parents and other members of their families, and likewise the general public, including physicians, nurses, and social workers, as well as the laity." As proof of the value of the work that may be done in a preventorium like Prendergast, he compares 705 children admitted to that institution in the decade from 1922 to 1932, with 705 other children with similar tuberculosis experience who had not been to Prendergast but had been taken care of in their homes either by family physicians or doctors and nurses from a health clinic. In the Prendergast group of children it was found that only one had subsequently died of tuberculosis, and only three had developed the disease in clinical form, whereas in the other group ten had died from tuberculosis and forty had developed the disease.

The figures presented by Hawes represent a striking difference in morbidity and mortality in favor of the preventorium group of children. One is inclined to think the efforts of breaking contact in the nonpreventorium group could not have been very effective. However, if further observation of comparable groups continues to show similar results, then certainly a powerful argument exists justifying preventorium residence.

CONCEPTS OF TUBERCULOSIS

Fifteen years of longitudinal study of many thousands of children for tuberculosis have enabled the Lymanhurst workers to form a concept of the evolutionary course of tuberculosis as it occurs in the human being from the beginning of the first seeding of tubercle bacilli on normal preallergic tissues to disabling disease or death from chronic destructive pulmonary tuberculosis. Their observations have been presented so succinctly and so convincingly that probably the rank and file of physicians in this country are in agreement with their views. However, there is a substantial number of other well-known workers in the tuberculosis field, whose opinions command respect, who differ with some of the interpretations of the Lymanhurst group. Controversial questions center largely about the significance of allergy and immunity; about racial and individual resistance; about the reason for the infrequent appearance of phthisis before the age of ten; about the effect of the massiveness of the infecting dose of organisms; about the relative importance of endogenous and exogenous sources in causing reinfections; about the part played by a first infection in preventing or predisposing to later reinfection types of tuberculosis; and finally about whether it is more desirable to enter adolescent and adult years with a negative or with a positive reaction to tuberculin.

The impression should not be gained that these are the only problems remaining for solution in tuberculosis, but merely, that at the present time, they are the questions receiving most attention in the literature on tuberculosis in children.

In last year's review[7] the Lymanhurst interpretation of tuberculosis was presented in considerable detail. It may be advantageous to restate the high points of that concept here, to add further contributions which have been made during the year, and then to consider some of the views which approach the problem from other angles.

Recent articles by Myers and his associates[8] and by Stewart[4, 9] summarize their ideas on the evolutionary course of tuberculosis. According to these authors, there are two general types of tuberculosis, the first infection type and the reinfection type, both caused by the same organism, but differing so markedly in almost every other respect as to suggest they are separate disease entities. Concerning this statement there is almost universal agreement among tuberculosis workers, but it may be said to be unique in this respect.

First infection tuberculosis results when tubercle bacilli are seeded on nonallergic tissues, whereas reinfection type tuberculosis requires for its development that the tissues be allergic to tuberculoprotein when the bacilli are implanted. The one essential determining difference between the two types, therefore, is allergy, and this holds true regardless of the age of the patient as will be brought out later. First infection may occur in the lungs, abdomen, or cervical region, and the foci may be single or multiple, large or small. It is probable, too, that from the primary focus during the preallergic period bacilli are disseminated like particulate matter to various organs of the body thus setting up numerous other foci which may be of importance in the development of subsequent reinfection forms of tuberculosis. Proof is not available, but it is possible that this is the mechanism involved in the formation of the foci in the brain, from which bacilli escape to produce meningitis as has been shown by Rich and McCordock. Similarly, it is conceivable that bone and joint tuberculosis or renal tuberculosis may arise from hematogenous "rests" deposited in these structures at the time of the primary infection, which do not become activated for months or years afterward.

During the preallergic stage following the initial infection, symptoms and physical signs are completely absent, and diagnosis of the condition is impossible except by recovery of organisms by gastric lavage. However, Myers states that he is at present engaged in a study to determine whether or not there occurs in the peripheral blood sufficient of the leucocytic, monocytic, and lymphocytic activity occasioned by tubercle formation to be of diagnostic significance. The difficulty in knowing the exact time infection takes place in accidental exposures obviously stands in the way of the practicability of this means of early diagnosis.

In from three to seven weeks sensitivity develops, and coinciding with it perifocal allergic reactions may occur about some favorably situated primary pulmonary lesions so that they can be visualized in x-ray films. Many of these lesions acquire central areas of caseation at the time allergy appears, and a transitory fever of varying intensity and duration may occur during this period. However, only a small percentage of the children who become infected with tubercle bacilli for the first time develop lesions which are large enough to cast shadows in the x-ray film. In those who do develop such lesions it is believed that the defense mechanism of the body has not adequately surrounded the foci of bacilli before allergy appears, thus permitting a diffusion of tuberculoprotein into adjacent tissues which causes the collateral inflammation visible roentgenologically. In the majority of cases the defense mechanism is adequate, and no collateral inflammation occurs about the primary focus, which fact explains why the x-ray film is negative in such a high percentage of positive reactors. Cases of both types have been followed by serial x-ray study, and in both, at some subsequent time, calcium deposits have been observed to make their appearance.

To date 210 children with proved first infection tuberculosis (131 with pulmonary infiltration demonstrable roentgenologically) have been observed by the Lymanhurst group, and have been followed by serial x-ray study. One of these children died of tuberculous meningitis approximately a year after he had been sent to a first class sanatorium. All the others followed a surprisingly uniform course. For weeks or months no gross change occurred in the extent of the pulmonary infiltration. There then occurred a gradual progressive process of resolution which led in the course of months to two or three years, to a complete roentgenologic disappearance of the lesions, or to their reduction to trivial fibrosed scars or to calcium deposits. "The changes observed in these lesions," says Stewart, "illustrate on a large scale the evolution of all primary varieties of the disease, regardless of where the pathology is situated and irrespective of whether the lesions are large or small." Furthermore, this same course has been observed to follow when first infections have occurred in adults, thus disproving, in the opinion of the Lymanhurst authors, the popular belief that an adult who becomes infected for the first time nearly always develops rapidly progressive clinical tuberculosis. Also negro, Mexican, and Indian children have been observed who have resolved their first infections in the same manner as white children. This ability on the part of children of these races throws doubt upon the alleged destructiveness of primary infections in the adult members of such races. Such destructive forms are more likely to be reinfections.

In the centers of the calcareous foci virulent tubercle bacilli may remain alive throughout the lifetime of the individual, thus accounting for persisting sensitivity. Attempts on the part of nature to remove the calcified areas as foreign bodies by ossification and revascularization provide an opportunity for the freed bacilli to gain access to the blood stream, and hence to the potential establishment of reinfection forms of tuberculosis of endogenous origin.

According to the Lymanhurst interpretation, the term "reinfection type of tuberculosis" is applied to those forms of tuberculosis which develop as new lesions or which extend beyond the limits of the original primary pathology when such lesions develop after tuberculin sensitivity has become established, regardless of whether the complications occur a few weeks or many months after the first infection form of the disease was acquired. Thus tuberculous meningitis, miliary tuberculosis, tuberculous pleurisy with effusion, and bone and joint tuberculosis, as well as phthisis are all regarded as reinfection forms of the disease.

First infection tuberculosis is considered to be a relatively benign disease, which almost invariably undergoes resolution without any special form of treatment, whereas reinfection tuberculosis accounts for practically all of the serious disease manifestations and deaths. However, primary tuberculosis is not, in the opinion of these authors, a beneficial experience to the host in that it tends to create a degree of immunity against the later development of serious tuberculous disease. On the contrary, they consider it a double liability: first, because it is responsible for the production of allergy to tuberculoprotein which is an essential antecedent to the development of reinfection tuberculosis; and second, because its original foci may be the source of the bacillary metastasis which results in early or late, acute or chronic forms of reinfection tuberculosis. In substantiation of this viewpoint, they call attention to the failure of first infections to create immunity sufficient to protect against tuberculous meningitis, bone and joint tuberculosis, and miliary tuberculosis, and point out that an immunizing procedure for other communicable diseases which was equally ineffective would hardly be acceptable. Moreover, they have shown that phthisis is never the result of a first infection but is always the product of a reinfection. In a group of 131 children with pneumonic lesions of first infection type not one developed into phthisis, but in a group of 54 tuberculin-sensitive patients who developed reinfection pneumonic infiltrations years after they acquired their primary infections, the invariable outcome has been progressive disease typical of phthisis, resulting in death for a fourth of the group, and in advanced disease for some of the others.

First infection tuberculosis, then, in the Lymanhurst interpretation, is the introductory state of all clinical varieties of the disease. It not only fails as an immunizing force to protect against the subsequent acquisition of phthisis, but actually contributes the essential factor which makes possible its development. The prognosis as regards tuberculosis for patients who contract a first infection cannot be determined for many years. A few of them, but not nearly so many as was once thought, will develop acute forms of reinfection tuberculosis, such as meningitis, and miliary disease; a few will acquire tuberculosis of the bones and joints and of various viscera; and from 10 to 20 per cent of this group of tuberculin-sensitive children are destined later to develop chronic pulmonary tuberculosis either from endogenous or exogenous sources. A positive tuberculin reaction, then, in the opinion of the Lymanhurst workers, can only be considered as a distinct liability to the child entering the age group susceptible to phthisis. The conquest of tuberculosis for the human race is to be achieved through epidemiologic and preventive measures, as it has been for the bovine family, rather than by widespread tubercularization and survival of the fittest.

Attention may now be turned to a consideration of some of the contributions appearing in the literature of the past year which attempt to shed further light on why tuberculosis behaves as it does in human beings. Myers[10] draws upon the results obtained by numerous workers in animal experimentation to offer a reasonable explanation for the observed benignity of first infections. He refers to the work of Vorwald[11] who found that within an hour after the intravenous injection of virulent tubercle bacilli into rabbits polymorphonuclear leucocytes could be demonstrated in alveolar capillaries grouped about collections of tubercle bacilli, some of which had already been phagocytosed. Within three hours mononuclear exudate cells had collected in the walls of the capillaries surrounding the bacillus-laden polymorphonuclear leucocytes, and within a few hours more the exudate cells had taken on the function of phagocytosing tubercle bacilli and disintegrating leucocytes. Typical tubercle formation was evident at the end of a day. At the end of a week the typical predominating cells were the mononuclears, some of which could be recognized as epithelioid cells. By the end of a month the tubercles were macroscopic in size. Lymphocytes and plasma cells were concentrated about the tubercles, and central caseation was observed in some of the tubercles in which tubercle bacilli were found free. "This focalization and walling off of bacteria before sensitization appears may be an important factor in making primary tuberculosis a benign disease," states Myers.

He cites the studies of Lemon and Montgomery,[12] who show that the tissues of rabbits at first react with a nonspecific form of inflammation to bovine tubercle bacilli injected into the pleural space, as though they were foreign bodies of particulate type. The fluid and cellular parts of the resultant effusion are promptly resorbed, carrying with them the particulate material, which has been phagocytosed, and depositing it in regional lymph nodes and in remote organs. This preallergic nonspecific reaction of tissues is further illustrated by the experiments of Lemon and Feldman,[13] who compared the tissue reactions produced when particles of silica and virulent avian tubercle bacilli were introduced into the trachea of different rabbits. The early cellular reactions which developed about the particles of silica were essentially the same as those which appeared about the tubercle bacilli. Later, however, with the advent of sensitivity and in response to growth and multiplication of bacilli, the type of inflammation became specific in the tuberculous animals. Myers refers to various other studies which demonstrate that the injection of virulent tubercle bacilli into animals previously rendered allergic to tuberculin is followed by a more rapid and severe type of inflammation than that which results from an initial injection. For instance, Long[14] has shown that small doses of tubercle bacilli and their products have no immediate effect upon the cells of the testes of normal guinea pigs. However, when equivalent doses of tubercle bacilli are injected into the testes of animals which have previously been sensitized, degeneration of the cells begins almost immediately. And again Stewart, Long, and Bradley,[15] and Holst[16] found that leucocytes from animals which had not been infected with tubercle bacilli were not harmed when they were brought in contact with tuberculin, whereas leucocytes from animals with tuberculosis were definitely damaged under the same treatment. Also Seibert[17] sensitized normal guinea pigs and showed that a high degree of sensitiveness conferred no immunity or increased resistance to tubercle bacilli. On the contrary, it seemed to hasten and extend the lesion and to be associated with much more extensive necrosis and caseation than is found in unsensitized animals.

The events leading to the development of sensitivity of tissues in animals (and the reaction in humans is believed similar) following an initial infection with tubercle bacilli are described by Myers. "The first defense is offered by the neutrophiles when they phagocytose the tubercle bacilli in the blood stream. However, this defense is soon overcome, probably because of tuberculopolysaccharid which is toxic to neutrophiles. These sluggish or dead cells containing tubercle bacilli accumulate even to the point of completely obstructing some capillaries, thus focalizing tubercle bacilli. The next line of defense consists of monocytes which engulf the disintegrating neutrophiles, but a tuberculophosphatid apparently is partially responsible for the early conversion of the monocytes into epithelioid cells. Although some tubercle bacilli apparently are killed by the epithelioid cells, others not only live, but also multiply. From the dead and disintegrating bacilli, as well as from those proliferating, more products are given off which stimulate the local cells. The waxes cause a proliferation of fibroblasts, and the acetone-soluble fat stimulates proliferation of all connective tissue cells. In due time, tuberculoprotein results in an outpouring of plasma about the lesion and later causes sensitization of the body to such an extent that it can be detected by the tuberculin test.''

Thus, animal experimentation has been employed to show that a quick ''walling off'' of tubercle bacilli occurs following first infection, that no differentiation is made in tissue reaction between inanimate particulate material and tubercle bacilli until sensitivity occurs, and that tissue sensitivity is responsible for the development of specific destructive lesions. Correlating these findings with observations made on human beings Myers states, ''The entire early development of tuberculosis occurs in the human body without symptoms, abnormal physical signs, or x-ray findings. In many cases, apparently the tubercle becomes fibrosed, and no significant destruction of tissue occurs. In my observations on large numbers of students of nursing and medicine who developed the first infection type of tuberculosis after exposure to patients, I have never seen one who presented any symptoms before the tissues were sensitized. Moreover, I have seen none who presented symptoms subsequently except those who developed reinfection tuberculosis, such as pleurisy with effusion, peritonitis, destructive pulmonary disease, etc.''

Burke[18, 19] records an interesting study in animal experimentation, in which he produced primary and reinfection types of tuberculosis in rabbits and studied the resulting lesions by serial roentgenology, by roentgenograms of the excised lungs, and by pathologic examination.

The primary pulmonary tuberculosis produced in rabbits by the intratracheal injection of 1 mg. of virulent tubercle bacilli was comparable in many ways to primary pulmonary tuberculosis in children. The animals, like children with this type of tuberculous infection, were not ill and had no fever during the early progressive phases of the disease. The first roentgenograms to reveal shadows were those taken between the tenth and seventeenth days. The largest shadows were usually observed in the second month. Some of the films failed to show any shadows after the first three months, and commonly films made during the third and fourth months showed fewer and smaller shadows. In other instances, the shadows became dense and discrete and, having reached this stage, changed little during a period of years.

Both the roentgenograms taken during life and those of excised lungs failed in many instances to portray a true picture of the extent and location of disease demonstrable at pathologic examination.

Examination of the lungs of rabbits killed in later periods gave the author an unusual opportunity to observe successive stages in the healing of primary pulmonary tuberculosis. In seven of the twelve rabbits killed between the eighth month and fourth year the lungs and paratracheal lymph nodes showed no evidence of disease. Some of the lungs showed various stages in the healing of tuberculous lesions by resolution, fibrosis, and calcification. Cavities were found in the lungs of only five of the thirty-five animals killed between the end of the first month and the end of the fourth year. Caseous foci were observed to be small, differing in this respect from those seen in the animals with reinfection tuberculosis.

In the second part of his experiment Burke sensitized rabbits by injecting avirulent tubercle bacilli in the groin, and produced reinfection tuberculosis by subsequent injections of 1 mg. of virulent tubercle bacilli. The disease thus produced was comparable in many ways to the adult type of reinfection tuberculosis seen in man. Unlike the rabbits with primary pulmonary tuberculosis, these became ill for a week or two following the injections, and many had fever. Abnormal shadows were found in the roentgenograms as early as the first day, and usually reached their largest proportions during the second week. However, no shadow or combination of shadows was found in the chest roentgenograms or in the roentgenograms of the excised lungs which served to differentiate the lesions of reinfection from primary. Caseous foci were larger, and more cavities were found in the lungs of the killed rabbits with reinfection experimental tuberculosis than in the animals with primary tuberculosis.

The author concluded that the study demonstrated a striking similarity between primary and reinfection types of tuberculosis produced experimentally in animals by a measured dose of organisms and the same types of tuberculosis as they occur in human beings.

Another approach to the acquisition of further information concerning the pathogenesis of tuberculosis is advanced by Sweany,[20, 21] who has made an extensive study of tuberculous calcifications. According to this author, primary calcifications can be differentiated from reinfection calcifications by the fact that, in general, the former are more heavily encapsulated and show a much greater tendency to ossification. Moreover, transitions from one type to the other occur with the development of allergy.

As a result of a study of multiple calcifications selected from over 600 autopsies, Sweany[21] concludes that "calcifications may result from any type of encapsulated tuberculous focus; namely, multiple primary seedings, scattered foci occurring in a resolving benign type of tuberculous pneumonia, in a hematogenous seeding occurring in the acute allergic period of the secondary stage of the primary, in various transition types from the primary into reinfection, in hematogenous reinfection, and in the healing of any form of tuberculous nodule or infiltrate arising from bronchogenic spread.

"By correlating the history, antemortem and postmortem roentgenographic findings, and the pathologic changes in multiple calcified lesions, it is possible in many cases to determine not only the character of the lesions themselves, but also attain an idea of the mechanism of the process leading up to their formation."

Frequent reference has been made in the literature to the report published by Heimbeck[22] in 1928 that clinical pulmonary tuberculosis developed much more frequently among nurses who entered training on a tuberculosis ward in Oslo with a negative reaction to tuberculin, than occurred among those whose test was positive. This was interpreted as indicating that the nurses with the positive reactions were, as a group, more immune to tuberculosis than the negative group. Also, it is, or rather was until recently, the general impression that the acquisition of a tuberculous infection for the first time in adult life was likely to result in a severe form unusually resistant to treatment.

Myers' observations[23] on the development of tuberculosis among students of nursing and of medicine in the city of Minneapolis is of particular interest, therefore, in the bearing it has on these views. The students were tested to tuberculin upon entrance to the school and were usually retested at intervals of not greater than six months, since positive reactions known to have developed in such a short time possess diagnostic value in differentiating first infection lesions from reinfections which appear in x-ray films. When the interval between testing is a year or longer, this significance of positive tests is lost. Both the students of nursing and of medicine had opportunities for exposure to open cases of tuberculosis in their routine hospital work, and not infrequently the time and source of contagion could be ascertained quite accurately.

The individuals comprising the study are divided into six groups, on the basis of tuberculin reactions, and the type of lesions subsequently developed. Protocols are given for each patient.

Group 1 consists of two persons whose tuberculin reactions changed from negative to positive under observation and in whom erythema nodosum appeared.

In Group 2 are placed twenty-one persons whose tuberculin reaction changed from negative to positive and who developed a primary focus demonstrable by x-ray film examination. No other lesion was demonstrated. This is a significant group. They are adults never before infected with tuberculosis, but when they did become infected the resultant lesions were observed to run the same benign course as similar lesions which develop in infants and children. Over a period of time resolution went on to complete disappearance of the x-ray shadow or was reduced to fibrous strands or lime deposits. Symptoms were absent in the majority of these cases, and healing occurred without the employment of any special therapeutic measures. There was nothing characteristic about the x-ray shadows observed in these patients which served to differentiate between first and reinfection types of tuberculosis. (Compare with Burke's statement in experimental tuberculosis.) "It is only when one has carefully administered and interpreted tuberculin tests with sufficient frequency or has observed the lesions sufficiently long that such differentiation is possible," says Myers.

Group 3 is made up of nineteen cases whose tuberculin reaction changed from negative to positive and in whom primary parenchymal lesions were demonstrable by x-ray in some, and nondemonstrable in others. Pleural effusion also developed. This complication is looked upon by the author as a reinfection form of tuberculosis. The primary lesion sensitizes the tissues, and bacilli are transmitted to the visceral lymph channels from the lesion which frequently lies close to the surface of the lung. While pleurisy with effusion occurs occasionally in infants and children who have acquired a recent first infection, it apparently is more common in young adults.

Group 4 consists of twenty-five individuals whose tuberculin reaction changed from negative to positive and in whom clinical pulmonary tuberculosis later made its appearance, with or without demonstrable primary focus or pleurisy with effusion. Three of these patients have died from tuberculosis. In each of them the evolutionary course of the disease was followed from exposure to tuberculous patients to death with resultant lesions. The other patients have been treated by modern methods, and most of them have their lesions at least temporarily under control.

This is the group which, according to views once popular, should have developed severe and rapidly fatal tuberculosis. "However," states Myers, "their lesions are no more severe and respond just as well to treatment as the lesions which develop in adult life among persons who were infected in infancy or childhood."

In Group 5 are included 15 individuals whose tuberculin reactions were positive when observation began, but in whom no evidence of clinical tuberculosis could be demonstrated. Later reinfection forms of tuberculosis made their appearance. In this group, then, a positive tuberculin test, indicative of previous tuberculous infection, did not produce sufficient immunity to prevent the development of clinical tuberculosis when exposure to tuberculous patients occurred. "Moreover," says Myers, "as far as we have been able to observe, the lesions which this group developed have not differed in intensity or in response to treatment from those who developed clinical disease after having become positive to the tuberculin test while under our observation."

Group 6 consists of four persons who had had no previous tuberculin tests, but negative x-ray films. All of them later developed extensive pulmonary tuberculosis. These patients are included in answer to the statement sometimes made that during the teen-age period x-ray films of the chest will reveal evidence of any disease which may cause illness at a later time in life.

Among the conclusions which may justifiably be drawn from this excellent piece of work are:

1. First infection type of tuberculosis possesses the same benign characteristics whether it occurs in infancy and childhood or in adult life.

2. The evolutionary course of tuberculosis is the same whether the first infection takes place in childhood or is delayed to adult life. A certain number will be followed by reinfection types of tuberculosis in either event.

3. The differentiation of pulmonary first infection and reinfection types of tuberculosis in adults depends upon one's knowledge of how recently sensitivity to tuberculin was acquired or upon long-continued x-ray study of lesions, unless symptoms characteristic of the reinfection form make their appearance.

4. Chronic pulmonary tuberculosis acquired by adults who have not been infected in childhood is no more severe or less resistant to treatment than is pulmonary tuberculosis which develops in adult individuals who have had positive tuberculin tests since childhood.

In the above paragraphs the attempt has been made to present a concept of the evolutionary course of tuberculosis from its earliest beginning when leucocytes phagocytose tubercle bacilli in the capillaries to the development of the chronic reinfection form of tuberculosis and to include the essential evidence upon which such a concept is based. There remains now the necessity of recording some of the published opinions of those who hold other views.

First of all, attention may be directed to the recently expressed opinions of Wallgren,[24] of Gothenburg, Sweden, an author who has had an extensive experience with tuberculosis. Concerning the much debated question as to whether a first or primary infection equips the host with sufficient specific immunity to prevent the subsequent development of pulmonary tuberculosis, he advances the interesting theory that there are, or can be, two distinct types of immunity: one against exogenous reinfections and the other against the infection which is already in the body and which has produced pathologic changes. An analogous situation is found in syphilis, in which the syphilitic individual is immune against reinfection, but, nevertheless, if untreated, may die as the result of progressive activity of his original infection. The immunity to exogenous reinfections in tuberculosis, however, is only relative, but sufficient under ordinary conditions to protect a tuberculin-positive child from appreciable risk, if the child is subjected to new possibilities of infection. Under unfavorable conditions this relative immunity may be broken through, and reinfection may take place. But against the virus of the primary infection and development of disease from its foci, there is no noteworthy specific immunity.

Another significant point raised by Wallgren has to do with the definition of the term "reinfection." It is incorrect, he believes, and has led to much confusion, to speak of reinfection tuberculosis as including dissemination of bacilli from primary foci in the postallergic period. He would abandon the term "endogenous reinfection" and would restrict the meaning of reinfection to apply only to exogenous, or new infections from without.

To the question, "Is it advantageous to have passed through a primary infection?" he answers, "Yes and no." Were it possible throughout life to avoid with certainty the risk of virulent infection, then naturally, this would be best, for in this way could be avoided all tuberculous disease, including consumption. But obviously at present this ideal is not attainable, at least for the average city resident. It is, therefore, necessary to weigh the advantages of a first infection in childhood against its disadvantages.

The outstanding advantage of a successfully undergone primary infection is the relative specific immunity secured against exogenous reinfection pulmonary tuberculosis. But in the acquiring of the primary infection and for several months immediately following, particularly for young children, there is created a serious risk with reference to inception of tuberculous meningitis, miliary tuberculosis, pleuritis, and tuberculous peritonitis, all of which conditions are directly related to the primary infection. "Therefore," says Wallgren, "no one would in cold blood expose a previously noninfected child to a virulent tuberculous infection merely to let the child benefit later from the specific relative immunity which the primary infection creates.

The risks are too great. For this purpose there is, on the other hand, no risk in using Calmette vaccine, although the immunizing effect of this can possibly never be thought to compare with that of the virulent primary infection.'' But the child who is safely past the risk period must be considered to be in a more advantageous position from this standpoint than the child who has just been infected or who has not been infected at all. The point is illustrated by comparing a group of tuberculin-positive children with a group who are tuberculin-negative, all exposed to a consumptive teacher in a classroom. Nothing happens to the tuberculin-positive group, but some of the tuberculin-negative group will become ill, and one or more may succumb to meningitis or miliary disease.

If it be granted that the tuberculin-positive child has a degree of specific immunity toward exogenous reinfection and that he is past the risk period of meningitis, miliary disease, etc., there is yet a disadvantage arising out of the primary infection which merits serious consideration. In Wallgren's conception of the genesis of lung tuberculosis, he postulates the hematogenous dissemination of tubercle bacilli to various organs in the body very early in the course of the primary infection. Thus foci may be set up in the bones, joints, kidneys, peritoneum, pleura, and in the lungs at a point apart from the primary focus itself. Such foci create little or no tissue reaction, and they may remain in a state of latency until some special set of circumstances causes their activation. Tuberculosis of the bones and joints is generally understood to originate in this manner. And it is Wallgren's contention that pulmonary tuberculosis, or phthisis, not occasionally, but usually, is brought about in the same way. He says, ''Tuberculosis of the lungs according to this concept is usually not the immediate result of introduction of tubercle bacilli either from the outside or the inside into the allergic portion of the lung, but is rather the effect of activity by tubercle bacilli, which in most cases of lung tuberculosis have long remained in the same place, but have not been able to start a progressive process on account of resistance on the part of the organism and especially the lungs.''

Finally, he discusses the problem of why only 1 or 2 per cent of the general population develop pulmonary tuberculosis, and why it does not commonly make its appearance until the age of puberty has been reached. Neither variations in virulency nor dosage of organisms are responsible. Therefore, it must be due to variations in resistance in the infected organism and especially in the infected tissue that make it possible for some individuals to contract lung tuberculosis while others do not. The well-known fact that phthisis seldom occurs in children before the age of puberty suggests that allergy cannot be the sole factor responsible for the bringing about of lung tuberculosis, for the chances are that children who have been infected at an early age and thus have become allergic meet with reinfection as often as individuals in and above the age of puberty. That puberty shall have been reached, then, seems to be one of the essential requirements, and this in turn is probably intimately related to internal secretions. The most significant factor, according to Wallgren, however, in order that lung tuberculosis shall develop from a primary infection, is probably hereditary disposition. Resistance-reducing factors such as unhygienic living, infections, and diseases, are important, but are secondary. "The first prerequisite that a lung tuberculosis shall develop is a tuberculous infection and this regardless of whether the infection occurs during childhood or later. The second prerequisite that lung tuberculosis shall develop is a disposition, and among all the constitutional and conditional factors, which together constitute the concept of disposition to consumption, the most significant are heredity and that the age of puberty shall have been reached," states Wallgren.

Opie[25] expresses still a different conception of the pathogenesis of tuberculosis from either that of Wallgren or of the Lymanhurst group. He regards first infection as a progressive disease, starting with an area of tuberculous pneumonia somewhere in the lung, progressing to adjacent lymph nodes, disseminating of tubercle bacilli by way of the blood stream to distant organs, as the spleen, liver, and meninges, and leading in many instances to death from generalized miliary tuberculosis. All of these ramifications are part of, and characteristic of, the first infection. In infancy it is accompanied by a relatively high mortality rate, but is usually benign throughout childhood. Adult negroes often exhibit the essential features of first infection tuberculosis as it is seen in white infants.

The type of tuberculosis which develops in adolescence and adult life is entirely different from the first infection type and is not, in his opinion, a continuation of the first infection, but is a new exogenous reinfection. However, its localization in the lung and its chronicity are referable to the immunity conferred by the first infection. Anatomic studies have repeatedly shown that at the time when the infection of adult life is progressive, the lesion of first infection is encapsulated and healed and there is no evidence that the former spreads from the latter. In a comprehensive study of the spread of tuberculosis in a thousand families Opie[26] and his associates have shown that in white persons first exposed to tuberculosis after fifteen years of age, pulmonary tuberculosis with few exceptions has the characteristics of the adult or reinfection type of the disease. The marked increase in mortality rate over that of the general population occurring in persons over fifteen years of age exposed to open cases of tuberculosis is further evidence of its exogenous origin. Furthermore, recent roentgenographic study of married couples has given proof of the transfer of tuberculosis of the lungs from one to the other partner in nearly half the cases. Since this is a far greater rate than occurs in the general population, it can only be interpreted as indicating exogenous infection. Also, it was apparent in the study referred to above, that the severity of the disease in adolescents and adults as well as in children, varied, being more severe in the individuals exposed to open cases of tuberculosis than in those exposed to tuberculosis in which no dissemination of tubercle bacilli was demonstrable. Such variation is explainable on the basis of variation in the number of tubercle bacilli in the environment, which again shows that pulmonary tuberculosis is an exogenous infection.

It is apparent, therefore, that no unanimity of opinion concerning the pathogenesis of tuberculosis exists even among competent observers of wide experience. The lesions of first infection to one (Opie) become a closed chapter and, except for the immunity produced, bear no relation to the development of phthisis in adolescent and adult life. Phthisis results only from an exogenous infection, and only in those individuals in whom the massiveness of the infecting dose overcomes the immunity imparted by the first infection. To another (Wallgren) phthisis seldom if ever results from an exogenous infection. The immunity set up by the first infection prevents outside reinfection. Phthisis results from an activation of tubercle bacilli planted in the lung usually years before, when hematogenous dissemination of organisms from the primary focus took place. In a third interpretation (Lymanhurst) phthisis may be the result of either an endogenous or an exogenous reinfection. For its development it is essential that there has been a preexisting first infection which has sensitized the tissues to tuberculoprotein. The immunity feature of the first infection is negligible.

No conclusions as to which of these concepts expresses the true situation is possible. The literature of the past year contains many excellent discussions bearing upon this interesting phase of tuberculosis which have not been recorded here because of space limitation. To those interested, however, reference may be made to articles by Miller and Rappaport,[27] by Pinner,[28] and by Long.[29]

REFERENCES

1. Tuberculosis Survey, J. A. M. A. **105**: 1855, 1935.
2. Myers, J. A.: Treatment, Prognosis, and Prevention of First Infection Type of Tuberculosis, Journal-Lancet **56**: 24, 1936.
3. Myers, J. A.: Basic Changes in Tuberculosis Control, J. Florida M. A. **22**: 412, 1936.
4. Stewart, C. A.: The Lymanhurst Interpretation of Tuberculosis, J. Missouri State M. A. **33**: 103, 1936.
5. Pastor, J. R.: The Fight Against Tuberculosis in Puerto Rico, Journal-Lancet **56**: 199, 1936.
6. Hawes, J. B., Jr.: Are the Preventorium and Summer Camp Worth While? Tr. Nat. Tuberc. A., 1935.
7. Hill, L. F.: Tuberculosis in Children. Critical Review, J. Pediat. **7**: 840, 1935.
8. Myers, J. A., Harrington, F. E., Stewart, C. A., and Wulff, M.: First-Infection-Type Tuberculosis: Its Treatment and Prognosis, Am. Rev. Tuberc. **32**: 631,. 1935.
9. Stewart, C. A.: Tuberculosis: Its Evolution, Treatment and Prevention, Journal-Lancet **55**: 573, 1935.
10. Myers, J. A.: The First Infection Type of Tuberculosis: Its Pre-Allergic and Post-Allergic Stages of Development, Am. Rev. Tuberc. Am. Rev. Tuberc. **34**: 317, 1935.
11. Vorwald, A. J.: The Early Cellular Reactions in the Lungs of Rabbits Injected Intravenously With Human Tubercle Bacilli, Am. Rev. Tuberc. **25**: 74, 1932.
12. Lemon, W. S., and Montgomery, L. G.: Pleural and Pulmonary Lesions Resulting From Intrapleural Injection Into Rabbits of Mycobacterium Tuberculosis, Thoracic Surg. **3**: 612, 1934.
13. Lemon, W. S., and Feldman, W. H.: A Comparison of the Development of the Specific Nodule of Siliocosis and of Tuberculosis, Arch. Int. Med. **53**: 367, 1934.
14. Long, E. R.: The Inflammatory Reaction in Tuberculosis, Am. J. M. Sc. **185**: 749, 1933.
15. Stewart, F. W., Long, P. H., and Bradley, J. I.: The Fate of Reacting Leucocytes in the Tuberculin and Reinfection Reactions, Am. J. Path. **2**: 47, 1926.
16. Holst, P. M.: Studies on Effects of Tuberculin, Tubercle **3**: 249, 1922.
17. Seibert, Florence B.: Effect of Sensitization With Tuberculin Protein Upon Development and Course of Experimental Tuberculosis, Proc. Soc. Exper. Biol. & Med. **30**: 1274, 1932-33.
18. Burke, H. E.: A Comparison of the Roentgenological and Pathological Findings in Experimental Pulmonary Tuberculosis in Rabbits: Part I, Primary Tuberculosis, Am. Rev. Tuberc. **32**: 343, 1935.

19. Burke, H. E.: A Comparison of the Roentgenological and Pathological Findings in Experimental Pulmonary Tuberculosis in Rabbits: Part II, Reinfection Tuberculosis, Am. Rev. Tuberc. **32**: 382, 1935.
20. Sweany, H. C.: Studies on the Pathogenesis of Primary Tuberculous Infections: The Regressive Lesions, Am. Rev. Tuberc. **27**: 559, 1933.
21. Sweany, H. C.: Observations on Multiple Tuberculous Calcifications, Am. Rev. Tuberc. **32**: 73, 1935.
22. Heimbeck, J.: Immunity to Tuberculosis, Arch. Int. Med. **41**: 336, 1928.
23. Myers, J. A.: The Development of Tuberculosis in Adult Life, Arch. Int. Med. (In press).
24. Wallgren, A.: From Childhood Infection to Adult Type of Pulmonary Tuberculosis, Journal-Lancet **56**: 237, 1936.
25. Opie, E. L.: Present Concepts of Tuberculous Infection and Disease, Am. Rev. Tuberc. **32**: 617, 1935.
26. Opie, E. L., McPhedran, F. M., and Putnam, P.: The Fate of Persons in Contact With Tuberculosis: The Exogenous Infection of Children and Adults, Am. J. Hyg. **22**: 644, 1935.
27. Miller, J. A., and Rappaport, I.: Resistance in Tuberculosis, J. A. M. A. **107**: 471, 1936.
28. Pinner, M.: Pathogenesis of Tuberculosis, J. A. M. A. **107**: 475, 1936.
29. Long, E. R.: Acquired and Constitutional Factors in Resistance to Tuberculosis, Tr. Nat. Tuberc. A., p. 308, 1935.

704 Equitable Building

American Academy of Pediatrics

Proceedings

SIXTH ANNUAL MEETING OF THE AMERICAN ACADEMY OF PEDIATRICS

KANSAS CITY, MO., MAY 11 AND 12, 1936

Round Table Discussion on Recent Advances in Nutrition

Chairman: Dr. W. McKim Marriott, St. Louis.
Assistants: Dr. Samuel W. Clausen, Rochester, N. Y.
Dr. Philip C. Jeans, Iowa City, Iowa.

CHAIRMAN MARRIOTT.—The aim of the nutritionist is to provide in utilizable form those materials which are necessary for the building up and maintenance of a bodily structure which will be functionally adequate. This aim may, to a considerable extent, be frustrated by such factors as heredity, congenital anomalies, or disease.

As the pediatrician deals with the body during the growing period, he may be compared with the builder of edifices; the internist and the surgeon, with the repair men. Given a solidly constructed structure, it will last well, and the minimum of repair work will be required. We cannot alter the general plans of the architect, but we can see that the proper materials go into the construction. Two buildings of the same size and outward appearance may differ greatly, depending upon the care taken in construction; the one may approach perfection in structure and wear well, the other, because of the use of poor materials, will not withstand wear and tear. It is so with the child's body; the architectural plan of nature may be excellent, but with skimping on materials a poor structure may result.

Adequate nutrition implies far more than the attainment and maintenance of a certain body size and weight or a certain thickness of adipose tissue. A child may be of average stature for the age and have an average height-weight ratio, yet the nutrition cannot be considered as satisfactory if the child is anemic, has weak flabby musculature, poor posture, hypoplastic or carious teeth, or a colloid goiter, or if he suffers from atonic constipation or night blindness, has but little resistance to infection, and is incapable of sustained physical or mental effort.

The growing body must be supplied with the necessary building materials to perfect its structure and to provide adequately for functional activity. If the total fuel or caloric value of the food is inadequate to provide for the energy exchange, the laying down of body tissues is of necessity interfered with, or else tissues already formed are destroyed to meet the energy demands. On the other hand, with an entirely sufficient caloric intake but insufficient protein and mineral salts, muscle, blood, and bone development may fail to keep pace with weight gain. Without sufficient mineral salts, protein cannot be laid down as active protoplasmic tissue. When vitamin D is lacking, calcium and phosphorus may not be deposited as normal bone structure even though these elements are supplied in liberal amounts. When the diet is deficient in carbohydrate, the processes of metabolism are deranged with the accumulation of potentially harmful ketone bodies. Even an abundant intake of all known dietary essentials may not result in normal nutrition unless a certain balance is preserved. Thus with what would ordinarily be an adequate calcium supply, a great excess of phosphorus in the diet may interfere with the utilization of calcium, and a great excess of calcium may interfere with the utilization of iron, and vice versa.

Even after normal body structures have been formed, these may suffer functional impairment due to lack of certain essentials in the diet. For example, epithelial structures become keratinized and readily invaded by bacteria when vitamin A is deficient; the gastrointestinal tract becomes atonic and the appetite is lost when vitamin B is deficient.

The digestibility of the food must of course be considered, especially in the case of infants. In dealing with children, psychic factors must necessarily be taken into consideration. A balanced diet which may be relished by the laboratory rat may be refused by the child.

It is often stated that the instinct serves as a fairly reliable guide in the selection of foods, and examples are cited of primitive peoples with no knowledge of nutrition who instinctively choose well-balanced diets and even of young children who, given free selection, choose diets which meet their nutritional requirements. While, in general, the instinct may lead the individual to select a complete diet, this cannot always be relied upon. All primitive peoples are not well nourished, and, unless a very wide choice of foods is readily available, certain essentials may be omitted, and the diet as a whole may be poorly balanced.

The appetite serves, in general, as a good guide to the total amount of food needed, and, provided a suitable dietary mixture is offered, there is but little danger of under- or overfeeding when the amount of food taken is regulated by the appetite of a normal infant or child. A child who has been underfed for a time will often take large amounts of food when given a free choice and gain at an extraordinary rate, but, as the nutrition improves and the weight approaches the norm for the age and the body build, the appetite falls off and the rate of gain becomes less. Normal infants and children, given all they wish to eat of a well-balanced diet, are not likely to become overnourished. It is true that infants fed on the more modern concentrated formulas and given about all that their appetites demand are, as a group, larger and heavier than the accepted averages. They are not excessively fat. The fact that they are larger and heavier and have retained more calcium, phosphorus and nitrogen is not to be interpreted as meaning that they are oversized or overfed. Such infants may be considered as approaching *ideal* body standards, which from the very nature of the case differ from *average* standards. It should be the aim of the pediatrician to have the child's nutrition approach the ideal rather than to keep it to the average.

It has been customary to consider the breast-fed infant as the ideal and breast milk as the only perfect food; yet all breast milk is not perfect; nor do all mothers have a sufficient amount for their offspring. Breast milk is subject to greater daily variations than mixed herd cow's milk. There may be alterations in the total amount and in the calcium, fat, and vitamin contents, depending upon the mother's diet and living conditions. Breast milk, although adequate for the normal infant, does not contain sufficient protein for the special requirements of the premature or undernourished infant. Infants who nurse at the breast are likely to take considerably larger volumes of food than those offered carefully measured amounts of a formula from a bottle and hence they grow more rapidly. Given a good cow's milk formula under sanitary conditions, the ultimate results may, by all standards, be as satisfactory as those obtained with breast feeding.

Certain individual constituents of the diet require special consideration. In the case of the infant and the growing child, there is an especially high requirement for protein because of the laying down of new body tissue. The breast-fed infant receives about 10 per cent of the total calories in the form of protein, or approximately 2 gm. per kilogram of body weight. In the case of the infant receiving cow's milk, however, a larger amount of protein is needed because of its poorer nutritional value. A suitable allowance is 15 per cent of the total calories, or 3.5 gm. per kilogram of body weight per day. This corresponds to 1.5 oz. of cow's milk per pound of body weight per day. Infants receiving protein at higher levels grow somewhat more rapidly and have more solid tissues. A protein intake somewhat in excess of the average amounts mentioned above does little or no harm. The idea that moderately high protein feeding damages the kidneys of the human has failed of substantiation. A high protein diet does cause some hypertrophy of the kidneys but no pathologic changes. An insufficient amount of protein, on the other hand, results in slow growth and anemia. When the protein of the diet is low, the serum proteins are diminished in amount, and when, as the result of this, the colloidal osmotic pressure of the plasma falls below a certain level, nutritional edema of a greater or lesser degree occurs. As judged from clinical evidence, a low serum protein level is associated with decreased resistance to infection, possibly as the result of a lowering of the globulin fraction. Although animal proteins may more quantitatively be converted into body protein, satisfactory nutrition may be maintained through a proper selection of vegetable proteins; excellent results have been accomplished with the proteins of soy beans and of almonds. Some idea of the protein needs of the individual may be gained by consideration of the creatinine output. This phase of the subject will be discussed subsequently by Dr. Jeans.

The particular physical property of milk casein in forming curds during the processes of digestion has claimed a great deal of attention. One of the chief disadvantages of cow's milk for the feeding of the infant has been assumed to be the character of the casein, in that it forms large curds in the stomach. This particular disadvantage may be so easily obviated by heat treatment, acidification, or by other methods that it need not give us serious concern.

Fat is not as essential in the dietary as protein. Certain unsaturated fatty acids, such as linoleic acid, appear to be necessary for normal nutrition, but the amounts required are minimal. Linoleic acid may be considered in about the same category as the vitamins. Most natural fats carry small but adequate amounts of this fraction. The two important vitamins A and D are associated with the fats in natural foods. It is for these reasons that diets very low in fat are likely to be unsatisfactory unless especially supplemented so as to provide the essentials mentioned. In the average dietary about 35 per cent of the calories may to advantage be supplied by fat, but great variations in this amount may be made without noticeable effect on the nutrition. The most comprehensive study of the metabolism of fat, especially in infants, has been made by L. Emmett Holt, Jr., and associates.[1] They have shown that the size of the globules in milk has little or no influence on digestibility and that digestibility is more related to the structure of the fat than to its melting point. Special fat mixtures designed to replace butter fat were shown to possess no particular advantages. An interesting reciprocal relationship between fats and mineral constituents of the diets was demonstrated, an excess of fat resulting in loss of certain minerals from the system and an excess of certain minerals leading to diminished fat utilization.

Carbohydrate is the most economical food both from the financial and metabolic standpoints. With self-selection of diets by older children and adults, approximately 50 per cent of the calories are ordinarily taken in the form of carbohydrate, and of this about one-half is starch and the remainder sugar. In the case of the young

[1]Holt, L. Emmett, Jr., Tidwell, Herbert C., Kirk, Claude M., Cross, Dorothea M., and Neale, Sarah: Studies in Fat Metabolism: I. Fat Absorption in Normal Infants, J. Pediat. 6: 427, 1935.

infant, sugars are the sole source of carbohydrate until starch is fed. When cow's milk is used for infant feeding, it has been empirically determined that a suitable amount of added carbohydrate is between 5 and 10 per cent of the amount of milk. Taking as an average 8 per cent, this will mean one-half as many calories are added as carbohydrate as are furnished by the milk. Too little carbohydrate necessitates excessive intake of fat and protein. Too much carbohydrate, on the other hand, may result in insufficient intake of protein. An additional disadvantage of high carbohydrate feeding, particularly of sugar, is that of intestinal fermentation. Starch is more slowly digested and absorbed than sugar, hence does not flood the blood with glucose. As to the advantages and disadvantages of the individual sugars in infant feeding, experimental observations are conflicting. The normal infant appears to do about equally well when fed lactose, sucrose, or dextrin-maltose mixtures. Sucrose leads to more rapid gain in weight than lactose and to more fat formation than the dextrin-maltose mixtures. Lactose is rather slowly absorbed and tends to change the bacterial flora of the large intestine to a type resembling that of the breast-fed infant. There is some evidence that lactose feeding favors calcium absorption, possibly because of the formation of lactic acid in the lower portions of the intestinal tract. The monosaccharides, dextrose and levulose, are the most quickly absorbed of the sugars and require no digestive effort; they are, however, in concentrated solutions, more irritating than the disaccharides and much more so than dextrin. Dextrose and levulose are capable of absorption and utilization in patients with celiac disease who are unable to tolerate starch or the disaccharides.

The mineral constituents of the diet assume especial importance during the growing period. Adequate amounts of sodium, potassium, magnesium, sulphur, and chlorine are likely to be contained in any average diet, and it is not usually necessary to make additions of these elements. Calcium, phosphorus, iron, and iodine may, on the other hand, be deficient unless the diets are especially selected or these elements added in inorganic form. Calcium and phosphorus seem to be better absorbed when given in the form of milk than in any other form, but, in general, minerals may be as satisfactorily supplied as simple inorganic salts as in specially selected diets. There would appear to be very little reason for taking large amounts of foods containing a few milligrams of iron or iodine per pound when simple inorganic salts will supply every need. When cod liver oil is given to infants and children, a fair amount of iodine is supplied at the same time. Only a few natural foods contain significant amounts of iron, and the much vaunted spinach may when fed actually rob the body of iron. The metabolism of iron, of calcium, and of phosphorus will be discussed further in this symposium by Dr. Jeans.

The importance of the selection of foods providing an alkaline ash has been overrated. A diet having an ash approximating neutrality is perhaps the best, but a moderate variation on either the acid or alkaline side is practically without effect. Following severe diarrhea or vomiting, the acid-base balance may be greatly altered, and the same is true in the presence of diabetes or nephritis, but this does not concern us in considering the nutrition of the normal child.

Recent advances in our knowledge of the vitamins will be discussed by Dr. Jeans and Dr. Clausen and thus will not be referred to at this time.

The state of nutrition may be influenced not only by the diet but by intrinsic body factors, such as heredity and the interrelationship of the various endocrine hormones, especially insulin, epinephrine, thyroxin, and numerous pituitary hormones. A detailed consideration of these would be beyond the scope of the present discussion.

It is not to be assumed that all factors influencing nutrition are as yet known. Certain foods, especially fruits, seem to have somewhat specific effects which it is difficult to explain on the basis of what we know of the individual factors present. The severe digestive and nutritional disturbance known as celiac disease is still obscure so far as etiologic factors are concerned, yet it may be controlled by dietary means.

The discussion as related to certain specific factors in nutrition will be continued by Dr. Jeans.

Specific Factors in Nutrition

Philip C. Jeans, M.D., Iowa City, Iowa

Nitrogen Metabolism and Muscle Growth

At the time of birth and throughout the first year of life muscle tissue, according to Scammon, comprises approximately 25 per cent of the total body mass; at twelve years of age and thereafter the proportion is 40 per cent. Thus the muscle tissue undergoes not only an absolute, but also a relative, increase in relation to the remainder of the body. The time at which the relative increase occurs has not been determined.

It has long been known that creatinine excretion is proportionate to muscle mass. A study of creatinine excretion at various age levels should give information concerning the age period at which the relative increase in muscle mass occurs. It has been found that the creatinine excretion of the breast-fed baby is approximately 10 mg. per kilogram and that of the artificially fed baby who is receiving an abundance of food is 12 to 13 mg. per kilogram. The level of creatinine excretion per kilogram for the adult is approximately the same as that for the child of twelve years, viz., 20 mg. per kilogram. When the creatinine excretion per kilogram is determined at various age levels, it is found that the values remain practically constant until the age of three years. At approximately three years of age the values rise rapidly. This rapid rise continues until about nine years. After nine years of age the curve of increase becomes much less steep and before twelve years of age reaches the maximum level which is maintained thereafter. From these observations it may be concluded that the period of most rapid muscle increase in relation to the body mass occurs between three and nine years of age.

In the first year of life the relative amounts of creatinine excreted indicate that the artificially fed baby who is receiving ample food has a more rapid muscle growth than the breast-fed baby. The proportion of muscle weight to total body weight, though greater than that of the breast-fed baby, is maintained at a constant ratio throughout infancy.

This discussion has considered only the changes in muscle mass in relation to its proportion of the total mass of the body. Total growth is rapid in infancy and slows very definitely before three years of age, when the changed relationship between muscle and the remainder of the body begins. The absolute increases in muscle tissue are reflected in the nitrogen retentions. During the period of rapid growth in the first year, approximately 27 per cent of the ingested nitrogen is retained. From the age of one to three years, with the same nitrogen intake, the retention is only one-third of this value, representing a definite slowing in the speed of total growth, while at the same time the muscle mass remains the same proportion of the total body weight. Between four and nine years, while the muscle mass is increasing out of proportion to the total body weight, from 14 to 15 per cent of the ingested nitrogen is retained, even though the rate of total growth is less than it is between one and three years. After nine years of age the percentage of nitrogen retained again decreases. Thus the nitrogen retentions offer further evidence that the period of greatest relative increase in muscle is between three and nine years of age.

Many physicians are disturbed over the apparent loss of appetite between one and three years of age. Regardless of intake, children at this age retain less calcium, phosphorus, and nitrogen than at any other age period from birth to twelve years. From these facts it may be interpreted that the lessened food intake is physiologic and is not to be considered abnormal. The evidence seems equally clear that children from three to nine years of age need a high protein diet as much as do those in the period of adolescence.

Effect of Sugars on Calcium and Phosphorus Utilization

Animal experiments have indicated that conditions in the intestinal tract are much more favorable for the absorption of calcium and phosphorus when the food contains lactose than when it contains other sugars commonly used in infant feeding. On the basis of these experimental results many have assumed that in the artificial feeding of infants lactose would have the same favorable influence. The animal experiments were conducted with a relatively low intake of calcium and phosphorus, whereas the observations on infants have been made with a relatively high intake of these substances. The formulas consisted of undiluted milk with 6 per cent added sugar. With calcium and phosphorus retentions used as the criterion, no difference could be detected between the results with lactose and those with dextrin-maltose preparations. The same calcium retentions were observed with corn syrup as with the dry dextrin-maltose preparations. However, when dextrose was the added sugar in the formulas for infants under five months of age, the retentions were slightly but significantly lower than with the other sugars mentioned.

From a group of infants from eight to thirteen months of age whose retentions had been under continuous observation previously, those were chosen who had the lowest retention values. For this group of selected infants lactose was substituted in the formula for the dextrin-maltose mixture previously used. In the thirteen studies made, no increase in retentions was observed as a result of the substitution. It is possible that some difference might have been found had the amount of milk been less or the amount of added sugar greater, but the proportions used were those commonly employed in infant feeding.

From these observations it may be concluded that no significant difference is to be observed in calcium retentions when comparison is made between feeding formulas containing lactose and those containing dextrin-maltose mixtures when the formula consists of undiluted milk with 6 per cent added sugar. Under these same conditions the use of dextrose as the added sugar apparently permits significantly smaller calcium retentions than those obtained with the other sugars mentioned.

Dextrose in Malnutrition

In the condition known as celiac disease, a diet high in protein and in monosaccharides and low in fats and complex carbohydrates has proved uniformly successful. Since one of the prominent symptoms of children with celiac disease is malnutrition, it seemed possible that children with malnutrition from other causes might benefit from this same type of diet. When this idea was put to the test of trial, it was found that malnourished children utilize the celiac type of diet far more efficiently than either the average normal diet or one high in fat.

Children who were markedly underweight did not make consistently good gains on the average diet until the energy intake reached 50 calories per pound. At this level fair gains were made also with a diet high in fat, but these were not as satisfactory as those with the average diet. However, when the celiac type of diet was administered at the level of 50 calories per pound, the gains were very rapid, some children increasing their weight at the rate of a pound a day for considerable periods.

When the energy intake was maintained at approximately 35 calories per pound, children receiving the celiac type of diet made fair gains, whereas with the average diet and the high fat diet at this level no gain was observed. When malnourished children are receiving a high fat diet in sufficient quantity to permit gain in weight, a greater gain in weight will be observed if the energy intake is reduced by 500 calories and the celiac diet substituted for the high fat diet.

Certain fruits are relatively rich in monosaccharides. Equivalent amounts of these fruits may be substituted for dextrose in the celiac diet, and the results are the same. Substitution of bananas in this manner gave results identical with those described for dextrose. In the celiac, or high dextrose, diet the amounts of dextrose varied from 250 gm. daily for a child of six or seven years to 500 gm. for a child of twelve or thirteen years.

It might be assumed that weight gains made as a result of a high sugar diet would consist largely of water. It is possible that this is true for the rapid gain of the first few days of the diet. However, metabolic observations have demonstrated conclusively that the net result is a substantial increase in useful tissue rather than water. This was indicated by the high retentions of nitrogen, calcium, and phosphorus and by the increased excretion of creatinine. It was observed that when the weight increased 20 per cent, the creatinine excretion increased 35 to 40 per cent.

These observations demonstrate that the malnourished child utilizes a high dextrose, low fat diet much better than the average normal diet and far better than a high fat diet. The same is true to a far greater degree with a child with celiac disease. It seems entirely possible that malnutrition itself may be an important determining factor in the production of celiac disease.

Malnourished children practically always are ingesting a diet which provides considerably less energy than the requirement. It is entirely logical to think of such a child in terms of a greater food intake. It may be logical also to think of cream and other fats as providing the additional energy in small bulk. With great frequency one finds that dietary increases have been advised along these lines. The observations of the preceding discussion demonstrate the fallacy of this type of advice. Much greater success will be attained with the high dextrose diet and at a lower energy intake.

Iron

The infant at the time of birth has a small store of iron. The amount varies greatly but does not average more than approximately 15 mg. or an amount which would be necessary for the formation of about 50 c.c. of blood. For approximately two months after birth a rapid destruction of hemoglobin occurs. As a result, from 150 to 200 mg. of iron is liberated. It is the general concept that all of this iron is stored for use in hemoglobin formation and that this amount is sufficient to supply the iron needs of the infant until six months of age. On a theoretical basis it is true that if all of this iron were conserved, the supply would be just sufficient for the needs up to six months. However, about 30 per cent of the iron freed from hemoglobin during the first two months is lost. During the period of hemoglobin destruction all infants are in negative iron balance. The diet supplies approximately 0.75 mg. of iron daily and the excretion varies from 1.5 to a high value of 4 mg. daily, producing an average negative balance of 1.35 mg. of iron daily. The stored remainder, equivalent to 300 to 375 c.c. of blood, would be sufficient to supply the iron needs until the age of about 4.5 months only if it were well conserved. However, babies receiving the usual milk formulas without additional iron are in negative iron balance during this period, and the reserve supply is exhausted before the theoretically calculated age. On this basis it becomes obvious that the diet of the infant requires consideration as regards iron considerably before six months of age.

The amount of hemoglobin present during infancy is less than at a later time. It is the general custom to consider this condition as normal. When statistical surveys are made and averages determined, these averages do not necessarily represent the normal. The finding of dental caries in 80 per cent of all school children would not be considered normal merely because it is an average of existing conditions. Elvehjem has found that, by giving an abundance of iron-containing foods to a selected group of infants, the average hemoglobin was more than 1 mg. to 100 c.c. greater throughout infancy than usual average values.

In order to maintain an infant in iron equilibrium, it has been found that the daily ingestion of 0.5 mg. per kilogram in the form of readily available iron is necessary. It has been calculated that an average retention of 0.75 mg. daily is necessary to maintain normal hemoglobin formation. In order to attain this amount of retention, an average intake of 0.7 mg. per kilogram is necessary. These statements apply at all ages from seven weeks to one year of age. A general impression that babies under six months of age do not use ingested irons seems to be erroneous. Intakes of iron greater than 0.7 mg. per kilogram lead to greater retentions up to an intake of approximately 1 mg. per kilogram, above which amount little or no increase in retention is to be observed. Ingestion of iron in excess of this amount not only is without benefit, but may be actually harmful. It has been shown quite definitely for the chick that the feeding of iron in amounts comparable to the high dosages recommended at times by physicians for severe anemia produces within 1 to 2 weeks severe low phosphorus rickets, with death of all the chicks within three weeks.

On the basis of the preceding discussion the iron requirement of the infant may be met satisfactorily by the ingestion of 5 mg. daily from three to six months of age and 10 mg. daily from six to twelve months. These amounts will permit an average retention of 0.75 mg. daily, an amount calculated to be necessary.

Cow's milk varies greatly in its iron content, depending on the method of handling. As the milk comes from the cow, it contains approximately 0.2 mg. per liter. With transport in tinned iron containers it may acquire a content of 2.5 mg. per liter. The average of values obtained by six different observers is 0.6 mg. per liter. The usual milk formula of the artificially fed baby, including the customary orange juice supplement, may be relied upon to supply approximately 1 mg. of iron daily. If no other source of iron is made available, the infant will have a definite and often a marked deficiency by six months of age.

It is the custom of many to add egg yolk to the diet at the fourth month or even earlier. An egg yolk contributes approximately 1 mg. of iron. This amount in addition to the formula would still leave a deficit, even if the iron of the egg were all utilized. Balance experiments have shown, however, that the iron balance when egg yolk is fed is little different from that of the same diet without egg. The reason for this is not clear, unless it may be accounted for by the sulphur content.

Vegetables have had an extensive usage in infant feeding. One of the functions is to supply iron. They are often added to the diet at a relatively early age. It is necessary to concede to vegetables a certain usefulness. However, in the case of spinach we seem to have a product of overestimated value. Canned puréed spinach ready for use contains approximately 0.35 mg. of iron to the ounce. With a large serving of spinach the amount of iron obtained by an infant would be from 0.5 to 1 mg. This amount of iron would not contribute greatly to the total requirement even if it were all utilized. Balance experiments have shown that not only is the iron of spinach not utilized, but the already negative balance of the infant is made greater. Presumably this effect is produced by the oxalate content. Spinach has the same effect on the calcium balance, probably for the same reason. Spinach seems to serve little useful purpose in supplying the mineral needs of the body, Popeye to the contrary notwithstanding.

The proprietary cereal food pablum contains 6.8 mg. of iron to the ounce of dry preparation. This is a higher proportion of iron than is found in any of the natural foods. Much of this iron is in the powdered alfalfa content. Balance experiments show that the iron of pablum is well utilized. The utilization is better than that with egg yolk and the same as that with ferric ammonium citrate.

It has long been recognized that iron ammonium citrate is well utilized. This material is not a definite crystalline substance, but varies somewhat in its iron content. One cubic centimeter of a 1 per cent solution contains 1.5 to 2 mg. of iron. In order to meet the iron requirement of the infant up to one year of age,

5 c.c. of a 1 per cent solution is ample. This supplies from 7.5 to 10 mg. of iron. More than this amount is unnecessary and amounts greatly in excess are likely to be definitely harmful. Though babies need more iron than most of them get, the overzealous administration of iron will do more harm than good.

Vitamin D

Vitamin D as it occurs in nature or is produced by irradiation is of two varieties, one of animal origin related to cholesterol and the other of vegetable origin related to ergosterol. On a rat unit basis these two varieties have markedly unequal values for the chick and to a lesser degree for the human infant. The evidence may be interpreted to indicate that approximately 1.5 times as many rat units of vegetable source vitamin D are required as of animal source vitamin D to produce the same effects in the human.

The smallest amount of vitamin D recommended to the public as being adequate is the amount found in irradiated milk, which contains 135 U. S. P. units to the quart. This amount of vitamin D will prevent and ultimately cure rickets in most instances. It has been found also that cod liver oil concentrate dispersed in milk and cod liver oil separately have the same effects as irradiated milk when administered on an equal rat unit basis.

Rickets prevention has had almost universal acceptance as a criterion of adequacy of vitamin D. If this is an acceptable criterion, 60 to 135 units of animal source vitamin D constitutes an adequate amount, instead of the 1,000 units or more in the recommended dose of 3 teaspoonfuls of cod liver oil. The discrepancy between these two recommendations is more than 600 per cent.

Evidence has been produced to show that rickets prevention is not a criterion of sufficient vitamin D. Babies receiving irradiated milk or its equivalent do not grow as well as those receiving a larger amount of vitamin D. Balance experiments show significantly smaller retentions of calcium and phosphorus with irradiated milk than when the amount of vitamin D in 1 teaspoonful of cod liver oil is administered. If babies receiving irradiated milk have inferior growth and inadequate calcium retentions, this amount of vitamin D cannot be accepted as satisfactory.

The minimum amount of vitamin D which will permit satisfactory growth and calcium retentions has not been determined, but it has been shown that the amount in 1 teaspoonful of cod liver oil is ample and perhaps in excess of the minimum requirement. It is indicated also that amounts of cod liver oil greater than 1 teaspoonful will cause no further increase in growth or in calcium retention. Apparently the maximum beneficial effect is obtained with a 1 teaspoonful daily dose.

Vitamin A

The general impression has obtained that vitamin A deficiency is infrequent in our general population. This opinion has been based on the relative infrequency of xerophthalmia and of night blindness. Apparently xerophthalmia depends on an extreme deficiency, and it is not surprising that this condition is uncommon. Because of the necessity for a marked deficiency in order to produce xerophthalmia, this condition could not be used as a criterion for lesser but significant degrees of vitamin A deficiency. Similarly, night blindness of sufficient degree to be a cause of complaint cannot be a good criterion. Conclusions based on questionnaire surveys concerning the frequency of night blindness must take into consideration the fact that routine ophthalmologic examinations do not detect night blindness. It is diagnosed usually only after complaint is made and special tests applied. It seems probable that significant degrees of night blindness of which the subject is aware are more common than is usually assumed. It is certain that moderate degrees of night blindness of which the subject may be unaware are exceedingly common.

When a special test for dark adaptation is applied, departures from the normal are found with considerable frequency. It is easily demonstrated that at least in the great majority of instances these abnormal results are dependent on vitamin A deficiency; when vitamin A is administered, the subjects develop normal dark adaptation. The great frequency with which vitamin A deficiency is found by this procedure would seem to demand attention. If anything like half of the children of this country are ingesting diets deficient in this respect, some kind of educational propaganda is indicated. It has been determined that a good diet containing ample vitamin A can easily be selected from common readily available foods. When such a diet is used, apparently vitamin A concentrates are not necessary. This fact being recognized, what should be the status of vitamin A concentrates? Should they be recommended for routine use or should their use be discouraged? Should vitamin A additions to foods be permitted?

Educational propaganda directed by nutritionists and physicians to the mass of people at large has had and for a long time may be expected to have only a very limited effect. Propaganda sufficiently extensive to be effective is economically impracticable, and to a considerable extent an urgent incentive is lacking. If we await optimistically the time when all of the people will select good diets because of this type of instruction, many will continue to have dietary deficiencies indefinitely.

On the other hand, if we accept and encourage the commercial exploitation of this need, a potent incentive with economic backing and considerable initiative immediately comes into the picture. Results will be more far-reaching and will be attained more quickly. If people persist in selecting foods containing little or no vitamin A, what possible harm can come from additions of this substance to certain of the most common foods selected for this purpose because of their appropriateness as a vehicle for vitamin A and because of their widespread use?

Observations on the Anti-Infective Action of Vitamin A and on Moderate Deficiency of Vitamin C

S. W. Clausen, M.D., Rochester, N. Y.

Within the past few years, exact knowledge of the chemical and physical properties of vitamins A, B_1, C, and D has accumulated with breathless speed. Methods for quantitative chemical estimation of carotene, the precursor of vitamin A, for vitamin A and for vitamin C are now available, methods which surpass in delicacy, exactness, and speed the biologic methods. For these reasons, workers sometimes ignore the fact that the chemical and physical methods are specific for the substances in question only when certain criteria are met. If not, conclusions based upon the use of the newer technic will be fallacious. Under properly controlled conditions, however, clinical results otherwise unattainable must result. With the pure vitamins now available, we shall be able eventually to settle with certainty questions of specificity; to determine the actual requirements of these vitamins under various conditions of age, sex, and disease; to discover states of "subclinical" deficiency; and to ascertain the upper limits of safe dosage. Moreover, with pure vitamins, it is possible to avoid the untoward effects which may result from substances which accompany the vitamins in nature.

Our own work has been concerned with the analysis of fluids and tissues of the body for carotene, xanthophyll, vitamin A, and vitamin C. Two questions will be considered: (1) the anti-infective action of vitamin A, and (2) the application of the newer methods to the study of deficiency of vitamin C.

The Anti-Infective Action of Vitamin A

McCollum in 1917 first showed that rats with xerophthalmia were liable to spontaneous infections. This work has been confirmed and extended by many other workers. It has been shown that the spontaneous infections of the respiratory tract are associated with the metaplasia of the respiratory epithelium characteristic of severe deficiency of vitamin A. The lowering of resistance to experimental infection with the paratyphoid group of organisms in rats may be due in part to metaplasia of epithelium; but, since the barriers of the liver, spleen, and bone marrow failed to prevent bacteremia in the feeding experiments of Lassen, it is evident that some factor other than epithelial metaplasia must be involved. In these experiments the infections were induced after the deficiency had fully developed. Bradford and Boynton, and later McClung and Winters, showed that rats receiving diets deficient in vitamin A became susceptible to infection before loss of weight or any other sign of deficiency developed. This suggests that mild forms of vitamin A deficiency may be a cause of susceptibility to infection. This suggestion receives support from the studies of Webster and Pritchett, who showed that mice raised for generations on a diet hitherto considered adequate were less resistant to inoculation with mouse-typhoid bacilli than were other mice whose diet was supplemented by the addition of cod liver oil or butter. Topley, Greenwood, and Wilson were apparently unable to confirm this work, but in their experiments, the deficient diets were not begun until relatively late in the lives of the mice. In all the work so far mentioned, no analyses were made of the tissues for vitamin A. Some observations of McCoy and McCoord may serve to reconcile the different conclusions of the authors mentioned. In their work, rats of varying age were depleted of vitamin A, as shown by a negative Price-Carr test for vitamin A, and then infected with trichinosis. The young rats were invariably more susceptible than the controls which received supplements of halibut liver oil. The older rats—even though their livers were devoid of vitamin A—were only slightly more susceptible than the controls. More work must be done, using other infecting organisms, various portals of entry, and other hosts. The study of the effect of a deficiency in fetal life or in early infancy, followed by normal diet, would also be of great clinical significance. The experimental work may be summarized by the statements: Frank deficiency of vitamin A in most animals leads to increased susceptibility to spontaneous and to artificial infections. There is no evidence that animals with adequate stores of vitamin A may be rendered more resistant to infection by administering carotene or vitamin A, although there is some evidence that some of the standard diets in use may be so improved.

With this brief discussion of experimental results, we may now consider the evidence for the anti-infective action of vitamin A in man. Bloch in 1928 reported his very extensive observations of xerophthalmia in Denmark and called attention to the frequency of severe infection in his 109 patients. Later he stated his belief that the liability to infection persisted even after cure of xerophthalmia. A liability to infection in xerophthalmia is, however, not evident in the reports of Spense or of Blackfan and Wolbach. Efforts to lessen the incidence and severity of infections in infants without xerophthalmia by the administration of cod liver oil, concentrates of vitamin A, or carotene have on the whole been unsuccessful. Erben reports success; Barenberg and Lewis, and Hess, Lewis and Barenberg report complete failure. Helen McKay finds no increase in resistance to respiratory infections but reports a decrease in infections of the skin. We have noticed in the reports of the work of Hess and his colleagues that only 7 per cent of the infants were under the age of six months and that the diet in very early infancy was not described. Therefore, we have analyzed in our own cases the feeding histories from the age of two months. We find that the addition of cod liver oil to the diet by the age of two months confers no increase of resistance to infection during the first six months of life but that the addition of cod liver oil by the age of two months and the inclusion of vegetables after the age of five months appears to confer considerable resistance between the ages of six and twenty-four months. This effect disappears in large part after the age of two years. The criticism that the control cases may not be comparable with those receiving additions of vitamin A is difficult to meet, for these cases are largely children of families who failed to follow all kinds of advice. The results, however, suggest that the infant in early life may require very much larger amounts of vitamin A than in later life. Our own work confirms the findings of several other workers that the liver at birth, especially in the case of premature infants, contains very little vitamin A and that colostrum is exceptionally rich in carotene and in vitamin A. We are at present studying the vitamin A requirements of the fetus. The blood of the umbilical vein always contains more carotene than does that of the umbilical artery, whereas the average concentrations of vitamin A in vein and artery are equal. A conservative, if not very accurate, estimate shows that at the time of birth, the fetus may be receiving 1000 international units of vitamin A as carotene per kilogram of weight each day. We are planning to study the effects of early administration of vitamin A upon subsequent tendency to infection in a carefully controlled series of cases.

The influence of administering vitamin A to older children and adults upon resistance to infection has been the subject of many conflicting reports. Mellanby and his coworkers in 1931 claimed that a preparation of vitamins A and D would lessen the incidence of postpartum fever and applied to vitamin A the unfortunate adjective "anti-infective." The term "anti-infective vitamin" has served to stimulate the publication of much uncritical work. Holmes, Pigott, Sawyer, and Comstock administered one tablespoonful of cod liver oil a day to a volunteer group of industrial workers. The incident of common colds and the loss of time from work was less than in a group of "controls" who refused to take cod liver oil. Ellison administered a concentrate containing vitamins A and D in 600 alternate cases of measles. Although the incidence of pneumonia and of otitis media was the same in both groups, the mortality was 3.7 per cent in the group receiving the vitamins and 8.7 per cent in the other. The fact that the two groups occupied separate wards renders the evidence less convincing. Recently several other authors have claimed that the administration of carotene lessened the incidence and severity of respiratory infections.

Equally impressive evidence has been recorded that the administration of vitamin A during an infection does not lessen its severity. Sutliff, Place, and Segod administered 400,000 U. S. P. units of vitamin A per day to 509 children with scarlet fever. The incidence of otitis media was 9.4 per cent. The expected incidence was 11.3 per cent. Alternate cases were not treated.

We have made a similar study, using carotene in scarlet fever, with no beneficial results. Studies of the blood showed that the carotene had been absorbed, although the level of blood carotene was less than that which was produced by the same dose in convalescent children.

For several years we have administered carotene in children living in foster homes. An effort has been made to keep the experimental and control groups as nearly alike as possible. We have been unable to observe any lessening of the incidence of infection or any decrease in its severity in the treated children.

Two chief criticisms can be directed against the clinical reports: (1) It is difficult to be certain that the experimental and the control groups are comparable; and (2) criteria have not been furnished that a deficiency of vitamin A existed in the subjects. From a study of carotinoid pigments of the blood in a large group of children, together with clinical histories of susceptibility to colds, we have concluded that not more than 5 or 10 per cent of the children *might* have been benefited by the administration of carotene. It is obvious that if subjects for the administration of carotene are selected at random, any beneficial effects may not appear on statistical analysis. We need an extensive experiment in which children with habitually low blood carotene are selected for a controlled test. Analysis of the liver, which is the great storehouse of vitamin A, often shows a marked decrease in persons who have died of severe infection. This decrease in vitamin A is not sufficient evidence that these persons had suffered from a deficiency of vitamin A before the infection. We have found that the stores of vitamin A in the livers of rats are depleted by infection and that the degree of depletion depends upon the severity and the duration of the infection.

It may be concluded that the administration of carotene or of vitamin A cannot be expected to increase resistance to infection in older persons who are not suffering from deficiency of vitamin A. Sufficient studies have not been reported of the anti-infective value of vitamin A in persons who actually are deficient. On the other hand, there is evidence that the young and rapidly growing infant may require abundant vitamin A in order to develop resistance to infection in early life. The actual requirements of vitamin A for this purpose are not known.

Test for Deficiency of Vitamin C

In clinical conditions supposed to be due to deficiency of vitamin C, four diagnostic tests have been proposed:

1. *The "Therapeutic Test."*—The condition must be relieved by the administration of vitamin C. The therapeutic test may be carried out with pure cevitamic acid. A number of reports have appeared on the cure of scurvy and the relief of prescorbutic symptoms by this method. Some years ago, Theobald Smith observed that guinea pigs during the winter were subject to pneumonia, which tendency disappeared as soon as fresh fodder was available. These experiments have been extended by von Euler, who has been able to show that fresh vegetables and fruits contain the anti-infective agent even after the vitamin C in them has been destroyed. These experiments are mentioned in order to show that relief of symptoms with fruit juices may not be proof that these symptoms are due to deficiency of vitamin C.

2. *The Capillary Resistance.*—Göthlin and his coworkers, using a standardized technic for the Leeds-Rumpel test, report decreased capillary resistance in persons consuming a diet low in vitamin C. Dalldorf, using measured negative pressure, reaches the same conclusion. Both investigators find that the administration of vitamin C increased capillary resistance. The reports of Greene and of Toverud fail to confirm the claims of these authors. Abt, Farmer, and Epstein find no relationship between the capillary resistance and the level of reduced cevitamic acid in the plasma. Hawley, Stephens, and Anderson, using a modification of the negative pressure method, observed no increase in capillary resistance in subjects after receiving large amounts of orange juice or of cebione (Merck). In these studies the daily output of cevitamic acid in the urine was measured. Hawley has observed one case of scurvy in which a marked and prompt increase in capillary resistance followed the oral administration of cebione and another, in which the capillary resistance was normal. She has also observed one case of thrombopenic purpura in which there was a close correlation of capillary resistance with the intake of vitamin C over a period of many months. In several other cases of purpura no such correlation was observed. Her observations seem to indicate that the discordant reports in the literature are not due to differences in technic or interpretation, but depend upon factors not understood. It is obvious that the tests of capillary resistance are not reliable indicators of vitamin C deficiency at the present time.

3. *Chemical Analysis of Urine for Vitamin C.*—Under proper conditions, titration of urine with the indicator 2:6-dichlorphenolindophenol is an accurate measure of its content of vitamin C. The iodine titration, reliable for certain fruits and vegetables, gives high results with urine, mainly owing to the presence of sulphur compounds. Using the dye method, Harris and his colleagues have shown that the urinary output of vitamin C is an accurate measure of the intake of vitamin C. The claim of Beszonoff that infants under four months of age are able to synthesize vitamin C appears to be unfounded. Abt and his colleagues believe that the excre-

tion of vitamin C, observed by Beszonoff, is wholly explained by the slow elimination of the stored vitamin. Hawley is at present engaged in a study of the vitamin C content of human colostrum and milk. She has shown that an increase follows within an hour after the ingestion of orange juice. She is also observing the output of cevitamic acid in the urine of infants on various analyzed diets and finding a close correlation between intake and output. She finds no evidence that the young infant is able to synthesize its own vitamin C. We have observed that patients receiving diets for gastric ulcer are invariably undersaturated with vitamin C. In nephritis the output of vitamin C is likely to be low. This is in part due to the rapid disappearance of vitamin C in the urine itself. The acid-base balance of this diet also affects the output of vitamin C when the intake is constant. Hawley and her coworkers have conducted an extensive experiment showing clearly that the measured output of vitamin C is reduced when the urine is alkaline. They have shown that the loss of vitamin, due to its destruction of oxidation in a medium as alkaline as the urine in question, does not wholly explain their results. An experiment involving the analysis of tissues of guinea pigs on various diets is in progress in the attempt to account for the findings. It is apparent that analysis of urine is an important and reliable method of investigation.

4. *Analysis of Blood and Tissues.*—The reports of Abt and his colleagues indicate that analysis of blood may become a satisfactory method for diagnosis of scurvy and prescorbutic conditions. Our own observations, few in number, fully confirm this opinion. Unpublished results of Clayton show that the tonsils contain abundant cevitamic acid and that the concentration depends upon the previous diet. She has observed a decrease in chronic infections but has not been able to show exceptionally low values in rheumatic fever.

Conclusions

The newer chemical and physical methods for quantitative estimation of vitamins A and C afford useful tools for the investigation of clinical problems. They will prove most fruitful as a supplement to accurate clinical observation.

GENERAL DISCUSSION

DR. JOHN ZAHORSKY (St. Louis).—I desire to bring up the question of overgrowth in infants. The high protein content of modern milk mixtures fortified by concentrated vitamin has a distinct tendency to product an overgrowth. It is very common now to obtain the same growth in the first year which we formerly believed required two years. Moreover, the fontanel is closed in so many of these infants at one year or less. The brain, however, does not quite keep pace with this somatic growth. The question whether this overgrowth during infancy is ultimately advantageous or detrimental to the child requires serious consideration. In animals the growing period to maturity can be shortened by heavy feeding. Are we going to shorten the period of childhood by this superalimentation?

In a study of 50 infants who were overgrown, we find a distinct tendency for the weight to approach the normal after the infant is eighteen months old. This makes it necessary that the child stop growing and, I believe, is the prime impulse in the nervous anorexia so common at this period. The administration of vitamins A and C regardless of the rate of growth seems entirely irrational. The child stops eating but he has to swallow viosterol. I am discouraging the routine use of the concentrated vitamin during the summer months and after the third year.

CHAIRMAN MARRIOTT.—Dr. Zahorsky is to be congratulated on the excellent nutritional results he obtained. The good nutritional results with generous feedings last to adult life.

The observations of Gray on boys in a private school showed that children of the better classes, well fed from the age of infancy, averaged distinctly larger than accepted normal standards. We know further that children today with better methods of nutrition are decidedly taller and heavier than the children of ten or fifteen years ago.

DR. JEANS.—Mental tests show higher ratings for babies who grow well. For several seasons it has been observed that babies kept on low vitamin D intake for experimental purposes did not do well. I think that 1 dram of cod liver oil is enough even under poor conditions if the food is good.

DR. JAMES A. WHEELER (NEWTON, KAN.).—Dr. Zahorsky stated that he wonders what will happen to the mental side of children by the newer feeding standards. I have been informed by several men who have worked in the child guidance centers that the problem is not strictly confined to the child but is mainly one with the parents. Most of these parents were fed under earlier methods.

DR. JOHN R. VONACHEN (PEORIA, ILL.).—Since Dr. Marriott mentioned the possible relationship between a high protein intake and premature senility, it occurred to me that there might be some connection between this and progeria. I remember the case of progeria because of its unusualness in that this child had taken between two and three quarts of lactic acid milk up to the age of almost three years. I saw her when she was about twelve years of age, not because of the high lactic acid milk intake but for the progeria. This child was so fond of the lactic acid that she preferred it to other milks. I mention this because of its unusual occurrence rather than it had anything to do with the progeria. However, I would like to ask Dr. Marriott if there could be any possible relationship.

CHAIRMAN MARRIOTT.—I doubt if there could be any relationship.

DR. MAURICE L. BLATT (CHICAGO).—What is the advantage of excess weight with monosaccharides?

DR. JEANS.—The large gains reported were in children who were 20 to 30 per cent underweight. Gains can be made better with a high dextrose diet than with fat. The increased gain tended to cease when the child had attained normal weight.

DR. BLATT.—In considering the weight of a child, its chronologic age, its height, whether it was premature or full term, and its build have to be taken into consideration. Children usually resemble their ancestors in stature. It does not seem important that a child be given additional food for no other purpose than to put on weight. In my experience, thin children enjoy quite as good health and are quite as long lived as are fat ones. Lack of weight due to disease is, in my opinion, not well treated by feeding carbohydrate for the purpose of increasing weight. A gain in weight occurring in a child ill with an infection is usually an indication of the child's general improvement.

DR. ARTHUR F. ABT (CHICAGO).—What significance does Dr. Marriott attach to the relationship, stressed by L. F. Meyer of Berlin, between fat and carbohydrate which is a 1 to 2 ratio in breast milk? Meyer contends that the failure of every effort with straight cow's milk has been solely due to its 1:1 ratio. He further believes that fat restricts, while carbohydrate favors, water retention and that for the normal metabolism of the human infant the 1:2 ratio of fat to carbohydrate is necessary.

CHAIRMAN MARRIOTT.—Most infants do somewhat better when the proportion of carbohydrate exceeds that of fat, but that this is not necessarily the case has been repeatedly demonstrated in the case of diabetic infants and children, in whom excellent nutrition has been maintained on high fat diets containing a minimum of carbohydrate.

DR. JAY I. DURAND (SEATTLE, WASH.).—How much milk should a child take?

CHAIRMAN MARRIOTT.—I do not know. It depends upon the child. If one refers to the experiments of Dr. Clara Davis and the experience of children in the tropics, it is recognized that one gets good results with a varied diet.

DR. JEANS.—The criterion may be the calcium intake rather than other food. Milk is the chief source of calcium.

DR. EVON ROSENSTERN (BERLIN, GERMANY).—At one time our children were getting a liter or more of milk. They were fat and had poor resistance. Lately we have given less milk, one-half liter, and more vegetables. The state of health on this schedule is better. The height of the population in Germany during the last fifty years has increased about 5 cm. In recent years the height of children was lessened. There were various theories as to the cause of that. It was thought to be due to lack of food after the war or due to rickets that many children developed before and after the war. We studied the growth of breast-fed and artificially fed babies and noted that the calcification centers developed earlier with artificial feeding.

DR. ZAHORSKY.—Does the incidence of rickets in infancy and early childhood have a tendency to produce shorter adults? I have a distinct impression that moderate rickets without deformity has no effect on the final height of the person. Or is this due to the fact that rickets occur generally in the infant who has a natural tendency to be tall?

CHAIRMAN MARRIOTT.—Many individuals who have had severe rickets during infancy and early childhood remain permanently dwarfed.

DR. JEANS.—I think that growth will be compensated later if the rickets was not too severe. I am not sure that the improvement in children referred to by Dr. Rosenstern is due to less milk or to other food given.

DR. B. FEINBERG (PROVIDENCE, R. I.).—I wonder whether Dr. Marriott has had any experience with small doses of thyroid in premature infants?

CHAIRMAN MARRIOTT.—We have not had any experience in the use of thyroid in normal premature infants.

DR. MARTHA M. ELIOT (NEW HAVEN, CONN.).—1. Dr. Jeans has indicated the efficacy of vitamin D in relation to growth. Does he think 1 teaspoon of cod liver oil will provide a sufficient margin of safety?

2. If 400 units are believed to be necessary for optimum calcium retention, should additional vitamin D be given to infants and children besides that contained in irradiated milk?

3. What is the easiest way to give the required amount of iron to infants? Is ferric ammonium citrate the best form? Should it be recommended routinely in well baby conferences, or should it be considered as a drug to be prescribed only by physicians? Would it be your opinion that the Children's Bureau should recommend the prophylactic use of iron in their publications?

DR. JEANS.—1. From our data it is indicated that when 1 teaspoonful of cod liver oil is ingested, the retention of calcium and phosphorus approaches closely or equals the maximum to be obtained. Presumably nothing is to be accomplished by larger amounts of vitamin D, and 1 teaspoonful of cod liver oil provides a sufficient margin of safety.

2. It is my opinion that the amount of vitamin D in irradiated milk as now produced is insufficient for the best nutrition of the infant and that additional vitamin D should be given. The requirement of the child past infancy is not known. It is the general belief that the child requires less than the infant, but the evidence for any belief is meager.

3. Much thought must be given to the infant's diet in order that sufficient iron may be obtained from food sources alone. It would seem a measure of safety to add one of the iron salts. Iron in the amount we have discussed could scarcely be considered harmful. Probably iron and ammonium citrate should not be stated as the best preparation, but it has seemed entirely satisfactory. The use of iron in the manner discussed should be considered from the nutritional point of view and could be recommended appropriately by anyone competent to give nutritional advice. I know of no reason why the Children's Bureau should not recommend the prophylactic use of iron if the director so desires.

DR. FRANK H. DOUGLASS (Seattle, Wash.).—When can we stop giving cod liver oil? When does rickets stop?

DR. JEANS.—It is our own preference to continue the use of cod liver oil throughout the period of childhood. The additional amount of both vitamins A and D may be considered advantageous.

Though rickets of the type caused by vitamin D deficiency is uncommon after two years of age, increased, and presumably more desirable calcium retentions are obtained, at least during the winter months, when cod liver oil or some equivalent is ingested. Increased calcium retentions appear to have a direct relationship to the prevention of tooth decay, which is so prevalent in childhood.

DR. FEINBERG.—1. What are the relative merits of vitamin D present in certified milk from cows on a ration of irradiated yeast and milk irradiated directly?

2. Do you feel that additional vitamin D in form of cod liver oil is necessary?

3. Do vitamin D concentrates have the same effect as vitamin D in the form of cod liver oil?

4. The iron question is very interesting. Do you feel that the comparatively small dose of iron and copper, such as is present in some of the proprietary sugars, as Abbott's cofron-maltose, is sufficient to prevent a negative iron balance during the first few months of life?

5. Are large doses of iron given to the mother during the latter months of pregnancy effective in preventing nutritional anemia in the infant?

DR. JEANS.—1. Yeast milk is usually produced with 430 U. S. P. units of vitamin D to the quart and irradiated milk, with 135 units to the quart. Some have considered that the relative value of these two milks is directly proportionate to the vitamin D unitage. Even if yeast milk proves to be less potent than irradiated milk, on a unit-for-unit basis, the difference is not great and a marked advantage still exists in favor of yeast milk because of the greater vitamin D content.

2. It is my opinion that the amount of vitamin D in irradiated milk is not sufficient to meet the needs of the infant and consequently additional vitamin D from some source is indicated. The amount of vitamin D in yeast milk probably is sufficient.

3. For all practical purposes, it may be stated that vitamin D concentrates have the same effect as the vitamin D of cod liver oil. When the dose is reduced to minimum levels the probability that vitamin D of vegetable source is less potent than that of animal source must be considered. It is generally agreed that at the minimum effective level more units as viosterol are required than as cod liver oil. With customary dosages, however, this difference need not be considered because both materials are commonly administered above the level which produces the maximum physiologic effect. In considering a choice among vitamin D preparations, one should not lose sight of a possible need for vitamin A.

4. I do not know the iron content of cofron-maltose, but if it supplies 10 to 25 mg. of iron a day, as I believe it does, this amount of iron is ample not only to prevent a negative balance but also to allow a good retention after two months of age. A negative balance during the period of hemoglobin destruction in the first two months does not have the same significance as it does later.

5. The store of iron in the liver at birth depends appreciably upon the iron intake of the mother. When the mother's intake has been low the store of the infant may be negligible and also the amount of hemoglobin less than normal. On the other hand, the liver storage is not great under the most favorable conditions. The later storage from hemoglobin destruction is always greater and therefore more important than the amount present at birth. It has been found that ingestion of 20 mg. of iron daily by the mother during pregnancy permits ample storage for her and the infant.

DR. EARL W. MAY (DETROIT).—1. Dr. Jeans, have you used irradiated milk higher than 135 units?

2. We have been using irradiated milk with 150 units and have found it most effective in the prevention of rickets and the maintenance of normal growth in the normal full-term infant.

DR. JEANS.—1. We have not. Such a milk has not been available to us.

2. The difference between 135 and 150 units to the quart is not great, and a marked difference in results would not be expected.

What is normal growth? The growth curves of Stuart published in 1933 and of Kornfeld published in 1929 show greater rates of growth than those published by Baldwin in 1921. This indicates that nutritional conditions are improving. Even the more recent studies of Kornfeld and Stuart have included individuals who had been receiving poor nutritional care, as well as those whose care had been good. Perhaps we should think of the ideal growth curve only in terms of good nutritional and hygienic care. In such case the rate of growth will be greater than that recorded in the Stuart and Kornfeld studies. Thus, good or optimal growth represents more rapid growth than the published averages now available.

DR. BLATT.—Three children in my practice receiving vitamin D milk have had gastrointestinal disturbances associated with diarrhea. Their diarrhea ceased on ordinary pasteurized milk, but they did not progress as satisfactorily as do most of the children whom we feed without the use of this irradiated product. They were more irritable, muscle and bone development was not as satisfactory, nor did they have the regularity of weight curve increase which I am accustomed to see in my practice.

DR. JEANS.—We have had no experience with irradiated milk causing diarrhea.

DR. ROGER MOORE (ST. JOSEPH, MO.).—Dr. Jeans stated that 1 dram of cod liver oil was sufficient. Will there be a deficiency of vitamin A in such a dose?

DR. JEANS.—I do not know the infant's requirement for vitamin A, but there has been no obvious evidence of vitamin A deficiency with such a dose.

DR. F. W. SCHLUTZ (CHICAGO).—What is the comparative prevalence of night blindness in urban and rural children, and what relation has this prevalence to the diet?

DR. JEANS.—In our survey of Iowa children subnormal dark adaptation was found in 26 per cent of the strictly rural group, 53 per cent of the village group, and in from 56 to 79 per cent of the urban group, the variation in the last group depending upon the economic level. It may readily be assumed that the prevalence found has a direct relationship to the type of diet, inasmuch as improvement in the diet nearly always corrects the difficulty.

DR. BLATT.—1. Is night blindness higher in cases with infection?

2. Does carotene drop in the winter?

DR. CLAUSEN.—1. Cases with infection have a low carotene perhaps due partly to lack of appetite.

2. Carotene is low in the winter and rises in March and April to a plateau with a slight rise and then a fall to January.

DR. DURAND.—1. How old were the children with night blindness?

2. Did any children with night blindness get cod liver oil?

3. Did you find more infection in the group with night blindness?

DR. JEANS.—1. The ages of the children with night blindness ranged from six to fourteen years. Children at other ages were not examined.

2. None of the children with night blindness were receiving cod liver oil.

3. No observations were made concerning the incidence of infections in children with night blindness.

DR. WHEELER.—I should like to ask Dr. Jeans if after further observation on vitamin A experimentation he is still of the opinion that mineral oil destroyed the absorption of vitamin A in the intestine.

DR. JEANS.—Mineral oil has a very decided effect in depleting the body of vitamin A, particularly when the intake of vitamin A is low or borderline as compared to the probable requirement.

DR. WHEELER.—Can the photometer test be used as a standard for determining vitamin A deficiency?

DR. JEANS.—The photometer is used as a means for detecting abnormal dark adaptation. Poor adaptation is caused by vitamin A deficiency in most, but not in all, instances. With these few exceptions, which are recognizable by ophthalmologic examination, the photometric test can be used as a standard for determining vitamin A deficiency. A new photometer is now available, which permits greater precision and ease of use than the one formerly employed.

DR. DOUGLASS.—What is carotene besides vitamin A and pigment? I ask this question because of the favorable results we have seen in cases of albinism in which the administration of carotene in oil has increased the color of the retina. Is it due to pigment or vitamin A?

DR. CLAUSEN.—The several isomeric carotenes are produced only by plants. They are hydrocarbons with the formula $C_{40}H_{56}$. One molecule of beta-carotene is transformed in the animal into two molecules of vitamin A, an alcohol with the formula $C_{20}H_{29}OH$. It is not yet known whether carotene as such performs any special function in the animal body aside from its function as precursor of vitamin A. When large quantities of carotene are ingested, especially when the carotene is not destroyed, the skin may become pigmented; it is possible that the retina may share in this pigmentation and that the process would be more apparent in an albino than in a normal person.

DR. MARGARET NICHOLSON (WASHINGTON, D. C.).—Is cod liver oil better than viosterol? Does the absence of vitamin A in viosterol make a difference?

DR. CLAUSEN.—Comparative studies by Hess and Lewis indicated that infants receiving cod liver oil had about as frequent and severe infections as infants receiving viosterol and that large additions of vitamin A to the diet in the form of carotene or halibut liver oil conferred no increase of resistance to infection. They concluded that the milk of the diet furnished enough vitamin A. However, most of the infants studied by them were over six months of age. We have, therefore, compared the incidence and severity of infection in infants who received cod liver oil at least from the third month with the incidence and severity of infection in infants who did not, and we have found an apparent considerable increase of resistance during the latter half of the first year of life. Our work is open to the criticism that other factors than lack of vitamin A may play rôles in the control group of infants. I feel that your question can be answered only when we know more about the requirements for vitamin A in the early months of life.

DR. MAURICE J. LONSWAY (ST. LOUIS).—I should like to ask Dr. Jeans if he has seen any bad effects with larger doses of iron. We give larger doses than he advises to premature infants, and it is our impression that they do quite well with no observable ill effects.

DR. JEANS.—Doses in excess of 25 mg. a day probably will do no good. We have observed no actual harm from larger amounts, but we have not studied the metabolic effects in detail.

DR. BLATT.—Do premature infants retain iron?

DR. JEANS.—They break down hemoglobin during the first two months and do not need iron during this period. The prematurely born infants we have studied have retained ingested iron after two months of age.

DR. ABT.—1. Do you still believe in Bunge's conception of the iron reservoir in the liver at birth?

2. Were the children who had a negative iron balance on breast milk or cow's milk?

3. Was the specific dynamic action of protein taken into account in the values you gave for creatinine excretion?

4. Are there any references in the literature as to the absorption of cod liver oil? It is not an uncommon experience, in calling at the homes of my patients, to have the mother show me the baby's diaper containing the stool and often a distinct separate oily substance which looks and smells like cod liver oil. When we state the optimal dose, must we not then allow for the amount of nonabsorbed oil (if a portion of the oral dose is not absorbed)?

5. Are there any other experiments recorded in the literature besides those which Dr. Jeans mentioned which substantiate the statement that spinach is a demineralizer?

DR. JEANS.—1. Apparently a small store of iron exists normally in the liver at birth. However, this store is relatively unimportant when compared to the amount of iron which becomes available from the destruction of hemoglobin in the early weeks after birth.

2. The infants with a negative iron balance were receiving cow's milk.

3. No, this was not considered. It is probable that this factor relates more closely to creatine than to creatinine excretion.

4. I am not familiar with the literature on this subject. My statements concerning the dose of cod liver oil were based on the usual or average utilization. In my own experience, failure of utilization has been exceptional. In such a case it seems doubtful that increase of the intake will increase the absorption. Some other source of vitamin D would seem indicated.

5. Dr. Schlutz and his coworkers have pointed out the lack of value of spinach as a source of iron for infants (J. PEDIAT. 3: 225, 1933).

DR. H. G. PONCHER, CHICAGO, ILL.
Recorder.

Academy News

The annual meeting of Regions I and II of the American Academy of Pediatrics will be held in Baltimore, Md. The headquarters will be at the Belvedere Hotel, Charles and Chase Streets. The following men are in charge:

Louis C. Schroeder, New York, N. Y., Chairman, Region I; Phillip Van Igen, New York, N. Y., Acting Chairman, Region I; Edward Clay Mitchell, Memphis, Tenn., Chairman, Region II; Baltimore Committee on Arrangements, Fred B. Smith, Chairman, L. Emmett Holt, Jr., C. Loring Joslin, J. H. Mason Knox, Jr., D. C. Wharton Smith.

The following program has been announced:

MONDAY, NOVEMBER 16

9:30 A.M. Hurd Auditorium, Johns Hopkins Hospital.

An Unusual Type of Bone Dystrophy Resembling Paget's Disease, With Presentation of a Case—Dr. Laslo Kajdi.

Presentation of Two Cases of Porphyria—Dr. Harriet G. Guild.

Certain Aspects of Serum Therapy in Meningococcus Meningitis—Dr. Francis F. Schwentker.

A Study of the Rate of Growth and Osseous Development in Hypothyroidism and Dwarfism—Dr. Lawson Wilkins.

Newer Concepts of the Achondroplastic State—Dr. Walter Block.

The Treatment of Gonococcal Vaginitis With Amniotin—Dr. Richard W. TeLinde.

The Cause of Icterus Neonatorum—Dr. Nicholson J. Eastman.

Observations on Hypertension in Childhood, With Particular Reference to the Rheumatic State—Dr. Helen B. Taussig.

Renal Hyperparathyroidism—Dr. Edwards A. Park.

Child Hygiene Program in Maryland—Dr. J. H. Mason Knox and associates.

12:30 NOON. Luncheon and meeting of state chairmen, Belvedere Hotel.

1:00 P.M. Luncheon at Welch Memorial Library.

2:00 P.M. X-ray Changes and Prognosis in Pulmonary Tuberculosis in Young Children—Dr. Miriam E. Brailey.

Experiences With Suipestifer Infection in Childhood—Dr. John A. Washington.

A Study of Chronic Nephritis in Childhood—Dr. Alexander J. Schaffer.

Experiences With Esophageal Injury Following the Ingestion of Corrosives—Dr. R. Campbell Goodwin.

The Surgical Treatment of Bronchiectasis—Dr. William F. Rienhoff, Jr.

The Possibilities of Active Immunization Against the Pneumococcus in Different Age Groups—Dr. Lloyd D. Felton.

Congenital Reading Disability—Dr. Leo Kanner and Dr. Angus L. McLean.

The Study of the Anemic Child—Dr. Hugh W. Josephs.

A Study of the Causes of Xanthochromia in Spinal Fluid—Dr. Frank H. Robinson, Jr.

Essential Familial Lipemia—Dr. Francis X. Aylward and Dr. L. Emmett Holt, Jr.

7:00 P.M. Annual banquet at Belvedere Hotel.

TUESDAY, NOVEMBER 17

9:30 A.M. Wilson Memorial Amphitheatre, University of Maryland Hospital.

Intracranial Hemorrhage of the Newborn: With Presentation of Cases Previously Treated—Dr. C. Loring Joslin.

Clinical-Pathological Discussion of Birth Hemorrhage—Dr. Charles Bagley.

Hypertension Associated With Embryonal Adenosarcoma: A Report of Three Cases—Dr. J. Edmund Bradley.

A Study on the Feeding of Whole Milk, Acidified Milk, and Gelatinized Milk, With Especial Reference to Calcium and Phosphorus Absorption—Dr. I. Meranski.

Banana Therapy in Diarrheal Diseases—Dr. Thomas A. Christensen.

Acute Empyema in Children—Dr. Cyrus Horine.

Xanthomatosis of Bone—Dr. Allen Voshell.

The Vitamin B Complex: An Experimental and Clinical Study With Special Reference to Growth and Constipation—Dr. A. H. Finkelstein.

Complications of Accessory Nasal Infections in Children—Dr. Edward A. Looper.

Presentation of a Case of Spontaneous Pneumothorax—Dr. Edgar Friedenwald and Dr. Bowers Mansdorfer.

Persistent Pyuria, Due to Congenital Urethral Malformation: A Case Report—Dr. Fred B. Smith and Dr. A. J. Gillis.

2:00 P.M. Regional business meetings to be held separately. There are a number of important questions to be decided. This is probably the most important session of the regional meeting. It is earnestly requested that all members in attendance at the general meeting be present.

The annual meeting of Region III will be held in Cincinnati, Ohio, Nov. 20 and 21, 1936, with headquarters at the Netherland Plaza Hotel. In addition to the scientific program given in three sessions, there will be a dinner on Friday evening at the Netherland Plaza Hotel with an interesting program.

The following scientific program has been announced:

FRIDAY, NOVEMBER 20

10:00 A.M. to 12:00 NOON. Netherland Plaza.

Use of Supravital Technic in Studying Children's Diseases—C. R. Rittershofer.

Significance of Albumin-Globulin Ratio in Nephrosis—H. W. Robinson.

Relation of Hemoglobin Content and Red Cell Size to Age and Nutritive Condition—George M. Guest.

Hypoglycemia Versus Hyperinsulinism—Stanley Dorst.

Stimulation With Histamine on Gastric Flow—Leon Schiff.

On Significance of Repeated Tuberculin Tests—Waldo E. Nelson.

Alkalosis—Glenn E. Cullen.

2:00 P.M. to 4:45 P.M.

Diagnosis and Treatment of Irritative Symptoms of the Central Nervous System of the Newborn—Harold F. Downing.

The Premature Department of the Cincinnati General Hospital—Edward A. Wagner.

Behavior Problems of Children—E. A. North.

Possible Relation of Various Types of *B. Coli* to Enteritis—Merlin L. Cooper.

Benigu Lymphocytic Meningitis (Aseptic Meningitis)—Frank E. Stevenson, Robert A. Lyon, and Clyde Dummer.

Epidemic of Pleurodynia in Children in the Summer of 1935—Robert McDonald, Barbara Hewell, and Merlin L. Cooper.

Pellagra in Children and Present Status of Pellagra—Tom D. Spies.

Vitamin D Content of Serum—Josef Warkany.

Relation of Liver to Ketosis—I. Arthur Mirsky.

SATURDAY, NOVEMBER 21

10:00 A.M. to 12:00 NOON. Children's Hospital Research Foundation Auditorium.

A Case of Congenital Heart Disease With Familial History—Robert H. Kotte.

Method of Blood Matching for Transfusions—Paul Hoxworth.

Report of an Unusual Condition Involving the Bones in a Ten-Year-Old Boy—Leo S. Friedman.

A Case of Unilateral Communicating Hydrocephalus Improved by Ureteral Dural Anastomosis—J. Victor Greenebaum and Henry Freiberg.

Connection Between Pyarthrosis of the Hip Joint and Pelvic Abscesses—Albert H. Freiberg and Joseph A. Freiberg.

The Diagnostic Use of Specific Antiserum in Intradermal Tests—Lee Foshay.

Relation of Endocrine Disorder to Hereditary Deviations—Josef Warkany and A. Graeme Mitchell.

The fifth annual meeting of Region IV was held on Oct. 22 to 24, 1936, in San Francisco, Calif. An interesting scientific program was presented, and a business meeting for the Region was held. Dr. Karl F. Meyer was invited to speak on "Neurotropic Viruses and the Diseases Caused by Them."

Dr. Dorman E. Lichty, of Ann Arbor, Mich., has just been elected a member of the Academy.

Dr. N. N. Allen, of Houston, Texas, died on Sept. 22, 1936. Dr. Allen was a fellow of the Academy and was one of the pioneers in pediatrics in Texas. He was very much loved in Houston and was a great friend of the young men.

Dr. Charles Schott, of Chicago, Ill., died Oct. 1, 1936. He was a fellow of the Academy of Pediatrics.

Dr. Robert K. Rewalt, of Williamsport, Pa., a well-known pediatrician of that state, died suddenly July 27, 1936. Dr. Rewalt was a fellow of the Academy of Pediatrics.

The following appointments have been made by the Executive Board:

Dr. A. Graeme Mitchell, of Cincinnati, to the chairmanship of the Committee on Nursing Education. Dr. Lucas resigned the chairmanship but remains on the committee.

To the Committee on Medical Education, Subcommittee on Postgraduate Education: Dr. George M. Lyon, Huntington, W. Va., chairman; Dr. Horton Casparis, Nashville, Tenn.; and Dr. Hugh L. Dwyer, Kansas City, Mo.

The Michigan Section of the American Academy of Pediatrics held its fall meeting on Sept. 24, 1936. The members attended the meetings of the Pediatric Section of the Michigan State Medical Society on September 24 and 25.

Preceding the meeting a dinner was held at the Hotel Statler in Detroit. Thirty members were present to honor R. Cannon Eley, of Boston, who was in Detroit to speak before the Michigan State Medical Society. Following dinner, reports of the committee appointed to cooperate with the State Health Department on matters pertaining to the Social Security Act and the Committee on Postgraduate Education were read and approved.

The members decided to hold the next meeting in January in conjunction with the meeting of the Detroit Pediatric Society.

Edgar E. Martmer, chairman for Michigan, announced the complete reorganization of the department of pediatrics at Wayne University, Detroit, and the acceptance of the position as head of the department of pediatrics by Thomas B. Cooley, past president of the American Academy of Pediatrics.

News and Notes

A bulletin announces the postponement of the **Fourth International Congress in Pediatrics.** The date is now definitely set for Sept. 27, 28, 29, and 30, 1937. The Congress probably will be followed immediately by the Second International Congress for the Protection of Infancy. Dr. L. Emmett Holt, Jr., Baltimore, is secretary of the American committee.

The **Central New York Pediatric Society** held its fall meeting in Schenectady on October 1. A clinical program was presented at the Ellis Hospital, and after a business meeting at the home of Dr. Frank Van Der Bogert, president of the Society, a dinner was served at the Mohawk Club. Dr. Whitney, of the General Electric Company, addressed the dinner meeting.

Pediatricians from Rochester, Auburn, Watertown, Utica, Schenectady, Albany, Troy, and Syracuse were present.

On September 19 the **Subcommittee on Child Hygiene of the Committee on Public Health and Medical Education, New York State Medical Society,** held a meeting in New York City with Dr. E. S. Godfrey, commissioner, state department of health, several officers of the state Society, and a small group of pediatricians.

The plan of the meeting was to outline a program on child hygiene through the various county societies.

A radio forum entitled "Growth and Development of the Child" will be given under the joint auspices of the **National Congress of Parents and Teachers,** the **American Academy of Pediatrics,** and the National Broadcasting Company.

COMMITTEE

Mrs. B. F. Langworthy, president, National Congress of Parents and Teachers, Chicago; C. A. Aldrich, M.D., Winnetka, Ill., and Henry F. Helmholz, M.D., Rochester, Minnesota, representing the American Academy of Pediatrics; Miss Judith C.

Waller, director of education, central division, National Broadcasting Company, Chicago; Mrs. John Sharpless Fox, Chicago, representing the radio forum committee of the Congress.

1.	Oct. 21, 1936	Introductory: What Is Growth?—Lawrence K. Frank.
2.	Oct. 28, 1936	Prenatal Growth—George L. Streeter.
3.	Nov. 4, 1936	Growth of Infants—Harry Bakwin.
4.	Nov. 11, 1936	Growth of the Adolescent—Horace Gray.
5.	Nov. 18, 1936	Growth of Organs—R. E. Scammon.
6.	Nov. 25, 1936	Our Ancestors—E. A. Hooton.
7.	Dec. 2, 1936	Does Like Beget Like?—Amos H. Hersh.
8.	Dec. 9, 1936	Measurements of Growth—Harold C. Stuart.
9.	Dec. 16, 1936	Individual Variations in Infants and Children—Alfred H. Washburn.
10.	Dec. 23, 1936	Foods and Growth—E. V. McCollum.
11.	Dec. 30, 1936	Chemical Elements and Their Part in Body Growth—S. Z. Levine.
12.	Jan. 6, 1937	Energy and Growth—A. A. Weech.
13.	Jan. 13, 1937	Our Glands—R. G. Hoskins.
14.	Jan. 20, 1937	The Action of Glands on Growth—Oscar Riddle.
15.	Jan. 27, 1937	Effects of Light, Sun, and Other Rays on Growth—Otto Glasser.
16.	Feb. 3, 1937	Heredity or Environment?—E. C. MacDowell.
17.	Feb. 10, 1937	How the Mind Grows in Infancy—Arnold Gesell.
18.	Feb. 17, 1937	How Children's Minds Grow—Walter R. Miles.
19.	Feb. 24, 1937	The Importance of Music for Growing Children—Walter Damrosch.
20.	Mar. 3, 1937	Emotional Development in Children—John E. Anderson.
21.	Mar. 10, 1937	The Connection Between Mind and Body Growth—Bert I. Beverly.
22.	Mar. 17, 1937	Fitting the Course of Study to the Child's Mental Development—Carleton Washburne.
23.	Mar. 24, 1937	Education and Mental Growth—Frank N. Freeman.
24.	Mar. 31, 1937	Athletics, Exercise, and Fatigue in Growing Children—D. B. Dill.
25.	Apr. 7, 1937	Physical Education for Growing Children—C. W. Savage.
26.	Apr. 14, 1937	Disease and the Doctor's Side of Growth—Joseph Brennemann.
27.	Apr. 21, 1937	The Effects of Family Income on a Child's Growth—Martha M. Eliot.
28.	Apr. 28, 1937	The Effect of Child Labor on Growth—Richard A. Bolt.
29.	May 5, 1937	Growth of Children During Wars and Depressions—Carroll E. Palmer.
30.	May 12, 1937	Health Hazards in the Period of Growth—Louis I. Dublin.
31.	May 19, 1937	Old and New Thoughts About Growth—Henry E. Sigerist.

Editor, Norman C. Wetzel, M.D., Babies and Childrens Hospital, Cleveland, Ohio. Music selected and arranged by Leon Machan, pianist, Cleveland Symphony Orchestra.

Dr. R. Langley Porter retired as dean of the School of Medicine, University of California, San Francisco.

Dr. W. McKim Marriott, of St. Louis, was appointed dean of the School of Medicine and professor of experimental research, University of California, San Francisco. Dr. Marriott, who succeeds Dr. Porter, assumed his duties on July 1, 1936.

Dr. Alexis F. Hartmann, of St. Louis, was appointed professor of pediatrics, School of Medicine, Washington University, and chief of staff of the St. Louis Children's Hospital. Dr. Hartmann succeeds Dr. Marriott. Dr. Hartmann assumed his duties on July 1, 1936.

The American Pediatric Society will hold its next annual meeting at University, Virginia on April 29, 30, and May 1, 1937.

The following men have been certified by the **American Board of Pediatrics** since the last report.

Harry S. Altman, New York, N. Y.
Louis Barash, New York, N. Y.
Walter Douglas Brown, Beaumont, Texas
Fred W. Bush, Rochester, N. Y.
Nicholas Boddie Cannady, Dothan, Ala.
Charles Rowse Dengler, Jackson, Mich.
R. Bruce Eldredge, Omaha, Neb.
Edward Porter Essertier, Hackensack, N. J.
George Julius Feldstein, Pittsburgh, Pa.
Alfred Elias Fischer, New York, N. Y.
Edward O. Fitch, Houston, Texas
James LeRoy Foster, Pittsburgh, Pa.
Hugh C. Graham, Tulsa, Oklahoma
Theodore P. Herrick, Cleveland, Ohio
George Russell Irving, New York, N. Y.
Sidney David Kramer, Brooklyn, N. Y.
Alfred Gustav Langmann, New York, N. Y.
George P. Laton, Los Angeles, Calif.
Mathilde Loth, New York, N. Y.
Mary Schwartz Newman, Brooklyn, N. Y.
Maurice J. Searle, Tulsa, Okla.
Harry M. Shapiro, New York, N. Y.
Edwin August Socola, New Orleans, La.
Edwin B. Weldon, Bridgeport, Conn.

Book Review

The Adopted Child. Eleanor G. Gallagher, New York, 1936, Reynal and Hitchcock, p. 291. Price $2.50.

This is a disappointing book. As a "first book" on an important subject frequently brought to the pediatrician for discussion, it merits more of a review than the book inherently justifies. According to the cover blurb, it is a "complete book" for the general reader, as well as a "handbook" for social workers, adoption agencies, etc. It fails to fulfill in a satisfactory way any one of these purposes, let alone all. There are a number of excellent chapters, as the historical introduction and the summary of state laws relating to adoption in the appendix. Rather than the sound critical discussion which we are led to expect, the book as a whole turns out to be a somewhat emotionally biased special plea for the immediate separation of the illegitimate child from the mother, its immediate placement in an adoption nursery, and its placement into the adopting home when the baby is a few weeks old. There is much to be said in favor of this, but there is another viewpoint held by many intelligent and experienced people. Rather than critically presenting the other viewpoint, which should be done in a "complete book" on the subject of adoption, the author indulges in an uncalled for tirade against trained social workers and cites a few stupid actions of trained workers to prove their incompetence as a whole, simply because they disagree with the author's viewpoint—a fallacious and silly argument, as an equal number of stupid actions could be cited in regard to volunteer workers. Since some trained workers do not agree with the author's views and are responsible, in her opinion, for laws requiring maternal nursing for a few months, away with the whole tribe of them. Since intelligence tests are not available for young infants, the author attempts to show intelligence tests are of no value and simply displays a rather limited appreciation of their value and functions. By a few citations from literature she attempts to show that artificial feeding is the equivalent or even superior to maternal nursing. Thus the book becomes a special plea to uphold a viewpoint rather than a sound balanced discussion of the subject of adoption.

We are not informed as to the author's training, qualifications, and connections, except that we are told that she has had many years of experience in adoption work. The reviewer would hazard from the text that it has been in connection with the Cradle in Chicago. The excellent work of the Cradle is well known and scarcely needs the defensive attitude of the author. She further refers to the splendid work of Dr. Chapin and his wife in New York and the Spence organization, and then rather naïvely remarks that, although there are many other adoption nurseries scattered throughout the United States, she is unfamiliar with them. Excellent as the work of the Cradle undoubtedly is, it scarcely gives a broad enough background to cover the entire field of adoption with its many problems. The chief criticism against the adoption nurseries is that so far they have not taken advantage of their unique opportunity to make a careful critical scientific study of the development of the infants they have placed. Such a study would do more to show the value, or weakness, of the ideas the author defends than these many pages of personal opinion.

The value of giving in detail the Dick technic is decidedly questionable in a book for the parent or general reader. Physicians will agree with the author that the child should be told it is adopted. The child, however, should have been told long before he could have understood the "precious" letter with which the author concludes the discussion of this topic.

The book is neither fish, flesh, nor fowl. If the emotionalism and non-germane controversial matter had been omitted and the title changed to "Adoption Nurseries" the book would have a place. But labeled as a "complete book" on the subject of adoption, it goes under false colors, and the reviewer feels it an unwise book for physicians to recommend to uncertain-minded and noncritical parents who are considering the problem of adoption.

Errata

In the article by Martha M. Eliot et al. entitled "A Study of the Comparative Value of Cod Liver Oil, Viosterol, and Vitamin D Milks in the Prevention of Rickets and of Certain Basic Factors Influencing Their Efficacy" in the September issue, the following corrections should be made.

On page 361 the last sentence above the illustration should appear as the last sentence of the first footnote.

On page 363 the following paragraph should be inserted after line 11:

"It should be pointed out that the incidence of rickets among the colored infants is consistently lower than among the white infants when the total groups given the different types of antirachitic agents are considered and that the same tendency exists with few exceptions at the different dosage levels for each agent."

On page 371 the footnote to Table X should read:

"Code: A_1–, B_1–, very slight," etc.

In the article, "The Problem of Dental Caries With Relation to Bacteria and Diet," by Philip Jay, M.S., D.D.S., which appeared in the June, 1936, issue of the JOURNAL, on page 729, line 44, the word "negative" should be "positive"; thus the sentence should read: "It was subsequently observed that the same proportion of caries-free individuals contained *L. acidophilus* agglutinins in the blood serum, whereas 70 per cent of the susceptible persons tested yielded positive skin tests and contained either no demonstrable acidophilus agglutinins or else agglutinin titers which were much lower than was ordinarily found in the caries-free."

In the article, "The Premature Infant," by William W. Swanson, M.D., Vernon E. Lennarson, M.D., and Fred L. Adair, M.D., which appeared in the July issue of the JOURNAL, the reference to Dr. Blackfan on page 15, line 41, is incorrect. His name should not have been mentioned in connection with the treatment by injecting whole blood intramuscularly.

The Journal of Pediatrics

Vol. 9 DECEMBER, 1936 No. 6

Original Communications

A STUDY OF 244 PREMATURELY BORN INFANTS

ETHEL C. DUNHAM, M.D.,
WASHINGTON, D. C.

AND

PAUL F. MCALENNEY, JR., M.D.,
NEW HAVEN, CONN.

SCOPE AND METHOD OF STUDY

THIS study has been made in an effort to determine the abnormal conditions that occurred in a group of prematurely born infants, especially the conditions that caused death, and to study the possible effects on these infants of complications of their mothers' pregnancy. The study was based on the medical records of all infants prematurely born in the New Haven Hospital during the ten-year period 1924-1933, and included every liveborn infant who was described in the medical records as "premature" and who weighed at birth 2,500 gm. or less. There were 244 such infants.* Sixty-six of them died before discharge from the hospital and 178 were alive at the date of discharge.† Of the 244 infants 112 were males, 132 females; 218 were white, 26 colored. Seventy were patients of private physicians and 174 were ward patients.

One hundred and ninety-four infants were the result of single pregnancies (79 per cent) and 50, of multiple pregnancies (21 per cent). The infants of multiple birth included one set of triplets, 21 pairs of twins, and 5 single twins.‡

Although infants of multiple birth are usually considered in the same category with single born infants with regard to prematurity, provided the birth weight is 2,500 gm. or less, many of them are born close to

*Twelve additional infants were described in the hospital records as premature, but their weights were not known and therefore these infants were not included in the study.

†The information with regard to these 244 infants was obtained only for the period of hospitalization. For the 66 infants who died in the hospital the information covers the entire period from birth to death; for the 178 infants discharged alive, the period from birth to discharge.

From U. S. Department of Labor, Children's Bureau, Washington, D. C., and Department of Pediatrics, Yale University School of Medicine, New Haven, Connecticut.

‡In each of these 5 cases the other twin weighed more than 2,500 gm. and therefore was excluded from the study.

term or even at term and have had a longer period of gestation than single born infants of the same weight, are therefore more mature and so are better prepared for extrauterine life. For this reason, although infants of multiple birth have been considered in this study as part of the *total number* of prematurely born infants, they have been dealt with as a special group also when mortality was studied.

Since it is well known that morbidity and mortality of prematurely born infants are closely related to birth weight, consideration of such infants in groups according to birth weight has become customary. Ylppö,[1] for example, separated the prematurely born infants that he studied into four groups according to weight at birth:

1. Infants weighing from 600 to 1,000 gm.
2. Infants weighing from 1,001 to 1,500 gm.
3. Infants weighing from 1,501 to 2,000 gm.
4. Infants weighing from 2,001 to 2,500 gm.

This grouping has been adopted almost universally in the literature.

In the present study the number of cases is small; therefore the infants have been divided into two large groups according to birth weight, as well as into the four smaller groups according to the plan used by Ylppö. These two large groups, which will be referred to throughout this paper as the "lower weight group" and the "higher weight group," are

1. Infants weighing 1,500 gm. or less (60 infants, 25 per cent of the cases).
2. Infants weighing 1,501 to 2,500 gm. (184 infants, 75 per cent of the cases).

The four smaller groups have been used in this study only for the purpose of studying mortality; the two larger groups, for studying various other factors as well as mortality.

WEIGHT OF INFANTS AT BIRTH

Of the 66 prematurely born infants who died in the hospital 43 were in the lower weight group and 23 in the higher. In Table I the mortality is shown for Ylppö's four weight groups and also for the two groups used throughout this study. The mortality of the infants was found to vary inversely with the birth weight, being 100 per cent among those weighing 1,000 gm. or less; 62 per cent among those weighing 1,001 to 1,500 gm.; 22 per cent among those weighing 1,501 to 2,000 gm., and 6 per cent for those weighing 2,001 to 2,500 gm. When the mortality of the infants was considered according to the two large weight groups used in this study—(1) 1,500 gm. or less and (2) 1,501 gm. to 2,500 gm.—it was found to be more than five times as high among the infants in the lower weight group (72 per cent) as among infants in the higher weight group (13 per cent).

TABLE I

MORTALITY OF PREMATURELY BORN INFANTS BY WEIGHT AT BIRTH

BIRTH WEIGHT	TOTAL	INFANTS WHO DIED		INFANTS WHO LIVED	
		NUMBER	PERCENTAGE	NUMBER	PERCENTAGE
Total	244	66	27.0	178	73.0
1,500 gm. or less	60	43	71.7	17	28.3
1,000 gm. or less	15	15	*	–	–
1,001-1,500 gm.	45	28	*	17	*
1,501 to 2,500 gm.	184	23	12.5	161	87.5
1,501-2,000 gm.	78	17	21.8	61	78.2
2,001-2,500 gm.	106	6	5.7	100	94.3

*Percentage not shown because the number of cases was less than 50.

SINGLE AND MULTIPLE BIRTHS

The mortality for infants who were the result of multiple pregnancies was much lower than for single born infants—16 per cent among the infants born of multiple pregnancies and 30 per cent among the single-born. This difference is similar to that noted by Ylppö,[1] who investigated a much larger group of cases, and probably is due to the greater maturity of the infants of multiple birth.

AGE OF INFANTS AT DEATH

The age at death of the 66 infants who died in the hospital is shown in Table II. Thirty-seven (more than half of them) died in the first twenty-four hours after birth. Eleven infants died in the next four days, 12 in the period between the fifth day and the thirtieth day, and 6 after they were one month old. When the mortality at each of these age periods up to one month was considered in the two weight groups, it was found to be definitely higher in the lower weight group than in the higher, as would be expected.

PRIVATE AND WARD CASES

Among the private cases the mortality for the total group of infants was 30 per cent; among the ward cases, 26 per cent, a difference that is

TABLE II

AGE AT DEATH OF 66 PREMATURELY BORN INFANTS

AGE AT DEATH	WEIGHT AT BIRTH		
	TOTAL	1500 GM. OR LESS	1501 TO 2500 GM.
Total	66	43	23
Less than 24 hours	37	25	12
24 hours, less than 5 days	11	7	4
5 days, less than 1 month	12	8	4
1 month or more*	6	3	3

*Includes one child who died at fifteen months. She was in the hospital during entire period of her life.

not significant statistically. In connection with the similarity in the mortality, it is of importance that in recent years the premature infants born in the private rooms have been transferred for treatment to the special units for premature infants in the pediatric wards and, therefore, both groups receive the same general treatment.

CONDITION OF MOTHERS

The mothers' records* were analyzed to determine:

(1) factors that might have influenced the premature onset of labor, and

(2) factors that might have influenced the fate of the offspring.

Parity.—The parity of the mothers did not seem to affect the weight of the infants or their mortality, for the proportion of infants in the two weight groups was practically the same for the infants of primiparas and of multiparas, and the mortality also was practically the same. The number of primiparas among the mothers was about the same as the number of multiparas.

Complications of Pregnancy.—The possible effects on the infant of the complications of the mother's pregnancy were studied. In 169 of the 244 cases the mothers had had complications of pregnancy; 126 had had one complication only; and 43 had had more than one complication. The cases have been grouped, as shown in Table III, according to the complication which, from the point of view of its severity and the period of pregnancy in which it occurred, was considered the most important in its effect on the infant. For example, a mother who had pyelitis and multiple pregnancy is included in the group of cases with infection.

Toxemia occurred in 73 cases; bleeding in 28; infection in 27; multiple pregnancy alone in 23†; and other complications in 18. A detailed list of the complications, grouped under four main headings, is given in the footnote to Table III.

The mortality of the infants among mothers who had had complications was approximately the same as that among mothers who had had no complication (28 and 24 per cent, respectively). When the infants were considered in the two weight groups, however, it was found that in the higher weight group the proportion of infants who died was about the same when the mothers had had complications as when they had had none (14 and 10 per cent respectively), whereas in the lower weight group the proportion who died was smaller when the mothers had had complications than when they had had none (67 and 86 per cent respectively). The proportion of infants of very low birth weight (1,000

*When prenatal and natal factors were studied, the mother of triplets was counted as three cases; the mother of twins as two cases whenever both twins were included in the study, as one case when only one of the twins was included.

†Twenty-seven additional cases in which multiple pregnancy occurred are included under other groups of complications as in these cases the multiple pregnancy was considered relatively unimportant.

TABLE III

COMPLICATIONS OF PREGNANCY* OF MOTHERS OF PREMATURELY BORN INFANTS BY MORTALITY OF INFANTS IN TWO WEIGHT GROUPS

COMPLICATIONS OF PREGNANCY	BIRTH WEIGHT OF INFANTS: TOTAL			1500 GM. OR LESS			1501 TO 2500 GM.		
	TOTAL	INFANTS DIED	INFANTS LIVED	TOTAL	INFANTS DIED	INFANTS LIVED	TOTAL	INFANTS DIED	INFANTS LIVED
Total	244	66	178	60	43	17	184	23	161
No complications	75	18	57	14	12	2	61	6	55
Complications	169	48	121	46	31	15	123	17	106
One complication only	126	36	90	35	24	11	91	12	79
Toxemia	51	11	40	12	6	6	39	5	34
Multiple pregnancy only	23	2	21	2	-	2	21	2	19
Bleeding	22	10	12	10	9	1	12	1	11
Infection	18	4	14	3	1	2	15	3	12
Other	12	9	3	8	8	-	4	1	3
More than one complication	43	12	31	11	7	4	32	5	27
Toxemia and other	22	8	14	8	5	3	14	3	11
Bleeding and other	6	1	5	1	-	1	5	1	4
Infection and other	9	1	8	1	1	-	8	-	8
Other (2 or more)	6	2	4	1	1	-	5	1	4

*The detailed list of complications of pregnancy is as follows:

Toxemia, total ---- 73
- Toxemia alone ---- 51
  - Toxemia, type not specified 23
  - Nephritic ---- 15
  - Preeclamptic ---- 6
  - Eclamptic ---- 7
- Toxemia and other complications ---- 22
  - Toxemia and multiple pregnancy ---- 9
  - Toxemia, multiple pregnancy, and hydramnios 2
  - Toxemia, multiple pregnancy, and heart disease ---- 2
  - Toxemia and heart disease 1
  - Toxemia, heart disease, and ectopic pregnancy- 1
  - Toxemia and pyelitis ---- 4
  - Toxemia and anemia ---- 1
  - Toxemia and myomas ---- 1
  - Toxemia and bleeding---- 1

Bleeding, total ---- 28
- Bleeding alone ---- 22
  - Bleeding, type not specified 10
  - Placenta previa ---- 4
  - Premature separation of placenta ---- 8
- Bleeding and other complications ---- 6
  - Bleeding and multiple pregnancy ---- 2
  - Bleeding and fall---- 1
  - Bleeding and syphilis---- 1
  - Bleeding and bronchitis---- 1
  - Bleeding and abscess of Bartholin's gland---- 1

Infection, total ---- 27
- Infection alone ---- 18
  - Gonorrhea ---- 1
  - Pyelitis ---- 5
  - Chronic cervicitis ---- 2
  - Syphilis ---- 4
  - Pneumonia ---- 2
  - Appendicitis ---- 1
  - Rheumatic heart disease ---- 1
  - Measles ---- 1
  - Tuberculosis ---- 1
- Infection and other complications ---- 9
  - Pyelitis and other ---- 4
    - Pyelitis and rheumatic heart disease ---- 1
    - Pyelitis and chronic arthritis ---- 1
    - Pyelitis and multiple pregnancy ---- 2
  - Syphilis and other---- 3
    - Syphilis, gonorrheal vaginitis, and myomas---- 1
    - Syphilis and multiple pregnancy ---- 2
  - Rheumatic heart disease and other ---- 2
    - Rheumatic heart disease and multiple pregnancy 2

Other complication, total---- 18
- One complication ---- 12
  - Brain tumor ---- 1
  - Diabetes ---- 2
  - Psychosis ---- 3
  - Lacerated cervix ---- 2
  - Fall ---- 1
  - Anemia ---- 1
  - Hydramnios ---- 2
- More than one complication- 6
  - Hydramnios and multiple pregnancy ---- 5
  - Psychosis and multiple pregnancy ---- 1

gm. or less) was slightly greater among the mothers with no complications. It was found, moreover, that a greater proportion of these mothers had had previous abortions and premature infants. In the total group and in the groups according to birth weight the numbers of infants are small, and the findings are merely suggestive.

The mortality of the infants was not studied according to the different groups of complications because the number of cases in each group was too small. The mortality of the infants, however, appeared to be highest among the mothers with bleeding as a complication (with or without other complications) and lowest among the mothers with multiple pregnancy as the only complication. As would be expected, the largest proportion of infants of low birth weight was found among the mothers in the former group, the smallest among those in the latter.

Complications of Labor and Delivery.—Labor occurred spontaneously in 149 cases and was induced in 61.* When the onset of labor was spontaneous, 29 (19 per cent) of the infants died; when it was induced, 22 (36 per cent) died.

The proportion of infants in the lower weight group was much greater among the mothers whose labor had been induced than among those whose labor had been spontaneous. The proportion of infants in the lower weight group who died was slightly greater also among the mothers whose labor was induced. Labor was generally induced on account of complications of pregnancy.

In 51 cases premature rupture of membranes occurred. In 13 of these cases the infant died. In only 7 of these 13 cases was the death of the infant ascribed to infection (general septicemia, 2 cases; respiratory infection, 3; diarrhea, 2). Only one of the 38 infants who lived had an infection (gonorrheal ophthalmia).

The total duration of labor† (first and second stages combined) was known in 190 cases. *Precipitate or prolonged labor* occurred in 42 cases (22 per cent); the labor was regarded as of normal duration in 148 cases (78 per cent). Among the 190 cases primiparas and multiparas were about equally represented (93 of the former, 97 of the latter). The frequency of normal labor was practically the same among primiparous and multiparous women (51 and 49 per cent, respectively). The proportion of infants who died was about the same among the group of mothers in whom labor was normal in duration as among those in whom it was abnormal (20 and 21 per cent, respectively).

Among the mothers whose labor was of normal duration, the deaths of their infants occurred in about the same proportion in the primiparas

*In 15 cases there was no labor (cesarean section); in 19 cases the type of labor was not recorded.

†Labor was regarded as normal if its duration was more than three but less than thirty hours; abnormal, if three hours or less, or thirty hours or more. The number of cases was insufficient and the data inadequate to permit study of the first and second stages of labor separately.

and in the multiparas (21 and 18 per cent, respectively). Among the mothers whose labor was of abnormal duration, however, the deaths of their infants occurred about three times more frequently in the primiparas than in the multiparas (35 and 12 per cent, respectively). Twenty per cent of the infants born after a normal duration of labor were in the lower weight group, 80 per cent in the higher. These proportions were practically the same for infants born after an abnormal duration of labor.

When the duration of labor was normal, nearly two-thirds of the infants in the lower weight group died (19 of 30 infants); in the higher weight group a very small proportion of the infants died (10 of 118 infants). On the other hand, when the duration of labor was abnormal, a larger proportion of infants in the lower birth weight group died (6 of 8 infants), but the proportion of deaths among infants in the higher weight group was the same (3 of 34 infants).

Abnormal pelvis was found in 19 cases, recorded as "contracted" in 9 cases, "rachitic" in 3, "funnel" in 5, and "simple flat" in 2. In 3 of the 19 cases the infant died; 2 of these infants were in the lower weight group and 1 in the higher. Sixteen of the infants lived; 1 was in the lower weight group and 15 in the higher. In none of the 19 infants were evidences of birth injury found.

Type of Delivery.—There were 165 cases of *spontaneous delivery* and 79 of *operative delivery*, as shown in Table IV. Of the infants born spontaneously, 45 (27 per cent) died; of those born by operative procedure, 21 (27 per cent) died. Thus mortality among these premature infants did not appear to depend upon whether delivery was operative or spontaneous. Of the infants born spontaneously, more than one-fourth were in the lower weight group; of the infants born by operative procedure, one-fifth. The number of cases was too small to permit statistical study of the mortality of the infants in relation to the different types of operative delivery. The largest proportion of infant deaths, however, occurred when the mother had been delivered by cesarean section.

TABLE IV

TYPE OF DELIVERY OF MOTHERS OF PREMATURELY BORN INFANTS BY MORTALITY OF INFANTS IN TWO WEIGHT GROUPS

TYPE OF DELIVERY	TOTAL	BIRTH WEIGHT OF INFANTS: 1500 GM. OR LESS			BIRTH WEIGHT OF INFANTS: 1501 TO 2500 GM.		
		TOTAL	INFANTS DIED	INFANTS LIVED	TOTAL	INFANTS DIED	INFANTS LIVED
Total	244	60	43	17	184	23	161
Spontaneous delivery	165	44	29	15	121	16	105
Nonspontaneous delivery	79	16	14	2	63	7	56
Forceps	25	1	1	-	24	1	23
Cesarean section	20	5	5	-	15	3	12
Version and extraction	17	5	4	1	12	2	10
Breech extraction	17	5	4	1	12	1	11

CAUSES OF ILLNESS AND OF DEATH OF INFANTS

In Table V are shown the principal causes of death of the 66 infants who died, divided into the two weight groups.

TABLE V

PRINCIPAL CAUSE OF DEATH OF 66 PREMATURELY BORN INFANTS

CAUSE OF DEATH	WEIGHT OF INFANT		
	TOTAL	1500 GM. OR LESS	1501 TO 2500 GM.
Total	66	43	23
Prematurity alone	34	27	7
Infection	16	8	8
Intracranial hemorrhage	11	6	5
Congenital defect	3	1	2
Other	2	1	1

Premature birth was considered the principal cause of death* of 34 infants (27 of these were in the lower weight group and only 7 in the higher). Four of these 34 infants were the result of multiple pregnancies (3 in the lower weight group and 1 in the higher). In 14 of the 34 cases postmortem examinations had been made and in each case no cause of death other than the incomplete development of the infant was reported.

Infection was considered the principal cause of death in 16 infants (pneumonia, 6 cases; septicemia, 5; respiratory infection, 2; diarrhea, 2; meningitis, 1); 8 of these infants were in the lower weight group and 8 in the higher. Three of the 16 infants were the result of multiple pregnancies (1 triplet and 2 twins); 1 was in the lower weight group and 2 in the higher. Postmortem examinations were made in 11 cases, and evidence of infection was found in 9 of them.

Intracranial hemorrhage, the result of birth injury, was considered the principal cause of death in 11 infants. Six of these were in the lower weight group, 5 in the higher; 1 of the infants in the higher weight group was a twin. Postmortem examinations confirmed the clinical diagnosis in every case. The deliveries were spontaneous in 10 cases, operative in 1.

Congenital defects were considered the principal cause of death of only 3 infants. One infant, weighing 960 gm. at birth, was an anencephalic monster; 1, weighing 1,625 gm., had multiple malformations of the skeletal and muscular systems; 1, weighing 1,790 gm., had a defect of the abdominal wall with herniation of the viscera. All these infants were single born. Postmortem examinations were not made in any of these cases.

Other conditions not classified in the groups mentioned in the preceding paragraphs caused the death of 2 infants, both of whom were single born. One of them, an infant weighing 1,960 gm. at birth, died of

*Diagnosis based on clinical or pathologic examinations or both.

peritonitis following rupture of a gastric ulcer; the other, weighing 1,282 gm. at birth, died of hemorrhagic disease. Postmortem examinations confirmed these diagnoses.

In no case was the principal cause of death *atelectasis.* Thirty of the 66 infants who died had atelectasis, diagnosed in 22 infants by clinical examination; in 8 of these the diagnosis was confirmed by postmortem examination. Atelectasis was found at postmortem examination in 8 additional infants in whom it was not found clinically. Among these 30 infants more than three times as many were in the lower weight group as in the higher. There were no multiple births in this group of infants.

An effort was made to find out the effect on the onset of respiration in the infant when *morphine* was given to the mother. In 188 cases the history showed whether or not the mother had received morphine after admission to the hospital. Of the 63 infants whose mothers had received one or more doses of morphine, 38 per cent died; and of the 125 infants whose mothers had received no morphine, only 23 per cent died, in spite of the fact that among the infants who died the proportion of infants of low birth weight was slightly greater among the infants of mothers who had had no morphine. When the mother had received morphine, the onset of respiration in the infant was delayed in 41 per cent of the cases; when the mother had not received morphine, in only 16 per cent.

Among the 178 surviving infants, there were 100 who during the period in the hospital had no abnormal conditions nor illnesses (94 of these were in the higher weight group, 6 in the lower) and 78 in whom abnormal conditions were found—101 conditions altogether. Those found most frequently were infection, 32 times; atelectasis, 23 times; congenital defects, 18 times; birth injuries, 5 times; hemorrhages other than intracranial, 2 times; miscellaneous conditions, 21 times.

The surviving infants were discharged from the hospital after various periods of time, whenever the medical staff considered that they might be treated as normal full-term infants. The period in the hospital varied considerably, the average being forty-three days. There were no surviving infants in the lower weight group who remained in the hospital less than eight weeks, but 93 per cent of those in the higher weight group were discharged in less than eight weeks.

Sixty-two per cent of the infants weighed 2,500 gm. or more when discharged; 14 per cent of these had been in the lower weight group at birth and 86 per cent in the higher.

Although these infants may have made return visits to the pediatric clinic following their discharge from the hospital, the records of these visits have not been analyzed for this study nor have records of mental tests been obtained.

METHODS OF CARING FOR INFANTS

The methods used in the care and treatment of the prematurely born infants included in the study varied widely in the ten-year period covered. The methods have been evolved gradually, and there is no sharp line of demarcation between the periods when different methods of treatment were used. In the early years very few prematurely born infants were transferred from the private pavilion to the pediatric service; now nearly all such infants are so transferred. Air-conditioned rooms were installed in 1928, and other details of treatment have been changed from time to time. For these reasons, it is not possible to compare the results of one method of care and treatment with another in this series of cases. The mortality for the first five-year period was the same as that for the second (27 per cent). Moreover, when the mortality was studied in the two periods for each of the two weight groups, no significant difference was found.

The method used in the most recent period for caring for prematurely born infants in the New Haven Hospital is as follows: A house officer who is a member of the pediatric staff is present at all premature deliveries. The infant is placed immediately after birth in a Hess bed heated to 80° F., which is always kept in readiness in the delivery room. When the house officer considers that the infant's condition will permit a change, the infant is transferred, usually in a Hess bed, to one of the special rooms of the pediatric ward. These rooms, about 10 by 14 feet in size, are air-conditioned, the temperature being automatically maintained by the Yaglou apparatus at about 75° F., and the moisture at about 68 per cent. Efforts are made to maintain the infant's temperature at 37° C., usually by regulation of the temperature of the Hess bed. Nurses and doctors are the only persons admitted to the room; isolation technic is used; hands are washed, and gowns are worn. Nursing care is given by student nurses under the supervision of the head nurse of the pediatric service. The infants are handled as little as possible. Oil baths are given every other day.

The infant is fed in the Hess bed (with the head end of the mattress raised) by means of a medicine dropper with a soft rubber catheter tip or a bottle and nipple of small size. Gavage is resorted to only in very exceptional cases. The feedings consist of breast milk, if it is available, otherwise of modified cow's milk (skimmed or half skimmed) with 5 to 10 per cent dextrimaltose added. The feeding interval is usually two hours. The general principle is to give small feedings at first, and to increase the feedings gradually both in amount and caloric value to an upper limit of about 150 calories daily per kilogram of body weight. Water is given with a medicine dropper between feedings, the total fluid intake being estimated on the basis of about 150 c.c. daily per kilogram of body weight. If the infant cannot take this amount of fluid by mouth, saline solution is administered by hypodermoclysis. Transfusions of blood are given repeatedly if the infant is not doing well or if evidences of infection or other pathologic conditions appear.

Viosterol, 10 to 15 drops daily, and orange juice, 8 c.c. daily, are started near the end of the second week; cod liver oil, 4 c.c. daily, at one to two months of age.

Anti-anemic therapy is not given as a matter of routine.

SUMMARY

This study was based on the medical records of all infants born prematurely in the New Haven Hospital during a ten-year period, and included every liveborn infant who was described in the medical records as "premature" and who weighed at birth 2,500 gm. or less. There were 244 such infants, of whom 66 died without having been discharged from the hospital and 178 were discharged alive. More than half the deaths occurred within twenty-four hours of birth.

The mortality was five times as high among the infants weighing 1,500 gm. or less as among those weighing 1,501 to 2,500 gm. It was nearly twice as high among single born infants as among those the result of multiple pregnancy.

The mortality among the infants of the mothers who had had one or more complications of pregnancy was not significantly higher than among the infants whose mothers had not had complications.

The infant mortality did not seem to be influenced by the duration of labor—normal or abnormal; nor by the type of delivery—spontaneous or operative; but it was higher when labor had been induced than when it had occurred spontaneously.

More than half the infant deaths were reported as caused by prematurity, about one-fourth by infection, and about one-sixth by intracranial hemorrhage.

Atelectasis occurred in nearly half of the infants who died and in about one-seventh of those who survived.

The effect on the fetus of morphine given to the mother was shown by the fact that of the 63 infants whose mothers had received morphine, 38 per cent died; and of the 125 whose mothers had not received morphine, only 23 per cent died, in spite of the fact that among the infants who died the proportion of infants of low birth weight was slightly greater among the infants of mothers who had had no morphine. When the mother had received morphine, the onset of respiration in the infant was delayed in 41 per cent of the cases; when the mother had not received morphine, in only 16 per cent.

In studying the effects on the infant of complications of the mother's pregnancy, labor, and delivery and the results of various abnormal conditions in the infants, the birth weights of the infants should always be taken into consideration and the proportion of those of higher or lower weight known.

REFERENCE

1. Ylppö, A.: Ztschr. f. Kinderh. 24: 1, 1919.

THE LIPOID FACTOR IN GLYCOGEN STORAGE DISEASE

Cecil Krakower, M.D.
Boston, Mass.

Although quite a number of clinical reports dealing with glycogen storage disease have appeared in recent years, there are relatively few anatomic observations. In the latter, concomitant fatty disturbances have not been emphasized. In a disease characterized by abnormal storage of glycogen with impaired glycogenolysis, manifesting itself by a very low fasting blood sugar, with practically no response to adrenalin, but with marked sensitivity to insulin, it might be expected that fat metabolism would also be affected. Particularly would this be true in the fasting state or when metabolic activity was increased. That this is so is evident from observations obtained from convincing clinical cases, as well as from those in which the diagnosis was established by biopsy or by necropsy. Acidosis and acetonuria are frequent, especially in the fasting condition. Likewise, elevated values for the blood lipoids have frequently been reported. It is also known that, following the ingestion of a fatty test meal, there is a prolonged, elevated blood lipoid curve. This has been emphasized in distinguishing this disease from other forms of hepatomegaly, particularly in cirrhosis of the liver (Beumer and Loeschke,[1] Unshelm[2]).

At present, there is reason to believe that this disease may occur without hepatonephromegaly as originally described by von Gierke,[3] hence the use of the broader term "glycogen storage disease." There have been types with greatly enlarged hearts (formerly included with idiopathic hypertrophy of the heart in infancy) due to massive deposits of glycogen. In most instances these have been associated with simultaneous abnormal storage in other organs, unaccompanied, however, by any degree of enlargement. Whether in these, biochemical changes similar to those of the hepatomegalies will be found remains as yet to be determined. They have only been recognized at autopsy without previous complete studies.

In the first of von Gierke's two cases of hepatonephromegaly (aged eight years) in addition to massive glycogenic infiltration, there was a considerable amount of fat in the liver. This was present in the form of smaller and larger droplets, infrequently larger than half the cell and often absent in many cells, particularly periportally. These droplets stained positively with sudan, were red with nile blue sulphate and did not stain with Smith-Dietrich or Ciaccio stain. In his second

From the Department of Pathology, Harvard Medical School and The Children's and Infants' Hospitals, Boston, Massachusetts.

case (aged four years) there were larger fatty droplets in the pericentral cells but in all less stainable fat than in the first. In Loeschke's[4] living case of hepatomegaly (aged three years) a biopsy of the liver was obtained. Putschar's description of this deals solely with the deposition of glycogen, intimating that there could not be much fat in view of the amount of the former substance. Schmincke examined a biopsy of the liver in one of Schall's cases[5] (aged eight and one-half years). Fat is not mentioned in the description although there was considerable glycogen in the cells and nuclei. Putschar[6] reported a case (aged four months) with marked glycogenic infiltration of the heart (greatly enlarged) associated with mild deposition in the slightly enlarged liver and moderate in the kidneys. There was no demonstrable fat in the heart or the kidneys, but there was some in the liver, with more or less uniformly distributed medium sized droplets. In Kimmelstiel's case[7] (aged one and two-thirds years) there was abnormal glycogen storage in the liver, brain, striated and cardiac muscle, and to a lesser degree in the kidneys. There was a moderate amount of fat in the liver in the form of large droplets. In Pompe's case[8] of cardiac hypertrophy (aged seven months), there was less stainable glycogen in liver and kidneys. Fatty changes are not mentioned except their absence in the heart. Antopol, Heilbrunn, and Tuchman[9] described a case (aged four and one-half months) similar in many ways to that of Pompe's. There were large fat-containing vacuolated cells in the periportal areas of the liver. There was no fat in the hypertrophied cardiac musculature except for some in the interstitial tissues. There was little fat in the livers of 3 cases (four, five, and eight months, respectively) reported by Humphreys and Kato[10] in which cardiac hypertrophy due to glycogen storage was the main finding. Lastly in Faber's case[11] of hepatonephromegaly (aged one month) there were occasional fat vacuoles, not exceeding the size of the nucleus in the pericentral cells of the liver. There were medium sized fatty droplets in the cells of the convoluted tubules and Henle's limbs of the kidney, always situated at the basal end of the cell, between the nucleus and the basement membrane.

Except in Humphreys and Kato's third case, in which large pale cells were observed in the corpuscles and pulp of the spleen, there is no reference to similar findings in that organ or elsewhere by any of the others.

Although it is realized that the liver ordinarily contains a variable amount of fat, its wide distribution in a greatly enlarged organ would exceed the usual quantitative variables. In two of the instances to be reported here, there were also apparently fat-laden monocytes in spleen and bone marrow, and in one, to a degree comparable with that encountered in diabetic lipemias.

Case 1.—B. S., aged five months, was born after a difficult instrumental delivery. He fared poorly the first few days but rapidly recovered thereafter. The family history was irrelevant. There was another sibling, ten years of age, who was apparently normal. The parents had noted that the patient's abdomen had been large since birth and had progressively increased in size. Two months prior to the present admission he had a cough and nasal catarrh from which he recovered after two weeks of treatment. He had another upper respiratory infection a week before admission. Physically the child was well developed and nourished. His breathing was labored and rapid with an occasional cough. He was perspiring profusely. There were diffuse coarse moist râles throughout both lung fields with harsh breath sounds everywhere. The heart was not enlarged. The sounds were regular, rapid, and of good quality. The abdomen was greatly enlarged. The liver occupied practically the whole right side to within one inch of the pelvic brim and extended over to the left for 5.5 cm. below the costal margin. The spleen was questionably palpable. There was a diffuse fine maculopapular skin rash. There were palpable small cervical glands bilaterally.

The temperature rose from 100° F. on the day of admission to 108° F. terminally on the third day. During this time, he showed signs of marked acidosis, with considerable respiratory embarrassment. There was a note on the third day that blood withdrawn for chemical analysis was creamy and opaque grayish yellow in color.

There were the following additional findings: body weight, 12.3 pounds; height, 25½ inches; circumference of the head, 17¼ inches; circumference of the chest, 17 inches; and circumference of the abdomen, 19½ inches; blood pressure, 132/60; red blood cells, 3,510,000 with 63 per cent hemoglobin; white blood cells, 17,300 to 24,900 with 50 per cent polymorphs, 42 per cent lymphocytes, 7 per cent monocytes, 1 per cent myelocytes; fasting blood sugar, 51 mg. per cent; carbon dioxide, 24 volumes per cent; nonprotein nitrogen, 48 mg. per cent; serum protein, 8.4 gm. per cent; chlorides, 102 c.c.N/10, Cl/100 c.c.; cholesterol, 394 mg. per cent; calcium, 13 mg. per cent; ionized calcium, 5.3 mg. per cent; phosphorus, 7 mg. per cent; sodium, 136 milliequivalents / liter. The urine contained acetone with a very slight trace of albumin. There was no sugar. X-ray films of the extremities revealed transverse bands 2 to 3 mm. from the ends of the long bones and of the chest accentuated peribronchial markings.

Necropsy was performed ten hours postmortem. There was a slight amount of pitting edema over the lower legs and ankles. The subcutaneous fat was pale yellow in color and approximately 4 mm. in thickness. There was no free fluid in the peritoneal cavity. The serosal surfaces were smooth and glistening. The liver was markedly enlarged (Fig. 1), extending far over to the left and lying within the iliac fossa in the right axillary line. The stomach and intestines were pushed inferiorly and to the left. The spleen was not enlarged and was well above the costal margin. The kidneys, as seen in situ, appeared large. Pleural and pericardial cavities were not remarkable.

**Heart* weighed 35 gm. (29). There was very little epicardial fat. The myocardium of the left ventricle was somewhat thickened, measuring on the average 0.9 cm. (average normal at this age, 0.7). It was pale reddish brown in color. Except for dilatation of the tricuspid ring (5 cm. as compared with average normal of 4 cm.), the heart was otherwise not very remarkable.

Lungs.—The right lung weighed 64 gm. (38); the left, 42 (35). The dependent and posteroinferior portions of both lungs were deep dark purplish red in color, and only slightly aerated. The cut surfaces were moist and from them a small amount of serosanguineous fluid could be scraped. The anterior portions of the lungs were

---

*Here and in the remainder of this paper the figures in parentheses will represent average weights for the organs as given in the tables of Coppoletta and Wolbach (Am. J. Path. 9: 55, 1933).

pink, dry and air containing. The bronchi contained a small amount of serosanguineous frothy fluid. Their mucosal surfaces were pale yellowish white in color.

Spleen weighed 15 gm. (16). It was firm in consistency with a thin transparent finely wrinkled capsule. The cut surfaces were pale yellowish red with numerous coarse purplish markings.

Liver weighed 705 gm. (188). It was firm with a smooth, thin and transparent capsule. Both the external and cut surfaces were strikingly pale yellowish in appearance, resembling that of a marked fatty liver, with these differences, however: the surfaces were wet; from them a grayish fluid could be scraped; and the liver substance was less friable. The usual markings were in great part obscured. The

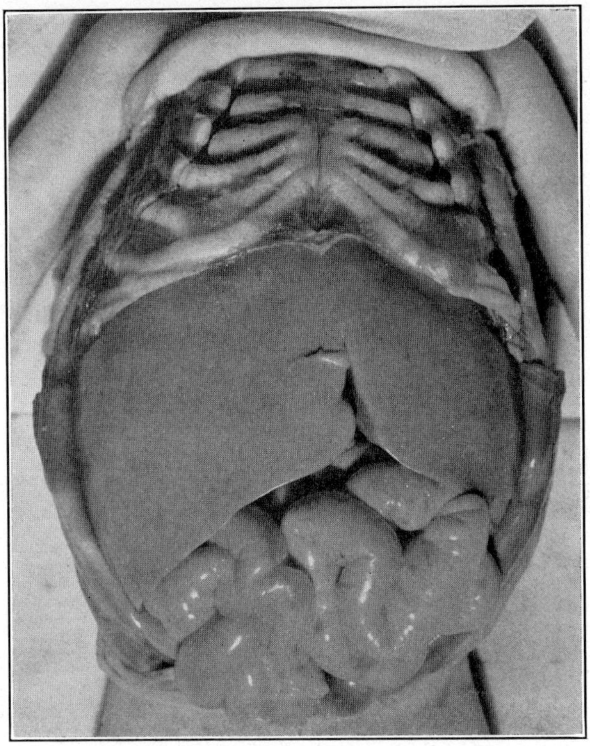

Fig. 1.—The greatly enlarged liver occupying both upper quadrants and lying in the iliac fossa on the right.

gallbladder was small and contained approximately 1.5 c.c. of golden brown bile. Its wall was thin and the mucosa, smooth and velvety. The biliary ducts were not remarkable.

Kidneys.—The right kidney weighed 46 gm. (25), the left, 48 gm. (25). They were firm, surrounded by a moderate amount of fat, and covered by thin capsules which could readily be stripped. Both the smooth external, as well as the cut, surfaces were strikingly pale in appearance. The usual markings were preserved.

Brain weighed 655 gm. (422). Except for mild convolutional flattening and a moderate pressure cone, the brain, meninges and calvarium were not remarkable.

Gastrointestinal Tract.—Pancreas weighed 8 gm.; adrenals (combined weight), 5 gm.; thyroid, 2 gm.; thymus, 12 gm.; pituitary, pineal, middle ears, air sinuses, bones, and aorta were grossly not remarkable.

Portions of liver, kidney, heart, spleen, pancreas, adrenal, skeletal muscle, brain, and lung were fixed in absolute alcohol. These were stained by Best's stain for glycogen. Representative samples of the above and other organs were fixed in formalin and Zenker's solution and subsequently stained with hematoxylin eosin. Various other stains were employed, using when necessary the material fixed in the three solutions and applying them to the organs indicated in the histologic description: for connective tissue, Mallory's aniline blue and phosphotungstic acid hematoxylin; for fat, scharlach R, nile blue sulphate, Smith-Dietrich, osmic acid, Fischler, Schultz, and Ciaccio; for glycogen, Langhan's iodine; for calcium, von Kossa; for iron, Tirmann's Turnbull blue, Mallory's ammonium sulphide, and potassium ferricyanide, Hueck's modification of Turnbull's blue; for bacteria, Gram and Giemsa; Foot's stain for reticulum; and a modified aniline blue, to bring out the granular qualities of the isletal cells of the pancreas.

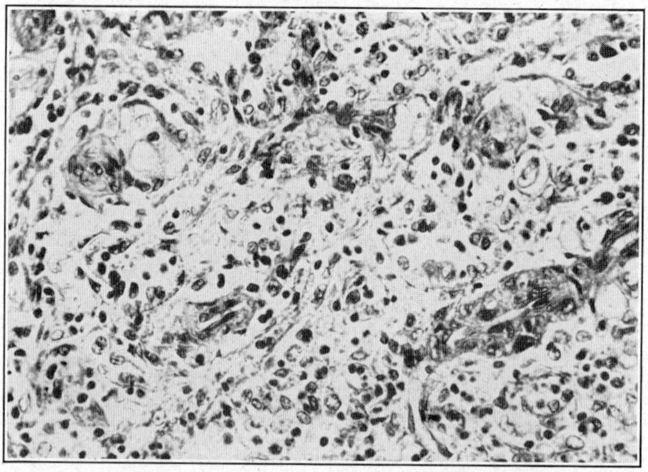

Fig. 2.—Spleen (hematoxylin and eosin). Note the large pale cells surrounding and compressing the arterioles. These were histochemically inert, staining neither for glycogen nor for fat. (×1250.)

Microscopic Examination

Heart.—The muscular fibers were of fairly uniform thickness with, in many, clear, large perinuclear spaces. These in instances contained pigmented granules. Only occasional fibers, but many leucocytes, contained glycogen. There was no iron or fat.

Lung.—There was only one lobular area of pneumonia with seropurulent exudate. Here were few scattered intracellular bacterial rods and cocci. Elsewhere there was moderate atelectasis with dilated bronchioles and areas of emphysema. There were scattered areas of alveolar hemorrhage and in others monocytes and occasional polymorphonuclears. The alveolar septal capillaries were congested and tortuous with increased numbers of polymorphonuclears and monocytes. There was no glycogen, except in an occasional polymorphonuclear. The free alveolar monocytes contained fine fatty droplets and only rarely hemosiderin granules.

Spleen (Fig. 2.).—There were many large pale cells, intimately associated with the intralobular arterioles, occurring singly and far more frequently in groups, within the pulp cords as well. These cells varied from 13.5 to 19.7 $\mu\mu$ in diameter. They were spherical or oval in shape with fairly sharply defined borders. The cytoplasm was frequently finely honeycombed with, in instances, larger vacuolated spaces. At times the cytoplasm appeared clear with a few strands attached to the nucleus.

The latter was usually single, rarely double, eccentrically placed in the cell, oval or spherical in shape, although occasionally wrinkled or slightly lobated and contained fine chromatin threads. These cells were incorporated in the parietes of intralobular arterioles, often disorganizing the muscular fibers and lying in juxtaposition to the endothelium, or compressing the muscular coat and thereby enlarging the adventitial portion of the vessel. In almost all instances the lumen was

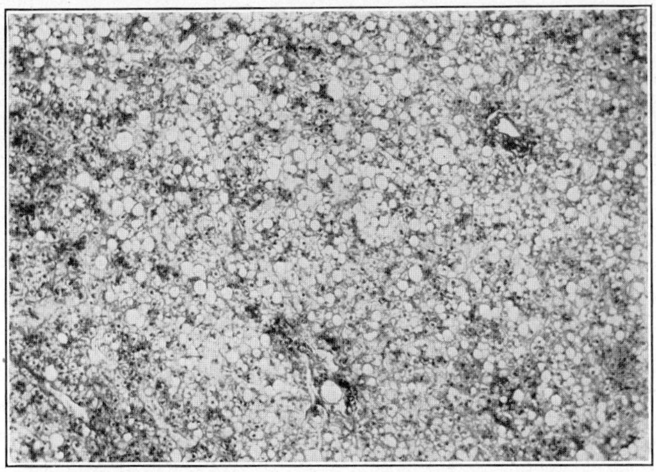

Fig. 3.—Liver (hematoxylin and eosin). An average field. Note the sharply bordered polygonal cells and the many large vacuolated ones. There was marked infiltration of the cells with glycogen and fat. (×150.)

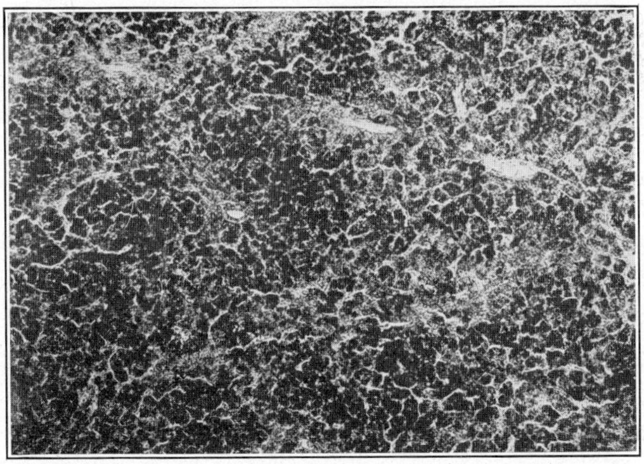

Fig. 4.—Liver (scharlach R). Note the abundance of fat. (×80.)

compressed or obliterated. Where related to these vessels, these cells were surrounded by fine collagenous fibrils. In all instances they were histochemically inert. Neither stains for glycogen nor repeated and varied stains for fat were to the slightest degree positive. They were not birefringent. There was very little blood in sinusoids or pulp cords. The former, however, were patent with prominent, almost columnar, lining endothelial cells. The subendothelial reticulum was prominent. There were large numbers of hemosiderin-laden monocytes, concentrated chiefly about trabeculae and intralobular vessels, so that with iron stains their distribution almost defined irregular lobelike areas. Here and there were increased numbers of polymorphonuclears. The corpuscles were of medium size with fairly large reactive central foci, made up of phagocytic reticular cells with included and scattered nuclear débris. These cells frequently contained sudanophilic granules.

Pancreas.—The islets were abundant and generally large. The cells were in general larger than in a control series of the same age. There were not infrequent cells with very large giant nuclei, from two to three times normal size, which were rich in chromatin. There was also moderate variation in nuclear size of the other cells. With modified aniline blue most of the cells stained light red, some deeper red, and fewer deep blue. The proportions of these were about the same in the control group. The cells with the larger nuclei, for the most part, stained blue. The parenchymal elements were not remarkable except for rare intracytoplasmic inclusion bodies. In some blood vessels and some polymorphonuclears there were deposits of glycogen. Occasional monocytes in the interlobular tissues were strongly positive for iron.

Liver (Figs. 3 and 4).—The lobular outlines were rather poorly defined. The central veins were frequently not seen or were irregularly related to the lobules. There was no increase in portal connective tissue, but there were collagenous fibrils radiating away from these compressed and elongated portal zones. Similar stellate projections of collagen extended from the adventitia of the hepatic veins. The reticular framework was not altered to any degree. The portal and hepatic veins were moderately congested. The sinusoids were narrowed and compressed. The bile ducts and capillaries were here and there dilated but were free of inspissated contents. The liver cells were generally large, plantlike in type, with thick-rimmed, sharply defined borders. They were polyhedral in shape and occasionally so arranged as to form pseudoacinar or tubular structures. There were frequent groups of larger vacuolated cells. The others had a fine threadlike and granular cytoplasm with variable numbers of smaller and larger vacuolated spaces. There were numerous fine granules of glycogen throughout the cytoplasm, occasionally larger in size or in laked form. In the large vacuolated cells, the deposits of glycogen either skirted the periphery or lay within a peripheral rim of cytoplasm surrounding an unflattened nucleus. Occasionally they formed a distinct film about the vacuole. There was massive fatty infiltration in many sections taken from different parts of the organ. Here and there periportal or perivenous (hepatic) areas were spared. The fat was deposited both small and medium sized droplets, and in the large cells as a single conglomerate sphere. It stained deep red with scharlach, rose violet to violet blue with nile blue sulphate, and not at all with the other stains. The nuclei of the cells were moderately large, spherical and more frequently eccentrically placed. Most of them were fairly densely chromatic. There were many, however, that were large and vacuolated, particularly periportally. These often contained glycogen in laked or in spherical form. Occasionally the liver cells were binucleated and, at times, one nucleus was large and vacuolated, the other of normal size and appearance. There was diffusion of glycogen into vascular spaces. There were rare small foci of necrosis with polymorphonuclear infiltration. These cells, as well as polymorphonuclears elsewhere, contained glycogen. The Kupffer cells were not particularly active, often were positive for iron, and occasionally contained sudanophilic granules.

Kidney (Fig. 5).—The cells of the convoluted tubules were of plantlike type. They were of increased height with thick, sharply defined cytoplasmic membranes, appearing in all quite rigid, although occasionally indented. Their central ends were rounded. They appeared hollow (hematoxylin and eosin) with, however, transitional forms, where the vacuolation appeared to start toward the central end of the cell, gradually effacing the acidophilic granular cytoplasm supra- and subsequently subnuclearly. The cells of the distal convoluted tubules were in all more involved than those of the proximal. The nuclei were basally placed, not flattened but spherical, with fairly thick membranes and compact chromatin. They were rarely enlarged and vacuolated. All these cells were stuffed with glycogen in the form of small and medium sized granules. Extending from the cortex well into the medulla, there was considerable glycogen in the lumina and cells of the limbs of Henle. There were deposits of urates in some of the terminal collecting tubules and hyaline casts, staining positively for calcium within small atrophic tubules, adjoining atrophic glomeruli. In the medulla there were occasional fibrosed areas, distorting adjoining collecting tubules and containing amorphous débris. There were fairly frequent fatty droplets within the convoluted tubular epithelium and occasionally within a glomerular tuft as a spherical mass probably occupying the lumen of a capillary. Many of the glomeruli were of fetal form, the others were not remarkable. Some of the pelvic epithelial cells contained glycogen.

Adrenals.—The adult cortex was regular and moderately thick. There was a greater amount of fat in the glomerular than in the fasiculate zone, but in all a goodly degree of lipoid depletion. The fetal cortex was almost completely involuted,

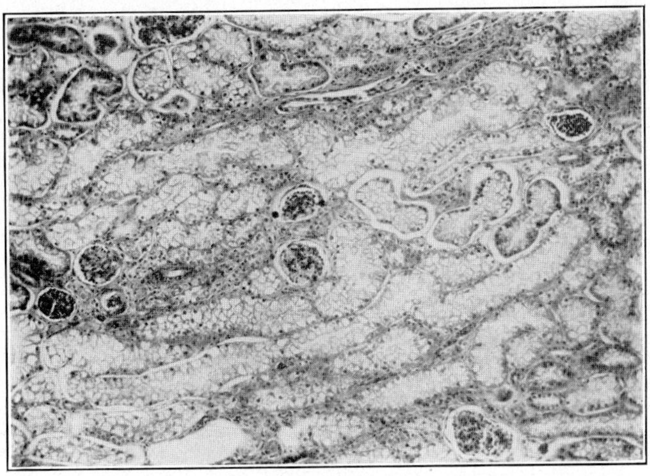

Fig. 5.—Kidney (hematoxylin and eosin). Note the thick, sharp bordered, rigid appearing, and clear cells of the convoluted tubules. These were massively infiltrated with glycogen. (×170.)

represented only by a highly vascularized fibrillar stroma in which there were many histiocytes laden with fat and hemosiderin.

Lymphoid Tissues.—There were large reactive foci in the primary follicles of the tonsils, paratracheal, mesenteric and peripancreatic lymph nodes, resembling those of the splenic corpuscles. In the tonsil there was a hyaline thrombus in one subepithelial venule and recent mural thrombi in some of the deeper-seated blood vessels. In one small paratracheal lymph node, there were many monocytes, some with a finely honeycombed cytoplasm resembling the pale cells in the spleen. In all nodes there were variable numbers of actively phagocytic monocytes. Some of these and the reticular cells of the reactive foci contained sudanophilic granules.

Thymus.—There was practically no involution. There were relatively few phagocytic monocytes. Within these, Hassall's corpuscles, and in many blood vessels there were deposits of fat. Eosinophilic myelocytes were frequent within the interlobular stroma and scattered throughout the lobules.

Thyroid.—The acini were smallish with little pale staining, at times vacuolated, colloid. The epithelium varied in height, being rather tall, with pale, almost vacuolated, cytoplasm at times, and with moderately chromatic nuclei occupying the greater part of the cell. There was no demonstrable fat.

Pituitary.—It was essentially normal, with abundant, acidophilic and chromophobe cells, but fewer basophiles (modified aniline blue).

Adipose Tissues.—In general there was mild to moderate atrophy of the retroperitoneal and mesenteric fat, with smaller lobules and cells.

Osseous System.—Sections of rib and vertebrae were studied. In the former there was a series of transverse bony bars (arrest of growth), one next to the epiphyseal zone. At this zone there was fairly active and regular penetration of the cartilaginous columns by vascularized marrow with, however, slight retardation in osteoid deposition. The nuclei of the cartilage cells in the hypertrophic zone were in instances prominently vacuolated and enlarged. There was some evidence of irregular absorption of the bony trabeculae of the shaft. Periosteum and cortical bone were not remarkable. In the marrow of both ribs and vertebrae there were many large pale cells, identical with those of the spleen. In addition there were occasional actively phagocytic histiocytes. The marrow elements were abundant, chiefly granulocytic, with many lymphocytoid cells, presumably red blood cell precursors. There were relatively few mature myeloid or erythroid forms. There were many megakaryocytes.

Brain and Cord.—The meninges were congested and lightly infiltrated with lymphocytes, monocytes, and an occasional polymorphonuclear. Except for a small area of red blood cell extravasation in the medulla, with mild congestion and edema in all sections, there were no unusual features. There was no demonstrable glycogen.

Pineal.—It appeared to be consistent in development with the age of the child.

Testes and aorta were not remarkable. There were stainable granules of glycogen in some of the striated fibers of the tongue and skeletal muscle. There was a mild degree of inflammatory reaction involving the mucosa of the trachea.

Anatomical Diagnosis.—Glycogen infiltration of liver and kidneys, marked; fatty infiltration of the liver; lobular pneumonia, mild; probably lipoid-storing cells in spleen and bone marrow; mild acute tracheitis; focal liver necroses; toxic reactive changes in lymphoid tissues generally; hemosiderosis of spleen, marked; mild peripheral and cerebral edema; lipoid depletion of adrenal.

CASE 2.—R. R., aged one year (Jewish), was admitted to the hospital for investigation of a large abdominal mass. At the age of two months, a midline dermoid tumor of the scalp was removed. Again at six months, he was seen in this hospital for hoarseness. On both these occasions there were no unusual physical findings. He had not been seen again until two days prior to the present admission. For the preceding six months, however, he had been almost constantly hoarse and had had frequent colds. The pertinent physical and laboratory findings were: rapid respirations; temperature, 100.2° F.; protuberant abdomen with a regular mass, presumably liver, filling the right flank and upper quadrant, extending to within 1 inch of the umbilicus and well over to the left; light trace of albumin in the urine with 3+ acetone (which was always present in subsequent specimens); moderate anemia. On the second day after admission, he was markedly hyperpneic and vomited several times. He died on the third day.

Necropsy was performed one hour postmortem. The incision was restricted to the abdomen. The body was well developed and nourished, measuring 73 cm. in length (normal). The head measured 17 inches in circumference; the chest, 17.5 inches; the abdomen, 20 inches. There was no free fluid in the peritoneal cavity. The liver was greatly enlarged, extending below the level of the crest of the ileum on the right to within 3 cm. of the umbilicus in the midline and disappearing behind the costal margin in the left midclavicular line. The spleen was not enlarged. Both kidneys, however, were greatly increased in size. The pleural and pericardial cavities were not remarkable.

Lungs.—The right lung weighed 104 gm. (64); the left, 74 gm. (57). Both lungs were firm and nodular in the dependent and juxtahilar regions, with dry purplish gray cut surfaces. The larger bronchi were not remarkable. From the smaller branches a serohemorrhagic fluid escaped.

Spleen weighed 32 gm. (26). The capsule was thin and smooth. The cut surfaces were brownish purple in color with prominent lymphoid markings.

Liver weighed 1213 gm. (288). It was firm with a thin, smooth, glistening capsule. The inferior edge was blunted with a deep prominent notch just medial to the gallbladder fossa. Both external and moist cut surfaces were pale yellow in color, and from the latter a grayish fluid could be expressed. The usual markings were obscured.

Kidneys.—The right kidney weighed 77 gm. (36); the left, 67 gm. (35). They were moderately firm. The capsules were thin and stripped readily, exposing smooth, pale pink, external surfaces. The cut surfaces were pale with well-defined markings, however.

Thymus weighed 22 gm. It was large, soft and pulpy, grayish white in color with little interlobular connective tissue.

The mesenteric, mediastinal and pulmonary hilar lymph nodes were large softish and pale yellowish gray in color. Heart weighed 50 gm. (64); pancreas and adrenals (combined weight), 9 gm.; gastrointestinal tract, bone and spinal cord were grossly not remarkable.

Only sections of liver, kidney, spleen, thymus and spinal cord were fixed in absolute alcohol at the time of autopsy.

Microscopic Examination

Lung.—There was an extensive pneumonia. The exudate varied from serous to frankly purulent with hyaline membranes in one subpleural area. Many gram-positive lancet-shaped diplococci were present within the polymorphonuclears and monocytes of the exudate. The bronchioles were variously involved, with ulceration, vascular thrombosis, and hemorrhage in some, as well as purulent exudate in the lumina of many. The fibers of their muscular coats appeared clear and vacuolated. The pleura, interlobular septums and subendothelial venous walls were mildly involved in the inflammatory process.

Spleen.—There were the same large pale cells as in the previous case, but far fewer in number. Here, too, they were histochemically inert. There was mild passive congestion with less endothelial hypertrophy. The pulp cords were cellular, chiefly due to lymphocytes. There were occasional actively phagocytic histiocytes but in all with little recognizable hemosiderin. There were large ''toxic'' reactive foci in the corpuscles. There were Best-positive granules in many of the polymorphonuclears and in eosinophilic myelocytes.

Pancreas.—The islets were abundant and of moderate size. There were only rare isletal cells with large nuclei, but there were many irregularly polyhedral or pyramidal atrophic forms. The cytoplasm of these was deeply acidophilic and their nuclei were dark staining, small, pleomorphic, and pyknotic. The parenchyma was not remarkable.

Liver (Figs. 6 and 7).—These sections were almost identical with those of the former case, with the following differences: there was more portal connective tissue, tending at times to outline lobules and occasionally surrounding islands of liver cells. The latter were a little more uniform and smaller in size with, in all, fewer large vacuolated cells. The cytoplasm of the smaller cells, however, contained many discrete small fatty droplets with less tendency to become confluent than in the previous case. Comparing the sections of both cases, one gained the impression that there was about the same amount of stainable glycogen but slightly less fat in this case. The liver in this case was, however, much larger than that in the former, so that quantitatively there possibly was more fat in the liver as a whole. The same probably applies for glycogen.

Kidney.—It was the same as in the previous case except for more frequent vacuolated nuclei, containing glycogen in the cells of the convoluted tubules, larger granules of glycogen in the cytoplasm of the cells, a lesser amount of stainable fat, and no evidence of calcification.

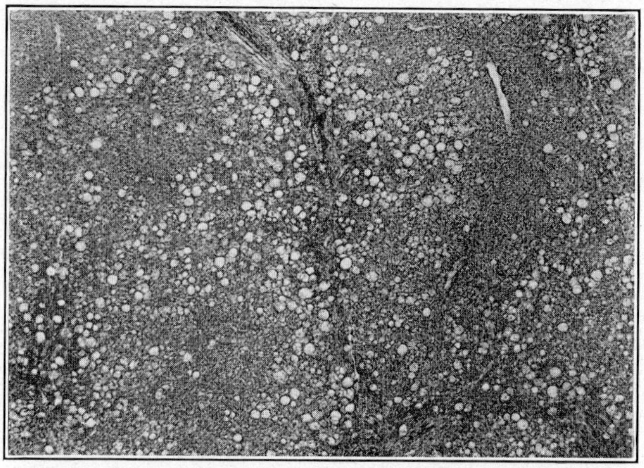

Fig. 6.—Liver (Best). There is considerable glycogen but also many large vacuolated cells. (×80.)

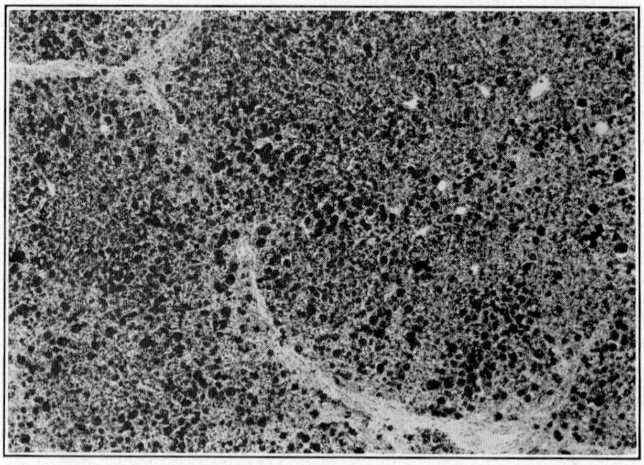

Fig. 7.—Liver (scharlach R). Note the large amount of stainable fat. An average field in a number of sections from several blocks. (×80.)

Adrenals.—The sections were identical with those of the former case particularly with reference to the degree of lipoid depletion and its distribution. There were fewer histiocytes in the medulla and the sympathochromaffin elements were more abundant.

Thymus.—Here again there was practically no involution but persistence of myelopoiesis. There were Best-positive granules in the polymorphonuclears infiltrating necrotic Hassall's corpuscles and in some of the myelocytes.

Lymph Nodes.—In those from the mesentery there were dilated sinusoids containing lymphocytes, monocytes and polymorphonuclears. In the cortical follicles there were large reactive foci, like those in the corpuscles of the spleen. The pulmonary hilar nodes presented more acute inflammatory changes.

Osseous System.—The sections of rib and vertebrae were identical with those of the former case except that the large pale cells were scarce in the rib but plentiful in the vertebrae.

Of the other sections there were chronic inflammatory changes in the esophagus with early mild ulceration and congestion of the small intestine with intramucosal lymphoid follicles containing ''toxic'' reactive foci. Heart, testes, and spinal cord were not remarkable. The adipose tissue was more abundant than in the former case, but there were areas of early atrophy in some of the larger fatty lobules, and in general the fat cells themselves were smallish.

Anatomical Diagnoses.—Glycogenic infiltration of liver and kidney; marked fatty infiltration of the liver; probably lipoid-staining cells in spleen and bone marrow; bronchopneumonia, marked; ''toxic'' reactive changes in lymphoid tissues generally; chronic passive congestion of the spleen; chronic esophagitis; lipoid depletion of the adrenal.

A third case will be described briefly, in which liver, skin, and muscle were obtained by biopsy, but in which postmortem examination was refused.

CASE 3.—E. P., aged eight years two months, had been noted to have an enlarged abdomen ever since six months of age. One sister died at the age of four years with apparently a similar condition. There was another younger sister living and well. This patient had been seen in the Out-Patient Department of this hospital on several occasions from the time she was one and two-thirds years old. Her physical development was tardy, and at the present hospital admission she appeared to be no more than five years old. The liver was always greatly enlarged. The spleen was not palpable. She had never been jaundiced. She had occasional epistaxis. For the past year she complained of fatigue. Three weeks before admission she developed extreme dyspnea and anorexia. The pertinent physical and laboratory findings were: delicate slender extremities, meager subcutaneous tissues elsewhere although full cheeks, dullness at the bases of both lungs with many moist râles; markedly protuberant abdomen with a palpable liver 10 cm. beyond the midline to the left and well below the iliac crest on the right. There was acetonuria on two occasions, red blood cells 2,520,000 with 29 per cent hemoglobin, white blood cells 7,750 with 50 per cent polymorphs, 11 per cent lymphocytes, 22 per cent young forms, and 14 per cent macrocytes. Fasting blood sugar levels varied from 51 to 72 mg. per cent. There was practically no response to adrenalin. The glucose tolerance curve rose from 72 to 166 after two hours and fell to 85 on the third hour. Serum calcium was 10.2 and phosphorus, 2.3. The nonprotein nitrogen was 18 and cholesterol, 184. She ran a constantly elevated temperature and died within a month of admission.

Biopsy Examination

Liver.—It was practically identical with that of the second case. There was, however, mild lymphocytic and polymorphonuclear infiltration of the portal areas. There was a large amount of glycogen and also fat. The latter was present in the form of smaller droplets, with, in frequent areas, larger cells with large globular masses of fat.

Skin.—There was mild perivascular lymphocytic infiltration with histiocytic proliferation. The endothelial cells of the small blood vessels were prominent. There was mild edema of the papillary layer of the corium. The coil glands were dilated. The smooth muscles of the subcutaneous arteries were enlarged and vacuolated. The subcutaneous fat was well developed. There was no stainable glycogen in the epidermis, but this substance was abundant in the epithelium of the hair shafts, the smooth muscle of the subcutaneous arteries, and mildly in the epithelium of the ducts of the sudoriferous glands, the fat cells of one small atrophic lobule, occasional polymorphonuclears, and rare fibrocytes or monocytes.

Muscle.—There was mild infiltration of the muscle fibers with glycogen.

In spite of several months of fixation in Pick's solution (ii), the liver and kidneys of the first case contained respectively 3.04 per cent and 11.5 per cent of glycogen in terms of dry weight.[12] This compares favorably with the findings of others in this disease, due consideration being paid to the duration of fixation. In von Gierke's first case, there was 33.72 per cent glycogen for dry weight of liver and 36.82 per cent for the kidney, fresh material being employed for chemical analysis (twenty-four hours postmortem). Kimmelstiel reported 16.5 per cent for wet weight of liver after five days in the ice chest and Antopol and his coworkers, 3.25 per cent and 4.34 per cent for liver and kidney, respectively, in formalin-fixed material four weeks after autopsy. Faber found 15.3 per cent glycogen for wet weight of liver and 5.9 per cent for the kidney twenty-eight hours postmortem. Popper and Wozasek[13] give the following values for glycogen in man: with slow agonal death 0.3 to 1.2 per cent for the liver; in sudden deaths, 2.42 to 6.17 per cent. The kidneys ordinarily contained 0.29 to 0.69 per cent rising to 0.97 and 1.64 per cent in diabetics. They reported elevated glycogen values for the liver in children with diabetes and alimentary intoxication. It is obvious that the values for the two organs here exceed by far those of the normal range.

Even more striking was the finding of a total fat content of 52.3 per cent for the dry weight of liver.[14] There are very few reported analyses for the fat content of this organ in different diseases. Hoppe-Seyler's figures[15] are given in terms of dry weight in the following:

Accidental death by drowning	9.6%
Passive congestion	2.8%
Acute yellow atrophy	27.4%
Acute yellow atrophy with mild cirrhosis	9.5%
Atrophic cirrhosis	7.3 — 27.9%
Atrophic cirrhosis with diabetes	7.3%
Large cirrhotic fatty livers (Zirrhotische Fettleber)	50.3 — 74.4%
Hypertrophic cirrhosis	46.7%

The ages of the individuals from whom these were obtained varied from twenty-three to sixty-two years. In reviewing the weights of frankly fatty livers from the autopsy files of this hospital, it was of interest that a number fell below the given average, that many were within or slightly above the average, with relatively few approaching double the normal weight. A very large percentage of these occurred in infants with nutritional disturbances, in whom, depending upon the duration of the disease and accompanying marasmus, there was in general goodly visceral atrophy. This might account for the above observations where with massive fatty infiltration there was for the most part an inappreciable elevation in weight of the liver. It is regrettable that there are no known fat values for these, but, even if one assumes that the percentage for the dry weight of them approximated that of the large cirrhotic fatty livers, there probably would be less total fat than in an organ some three and one-half times normal weight. Whether the fat factor here, even as in the enlarged livers of juvenile diabetics, contributes in any way to the hypertrophy of the organ is quite uncertain. In view of the antagonistic hydration tendencies of glycogen and fat, the former being high, the latter low, it might be expected that the fat in cells filled with stable glycogen would tend in all to be of finer dispersed form. Hence from histologic observations alone, the fat factor may appear to be inappreciable. One, therefore, gains the impression that with future chemical analyses the livers in this disease will be found to contain a considerable amount of fat, even exceeding at times those of the above mentioned type in which almost all the liver cells are stuffed with lipoids and the appearance is almost one of adipose tissue.

Associated with the marked degree of fatty infiltration of the liver also noted in the two other cases in which there were no chemical analyses, there were, clinically, a distinct lipemia, with a serum cholesterol of 394 mg. per cent, acidosis with a carbon dioxide combining power of 24 volumes per cent and acetonuria. Another unusual morphologic finding was the presence of large vacuolated cells in the spleen and bone marrow of both this and the second case. These failed to stain for fat or glycogen, although various methods were employed. Yet there is no reason to believe that they contained glycogen in view of the apparent stability of this substance in this disease and therefore little chance of complete lysis having occurred here and not elsewhere, as well as the fact that the leucocytes in the same organ contained granules which stained readily with Best's stain and iodine. There is far more reason to believe that they stored lipoids. Morphologically they resembled fat-laden monocytes without, however, any of the characteristics of the Gaucher cell. Furthermore, Warren[16] states that "aside from this fairly common finding of rare lipoid-containing cells in the spleen, there are a few cases of diabetes with lipemia recorded, in which very marked hyperplasia of these cells occurs, and the lipoid present does not as a rule give the staining reactions usually encountered." It is possible that here one is dealing with a complex combination of fats of which poorly stainable or nonstainable chemical forms may be present.

This leads one to draw an analogy between this disease and diabetes mellitus, at least from the point of view of fat metabolism. If it is true, in a physiologic sense, that diabetes is characterized by excessive, and this disease by diminished, glycogenolysis, then in both, fats will be excessively burnt, particularly when there is greater metabolic activity. In both, therefore, there may be lipemia and ketosis. But, whereas in diabetes there are hyperglycemia and glycosuria, here there are hypoglycemia and no glycosuria. Furthermore, enlarged fatty livers in juvenile diabetics, particularly, are not at all infrequent, and in instances with lipemia, they too have had fat-laden monocytes in the spleen.

In the review of the histologic observations of fat in the liver reported in the literature in this disease and cited elsewhere in this paper, as well as in the present cases, it is obvious that the amount of fat in the organ can be quite variable. Recently there have appeared several reports dealing with hypertrophy of the liver in infancy, said to be due to massive fatty infiltration. Bjorum[17] in 1926 reported in the same family four cases with greatly enlarged livers, which he diagnosed as adipositas hepatis, at postmortem. Debre and Semelaigne[18, 19] have placed four of their living cases of hepatomegaly into the same category, on the basis of a single biopsy from one. The clinical aspects of their cases agree favorably with those of glycogen disease. Van Creveld[20] has emphasized that variations in clinical behavior and laboratory findings are to a degree to be expected. In both these reports there were no histochemical studies for glycogen. It is to be emphasized that fat and glycogen may coexist abundantly in the same organ and in the same cell. There is, however, one puzzling report by Kramer, Grayzel, and Solomon,[21] which appears to stand alone in this respect. It is that of a child, eight months of age, with hepatomegaly, marked hypoglycemia, no response to adrenalin, and no acetonuria. There was extensive fat replacement of the liver and with Best's stain no evidence of glycogen. Whether in the group of hepatic hypertrophies in infancy and childhood, excluding the cirrhoses and other well-defined lesions, and of which glycogen storage disease at present forms a well-recognized division, that of pure massive fatty infiltration alone, will also form a distinct group is not as yet entirely clear. There have been clinical descriptions of instances without anatomic studies where the disturbance in carbohydrate metabolism has been considered to be of the nature of absence or disturbed glycogenesis (*azoomylie* and *dyszoomylie* of the German literature). It may be that, in these, future pathological studies may reveal that the accompanying enlarged livers in such instances are due to fatty infiltration alone with no abnormal glycogen storage in this or other organs.

Lastly, in the first two cases there were several features in common, viz., considerable depletion of the lipoids of the adrenal as described by Goldzieher[22] in diabetic lipemias; practically no involution of the thymus with, however, persistent myelopoiesis; evident lines of arrest of bony growth characterized histologically by the persistence of transverse bony trabeculae; and some degree of atrophy of the adipose tissues in general.

CONCLUSIONS

Two cases of glycogen storage disease with autopsy findings and one with biopsy of the liver are described.

Disturbances in fat metabolism, accompanying this disease, are stressed, and an analogy is drawn between glycogen storage disease and diabetes mellitus from that standpoint.

I wish to acknowledge my thanks to Dr. William Salter for the glycogen analyses and to Dr. Allen M. Butler for the fat determinations.

REFERENCES

1. Beumer, H., and Loeschke, A.: München. med. Wchnschr. **80**: 377, 1933.
2. Unshelm, E.: Deutsche med. Wchnschr. **17**: 633, 1934.
3. Von Gierke, E.: Beitr. z. path. Anat. u. allg. Path. **82**: 497, 1929.
4. Loeschke, A.: Ztschr. f. Kinderh. **53**: 553, 1932.
5. Schall, L.: München. med. Wchnschr. **79**: 2078, 1932.
6. Putschar, W.: Beitr. z. path. Anat. u. allg. Path. **90**: 222, 1932.
7. Kimmelstiel, P.: Beitr. z. path. Anat. u. allg. Path. **91**: 1, 1933.
8. Pompe, J. C.: Ann. d. anat. path. **10**: 23, 1933.
9. Antopol, W., Heilbrunn, J., and Tuchman, L.: Am. J. M. Sc. **188**: 354, 1934.
10. Humphreys, E. M., and Kato, K.: Am. J. Path. **10**: 589, 1934.
11. Faber, V.: Frankfurt. Ztschr. f. Path. **47**: 443, 1935.
12. Slosse, A.: Compt. rend. Soc. de biol. **97**: 1810, 1927.
13. Popper, H., and Wozasek, O.: Wien. med. Wchnschr. **79**: 456, 1929.
14. Kirk, E., Page, I. H., Van Slyke, D. D.: J. Biol. Chem. **106**: 203, 1934.
15. Hoppe-Seyler, G.: Cited by Rossle, R., in Henke-Lubarsch: Handbuch der Speziellen Pathologischen Anat. und Histologie, Berlin, 1930, Julius Springer, 5,[1] p. 394.
16. Warren, S.: The Pathology of Diabetes Mellitus, Philadelphia, 1930, Lea & Febiger, p. 94.
17. Bjorum, A.: Acta Paediat. **6**: 225, 1926-1927.
18. Debre, R., and Semelaigne, G.: Presse méd. **101**: 1742, 1930.
19. Debre, R., Semelaigne, G., and Nachmansohn, Gilbrin: Bull. et mém. Soc. méd. d. hôp. de Paris **50**: 1023, 1934.
20. Van Creveld, S.: Arch. Dis. Child. **9**: 9, 1934.
21. Kramer, B., Grayzel, H. G., and Solomon, C. I.: J. Pediat. **5**: 299, 1934.
22. Goldzieher, M. A.: The Adrenals, New York, 1929, The Macmillan Co., p. 263.

ANGIOMAS IN PREMATURE INFANTS

Alwin C. Rambar, M.D.
Chicago, Ill.

Tumors of the blood vessels are the most common type of neoplasm occurring in infancy. This communication deals only with angiomas of the skin in premature infants seen in the premature clinic of the Sarah Morris Hospital in the three-year period, 1932 to 1935. Although these lesions are by no means rare in either full-term or premature infants, their incidence according to the author's knowledge has not been previously computed. Of 344 premature white infants observed during this period, 40, or 11.64 per cent, were so affected. In 78 premature negro infants seen during the same period, no angiomas were noted.

VARIETIES OF TUMORS AND TIME OF APPEARANCE

Thirty-five of the infants had angioma simplex, so-called strawberry marks; 4 had cavernous angiomas; and 1 had a nevus flammeus, or port-wine stain. These diagnoses are clinical, based only on their appearance, as it is impossible to classify accurately the character of the tumor without histologic examination. In only 7 instances were these marks noted at birth, and in each case the lesion developed into a comparatively large tumor. The nevus flammeus noted was also present at birth. In all of the other instances, the lesion first made its appearance between the first week and the second month of life. The angiomas first appear as slight irregular discolorations, of the skin, which rapidly enlarge and become elevated until they assume their characteristic red spongy appearance. According to Bland-Sutton,[1] an angioma may be present at birth, but much more frequently it appears in the first few weeks of life. Fitzwilliams[2] stated that this was a widely believed fallacy, and he presented figures in 645 cases showing 537, or 83.2 per cent, of the lesions present at birth. His investigation showed that the marks were usually noted at the twelfth to fourteenth day of life and concluded that this was the first day that the mother bathed the baby and thus saw it undressed for the first time. He therefore felt that the figure of 83.2 per cent underestimated the true facts, and that practically all vascular nevi were present at birth. Culver,[3] in reporting a series of 23 infants with angiomas, found that 14 were present at birth. Other authors agree that the lesions are either present at birth or may appear at any time up to the first several months of life.

In the 40 infants in whom lesions were found, there were 60 angiomas noted. Twelve had multiple lesions, 7 being the greatest number found

From the Department of Pediatrics, Michael Reese Hospital.

in any one infant. No convulsions, spastic hemiplegias, or mental deficiency which might be referable to associated angiomas of the brain have occurred.[4]

LOCATION OF TUMORS

Scalp	3		
Face	8	15	25.0%
Neck	4		
Upper extremities	12	19	31.6%
Lower extremities	7		
Anterior thorax	7		
Back	9	26	43.3%
Abdomen	8		
Genitals	2		

These tumors differ in location from the usual sites reported by other observers. In this series, 15 (25 per cent) were on the head and neck;

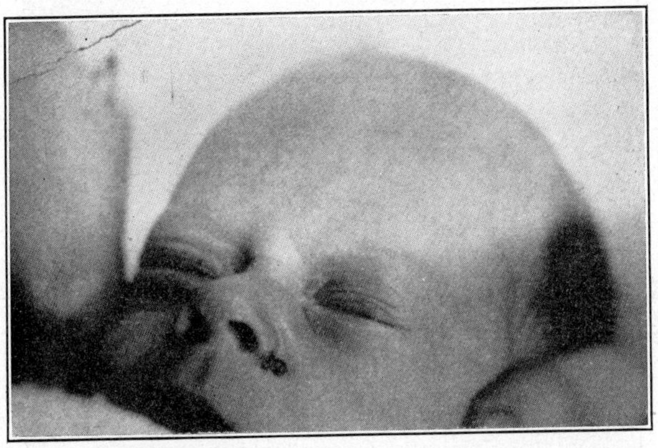

Fig. 1.—A. S., aged six weeks. Angioma simplex at side of nose first appeared at the age of nineteen days.

19 (31.6 per cent) were on the extremities; and 26 (43.2 per cent) were on the trunk or genitals. In Fitzwilliams' series[2] of 645 cases, 49.3 per cent were found on the head and neck, 21.2 per cent on the extremities, and 29.2 per cent on the trunk. Taylor,[5] in reviewing all the cases treated at Huntington Memorial Hospital from 1914 to 1925, found that in the 193 patients seen, 167 lesions were on the head and neck, 19 on the extremities, and 15 on the trunk. In Rulison and McLean's series[6] of 33 patients with 43 lesions, 60.5 per cent were on the head; 18.6 per cent were on the extremities; and 20.3 per cent were on the trunk. In Culver's series[3] of 29 angiomas in 23 infants, there were 25 about the head, mostly on the face. In Robinson's series[7] of 276 infants with 297 angiomas, there were 76 per cent on the head and neck, 13.1 per cent on the extremities, and 10.8 per cent on the trunk. Geschickter[8] noted that the distribution of 370 cutaneous angiomas was as follows: head and neck, 201; extremities, 110; trunk and genitals, 59. He stated that

his study included only lesions based on surgical and autopsy records and did not consider the very common angiomas on the surface of the body which escaped clinical and pathological study. MacCollum[9] recently reviewed 697 angiomas seen at Children's Hospital in Boston and noted that 469 (67 per cent) were on the head and neck.

The above statistics were compiled mainly by consultants to whom these patients were referred for treatment. This fact probably accounts for the prevailing statement in the literature that angiomas predominate on the head and neck. Since angiomas in other locations are not as objectionable from an esthetic viewpoint, they do not reach the attention of a consultant as commonly, and hence are not included in these authors' statistics.

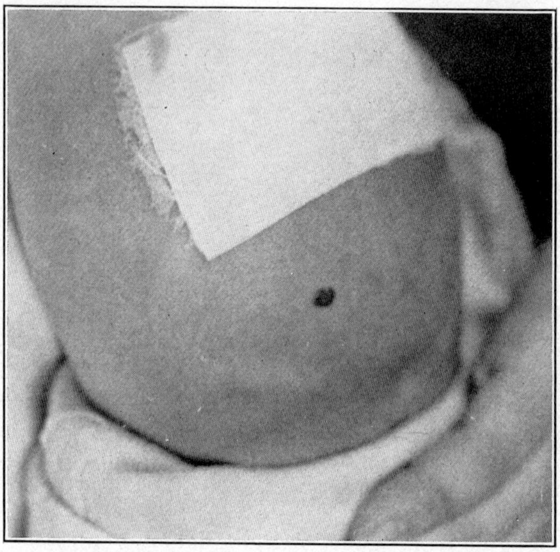

Fig. 2.—B. T., aged six weeks. Angioma simplex on abdomen first appeared at the age of twenty days.

RELATION TO SEX

Twenty-six of the infants (65 per cent) were female, and 14 (35 per cent) were males. These figures correspond exactly with those of Fitzwilliams,[2] who found 65.2 per cent in females and 34.7 per cent in males. In Robinson's series[7] there were 68.1 per cent females and 31.9 per cent males. MacCollum[9] found 69 per cent females and 31 per cent males. This constitutes a rather striking similarity of figures in both large and small groups of infants.

RELATION TO BIRTH WEIGHT

In an incomplete review of the same group of premature infants which I am reporting, Mohr[10] previously noted that angiomas and other nevi are more common among the prematurely born than among their siblings. He stated that in this group these conditions were observed to occur only among the children with low birth weights, none of the infants having weighed as much as 2,000 gm. at birth. A study of the birth weight of the 40 infants making up this series shows that 9 infants weighed between 1,000 and 1,500 gm. at birth, 19 weighed between 1,500 and 2,000 gm., and 12 weighed over 2,000 gm.

EMBRYOLOGY AND HISTOPATHOLOGY

The primitive circulatory system develops from the mesoderm overlying the yolk sac at the junction of the foregut and hindgut. Blood islands, isolated areas of formative tissue, occur here and by joining to-

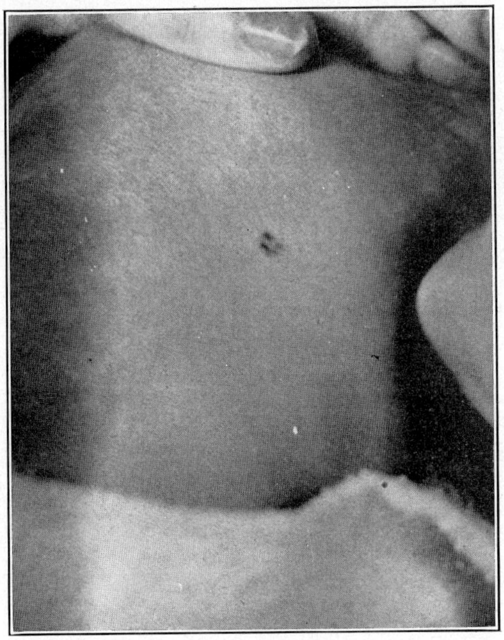

Fig. 3.—M. M., aged seven weeks. Angioma simplex on back first appeared at the age of twenty-three days.

gether develop a network of vessels over the yolk sac. From this mesenchymal network the circulatory system grows by extension. Proliferative growth of the endothelial lining links the vascular spaces into continuous channels, which further expand by independent sprouting.

Three clinical forms of angiomas are recognized: 1. The simple raised type, angioma simplex, or strawberry mark, is composed of endothelial lined spaces of varying sizes. Both venules and arterioles may form the constituents. There appears to be an endothelial proliferation of the intima in the form of outbuddings of a parent vessel. Histologically these vessels are separated by a narrow strip of connective tissue, or are freely connected with each other by a system of vessels.

2. Cavernous angiomas are deep seated. They are either venous or arterial in origin, and are usually deep purple in color, having the same structure as erectile tissue. Histologically they contain larger vessels than the angioma simplex.

3. Nevus flammeus, or port-wine stain, usually occurs in the upper layer of the corium. Here are formed a large number of dilated capillaries which are distinctly elongated and extend in various directions. These are particularly of the venous type.

THEORIES OF CAUSATION

Unna[11] believed that abnormal pressure during fetal life was the genetic factor in the production of angiomas. Ribbert's theory[12] was that these tumors develop from embryologic rudiments. Virchow[13] believed that these tumors result from the action of local irritation on imperfectly formed vessels, as those found in embryonal fissures. According to Ewing,[14] their origin lies in a developmental anomaly in the structure of certain vascular segments which retain embryologic characters. He states that the congenital origin of the great majority of angiomas speaks strongly in favor of a tissue predisposition as a prominent factor in their genesis. Some authors[2, 15, 16] believe that there is a relationship of these lesions to the distribution of the peripheral nerves. Laidlaw and Murray[17] have extended the theory that angiomas may be phylogenetic remnants of early vascular tufts that served as accessory lung tissue in the skin of reptiles and lower forms. Their occurrence in man might then be compared with the appearance and disappearance of the gill arches, suggesting that such tumors may be the remains of the vascular tufts that did not disappear in early embryonic life.

Because of the greater incidence of these lesions in premature infants, the author suggests that there is a relationship between the production of angiomas and the peripheral vascular needs of the body. Thus, these lesions appear at a time of rapid growth, when the body surface is expanding and has a demand for increased blood supply. During part of this period the temperature mechanism of the premature infant is poorly regulated, and the skin temperature is lower than normal. The blood pressure at this time is increasing with the growth of the infant.[18] Thoma[19] has stated that increase of blood pressure tends to excite new growth of blood vessels, although Leader[20] believes that this would cause an increase in the size of vessels already present rather than overproduction.

COURSE AND TREATMENT

With the exception of the nevus flammeus and small vascular papules that remain stationary in size, all of these angiomas have shown signs of rapid growth immediately following their appearance. In a few of these infants who were untreated for various reasons, the growth persisted until about the age of six months, when its maximum size was reached. Seven infants had lesions so small that no treatment was deemed necessary. Five infants failed to return for observation. In four infants with moderately large lesions spontaneous regression after six months has occurred. Twenty-four patients have received treatment by exposure to radium.

The optimum time to begin treatment and the type of treatment advised have long been subjects of considerable controversy. Many forms of therapy have been reported with varying success, mainly radium, x-ray, freezing with carbon dioxide snow, removal by surgery, cautery, injection of various substances from boiling water to sodium morrhuate, chemical caustics, etc.

Traub[21] recently reviewed the subject of whether vascular nevi should be treated, by questioning 117 members of the American Dermatologic Association. Sixty-three per cent of the answers indicated that the authors had seen an infrequent spontaneous disappearance (1 to 2 cases each). From the answers he concluded that it is best to wait for a very short time only in stationary angiomas, but in progressive lesions immediate measures are advisable. He further states that today, probably more men prefer radium than any other method of treatment. Culver[3] states that a baby can receive treatment at any age with complete safety. Simpson[22] believes that treatment should be begun in earliest infancy. Rulison and McLean[6] conclude that the younger the patient the better and more rapid are the results under radium therapy. Schamberg and Bradley[23] were of the same opinion and stated that their best results were obtained in infants in whom treatment was started between the fourth and tenth week. Authors advising other types of treatment, namely, x-ray and carbon dioxide snow, believe that treatment should be started as early as possible. MacCollum stresses the use of endothermy coagulation in raised lesions, emphasizing, however, that in many instances no one method is sufficient.

In this group of infants radium* has been applied at the age of three to six months, although I believe that it may be used earlier with safety. The cavernous angiomas have been treated by means of interstitial radiation. Monel needles containing platinum cells are inserted for periods varying from twenty-four to forty-eight hours. The other angiomas have been treated by means of external radiation with radium plaques. The treatments have been administered in divided doses. From 4 to 12 applications at one-month intervals have been necessary, depending upon the size of the lesion. In this manner local reactions are completely eliminated.

The response of the lesion to such treatment is slow and occurs over a period of months. It is believed that this form of regression represents

*Radium therapy was administered by the tumor clinic under the direction of Dr. Max Cutler.

the ideal in the treatment of these lesions, and it is the purpose of the technic employed to cause a slow regression without violent reactions in normal tissues.

CONCLUSIONS

1. Of 344 premature white infants 40 (11.64 per cent) developed angiomas. In 78 premature negro infants no angiomas occurred.
2. Thirty-five of the infants had angioma simplex, 4 cavernous angiomas, and 1 nevus flammeus.
3. Fifteen (25 per cent) of the lesions occurred on the head and neck, 19 (31.6 per cent) on the extremities, and 26 (43.3 per cent) on the trunk; 26 (65 per cent) of the infants affected were females, and 14 (35 per cent) were males.
4. It is suggested that there is a relationship in the development of the angiomas to the peripheral vascular needs of the infant.
5. Radium has been used successfully in the eradication of these lesions with no local or general reactions.

REFERENCES

1. Bland-Sutton, John: Tumours, Innocent and Malignant, ed. 3, Chicago, 1903, W. T. Keener & Co., p. 156.
2. Fitzwilliams, D. C. L.: Brit. M. J. **2**: 489, 1911.
3. Culver, George D.: Arch. Dermat. & Syph. **8**: 769, 1923.
4. Yakovlev, P. I., and Guthrie, R. H.: Arch. Neurol. & Psychiat. **26**: 1145, 1931.
5. Taylor, Grantley W.: Boston M. & S. J. **195**: 717, 1926.
6. Rulison, R. H., and McLean, Stafford: Am. J. Dis. Child. **25**: 359, 1923.
7. Robinson, G. Allen: Arch. Pediat. **44**: 660, 1927.
8. Geschickter, C. F., and Keasbey, L. E.: Am. J. Cancer **23**: 568, 1935.
9. MacCollum, Donald J.: Am. J. Surg. **29**: 32, 1935.
10. Hess, Julius H., Mohr, George J., and Bartelme, Phyllis F.: The Physical and Mental Growth of Prematurely Born Children, Chicago, 1934, The University of Chicago Press, p. 190.
11. Unna, P. G.: The Histopathology of Diseases of the Skin, Edinburgh, 1896, Wm. F. Clay, p. 1168.
12. Ribbert: Virchows Arch. f. Path. anat u. Phys. u. f. klin. Med. **151**: 26, 1898.
13. Virchow, R.: Arch. f. path. Anat. **3**: 425, 1851.
14. Ewing, James: Neoplastic Diseases, ed. 3, Philadelphia, 1928, W. B. Saunders Co., p. 243.
15. Cushing, H.: J. A. M. A. **47**: 178, 1906.
16. Stewart, S. F., and Bettin, M. E.: Surg. Gynec. Obst **39**: 307, 1924.
17. Laidlaw, G. F., and Murray, M. R.: Am. J. Path. **9**: 827, 1933.
18. Londe, Sol.: Am. J. Dis. Child. **44**: 110, 1932.
19. Thoma: Quoted by Ewing.[14]
20. Leader, Sidney: Personal communication to the author.
21. Traub, Eugene F.: Arch. Pediat. **50**: 272, 1933.
22. Simpson, Frank Edward: Surg. Gynec. Obst. **38**: 407, 1924.
23. Schamberg, Jay Frank, and Bradley, R. A.: Surg. Clin. North America **7**: 103, 1927.

1525 East Fifty-Third Street

SODIUM CHLORIDE IN THE TREATMENT OF NOCTURNAL ENURESIS IN CHILDREN

William Rosenson, M.D., New York, N. Y., and
Rebecca Liswood, M.D., Brooklyn, N. Y.

The treatment of nocturnal enuresis in children has been a rather desultory and haphazard procedure. In the management of a case one method after another has usually been tried in the hope of finding something eventually that would control the bed-wetting. From the physical standpoint, perhaps the most satisfactory results have been obtained by the limitation of the fluid intake toward the end of the day in conjunction with the administration of some form of atropine. From the mental aspect, the condition not infrequently has responded to the simple use of suggestion or to the more complex analytic approach. But in many instances, all measures have proved unsuccessful.

Quite by accident, Krasnogorski[1] came upon a new and interesting idea for the control of this condition. In 1927 he and his coworkers, Gantt and Harbedia, were engaged in experimental work upon the salivary glands. They were trying to determine what factors influenced the quantity of secretion from these bodies. Neither the elimination of water from the diet nor the production of a profuse perspiration by sun baths decreased the amount of secretion except in one group of children. At first this seemed puzzling, but further investigation disclosed that this group in whom water was eliminated from the diet happened to have had a breakfast which included salt ham and herring. This suggested a possible association of the salty diet with the diminution of the secretion. Subsequent experimental work along this line revealed that sodium chloride if given in sufficient amounts invariably reduced the amount of salivary flow. Later this lessening of secretion by an increased salt intake was even more strikingly demonstrated in relation to the pancreatic juice.

Krasnogorski then decided to apply this principle to the secretion of urine in cases of nocturnal enuresis in children. The salt was given in the form of a caviar or ham sandwich when the child was already in bed and about ready to go to sleep. This arrangement left no time for the development of thirst while awake. Children can sleep all night in spite of a slight or moderate thirst. In addition, the routine care included the elimination of fluids after four o'clock in the afternoon and a strictly dry supper. Under this plan of procedure, Krasnogorski reported consistently good results.

From the Department of Pediatrics, Sea View Hospital, New York, and private practice. Read before the Metropolitan Medical Society, New York, Dec. 11, 1935.

About two and one-half years ago at the suggestion of Dr. Béla Schick, we decided to try this method on two groups of children suffering from nocturnal enuresis. One of us (Rosenson) planned to follow the results of its application in private practice; the other (Liswood), in an institution. The pediatric service at Sea View Hospital was well adapted for this latter study.

Sea View Hospital is an institution devoted to the care of tuberculous patients and affords ample opportunity for long periods of observation. Among the children there is the usual quota of enuretic cases found in any child-caring institution. The patients selected for the study were ambulatory cases showing no evidence of open tuberculosis. There were eighteen such cases with nocturnal enuresis. Their ages ranged between four and seven years. There were eleven boys and seven girls. Physical examination and repeated urine tests failed to reveal an organic basis for the enuresis in any of the cases.

Before inaugurating the new treatment, a control period of a week during which all fluids were withheld from the children's diet after 4 P.M. was instituted. The mere elimination of liquids in this way did not seem to control the enuresis in any of the cases. No other treatment for the bed-wetting as far as is known had been previously tried on any of these hospital patients.

The cases observed in private practice were for the most part brought for the treatment of the annoying and troublesome bed-wetting. Ten children were included in this group. As far as could be determined by physical examination and urinalysis, the nocturnal enuresis in these cases, too, was functional in character. The youngest child was four and the oldest ten years. There were six girls and four boys.

Various methods had been tried among this private group of children. The curtailment of liquids before retiring, the administration of tincture of belladonna, awakening of the child at intervals to urinate during the night, the psychologic approach including suggestion and the awarding of gold stars and prizes; all these time-honored procedures had been employed without producing any lasting successful results for the control of the nocturnal enuresis.

THE DAILY REGIME FOR THE CONTROL OF NOCTURNAL ENURESIS

During the day the child is given his regular diet. Until 12 o'clock noon, he is allowed to take as much fluids as he desires; after that, fluids are somewhat limited until 4 P.M. At that time he is offered his last drink of water or milk until the following morning. For supper at 5:30 he is served with food containing as little water as possible. Such dry food includes meat, fish, egg, bread, butter, cheese and crackers. No vegetables, fruit, or cereal are offered.

When the child is already in bed for the night and all his wants and requests have been attended to, he is given the salty sandwich. To satisfy differences of taste and to vary the monotony of repetition in food, we concocted a number of salty sandwiches. Krasnogorski found that about 5 gm. of salt are needed to obtain a therapeutic result. With some slight variations we have kept to this amount. It is important to mention here that in Krasnogorski's original publication there was a serious typographical error. The amount of salt required was given as 5 mg., when it should have been 5 gm. This was made clear to us in a personal communication.

The salt is given most effectively when combined with fat or meat abundant in binding tissue. Under such conditions the salt is absorbed gradually and the restraining influence upon the discharge of urine is prolonged. Caviar is rich in salt, but its general use here is obviously precluded. For our various sandwich fillings we used measured quantities of salt butter, ham, bacon, boned herring, boneless salt codfish, Swiss cheese, smoked salmon, and salt. To make the herring or fish more palatable, chopped hard-boiled egg or raw scraped apple was added.

The following is a list of recipes which we used for the filling of sandwiches:

SANDWICH FILLINGS	QUANTITIES	GRAMS OF SALT
Bacon	6 strips	3
Salt butter	2 teaspoonfuls	0.5 to 1
Salt	¼ teaspoonful	2
Boned herring	30 gm.	5
Salt butter	2 teaspoonfuls	0.5 to 1
(Chopped hard-boiled egg)		
Ham	45 to 50 gm.	2
Swiss cheese	30 gm.	2
Salt butter	2 teaspoonfuls	1
Salt	¼ teaspoonful	2
Boneless salt codfish	35 gm.	4 to 5
(Raw scraped apple)		
Salt butter	2 teaspoonfuls	0.5 to 1
Smoked salmon	45 to 50 gm.	4 to 5
Salt butter	2 teaspoonfuls	0.5 to 1

At the end of about two months of this regime a more varied evening meal was offered. Cereal, vegetables, and some fruit were gradually added. This more liberal plan was continued for two months longer, after which the salt was slowly decreased by reducing the size of the sandwich by one-quarter at intervals of about two or three weeks until it was entirely discontinued. The length of these intervals varied in individual cases in accordance with the response of the child to the decrease in the amount of salt. If at times bed-wetting occurred on the reduction of the salt intake, it became necessary for a while to order a larger portion of salt sandwich. In most cases, the reduction of the salt intake was gradually accomplished without any recurrence of the nocturnal enuresis.

In the study of our institutional cases, the ward nurses were given detailed directions for the carrying out of the plan and were asked to watch carefully through the night for any evidence of bed-wetting. Each such instance was charted.

RESULTS

Little difficulty was encountered in feeding the children the salty sandwiches. Their sleep was not disturbed by any undue thirst. In seventeen of the eighteen institutional cases, prompt cessation of the nocturnal enuresis occurred. In three of these cases there was a temporary relapse during the second week when two instances of bed-wetting were scored against one child and one instance against two children. From then on there followed an unbroken succession of nights with no bed-wetting. This group of cases has been followed for two years or longer and has remained free from the undesirable habit. One child failed to respond to the dietetic regime. This child, who often refused to comply with routine orders, was afflicted with epilepsy.

The cases studied in private practice were treated at home. The mothers were given full written instructions, including the list of recipes for the salty sandwich fillings. Emphasis was laid upon the importance of carrying out every detail of the plan. In the cases where complete cooperation was secured, the nocturnal enuresis promptly stopped. In two of the children a temporary lapse occurred during the third month of treatment, which was overcome by an increase in the salt intake. The treatment was entirely discontinued after six months and the children have remained free from bed-wetting up to the present time. Urine examinations showed no evidence of kidney irritation at any time.

CONCLUSIONS

Among twenty-eight cases of nocturnal enuresis treated with sodium chloride, successful results were obtained in all but one. Our inability to control the enuresis in this instance was due to the child's refusal to cooperate.

The cases followed are too few to draw any statistical conclusions. Krasnogorski, in a recent personal communication, reports 78 per cent of successful results among 125 cases treated.

Our study suggests that nocturnal enuresis in children can be controlled, in a large proportion of cases, by the dietetic regime described. However, before applying this regime in any given cases, an effort should be made first to find and treat any underlying physical or psychologic condition that might account for the bed-wetting. If such attempts fail, the sodium chloride treatment, as outlined, offers an effective method.

REFERENCE

1. Krasnogorski: Monatschr. f. Kinderheilk. **57**: 252, 1933.

142 West 87th Street
8415 Bay Parkway, Brooklyn

THE CONTINUOUS INTRAVENOUS METHOD OF SERUM ADMINISTRATION

CASE REPORTS

NELLES SILVERTHORNE, M.B. (Tor.)
TORONTO, ONTARIO

FOR many years the continuous intravenous injection of 5 per cent glucose in physiologic saline in the treatment of infants and children with toxemia or infections involving the meninges has been used extensively at the Hospital for Sick Children. The administration of large doses of antitoxin in the treatment of tetanus[1] and meningococcic infections has been carried out by injecting the therapeutic antiserum by means of the continuous intravenous apparatus with the glucose-saline solution. The method employed, with a diagram, is described in detail by Brown and Tisdall.[2] Results of the continuous intravenous administration of glucose saline as a therapeutic agent in the toxicosis of infants were reported by Schick and Karelitz.[3] Chargin, Leifer and Hyman[4] reported a series of cases in which large doses of neoarsphenamine were administered in a similar manner. This method is one which may with advantage be adopted in the administration of large amounts of serum to patients.

There is not infrequently some hesitation on the part of physicians in administering antitoxic horse serum intravenously. In recent years various types of antitoxin have, nevertheless, been injected into the veins of critically ill patients suffering from a variety of diseases. The serum is usually given by direct venipuncture. The use of foreign protein (i. e., horse serum), so given in from 15 c.c. to 50 c.c. doses, may produce a marked reaction. The patient has a rise in temperature, rapid respiration, profuse perspiration, cyanosis, and chills, a sequence of events which often causes anxiety on the part of the attending physician. Yet the intravenous method of therapy is undoubtedly the most rapid and effective way of neutralizing toxins in the blood stream. In the present communication a method is described for the administration of antitoxic horse serum which we feel materially reduces the incidence of immediate serum reactions. A summary of the different types of disease which have been treated and the final outcome will be outlined.

METHOD OF THE INTRAVENOUS USE OF ANTITOXIN

The usual apparatus for the continuous intravenous administration of glucose saline is set up with the gold cannula tied in the internal saphenous vein of the leg. The rubber tubing above the drip bulb is

From the wards and laboratories of the Hospital for Sick Children, the Department of Paediatrics and the Connaught Laboratories, University of Toronto.

well scrubbed with an alcohol sponge, and the antitoxin to be administered is injected by needle and syringe at this site. The first dose thus introduced is 0.5 c.c. This is followed in from one-half to one hour with 1 c.c. and increased by 1 c.c. each hour until a total of 5 c.c. at hourly intervals is given. The antitoxin is given in this manner until the total dosage required is used.

The following charts summarize the case histories of patients suffering from tetanus and from streptococcic infections who were treated by this method, using tetanus antitoxin and scarlet fever antitoxin, respectively.

TABLE I

CASES OF TETANUS

NAME	AGE	ANTITOXIC UNIT PER C.C.		TOTAL AMOUNT A.T. UNITS	REACTION	RESULT
		BEFORE A.T.*	DURING A.T.			
B. J.	7 days	<0.001	-	14,000	None	Died
R. H.	11 days	-	>50	108,500	None	Recovered
D. C.	6 yr.	-	-	1,150,000	None	Recovered
H. M.	12 yr.	<0.001	>25	9,000	None	Recovered
J. H.	3½ yr.	<0.001	>75	214,000	None	Recovered
G. B.	12 yr.	-	-	135,812	None	Recovered

*Antitoxin.

It will be noted that in cases of tetanus in which samples of blood were taken, the antitoxic unit per cubic centimeter was negligible before the use of serum and was raised to from 25 to 75 units per cubic centimeter after antitoxin administration. In all of these patients no immediate reaction to serum occurred although in certain instances very large doses were administered. An infant, eleven days old, made a complete recovery after the administration of 108,500 units of tetanus antitoxin.

TABLE II

CASES OF STREPTOCOCCIC INFECTIONS

NAME	AGE (YEARS)	TYPE	TOTAL AMOUNT A.T.* INTRAVENOUSLY	REACTION	RESULT
G. G.	7	Meningitis	188 c.c.	None	Died
R. G.	8	Meningitis	155 c.c.	None	Died
S. A.	2½	Meningitis and septicemia	164 c.c.	None	Died
J. S.	7	Meningitis	100 c.c.	None	Died
M. M.	7	Meningitis	101 c.c.	None	Died
M. J.	13	Meningitis and septicemia	270 c.c.	None	Died
W. T.	7	Septicemia	150 c.c.	Febrile	Recovered
K. McC.	10	Septicemia	70 c.c.	None	Recovered

*Antitoxin.

From Table II it will be observed that although there were no recoveries with the intravenous or intrathecal use of scarlet fever antitoxin in cases of meningitis, no reaction to serum occurred. Most of these children died as a result of meningitis some few days after antitoxin administration had been discontinued. It is also noteworthy that two patients with septicemia made a complete recovery. In one of these children several forms of treatment had been tried for a week before the administration of antitoxin.

DISCUSSION

In the series of cases reported there have been spectacular results as well as failures, which are inevitable, with present methods of prevention and treatment. The observation was that the majority of these patients had no immediate direct reaction to serum. In one instance sensitivity to horse serum was noted by the presence of an urticarial-erythematous reaction in the skin. This patient received horse serum intravenously without the slightest sign of systemic reaction. Often, not even a febrile response was noted, although many of the patients had some fever with their infection. In one instance the child was admitted in a critical condition. His temperature was 107° F. He was pulseless, cyanosed, and in a moribund condition. A continuous intravenous injection was commenced immediately, and scarlet fever antitoxin was given by this method. In spite of the septicemia and meningitis due to the *Streptococcus hemolyticus* he lived for nine days after admission, and his temperature remained at a lower level than before the administration of antitoxin. It is noteworthy that there was no difference in the incidence of serum disease from that usually found after the use of horse serum by other methods.

In conclusion, the author believes that a reasonably effective method of administering antitoxic horse serum to infants and children, which produces minimal or no reaction, has been outlined. Large quantities of serum well diluted with glucose in normal saline may be given within very few hours by use of the continuous intravenous method. This method of therapy has been applied to a variety of clinical conditions for a period of two years with no general reaction following the use of large doses of antitoxic horse serum intravenously.

The author is indebted to Dr. E. G. Kerslake for blood antitoxin studies.

REFERENCES

1. Silverthorne and Hart: Canad. Pub. Health J. **22**: 181, 1931.
2. Brown and Tisdall: Common Procedures in the Practice of Paediatrics, Toronto, 1932, McClelland & Stewart.
3. Schick and Karelitz: Am. J. Dis. Child. **42**: 781, 1931.
4. Chargin, Leifer, and Hyman: J. A. M. A. **104**: 878, 1935.

PUBERTY MASTITIS

Philip Rosenblum, M.D.
Chicago, Ill.

WITH the increase of public education in the field of cancer and allied medical subjects, it is my impression that parents are often unnecessarily alarmed over a condition that occurs in children at or just before puberty, frequently in girls but not infrequently in boys. This is a tumorlike enlargement of one or both breasts known as *mastitis adolescentium* or puberty mastitis.

While this condition is familiar to pediatricians, the general physician is not as well acquainted with it as he should be to prevent often unnecessary operations and much needless worry. There are very few references to the condition; practically none in the pediatric literature, and the few descriptions in textbooks on pathology and surgery are rather indefinite and at variance with each other, so that there seems to be no unanimity of opinion about it.

The very scanty reference to this more or less physiologic process was noted by Still, who quotes Underwood as giving the first description of mastitis occurring in children at a variable time before puberty. A condition, which Still remarks, is so little known that he has more than once known operations proposed for it because of the mistaken idea that it was a malignant growth. In Underwood's early description, "Induration of the Breasts," he says: "It would be improper to pass over the slightest affection that has on many occasions exceedingly alarmed parents and sometimes perplexed the younger part of the profession. Of this kind, are affections of the breasts in female children previously to, or about the time of, their beginning to enlarge. At this period they sometimes become very painful and upon examination a hardness and swelling are discovered and in some instances sharp points may be felt, which are very painful when pressed. The hardness is deep-seated, around and behind the nipple and is sometimes loose and at other times fixed and attended with severe lancinating pains which have given rise to disagreeable suspicions in regard to the probable nature of the complaint, and would indeed at a more advanced age claim serious attention. When happening in families addicted to scrofula, that disorder is naturally suspected, and sometimes a morbid scirrhus has been feared."

Underwood further states: "In some instances only one of the breasts is affected and after some months the other or sometimes both nearly at the same time. Yet no evil consequence in any instance under my eye has

From the Sarah Morris Children's Hospital of the Michael Reese Hospital.

ever ensued in patients at the above-mentioned age nor have I heard of any from other practitioners though it has sometimes been seriously apprehended."

This gives a fairly clear picture of the condition, and is more accurate than the few references I have seen in modern textbooks.

Some eighteen or twenty years ago I saw my first patient with this condition. The mother was very much alarmed about the swelling of her child's breast just behind the nipple. I could find practically no reference to the condition in any pediatric text. Since then I have seen, like all pediatricians, many children with similar swellings.

Two years ago I was prompted to write this paper when a mother brought her ten-year-old daughter to me with a story that she had a breast removed six months previously and now had, she was sure, a similar swelling in the other breast. I found it a typical case of mastitis adolescentium.

The breast is a modified sudoriferous gland and physiologically is related rather intricately to the reproductive system. The epithelial lining of the ducts and alveoli is derived from the ectoderm and the supporting connective tissue from the mesoderm.

Each breast consists of fifteen to twenty lobes, which are themselves branched saccular glands whose lactiferous ducts open on the surface of the nipple near its apex. The main lactiferous ducts subdivide into many interlobular ducts about which are clustered the group of secreting acini. Each group forms one of the many lobules included in one lobe of the gland.

At puberty, and again at the end of pregnancy, marked enlargement of the gland and the development of additional lobules and acini take place. There is also an increase in the deposit of adipose tissue at puberty.

Goltz and Evald have shown that the development of the mammary glands at puberty is due to the action of ovarian hormones, both follicular and luteal. C. W. Lurner has demonstrated that the follicular hormone stimulates the development of the duct system, and the corpus luteum the alveoli. The anterior pituitary gland is also active and important in the production of lactation (Stueker and Grueter).

Cheatle and Cutler[2] regard puberty mastitis as a result of some aberrance in the physiologic hyperplasia of the mammary tissues, probably an overactivity of the tissues in response to an excess of growth-stimulating substances.

Muir[3] speaks of mastitis adolescentium as a nonsuppurative acute inflammatory condition similar to puerperal mastitis.

Rose and Carless[4] write of mastitis adolescentium as being a condition similar to mastitis neonatorum, which it does resemble very closely.

Kaufmann[5] states that puberty mastitis is probably the result of irritation of the ducts due to the retention of the material secreted by the ducts. This secreted material provides a favorable medium for the growth of organisms.

Walther[6] remarks that the enlargement of the breasts in puberty very often coincides with the presence of a positive tuberculin reaction. In other words, he believes that this type of mastitis is a manifestation of a tuberculous infection. The connective tissue proliferation is explained on an allergic basis.

Ochsenius,[7] although not completely contradicting Walther, reports three cases in which the tuberculin reaction was negative.

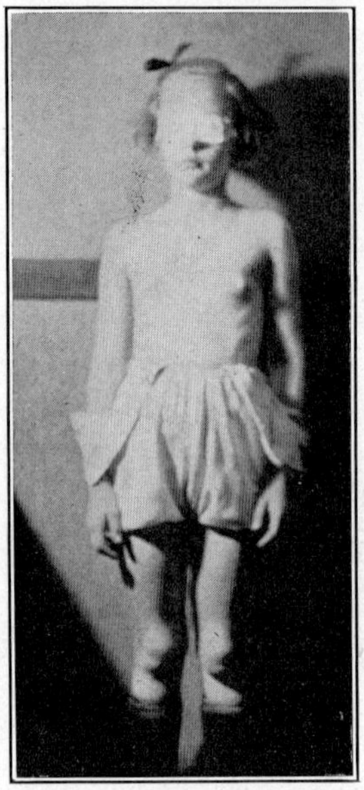

Fig. 1.

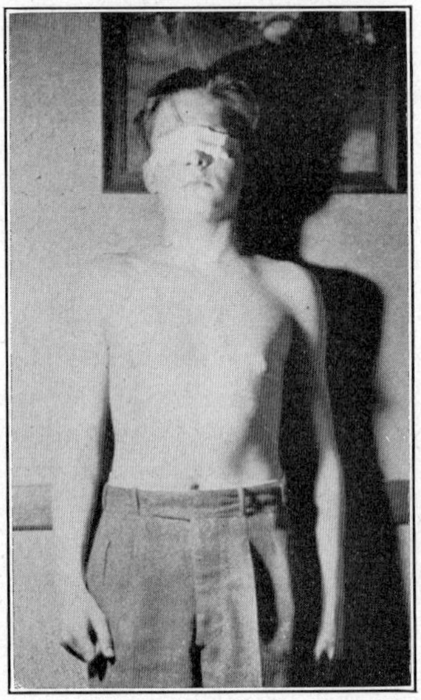

Fig. 2.

Fig. 1.—Girl, nine years old. Swelling of left breast for one month. Typical tumorlike enlargement behind nipple. Mass completely disappeared in four months. This girl had a severe eczema and asthma.

Fig. 2.—Boy, sixteen years old. Swelling of both breasts but more marked in left. Location typically behind nipple. Complete disappearance in five months.

In none of my patients was there a positive tuberculin reaction, and I feel definitely there is no relationship. Of the ten or twelve cases I have seen in the last two or three years, five or six had a definite allergy characterized by a severe eczema, asthma, or both.

Harbeson[8] describes a case of mastitis adolescentium in which the tumor began in the upper outer quadrant of the left breast. Then two months later another tumor developed in the same location. Soon afterward, the right breast was the site of a similar tumor. The location, relative to the nipple, was not mentioned, and the last note several months later stated that the tumors were smaller but still present. They were probably fibroadenomas. Harbeson thinks it is due to a preponderance of luteal hormone which produces an overstimulation and rapid development of the acini before development of the ducts.

The children I have seen with this tumor in the breast all had characteristics similar to those described by Underwood one hundred and fifty or more years ago. They occur more frequently between the ages of eight or nine and fifteen or sixteen years. The majority are found between the ninth and eleventh years in girls. One or both breasts may be involved, and one side may precede the other by as long as a year or more. The areola becomes darker in color and, as Cheatle and Cutler described, the lesion assumes definite and very characteristic features.

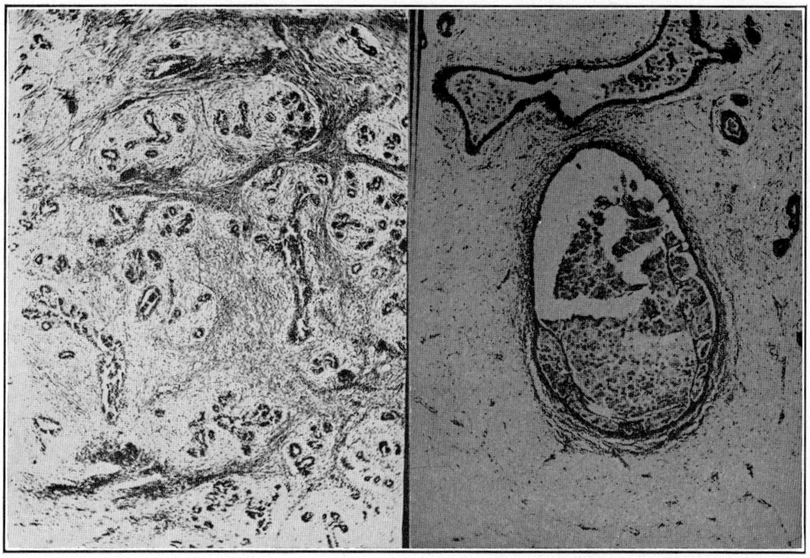

Fig. 3. Fig. 4.

Figs. 3 and 4.—Periacinous and pericanalicular infiltration and epithelial hyperplasia. (Fig. 3, ×90; Fig. 4, ×150.) (These photomicrographs were kindly lent by Dr. Max Cutler, of Michael Reese Hospital.)

The swelling forms a firm disklike or spherical tumor varying from 3 to 5 cm. in diameter, which is painful on pressure only. It is situated directly behind the nipple, which usually is flattened and often slightly inverted by the enlargement. Occasionally a few drops of an opaque serous fluid may be expressed from the nipple. The location in those I have seen is always behind the areola, and this differs from most of the other possible tumors of the mammary gland.

Puberty mastitis is not a true inflammation, but is due to an increased physiologic hypertrophy of the pericanalicular and periacinous connective tissue. The proliferative changes closely resemble those which are produced by the injection of estrin (as shown by Lacassane). It is possible that trauma may aggravate it or be responsible for its appearance in only one breast. Usually the induration disappears as the breast develops fully. Some disappear in a few weeks while others require months.

In the male sex this condition begins at the earliest in the fourteenth or fifteenth year of life, and it may be so marked as to constitute a true fibrous tumor. Zappert is of the opinion that in the male this state is associated with an advanced development of the genital glands.

This condition is not to be confused with certain tumors which may arise only occasionally in breasts of children.

In all the children I have seen with puberty mastitis, the mothers were worried because they feared a cancer or tumor. The age, location and characteristics outlined will be sufficient readily to differentiate it from other pathologic entities.

SUMMARY

Puberty mastitis (mastitis adolescentium) has definite characteristics. It is always behind the nipple and occurs in girls between eight and twelve years of age and in boys between fourteen and eighteen years.

It is probably caused by some endocrine dysfunction and local trauma may play a rôle.

Pathologically it is a pericanalicular and periacinous infiltration with connective tissue and lymphocytes, together with epithelial hyperplasia.

The condition is benign and disappears within a few months.

REFERENCES

1. Underwood: ed. 4, Vol. II.
2. Cheatle, G. Lenthal, and Cutler, Max: Tumours of the Breast: Their Pathology, Symptoms, Diagnosis and Treatment, Philadelphia, 1931, Lippincott.
3. Muir, R.: Text Book of Pathology, Philadelphia, 1924, Lippincott, p. 710.
4. Rose and Carless: Manual of Surgery, ed. 11.
5. Kaufmann, E.: Lehrbuch der speziellen pathologischen Anatomie für Studierende und Ärzte, Band I, 1931, Ninth-Tenth Edition.
6. Walther, E.: Monatschr. f. Kinderh. **58**: 452, 1933.
7. Ochsenius, K.: Monatschr. f. Kinderh. **59**: 120, 1934.
8. Harbeson, A. E.: Canad. M. A. J. **30**: 648, 1934.

104 S. Michigan Avenue

SIGNIFICANCE OF THE DIMINUTION OF THE SPINAL FLUID SUGAR IN TUBERCULOUS MENINGITIS

MANFRED WEICHSEL, M.D., AND GERTRUD HERZGER, M.D.
NEW YORK, N. Y.

THE present paper is a report of studies carried out to determine the diagnostic value of quantitative sugar determinations of the spinal fluid in cases of tuberculous meningitis. At the same time an attempt was made to ascertain the possible mechanism influencing the reduction in sugar content.

In the course of our studies more than one hundred cases of tuberculous meningitis were observed. The diagnosis in most cases was based on clinical signs, bacteriologic examination, as well as autopsy examination. The method used for the examination of the spinal fluid sugar was that of Jensen and Hagedorn. It should be stated that, according

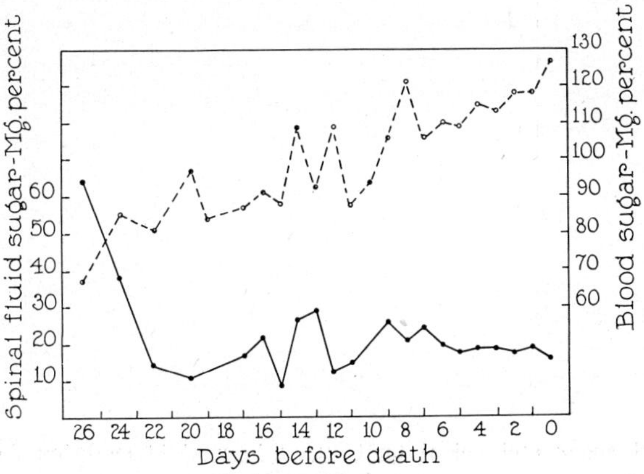

Fig. 1.—Blood sugar and spinal fluid sugar in tuberculous meningitis: 130 tests in 80 children.

to this method, the amount of sugar in the cerebrospinal fluid of fasting infants and children ranges from 35 to 60 mg. per cent. It has been shown that the reducing substance in the cerebrospinal fluid consists almost exclusively of dextrose.[1, 2] It is important, in all cases in which a quantitative estimation of the spinal fluid sugar is being made, to precede the spinal puncture by an examination of the blood sugar level. Spinal fluid drainage in itself is sufficient to cause a rise in the level of blood sugar.[3]

Figure 1 represents graphically blood sugar and spinal fluid sugar determinations of eighty children suffering from tuberculous meningitis.

The curve shows a progressive diminution of the spinal fluid sugar from the time of first observations to the fatal terminations of the cases.

From the Children's Hospital of the University of Leipzig.

In this decline there is, in many cases, a slight increase about two weeks before death, and then a final drop of the sugar content. This peculiar curve seems to be very characteristic in tuberculous meningitis although it was not observed in every patient.

We feel that the diminution of the spinal fluid sugar is an early diagnostic sign since in several cases the value of the sugar showed a decline twenty-five to thirty days before the death of the patient. In most cases the decrease in the sugar content follows a rise in globulin and an increased cell count.

Figure 1 shows, not only the gradual diminution of the amount of sugar in the spinal fluid, but also a progressive and concomitant increase of the blood sugar. This occurred in most of the single cases in which repeated examinations were made. This is surprising, in view of the fact that most of the patients suffered from malnutrition.

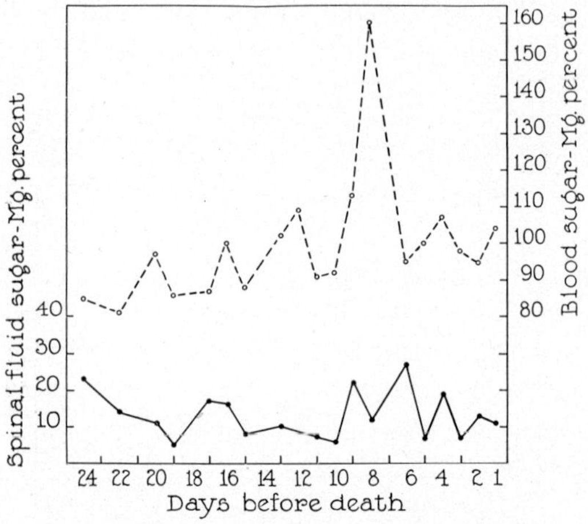

Fig. 2.—Blood sugar and spinal fluid sugar in a child suffering from tuberculous meningitis.

In observing single cases we encountered the difficulty that most patients did not come under observation until three weeks before death, so that in the average case not more than four to six examinations of the spinal fluid could be made. A few patients were observed from the onset of the disease, some with other tuberculous lesions and others free from tuberculosis when admitted to the hospital. The quantitative blood and spinal fluid sugar determinations of one of these children is shown in Fig. 2, demonstrating the diminished spinal fluid sugar level as it occurred twenty-four days before death.

In one patient, tuberculous meningitis developed following tuberculous spondylitis. When the first meningeal signs were observed, the spinal fluid revealed tubercle bacilli, but a normal sugar content, 59 mg. per cent (blood sugar, 94 mg. per cent), and only a slightly increased cell count and protein content. Five weeks later (five weeks before death) the spinal fluid sugar dropped to 27 mg. per cent, when the first signs of meningeal irritation were observed in the spinal fluid, as revealed by increased cell counts and strongly positive protein reactions. The clinical picture in this case was always doubtful as to the presence of a basilar meningitis, since the patient was suffering from Pott's disease, with spasms of the lower extremities.

In another exceptional case the disease lasted eighteen weeks. One hundred three days before the death of the child, the spinal fluid sugar dropped to 19 mg. per cent. This value remained approximately on the same level until the fortieth day before death. Four days later the sugar was 8 mg. per cent, rising to 24 mg. per cent in the fifteenth day before death and finally diminishing again. The autopsy in this case, in contrast to the usual finding, revealed a definite productive leptomeningitis.

The question arises whether a low spinal fluid sugar in itself in cases of tuberculous meningitis would indicate invariably a fatal prognosis. As we have not observed any recoveries from this condition, we cannot definitely state this to be a fact. We may, however, reason from cases with purulent meningitis in which we have observed the return of the spinal fluid sugar level to a normal value with recovery.

In syphilitic meningitis of infants, in whom the values of spinal fluid glucose in some cases show a considerable diminution, a progressive increase in the sugar content accompanied the clinical improvement.

From a therapeutic standpoint it seemed of interest to attempt to raise the lowered spinal fluid sugar in cases of tuberculous meningitis. We injected glucose into the spinal canal in order to observe whether such injections would perhaps maintain the spinal fluid sugar at higher levels. Repeated examinations of the spinal fluid in children who were so treated showed that on the day following the injection the spinal fluid sugar had returned to the same low level as previously. Since no intraspinal glucose injections have been carried out on normal children, we have no means of determining whether a similar decrease ensues.

However, the injection of 5 per cent glucose intraspinally in children suffering from tuberculous meningitis did produce another result. We observed that there was a response in blood sugar following such injections, which can be compared with that found after intramuscular injection or after absorption of sugar from the intestinal tract.

Table I shows the rise and fall of the blood sugar after the intraspinal injection of 5 per cent glucose (30 c.c.) in a patient with tuberculous meningitis. An equal amount of fluid had been withdrawn before the injection. This may perhaps indicate that in cases of severe tuberculous meningitis the sugar center in the brain responds to the intraspinal injection of glucose with an initial intense increase and a subsequent slow decrease of the blood sugar. Regardless of whether this change in blood sugar is a specific sequela of the sugar injection or, what is more likely, is due to the intraspinal procedure itself, it would seem that the blood sugar center in the brain can easily be influenced.

TABLE I

RESPONSE IN BLOOD SUGAR FOLLOWING THE INTRASPINAL INJECTION OF 5 PER CENT GLUCOSE

	BEFORE INJ.	½ HR. AFTER INJ.	1 HR.	1¼ HR.	2 HR.	3 HR.
Blood sugar in mg. per cent	114	201	220	222	194	148

The rapid increase of the blood sugar following intraspinal injection of glucose would tend to indicate that in tuberculous meningitis, as well as in normal individuals, substances brought into the subarachnoid space are likely to enter the brain tissue itself, or to come into such close contact as to produce an irritative effect. The presumption is that the pressure within the subarachnoid space is high enough to allow a substance to pass into the perivascular spaces of Virchow-Robin, as well as into the directly communicating perineuronal spaces.

The question arises as to whether the low content of the sugar in the spinal fluid can be explained by actual splitting up of sugar within the ventricular system or spinal canal, either by the cells themselves or by the disease-producing organisms. This has been shown to be the cause for the decrease of sugar in cases of purulent meningitis, in which both cells and bacteria are able to break down glucose. Experiments of Mader[4] have shown that a considerable decline of the spinal fluid glucose occurs after the addition of bacteria.

An indirect proof of the breaking down of glucose in the spinal fluid has been demonstrated by some investigators by showing an increase of lactic acid. However, Fasold and Schmidt[5] showed that this increase in tuberculous meningitis is not high enough to explain the diminution of the spinal fluid glucose by the breakdown of sugar. The studies of Fasold and Schmidt, as well as our own, have also shown that, when suspensions of tubercle bacilli are added to normal spinal fluid, or when spinal fluid from patients with tuberculous meningitis is incubated for from one to fourteen days, there is no breaking down of glucose. It has been shown that normally the sugar content of the ventricular cerebrospinal fluid is higher than that of the subarachnoid fluid, because of the utilization of the glucose by the brain itself or its nervous elements. The irritation of the cells of the brain in tuberculous meningitis, resulting in an increased utilization of glucose, may account partially for the diminution of the sugar.

Is there another mechanism for the decrease in the sugar of the spinal fluid in cases of tuberculous meningitis? In studying this question the sugar content of the spinal fluid was examined in some cases of tuberculous meningitis at the beginning and at the end of a spinal puncture after removing a large amount of fluid. In other patients the examination of the spinal fluid sugar was repeated after one hour. If it is assumed that the spinal fluid is produced in the choroid plexus with normal glucose value and then is reduced in sugar concentration by the action of bacterial enzymes, a period of time greater than the duration of a spinal drainage would be necessary to yield this reduction. Therefore, the sugar concentrations of specimens removed after withdrawal of large amounts of fluid would certainly be normal or at least greater than the original value at the beginning of the drainage. Our observations, however, showed that the sugar content at the end of a spinal puncture gave almost the same value as at the beginning and that a repetition of the puncture after one hour usually gave no higher amounts. Therefore, the possibility of glycolytic enzymes having been the sole cause of the diminution seems unlikely.

If the increased splitting up of sugar is not the only cause of the diminution, we must assume that in cases of tuberculous meningitis the spinal fluid primarily contains a lower sugar content. It seems possible to explain this low content of glucose on the basis of a diminished passage of sugar through the barrier between blood and spinal fluid. Apparently in tuberculous meningitis this threshold is raised, and instead of a normal relation of blood to spinal fluid sugar of 2:1, we find a relation of 8:1, 10:1, or even 12:1. Walter[6] states that especially in inflammatory processes of the meninges the passage for certain substances, such as protein and the bromides, is increased, but that, on the contrary, the threshold for sugar is higher.

A series of experiments was made to test the assumption that in cases of tuberculous meningitis the barrier between blood and spinal fluid is disturbed with respect to glucose. We raised the level of blood sugar in normal patients and in those suffering from tuberculous meningitis by the injection of adrenalin, or by feeding glucose and cane sugar, or by the injection of glucose intravenously.

We know that a parallel rise in spinal fluid sugar of the normal individual accompanies an artificial increase of blood sugar. We also know that the relation of the blood to spinal fluid sugar is maintained in diabetes in which we find values of 100 to 200 mg. per cent in the spinal fluid corresponding to amounts of 200 to 400 mg. per cent in the blood.

Different opinions have been expressed in the literature as to when the spinal fluid sugar reaches its maximum following augmentation of the blood sugar. Table II gives a survey of our experiments on two normal cases of our series.

The results show the response of the spinal fluid sugar to an increase of blood sugar, indicating that the increase of sugar in the normal spinal fluid follows that of the blood sugar closely. The spinal fluid remains

TABLE II

RESPONSE OF BLOOD SUGAR AND SPINAL FLUID SUGAR FOLLOWING THE ORAL ADMINISTRATION OF GLUCOSE IN NORMAL CHILDREN

		SPINAL FLUID SUGAR IN MG. PER CENT	BLOOD SUGAR IN MG. PER CENT	SUGAR ORAL
Case 1	Before feeding	58	91	
	After 1 hr.	93	165	100 gm.
Case 2	Before feeding	51	99	
	After 1 hr.	144	252	50 gm.
	After 2 hr.	144	171	

high even after the blood sugar has decreased. As it was not feasible to puncture normal children more than two to three times without any clinical indication, we cannot state how long the cerebrospinal fluid sugar would remain high and how long the increase would be maintained.

Table III gives the data of a few cases of tuberculous meningitis with a diminished content of spinal fluid sugar which we attempted to raise by

TABLE III

RESPONSE OF BLOOD SUGAR AND SPINAL FLUID SUGAR FOLLOWING THE ORAL AND INTRAVENOUS ADMINISTRATION OF GLUCOSE IN CHILDREN WITH TUBERCULOUS MENINGITIS

CASE		SPINAL FLUID SUGAR IN MG. PER CENT	BLOOD SUGAR IN MG. PER CENT	GLUCOSE
1	Before feeding	14	116	50 gm. oral
	After 1 hr.	36	256	
2	Before feeding	17	142	50 gm. oral
	After 1 hr.	35	211	
	After 1½ hr.	49	146	
	After 2 hr.	39	133	
3	Before feeding	7	100	50 gm. oral
	After 1 hr.	14	220	
4	Before injection	8	109	20 c.c. 25%
	After 10 min.	11	300	intraven.
5	Before injection	8	118	20 c.c. 25%
	After 30 min.	10	140	intraven.
	After 1½ hr.	9	105	

giving dextrose by mouth or by intravenous injection. In Case 1, after the ingestion of 50 gm. of glucose, the spinal fluid sugar showed an increase in the same proportion as the blood sugar. The percentage of increase as compared with the rise in blood sugar seems to be normal, or at least not less than that of normal individuals who show an increase in blood sugar. The absolute augmentation (7 mg. per cent in Case 3), however, is very low. Similar results were obtained after the injection of adrenalin. Thus we see that the absolute increase of spinal fluid sugar is in proportion to the original amount of sugar. Case 2 shows that the maximum of the rise in the spinal fluid sugar follows that of the blood sugar, but it is interesting to note that after one hour the value was doubled. Two hours after the feeding the spinal fluid sugar began to fall. The augmentation of the blood sugar content, therefore, does not help much in maintaining a higher spinal fluid sugar.

These observations do not favor the theory of increased destruction of glucose, because, if we assume the decrease in spinal fluid sugar to be the consequence of glycolysis by tubercle bacilli, we would not expect such a rapid diminution within one hour after the passage of sugar into the spinal fluid. On the other hand, a careful study of the above tables shows that the original ratio between blood and spinal fluid sugar remains approximately the same. In other words, if we increase the blood sugar to double the amount, the spinal fluid sugar rises in the same proportion.

Since the mechanism of the production of the normal spinal fluid has not definitely been established, it is difficult to draw a conclusion from the results in pathologic conditions. The question has not been decided whether the spinal fluid is to be considered a dialysate or an ultrafiltrate alone or whether it is produced by active work of the cells. The results of our experiments in cases of tuberculous meningitis could hardly be explained by ultrafiltration of sugar. Evidently, in such advanced conditions as cited, the barrier between blood and spinal fluid is not entirely closed, but partially blocked so as to allow only a small percentage of sugar to pass, at least less than the normal amount of 50 per cent. If we increase the amount of glucose in the blood, the barrier allows more sugar to pass, but an amount much smaller than normal. We feel that an active secretion by the cells within this barrier is to be held responsible for this phenomenon.

Another possible explanation is that the cells within the membranes representing the barrier and regulating the passage of sugar are so definitely disturbed in tuberculous meningitis that only a small percentage of sugar can enter the spinal canal but that after a considerable increase of the blood sugar a local production or secretion of sugar follows.

Experiments have shown that the increased passage of one substance from the blood into the spinal fluid does not necessarily prove that the passage for all substances is enhanced. The passage of one of these substances, which may be crystalloids, colloids, or nonelectrolytes in molecular dispersion, such as sugar or urea, is independent of the others. According to Walter,[6] the barrier may allow crystalloids and nonelectrolytes in molecular dispersion to pass without increased passage of proteins. On the other hand, in some pathologic conditions of the central nervous system, in which the protein passes in larger amounts, the permeability for crystalloids is regularly increased. This tends to prove that in all probability specific functions of the cells regulate the passage of the sugar and that pathologic conditions affecting these functions can produce definite disturbances of the barrier leading to a primarily decreased sugar content of the spinal fluid.

SUMMARY

1. The spinal fluid sugar in more than one hundred children with tuberculous meningitis revealed a progressive diminution from the time of the first observations to their deaths. In this decline there was in many cases a slight increase a few days before death, followed by a final decline.

2. Most of these children showed a marked progressive increase of the blood sugar.

3. Following the intraspinal injection of glucose in children with tuberculous meningitis, a response in blood sugar was observed, which can be compared with that found after intramuscular injection or after absorption of sugar from the intestinal tract.

4. The sugar content of the cerebrospinal fluid at the end of a spinal puncture gave almost the same value as at the beginning, and a repetition of the puncture after one hour usually gave no higher amounts.

5. After an artificial increase of the blood sugar, the ratio between blood and spinal fluid sugar remained the same, the absolute augmentation of the glucose in the cerebrospinal fluid being very low.

6. These experiments tend to show that the chief cause of the diminution of sugar is not an increased glycolysis, but rather a disturbance of the barrier between blood and spinal fluid.

REFERENCES

1. Schloss and Schroeder: Am. J. Dis. Child. **11**: 1, 1916.
2. Geldrich: Jahrb. f. Kinderh. **124**: 159, 1929.
3. Schoenfeld, H.: Jahrb. f. Kinderh. **138**: 74, 1933.
4. Mader, A.: Jahrb. f. Kinderh. **126**: 187, 1930.
5. Fasold and Schmidt: Klin. Wchnschr. **8**: 1532, 1929.
6. Walter, F. K.: Die Blutliquorschranke, Leipzig, 1929, Georg Thieme.

TWISTED OVARIAN CYSTS IN CHILDREN

Report of a Case in a Ten-Year-Old Child

M. S. Mazel, M.D., and L. J. Halpern, M.D.
Chicago, Ill.

Ovarian tumors in childhood are relatively uncommon. The literature contains a moderate number of references to this condition. The seriousness of the condition when present and, more particularly, its early recognition and surgical treatment are of sufficient importance to report a case.

J. S., a white girl, ten years of age, was admitted to the Edgewater Hospital, Jan. 15, 1936, because of cramplike pains in the abdomen. Her past history was essentially negative except for a similar attack of pain experienced for the first time on Dec. 15, 1935. At that time she was awakened at night by the pain in the lower left side of her abdomen. There were no other associated complaints. An enema administered by her mother produced relief from pain in about an hour, and the child returned to school the next day.

On December 17 and December 30, 1935, she again had similar attacks of pain. The latter were associated with vomiting of undigested food, and the pains were more severe and persistent. However, the administration of enemas again produced the same relief as was effected on previous occasions, with complete absence of pain in the interim. After the last attack, medical consultation was sought, and a diagnosis of spastic colitis was made. A bland diet and medication were prescribed. After freedom from the attacks for the next two weeks, the patient was suddenly seized with severe abdominal cramps again and brought to the hospital where she was seen by us for the first time.

It seemed that the child had departed from the prescribed diet for the past twenty-four hours and the repeated vomiting attacks, both at home and at the hospital, revealed undigested foods. The administration of an enema by the mother failed to effect the usual relief from pain during this attack.

Physical Examination.—The child cried almost continuously because of pain in the lower left side of her abdomen. At times she was entirely free from pain for short intervals. She was well nourished and did not appear acutely ill or toxic. The temperature on admission was 98.6° F.; pulse, 88; and respirations, 22. Regional examination was essentially negative.

The abdomen was soft, no masses were palpable, and the only essential finding was definite tenderness to palpation in the lower left quadrant.

The blood, on admission, showed 8,850 leucocytes, 62 per cent polymorphonuclears, and 38 per cent small and large lymphocytes. The urine was entirely normal. The condition was considered nonsurgical for the time being, and the patient was placed in semi-Fowler's position, and an ice bag was applied to the abdomen. Sedatives were administered for the pain without much effect.

Course of Illness.—The patient continued to be afebrile the next day, and the pulse ranged between 88 and 108. Repeated blood examination revealed a rise in leucocytes to 14,000 with 92 per cent polymorphonuclears. She did not appear toxic or acutely ill. Pain and vomiting of undigested food continued, and enemas produced no results. Rectal examination at this time revealed a somewhat firm and tender mass the size of a small orange in the culdesac. A flat x-ray film of the abdomen taken on admission visualized a mass which was interpreted by the roentgenologist to be a full urinary bladder. Evidences of intestinal obstruction or urolithiasis were not visualized (Fig. 1).

The possibility of ovarian tumor was now considered, but in view of all findings it was deemed better to observe the patient further since the abdominal findings and her general condition had remained unchanged.

The following morning the whole clinical picture had abruptly changed. The patient appeared acutely ill. The pain had increased in severity and was continuous. Vomiting of clear fluid continued. The legs were drawn up toward the abdomen. There were signs of mild toxicity, but still the patient remained afebrile while the pulse ranged between 110 and 128. The abdomen was tender throughout, but more so over the pubic region and both lower quadrants, where there was definite muscular resistance to palpation. No mass could be palpated. Rectal examination at

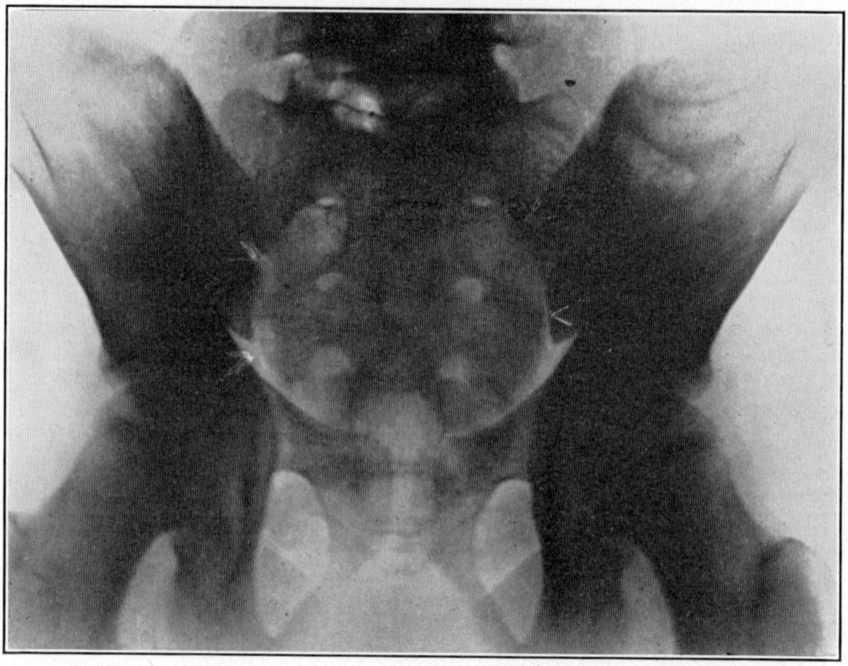

Fig. 1.

this time revealed the previously felt mass now markedly increased in size, excruciatingly tender to palpation, and of a semifluctuant consistency. A definite diagnosis of twisted ovarian cyst was now made, and surgical procedure instituted.

Treatment.—The abdomen was opened in the midline, and at once we were confronted with a dark, bloody fluid within the peritoneal cavity. On the left side was a large dark mass which appeared almost gangrenous and which had become so engaged in the pelvis that we had considerable difficulty in disengaging it from the pelvic cavity. Grossly, the mass was dark red, hard, and had cystlike areas. It was noted that this mass had become twisted on itself and had five definite twists around the pedicle, which accurately coincided with each attack of pain. The mass was removed easily by means of two clamps at its base and ligated.

Examination of the opposite tube and ovary showed them to be small and normal in appearance. The appendix was removed at the same time. The abdomen was closed in the usual manner.

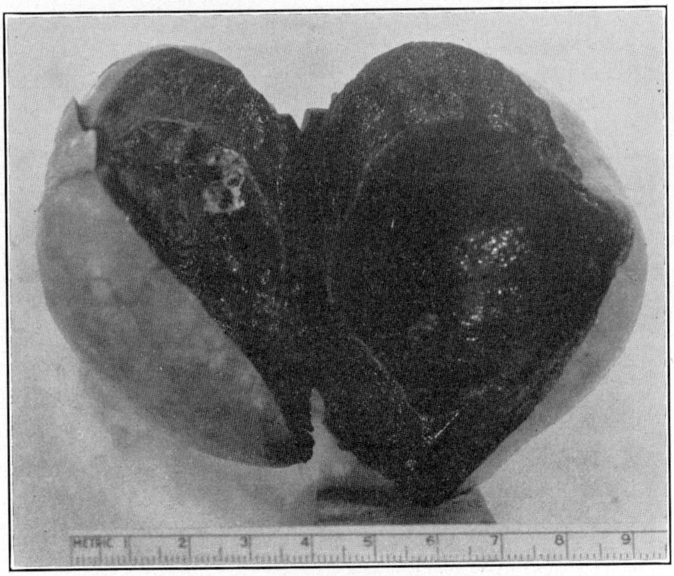

Fig. 2.

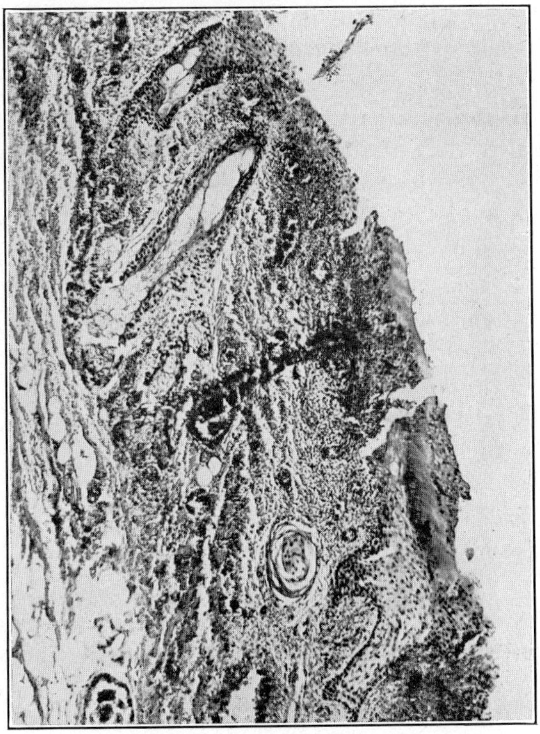

Fig. 3.

Pathologic Report.—Gross Examination: The mass was 7 by 5 by 5 cm. and globular in shape (Fig. 2). The surface was smooth and deep purple in color. A short twisted pedicle was attached. Section revealed a smooth-walled sac 5 cm. in diameter filled with serosanguineous fluid. The portion of the wall adjacent to the pedicle was thickened to 15 mm. in diameter, the remainder being thin and comprising the wall of the sac. Portions of the thickened wall contained small sacs filled with cheesy white material and hair.

Microscopic Examination: Section revealed a fibrous tissue wall so densely infiltrated with blood elements as to obscure almost completely the cellular structure. The thickened portion of the wall has a similar dense extravasation of blood with areas revealing squamous epithelium with cornification and a few typical hair follicles and sebaceous glands (Fig. 3).

Diagnosis.—Dermoid cyst with recent hemorrhage from torsion.

The child made an uneventful recovery and left the hospital on the tenth day. She has since been entirely free from pain and symptoms, except for a slight menstrual flow which appeared for one day.

COMMENT

Previous to 1905 about sixty cases of various tumors of the ovary in children had been reported, and since that time another thirty-eight have been added.[1] It is of importance to note that 60 per cent of these tumors were considered benign until 1912, but with improved histologic study it has been shown since that 60 per cent of them are malignant.[2] This finding is of importance in the consideration of the subject. The greatest number of tumors of the ovary in children occur between the ages of ten and fourteen years. Their earlier occurrence may be associated with signs of sexual precocity. The earliest reported case was that of Doran in a seven-month premature living infant.[3]

The history and clinical course of the case reported here, until marked torsion of the pedicle of the ovary took place, could easily have been attributed to a number of conditions which occur in childhood. Certainly ovarian tumor would be the least likely. Indigestion associated with dietary indiscretions, spastic colitis, left-sided appendicitis, appendiceal abscess, and the less likely conditions such as urolithiasis, and incomplete intestinal obstruction, intussusception, mesenteric adenitis were to be considered. The roentgenologic report offered no aid, although the fact was immediately appreciated after surgery that had the urinary bladder been emptied before the flat plate of the abdomen was taken, the evidence of the ovarian mass could have been suspected by visualization. This point is of great importance. In the face of the nonsurgical clinical course of our patient, the one great aid to the correct differential diagnosis lay in the rectal examination which, together with a correct x-ray interpretation, might have made possible an earlier recognition of the condition encountered here. The absence of toxicity, of abdominal surgical findings, and of fever justified medical observation with a view toward evaluating the mass palpated rectally. Twisting of the pedicle within the following twelve hours produced an increase in the size and tenderness of the mass, with symptoms of toxicity of the patient, which clarified and substantiated the correct diagnosis, thus leading to immediate surgical intervention.

CONCLUSIONS

1. Repeated attacks of abdominal pain in children justify a complete and careful study comparable to that afforded adults. It is wrong to assume that such attacks are probably insignificant, or to ascribe them to the large mass of indefinite conditions headed by the much abused term "colitis."

2. Rectal examination done carefully and repeatedly is of utmost importance in all children with abdominal pain. This statement cannot be repeated too often.

3. The roentgenologist may be of definite assistance in the visualization of the ovarian mass quite early in the course of its development if a series of flat plates of the abdomen are taken before and after the urinary bladder is emptied.

4. Surgical treatment should be instituted as soon as the diagnosis is made, particularly because of the high frequency of malignancy encountered in tumors of the ovary in childhood.

REFERENCES

1. Secor, W. L.: J. A. M. A. **87**: 940, 1926.
2. Downes, Wm. A.: J. A. M. A. **74**: 443, 1921.
3. Abt: Clinical Pediatrics, Ovarian Cysts in Children.

SPONTANEOUS RUPTURE OF THE LIVER IN A CHILD WITH COMPLETE RECOVERY

C. E. Bradley, M.D., and D. L. Garrett, M.D.
Tulsa, Okla.

TRAUMATIC rupture of the liver is comparatively rare, but spontaneous or hemorrhagic rupture is even more rare. There is no doubt regarding its occurrence in certain cases, some patients having been confined to bed under close observation for some time previous to the rupture. These spontaneous ruptures may be differentiated from traumatic ruptures by the fact that they are intracapsular. Anatomically the rupture is due to a hemorrhage, which may be secondary to old lesions of the hepatic parenchyma, such as secondary tumors, syphilitic lesions, or lesions of obliterating arteritis, which have been demonstrated histologically in some of these cases. According to Devic and Beriel,[2] spontaneous rupture is due to lesions of arteritis. This is an infarct at first, followed by increased vascularization at the periphery and rupture of a vessel causing an intrahepatic hemorrhage. This is followed by rupture of the glandular tissue with the production of a subcapsular hematoma. There may result a degeneration of the parenchyma and connective tissue, particularly in cases of central rupture, which are, of course, difficult to diagnose, with the formation of secondary abscesses. The classical symptoms and signs of spontaneous rupture are as follows:

Sharp pain in the right hypochondrium
Vomiting
Pallor
Anemia
Slow pulse early with rapid pulse as peritoneal irritation sets in
Jaundice
Leucocytosis
Cullen's sign of bluish discoloration at the umbilicus
Shock
Right hypochondriac mass—tense, tender, resilient
Tympanites
Rigidity
Blurring of the pleural sinus
Negative gastric, renal, and pulmonary signs.

Death may occur in a few minutes, an hour or two, a few days, or occasionally after a week or more. So far as we have been able to determine, no patient with true spontaneous rupture of the liver has ever recovered.

Mast and Streamer[1] reported a case of spontaneous rupture of primary carcinoma of the liver, which was probably brought on from a jar while the patient was driving a tractor. Devic and Beriel[2] reported eleven cases gleaned from the literature; three of these cases were definitely due to syphilis, as no doubt were some of the others; one was due to cancer; three were uncertain or incomplete; and in four there was no history of injury, and no definite cause for the rupture was discernible. Since we have been unable to get a copy of their original article, it is impossible for us to determine whether or not some of the cases which they discussed are duplicated in the cases which we have been able to locate in the literature. Nauwerck[3] reported two cases of rupture of the liver due to stasis of bile. Genell[4] reviewed three of the four known cases of rupture of the liver in the newborn and added three cases of his own. He suggested that two accidentally coinciding lesions, both of which are individually rare, that is, a mechanical traumatic factor, contracted or distorted pelvis, plus an abnormal tendency to bleed, pseudohemophilia of the newborn, are responsible for the ruptures in these cases. Steiger,[5] Andersson,[6] Furtwaengler,[7] and Aldridge[8] each reported a case of rupture of the liver due to trauma. Watzold[9] reported a case due to syphilitic aneurysm, and Carnable[10] reported a case of spontaneous rupture of the liver in a twenty-six-year-old male, in which the direct cause was obscure. Ecarius[11] reports three cases: one due to trauma, one due to adenoma, and one due to an aneurysm.

With the exception of the cases of rupture of the liver in the newborn, which were all due to trauma, the few cases recorded in the literature were all adults; moreover only four of these were not due to trauma, syphilis, carcinoma, or adenoma; and recovery in a case of spontaneous rupture of the liver has so far as we can ascertain not been reported. We present a case of spontaneous rupture of the liver in a three-year-old child, who recovered and has remained in good health for more than two years.

Family History.—The mother, aged thirty-four years, father, aged sixty years, one half sister, aged forty-two years, and two half brothers, aged thirty-four and forty years, respectively, were all living and well. The family history was negative, so far as the immediate family knew, for syphilis or blood dyscrasias.

Patient's History.—M. A. G., a female child, three years of age, was born normally at full term. She was fed goat's milk modified with dextrimaltose until she was nine months of age. Then she was fed table food. At nine months of age she had a mild attack of measles without complications. She had had no illness since; no colds, coughs or sore throat, and no constipation. She had never had an intestinal disturbance of any kind until Feb. 8, 1934.

That morning the child was up at the usual hour and played about the room a few minutes before breakfast. Shortly after beginning the morning meal, she became ill and vomited immediately, before being taken away from the breakfast table. She was placed in bed and appeared exhausted. During the morning, she developed a temperature of 103° F. and was exceedingly pale. She was given castor oil and chicken broth; and orange juice and water were given freely. Her temperature was not taken at regular intervals until February 11, when the parents became alarmed at her extreme pallor, marked distention of the abdomen, and restlessness.

A physician was called, and she was given pituitrin, hot turpentine stupes, and enemas without relief of tympanites. At that time her temperature was 103.6° F.;

pulse, 152; and respiration, 36. For the next three days her temperature ranged from 102° F. in the morning to 104° F. about the middle of the afternoon.

When one of us saw the patient for the first time, six days after the onset, at 11 P.M., Feb. 14, 1934, she presented the following appearance.

A well-nourished, three-year-old female was resting quietly. Respiration was regular and not rapid. The head was negative; facies, anxious; skin, very pale; ears, waxy. The mucous membranes of the mouth, lips, and conjunctiva were very pale. The sclera was blue white; the pupils were equal and reacted to light. The chest was well developed; expansion was equal; and respiration was regular. Lungs were normal to auscultation and percussion. *Heart:* Apex beat was heard in the fourth interspace, 1 cm. inside the nipple line; a soft blowing systolic murmur was heard loudest just to the left of the sternum, and in the second, third, and fourth interspaces. The murmur was considered functional. The heart sounds were muffled and were not of good quality. *Abdomen:* There was a good abdominal wall, with generalized tenderness, most marked in the upper right quadrant. The liver was palpable four fingerbreadths below the costal margin and to the left of the midline. The liver's edge was rounded, soft, and tender on slight pressure. No other palpable masses in the abdomen. There was a bluish discoloration around the umbilicus. The genitals and extremities were negative.

The patient was hospitalized the following day. *Progress:* As Table I shows, her hemoglobin level at that time was 20 per cent (Dare); the red blood cells numbered 1,800,000, and the white cells, 29,150. The leucocytosis was due to an increase in young forms of polymorphonuclear leucocytes. At 11:35 A.M., a transfusion of 250 c.c. of whole blood was given by the syringe method.

Radiologic examination of the abdomen, Feb. 15, 1934, showed the liver shadow to be very much enlarged, mainly from the lower aspect, probably due to liver abscess. The abdomen was otherwise negative.

Nourishing food, plenty of fluids, medication to produce rest, and temperature sponges were given the next two days. A stool examination on the seventeenth was normal with the exception of a slight increase in mucus. Urine examinations on February 16 and 17 were normal. The patient's pulse was more feeble on February 17, but she was less toxic, and the mass had not enlarged. A blood count showed some improvement, although the hemoglobin was only 30 per cent.

On February 18, a transfusion of 210 c.c. of whole blood was given. The mass in the upper right quadrant was softer, more rounded, and extended 1 cm. lower than it had before. The left chest was more resonant to percussion, and edema of the lid of the right eye was present.

On February 20 the hemoglobin showed some improvement, and there was an even greater elevation in the white and polymorphonuclear counts; however Cooke-Ponder's index was slightly lower. There was a macular rash over the extremities, neck, and back. The temperature averages were lower, and the patient looked less toxic. There was no change in the mass.

On February 21, the patient's sclera had developed a yellowish tint, but she looked less toxic. The mass was rounded and not so tense. Neoskiodan was given intravenously, and the report of the pyelography was as follows:

On February 21, intravenous pyelography after injection of neo-iopax showed incomplete filling of the calyces of both the right and left, but good filling of both pelves. The entire right kidney was well outlined, the left not so well. The ureters were not filled well enough to make any further statement of their condition. The bladder was apparently normal.

The blood count showed improvement in that the hemoglobin was 55 per cent.

On February 22 a transfusion of 250 c.c. of whole blood was given by the syringe method.

On February 23 a hypodermatoclysis of 500 c.c. of normal saline was given.

TABLE I

BLOOD

Date	2/15/34	2/15/34 Transfusion 250 c.c. Whole Blood	2/17/34	2/18/34 Transfusion 210 c.c. Whole Blood	2/20/34	2/21/34	2/22/34 Transfusion 250 c.c. Whole Blood	3/5/34
Red blood cells	1,800,000							
Hemoglobin	20%		30%		40%	55%		60%
White blood cells	29,150		20,000		21,200	17,200		
Coagulation time	9 minutes		6 minutes		8 minutes			
Differential								
Neutrophiles	71%		72%		82%	87%		
Arneth and Shilling: Myelocytes	1%		0		3%	1%		
Juvenile	1%		3%		7%	1%		
Band	42%		47%		38%	37%		
Segmenters	27%		22%		34%	48%		
2 segmenters	19%		20%		29%	35%		
3 segmenters	6		2%		5%	11%		
4 segmenters	2		0		0	2		
5 segmenters	0		0		0	0		
Lymphocytes	29%		24%		15%	11%		
Mononuclears	0		4%		1%	2%		
Eosinophiles	0		0		2%	0		
Basophiles	0		0		0	0		
Platelets								
Malaria								
Cooke-Ponder Index	1.52		1.33		1.47	1.69		
Polychromatophilia	slight		moderate		slight	slight		
Normoblasts	few		occasional		occasional			
Basophilic degeneration	occasional							
Karyorrhexia	slight							
Pyknosis						moderate		
Deliquescence			marked					

Blood Culture: Taken Feb. 16, 1934, negative on February 17, 19, 21, 26, March 12, 17, and 30.

Urinalysis: February 16, normal; February 17, normal; February 21, normal with exception of positive acetone and diacetic acid.

Feces Analysis: Feb. 17, 1934.

Amount: 10 gm.
Character: soft
Odor: pungent
Mucus: moderate excess
Blood (occult): very slight trace
Ova and parasites: none found

Bacteria: gram-positive and gram-negative bacilli

The sclera continued to have a yellowish tint. The entire body presented a peculiar and striking appearance, that is, a color which was midway between the appearance of the skin in hemolytic jaundice and in biliary jaundice—a most peculiar and definite coppery shade.

Radiologic examination of the chest showed an absence of a line of demarcation between the liver and lung, generalized increase in density over the entire right field due to pleural fluid and compression of the lung.

On February 24 laparotomy was performed and a hematoma of the right lobe of the liver was removed and packed as follows. A high right rectus incision was made and the peritoneal cavity opened. Immediately below the incision the enlarged liver presented, with a bluish mass beneath the thin capsule, which was covered with a thin layer of fibrin. The capsule was ruptured, and the liver, which seemed to have ruptured previously, now inclosed a large clotted mass. As much as could be safely removed was taken out, leaving a transverse irregular crater in the right lobe of the liver. The opening in the liver was packed with two gauze packs, the ends of which were brought out through the incision, which was closed in layers in the usual manner.

On February 26, although the temperature was lower than it had been in the past twenty-four hours, there was an occasional râle in the upper left lung, but no bronchophony. The general condition was good.

On February 28 a small area of bronchophony was found in the base of the right lung posteriorly. There was slight dullness over the entire right half of the chest. The yellowish cast of the sclera was clearing, and the skin was less bronzed. The roentgenologist reported that radiologic examination of the chest showed the entire right side exhibiting a density due to compressed lung, surrounded peripherally by fluid. The diaphragm shadow was completely obliterated. The heart and the mediastinum were not displaced to the left.

On March 1, bronchophony from the sixth interspace to the base of the right posteriorly and bulging of the intercostal spaces from the sixth rib downward with a beginning cellulitis, were noted. The apex beat was heard just to the left of the nipple, fifth interspace. Expansion of the right lung much less than the left. Respiration was rapid.

On March 2 bronchophony was more pronounced and over a greater area. Percussion note was not so flat, and there were no râles.

On March 3 the area of dullness had increased. There was less bronchophony, and no râles. Apex beat just to the right of the nipple line.

On March 6, 180 c.c. of fluid aspirated from the right chest.

Convalescence from the operation of the liver was more or less uneventful. The removal of the packs was accomplished after thirteen days, with some trepidation and difficulty, but no untoward results. On March 8, there was no increase in dullness since aspiration. Apex beat was in normal position.

On March 13, 1934, she was dismissed from the hospital.

CONCLUSION

A three-year-old female child, presenting a history of sudden onset of acute intestinal distress, with marked pallor and distention of the abdomen due to a mass in the upper right quadrant (which was definitely felt to be an enlarged liver), and a striking bronzing of the skin with blue discoloration around the umbilicus which led to a diagnosis of spontaneous rupture of the liver, was successfully operated upon, after the general condition of the child had been improved; she has remained in good health for over two years.

We present this case because of the rarity of the condition, the rarity of diagnosis without benefit of autopsy, and because of the gratifying outcome of our efforts, hoping that, as these rare cases are reported, sufficient data will be accumulated to reduce the difficulty in diagnosis.

REFERENCES

1. Mast, William H., and Streamer, Charles W.: J. A. M. A. **100**: 1648, 1933.
2. Devic, E., and Beriel, L.: Ann. de dermat. et syph. **7**: 642, 1906.
3. Nauwerck: München. med. Wchnschr. **52**: 931, 1905.
4. Genell, S.: Acta Obst. & Gynec. Scandinav. **9**: 100, 1930.
5. Steiger, W.: Wien. klin. Wchnschr. **38**: 1308, 1925.
6. Andersson, L.: Beitr. z. klin. Chir. **135**: 696, 1926.
7. Furtwaengler, A.: Krankheitz-forschung, Leipz. **4**: 349, 1927.
8. Aldridge, A. R.: Lancet **1**: 1616, 1898.
9. Watzold: München. med. Wchnschr. **53**: 2107, 1906.
10. Carnable: Bull. et mém. Soc. de chir. de Bucarest **2**: 110, 1899.
11. Ecarius: Arch. f. klin. Chir. **172**: 755, 1932.

Mazel: Rev. de méd. leg. **20**: 238, 1913.

FURTHER ROENTGENOGRAPHIC STUDIES OF THE SELLA TURCICA IN ABNORMAL CHILDREN

Murray B. Gordon, M.D., and A. L. Loomis Bell, M.D.
Brooklyn, N. Y.

The roentgenographic findings as to the sella turcica in 104 normal children were reported in May, 1921.[1] That study was undertaken as an attempt to establish, if possible, normal sellar appearance and formation as a basis for comparison with the changes in abnormal children. The conclusions reached were briefly as follows:

1. The shape of the sella turcica in normal children falls in a general way into three groups: A, circular; B, oval; and C, flat or saucer shaped, with modifications in each.

2. There is a marked variation for each age, in both the height and length of the sella for that particular age. The average height and length of the sella show comparatively rapid increase in the first two years with gradual yet irregular increase from then on up to the age of twelve years.

3. There is no relationship between the shape of the sella and the size of the head except in the case of the flat type which was always found in small heads. It does not necessarily follow that all small heads exhibit this type.

4. There is apparently no influence of sex on either the appearance or formation of the sella.

5. There is apparently no relationship between the size of the sella and the size of the head.

Our results in this series of normal children serve as controls in the series herein reported. Although the literature abounds with numerous statements as to the appearance or formation of the sella turcica in various diseases, there have been very few control studies of normal sellae.

The present report deals with four problems:

1. Does the shape of the sella turcica in abnormal children differ from that in normal children?

2. Are there any characteristic differences in the formation of the sella in various types of abnormal children?

3. Is there a difference in size of the sella in normal and abnormal children?

4. Has the appearance, formation, or size of the sella any clinical or diagnostic significance?

From the Department of Pediatrics and Radiology, Long Island College Hospital and Department of Pediatrics, Israel Zion Hospital, Brooklyn, N. Y.

Number VII in the series, "Endocrine Studies in Infants and Children."

From a roentgenographic viewpoint, the changes in different sellae are those of general shape, changes in the development and shape of the posterior clinoid processes and dorsum sellae, and changes in the development and shape of the anterior clinoid processes. The middle clinoids are more nearly constant.

The technic used in a study of this kind is important, not so much the exact technic used, but the constancy with which it is followed. In adults, teleroentgenography is, of course, the most exact method, but in children the long exposures necessary in this technic are not practical. We have therefore selected a tube film distance of 26 inches and have, by using a high penetration and milliamperage, been able to obtain good films with ⅛-second exposure. The tube carrier is so adjusted that the central ray passes along a line tangent to the cornea of both eyes and is then moved backward until the central ray passes through the head at a point about one-third of the distance from the external auditory meatus to the glabella. In most instances this technic gives a good projection of the sella. One can readily imagine that in some rather badly trained infants the following of any technic would be difficult even when only an ⅛ of a second immobility is required. Duplitized films and screens were used.

SHAPE OF THE SELLA

In our normal series the circular or round sella was more frequently noted. Camp,[6] who utilized our classification in a study of 1,000 sellae, mostly of adults, also found that the circular and oval predominated, but in a different ratio from ours: namely, circular, 22.5 per cent; oval, 67 per cent; flat, 15 per cent. This demonstrates that there is little difference in the occurrence of the three groups in normal and abnormal individuals. Both the circular and oval predominate and the flat shape occurs the least frequently of all. No one shape predominated in any individual disease.

TABLE I

COMPARISON BETWEEN SELLAE OF NORMAL AND ABNORMAL CHILDREN

	NO. OF CASES	SHAPE OF SELLA			PRESENCE OF SLIT		
		A ROUND %	B OVAL %	C FLAT %	NOT PRESENT %	PRESENT UNCOVERED %	PRESENT COVERED %
Normal children Series I	104	66	24	10	22	39	38
Abnormal children Series II	64	43	42	15	18	33	48
Abnormal children Series III (present)	168	42	48	10	11	32	57
Abnormal children Series II, III	232	43	46	11	13	32	55

The findings in the present and previous studies on abnormal children in comparison with those of normal children are given in Table I. They confirm our previous conclusions.

FORMATION OF THE SELLA

To appreciate properly the formation of the sella turcica as depicted on an x-ray film, it is necessary to visualize the anatomic relations. The sella exists as a depression in the superior surface of the body of the sphenoid, limited anteriorly by the middle clinoid processes and posteriorly by the dorsum sellae, which carries the posterior clinoid process on either side of its tip. The middle clinoids are directly lateral and posterior to the olivary eminence. The sella is covered by an extension of the tentorium cerebelli (the diaphragma sellae) which is attached to the middle and posterior clinoid processes. All of the pituitary body with the exception of the base of the infundibulum lies below this tentorial extension. The anterior clinoid processes are formed by the medial ends of the posterior border of the lesser wings of the sphenoid; they are located at a considerable distance lateral to and above the sella turcica. The olivary eminence and the optic chiasmal groove are both extrasellar since they lie anterior to the middle clinoid processes. Differences then in configuration of the sella caused by the difference in position of the anterior clinoid processes and variations in height of the olivary eminence can mean absolutely nothing referable to the pituitary body.

In our first paper on normal children we found that "in some instances the anterior clinoids are raised above the level of the middle clinoids and are very long. In these latter cases a slit is seen running anteriorly from above the middle clinoid processes under the anterior clinoids. This slit is no way a part of the sella."

This excavation is made up below of the optic chiasmal groove anteriorly and the olivary eminence posteriorly, above by the posterior por-

TABLE II

COMPARISON BETWEEN SELLAE OF ABNORMAL CHILDREN

DISEASE	NO.	SHAPE OF SELLA: A CIRCULAR %	B OVAL %	C FLAT %	PRESENCE OF SLIT: NOT PRESENT %	PRESENT UNCOVERED %	PRESENT COVERED %
Mongolism	28	41	48	1	11	57	32
Adiposogenital dystrophy	79	44	47	9	8	30	62
Anterior pituitary deficiency	11	36	45	19	10	80	10
Mental retardation	74	41	50	9	23	29	48
Hypothyroidism	28	45	42	13	32	7	61
Hyperthyroidism	4	50	25	25	25	0	75
Hypogonadism	4	50	25	25	0	25	75

tion of the inferior surfaces of the lesser wings of the sphenoids, the tips of which are the anterior clinoid processes. We have designated the excavation as being uncovered or covered. By an uncovered excavation is meant one in which the lesser wings of the sphenoid are high enough to permit a visualization of the slit in the lateral view. In a large number of cases, both normal and abnormal, the slit is easily discernible, but it is partly covered by the lesser wings of the sphenoid—this we have termed a covered slit.

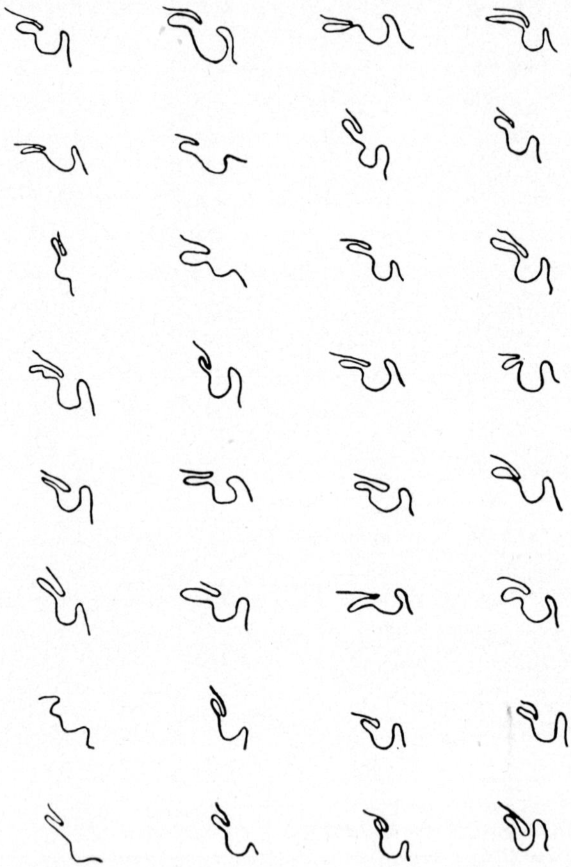

Fig. 1.—Normal children. Contour of sella turcica and uncovered slit below anterior clinoid process.

Timme in 1921[5] reported the presence of an excavation under the anterior clinoid process in 23 out of 24 mongolian imbeciles. He believed that there was some link between the appearance of the anterior process and this disease and further stated that "the excavation is seen occasionally in persons who have not mongolian characteristics but who have isolated symptoms and signs due to anterior lobe disturbances, namely, growth and genital abnormalities." This belief has not been confirmed by others who studied the subject on a large series. Clift[2] and Stevenson and Stultz[3] state that this appearance is not characteristic of mongolianism but that it may be a corollary of the peculiar facial arch present in that disease.

Tables I and II show the incidence of each type of excavation in each individual disease studied and also in normal children. A covered or uncovered slit is noted in 87 per cent of the abnormal children and in 77 per cent of the normal. An uncovered slit is found most frequently in the following conditions in the order named: anterior pituitary de-

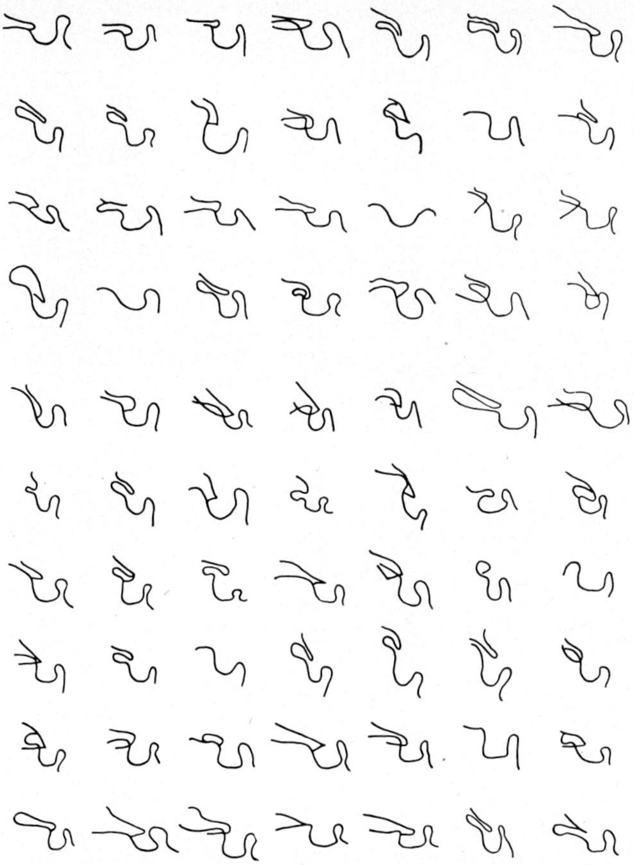

Fig. 2.—Adiposogenital dystrophy and obesity. Sella turcica shows variations in size and shape of all processes. Examples are seen of slit (*5, 6*), covered slit (*1-4*), and absent slit (*13, 19*).

ficiency, mongolian imbecility, normality, adiposogenital dystrophy, mental retardation, hypogonadism, and hypo- and hyperthyroidism. We feel that the small number of sellae studied in each disease entity prevents us from arriving at any definite conclusion as to the significance of the order of frequency. We are justified, however, in stating that its presence is not pathognomonic of any particular disease.

The shape of the slit is certainly not characteristic of any of the diseases studied as can be seen by even a casual examination of Figs. 1, 2,

3, and 4. In fact it is impossible to differentiate by means of this excavation between the sellae in the various abnormal conditions: mongolian imbecility (No. *6, 10, 11,* Fig. 3), mental retardation (No. *15, 21,* Fig. 3), childhood myxedema (No. *5, 14,* Fig. 4), hypogonadism (No. *24,* Fig. 4), lipodystrophy (No. *29,* Fig. 4), hydrocephalus (No. *40, 42,* Fig. 4), adiposogenital dystrophy (No. *5, 6, 7, 8, 34, 36,* Fig. 2). Similarly, every variation and type of the abnormal group is duplicated in the normal (Fig. 1). Comparison of the covered excavations shows that it is also impossible to differentiate between normal and abnormal (Figs. 1, 2, 3, and 4).

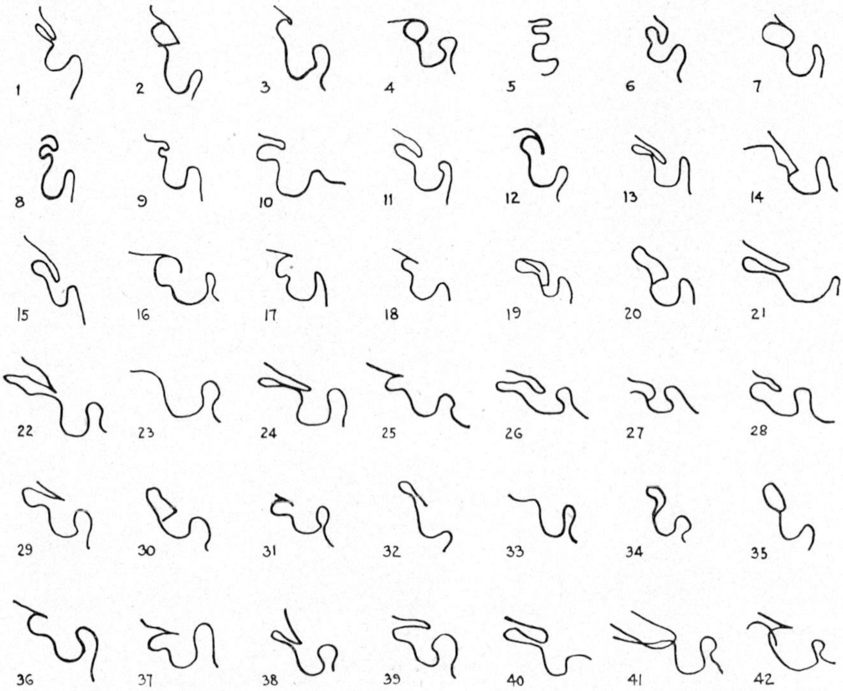

Fig. 3.—Sella turcica in mongolian imbecility (*1-14*) and mental retardation (*15-42*). Example *5* is of seven-week-old infant

The type of sella without any excavation occurs in 22 per cent of the x-ray films of normal children and in from 8 to 32 per cent of the abnormal. Here also every variation of formation and contour appearing in the abnormal children is duplicated in the normal.

The characteristics of the anterior and posterior clinoid processes are not constant in any particular disease as may be noted in studying Figs. 1, 2, 3, and 4. They show similar variations in size, shape, and development in both normal and abnormal children. The dorsum sellae, which is of more importance in this discussion than the anterior clinoid process, which is extrasellar, may be broad with rounded or bulbous posterior process, narrow with long process, or pyramidal shaped with an apical clinoid. It may be long or short and point forward, upward, or backward. It may be well developed or poorly developed.

The dorsum sellae in adiposogenital dystrophy tends to be broad and well developed with at times a bulbous posterior clinoid process. In a few instances, the dorsum sellae and posterior clinoid may be poorly developed. The well-developed dorsum sellae is found more frequently in all of the diseases studied than the poorer developed form (Table III). In mongolian imbecility the broad dorsum sella is infrequent as compared to the pyramidal type and the long, curved narrow process.

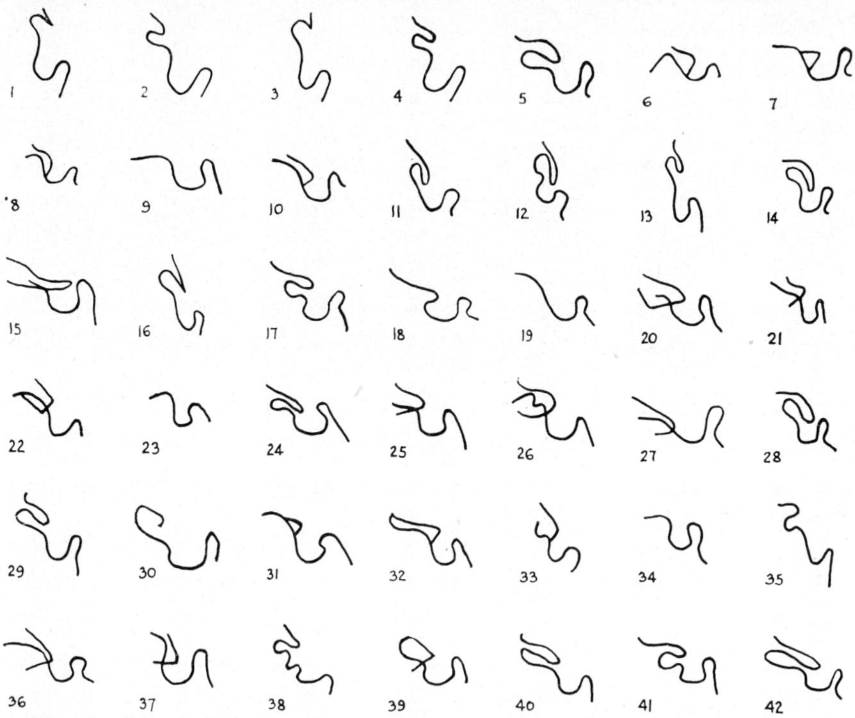

Fig. 4.—Sella turcica in various conditions. Childhood myxedema and hypothyroidism (*1-17*); anterior pituitary deficiency and infantilism (*18-23*); hypogonadism (*24-28*); lipodystrophy (*29*); achondroplasia (*30-31*); diabetes insipidus (*32*); microcephalus (*33-35*); hyperthyroidism (*36-37*); hydrocephalus (*38-42*).

Bridging and near bridging, that is approximation of the anterior and posterior clinoid processes, was encountered in only 8 instances in the series, all in the obese group.

SIZE OF THE SELLA

The dimensions of the sella turcica on x-ray films are generally expressed in terms of vertical and anteroposterior measurements. There is no uniformity, however, as to the points from which these measurements are taken. Camp[6] states that "the anteroposterior measurements are taken from the most dorsal point of the tuberculum sellae in the sagittal plane to the anterior edge of the dorsum sellae in the same plane. The vertical dimension or height is taken along a line dropped from the anteroposterior line to the deepest point on the floor of the sella.'' Royster and Rodman[7] consider the height to be ''a line drawn from the lower limits of the curves of the clinoid processes to the floor of the sella turcica.'' They do not designate the particular clinoid process, i.e., anterior or middle to the posterior, but evidently refer to the middle as their height dimensions are shorter than ours in the first series.

In our first two series[1, 4] we measured the sella as follows: the length, from the middle clinoid process to the farthest posterior part of the sella; the height, on a line joining the tips of the anterior and posterior clinoid processes, a perpendicular was drawn to the deepest portion of the sella.

In the present study we have changed our points of measurement, especially that of height since we feel that the anterior clinoid process is not a part of the sella per se and therefore should not be considered in the dimensions. In the present series the height is computed as follows: a line is drawn from the most anterior and upper point of the dorsum sellae forward to the nearest point of the dorsal aspect of the tuberculum sellae. From this line or its extension, a perpendicular dropped to the deepest part of the sella represents the height. The length is the longest anteroposterior diameter. We use Royster and Rodman's figures as normal averages for the present study as their measurements are practically the same as ours.

While our former measurements cannot be used as criteria for the present study, the general trends noted by us in the first two series, especially as to the relationships between the size of the sella and the size of the head and the increase in the size of the sella with age, are still valid.

TABLE III

APPEARANCE OF DORSUM SELLAE WITH POSTERIOR CLINOID PROCESS

	BROAD DORSUM SELLAE WITH ROUNDED POSTERIOR PROCESS			BULBOUS POSTERIOR CLINOID	POINTED POSTERIOR BROAD BASE DORSUM SELLAE	LONG CURVED NARROW POSTERIOR	POORLY DEVELOPED DORSUM SELLAE
	MEDIUM	SHORT	LONG				
Adiposogenital dystrophy	20	10	3	15	12	8	6
Anterior pituitary deficiency	3	3	0	2	2	0	1
Mental retardation	14	13	3	7	8	4	5
Mongolism	1	1	0	1	3	5	2
Hypogonadism	1	1	0	0	1	0	1
Hypothyroidism	2	3	0	3	1	0	1
Hyperthyroidism	0	0	1	1	0	0	0
	41	31	7	29	27	17	16 168

The variations in the normal series were so great that it was difficult to arrive at an average for any particular age. The same variations in size were noted in our first series of abnormal children, and it is therefore difficult to state whether they represent the normal variations. It seems that the type of disease has apparently no influence on the size of the sella per se, for the differences are not constant enough for any one disease to be of any diagnostic value. The average size of the sella turcica in various diseases is given in Table III. The sellae in the adiposogenital dystrophy group are slightly larger on the average than those in the other groups, but this increase in size is not great enough to be characteristic.

TABLE IV

AVERAGE SIZE OF SELLA TURCICA IN VARIOUS DISEASES COMPARED WITH THAT IN NORMAL CHILDREN

AGE	1-2-3 YR.	4-5-6 YR.	7-8-9 YR.	10-11-12 YR.	13-14-15 YR.	15 YR. +
*Normal**	6 × 4 mm.	7.7 × 5.4 mm.	8.4 × 6.2 mm.	9.3 × 6.0 mm.	9.6 × 6.8 mm.	mm.
Adiposogenital dystrophy		6.2 × 5.5	8.9 × 7.1	8.7 × 7.3	9.0 × 7.7	7.7 × 7.7
Mental retardation	6.8 × 6.0	8.7 × 7.0	8.3 × 8.7	8.4 × 7.4	8.0 × 6.0	
Mongolism	5.5 × 5.5	7.5 × 7.3	7.7 × 7.0			
Hypothyroidism	8.5 × 7.0	9.2 × 7.7	7.0 × 5.0 (1)		10.0 × 9.0 (1)	
Anterior pituitary deficiency		8.0 × 5.5	5.0 × 6.0 (1)	8.5 × 8.5	7.5 × 7.5	11 × 4 (17 yr.) 8 × 9 (18 yr.)
Hypogonadism			7.5 × 6.5	12.0 × 10.0 (1)	11.0 × 8.0	

*Averages taken from Royster and Rodman.[7]

One expects to find smaller sellae in children with anterior pituitary deficiency of growth, but in the present series five are below the average for the respective age, three are normal, and one is exceedingly large (10 mm. by 5 mm. in a five-year-old child).

To emphasize our statement that there is no relationship between the size of the sella and the size of the head, we note that in a microcephalic idiot ten years of age the size of the sella is 10 mm. by 10 mm., which is greater than the average for that age, while a child with hydrocephalus in the same age group has a sella which measures 8 mm. by 7 mm.

The average size of the sella in microcephalus is 7.5 mm. by 7.3 mm., irrespective of the age, while that in hydrocephalus is 8 mm. by 7 mm.

The size in nonendocrine mental retardation falls fairly within the normal limits with slight upward or downward trends in different age groups. The same tendencies are noted in hypothyroidism. The trend in mongolian imbecility is toward a smaller sella than the normal. In two cases of achondroplasia the sellae are both much larger than the average for the respective ages.

SUMMARY

Studies were carried out on the sella turcica of 168 abnormal children suffering from adiposogenital dystrophy, obesity, anterior pituitary deficiency, hypothyroidism, mongolian imbecility, mental retardation, etc., and the findings were correlated with those of 64 abnormal children and 104 normal children previously studied. We are able to confirm our previous findings that the shape of the sella does not differ significantly in normal and abnormal children. The type of disorder is not correlated with the shape of the sella. Round and oval shapes predominate both in normal and abnormal children, and flat sellae are the least frequent.

The formation of the sellae does not differ in abnormal children from those in the normal children, nor is there any formation characteristic of any individual disease. The excavation beneath the anterior clinoid process is extrasellar and is not significant of mongolian imbecility nor of any other disorder studied in this series. The size of the sella is not influenced by any of the diseases. There is no relationship between the size of the sella and the size of the head.

REFERENCES

1. Gordon, M. B., and Bell, A. L. L.: New York State J. Med. **22**: 54, 1922.
2. Clift, M. W.: Am. J. Roentgenol. **9**: 420, 1922.
3. Stevenson, G. S., and Stultz, A. D.: Arch. Neurol. & Psychiat. **10**: 299, 1923.
4. Gordon, M. B., and Bell, A. L. L.: Endocrinology **9**: 265, 1925.
5. Timme, W.: Arch. Neurol. & Psychiat. **5**: 568, 1921.
6. Camp, J.: Am. J. Roentgenol. **12**: 143, 1924; Radiology **1**: 65, 1923.
7. Royster, L. T., and Rodman, N. F.: Tr. Am. Pediat. Soc. **34**: 246, 1922.
Royster, L. T., and Moriarty, M. E.: Am. J. Phys. Anthrop. **14**: 451, 1930.

MENINGITIS DUE TO THE MORGAN BACILLUS

Report of a Case

Reginald H. Mitchell, M.D.
Washington, D. C.

NUMEROUS bacteria have been reported as causative organisms in meningitis. In a review of the literature but one report of meningitis due to the Morgan bacillus has come to my attention. The following is believed to be the first case of this type of meningitis to be reported in the American literature.

The patient, a colored male, aged eleven months, was admitted to the Children's Hospital on June 13, 1935, with a history of cough and rhinitis of two weeks' duration, listlessness, and anorexia. Three days before admission he developed a discharge from his right eye and the day following he vomited once. At all times his bowels were regular, and the stools were of normal consistency.

The past history of the child was essentially negative. He was a full-term baby, having an uneventful birth and a birth weight of 6 pounds and 7 ounces. He was never ill and was given orange juice but no cod liver oil for rachitic prevention.

The physical examination on admission revealed an acutely ill colored male of about one year of age. The head examination presented a discharge from the right eye, hypertrophied tonsils, and an injected pharynx. The chest showed diminished breath sounds and a percussion note over the right base posteriorly. The heart and abdomen were essentially negative, as was the neurologic examination. The admission diagnosis was a rhinopharyngitis, catarrhal conjunctivitis, and a possible early pneumonia.

For several days the chest signs remained unchanged, and three days after admission the temperature, which was 101° F., reached 104° F. rectally. It continued to vary between 99° and 103° F., and four days after admission an x-ray plate of the chest disclosed the heart, lungs, and thymus to be normal. Smears from the eye were negative until June 15, when an organism having the morphology of the Koch-Weeks bacillus was reported.

Throughout this time the bowels had been moving only once or twice a day, and the stools were quite normal in character. The blood count gave a 44 per cent hemoglobin (Newcomer), 3,820 red blood cells, 21,000 white blood cells with 81 per cent polymorphonuclear leucocytes including 42 bands, 27 lobulated, and 2 young forms. There was a marked achromia, anisocytosis, and poikilocytosis.

On June 24 the temperature, which had slightly dropped to an average of 101° F., again rose to 104° F. At this time a bulge of the anterior fontanel was noted, and another neurologic examination was entirely negative. A spinal puncture was done, the fluid being removed under a pressure of 24 mm. of mercury, rising to 30 mm. under jugular compression with the child crying during the examination. The fluid was colorless but had a granular appearance. That evening 130 c.c. of slightly cloudy spinal fluid was withdrawn, and 30 c.c. of antimeningococcus serum was given intraspinally. Thereafter a daily spinal tap was done.

The laboratory report on the first spinal fluid showed a cell count of 250 per c.mm. with 8 per cent lymphocytes and 92 per cent polymorphonuclear leucocytes. There

From the Medical Service of the Children's Hospital, Washington, D. C.

was a normal reduction of Benedict's solution, and the globulin was not increased, although the second specimen showed an abnormal amount. Examination of the culture of the first specimen of spinal fluid disclosed the finding of a gram-negative bacillus. Later the laboratory reported that this organism appeared to belong to the salmonella group and might be the *Salmonella morgani.* From the time of the first culture until the third week before discharge the cultures for this organism were consistently positive. Throughout the course of the illness there was a wide variation of the differential cell count of the spinal fluid. The lymphocytes ranged from 10 per cent to 90 per cent with a corresponding change in the polymorphonuclear leucocytes and the total count varied from 170 per c.mm. to 2,000 per c.mm. A number of blood cultures were taken and were all negative. Stool cultures were consistently negative as were several nose and throat cultures.

On July 15 the intraspinal administration of an autogenous vaccine was begun, 0.1 c.c. of the vaccine being given, the dose being increased 0.1 c.c. daily until 1.0 c.c.

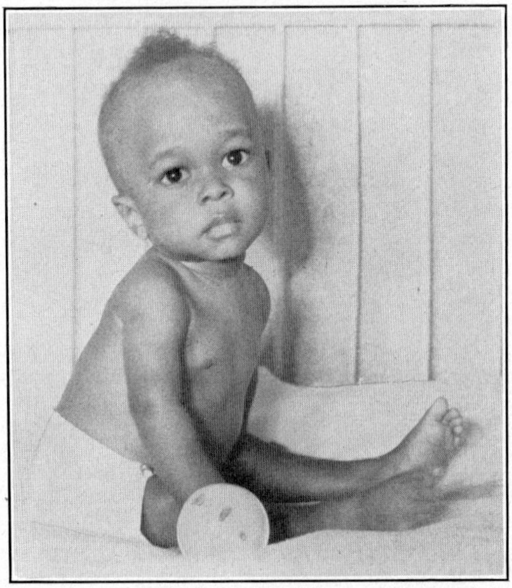

Fig. 1.—Morgan bacillus meningitis. Photograph taken five weeks after admission. The spinal fluid cell count at this time was 1,700 per c.mm.

was given. The cell count rapidly rose to 1,400 per c.mm. and then the vaccine was stopped. The count receded until the last puncture was done on August 5 when it was 160 per c.mm. In general the patient looked well and was discharged August 13, two months after admission, as cured. The child was seen several times about two months later and seemed to be in the best of health.

COMMENT

As we review the case we are impressed with several striking features. One is that, in a case of meningitis with a spinal cell count mounting to 2,000 per c.mm., at no time did the child ever have any of the neurologic symptoms of meningeal infection, in fact, the child was never acutely ill. During the course of his illness he learned to stand and even walk a few steps. The picture of the patient was taken five weeks after admission, and at the time his spinal fluid cell count was 1,700 per c.mm.

Another interesting fact was that the stool cultures and the blood cultures were repeatedly negative. One can rule out infection of the spinal tract from lumbar puncture by the obtaining of the positive culture from the very first specimen of spinal fluid.

To check the diagnosis of a Morgan bacillus infection further, a specimen of the spinal fluid and one of the laboratory's cultures were sent to the National Institute of Health. Their examination showed the presence of gram-negative motile rods. The fermentation reactions were studied on twenty-five different sugars and a number of media. The organisms studied produced acid and gas in dextrose, galactose, levulose, mannose, and a trace of acid in glycerin. After seven days the following were completely negative: adonitol, amygdalin, arabinose, dulcitol, dextrin, erythritol, inositol, inulin, lactose, maltose, mannitol, raffinose, rhamnose, saccharose, salicin, sorbitol, starch, trehalose, and xylose. The methyl red reaction was positive. Gelatin was not liquefied and litmus milk was neither acidified nor coagulated. Indol was formed and lead blackened. The nitrates were reduced. Agglutination serums for the Morgan bacillus were not available but ''cartrol'' agglutination tests with serums for the typhoid, dysentery, and various salmonella strains were all negative. In the opinion of Dr. Branham, of the National Institute of Health, agglutination by specific serums was entirely unnecessary as the organisms had such clear-cut cultural and biochemical characteristics. The lack of maltose fermentation and positive reduction of nitrates were the only deviations from the classic strains first described by Morgan.

A review of the literature reveals only one other case of a Morgan bacillus meningitis.[1] The symptoms in this case were those of a typical meningitis ending fatally. The Morgan bacillus is primarily a habitant of the intestinal tract both normally and in the presence of a diarrhea.[2] It has often been reported as a common cause of diarrhea in infants,[3] especially in the summer time.[4] The extent of the infection of the Morgan bacillus is not limited to the intestinal tract. Magath and Jackson[5] in 1924 reported a case of a fatal septicemia due to this organism, and similar infections have also been reported by others.[1] It has been known to produce pyelitis,[6, 7] ulcerative colitis,[8] and a fatal cholecystitis[9]; d'Aunoy[10] also reports colitis and pyelitis. Through a series of thirteen cases Havens and Ridgway[11] studied the pathogenicity of the Morgan bacillus and its wide range of infection. The organism occasionally gives rise to a diarrhea similar to a paratyphoid infection[12] and the patient's serum gives a positive agglutination with the Morgan bacillus.

In general, the Morgan bacillus[13] is seen to be a gram-negative motile rod which ferments only glucose, levulose, and galactose. It causes a strong indol reaction in peptone water and will not cause any growth in uric acid or citrate media. In Jordan's citrate medium it causes an acid reaction in the butt and slant. This organism has been observed to be nonpathogenic for laboratory animals if obtained from healthy individuals and fatal to them if obtained from persons ill with the disease. The Morgan bacillus has been seen not only in man, but also in cows, monkeys, mice, snakes, parrots, and even roaches, and has been obtained from the soil and water.

It can thus be seen that the distribution of the Morgan bacillus and its infectiousness is not limited to the gastrointestinal system. It has even been seen in conjunction with mastoiditis[14] and with mental disease.[15]

SUMMARY

1. A case of Morgan bacillus meningitis is presented, and it is believed to be the only case reported in the American literature.

2. There is a brief review of the extent of the infectiousness of the organism.

3. The cultural and biochemical characteristics of the Morgan bacillus of the case are presented.

The author wishes to express his appreciation for the help given him by Dr. H. A. Ong, Dr. C. B. Conklin, and Dr. E. C. Rice, of the Children's Hospital attending staff. He also wishes to thank Dr. Sara Branham, of the National Institute of Health, for her work in confirming the recognition of the organism under discussion.

REFERENCES

1. Gittens, R., and Hawksley, J. C.: Lancet **1**: 1040, 1932.
2. Lewis, C. J.: Great Britain Loc. Gov. Bd. Rep., Med. Supp., Appendix B, No. 3, p. 375, 1912-13.
3. Logan, W. R.: Lancet **2**: 824, 1916.
4. Mackenzie, G. M., and Batt, L. M.: J. Immunol. **19**: 371, 1930.
5. Magath, T. B., and Jackson, E.: Med. Clin. North America **8**: 1381, 1925.
6. Riding, D.: Brit. M. J. **7**: 183, 1927.
7. Riding, D., and Ridgway, C.: J. Prevent. Med. **3**: 159, 1927.
8. Thjotta, T.: J. Bacteriol. **5**: 159, 1920.
9. Thjotta, T.: J. Infect. Dis. **43**: 249, 1928.
10. d'Aunoy, R.: Am. J. M. Sc. **178**: 834, 1929.
11. Havens, L. C., and Ridgway, C.: J. Prevent. Med. **3**: 159, 1929.
12. Havens, L. C., and Mayfield, C. R.: J. Prevent. Med. **4**: 179, 1930.
13. Jordan, E. O., Crawford, R. R., and McBrown, J.: J. Bacteriol. **29**: 131, 1935.
14. Dick, G. H., and Williams, J. L.: Am. J. Dis. Child. **35**: 955, 1928.
15. Stewart, F. H.: J. Ment. Sc. **74**: 269, 1928.

CITRATED TRANSFUSION IN INFANTS AND CHILDREN

SIDNEY HIRSCH, M.D.
NEW YORK, N. Y.

RECENTLY I described an automatic two-way valve for use in transfusions and other therapeutic procedures. I wish to report its successful use in over 125 transfusions since January, 1935, on the pediatric service of Mount Sinai Hospital. Here it is employed for citrated transfusions in infants and young children. Experience with the unit in these cases emphasized the ease and desirability of utilizing this automatic device. It facilitates the injection of the citrated blood into the recipient under pressure. This permits the use of a fine hypodermic needle of a 23 or 25 gauge, thus eliminating in most of the cases, the necessity of cutting down to enter the vein. In the series of cases here

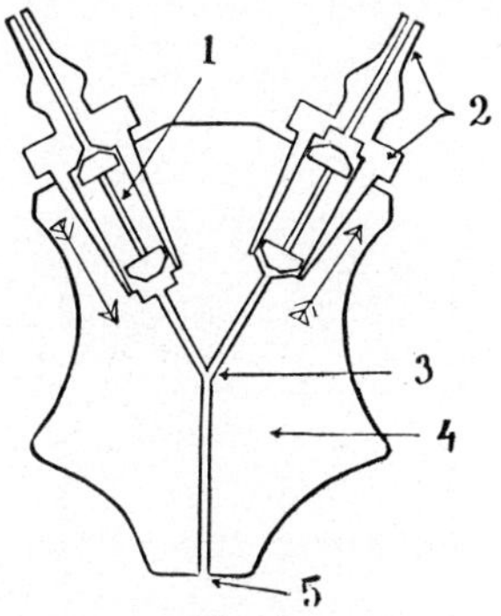

Fig. 1.

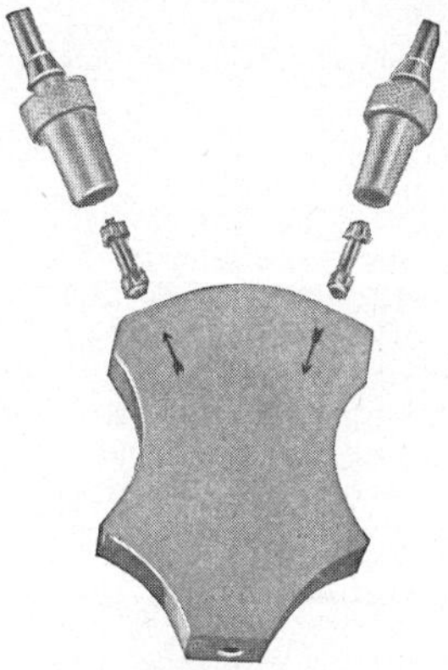

Fig. 2.

Fig. 1.—Cross-section. *1*, Automatic valve without washers or packing. *2*, Fitting with knurled nut and end tapered for needle or rubber hose. *3*, Flow of fluid in "Y" arrangement. *4*, Stainless steel body with finger grips. *5*, Inlet for adapters for either Luer or Record syringe or for Luer syringe itself.

Fig. 2.—Apparatus taken apart.

reported 3.8 per cent gave reactions (chill or fever). It is desirable that even this small incidence of reactions should be avoided if possible. The cleaning of the apparatus after transfusion is a little more difficult than the cleaning of a needle. I am experimenting in altering the cleaning technic and in changing some little details of the apparatus with the hope that the number of reactions will be reduced to a negligible figure.

The apparatus is constructed entirely of stainless steel. Its five parts, body, two valves, and two fittings, are easily taken apart, making for thorough cleaning and sterilization of the individual parts. The valves

From the pediatric service of Mount Sinai Hospital.

are interchangeable and reversible making them foolproof. The fittings are tapered for either needles or rubber tubing. The shape of the apparatus is especially adapted for easy grip with the fingertips. The attachment for the syringe permits the use of a lock type syringe, thus preventing the separation of the syringe and apparatus during the operative procedure. The device has arrows stamped on both sides of the body to indicate the direction of the flow.

Figure 1 shows a cross-section of the apparatus, and Fig. 2 shows the apparatus taken apart.

Figure 3 shows the set-up for the extremely simple method of transfusing citrated blood. The blood is first collected from the donor,

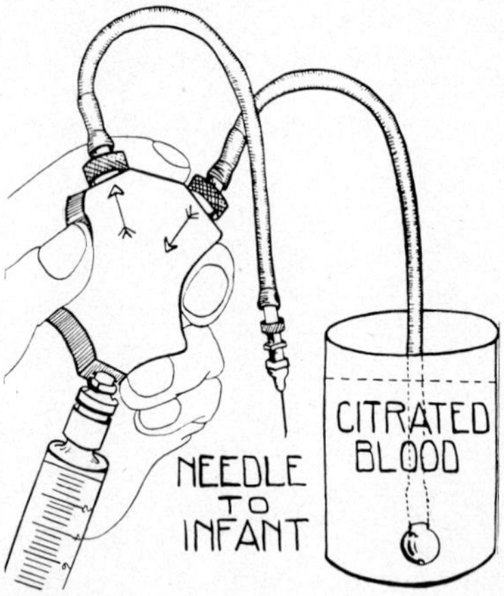

Fig. 3.—Set-up for infant transfusion using citrated blood and a small hypodermic needle with lock type syringe and the automatic two-way adapter.

using 1 c.c. of 2.5 per cent sodium citrate solution for each 10 c.c. of blood to prevent clotting. Then the needle is connected to the recipient as illustrated, and the transference of the blood begins.

In operating the instrument, one merely grips it with the fingers of the left hand in the curves especially made for convenient holding, while the syringe lies in the palm of the left hand. The upstroke of the piston automatically opens the inlet valve and closes the outlet valve filling the syringe with citrated blood from the beaker; conversely the downstroke closes the inlet valve and opens the outlet valve injecting the blood in the syringe into the recipient.

609 Broadway,
Cedarhurst, L. I.

Critical Review

NEUROLOGIC CONDITIONS IN INFANTS AND CHILDREN

R. Cannon Eley, M.D.
Boston, Mass.

THE complications of the central nervous system that may occur during the course of some of the exanthems were reviewed[1] last year and at that time the similarity of both the gross and microscopic pathology was discussed and the various opinions as to the possible etiologic factors were considered. As the same questions are pertinent to the complications of the common contagious diseases which were not included in the previous review, it appears appropriate to consider them at this time.

Smallpox.—Complications of the central nervous system have been observed during the course of variola since the earliest recognition of the disease. Yet the frequency with which these conditions arise has been variously stated: Rolleston[2] found only 25 cases among 10,000 patients; Shamberg and Kolmer[3] observed 8 instances among 3,000; Troup and Hurst[4] report that in 51,243 cases of variola occurring in England and Wales from 1925 to September 30, 1929, there were only 140 deaths, and of this group "central nervous system complications contributory to death" appeared on the death certificates of only 25 patients. The variability in the frequency with which these complications are encountered would suggest that they occur more often during endemic or epidemic appearances of the disease than during those periods when it appears in a sporadic manner.

Clinically, the neurologic complications may vary from a peripheral neuritis (such as the case described by Putnam,[5] in which there was paralysis and subsequently atrophy of the serratus magnus alone) or hemiplegia[6] to severe and often fatal instances of encephalomyelitis.[7, 8] However, either the encephalitic or spinal types of disturbances can usually be recognized according to the predominance of the symptoms. The onset of these manifestations, which usually develop between the fifth and thirteenth day after the appearance of the rash and bear no relationship to the severity of the infection, may be sudden or may be heralded by the gradual development of somnolence, headache, unsteady gait, and alterations in behavior, or by severe pains in the abdomen, extremities, and back. In the encephalitic group the onset is usually preceded by inability to enunciate distinctly and a somnolence which rapidly passes into coma and terminates within a few hours in death. This is well exemplified in the case reported by Marsden[7] of a seventeen-year-old boy who on the seventh day of the rash complained of headache and was unconscious at the end of twenty-four hours. Death occurred forty-eight hours after the initial symptoms. However, should the patient survive the acute phase of

From the Infants' and the Children's Hospitals of Boston and the Department of Pediatrics, Harvard Medical School.

the disease, recovery may be expected although the patient may remain unconscious for days or weeks. In the spinal type of involvement paralysis of the extremities constitutes the chief clinical sign. The paralysis is usually preceded by the development of stupor, severe pains in the extremities, the abdomen, or in the back, nausea, vomiting, and progressive loss of sensation and sphincter control. In the majority of instances the drowsiness or stupor disappears after a few days, but the paralysis may be present for months before recovery is made. Some of the reported instances of transverse myelitis[9, 10] would suggest a form of Landry's paralysis, such as the case of Gross[9]: A woman, fifty years of age, first developed weakness of the lower extremities, followed by involvement of the respiratory muscles, upper extremities and swallowing; death occurred at the end of seventy-two hours. The prognosis in either of the two types, i.e., spinal or encephalitic, is poor but tends to be grave in the latter group.

Unfortunately, the literature contains very little information in regard to the alterations which may occur within the *cerebrospinal fluid.* The observations of Marsden and Hurst,[11] however, would indicate that very early in the course of the disease there is a pleocytosis of either lymphocytes or polymorphonuclear leucocytes but that later the cytology is practically entirely of the lymphocytic series. Usually there is no increase in either the sugar or protein content of the fluid; bacteriologic studies have been uniformly negative.

Although the pathology of encephalomyelitis occurring in the course of certain of the exanthems has been carefully studied and is now generally recognized as possessing characteristic features, yet the etiologic factor remains debated. In fact, there appear to be two very divergent views: One group expresses the opinion that the disturbance is due to the virus of the specific disease, while the other is of the opinion that the complication is secondary to an inflammatory process initiated by the activation of a neurotrophic virus which under normal conditions remains dormant. The same controversial situation arises in the discussion of encephalomyelitis following vaccination. Thus Troup and Hurst,[12] after a careful study of the literature and a case of their own, concluded that the demyelinization, perivascular infiltration, and degeneration occurring in postvaccinal encephalitis were indistinguishable from those changes encountered in disseminated encephalomyelitis following measles or smallpox. McIntosh and Scarff[13] in 1930 concluded that the virulent strains of the virus of smallpox when injected intracerebrally, intravenously, or intradermally into rabbits produced a definite meningoencephalitis and that the lesions produced were comparable to those observed in postvaccinal and postvariola encephalitis in man. Jorge[15] in a recent review of this type of encephalitis and other allied conditions has discussed both views concerning the etiology of postvaccinal encephalitis and has concluded that the experimental evidence is not yet conclusive.

Greenfield[15] has emphasized the marked similarity in the pathologic findings in postvaccinal encephalitis, encephalitis following variola, and encephalomyelitis following measles and considers that the observations support the theory "that both the postvaccinal and other forms of encephalitis which follow eruptive fevers are not directly due to the virus of the preceding fever, but to another virus which is either stimulated to activity, or is directed against the nervous system by the exanthema." Zimmermann and Yannet[16] have described the histopathologic changes of the central nervous system in two fatal cases of encephalitis occurring during the course of chickenpox and noted that the alterations did not possess any specific or characteristic features which might differentiate them from the pathologic changes noted in variola. After a very careful study, Marsden and Hurst state: "If, therefore, we find the same clinical and pathologic conditions following after a roughly similar 'incubation period' such different predisposing causes as smallpox, measles, antirabic treatment, etc., the conclusion seems inevitable that we are dealing with an independent malady activated by the conditions mentioned and not with one resultant upon some change in virulence or other property of the virus of the primary infection.

Turnbull,[15] on the other hand, has studied the pathology occurring in fatal cases of encephalitis following variola and has concluded that the virus or vaccina is the etiologic factor. After an experimental and pathologic study of the various forms of encephalitis seen following the exanthems, McIntosh[17] decided that the pathology of variola was not only specific in its nature but also in its etiology. He did not concur with those who felt that the various forms of encephalitis developing during the course of the eruptive fevers were due to the activation of a dormant virus. However, from the literature alone one receives the impression that the general opinion is in accord with that as expressed by Greenfield[15] and Marsden and Hurst[11] as quoted above. From the clinical point of view it does appear difficult to understand why the mortality rate and the morbidity rate of the neurologic complications of the exanthems should be so different if the etiology and pathology are the same; for example, the mortality rate in encephalitis complicating measles is 10 per cent, whereas in postvaccinal encephalitis the mortality rate is 58 per cent.

Varicella.—The general tendency is to consider chickenpox as a relatively minor disease and one that more often proves itself to be annoying by virtue of its period of quarantine rather than by the seriousness of its complications. This fact is well illustrated by the short statement of Ker,[18] "There is little to be feared in the way of complications." However, such a statement should not be accepted without consideration, as complications of a most serious nature are not unknown.

The *incidence* with which these complications occur is fortunately low. Bullowa and Wishik[19] reported only five cases of encephalitis and three cases of meningitis occurring among 2,534 patients with chickenpox. Such factors as age, sex, seasonal distribution, and severity of the infection do not appear to exert any direct influence upon the development of disturbances of the central nervous system. As one might expect, secondary infections of the cutaneous manifestations with subsequent development of septicemia may occur, but such complications as these cannot be directly attributed to the etiologic agent causing the primary infection.

Classifications of the various types of neurologic disturbances which may occur during the course of chickenpox have been offered by several observers and have usually been based on either (a) the suggested pathologic lesions or (b) upon the predominant clinical signs and symptoms. As the clinical manifestations of any central nervous system disturbance in which the lesion is of a diffuse nature are seldom comparable to those encountered when there is a well-localized pathologic condition, it becomes apparent that a classification based entirely upon symptomatology cannot be too rigid. The recent classification offered by Underwood[20] has been based upon both the expected pathologic lesion and the clinical manifestations dividing the cases into "the four main sections of the nervous system—meninges, brain proper, spinal cord, or peripheral nerves—which may be involved." However, in this review no attempt will be made to consider the detailed classifications as the disturbances will only be referred to in general terms.

Encephalitic manifestations occurring in the course of varicella are not uncommon as numerous case reports may be found in the literature.[21-30] The clinical manifestations are usually observed between the fourth and fourteenth day after the appearance of the eruption and are accompanied by muscular weakness and paralysis. The temperature is rarely above 100° F.; stupor and mental dullness are rare, while irritability and delirium are common. During the period of these manifestations definite changes within the cerebrospinal fluid can usually be demonstrated; they consist of an increase in the globulin content and a lymphocytic pleocytosis, the total cell count varying between 5 and 71 cells per cubic centimeter. In the majority of instances the clinical manifestations of the central nervous system disturbance gradually subside, the patient making a complete recovery in the course of eight to ten days.

Complications such as hemiplegia,[31] paraplegia,[32] and ataxia[33-38] developing during the course of the acute phase of the disease or during the period of convalescence have been reported in the literature. Waldman[39] has reported the case of a patient who on the tenth day of her illness developed acute ascending myelitis, and Heller[40] has recorded the occurrence of a fairly typical case of complete transverse myelitis occurring during the course of chickenpox.

Varicella lesions appearing on the cornea have been noted by Terson[41] and Wyler,[42] but impairment of vision or temporary blindness is extremely rare. In 1925 Ratner[43] reported a patient who on the ninth day of illness complained of impairment of vision which became progressively worse and was soon followed by complete loss of sight. Ophthalmoscopic examination revealed marked optic neuritis. Ten days after the onset these changes entirely disappeared, and the patient made a complete recovery.

In the majority of instances the *prognosis* is good although death or a persistence of the clinical manifestations may occur. In a study of 120 cases of which number information concerning 109 patients was available, Underwood found that 12 died, 80 recovered completely, and that 15 recovered with sequelae of some type. As this author points out, some of the sequelae were of little, if any, significance and should these be disregarded, the total number of patients who made a complete recovery would be increased.

Zimmermann and Yannet[16] have described in detail the pathologic changes involving the central nervous system in one of their patients, and as shown by the following quotation, the pathology does not appear to be characteristic: "Widespread, noncharacteristic, degenerative lesions of the ganglion cells with a perivascular destruction of the myelin sheaths in the white matter of the parietal and occipital lobes. There was an extensive phagocytosis of fat in these regions and collections of fat granules in the leptomeninges. Small focal hemorrhages were scattered in the cerebral cortex."

Scarlet Fever.—Complications of the central nervous system are rare in this disease and when they do occur are usually secondary to otitic infections or to infections of the paranasal sinuses. Gordon and Top[44] have recently reported nineteen cases of generalized streptococcus meningitis occurring among 17,311 consecutive hospital patients with scarlet fever. In thirteen of these patients the infection originated from a primary infection of the middle ear, in four from the paranasal sinuses, and in two from suppurative joint infections with subsequent infection of the blood stream. The clinical course of this complication is usually rapid and, except in rare instances, terminates fatally regardless of what form of therapy is employed. In Gordon and Top's group there was only one recovery; Neal and Jones[45] have reported a case with recovery following the intraspinous administration of anti-streptococcus serum. Rosenberg and Nottley[46] collected from the literature forty proved cases of streptococcus meningitis with recovery and to this group added one of their own. Although numerous and sundry types of treatment have been employed, yet no particular one has appeared to be of greater value than another. In brief, one might say that general supportive measures plus removal of the original focus of infection (when possible) and repeated drainage of the cerebrospinal canal have offered as good, if not better, results than the less conservative and more drastic procedures. Specific or would-be specific measures have been rather disappointing.

Encephalitic complications are less frequently encountered than are the purulent infections and, as this statement would infer, are extremely rare. Mornet and Vezin[47] have recently reported a patient who developed the clinical manifestations of encephalitis during the course of scarlet fever as evidenced by stupor, pharyngeal paralysis, coma, and alterations within the chemical and cytologic reactions of the cerebrospinal fluid. This patient made a complete recovery. The patient of Dagnelie and Dubois[48] who developed ataxia, slow speech, and intention tremor, died, and at the postmortem examination diffuse perivascular infiltration, demyelinization, and edema of the brain were noted. Both Rossi[49] and Dubois[50] have cited cases of ataxia following what clinically appeared to be encephalitis, and Van Bogaert[51] has admirably discussed the nervous manifestations that may be observed during the course of scarlet fever. Rolleston[52] had under his care a boy, three and one-half years old, who on the thirty-third day of severe septic scarlet fever developed aphasia and hemiplegia. The boy subsequently made a complete recovery from the aphasia and some improvement from the hemiplegia. The above author has collected from the literature seventy-five cases of hemiplegia following this disease and has suggested four possible etiological factors: (a) cardiac involvement with embolism; (b) uremia; (c) encephalitis; and (d) cerebral atrophy and sclerosis. A case similar to the one reported by Rolleston has recently been noted by Moschini.[53] If we are to accept the statistics which may be obtained from the literature, it would appear that complications involving the central nervous system are rare in scarlet fever and when they do occur usually manifest themselves in the form of purulent infections.

Diphtheria.—The neurologic complications which may appear during the course of, or following, diphtheria[54-58] are so well established and recognized that a discussion of them at this time would simply be repetition. However, a few of the facts relative to these disturbances may be of interest. It has been the general impression, and statistics would indicate, that a larger number of patients with postdiphtheritic paralysis are encountered today than were encountered before the institution of serum therapy. However, this does not question the efficacy of specific treatment in any way, as the increased incidence can readily be accounted for by: (a) an increase in the total number of cases diagnosed as diphtheria by means of bacteriologic methods (cases which formerly were not recognized); and (b) a larger number of the very severe cases with survival and therefore with a greater opportunity for the development of paralysis.

Although paralysis is more frequently encountered in the severe forms of the disease, its occurrence with mild forms of faucial or even nasal diphtheria is not unknown, and particularly is this true if the disease has been unrecognized and therefore untreated. It would appear that the anatomic location of the infection plays some part in the incidence of the complications as they are more likely to occur in those cases in which there is both faucial and nasal involvement than in those in which the larynx and trachea are involved alone. At this point it might be well to call attention to the fact that paralysis has been observed among those individuals who have had cutaneous infections alone,[59] such as diphtheritic infections of the conjunctiva, umbilicus, penis, or wounds.

The distribution of the paralysis cannot be stated in a categorical manner, for not infrequently the neuritis may entirely subside in one area only to reappear in a remote group of muscles. However, the situation most frequently involved is the soft palate, for here paralysis has been observed as early as the fourth day and often makes its appearance by the end of the second week. Paralysis of the ciliary muscle with resultant loss of the power of accommodation probably occurs second to palatal paralysis as far as frequency is concerned, although there is some question as to whether or not involvement of the lower extremities should not be entitled to this position. Except for cardiac failure, paralysis of the respiratory muscles, either the intercostal muscles or the diaphragm, offers the most serious complication. Fortunately, this type of involvement is not very common as it usually appears only in those instances in which there is generalized paralysis.

Although the diagnosis can usually be established without difficulty, yet not infrequently other diseases may so closely simulate postdiphtheritic paralysis that confusion arises. This is particularly likely to occur when a definite history of infection cannot be obtained or when there has been some vague or indefinite preceding illness. Paralysis occurring as a result of poliomyelitis or in the course of chronic lead poisoning may produce a clinical picture comparable to that of diphtheria. Furthermore, since loss of sphincter control, paresthesia, and analgesia may be present when the lower extremities are involved, one can easily see how tumors of the spinal cord may at times prove confusing. However, the course of the disease with its tendency toward gradual improvement and the inability to demonstrate the presence of other conditions will usually establish the diagnosis.

The prognosis in postdiphtheritic paralysis is usually good, as the general tendency is toward a slow but complete recovery. The respiratory and pharyngeal muscles regain their function at a very early date, although the palatal muscles and the muscles of the extremities may require several weeks or even months before their function returns.

REFERENCES

1. Eley, R. Cannon: J. PEDIAT. 7: 248, 1935.
2. Rolleston, J. D.: Acute Infectious Diseases, ed. 2, London, 1929, William Heinemann, p. 379.
3. Shamberg, J. F., and Kolmer, J. A.: Acute Infectious Diseases, Philadelphia, 1928, Lea and Febiger, p. 241.
4. Troup, A. G., and Hurst, E. W.: Lancet 1: 566, 1930.
5. Putnam, James J.: Boston M. & S. J. 89: 125, 1874.
6. Rice, R. M., and Carey, M. J.: J. A. M. A. 100: 817, 1933.
7. Marsden, J. P.: Lancet 2: 871, 1934.
8. Aldrich, C. J.: Am. J. M. Sc. 67: 198, 1904.
9. Gross, F. W.: Boston M. & S. J. 88: 464, 1873.
10. Brouwer, B.: Rev. neurol. 2: 446, 1931.
11. Marsden, J. P., and Hurst, E. W.: Brain 55: 181, 1932.
12. Troup, A. G., and Hurst, E. W.: Lancet 1: 566, 1930.
13. McIntosh, J., and Scarff, R. W.: J. Path. & Bacteriol. 33: 483, 1930.
14. Jorge, Ricardo: Lancet 2: 215, 1932; Lancet 2: 267, 1932.
15. Turnbull, H. M.: Brit. M. J. 2: 331, 1928.
16. Zimmermann, H. M., and Yannet, Herman: Arch. Neurol. & Psychiat. 26: 322, 1931.
17. McIntosh, J.: Brit. M. J. 2: 334, 1928.
18. Ker: Infectious Diseases, London, 1929, Oxford University Press.
19. Bullowa, J. G. M., and Wishik, S. M.: Am. J. Dis. Child. 49: 923, 1935.
20. Underwood, E. A.: Brit. J. Child. Dis. 32: 241, 1935.
21. Winnicatt, D. W., and Gibbs, N.: Brit. J. Child. Dis. 33: 107, 1926.
22. Marfan, A. B.: Bull. et mém. Soc. méd. d. hôp. de Paris, 1893.
23. Coccia, G.: Rev. de clin. Pediat. 2: 817, 1904.
24. Miller, R., and Davidson, J. A.: Brit. J. Child. Dis. 9: 15, 1914.
25. Conrad, C. E.: Arch. Pediat. 46: 716, 1929.
26. Graham, S.: Arch. Dis. Child. 5: 146, 1930.
27. Fushiki, T.: Orient. J. Dis. Infants 6: 31, 1929.
28. Van Bogaert, L.: Rev. neurol. 1: 150, 1933.
29. Fry, F. M.: Canad. M. J. 32: 926, 1931.
30. Marfan, A. B.: Arch. de méd. d. enf. 1: 153, 1898.
31. Osler, W.: The Cerebral Palsies of Children, 1889.
32. Smith, D. C. W.: Am. J. Dis. Child. 10: 445, 1915.
33. Dagnelie, J., and Dubois, R.: J. de neurol. et de psychiat. 32: 630, 1932.
34. Nyrsen, R., and Vervaeck, P.: J. de neurol. et de psychiat. 30: 589, 1930.
35. Cornil, L., and Kessil, P.: Rev. Neurol. 1: 169, 1930.
36. Wilson, R. E., and Ford, F. R.: Bull. Johns Hopkins Hosp. 40: 337, 1927.
37. Krabbe, E. H.: Brain 48: 535, 1935.
38. Galli, P.: Pediatria 33: 681, 1924 (abst. J. A. M. A. 85: 781, 1925).
39. Waldman, D. P.: J. A. M. A. 85: 1612, 1925.
40. Heller, N. B.: J. M. Soc. New Jersey 26: 700, 1929.
41. Terson, A.: Clin. Ophth., Paris 10: 192, 1904.
42. Wyler, J. S.: J. A. M. A. 58: 1476, 1917.
43. Ratner, B.: M. Clin. North America 9: 809, 1925.
44. Gordon, J. E., and Top, F. H.: J. PEDIAT. 6: 770, 1935.
45. Neal, Josephine, and Jones, A.: Arch. Pediat. 44: 395, 1927.
46. Rosenberg, L., and Nottley, H. W.: Ann. Int. Med. 4: 1154, 1931.
47. Mornet and Vezin: Bull. et mém. Soc. méd. d. hôp. de Paris 57: 378, 1936.
48. Dagnelie, J., and Dubois, R.: J. de neurol. et de psychiat. 32: 630, 1932.
49. Rossi, L.: Pediatria prat. 8: 327, 1931.
50. Dubois, R.: Rev. franç. de pédiat. 10: 320, 1934.
51. Van Bogaert, L.: Rev. Neurol. 1: 150, 1933.
52. Rolleston, J. D.: Proc. Roy. Soc. Med. (Sec. Dis. Child.) 21: 1, 1927.
53. Moschini, S.: Pediatria de med. prat. 10: 408, 1935.
54. Ker: Infectious Diseases, London, 1929, Oxford University Press.
55. Shamberg, J. F., and Kolmer, J. A.: Acute Infectious Diseases, Philadelphia, 1928, Lea & Febiger.
56. Park, W. H., and Dickson, A. J.: Abt's. Pediatrics, Vol. 6, Philadelphia, W. B. Saunders Company.
57. Park, W. H., Dickson, A. J., and Thomson, C. O.: Nelson's Loose Leaf Medicine, Vol. 1, New York, Thomas Nelson and Sons.
58. Holt: Diseases of Infancy and Childhood (Holt and McIntosh) ed. 10, New York, D. Appleton-Century Company.
59. Ronaldson, A. W.: Brit. M. J. 1: 1019, 1935.

American Academy of Pediatrics

Proceedings

SIXTH ANNUAL MEETING OF THE AMERICAN ACADEMY OF PEDIATRICS

KANSAS CITY, MAY 11 AND 12, 1936

Round Table Discussion on Allergy in Children

Chairman: Dr. Francis M. Rackemann, Boston, Mass.
Assistants: Dr. Bret Ratner, New York, N. Y.
Dr. Marion B. Sulzberger, New York, N. Y.

CHAIRMAN RACKEMANN.—Allergy may be defined as the abnormal reaction manifested by certain individuals toward certain substances which are harmless for normal persons. This definition includes the two main forms of allergy: the immediate response, urticarial in nature, which determines the pathology and the symptoms of hay fever, asthma and perhaps eczema; and the tuberculin reaction, inflammatory in character, which is closely concerned with the mechanism of many infectious diseases. There is evidence that these two reactions are related and that each one represents a phase in the development of the normal immunity. The immediate urticarial reaction is so characteristic and of such great importance clinically, and the individuals who manifest it comprise such a characteristic group that Coca has conceived of the term ''atopy'' with ''atopic'' reactions to ''atopens'' for the definition of this group.

How do certain people become allergic or atopic? Coca, Cooke, and others believe that heredity plays an important part. This heredity, however, applies more to the capacity for developing a specific reaction than for the particular reaction which occurs. Allergic individuals show as a group, certain general clinical characteristics, as follows:

1. They present the characteristic picture of hay fever, asthma, or eczema, or possibly others.
2. They have some other symptom along with the first.
3. They present positive skin tests.
4. They have a blood eosinophilia.
5. They have a positive family history of allergy.

Allergic or ''atopic'' individuals have then the capacity to develop sensitiveness. The particular form which this takes depends in most of the cases upon the patient's environment. If there are dogs, cats, feathers, or kapok, he may become sensitive to them. The occupational group in adults is particularly interesting here. In young children, new foods become new points of contact and sensitiveness often appears. Sometimes, however, and particularly in infants, these symptoms arise after the first contact. In these cases Ratner has demonstrated that the specific sensitiveness is transferred through the placenta or the breast milk. It is important, however, to distinguish this maternal transmission of allergens, or of antibodies, as the case may be, from the inheritance of the fundamental allergic state.

Our interest in allergy has so far been concerned chiefly with the diagnosis of the exciting cause. In this, the important method is not the skin test but the history. If true sensitiveness is present, the fact should be demonstrated by showing that symptoms appear on contact and disappear when contact is broken. Histories which include particular dates of changes in environment as well as of new symptoms, and which account for all the time, should contain enough evidence for the diagnosis. Skin tests themselves are interesting, but the discrepancies between skin tests and history are even more interesting. Many patients have skin tests without symptoms while others fail to react even though they are sensitive clinically. In each case, therefore, the skin tests must be correlated with the history so that the picture as a whole will make sense. The technic of skin tests and the choice of method are always important. Sometimes, the scratch test is negative when the intracutaneous test is positive, while in other cases the intracutaneous method shows such irritability of the skin that the results mean nothing. Eye tests, nasal tests, and patch tests are each useful in its special case.

DR. W. C. C. COLE (DETROIT).—Will you say more about the physiologic nature of allergy?

CHAIRMAN RACKEMANN.—How or why sensitiveness develops is unknown. It is a fundamental question. Heredity plays a part. The artificial sensitization which occurs after a dose of horse serum is more easily understood. After ten days or so, antibodies appear in the blood as precipitins and in the skin as a positive skin test. The circulating antibodies are temporary, disappearing within a few days or a week or two, while the skin test persists often for years, and this provides another illustration of positive skin tests which indicate the past history rather than the present illness. However, a latent sensitiveness also exists, and, if another dose of horse serum is given later on, the reaction may be violent. This mechanism is interesting because clinical sensitiveness is often acquired in patients who have the fundamental capacity to develop it. The particular substance to which sensitiveness is directed depends on the patient's contacts. Occupational asthma must arise in this way. One patient has horse asthma; another has orris powder rhinitis according to his or her previous contacts.

DR. RATNER.—Sensitiveness to foods no doubt arises in the same way—by repeated contact.

DR. SULZBERGER.—I agree that the fundamental causes for the varying degrees of susceptibility are still unknown. The quantitative factor in exposure is often evident, but it represents only one factor among the many important and unknown influences which terminate in the production of clinical hypersensitivity. There are many different forms of specific sensitization. Some are acquired regularly and represent a normal response. The regular production of tuberculin sensitivity is an example. In the production of abnormal sensitizations, there are, in addition to hereditary predisposition and the influence of infections, etc., other factors which may reduce resistance or favor sensitization under certain particular conditions, not always understood, but including the time and the duration of exposure of the given individual to the given allergen.

DR. LOUIS DIENES (BOSTON).—No doubt at certain times certain changes occur which predispose to sensitiveness. During infection, such as whooping cough, that part of the system which makes antibodies is much more irritable. Sensitiveness frequently follows infections.

DR. J. C. OVERALL (NASHVILLE, TENN.).—Why is the tuberculin test negative or reduced during and after an illness?

DR. SULZBERGER.—Tuberculin tests apparently become negative under two conditions: (1) during an overwhelming illness, or in a cachectic state—so-called negative anergy; and (2) as a result of progression toward immunity—as seen in the *positive* anergy found in sarcoids, for example. A negative tuberculin reaction is the rule in miliary tuberculosis; but here the skin, as a rule, ceases to exhibit reactions to other substances, such as trichophytin, typhoid vaccine, etc. This is apparently because the macroorganism is overwhelmed by the infection, and the skin has lost all power to react. This is, as I have said, the state of so-called negative or *nonspecific* anergy.

QUESTION.—How long does allergy persist?

DR. RATNER.—As a rule, allergy is not present throughout life. It is evanescent.

CHAIRMAN RACKEMANN.—I do not feel that way. Skin tests persist; symptoms do not. Clinical sensitiveness to particular substances may come and go. Egg sensitiveness is common in infants, rare in adults; and yet skin tests to egg may persist for many years before they fade. The fundamental allergy does, I believe, persist. I think of a boy who had infantile eczema due to eggs; now at the age of eighteen years, he has hay fever. He can eat eggs though his egg test is still there. His capacity to develop sensitiveness to foreign substances in his environment, that is to say, his ''allergy,'' remains with him.

The *diagnosis* of the exciting cause of symptoms is a problem of great practical importance. I would like to emphasize that in my own experience at least the *history* is of far greater value than the skin tests. In taking a history on a patient with hay fever, asthma, or eczema, there are two important points. One is to record dates: the date on which the attack began and the date on which it ended. It is often quite as important to discover the reason for recovery as it is to find the reason for the onset of symptoms. Other events, intercurrent diseases, operations, changes in residence or occupation, must be dovetailed into the history to make a consecutive story, arranged chronologically. The other point is to *account for all the time.* If the patient was free of symptoms for several months or years, the fact is important, and one should ask ''why.''

DR. SULZBERGER.—It is of the very greatest importance to get time and dates into the history. In the investigation of allergic disease, I should rather dispense with all skin tests than have to work without adequate and careful histories. Only the combination of exact and intelligent history-taking, and exact and intelligent skin testing can produce the optimum results in the search for causal excitants.

DR. OVERALL.—The mother's history may be as important as the child's history—especially the history of her pregnancy.

CHAIRMAN RACKEMANN.—*Skin tests* constitute the drama of allergy. There are several methods and a multitude of materials. The wise selection of each will save time and lead to better results. Skin tests should confirm the history, at least they must be correlated with it, to make sense. In a few instances they will suggest new possibilities and these too must be explained and correlated by the history or by clinical experiments with diet and environment. For routine use, the scratch method is satisfactory in children. Occasionally, the intracutaneous method must be employed, and here the technic is most important. When ragweed will cause a reaction in a dilution of one part in a million, the necessity for chemical as well as bacteriologic cleanliness becomes apparent. Separate syringes, scrupulously clean, each reserved for a particular allergen, must be used.*

*Rackemann and Simon: J. Allergy 6: 184, 1935.

The discrepancy between skin tests and history is often marked. On the one hand, we find positive skin tests which have no clinical significance. As indicated above, they often represent past history. I have patients who formerly had hay fever. Now their symptoms have disappeared, but their skin tests persist. On the other hand, we find negative skin tests in patients who are clinically sensitive. This is harder to prove, but there are clinical examples. If these two extremes are facts, is it not obvious that the interpretation of skin tests is always difficult?

DR. SULZBERGER.—The contamination of syringes is a most important factor of error. This is one reason why the use of scratch tests is preferable for all those who do not specialize in allergy. In quantitative tuberculin testing, in which high dilutions are used, the contamination of syringes becomes apparent at once. No syringe once used for a strong concentration may be employed later for a higher dilution. Traces of tuberculin defy removal, even by washing or sterilization of the glass. Such traces can entirely vitiate the results of tuberculin testing in high dilutions.

DR. W. A. McGEE (RICHMOND, VA.).—Do different extracts, glycerol or saline, for example, require different interpretation?

CHAIRMAN RACKEMANN.—No! Extracts, however made, should show reactions only in sensitive patients, never in normal controls.

DR. McGEE.—Do you test with fungi?

CHAIRMAN RACKEMANN.—In our clinic, tests with extracts of fungi are usually negative. The question reminds me of our recent experiences with kapok, cotton linters, and other vegetable fibers. As first brought out by Milton B. Cohen, we find that extracts of kapok which is new give positive tests in only a few patients. When, however, old used kapok, as found in mattresses and pillows, is employed, extracts give positive tests in a high percentage. This old kapok is moldy; it is the molds which cause the fibers to break down into a fine dust; and our present theory is that symptoms come from the action of the mold (which in itself is harmless) on a substrate of vegetable fiber (which in itself is also harmless). Changes in bedding and sometimes in other furniture or toys result not infrequently in a relief of asthmatic symptoms which is brilliant. Direct inspection by a visit to the house of the patient may lead to dramatic results.

DR. SULZBERGER.—Asthma may be due to many as yet unsuspected causes. As only one example, trichophytin fungi, or monilia fungi, harbored in an insignificant skin or nail focus, may be a cause of perennial attacks. In such (of course, rare) cases, I have seen attacks of typical asthma produced by injections of trichophytin or oidiomycin extracts.

DR. G. F. WEINFELD (RAVINIA, ILL.).—If the skin test for foods is negative, is there any value in elimination diets?

CHAIRMAN RACKEMANN.—Yes, clinical sensitiveness may exist even if the skin test be negative.

DR. J. C. MONTGOMERY (DETROIT).—How often is asthma in children due to food in cases in which eczema does not occur?

CHAIRMAN RACKEMANN.—That is an interesting question because food sensitiveness goes so often with eczema and dusts, with asthma. The opposites, however, do occur, though not commonly.

DR. R. D. HOSTETTER (DAYTON, O.).—Will an intradermal test sensitize the patient and lead to asthma?

CHAIRMAN RACKEMANN.—I know of no specific case, but I can remind you that Hooker found a considerable number of patients tested with toxin-antitoxin mixtures in the Schick test showed later a positive skin reaction to horse serum, and similarly Zinsser, Dienes, Simon, and others, working with both animals and man, have demonstrated the development of a positive skin reaction following repeated intracutaneous injections of the specific proteins, usually foreign serum. Symptoms, however, were not produced.

CHAIRMAN RACKEMANN.—Let us turn to *infection as a cause of asthma.* There are four ways in which infections influence allergy.

1. As Dr. Dienes has said, an acute infection alters that part of the system which makes antibodies. Asthma may often begin after whooping cough, measles, or other acute infection.

2. When allergy is established, the effect of an intercurrent infection will depend upon its severity. As Dr. Sulzberger has already noted in discussing the tuberculin reaction, an acute infection of relative severity may abolish the allergy temporarily. The allergic child who gets measles will lose his eczema or his asthma at the time of the intercurrent disease. This relationship is the principal basis for the use of nonspecific therapy.

3. An acute infection of mild severity like a head cold will aggravate the allergy. There are many children and adults who have positive skin tests to cat hair, kapok, or house dust, for example, and yet no symptoms from them until they ''take cold.'' The new infection brings the sensitiveness to the level of clinical symptoms.

4. ''Bacterial allergy'' is a common term, which implies that the individual may be sensitive to bacteria directly and have symptoms from the infection itself. Here again, processes both acute and chronic are concerned. There is a small group of individuals who have asthma only twice a year, in spring and fall, in attacks following acute colds. There is no change in their environment or diet; their skin tests show no reaction to common foods or dust. The new cold is the only evident cause of trouble. Another group of patients has mild chronic infections in teeth or sinuses which evidently cause trouble because the asthma is relieved when the focus is removed. A diagnosis of bacterial allergy seems inevitable in both groups.

DR. MONTGOMERY.—Will a tonsillectomy performed in the pollen season set up a sensitiveness?

CHAIRMAN RACKEMANN.—Yes, conceivably. Like new infections, surgical operations or injuries may change the resistance mechanism, so as to modify both the development of sensitiveness and the course of the process after it is established.

Asthma in Children

DR. RATNER.—Time does not permit a lengthy discussion of the problem of asthma in childhood. There are a few points that concern the pediatrician. It is generally conceded that in childhood asthma is, in many instances, preceded by eczema and the general syndrome of exudative diathesis first described by Czerny. As pediatricians, we must be on the alert, for this condition does come on insidiously. It is a mistake, however, to diagnose asthma on the basis of a single isolated attack of dyspnea accompanied by the objective finding of sibilant and sonorous râles. I would never tell a parent that a child has asthma after such an episode. It is only after repeated occurrences of such syndromes that one should begin to think of asthma. Repeated attacks of so-called colds without temperature or repeated attacks of vasomotor rhinitis may be forerunners of asthma. During the period of observation and before any definite diagnosis is made, much valuable data can be obtained by careful questioning with reference to the relation of the illness to particular foods; to environmental factors, such as a particular room, a visit, contacts with animals, the occupations of parents or other members of the household; and other possibilities that may eventually be pieced together and aid in detecting the actual cause of the allergic attacks if such they are. It might be intimated to the parents that allergy may be the cause of the child's illness.

Much harm is being done to the good name of allergy by a too hasty resort to protein skin tests. Many cases of allergy, diagnosed in an early stage, will give completely negative results at the inception of the disease. It requires repeated attacks to sensitize the skin and make it possible to obtain positive skin reactions. Furthermore, a child should not be subjected to skin tests in the early stages of asthma because in many cases the condition is evanescent and clears up spontaneously. Asthma, therefore, is a condition that should and can be adequately handled and controlled by the pediatrician, and it is only those cases which are complex and intractable that the allergist should be called upon to study thoroughly, which study means hundreds of skin tests, careful analyses of blood and urine, x-ray examinations, and a most careful study of the environment.

I have found that a large percentage of some of the severest cases of asthma give negative reactions to the ''ordinary'' skin tests but definitely positive reactions to extracts made from substances in the immediate environment of the child. I should like to cite an example: A child had been studied by several allergists and gave negative reactions to all the proteins used; I obtained similar results to the routine proteins, but, when we made extracts, he reacted positively to thirty-odd samples of stuffings from mattresses, pieces of furniture, comforters, and so on. These samples all turned out to be identical in nature, old cotton linters. The incriminating articles were either removed, replaced, or specially treated; the child has been free from asthma for a period of several years, with the exception of two attacks which were directly traced to contact with cotton linters in one instance at school and the second in the family's country home.

DR. A. B. C. HOYER (CINCINNATI).—Dr. Ratner, how did you treat the child?

DR. RATNER.—In these cases the child should sleep on a horsehair pillow, and, if possible, on a horsehair mattress. All the articles containing cotton linters that can be eliminated from the environment are discarded. Those articles of furniture which cannot be discarded should be thoroughly cleansed and reupholstered by covering with an impervious dustproof material, all the joinings being carefully sealed. Egyptian cotton is best, especially if a double thickness is used.

DR. OVERALL.—How about covering with rubber?

DR. RATNER.—Rubber is inadvisable because of the sweating and because it is not durable.

As to the infectious element in asthma, all the work done in the direction of bacterial allergy tends to prove beyond doubt that molds, bacteria, and viruses may very well produce asthma because of the proteins resident in them, for even the virus has recently been shown to be of protein nature. Infectious allergy is brought about by overwhelming contacts with particular parasites which sensitize the individual, and, when these organisms again come in contact with the host, allergic symptoms may result. Repeated invasions of streptococci may produce allergic phenomena in rheumatism or may account for acute upper respiratory infections. Repeated invasions of the tubercle bacillus in time may produce allergic tuberculous phenomena.

DR. S. H. ASHMUN (DAYTON, O.).—Is hypothyroidism common in allergy?

DR. RATNER.—For many years we have studied the ossification centers of all our children and have given thyroid to those children who had delayed ossification. The results in several cases of eczema were truly brilliant. Giving thyroid to certain asthmatic children, I believe, materially helped them in their general resistance.

I do not believe, however, that hypothyroidism per se plays a direct rôle in allergy. Obviously, every allergic patient who shows symptoms of hypothyroidism should receive the benefit of thyroid therapy.

DR. C. D. BUTLER (OAK PARK, ILL.).—Nothing has been said of the *psychic effect.* Does it play a part in the cause of asthma or allergy?

DR. RATNER.—The psyche unquestionably plays a certain rôle in asthma. It is not a primary one, however, and is the result of a "conditioned reflex." I have seen cases in children who have learned to simulate asthmatic attacks. These psychic episodes, which grow out of the desire of the child for attention, must be treated intelligently or else they may become fixed. The same circumstances may cause undue irritation and scratching in cases of eczema and contact dermatitis. Many cases could be cited to show how eczema can be prolonged by such psychic conditioning.

CHAIRMAN RACKEMANN.—No doubt the psyche is important. However, in asthma at least, nervousness and other disturbances of the psyche are more likely effects than causes of the asthma.

DR. SULZBERGER.—All disease processes are, to some degree, dependent upon the general state, and thus to some degree upon the psychoneurogenous mechanisms. There can be no denial that, particularly in reactions due to allergic hypersensitivity, the influence of the psyche may be most evident and, in some instances, may even play a leading part in the production or inhibition of reactions.

DR. F. P. GENGENBACH (DENVER).—How do you explain the fact that some individuals are more sensitive to flea or insect bites than are others?

DR. RATNER.—*The basis for sensitivity to insect bites* is exactly the same as the basis for other sensitivities, namely, that children who have been bitten may under certain circumstances become sensitized, and subsequently insignificant bites may produce marked reactions.

DR. SULZBERGER.—Even the normal skin reactions to insect bites represent an acquired type of skin hypersensitivity; in some instances responsible specific antibodies can be demonstrated by the Prausnitz-Küstner technic. Some of the cases of hypersensitivity to insect bites can be cured by specific hyposensitization measures. I have had several successes with such measures. This entire subject has been carefully studied. Those interested may begin reading up the voluminous literature by first studying the monograph and bibliography of O. Hecht.*

DR. BUTLER.—What part do *physical aspects, such as heat and cold,* play in the cause of asthma?

DR. RATNER.—I believe that heat and cold play a secondary, if any, rôle in the causation of asthma. There are some who assert that heat or cold are primary causes in certain cases. It is my impression that heat and cold may aggravate a particular attack but that the actual cause of the asthma is a sensitivity to some definite allergen.

I have been asked to discuss the question of *food hypersensitivity.* Children become sensitized to foods in one of several ways: The first contact is during fetal life; in the latter months of pregnancy, the mother, eating excessively of certain protein foods, may have enough undigested food proteins in her circulation which readily traverse the highly permeable placenta and thus sensitize the fetus. Second, infants may be sensitized during the newborn period by the passage of undigested protein, particularly milk, through the highly permeable intestinal tract. Third, overfeeding in early childhood may also lead to sensitization. It is, there-

*Hautreaktionen auf die Stiche blutsaugender Insekten und Milben als allergische Erscheinungen, Zentralbl. f. Haut- u. Geschlechtskr. **44**: 241, 1933.

fore, of paramount importance to control the diet of the pregnant woman and to introduce foods in early infancy in a partially denatured form and in small amounts, thus establishing a tolerance.

A question has been raised about sensitivity to egg. It is rather interesting that egg white is one of the most common offenders. The reason for this may be due partly to the fact that the molecular weight of egg white is rather small and to a larger extent to the fact that raw egg white escapes digestion and therefore enters the circulation in a native state more frequently than other proteins; this holds true for lactalbumin and possibly other food proteins. Egg white is prevalent in various food preparations so that very often a child may be getting it without the physician's even being aware of it.

DR. OVERALL.—How about using elimination diets as an aid in diagnosis if you do not use them in treatment?

DR. RATNER.—Elimination diets in the diagnosis of food allergy have been popularized by Dr. Rowe and used extensively in the past few years. These diets may be of great value in ferreting out the cause of food allergy in adults, and they are of value occasionally in childhood when the allergy is of a gastrointestinal nature, in which cases negative skin reactions are the rule. Because of the simplicity of the elements that enter into the young child's diet, however, it is of greater value to take very careful histories or to have the mother keep a diary. In the treatment of food allergy, the foods to which the child is sensitive or those that I suspect to be the cause of trouble should be eliminated. In creating a true elimination diet, one must not only remove the particular food itself but be certain to eliminate all forms of food that may contain even traces of the offending protein. At times it is necessary to eliminate such foods as fish, eggs, and nuts from the household because of the possibility of contamination of cooking utensils and other objects used in the preparation of foods.

DR. McGEE.—How about the methods of Dr. B. M. Keston, Dr. Irene Waters, and Dr. J. G. Hopkins, New York, N. Y., for oral desensitization?

DR. RATNER.—These methods have been used by others prior to them. I practically always desensitize my food-sensitive patients orally. Tolerance can be established in about six to nine months; but it is essential for the child to take moderate amounts of the foods to which he has been desensitized quite regularly after the point of tolerance has been reached. In rare instances in which one may not have the cooperation necessary for oral desensitization, I desensitize against foods by injection.

DR. McGEE.—What does one do with a child who is sensitive to rabbit hair?

DR. RATNER.—In such cases eliminate all rabbit hair furs, stuffings of pillows, fuzzy woolens and gloves, felt blankets and hats, and toys covered with rabbit hair. Do not attempt to desensitize toward this fur except in very rare instances in which you may give injections in very minute doses.

CHAIRMAN RACKEMANN.—How young do you start hay fever treatment?

DR. RATNER.—I never start hay fever desensitization in children who are very young. As a rule, pollen tests in children may be done when they give a history of seasonal sneezing, and this can be determined only after the second or third year of life. Such patients may be watched and taken to the seashore for the summer and treated seasonally with tincture of belladonna and an acid-forming diet. If, however, the case becomes pronounced, I then start perennial desensitization. It is necessary to adhere to doses that give practically no reaction. It is important to give very minute injections so as to avoid making the child more sensitive.

DR. McGEE.—Do you use epidermals in desensitizing children?

DR. RATNER.—In the overwhelming majority of cases, I prefer not to, as the wholesale use of injections is not well advised and at times dangerous because severe shock and even death may result. If the epidermal dust in the environment can be reduced or eliminated, it has been my experience that the child gradually becomes tolerant.

The pediatrician has within his power the reduction of the incidence of allergy in childhood by a most careful control of the environment and diet throughout infancy and early childhood. The fundamental principles of infant feeding have been evolved because of allergic reactions that have been variously diagnosed as exudative diathesis, colic, pylorospasm, cyclic vomiting, diarrhea, appendicitis, and anorexia nervosa. The regimens advocated by our most eminent pediatricians with their insistence upon the introduction of new foods in small and gradually increasing amounts, the use of well-cooked foods, boiled milk, evaporated milk, hard boiled eggs, etc., are part and parcel of the armamentarium of the allergist who advocates the use of denatured foods for food-sensitive patients and accomplishes desensitization by the use of gradually increasing amounts. As to the environment, the parent can be taught how to equip the nursery, to avoid such articles as down pillows, stuffed furniture, cotton mattresses, and stuffed toys.

DR. ESTHER B. CLARK (PALO ALTO, CALIF.).—Can any child become asthmatic without a family history of allergy?

DR. RATNER.—Yes, a child can become asthmatic without a family history of allergy. I have just completed a study over a period of many years on the inheritance factor in childhood allergy, and my conclusion is that inheritance per se has not been proved to play a rôle in allergy. We found that approximately 50 per cent of the family histories of allergic children were negative and, conversely, that 50 per cent of the families of *normal* children gave positive allergic histories. I believe that allergy is essentially an acquired condition, the same as infectious diseases. On the one hand, you are dealing with the invasion of an allergen, and on the other hand, with the invasion of a bacterium or virus.

DR. HOSTETTER.—How many tests do you do on household dusts and materials?

DR. RATNER. The patient is requested to bring samples of all of the pillows and other bedding, stuffed furniture, rugs, clothing, toys, in short, all dust-producing articles in his immediate environment. These samples are placed carefully in separate envelopes and labeled. They are analyzed and an extract of each is made for testing. The number may vary anywhere from a dozen upwards. The most common provocators are old cotton linters, old feathers, rabbit hair, wool, and silk.

DR. L. F. HILL (DES MOINES, IOWA).—Please tell of what value are allergen coverings that are commercially advertised.

DR. RATNER.—Their value depends upon the closeness of the weave of the material. Rubberized materials, as I have already explained, are the least valuable, and Egyptian cotton, the most desirable. Thoroughly cleaned and sterilized horsehair is the most desirable form of stuffing for pillows and mattresses of the allergic patient even if he is sensitive to horse dander.

DR. WEINFELD.—You discussed the inadvisability of feeding raw protein early. Have you seen the development of a sensitivity to egg albumen?

DR. RATNER.—It is inadvisable to give raw proteins in early infancy because there is a tendency for such proteins to escape digestion and enter the circulation through the highly permeable intestinal tract in a native state and thus produce hypersensitiveness. The question of sensitivity to egg albumen has been discussed.

The question of milk sensitivity has also been raised. Experimental studies show that evaporated milk is the best form of denatured milk to use. This conclusion is based on the fact that the whey proteins in evaporated milk are partially denatured; practically all milk-sensitive patients are sensitive to the whey proteins, and the casein plays a negligible rôle. Because the whey proteins are not chemically changed but only physically modified, the child in time develops a tolerance to the proteins of raw milk through the use of evaporated milk which, incidentally, can be fed indefinitely.

DR. T. F. REILLY (SPRINGFIELD, MASS.).—How can you say the reaction in cotton linters test is due to old cotton rather than to ordinary house dust?

DR. RATNER.—We are certain that the reaction to old cotton linters is due to age because the patient will give an absolutely negative reaction to fresh cotton linters and a positive reaction to an extract from old cotton linters from a used mattress or other old piece of furniture. Ordinary house dust is of little value for diagnostic purposes; it is important to determine exactly what ingredient in the house dust is responsible for the sensitivity.

DR. F. J. CORPER (CHICAGO).—I have had patients who were sensitive to pollen and who have desensitized themselves only to have the pollen sensitivity returned later. Does not our pollen injection sensitize rather than desensitize the individual?

DR. RATNER.—It is quite true that a pollen case may become desensitized spontaneously, and the condition then recur at a later period. This may result from an exposure to an excessive amount of pollen which induces a new sensitization. I do agree that pollen injections may sensitize rather than desensitize the individual if large enough injections are given to produce a local reaction; it is precisely for this reason that I strongly advocate the use of minimal dosages that are below the threshold of the patient's reactivity. One thus also avoids the danger of systemic reactions.

DR. CORPER.—What are your criteria for determining specific hypersensitivity?

DR. RATNER.—A carefully interpreted positive skin reaction or, in the case which gives negative skin reactions, a carefully interpreted clinical reaction to a specific substance.

DR. G. M. CLINE.—(BLOOMINGTON, ILL.).—Do you not think there is a lot more pollenosis in babies than we think is probable?

DR. RATNER.—I do not believe that there is a great deal of pollenosis in infancy, for as I have already stated it requires several years of contact before pollen allergy is established. For this reason, pollenosis begins to manifest itself as a rule only after the second or third year of life.

DR. H. F. HELMHOLZ (ROCHESTER, MINN.).—What do you think of the value of the eosinophile count as determining the degree of allergy?

DR. RATNER.—In a very careful study on eosinophile counts made on allergic children, we found that there is no direct correlation between the severity of the allergy and the eosinophile count. We found the widest variation in the count, not only in patients having varying degrees of allergy, but we also found a wide variation in the count in the same individual who would have a high count when he was free from allergic symptoms and a low count during the height of an attack. I should say, therefore, that the eosinophile count is of value in the diagnosis of the allergic state but not of its degree.

The Allergic Aspects of Eczema

DR. SULZBERGER.—I shall discuss only infantile eczema, i.e., the common eczematous eruptions in children from one month to two years of age. The first difficulty encountered in all studies and in all discussions of eczema is that this appellation does not constitute a diagnosis, but only a temporary pigeonhole into which, for the present, we place those itching and papulovesicular scaly and erythematous dermatologic odds and ends which await further classification. We shall not progress much further in the study of infantile eczema until investigators realize fully that the conditions thus designated are heterogenous and do not constitute an entity.

It would appear that, even today, the attempt to separate infantile eczemas into at least four categories were fully justified, and, with proper care, should meet with some measure of success. These four categories follow the present four classes of adult eczematous and eczematoid processes:

(1) atopic dermatitis; (2) contact dermatitis (true eczema); (3) seborrheic dermatitis; and (4) unclassifiable forms, which include intertrigos, fungus, and dyshidrotic eczemas, microtic eczemas of other types, etc.

In the first, the atopic group, the site of the hypersensitivity—i.e., what is called the "shock tissue"—is the superficial vascular net of the cutis, just as the vascular reaction is at the basis of urticarial reactions, of vasomotor rhinitis, of hay fever, and in all probability, also of asthma (Matthew Walzer). There is already sufficient clinical, histologic, and immunologic evidence to conclude that in atopic dermatitis the primary phenomenon is subclinical whealing, and that the eczematization and lichenification is usually secondary.

In the second group—the contact type dermatitis, and the one in which allergy has been demonstrated the most clearly—the "shock tissue" is probably predominantly the epidermis itself; and the vascular reactions, although always present to some degree, are considered as accompanying or secondary phenomena (J. Jadassohn, Br. Bloch, Darier, Civatte, W. Jadassohn, and many others).

The third and fourth groups—seborrheic and heterogenous eczematous or eczematized dermatoses—do not merit lengthy discussions here, for in most forms in this group the immunologic alterations are inadequately known, and strict evidence of a leading rôle played by allergy has not yet been submitted.

It must be stated at the outset that, in infantile eczemas, the contact type is surely much less important than in the adult, and I shall not, therefore, discuss this form here. I shall make no further reference to the rare cases of infantile eczema due to true contact allergens, such as simple dyes, chemicals, anesthetics, etc., and shall not discuss the patch test, which is so important in adult eczema; when I refer to "skin tests" in the remainder of this discussion, I mean the scratch or intracutaneous tests, with so-called protein allergens, which produce their wheal and flare reactions.

In addition to the common seborrheic form of dermatitis in infants, the atopic group ranks first in importance. This is the form associated with familial and personal hay fever and asthma, and with atopic dermatitis of childhood and adult life. Dr. Lewis Webb Hill, Dr. A. F. Coca, and I believe and have proposed that this form should be called "atopic dermatitis of infants."

These atopic skin manifestations are based, in all probability, upon true sensitization mechanisms and correspond to hay fever and asthma. Nevertheless, the best management of these cases still consists, first and foremost, in the proper selection of the correct topical remedies and above all, in their correct mode of application and bandaging (just as in all other infantile eczematous, eczematoid eruptions, and in many other dematoses in patients of any age).

From the allergic standpoint, elimination is much more important than skin testing. Skin tests are never capable of bringing absolute proof of the culpability or innocence of a given allergen. Their results simply indicate possibilities which must be verified or excluded by the essential clinical trials of elimination and reexposure. At my hands, the following have eventually proved themselves to be the best and most practical rule-of-thumb elimination measures in infantile atopic dermatitis.

1. Eliminate ali important inhalant allergens, and all the important environmental allergens which may in the infant pass through the epidermis and reach the sensitive superficial blood vessels (transepidermal route). This is done by re-

moving all possible dust-formers (pillows, mattresses, overstuffed furniture, carpets, orris-root-containing face powders, and cosmetics, etc.), and all dust-catchers (draperies, hangings, carpets, etc.). Let the child sleep on a cot in a bare room, on sterilized horsehair pillows and mattress (for double safety, these can be covered by so-called ''allergen-proof'' covers—remember, the baby carriage must here also bear scrutiny).

2. Denature foods as far as possible without harming the state of nutrition. Add vitamins in pure form if necessary. Here the elimination of eggs is important. Milk should be either the dried, evaporated form, or should be boiled for five minutes. Wheat and other cereals must be borne in mind as not infrequent causes. Change the form of source of carbohydrate (for example, from corn sugar to other sugar, or vice versa). See that the child is not overweight. If there is any tendency in this direction, a simple reduction of fat or carbohydrate calories may help the eczema with astonishing rapidity.

Unfortunately, many very important points cannot even be mentioned in this brief discussion. But it must be emphasized once again that correct detective work and elimination are more important than skin tests. The unreliability of skin tests—if one regards them as absolute guides to clinical management—is well illustrated by the fact that from 60 per cent to over 90 per cent of patients with infantile atopic dermatitis give strong wheal and flare reactions to skin tests with egg white and that many of these patients have reagins to egg white. Yet in many of these very same egg skin-test positive infants, the egg white cannot be causing the dermatitis, for in many of them the eczema has appeared without exposure to egg in any form and the dermatitis continues unabated, under protracted elimination of all possible exposure to egg, even under the most absolute and scientific exclusion of egg and egg products, including specially prepared formulas, prepared in special utensils in a laboratory in which no egg has ever been employed.

Furthermore, the administration of egg produces no exacerbation in some of these cases, even though they have the strongest reaction to egg white skin tests and even though they have egg white reagins in high titer. Those interested are referred to the discussion and literature on this subject (Moro, Worringer, and many others), which is mentioned by Hill and me (Arch. Dermat. & Syph. **32**: 451, 1935), and in my recent review, ''Allergy in Dermatology'' (J. Allergy **7**: 385, 1936).

It is unfortunate that the differential diagnoses, particularly of the various forms of infantile eczema, are rendered peculiarly difficult, and often frankly impossible, by the following factors which in the adult forms do not usually present the same difficulties:

1. The tendency to weeping and vesiculation on the part of infantile skins, as compared with adults; so that forms which in the adult can be differentiated because they are usually dry and scaly (seborrheic and atopic dermatitis), when they occur in infants often simulate the vesiculating and oozing contact types.

2. Secondary impetiginization and fungus infection, which are so likely to appear in infants; and thus often obscure beyond recognition and underlying original dermatosis.

3. The fact that in older children and adults the external contact with such substances, as feathers (Peck and Salomon), wool, silk, etc., rarely allow penetration to the sensitive cutaneous blood vessels through the adult type of epidermis. (While it is true that cases are seen in which transepidermal penetration takes place even in adults, these are surely the very greatest exceptions.) In infants such transepidermal penetration is the rule; so that external contact even with ordinary protein allergens may often lead to penetration of these allergens through the intact infantile epidermis to the vascular layers beneath and thus produce infantile atopic dermatitis (which, in my opinion, is both in adults and infants usually a form of submanifest whealing, with the shock tissue in the vessels of the upper cutis).

There are, of course, many mysteries still to be solved here, and our immunologic approach is still highly unsatisfactory in the majority of instances. It may be said, today, that the judicious choice and proper application of the correct dermatologic local measures, sometimes combined with a few superficial x-ray treatments, is by far the most successful method in managing most of these cases. It is here to be stressed that superficial x-ray therapy, properly administered and in proper dosage, is absolutely without danger, even in infants as young as six months.

Among the problems in infantile eczema are:

1. The significance of the egg white skin test reaction and of the egg white reagins.

2. Why do many of these cases improve rapidly in the hospital or in some other new environment—even in the house next door—and then rapidly get worse again at home? Is this due to environmental allergens and, if so, to which particular allergens?

3. Why are marked seasonal fluctuations to be observed in some cases? Is it because of pollens, of wool, or of sunlight?

4. What are the rôles of such physical factors as heat, cold, light, etc.?

5. What are the underlying systemic factors, the nervous influences, the hormonal factors, the metabolic, and other factors?

All these and many more questions will perhaps be answered some day. But I cannot emphasize too strongly that for the present, no real progress can be made until we meticulously analyze and subclassify the infantile eczema group, with its various different and essentially nonrelated components, and that we must all, therefore, now strive for greater clarity in differential diagnosis and for ultimate rational subdivision and clear-cut classification and nomenclature.

DR. McGEE.—What is the treatment when patch tests are positive?

DR. SULZBERGER.—In the case of oils, such as plant oils, desensitization is often effective. In the case of other substances, avoidance is, at present, the only practical measure.

DR. McGEE.—If a man is sensitive to wood or the oil out of wood, do you make a patch test with the sawdust?

DR. SULZBERGER.—Yes.

DR. GENGENBACH.—Certain foods like spinach will cause a contact dermatitis around the mouth.

DR. SULZBERGER.—The cases due to foods and with lesions occurring around the mouth are excellent examples of the transepidermal penetration of the allergen which, as I have said, may take place in infants and children. The reaction is often almost immediate, and of wheal and erythema type, followed by secondary eczematization. I also have a healthy respect for egg white skin test reactions, and know that the ingestion of egg may cause severe and even disastrous reactions in some of these cases. These reactions, however, do not occur in all of them. Nevertheless, some infants showing antibodies to egg, and with huge positive skin test to egg, will not improve with removal of egg, and they will not get worse when egg is administered.

DR. RATNER.—I do not agree with this. Children may not get egg in food, but there are other ways of contact, such as contamination of cooking utensils and dishes with egg white used by other members of the family and the ubiquitous presence of egg in many food substances which escape attention.

DR. McGEE.—How about the leucopenic index?

DR. SULZBERGER.—I have no personal experience with this form of test. It is an extremely old method, included among the first known manifestations of allergy (Widal's crisis), but it has heretofore never been considered a useful or reliable means of testing. I should consider it a difficult procedure and, at best, one which is very hard to evaluate correctly. Under normal conditions, the white count as made by present methods varies widely. It gives no constant and reliable figure.*

DR. McGEE.—Is milk a common cause?

DR. SULZBERGER.—Diet is the answer in only a small number of cases. Only a certain percentage of infantile eczemas is due to sensitization, and again in these only a small percentage is due to foods alone, while a greater proportion can be helped by elimination of both food and environmental allergens. Among the latter, inhalants (silk, wool, feathers, and even pollens, etc.) must be considered.

DR. GENGENBACH.—Where do you place intertrigo?

DR. SULZBERGER.—I place intertrigo among the eczematized and infected processes. It is not a true primary eczema, but here heat, friction, maceration, acid and alkali, fungi, and other microorganisms, plus the proper terrain, are the important factors.

DR. RATNER.—Why do most eczema cases clear up at about one year?

DR. SULZBERGER.—This spontaneous cure between the ages of one and two years is still a mysterious but undoubted fact. Many so-called therapeutic successes are those which have been assayed just at this time of spontaneous remission or during a remission due to change of environment (hospitalization). It is to be remembered, however, that there is often a later recurrence of the dermatitis, as Dr. Lewis Webb Hill and I have pointed out. As a child gets older, it becomes increasingly more difficult to find the cause of his dermatosis. This is due perhaps to the increasing number of factors in the environment and the greater variety of foods. The number of hypersensitivities often increases, and there is usually a shift from foods to inhalant and environmental substances. It is, however, most important in evaluating therapy to realize that in infants and children the majority of clinical food sensitivities disappear spontaneously. There is no real proof of successful active desensitization to foods by any known method in any representative series of cases.

DR. L. M. EARLE (Hollywood, Calif.).—I have had good results by giving large doses of raw linseed oil—three tablespoonfuls three times a day. Improvement began in five days. I did observe that most of the babies had loose stools on the treatment.

DR. CORPER.—I used oleic acid on a number of cases but without success.

DR. SULZBERGER.—As I have stated, we cannot evaluate therapy until we take full cognizance of the erratic natural course of infantile eczema, with its inexplicable spontaneous recoveries and its ready favorable response to simple change of environment, hospitalization, and even to changes of season. For all these reasons, we must continually insist upon an adequate control series of cases. Nor can we carry out reliable therapeutic studies until we learn to classify our cases and to separate the various entities now being promiscuously grouped under the head of ''infantile eczema.'' For example, I could well imagine that the unsaturated oil treatment might be useless in contact or atopic dermatitis, and that it might be excellent in seborrheic dermatitis.

CHAIRMAN RACKEMANN.—Gentlemen, I am sure that this discussion could be continued for several hours longer and with profit to everyone here, but I am sorry to say that our time is up. We thank you for your close and critical attention.

Dr. Benjamin C. Hoyer, Cincinnati, Ohio.
Dr. Norman T. Welford, La Grange, Ill.
Recorders

*See editorial in J. A. M. A. **106**: 1988, 1936

REPORT OF THE COMMITTEE ON HOSPITALS AND DISPENSARIES

Contagious Disease Hospitals

Part III

Committee on Hospitals and Dispensaries: Dr. Clifford G. Grulee, Chairman; Dr. George F. Munns, Secretary; Dr. Murray H. Bass, Dr. Laurence R. DeBuys, Dr. Henry Dietrich, Dr. Lewis Webb Hill.

REGION I

Forty-four hospitals returned answers to the questionnaire (Table I).

1. *Staff: Professional Staff—Attending Staff.*—Among 41 hospitals which reported as to whether ward patients were under the exclusive care of the attending staff, 23 answered "yes" and 18, "no" (Table II). In reply to whether community doctors may treat patients, 39 reported: 19, an unqualified "yes" and 16 an unqualified "no." In two only may private patients be treated in private rooms. In some cases the private doctor must be approved by the staff of the hospital; in others he need only be a physician in good standing. In one hospital (No. 24) any outside physician may treat a patient.

House Staff.—Forty hospitals replied. Ten have one or more full-time residents or superintendents; 22 have no full-time men; 3 failed to reply. Eighteen of the 40 receive some salary. Of these, several are part-time physicians serving as pathologists or roentgenologists. In some cases only the director is paid. Twenty-four have resident physicians; 1 hospital reports having assistant residents but no resident. Sixteen accept women as resident physicians; 21 pay salaries which vary greatly, the smallest stipend being $30 a month. Some pay $1,200 and $1,500 annually. The highest remuneration is $4,000 for a superintendent.

The qualifications for residents vary greatly. Only three hospitals demand that their residents be graduate physicians; 8 require one year's previous hospital experience; 3 require two years; 2 require three years, 5 require special experience in contagious diseases; 1 is filled by civil service examination. The length of residency varies from four months' service to an indefinite tenure of office. Two hospitals report permanent residents; 1 other reports an incumbent who has been on service thirteen years, another, fifteen years. Ten hospitals offer one year's residency. Only 6 hospitals require the resident to attend dispensary service.

Eight hospitals require the services of assistant residents; 5 accept women; 6 have one each; 2 hospitals require three; and 1 (No. 35) requires twenty-seven assistant residents.

The salary varies from $25 a month to $1,200 a year with maintenance. The qualifications vary from graduation from a grade A school to one year interneship. The length of service in all is one year. In 4 hospitals the assistant resident works in the dispensary. Nineteen hospitals have interneships; 5 hospitals have one interne each; 4 have two; 1 has three; 1 has four; 3 have six; 1 has seven; 1 has eight; 1 has nine; 1 has seventeen; 1 has thirty (No. 35); 15 admit women, and 4 do not.

Seven pay no salaries; the remainder pay from $10 to $50 a month. Most of the hospitals only require graduation from medical school as qualification for interneship though 4 ask for previous hospital service, and 1 requires one year's pediatric service (No. 14).

TABLE I

REGION I—HOSPITALS

KEY NO.	NAME
	Canadian Hospitals
1	Riverdale Isolation Hospital, Toronto, Ont.
2	Hospital Civique of Que.
3	Hospital Pasteur, Montreal, Que.
4	Alexandra Hospital, Montreal, Que.
5	Isolation Hospital, Edmonton, Alta.
6	Strathcona Hospital, Ottawa, Ont.
7	Vancouver General Hospital, Vancouver, B. C.
	Eastern Hospitals, United States
8	Garfield Memorial Hospital, Washington, D. C.
9	Doris Memorial Hospital (Wilmington General), Wilmington, Del.
10	Scranton Municipal Hospital, Scranton, Pa.
11	Hartford Municipal Hospital, Department of Communicable Diseases, Hartford, Conn.
12	Portland Isolation Cottage, Portland, Me.
13	Sydenham Hospital, Baltimore, Md.
14	Children's Hospital, Boston, Mass.
15	The Board of Health Hospital, Brookline, Mass.
16	Haverhill Contagious Hospital, Haverhill, Mass.
17	New Bedford Isolation Hospital, New Bedford, Mass.
18	Health Department Hospital, Springfield, Mass.
19	Belmont Hospital, Worcester, Mass.
20	Manchester Isolation Hospital, Manchester, N. H.
21	Essex County Hospital for Contagious Diseases, Belleville, N. J.
22	Hudson County Contagious Diseases Hospital, Laurel Hill, Secaucus, N. J.
23	Trenton Municipal Hospital, Trenton, N. J.
24	Municipal Hospital for Contagious Diseases, Camden, N. J.
25	Passaic Municipal Hospital, Passaic, N. J.
26	Municipal Hospital, Atlantic City, N. J.
27	Bide-A-Wee Hospital, Watertown, N. Y.
28	Jefferson County Hospital for Contagious Diseases, Calcium, N. Y.
29	Schenectady Isolation Hospital, Schenectady, N. Y.
30	Richmond Borough Hospital for Contagious Diseases, Staten Island, N. Y.
31	Queensboro Hospital, Jamaica, N. Y.
32	Syracuse City Hospital, Syracuse, N. Y.
33	Niagara Falls Municipal Hospital, Niagara Falls, N. Y.
34	Willard Parker Hospital, Manhattan, N. Y.
35	Strong Memorial Hospital and Rochester Municipal Hospital, Rochester, N. Y.
36	Binghamton City Hospital, Binghamton, N. Y. (general hospital)
37	Albany Hospital, Albany, N. Y.
38	Lakeview Hospital, Erie, Pa.
39	Municipal Hospital for Contagious Diseases, Pittsburgh, Pa.
40	Philadelphia Hospital for Contagious Diseases, Philadelphia, Pa.
41	Contagious Disease Hospital, Wilkes-Barre, Pa.
42	Municipal Hospital, Johnstown, Pa.
43	Charles V. Chapin Hospital, Providence, R. I.
44	Carpenter Isolation Hospital, Holyoke, Mass. (hospital closed)

The length of interneship is under six months in 6 hospitals, six months in 4 hospitals, one year in 6 hospitals, and indefinite in 2.

Educational Activities.—Thirty-seven hospitals replied to this section of the questionnaire (Table III). Only 9 are connected with medical schools: University of Toronto, McGill University, Johns Hopkins University, and the University of Maryland, Harvard University, Syracuse University Medical School, University of Rochester, Albany Medical College, University of Pittsburgh, Tufts Medical School. Clinics are given for medical students in 15 hospitals and students are on ward rounds in 13.

TABLE II

STAFF

				PEDIATRICS				OTOLARYNGOLOGY				ORTHOPEDICS			
HOSPITAL	WARD PTS. EXCLUSIVE CARE DRS. ON ATTENDING STAFF	COMMUNITY DRS. ALLOWED SEND PTS. AND TREAT THEM	QUALIFIED DRS. ALLOWED TO SEND PTS. AND TREAT THEM	NO. SPECIALISTS ATTENDING STAFF	MONTHS ON DUTY EACH YEAR	VISITS AT REGULAR INTERVALS	ON CALL ONLY	NO. SPECIALISTS ATTENDING STAFF	MONTHS ON DUTY EACH YEAR	VISITS AT REGULAR INTERVALS	ON CALL ONLY	NO. SPECIALISTS ATTENDING STAFF	MONTHS ON DUTY EACH YEAR	VISITS AT REGULAR INTERVALS	ON CALL ONLY
1	Yes	No treatment	Licensed and good standing	Yes			Yes	Yes	12	Yes					
2	Questionnaire not returned														
3	Yes	No		2	Full			2	Full						1
4	Yes	No treatment	Private cases	Yes	Yes	Yes		Yes	Yes	Yes		Yes	Yes	Yes	
5	No	No	Recommendation and appointment	4	3		Yes	6	2		Yes				
6	No	Yes		2	12		1	2	12		Yes				
7	No	Yes		Yes			Yes	Yes			Yes	Yes			Yes
8	Yes and consulting staff	Acceptable to staff	Class A hosps.	2	12	Yes	Yes	8	3	Yes	Yes	4	6	Yes	Yes
9	No	Yes		3	4	Yes		3	4	Yes		1	12		Yes
10	Yes	Yes		Yes			Yes	Yes			Yes	Yes			Yes
11	No	Yes													
12	No	Yes		No				No				No			
13	Yes	(Private rooms)	Good standing	Yes			Yes					1			Yes
14	No	No treatment	Approved by committee	Yes		Yes		Yes		Yes		Yes		Yes	
15	Yes	No treatment						Yes			Yes				
16	Yes	Yes		Yes			Yes	Yes			Yes				
17	No staff	Yes	No qualification												

TABLE II—CONT'D

18	No	Yes		Yes	Rotating	Yes		Yes			Yes	Yes			Yes
19	No	Yes	Good standing	Yes			Yes	Yes			Yes	Yes			Yes
20	No staff														
21	Yes	No		8	3	Yes		14	2	Yes		5	3		Yes
22	Yes	No treatment		Yes			Yes					Yes			Yes
23	Yes	(Private rooms)						Yes	Full		Yes	Yes	Full		Yes
24	Yes	No treatment	All Drs.	Yes 1	Full		Yes	Yes 1	Full		Yes	1	Full		Yes
25	Yes	No		1		Yes		3			Yes	1			Yes
26	Yes	No	None	Yes	Full		Yes	Yes	Full		Yes	Yes	Full		Yes
27	No staff	Yes													
28	No	Yes													
29	Yes	Yes		1	12	Yes	Yes	1	12	Yes	Yes	1	12	Yes	Yes
30	Yes	No		No				2	Full	Yes	Yes	1	Full	Yes	Yes
31	Yes	No						2			Yes	2			Yes
32	No	Yes		1 to 6	Full 2 mo. each	Yes		4	3 mo. each			3	4 mo. each	Yes	
33	No	Yes					Yes				Yes				
34	Yes	No		34	3	Yes		8	5	Yes		2	12		Yes
35	Yes	No													
36	Yes		Approval of attending staff	Yes	Full	Yes		Yes	Full	Yes		Yes	Full	Yes	
37	No staff	Yes													
38	Yes	Yes, restriction on treatment						1	Full		Yes				
39	Yes	Yes, no treatment		4	Full		Yes	7	4		Yes	3	Full		Yes
40	No	Yes	Good standing	Yes			Yes	Yes			Yes	Yes			Yes
41	No	Yes	None	2	6	Yes		2	6		Yes	1	12		Yes
42	Yes	No		16	3	Yes		7	3	Yes		3	4		Yes

Table II—Cont'd

HOSPITAL	OPHTHALMOLOGY				SURGERY				NEUROLOGY				PSYCHIATRY			
	NO. SPECIALISTS	ON DUTY	VISITS REGULAR	ON CALL	NO. SPECIALISTS	ON DUTY	VISITS REGULAR	ON CALL	NO. SPECIALISTS	ON DUTY	VISITS REGULAR	ON CALL	NO. SPECIALISTS	ON DUTY	VISITS REGULAR	ON CALL
1					Yes			Yes					Yes			Yes
2		No reply														
3	2	Full			1	Full						Yes				Yes
4	Yes	Yes	Yes	Yes	Yes	Yes	Yes		Yes	Yes	Yes		No			
5	6	2		Yes	4	3		Yes	2	6		Yes	1	12		Yes
6	1	12		Yes	2	12		Yes								
7	Yes			Yes	Yes			Yes	Yes			Yes	Yes			Yes
8	3	12	Yes	Yes	14	3	Yes	Yes	3	12	Yes	Yes	No			
9	1	12		Yes	3	4		Yes	1	12		Yes	1	12		Yes
10	Yes				Yes			Yes	Yes			Yes	Yes			Yes
11																
12	No				No				No				No			
13					Yes 2			Yes	2			Yes				
14	Yes			Yes	Yes		Yes		Yes		Yes		Yes		Yes	
15					Yes			Yes								
16	Yes			Yes	Yes			Yes	Yes			Yes	Yes			Yes
17																
18	Yes			Yes	Yes			Yes	Yes			Yes	Yes			Yes
19	Yes			Yes	Yes			Yes	Yes			Yes	Yes			Yes

TABLE II—CONT'D

20									Neurol. and psychiat. 3				Psychiat. and neurol. 3			
21	6	4		Yes	15	3	Yes					Yes				Yes
22	Yes			Yes	Yes			Yes								
23	Yes	Full		Yes	Yes	Full		Yes	Yes	Full		Yes	Yes	Full		Yes
24	1	Full		Yes	1	Full		Yes								
25	1			Yes	4			Yes	1				No			
26	Yes	Full		Yes	Yes	Full		Yes	Yes	Full		Yes	Yes	Full		Yes
27																
28																
29	1	12	Yes	Yes	1	12	Yes	Yes	1	12	Yes	Yes	1	12	Yes	Yes
30	By otolaryngologist				1	Full	Yes	Yes								
31	1			Yes	4			Yes	1			Yes				
32	1			Yes	4	6 mo. each	Yes		2	6 mo. each		Yes				Yes
33				Yes				Yes								
34	2	12		Yes	5	8		Yes	3	12		Yes				
35																
36																
37																
38	Yes	Full	Yes		Yes	Full	Yes		Yes	Full	Yes		Yes	Full	Yes	
39																
40																
41	2	Full		Yes	2	Full		Yes	2	Full		Yes				
42	Yes			Yes	Yes			Yes								
43	1	12		Yes	2	6										
44	4	6	Yes		2	12		Yes	10 and 3 psych.	6	Yes		See neurology			

TABLE II—CONT'D

HOSPITAL	PSYCHOLOGY				DERMATOLOGY				DENTISTRY				ORAL SURGERY			
	NO. SPECIALISTS	ON DUTY	VISITS REGULAR	ON CALL	NO. SPECIALISTS	ON DUTY	VISITS REGULAR	ON CALL	NO. SPECIALISTS	ON DUTY	VISITS REGULAR	ON CALL	NO. SPECIALISTS	ON DUTY	VISITS REGULAR	ON CALL
1	Yes			Yes					Yes			Yes				
2	No reply															
3				Yes								Yes				Yes
4	No				Yes	Yes	Yes		No				Yes	Yes	Yes	
5					1	12		Yes	12	1		Yes				
6					1	12		Yes								
7	No				Yes			Yes	Yes			Yes	Yes			Yes
8	No				3	12	Yes	Yes	3	12	Yes	Yes	1	12	Yes	Yes
9	1	12		Yes	1	12	Yes		2	6		Yes	2	6		Yes
10	Yes			Yes	Yes			Yes	Yes			Yes	Yes			Yes
11																
12	No				No				No				No			
13					1			Yes	1			Yes				
14	Yes		Yes		Yes		Yes		Yes		Yes		Yes		Yes	
15									Yes			Yes	Yes			Yes
16									Yes			Yes	Yes			Yes
17																
18	Yes			Yes	Yes			Yes	Yes			Yes	Yes			Yes
19					Yes			Yes								

TABLE II—CONT'D

20																
21	No				7	3	Yes		O.S. & O.H. 10			Yes	Dent. & O. H. 10			Yes
22					Yes			Yes	Yes			Yes				
23	No				Yes	Full		Yes	Yes	Full		Yes	Yes	Full		Yes
24									1	Full		Yes				
25	No				1				1				1			
26	Yes	Full		Yes	Yes	Full		Yes	Yes	Full		Yes	Yes	Full		Yes
27																
28																
29					1	12	Yes	Yes	1	12	Yes	Yes	1	12	Yes	Yes
30																
31					1			Yes	1			Yes				
32					2	6 mo. each		Yes	2			Yes				Yes
33																
34					3	12		Yes	1	11	Yes					
35																
36																
37																
38	Yes	Full	Yes		Yes	Full	Yes		Yes	Full	Yes		Yes	Full	Yes	
39																
40																
41					1	Full		Yes	1	Full		Yes				
42									Yes			Yes				
43					1	12		Yes								
44					4	3	Yes		1 & O.S.	12	Yes		See dentistry			

TABLE II—CONT'D

	ORAL HYGIENE				REONTGENOLOGY				PATHOLOGY				ALLERGY			
HOSPITAL	NO. SPECIALISTS	ON DUTY	VISITS REGULAR	ON CALL	NO. SPECIALISTS	ON DUTY	VISITS REGULAR	ON CALL	NO. SPECIALISTS	ON DUTY	VISITS REGULAR	ON CALL	NO. SPECIALISTS	ON DUTY	VISITS REGULAR	ON CALL
1																
2																
3					1	Full			1							Yes
4	No				Yes	Yes	Yes		Yes	Yes	Yes		No			
5					2	12		Yes	2	12		Yes	2	6		Yes
6	1	12		Yes					1	12		Yes				
7	Yes			Yes	Yes			Yes	Yes			Yes	No			
8	1	12	Yes	Yes	3	Full	Yes	Yes	3	Full	Yes	Yes	No			
9	2	6		Yes	1	12		Yes	1	12	Yes		4	3	Yes	
10	Yes			Yes	Yes			Yes	Yes			Yes	No			
11																
12	No				No				No				No			
13					1			Yes	2			Yes				
14	Yes			Yes	Yes		Yes		Yes		Yes		Yes			Yes
15					Yes			Yes	Yes			Yes				
16					Yes			Yes	Yes			Yes				
17																
18					Yes		Yes		Yes		Yes		Yes			Yes
19					Yes			Yes								
20																
21	Den. & O. S. 10			Yes	1	Part-time salary			Path. & Allergy 1	Part-time salary			Allergy and Path. 1	Part-time salary		

TABLE II—CONT'D

22					Yes			Yes								
23	No				Yes	Full		Yes	Yes	Full		Yes	No			
24									1	Full		Yes				
25	No				No				No				No			
26	Yes	Full		Yes	Yes	Full		Yes	Yes	Full		Yes	Yes	Full		Yes
27																
28																
29									1	12	Yes	Yes				
30					1	Full	Yes	Yes								
31					2			Yes	2			Yes				
32					1	Full	Yes	Yes				Yes				Yes
33								Yes								
34					2	12	Yes									
35																
36																
37																
38	Yes	Full	Yes		Yes	Full	Yes		Yes	Full	Yes					
39																
40																
41					1			Yes								
42					Yes			Yes	Yes			Yes				
43																
44					1	12	Yes		1	12	Yes					

Table III

Staff—Educational Activity

Hospital	Connected with Medical School	Name	Medical Students: Clinics Given	Medical Students: Ward Rounds or Walks	Physicians: Clinics Open	Physicians: Number and Character	Physicians: Ward Rounds or Walks Open	Physicians: Number and Character	Physicians: Definite Courses in Post-Graduate
1	Yes	U. of Toronto	Yes	Yes	Yes		Yes		Yes
2	Not returned								
3	No		No		On demand				No
4	Yes	McGill Medical School	Yes	Ward rounds	Yes	1 a week	Yes	1 a week	No
5	Yes	Alberta Univ.	Yes	Yes			Yes	Weekly rounds	No
6	No		No	No	May attend	10-15			No
7	No		Yes		Yes				No
8	No		Yes	Yes	Yes	Every branch also conference and presenting papers	Yes	Staff	No
9	No								No
10	No		No		Yes	Occasional	Yes	Daily	No
11	No		No		No		No		No
12	No	——	No	No	None		None		No
13	Yes	By agreement Johns Hopkins and U. of Md.	Yes	No			Yes		No
14	Yes	Harvard Medical School	Yes	Yes	Yes	Weekly	Yes	Weekly	No
15	No		No	No					No
16	No				No		Yes		No
17									
18	No		No	No	Yes	T. B. for exam. and diagnostic	Yes	Men on service only. Others are courtesy	No

TABLE III—CONT'D

19	No		Yes	Yes	Yes		Yes		
20									
21	No				No				No
22					No				No
23	No		No	No	No		No		No
24	No		No		No		Yes		No
25	No				No				No
26	No		No	No	No		Yes	Not regular	No
27	No		No						No
28									
29	No						Yes		
30	No		No	No	No		No		No
31	No				Yes	1 a yr. Auspices County Med. Soc.	No		
32	Yes	Syracuse U. Med. School	Yes	Yes	No		Yes		No
33	No		No	No	No		No		No
34	No		Yes	Yes	No		No		No
35	Yes	U. of Rochester Medical School	Yes	Yes	Yes	Practitioner 1 a month	Yes	Not regular	Yes
36									
37									
38	Yes	Albany Medical College	Yes	Yes	Yes	Daily	Yes	Daily	No
39	No				No		No		No
40	Yes	U. of Pittsburgh, Pa.	Yes	Yes				As desired by individual practicing Dr.	No
41	No		Yes	Yes	No		No		No
42	No		No	No	No		Yes	Anyone interested welcome	No
43	No				No		Yes	Daily	No
44	Yes	Tufts Medical School	Yes	Yes	Not regularly	Allowed to visit clinics	Not regularly	Allowed to visit	No

TABLE III—CONT'D

HOSPITAL	LIMITED TO	P. G. ENROLLMENT LAST YEAR	P. G. ENROLLMENT THIS YEAR	LENGTH OF COURSE	HOURS	INTERNES			
						CLINICAL CONFERENCES HELD	HOW OFTEN	PATHOLOGICAL COFERENCES HELD	HOW OFTEN
1								No	
2									
3						Yes	Monthly	Yes	Monthly
4						Yes	Weekly	Yes	Occasionally
5						Yes	Monthly	Yes	Monthly
6						Yes	Weekly	No	
7									
8						Yes	Monthly	Yes	Weekly
9									
10									
11						No		No	
12						No		No	
13						Yes	On interesting cases	Yes	On interesting cases
14						Yes	Daily	Yes	Weekly
15									
16									
17									
18									
19									
20									

TABLE III—CONT'D

21						Yes	3 times a week	Yes	Occasionally
22						None			
23						Yes	Monthly	No	
24						No			
25						No			
26						At A. C. Hosp. only		At A. C. Hosp. only	
27									
28									
29									
30						No		No	
31						Yes	Monthly	No	
32						No			
33									
34						Yes	Monthly	Yes	Monthly
35	50	50		1 wk.	9-5	Yes	Weekly	Yes	Weekly
36									
37									
38						Yes	Weekly	Yes	Weekly
39						No		No	
40						Yes	Daily	No	
41						No		No	
42						No		No	
43									
44						Yes	Monthly	Yes	Monthly

TABLE IV

STAFF (SPECIAL INFORMATION)

HOSPITAL	MEDICAL LIBRARY	NUMBER OF VOLUMES	FACILITIES AVAILABLE TO STAFF	DESCRIBE	RESEARCH IN COM. DISEASES ENCOURAGED	HOW LONG ALL CASES KEPT IN OBSERVATION	HOW LONG MAY THEY BE KEPT	PROCEDURES BEFORE ADMISSION TO WARDS
1	No				Yes	Diagnosed	Indefinite	
2								
3	At St. Luke Hosp.		Yes		Yes	15-20 days	Full time	Thorough exam. by resident
4	Yes	350	Yes	At McGill Med. Library	Yes	3 wk.	3 wk.	Examination
5	Yes		No		No	Varies	Definite diagnosis is made	
6	Yes	50	No		Yes	2 wk.		Throat, vaginal, careful physical
7	Yes		Yes		Yes	3 wk.	As long as desired	Examination by interne
8	Yes		Yes		Yes		As required	Isolation, etc.
9	Yes	125			Yes	24 hr.	21 days	
10	No		No		No	2 days	Indefinite	Consultation and clinical lab.
11	Yes	75	Yes	Experimental work for treatment comm. dis.	Yes	No observation ward		
12	No		No			None		None
13	Yes	200	No		No	None (plan for near future)	In isolation full time	Examination
14	Yes		Yes		Yes	None		
15	No		No		Yes	None		
16	No		Yes	Municipal Hosp. Lab., X-ray, etc.	No	Until positive diagnosis	As necessary	Positive diagnosis

TABLE IV—CONT'D

HOSPITAL	MEDICAL LIBRARY	NUMBER OF VOLUMES	FACILITIES AVAILABLE TO STAFF	DESCRIBE	RESEARCH IN COM. DISEASES ENCOURAGED	HOW LONG ALL CASES KEPT IN OBSERVATION	HOW LONG MAY THEY BE KEPT	PROCEDURES BEFORE ADMISSION TO WARDS
17								
18	No				No	1 wk.	As necessary	As follows
19	Yes	100	Yes	More when new bldg. is completed	No	None		
20								
21	Yes	150	Yes		Yes	None		
22	No		Yes		Yes	24-48 hr.	48 hr.	As follows
23	Yes	30	Yes	Clin. lab.	Yes	As needed	As needed	
24	Yes	40	No		Yes			In rooms after history and examination
25	No							
26	In A. C. Hosp.		No		No	None		
27	No					None		Exam. by attending physician
28								
29	Available nearby				Yes			
30	No		No		No	None		Diagnosis confirmed by board of health
31	No		No		Yes	Until diagnosed	Termination of case	Seen by health office
32	No		Clinical and statistical		Yes			Not positively diagnosed go in individual rooms

TABLE IV—CONT'D

HOSPITAL	MEDICAL LIBRARY	NUMBER OF VOLUMES	FACILITIES AVAILABLE TO STAFF	DESCRIBE	RESEARCH IN COM. DISEASES ENCOURAGED	HOW LONG ALL CASES KEPT IN OBSERVATION	HOW LONG MAY THEY BE KEPT	PROCEDURES BEFORE ADMISSION TO WARDS
33	No		No staff		No	24 hr. to 7-10 days	Indefinitely	
34	Yes	187	Yes	If not large expenditures collaborate with Health Dept.	Yes	At least 3 wk.	As necessary	Examination
35	Yes	35,000	Yes		Yes	No observation wards	Individual precaution at least 3 days	Exam. history
36								
37								
38	Yes		Yes	In all depts. of Med. School	Yes	Until diagnosed	Diagnosed or duration of disease	
39	No					24 hr.		
40	No		Yes	Limited lab. services	No	No observation		
41	Yes	85	Yes		Yes	Indefinitely	Indefinitely	Report from Dept. of Public Health
42	No		No		No	All private rooms		
43	No		No		No	Not at all		Admitted directly to wards
44	Yes	1,000	Yes	Clinical cases and records of 25 yr.	Yes	Indefinitely	Indefinitely	Physical exam. culture

(*Table IV continued on p. 836.*)

Special Information.—Thirty-three hospitals answered this section of the questionnaire (Table IV). In regard to the admission of patients, 13 answered that they have observation wards. Of the remainder several answered that they use the observation ward merely until the case is diagnosed; 5 keep the patient under observation for three weeks; 1, one week; 1, two weeks. Several merely answered "until diagnosed"; 5 kept patients under observation three weeks; 1, one week; 1, two weeks; 5, only twenty-four to forty-eight hours. Most hospitals keep the patient under observation until the diagnosis is positive.

Procedure before admission to wards varied greatly. Eighteen answered this question. In 4 cases the resident admits the patient; in 4 the diagnosis must be confirmed by the board of health; 31 require a throat culture for diphtheria on admission; 3 take this only if there is a suspicion of the disease; 19 take routine throat cultures for hemolytic streptococcus. Four replied that cultures are taken "if indicated." As to vaginal smears for gonorrhea, in 2 hospitals they are made routinely; in 1, only in girls under fifteen years; in 1, in girls under twelve years. Five reply "no," and the remainder, "culture only if indicated" or "on request."

Routine tuberculin tests are done in 9 hospitals; Wassermann tests, in 12; Schick tests, in 16; Dick tests, in 12. Routine blood counts are done in 18 institutions. History is taken in all and complete physical examination in all but 1.

Superintendent.—Twenty-eight hospitals are situated in better class districts; only 1 is in a tenement section. Five are in business districts; 7 are in noisy areas, near elevated railroads or noisy factories. Thirty hospitals are located on smooth paved streets; 1 is on a gravel road. The variation in the importance and size of these institutions is shown by the number of their buildings. Thirty-seven answered this section of the questionnaire; of these, 14 reported one building each; 13 reported two to five buildings; 8 reported five to fifteen; 1 reported nineteen, and 1 twenty-seven buildings (Table V). Some of the structures are very old, one dating back to 1876, but the great majority were constructed during the last twenty years. Fourteen have only one or two floors, but many are large with pavillions of six stories. Twenty-five hospitals report that their buildings are fireproof; 8 that they are not; 25 replied as to firestairs in the walls; of these 11 have them, and 14 have not. Twenty have outside fire escapes.

The cost of the buildings varies with the size of the institution, running from $3,250 to $5,000,000.

As to total bed capacity, 37 replied. The smallest institution has 12 beds, the largest, 907; 8 hospitals have over 250 beds; 14 have 50 beds or less. Thirty have cribs for children under two years, varying in number from 3 to 600.

Thirty-three hospitals answered that they have wards varying in number from 1 to 59. Of those replying, 25 had cubicles, and 8 did not; 5 hospitals report all their cases in cubicles, 1 having 310 bed capacity and another 155.

Thirty-five hospitals replied to the question of exclusion of certain contagious diseases; 20 accept any contagious disease; 5 exclude smallpox; 2 exclude erysipelas; 5 exclude gonorrhea and syphilis; 1 excludes pertussis; 2 exclude typhoid; 2 exclude diphtheria. Some exclude measles and chickenpox, unless complicated.

Contagious Disease Wards.—Thirty-two replied, all of which hospitals have wards but 1 (Table VI). The total number of beds is 2,511. The number of beds per ward varies from 1 to 50. Six have cubicles, 1 of which has as many as 297; 27 have separate rooms, about 225 beds in all. Thirty wards have sunlight; 22 have outdoor porches. In 21 hospitals adults and children are put in the same ward.

Admissions.—The number of cases of children's diseases handled by these hospitals varies, of course, according to size (Table VII). One hospital admitted 66, 60, and 69 cases in 1932, 1933, and 1934, respectively. The largest institution

TABLE IV—CONT'D

HOSPITAL	THROAT CULTURE: B. DIPH.	THROAT CULTURE: HEMOLYTIC STREPTOCOCCUS	VAGINAL SMEARS FOR GONOCOCCI	VON PIRQUET OR MANTOUX	WASSERMANN OR KAHN	SCHICK TEST	DICK TEST	ROUTINE BLOOD COUNTS	URINALYSIS	HISTORY TAKEN	COMPLETE PHYSICAL EXAMINATION MADE
1	Yes	Yes	Yes	Not always	When indicated	Yes	Yes	Yes	Yes	Yes	Yes
2											
3	If judged useful	If useful	If useful	If useful	If useful	If useful	If useful	Mostly	Admission and 1 or 2 a week	Yes	Yes
4	2 on admission	No	Occasionally	Occasionally	No	Yes	No	Yes	Every other day	Yes	Yes
5	Yes	Yes	Yes	Mantoux in T. B. suspect cases	Yes	Yes	No	Yes	Yes	Yes	Yes
6	Yes	No	Yes	When indicated	Not routine	If doubtful	If doubtful	If indicated	Biweekly	Yes	Yes
7	Yes		Yes				Yes	Yes	Yes	Yes	Yes
8	Yes	Yes	Yes		Yes	Routine	Routine	Routine	Routine	Routine	Routine
9	Yes	Yes	Yes	Yes	Yes	Yes	Yes	Yes	Yes	Yes	Yes
10	Yes	Yes	Yes	Yes	Yes	Yes	Yes	No	Yes	Yes	Yes
11	Yes	Yes	Yes	When indicated	When indicated	No	No	Yes	Routine	Yes	Yes
12	Yes	Not routine	No	No	No	No	No	No	No	Yes	No
13	Yes	Not routine	On girls under 12 yr.	Not routine	Not routine	Not routine	Not routine	Yes	Yes	Yes	Yes
14	Yes	Yes	No	Yes	Yes	Yes	Yes	Yes	Yes	Yes	Yes
15											
16	Yes		Yes	Yes	Yes	Yes	Yes	Yes	Yes	Yes	Yes

TABLE IV—CONT'D

17											
18	Yes	Yes	If suspicious		Yes			Yes	Yes	Yes	Yes
19											
20											
21	Yes	No	Yes	Not routine	Not routine	Not routine	Not routine	Yes	Yes	Yes	Yes
22	Yes	Yes	Yes	Yes	Yes	Yes	Yes	Yes	Yes	Yes	Yes
23	Yes	Yes	If requested	No	No	No	No	If advisable	Yes	Yes	Yes
24	Yes	Occasionally	If indicated	No	No	No	No	No	Yes	Yes	Yes
25	Yes	Yes	Yes	Yes		No	No	No			
26	If indicated	No	Yes	No	No	No	No	No	If necessary	Yes	Yes
27	No	If requested	No	No	No	No	No	No	No	Yes	Yes
28	Only on request of attending physician. Then at lab. of General Hosp.										
29	Yes	Yes	Yes		When suspicious	Yes	If in diagnosis		Yes	Yes	Yes
30	Yes	Yes	Yes	Yes	Yes	Yes	Yes	Not always	Yes	Yes	Yes
31			Yes	When necessary	When necessary	Yes	Yes	No	Yes	Yes	Yes
32	Yes	Yes	Yes	Not regularly	Not regularly	Yes	Yes	Yes	Yes	Yes	Yes
33	Yes	Yes							Yes	Yes	Yes
34	Yes	On order	Yes	On order	On order	Yes	Yes	Yes	Yes	Yes	Yes
35	Yes	Yes	Yes	Yes	Yes	Yes	Yes	Yes	Yes	Yes	Yes
36											
37											
38	Yes		When indicated	Yes	Yes	Yes		Yes	Yes	Yes	Yes
39	Yes	No	No	No	No	No	No	No	Yes	Yes	Yes
40											
41	Yes	Yes	Yes			Yes		Yes	Yes	Yes	Yes
42	Yes	Yes	Yes	When indicated	Yes	When indicated	When indicated	Yes	Yes	Yes	Yes
43	Yes	Yes	No	No	If indicated	No	No	No	Yes	Yes	Yes
44	Yes	Yes	Females under 15 yr.	When indicated	When indicated	When indicated	When indicated	When indicated	Yes	Yes	Yes

TABLE V

SUPERINTENDENT (GENERAL)

HOSPITAL	NUMBER BUILDINGS IN PLANT	DATE OF CONSTRUCTION	DATE OF ADDITIONS	NUMBER OF FLOORS	FIREPROOF	FIRE STAIRS IN WALLS	OUTSIDE FIRE ESCAPE	COST OF BUILDINGS (NOT LAND)
1	6	1891-3-2, 1910, '22, '27		3	1 yes 4 no	Yes	Yes	
2								
3	2	1933		Main—6, Nrs. hm.—4	Yes		Yes	$1,500,000
4	3	1906, '19, '14		3	Yes	No	Yes	$460,000
5	1	1923		3	Yes		Yes	
6	2	1903, '21	To hosp. 1910, '20	4, 3	No	Yes	Yes	$250,000
7	1	1925, '26		4	Yes	Yes		$250,000
8	14	1884, '87, '92, '93, '98 (3), 1902, '09, '12, '15, '25, '33		5—2 fl., 2—4 fl, 6—3 fl., 1—5 fl.	Built since 1909	Recent	Yes	
9	1	1931		3	Yes		2	$180,874.20
10	6	1915		1	No			?
11	5	4 bldg. 1914	1 fl. 1920	3—1 fl., 2—2 fl.	No	No	No	$99,906.83 $44,906.13 (addit.)
12	1	1919		2	No	No		
13	1	1923		3	Yes	Yes	No	
14	1	1931		4	Yes	Yes		$340,000
15	5			1—3 fl., 4—1 fl.	Yes			?
16	1	1914		3	Semi	No	Yes	$41,210
17								
18	4 2 in use	Main bldg. 1929		2	Yes	Yes		$100,000
19	12 1 T.B.	4—1896, 2—1907, 2—1913, 1—1921, 2—1925	1907		Yes			Approximately $1,500,000

TABLE V—CONT'D

20	4			2	Yes			
21	13	7—1908, 2—1922, 1—1929, 3—1932	Power plant and laundry, 1932	1—6 fl., 1—3 fl., 1—5 fl., 6—2 fl., 4—1 fl.	Yes	Yes	3 bldg. old	New unit $3,250,000
22	3	1931		1—4 fl., 2—2 fl.	Yes	No	No	
23								
24	3	1912, 1918, 1916		1—3 fl., 1—2 fl., 1—? fl.	No		Yes	$58,000
25								
26	1	1907		1	Partly	No	No	$132,000
27	1	1885		2	No	No	No	$3,250
28	1 and garage			2 and attic		No	No	$10,000 with land
29	1	1906	1926	2	Yes			
30	1	1929		1	Yes	No	No	
31	2	1916, '26		3	Yes		Yes	
32	1	1928		2	Yes			$270,000
33	3	2—1889, 1—1919		2	No	No	Yes	$60,000
34	19	Attached			Yes	1 bldg.	Yes	Attached
35	7	1925, 1933		2—6 fl., 1—3 fl., 3—2 fl. Power plant	Yes	Yes	Yes	$5,000,000
36								
37								
38					Yes	Yes	Yes	$1,523,050
39	2	1901, '27		2 and 3	Yes	No	Yes	$115,000
40	9	1902	Nurses' homes 1924	1—3 fl.	No	No	Yes	?
41	27	25—1909, 2—1922		12—1 fl., 10—2 fl., 5—3 fl.	Yes		Yes	$3,000,000
42	1	1918		1	Yes	No	No	
43	2	Rebuilt 1935		1	Yes	No	Yes	$100,080
44	10	6—1910, 1—1912, 3—1930	1932	3—3 fl., 2—1 fl., 1—4 fl., 4—2 fl.	Yes		Yes	

TABLE V—CONT'D

SUPERINTENDENT (B. BED CAPACITY)

HOSPITAL	TOTAL NUMBER BEDS	CRIBS (UNDER 2 YR.)	BEDS 2-14YR.	TOTAL NO. IN WARDS	HOW MANY IN CUBICLES	SPECIFY IF NOT ALL	BEDS IN EACH CUBICLE	ANY TYPES CONTAGIOUS CASES EXCLUDED	SPECIFY
1	400	None	Cots to 6 yr. then hosp. beds	54			1	No	
2									
3	310		310	8	All	Exc. 30 rms. of 2-4 beds. Iso. and pri. rooms	1	Yes	Smallpox
4	155	35	120	16-18 pts.	All ex. 1			Yes	Smallpox
5	100	20	80	30	2	Originally sep. for diph.	2	No	Accept measles, chickenpox, mumps, etc., wh. complications or transferred
6	145	90	55	4	2	Observ.	1 or 2		Ven. dis. only
7	117 36 for T.B.					Grd. fl. 9 each; 2 and 3 fl. 20 each	1		Ven. dis. only
8	311	42	50	3	1		1	Yes	Diph. and smallpox
9	30		14	4	4		4	Yes	Smallpox
10	50	10		None					Pertussis
11	65	25	40	3	None	1 to be		Yes	Impetigo, scabies, gonorr., and syph.
12	20	1-6	14-20	3	None			No	
13	74	Interchangeable		13	None			Yes	Typh., pneumo., ven. dis., tbc.
14	38	Interchangeable		2	All		1 and 2	No	
15	45	Interchangeable		3	None			Yes	Diphtheria
16	40	10	30	4	None			Depending on Bd. Hlth.	
17	6-12			1					
18	100	50	50	4	4		1	No	
19	150	Interchangeable							Ven. dis.

TABLE V—CONT'D

20		18	50	4	None			Yes	Diphtheria, sc. fever without reservation
21	550	To 7 yr. 120, 158 in new unit	7-14 yr. 66	22 wds. on ea. floor	Wds. in old bldg.	New unit in rooms	1 and 2	No	
22	176	100	76	14	None			No	
23								No	
24	110	35	75	2	All		4	Yes	Syphilis and typhoid fever
25									
26	60	4	56	2	None	Small rms. with 2 beds		No	
27	14	6	2 jr. 6 adult	2	None			No	
28	18	6	12	2	None			No	
29	35	8	27	3	1	Infants	1	No	
30	16	10	6		All rms.		1 in 12 2 in 2	Yes	Erysipelas
31			50	4	3	1 wd. in single iso. rooms	1	Yes	Smallpox (always), chickenpox and meas. (at times)
32	84	42	42	4				No	
33	38	6	32	4	2	Mixed inf. bldg.	1	No	
34	424			23	17½	12 in Pav. IV; 52 in II	1	Yes	Gonococcus inf., syphilis, erysipelas
35	519			21	18	Pri. floors	4	No	
36									
37									
38	550		To 12 yr. 36	59	2		Av. 4	No	
39	80	8	72	8	None			Yes	Confined to sc. fever and diph.
40	150	25	125	4	None			Yes	Certain types due to lack of isolation facilities
41	907	600	307	22	16	Ex. 6 cottages w. 10 pts. each	2-8	No	
42	12	3	9		12		1	No	
43	50	10	40	4	None			No	
44	265	65	100	9	2	2 wds., single rms.		No	

TABLE VI

SUPERINTENDENT (C. WARD CAPACITY DETAILS)

	OBSERVATION					CONTAGIOUS DISEASE WARDS							
HOSPITAL	SITUATED	NUMBER SEPARATE ROOMS	NUMBER BEDS IN EACH	DIVIDED IN CUBICLES	NO. BEDS IN EACH	NO. WARDS	BEDS IN EACH WARD	TOTAL NO. BEDS	NUMBER CUBICLES	NUMBER SEPARATE ROOMS	SUNLIGHT	OUTDOOR PORCHES	ADULTS AND CHILDREN IN SAME WARD
1	Easy access of adm. room				1	Foregoing information relates to contagious disease					Yes	Yes	No
2													
3	Ends of ea. fl.	60	16 sgl. 32 dbl. 12 4bd.	Yes	1						Yes	No	No
4		12	2	Yes	1 and 2	7	16	127	10		Yes	No	Yes
5	Grd. fl. ambulance entr.	8	1			5	8	40	4	8	Wards have sun gallery	No	No
6	No. and east wings	22	1 cot 1 bed	2	1 and 2	6	14	145	12	22	Yes	Yes	Females and children
7												No	Yes, sep. cub.
8	Cont. Pavl.	4	2 in 2 2 in 1			4	6	24		26	Plenty	Yes	No
9						4	4	30	4	Convertible	Yes	No	No
10		5	1	No		2	20	50			Yes	Yes	Yes
11						3	21, 22, 22	65	None	10	Yes	Yes	Yes
12		2	1-3	No		2	8	20	None	2	Yes	Yes	Yes
13						13	2-6	70	None	36	Yes	Visiting only	Adults and child. not same
14						2	12 rms. 2 bds. ea.	38		14	Yes	Yes	No
15						3		45	None	14	Yes	Yes	Yes
16	Sep. rms.	7	1	No		4	8	32	None	7	Yes	Yes	Yes
17													Yes
18						2	16	32	16	12	Yes	No	Yes
19													

TABLE VI—CONT'D

20													
21													No
22	1st and 2nd floors		3	None		10	14 & cribs	164	None	8	Yes	No	Yes
23		5	1 and 2	None		4			None	8	Yes	Yes	Rarely
24										14	Porches	Yes	No
25													
26		10	2	None		2	8	16	None	10	Yes	No	No
27						2	4	14		3 rms. may be used for 2 bd. wds. or pri.	Yes	Yes	No
28						2	5	10	None	3 semipri.	Yes	Yes	Yes
29						3	4 in 2 8 in 1		1 wd. with 8 cu.	19	Yes	Yes	No
30	All cub.	14	1 in 12 2 in 2	Yes		All cub.					Yes	No	No wds.
31	1st fl.	10	2			3	12	36	12			Yes	Yes
32						4	21	84		4 pri. on ea. wd.	Yes	Roof & yd. on occa.	Yes
33	2nd fl.	6	1	No		4	2-4 & 5	32	9	6	Yes	2	No
34	Pav. III, 1st Pav. IV	72	1	No		23	16, 10, 20	352	297	None	Yes	Yes	Yes, if no sep. room available for type of dis.
35						2	30 & 17	47	6	23	Occasionally	No	No
36													
37													
38		20	1	No		4		30	No	7	Yes	No	Yes
39	1st fl.	1	6	No		8	8	64		9	Yes	Yes	No
40						4	Av. 35	150	None	6	Yes	No	Yes
41	1 east end 2 west end	35	6 in 27 8 in 4 9 in 4			13	44 in 1 45 in 4 50 in 8	624	17	3	Sun parlors		Yes
42						None							
43						4	7-9		None	7	Yes	Yes	Sometimes
44						6	18-35	150		18	Yes	2 wards	Yes at times

TABLE VII

SUPERINTENDENT (D. ATTENDANCE)

HOSPITAL	PATIENTS ADMITTED			PATIENTS DISCHARGED			DIED IN HOSPITAL			NO. OF PATIENTS OPENING OF LAST YEAR	NO. OF PATIENTS CLOSE OF LAST YEAR	COLORED AND WHITE ACCEPTED	IF SO, SEGREGATED	LIMIT TO NO. COLORED CHILDREN AT ONE TIME
	1932	1933	1934	1932	1933	1934	1932	1933	1934					
1		971	963		910	938		29	30	103	105	Yes	No	Very few
2														
3			2,571			2,196			100	Hosp. opened 1/5/34	275	Yes	No	No
4		1,075	1,559		1,064	1,487			35	126	158	Yes	No	No
5			346			316			23	33	40	Yes	Yes	No
6	758	644	575	762	627	539	27	27	23	23	36	Yes	No	No
7	524	438	699	555	402	736				68	31	Yes	No	No
8			5,687			5,646			236	161	202	Yes	Yes	No
9	222	229	298	201	209	265	15	16	30	6	6	Yes	Yes	No
10	156	94	79	151	86	73	5	8	6	3	3	Yes	No	No
11	559	522	491	475	470	472	49	31	27	21	35	Yes	No	No
12												Yes	No	
13	1,453	1,382	1,423	1,369	1,311	1,312	84	71	111	65	65	Yes	Yes	Limited by amount of bed space
14	89	117	167	89	117	152	2	3	8	8	15	Yes	No	No
15	165	101	87	144	73	64	1	3	1	24	23	Yes	No	No
16	135	247	420				7	14	8	15	29	Yes	No	No
17	No answer													

TABLE VII—CONT'D

18	291	261	226	260	258	206	24	18	10	6	17	Yes	No	No
19	972	704	598	944	684	575	28	20	23	49	57	Yes	No	No
20	284	112	100	284	112	100	2	1				Yes		
21	2,701	3,296	2,272	2,559	3,198	2,175	105	122	84	137	147	Yes	No	No
22	729	675	646	799	652	639	12	10	9	59	48	Yes	No	No
23												Yes	If possible	No
24	738	493	402				23	19	18	42	20	Yes	Yes	No
25	91	57	68	94	60	66						Yes	Yes	No
26	Same	as 1934	45	Same	as 1934	45			None	2	5	Yes	No	No
27	57	280	99	46	276	101	2	3	3	8	3	Yes	Yes	No
28	65	118	63	60	117	64	2	4	1	6	4	Yes		
29	303	374	328	297	374	318			6	11	15	Yes	No	No
30	233	214	164	218	203	155	14	15	5	10	14	Yes	No	No
31	785	669	559	730	624	530	41	43	35	43	37	Yes	Yes	No
32	533	428	269	511	428	267	24	19	12	25	15	Yes	No	No
33	129	156	132	124	143	136	9	10	7	13	2	Yes	Yes	No
34	5,946	6,448	4,689	5,718	6,270	4,429	193	231	195	249	314	Yes	No	No
35		Strong and Roch. 11,357	Strong and Roch. 11,892					Strong and Roch. 556	Strong and Roch. 552	Strong and Roch. 362	Strong and Roch. 375	Yes	No	No
36														
37														
38	9,192	9,456	10,174	9,165	9,399	10,155	361	409	428	344	419	Yes	No	No
39	235	410	251	231	405	250	4	5	1	22	7	Yes	No	No
40	1,108	1,195	1,078	1,019	1,166	1,004	67	54	70	70	74	Yes	Yes	No
41	5,406	3,385	3,286	5,716	3.719	3,425	120	66	122	261	247	Yes	No	No
42	100	53	47	81	46	42	19	7	5	1	1	Yes	Yes	No
43	66	60	69	55	48	60	11	12	9	6	2	Yes	No	No
44	2,549	2,321	1,901	2,556	2,310	1,919	129	148	118			Yes	No	No
Totals	36,624	49,602	54,703	35,213	36,721	40,857	1,510	1,374	2,350					

TABLE VII—CONT'D

SUPERINTENDENT (D. ATTENDANCE)

HOSPITAL	GENERAL PROPORTION COLORED CHILDREN	NO. OF STRICTLY CHARITY BEDS	NO. OF STRICTLY PAY BEDS	NO. OF PRIVATE ROOMS FOR CHILDREN	NO. OF PRIVATE ROOMS FOR ADULTS	FACILITIES FOR MOTHERS TO STAY IN HOSPITAL WITH CHILDREN
1	4 in 1,000	380-385	to 15	Same	Same	No
2						
3	None in 1934	290	20			Yes
4	1 in a yr.	155	?	9	20	Yes
5	1 or 2 a yr.	0	All	6	1	1 suite suitable
6	Very few	120	20	10	10	When nursing
7	Not important enough	According to ability to pay or not				Yes
8	40%	About 30 used by community chest or part pay	239	Used as found necessary	110	Yes
9	10%	No distinction		6	Same as for children	
10	Very few	Municipally owned		5	Same	No
11	1-2%	None		10	Same	No
12		As occasion demands		No	No	No
13	1 to 7 or 8	Available to citizens without pay		According to demands		No
14			14	14		No
15	Rarely have one	45	0			No
16	Rarely 1 in 10 yr.	Interchangeable		7	7	No
17						
18				12 for adults and children		No
19	Few in a yr.	71% unpaid 1934	29% paid in 1934	Not operated for private patients		No
20	Very few	All				
21	1 to 5 white					No
22	2%	All	None	None	None	No
23						No

TABLE VII—CONT'D

SUPERINTENDENT (D. ATTENDANCE)

24	7.7%	All free to Camden res.	All outside Camden pay	None	None	No
25		25	5			No
26	⅓	90%	5%	Not limited		No
27	None admitted yet	None	None	3 for children or adults		No
28						Yes
29	Very few			Rooms for children and adults		Yes
30	1%	All	None	None	None	No
31	3%	All	None	None	None	No
32	1%	Maintained by city	As required			When children critically ill
33	0.1%	36	2	2	2	No
34	10.8%	Municipal Hosp. class not considered	None	None	None	No
35		Divided according to condition	If able to pay expected to do so	3	3	Noncontagious condition only
36						
37						
38		304	246	7	73	Not in contagious ward
39	2%	All pay bills if patients are able, otherwise free		9	9	Only in emergency
40	5%	150	None	None	None	No
41	10%	All	3	3 for both children and adults		No
42	4 in year	Collect whenever possible		12 when needed	9	Yes
43	Less than 5%	Based on ability to pay		7 for children and adults		Yes
44	2%	90%	10%	25	30	Not in wards

admitted 9,192, 9,456, and 10,174 in the three years. Four hospitals admitted about 100 cases annually. In nine hospitals the admissions were 1,000 or over.

The percentages of deaths for all hospitals were 4.1, 2.6, and 4.3 for the years 1932, 1933, and 1934, respectively.

Of 40 hospitals replying, all accept colored patients. In 12 cases the races are segregated. In no case is the number of colored patients limited. The percentage of colored inmates varies from 0.1 per cent to 40 per cent. In 24 of the 40 hospitals the colored patients were under 10 per cent of the total number of inmates.

In answer to the question of availability of charity beds, 33 hospitals replied, of which 5 replied that all their beds are charity beds. Five are city hospitals with free beds for citizens. Others apparently collect whenever possible. Two have 90 per cent charity beds. (In 6 instances the answer to the question of the number of strictly pay beds was "None.") In 1 instance all the beds are "pay beds."

Thirty hospitals replied to the question of private beds. Twenty-one have private rooms for children or for adults. With the exception of 2 hospitals none permit the mother to stay with her child unless the child is critically ill.

Finances.—Forty institutions answered the question concerning finance: of these 4 derived funds from the county only; 1 from state, county, and city; the remainder from the city only. Seven apparently derive only part of their income from this source. None are entirely endowed. Two receive support from the Community Chest.

The cost of running the hospital for a year naturally varies with its size, the lowest reported (19 replies) being $6,000, the highest being $391,144. The cost per patient per day, exclusive of interest on investment, varies from $1.32 to $6.53. The figures for food, nursing, and supplies per day varied so greatly as to indicate misunderstanding the question. In 24 hospitals the superintendent was a man; in 15, a woman. Nineteen of the men and 2 of the women were physicians. Thirteen of the women were trained nurses.

Nursing.—The number answering this was 41. Seventeen are affiliated with other hospitals as far as nursing is concerned. The number of nurses employed varies from 3 to 250 yearly. In some of the institutions the nurses are drawn from other hospitals, and their time of service varies, usually about three months. In 6 hospitals the term of service is three years. In 23 hospitals only graduate nurses are employed to care for the patients.

Thirty-one institutions require immunization of nurses against diphtheria; 19, against smallpox; 10, against typhoid. Out of 33 replies 4 stated that 4 nurses acquired diphtheria in 1934 and 46 contracted scarlet fever. In 10 hospitals other diseases were contracted by nurses (mumps, measles, chickenpox, and whooping cough).

Training.—The number of day nurses varies from 3 to 161, the night nurses from 1 to 32. The question as to their length of assignment to duty was not answered satisfactorily and will be omitted.

Operating Room.—Thirty-nine hospitals answered this section. Of these, 31 have operating rooms, 1 for emergency only. Seven have none. Five have student nurses definitely assigned to the operating room; they are assigned for periods varying from a week to a month. The number of operations varied, one of the largest institutions recording ninety-eight major operations, 62 citrate transfusions, and 46 direct transfusions. In some of the small institutions only one or two operations were performed.

Diet Kitchen.—Ten hospitals definitely stated that no student nurses were employed in the diet kitchen; 8 hospitals have from one to four. In four cases the food is prepared in a central kitchen which serves the whole general hospital.

Supervision.—Of the 33 hospitals replying, 26 have a nurse in charge of each ward. These are all graduates. Only 4 hospitals answered that undergraduates were also employed. In 21 there are graduate nurses in charge of the wards at night, but in 2 hospitals 1 nurse is responsible for more than one ward. Thirty hospitals replied that they have supervising nurses, usually 1 or 2, but in some cases as many as 12, 13, and 22. These nurses are graduates and there are about the same number of night supervisors.

The question of the occurrence of cross-infection was answered by 31 hospitals. Only 1 diphtheria infection was reported. Eleven hospitals reported scarlet fever cross-infection, as follows: 3 had one case each; 4 had two each; 2 had three each; and 1 had four. Eleven institutions had measles cross-infection; 2 hospitals reported one case each; 2 reported two cases; 2 reported four; 1 reported six; 1 reported nine; 1, thirteen; 1, eighteen; and 1, forty cases. Four institutions had pertussis cross-infection, one or two cases each. Ten reported varicella; 4 had one case each; 1 had three; 1 had five; 1 had twenty-one; 1 had twenty-four; and 1 reported ''several'' cases. Several reported mumps cases.

X-Ray.—Forty hospitals answered this section (Table VIII). Thirteen replied definitely that they had no x-ray facilities; 21 had their own x-ray plant. The remaining 6 send their patients to other hospitals if x-ray examination becomes necessary. There are full-time men in charge in 13 hospitals. In 19 the department is available at any hour of the day or night; 12 are equipped for high speed radiography with milliamperage as indicated in Table VIII. Twelve are equipped for superficial radiography with voltage as indicated in the table. Six are equipped for deep radiotherapy with voltage as indicated in the table. Fifteen have fluoroscopes; 13 can take stereoscopic plates; 18 have portable machines. In 3 hospitals internes take the radiographs. Only 3 hospitals take radiographs as a routine procedure. Twenty-three replied that x-ray facilities were adequate; 1 replied that they were ''fair.'' The x-ray serves the dispensary in 7 cases and outside physicians in 5. The figures given for the number of plates taken during the year vary greatly and run into such high figures that it is evident that the figures apply to general hospitals whose x-ray facilities are used by the contagious disease hospital. These figures are, therefore, of no value for this investigation.

Laboratories.—Forty-one hospitals answered this section completely or in part. Eighteen have a general director for all laboratories; 8 have none. The remainder have their laboratory work done at other institutions. In only 7 is the director a full-time man.

Pathologic Laboratory.—Thirteen hospitals have full-time directors of the pathologic laboratories. Apparently in many instances pathologic work is done at a general hospital. Twenty hospitals have full-time technicians varying in number from 1 to 7. In 16 hospitals the internes do laboratory work, in most cases just routine. In 1 instance autopsies are done by internes under supervision; in another, special mention is made of blood counting and typing of patients in the wards. Seventeen hospitals consider their pathologic laboratory equipment adequate; 4 do not: 2 need more technicians; 1 says space and equipment are limited; 1 complains of inadequately trained bacteriologists.

Twenty-five hospitals replied concerning deaths and autopsies. In 2 hospitals there were no fatalities in 1934. In 3 smaller institutions there was a total of 14 deaths with no autopsies. However, taking the series as a whole, a surprisingly large percentage of postmortems was obtained. The total number of deaths reported for 1934 was 1,857; the number of autopsies obtained was 1,173, 63 per cent. There are facilities for pathologic research in 11 hospitals.

Clinical Laboratories.—Sixteen hospitals are in the immediate charge of a director, a full-time man in 14 instances. Sixteen have full-time technicians, and in 15 the in-

TABLE VIII

X-RAY DEPARTMENT

HOSPITAL	DIAGNOSTIC FACILITIES	NO. FULL-TIME TECHNICIANS	FACILITIES ANY HOUR, DAY OR NIGHT	EQUIPPED FOR HIGH SPEED RADIOTHERAPY	SUPERFICIAL RADIOTHERAPY VOLTAGE	DEEP RADIOTHERAPY VOLTAGE	FLUOROSCOPY	TAKE STEREOSCOPIC PLATES?	PORTABLE X-RAY MACHINE	INTERNES DO X-RAY WORK	ROUTINE	SPECIAL
1	Gen. Hosp.											
2												
3	Yes	1	Yes	Yes	220	200,000	Yes	Yes	No	No		
4	Yes	Part time 1	Yes	No	No	No	No	No	Yes	No		
5	Yes	2	Yes	No	Yes 90-100 kv.	Yes 200 kv.	Yes	Yes	Yes	No		
6	Yes	2	24 hr.	No	No	No	No	No	Yes	Yes	Yes	No
7	Yes		Yes		Yes		Yes	Yes	Yes	No		
8	Yes	4	Yes	Yes 20 mlm.	Yes, high & low	Yes, high & low	Yes	Yes	Yes	Yes	Yes	
9	Yes	1	Yes	No	No	No	No	No	Yes	No		
10	No x-ray											
11	Yes	2	Yes	Yes 200 mlm.	Yes 85,000	No	Yes	Yes	Yes at Gen. Hosp.	No		
12	No x-ray											
13	Yes	0	Yes	No	No	No	Yes	No	No	Yes	Yes	No
14	Yes	0	Yes	Yes 80 mlm.	Yes 100 kv.	No	Yes	No	No	No	No	
15	Sent to outside technician											
16	Lab. work in Gen. Municipal Hosp.								Yes			
17	No x-ray											
18	Yes	1	Daily 8-4:30 on call at night	Yes 100 mlm.	No	No	No	Yes	No	No		
19	T. B. division has x-ray dept. New building will have its own								Yes			

TABLE VIII—CONT'D

20	No											
21	Yes	1	Yes	Yes 100 ma. 100 kv.	Yes 130 kv. 5 ma.	No	Yes	Yes	Yes	No		
22	X-ray in Hudson County Hospital											
23	Yes	1	Yes	Yes 100 ma.	Yes	Yes 200 kv.	Yes	Yes	No	No		
24	No x-ray											
25	No reply											
26	X-ray done through Atlantic City Hosp. when necessary											
27	No x-ray dept.											
28	No x-ray dept.											
29	Done at Ellis Hosp. or Health Center											
30	Yes		Yes	125 yes	Yes	Not used	Yes	Yes	Yes	No		
31	Yes	No	Yes	Yes	No	No	Yes	Yes	Yes	No		
32	Yes	1 Half time	Yes	Yes 30 ma.	No	No	No	No	Yes	No		
33	No											
34	Yes	Part time 1	Yes	No	Yes 120 kv.	No	Yes	Yes	Yes	No		
35	Yes	3, plus 2% res. staff	Yes	Yes 1,000 ma.		Yes 200 kv.	Yes	Yes	Yes			
36												
37												
38	Yes	2	Yes	Yes 100 ma.	Yes 76-130 kv.	Yes 200,000 kv.	Yes	Yes	Yes	No		
39	No x-ray dept.											
40	No x-ray dept.											
41	Yes	No	Day until 7:00 P.M.	No	No	No	No	No	Yes	No		
42	No	No	No	No	No	No	No	No	Yes on call	No		
43	No x-ray department											
44	Yes	1	Yes	No	Yes 125 k. v. p.	No	Yes	No	Yes	No		

TABLE VIII—CONT'D

HOSPITAL	SPECIFY IF SPECIAL	EQUIPMENT AND FACILITIES ADEQUATE	IF NOT, IN WHAT RESPECTS?	DEPARTMENT SERVE DISPENSARY	OUTSIDE PHYSICIANS	NUMBER OF X-RAY PLATES TAKEN LAST YEAR	NUMBER OF SUPERFICIAL TREATMENTS	NUMBER OF DEEP THERAPY TREATMENTS
1								
2								
3		Yes		No dis.	No	56	0	0
4		Yes		No dis.	No	43	0	
5		Yes		No	Yes			7,712
6		Yes		No dis.	No	33	0	0
7		Yes				Included in total of Vancouver General Hospital		
8		Yes		Yes	Yes	5,500	227	9,686
9		Yes						0
10								
11		Yes		Yes	No	197	0	0
12								
13		Yes		No dis.	No	962	0	0
14		Yes		Yes	Yes		0	0
15	Sent to outside technician							
16		Yes		No dis.	Yes			
17	No x-ray							
18		Yes		Yes	Occasionally	822		
19						2,396		
20								
21		Yes		No	No	2,016	40	0
22	X-ray in Hudson County Hospital							
23		Yes		No dis.		629	2	355
24	No x-ray							
25	No x-ray							
26	X-ray done through Atlantic City Hospital when necessary							

TABLE VIII—CONT'D

27	No x-ray department							
28	No x-ray department							
29	Done at Ellis Hospital or Health Center							
30		Yes		No			0	0
31		Yes		No	No	231	0	0
32		Yes				118	0	0
33		Portable x-ray of outside Roentgenologist available					0	0
34		Yes		Dis. for employees only	No	3,617	1	0
35	Assoc. res. radiol.; assist. res. radiol.	Yes		Yes	No	28,049	Total 3,352	
36								
37								
38		Yes		Yes	Yes	10,000	200	Installed in last 2 mo.
39		Yes		No				
40								
41		Fair		No		200	0	0
42		Yes	Send detailed x-ray studies to disp. Wilkes-Barre Gen. Hosp.	No		0	0	0
43								
44		Yes		Yes	No	3,600	40	0

TABLE IX

GENERAL INFORMATION (1934)

HOSPITAL	DIPHTHERIA		SC. FEVER		MEASLES		WH. COUGH		SMALLPOX		CHICKENPOX		EPIDEMIC CEREBRO-SPINAL MENINGITIS	
	CASES	DEATHS	CASES	DEATHS	CASES	DEATHS	CASES	DEATHS	CASES	DEATHS	CASES	DEATHS	CASES	DEATHS
1	18	0	647	9	18	0	91	1	0	0	65	0		
2														
3	213	23	772	24	823	7	391	34			96			
4	93	4	792	11	210	5	313	11			38	1	0	0
5	11	0	64	0	2	0	17	3	0		4	0	3	1
6	33	0	245	5	2	0	29	4			20	0	1	0
7	14	4	599	3	0	0	4	0	0	0	12	0	2	0
8	4	0	382	6	23	0	0	0	0	0	6	0	1	0
9	56		61		47		30						8	
10	6	3	43	1	11	1					3	1	1	0
11	18	0	235	2	3	0	14	2	0		6	0	2	1
12	4	0	165	1	18	0	394	1	0	0	574	0	2	2
13	66	6	552	7	294	43	110	26	0	0	11	0	4	1
14	6		31		33	1	19	2	0		7	1	1	1
15			34	0	6	0	1	0	0		0		0	
16	2		304	4	9		2	1	0		4		0	
17	No answer													
18	3	0	167	1	138	0	368	0	0	0	762	0	6	5
19	23	1	432	9	603	35	36	6	0		6	0	0	
20	0		66		0		0		0		0		0	
21	40	1	596	7	28	0	161	8	0		144	0	11	2

TABLE IX—CONT'D

22	71	2	71	1	3	0	32	1	0	0	40	0	4	1
23	1		181	1	9	1	5		0		1		1	
24	56	7	198	5	33	3	19	2	0		0		1	1
25	26	0	56	0	106	0	95	0	0	0	108	0	2	2
26	0	0	27	0	5	0	0	0	0	0	1	0	In A. C. Hosp.	
27			93	3	7									
28	0		63	1	0		0		0		0		0	
29														
30	14	0	95	4	1	0	16	0	0	0	13	1	1	0
31	64	11	366	3	12	2	60	7	0	0	4	1	2	1
32	5	1	143	4	17		52	1	0		5		5	1
33	0		89	1	3		2	2	0		1		0	
34	579	29	1461	8	372	5	505	24			454	0	13	2
35	7	1	141	7	8	0	36	6	0	0	11	1	1	0
36														
37														
38	31	4	54	0	4	0	19	1	0	0	16	2	0	0
39	12	1	238	0	0		0		0		0		0	
40	203	29	615	11	5	0	0		0		3	0	16	12
41	164	21	2348	22	307	34	137	29	0	0	70	1	0	
42	9	1	8	0	1	0	2	0	0		2	0	1	1
43	8	2	38	2	3	0	5	1	1	1				
44	39	1	196	3	13	0	98	7	0	0	19	0	2	1
Totals	1899	152	12,671	176	3783	103	3063	200	1	1	2506	9	91	35
Deaths %	8.0		1.3		3.1		6.5		100.0		0.35		38.3	

TABLE IX—CONT'D

GENERAL INFORMATION (1934)

HOSPITAL	TYPHOID FEVER		AMEBIC DYSENTERY		BACILLARY DYSENTERY		OTHER CASES		
	CASES	DEATHS	CASES	DEATHS	CASES	DEATHS		CASES	DEATHS
1	4	0	8						
2									
3							Erysipelas	84	6
							Mumps	47	
4							Erysipelas	58	8
5	6						Erysipelas	35	1
							Tuberculosis	43	8
6									
7	8	0					Mumps	5	0
							Enceph. lethargica	2	0
							Erysipelas	24	1
							Ant. poliomyelitis	4	0
							Leprosy	1	0
8			2	0	0	0	Erysipelas	1	1
9							Erysipelas	5	
							Poliomyelitis	8	
10							Scabies	9	0
11	1	0							
12	35	5					Influenza men.	2	2
							Influenza	7	0
							Pulmonary tbc.	38	18
							Others from tbc.	7	6
13					12	2	Erysipelas	31	3
							Acute polio.	8	0
							Mumps	6	0
							Gon. ophthalmia	25	0
							Others	304	23
14					1		Mumps	1	
15							Tuberculosis	41	1

TABLE IX—CONT'D

16									
17									
18	5	0							
19							Misc. dis. and doubtful diag.	11	1
20							Unclassified	34	
21	15	0	1	0					
22					4	0	Erysipelas	60	0
							Scabies	144	0
							Flu-pneumonia and grip	46	0
							Imp. contagioso	100	0
							Tetanus	2	2
23									
24							Other diseases	64	
25	3	1	1						
26							Poliomyelitis	1	0
							Erysipelas	5	0
							Croup	1	0
27							Erysipelas	1	
							Septic sore throat	2	
							Septic antrum	1	
28							Erysipelas	6	0
29									
30							Parotitis	6	0
							Pseudocroup	2	0
							Membr. tonsillitis	5	0
							Poliomyelitis	1	0
31									
32							Erysipelas	4	
							Mumps	15	
33									
34	2	0							
35	3	0	4	0	20	1			
36									
37									

TABLE IX—CONT'D

HOSPITAL	TYPHOID FEVER		AMEBIC DYSENTERY		BACILLARY DYSENTERY		OTHER CASES		
	CASES	DEATHS	CASES	DEATHS	CASES	DEATHS		CASES	DEATHS
38	4	1			6	1	Erysipelas	1	0
39							Mumps	1	0
40							Erysipelas	59	11
							Diphth. carrier	70	0
							Infantile paralysis	1	0
							Mumps	2	2
							Cellulitis	1	0
41							G. measles	15	0
							Anthrax	4	0
							Polio.	3	0
							Mumps	28	0
42							Tbc. meningitis	2	2
							Polio.	1	0
							Scabies	2	0
							Bronchopneumonia	1	0
							Erysipelas	10	1
							Strep. thr.	1	0
							Mumps	1	0
							V. angina	1	0
43							Influenza	1	0
							Scabies	2	0
							Tbc.	2	2
							Other diseases	6	1
44	7	0					Other diseases	393	29
Totals	93	7	16	0	43	4			
Deaths %	7.5		0		9.3				

ternes do the laboratory work, in most instances only routine. Nine hospitals have a "fume hood"; 13 have a colorimeter. Nine are equipped to determine basal metabolic rates; 17 consider their facilities adequate; 6 do not. The complaints are lack of facilities in the hospital: inadequate space, insufficient apparatus, and technicians. Eleven have research facilities.

Bacteriologic Laboratory.—Twelve hospitals have full-time directors; 11 have part-time directors. Seventeen have full-time technicians. In 17 the internes do routine work; in 3 they do special work. Eighteen have electric incubators, and 1 has a gas incubator. Fourteen hospitals keep animals for experimental purposes, and 12 are equipped for research work. Five hospitals replied that their facilities were not adequate.

Serologic Laboratory.—Out of 27 hospitals replying, 11 each had a director of the laboratory. In the remainder the work was done at other hospitals or by the board of health. Eleven have full-time technicians. In 6 the internes do laboratory work—only routine. Wassermann tests are done in 10 hospitals; Kahn tests, in 4. In 14 hospitals facilities are considered adequate; in 6 they are not. In 11 there are facilities for research.

Miscellaneous Facilities.—Fourteen hospitals have facilities for taking simple photographs; 18, for color photographs. Fourteen have electrocardiographs, of which 1 is owned by a staff physician.

Diet Kitchen.—Out of 39 replies, 19 report dietitians in charge of the diet kitchen. In some cases the person is simply a cook; in others, a nurse, a housekeeper, or a superintendent takes care of the diets. Of the 19 so-called dietitians, 14 apparently have had adequate training. In 27 hospitals the dietitian has entire charge of the menus. Standard special diets are drawn up by the medical personnel in 14 instances; by cooperation between dietitian and physician, in 6; in 12 instances, by the dietitian alone.

Social Service.—Only 13 hospitals out of 38 answering have social service departments. Eleven of the 13 have full-time workers in charge, of whom 9 have had special social service training. Eight hospitals have more than 1 full-time worker. Respective numbers are reported as 2, 6, 2, 3, 2, 3, 3, 2. In 13 institutions all cases are investigated. In all these the parents are interviewed at the hospital; supplementary home visits are made in the case of 10 hospitals. Home visits are made in all cases in 5 hospitals. In 10 hospitals histories are taken. Twelve hospitals answered "Yes" to the question of filing social service data on the history chart, abstracts being attached to the notes or filed with history in 14 cases.

The ability of the patient to pay for hospital service is investigated by the social service department in 12 institutions. In 1 this is done by the city collector; in another, by a "hospital adjuster."

In 13 hospitals the social service division arranges for convalescent care. Only 9 hospitals have convalescent homes available, 1 of which admits adults only. Convalescent institutions are used in 8 cases. Foster homes are available in 7 hospitals. Of these, 6 are used frequently; 1, "only rarely." Twelve hospitals complain that facilities for children's care are inadequate. One reports ability to give convalescent care only if a fee is available.

Eleven hospitals have routine follow-up service, and 7 follow cases only under special circumstances. In 10 hospitals the social service department assists in getting patients to return for follow-up. Three hospitals have volunteers for indoor work and for outdoor work. Seven social service departments are entirely supported by hospital funds; 1, only partially. Eight departments are supported by funds from the outside. Three hospitals have special social service committees, in 2 of which physicians are members. In 2 hospitals the committee is represented on the board of managers.

General Information (1934).—Table IX reveals the number of cases of the more usual contagious diseases admitted to these hospitals during 1934, together with total deaths and the percentage death rate in all hospitals for each disease. Information was also requested concerning cases of other diseases admitted by the hospitals, but the replies are too diverse and varied to warrant tabulating.

The mortality figures are of considerable interest, especially when compared with those reported in hospitals of Region III (J. PEDIAT. pp. 142, 143, July, 1936).

The lowest rate is found in chickenpox (0.35 per cent) and the next highest in scarlet fever (1.3 per cent). Measles is next (with 6.5 per cent); typhoid fever (7.5 per cent), and then diphtheria (8.0 per cent). In spite of all the propaganda for the eradication of diphtheria, the hospitals in Region I admitted 1,899 cases in 1934. It is of interest also that the largest number treated in any one institution was at the Willard Parker Hospital in New York City, where 579 cases were admitted. One of the most elaborate campaigns to popularize antidiphtheria vaccinations was carried on in New York City; nevertheless there is a considerable diphtheria morbidity with 29 deaths. The measles mortality is quite low as compared with that in the Middle West (3.1 vs. 6.3). The largest number of deaths reported for any one disease was 200 in the case of pertussis. The variability in the mortality percentage of cerebrospinal meningitis is well shown. Though the total mortality rate is 38.3 per cent, some hospitals had a much lower and others a much higher rate; in 1 institution out of 16 cases 12 died; in 1 hospital 5 out of 6 died whereas in another hospital out of 11 cases only 2 patients died. It is also striking that in all of these institutions there was only a single case of smallpox reported.

WILLIAMS McKIM MARRIOTT
1885-1936

Williams McKim Marriott, one of America's most distinguished pediatricians, died November 11 in San Francisco, Calif., of a streptococcic septicemia following an appendiceal abscess. Dr. Marriott was born in Baltimore, March 5, 1885. He attended the University of North Carolina from which he received the degree of B.S. in 1904. His medical training was at Cornell University from which he received his M.D. degree in 1910. In 1936 he was given the honorary degree of LL.D. by the University of Missouri. During his medical course at Cornell he served as an assistant in the department of biochemistry, and in 1910 he became instructor in biochemistry at Washington University School of Medicine, St. Louis. In 1914 be became interested in chemical problems in pediatrics and was appointed an associate of Dr. John Howland at the Harriet Lane Home of the Johns Hopkins Hospital and Medical School. In 1918 he returned to St. Louis as full-time head of the Department of Pediatrics in the School of Medicine of Washington University, and as pediatrician-in-chief of the St. Louis Children's Hospital. He was made dean of the medical school in 1924, holding these positions until July, 1936. Last spring Dr. Marriott decided to withdraw from active pediatric work and on July 1, 1936, he became the dean of the University of California Medical School in San Francisco, and the professor of research medicine.

He was greatly interested in chemistry and made numerous contributions to the clinical science of pediatrics. His administrative duties as dean had become so time consuming in the last few years that he was able to give less and less attention to pediatrics; and this led him to make such an important change this year. His most important work was in the field of infant nutrition. He possessed a rare and unusual faculty of applying the results of basic scientific research to clinical medicine. He was an excellent teacher and had a strong influence in the development of many of our younger leaders in pediatrics. He was a member of, and had been honored by, many medical societies, including the American Pediatric Society and the American Academy of Pediatrics. He served for many years as associate editor of the *American Journal of Diseases of Children.* His textbook, *Infant Nutrition,* has recently gone into a second edition. Dr. Marriott was one of the ablest of present-day pediatricians and his death at the age of fifty-one is a distinct loss to pediatrics as a whole, to the associates and assistants who have come under his influence, and to his many friends.

News and Notes

The following men have been certified by the **American Board of Pediatrics.**

Carl George Ashley, Portland, Ore.
Einor Hugo Christopherson, San Diego, Calif.
Herbert Everett Coe, Seattle, Wash.
Frank H. Douglass, Seattle, Wash.
Benjamin F. Feingold, Los Angeles, Calif.
Rafael Clarence Harris, Santa Ana, Calif.
Newell Linton Moore, Santa Ana, Calif.
Norman K. Nixon, Los Angeles, Calif.
William Anthony Reilly, San Francisco, Calif.
Arthur Edward Varden, San Bernardino, Calif.
Jerald Samuel Backstrand, Salem, Ore.
Mary Knott Bazemore, Merion, Pa.
Albert James Bell, Cincinnati, Ohio
Adrien Bleyer, St. Louis, Mo.
Maxwell Philip Borovsky, Chicago, Ill.
Julian Deigh Boyd, Iowa City, Iowa
William Leslie Bradford, Rochester, N. Y.
William L. Channell, Oakland, Calif.
Hugh Chaplin, New York, N. Y.
Arthur William Chapman, Glens Falls, N. Y.
Esther Bridgman Clark, Palo Alto, Calif.
Jean V. Cooke, St. Louis, Mo.
Clyde V. Croswell, Memphis, Tenn.
Leonard Tomb Davidson, New York, N. Y.
Leon De Vel, Grand Rapids, Mich.
Leroy Morgan Downing, Cedar Rapids, Iowa
Howard L. Eder, Santa Barbara, Calif.
Richard Cannon Eley, Boston, Mass.
Gertrude Felshin, New York, N. Y.
Manning C. Field, Brooklyn, N. Y.
Mark L. Floyd, Iowa City, Iowa
L. Fernald Foster, Bay City, Mich.
Henry E. Gallup, Brookline, Mass.
Henry John Gerstenberger, Cleveland, Ohio
A. Lawrence Gleason, Oakland, Calif.
Isidore H. Goldberger, New York, N. Y.
Harold G. Grayzel, Brooklyn, N. Y.
Ruth Alline Guy, Peiping, China
Paul György, Cleveland, Ohio
Jeanette Harrison, Los Angeles, Calif.
Alexis Frank Hartmann, St. Louis, Mo.
Walter Heymann, Cleveland, Ohio
Urius Himmelstein, New York, N. Y.
Luther Emmett Holt, Jr., Baltimore, Md.
Rieta Campbell Hough, San Diego, Calif.
Thomas D. Jones, Richmond, Va.
C. Loring Joslin, Baltimore, Md.
Katsuji Kato, Chicago, Ill.
Camille Kereszturi, New York, N. Y.
Thomas F. Krauss, Rockford, Ill.
Clifford Lanier Lamar, Birmingham, Ala.
Gilbert J. Levy, Memphis, Tenn.
Percy Edgar Luecke, Dallas, Texas
John D. Lyttle, New York, N. Y.
Howard Harris Mason, New York, N. Y.
William Patton McDowell, Norfolk, Va.
Preston A. McLendon, Washington, D. C.
Lionel N. Merrill, Detroit, Mich.
Marjorie F. Murray, Cooperstown, N. Y.
Harry A. Naumer, Brooklyn, N. Y.
John D. Nourse, Cleveland, Ohio
Gilbert Seymour Osincup, Orlando, Fla.
M. C. Overton, Lubbock, Texas
Paul L. Parrish, Brooklyn, N. Y.
K. C. Reese, Tulsa, Okla.
Irwin Rubell, Chicago, Ill.
Mitchell I. Rubin, Philadelphia, Pa.
Stanley Stewart Saunders, High Point, N. C.
Béla Schick, New York, N. Y.
A. Clement Silverman, Syracuse, N. Y.
David M. Siperstein, Minneapolis, Minn.
Eugene Herbert Smith, Ogden, Utah
Joseph Stokes, Jr., Philadelphia, Pa.
John A. Toomey, Cleveland, Ohio
Alexander Ashley Weech, New York, N. Y.
William Weston, Columbia, S. C.
T. Wistar White, St. Louis, Mo.
William R. Wilson, New Haven, Conn.
Mendel Zeligs, Cincinnati, Ohio

INDEX TO VOLUME 9

A

Abelson, Sol M., and Greengard, J., 483
Abt, Arthur F., and Frank, I., 68
Adair, Fred L., Swanson, W. W., and Lennarson, V. E., 11
Adrenal gland, carcinoma of cortex of, 62
Agglutinin response after pertussis vaccination with Sauer vaccine and with a toxin vaccine and in untreated clinical pertussis, 492
Aldrich, C. A., and Veeder, B. S., 323
Allergy in children (round table discussion), 804
  of nose and paranasal sinuses, 416 (Bk. Rev.)
American Academy of Pediatrics: committee on hospitals and dispensaries, report of, 125, 377, 818
    news, 146, 277, 709
    proceedings, 116, 125, 249, 377, 549, 689, 804, 818
    treasurer, report of, 145
Anemia, aplastic, hematology and pathology of, 433
  Cooley's (*see* Anemia, erythroblastic)
  erythroblastic, associated pigment abnormalities simulating hemachromatosis, 279
    observations on, morphology of erythrocytes in, 312
  of newborn, 427
Angiomas in premature infants, 744
Antigen, intranasal, treatment of pertussis with, 42
Appendicitis, basis for, mechanical lesions of appendix in children, 647
  round table discussion, 249
Appendix, mechanical lesions of, in children as a basis for appendicitis, 647
  rheumatic involvement of, 234
Atrophy, hemiatrophy, scleroderma with sclerodactylia and, 173

B

Bacillemia (*see* Blood, bacteria)
Bacilli, ''late lactose-fermenting'' coli-like, pathogenic significance of, 23
Barnes, Donald J., Eliot, M. M., Nelson, E. M., Browne, F. A., and Jenss, R. M., 355
Bell, A. L. Loomis, and Gordon, M. B., 781
Bell, E. T., Thompson, W. H., and McQuarrie, I., 604
Birch-Hirschfeld photometric test for vitamin A deficiency, 655
Blood, bacteria, dysentery, 167
  bactericidal property of, against meningococcus, 328
  intravascular clotting in abandoned fetal channels in newborn, 318
  transfusion, citrated, in infants and children, 795
  vessels, abandoned, fetal, intravascular clotting in, in newborn, 318
Bonar, Barnet E., 96
Boyd, Gladys L., 417
Bradford, W. L., and Dye, J., 312
—, and Whipple, G. H., 279
Bradley, C. E., and Garrett, D. L., 776
Brown, Alan, Drake, T. G. H., and Tisdall, F. F., 421
Browne, Florence A., Eliot, M. M., Nelson, E. M., Barnes, D. J., and Jenss, R. M., 355

C

Calcium and phosphorus, metabolism of, in case of intractable rickets, 56
Capillary resistance, test for, and its relation to vitamins C and D, 226
Carbon tetrachloride poisoning, 662
Carcinoma of adrenal cortex, 62
Castrovinci, Frederick, and Leopold, J. S., 620
Chamberlain, John W., 215
Childe, A. E., Wiglesworth, F. W., and Goldbloom, A., 331
Children, abnormal, roentgenographic studies of sella turcica in, 781
  adopted, 715 (Bk. Rev.)
  allergy in (round table discussion), 804
  ambulatory, follow-up study of, with tuberculosis infection, 467

Children—Cont'd
appendix, mechanical lesion of, as a basis for appendicitis in, 647
cysts, twisted ovarian, in, 771
enuresis, nocturnal, in, sodium chloride in treatment of, 751
lymphosarcoma, mediastinal, in, 331
neurologic conditions in (critical review), 797
protamine insulin in, 417
rheumatic heart disease in, 505
spontaneous rupture of liver in, with complete recovery, 776
transfusion, citrated, in infants and, 795
tuberculosis in (critical review), 672
typhoid fever, treatment of, 149
vaginitis, gonorrheal, treatment of, with estrogenic substances in, 240
vulvitis, gangrenous, with associated mouth and rectal lesions in, 75
Cholesterol, irradiated, antirachitic effect of, and cod liver oil, 421
Cod liver oil, comparative value of viosterol, vitamin D milk and, in prevention of rickets, and of certain basic factors influencing their efficacy, 355
antirachitic effect of, and irradiated cholesterol, 421
Coe, Herbert E., 513
Comments, 568
Committee report: hospitals and dispensaries, contagious disease hospitals, 125, 377, 818
Contagious disease hospitals, committee report on, 125, 377, 818
Cooke, Jean V., 641
Correspondence, 667
Critical review, neurologic conditions in infants and children, 797
newborn, 96
surgical pediatrics, 513
tuberculosis in children, 672
Crocker, Walter J., and Habel, K., 149
Cyanosis in newborn (panel discussion on), 262
Cysts, ovarian, twisted, in children, 771

D

Davison, Wilburt C., 209
Dawson, Helen L., 187
DeJong, Russell N., 203
Denenholz, E. J., and Gibson, S., 505
Deuell, William D., and Landon, J. F., 75
Diagnosis, pediatric, 209
Diarrhea, epidemic, and vomiting, 87
Diphtheria immunization, active artificial, 641
Dodd, Katharine, 486
Drake, T. G. H., Tisdall, F. F., and Brown, A., 421
Dunham, Ethel C., 17
—, and McAlenney, P. F., Jr., 717
Duryee, Margaret, Higgons, R. A., and West, T., 81
Dye, Jane, and Bradford, W. L., 312
Dysentery bacillemia, 167

E

Eczema, infantile, influence of breast and artificial feeding on, 223
Edema associated with hypogenesis of serum protein and atrophic changes in liver, and studies of water and mineral exchanges, 604
Eley, R. Cannon, 797
Eliot, Martha M., Nelson, E. M., Barnes, D. J., Browne, F. A., and Jenss, R. M., 355
Ellenberg, Samuel T., and Martin, A. T., 234
Encephalogram, interpretation of tuberous sclerosis, 203
Enuresis, nocturnal, sodium chloride in treatment of, in children, 751
Erythrocytes, morphology of, in erythroblastic anemia, 312
Estrogenic substances (*see* Hormones, sex)

F

Food, artificial, influence of, on infantile eczema, 223
breast, influence of, on infantile eczema, 223
Fothergill, LeRoy D., Krakower, C. A., and Freeman, D., 23
Frank, Ira, and Abt, A. F., 68
Freeman, Don, Fothergill, L. D., and Krakower, C. A., 23

G

Gallagher, Eleanor G., 715
Garrett, D. L., and Bradley, C. E., 776
Gibson, Stanley, and Denenholz, E. J., 505
Glycogen storage disease, lipoid factor in, 728
Goldbloom, Alton, Wiglesworth, F. W., and Childe, A. E., 331

Gonorrheal vaginitis, treatment of, with estrogenic substances, in childhood, 240
Gordon, Murray B., and Bell, A. L. L., 781
Greengard, Joseph, and Abelson, S. M., 483
Greenthal, Roy M., 87
Greenwald, Harry M., and Koota, J., 472
Growth, linear, effect of vitamin D on, in infancy, 1
Grulee, Clifford G., and Sanford, H. N., 223

H

Habel, Karl, and Crocker, W. J., 149
Halpern, L. J., and Mazel, M. S., 771
Hamilton, Bengt, and Highman, W. J., Jr., 56
Hansel, French K., 416
Heart disease, rheumatic, in childhood, 505
Hemochromatosis, pigment abnormalities simulating, associated with erythroblastic anemia, 279
Hemorrhage complicating deep pharyngeal infection, 68
Herzger, Gertrud, and Weichsel, M., 763
Heyl, Henry L., 662
Hieronymus, Ethel E., and Limper, Margaret A., 240
Higgons, Reginald A., West, T., and Duryee, M., 81
Highman, Walter J., Jr., and Hamilton, Bengt, 56
Hill, Lee Forrest, 672
Hirsch, Sidney, 795
Hoffmann, Erich, 569
Hormones, sex, treatment of gonorrheal vaginitis in childhood with, 240
Hospitals, contagious disease, committee report, 125, 377, 818
Huenekens, E. J., 427
Hyperpyrexia of unknown etiology of sixteen months' duration, 472
Huntington, Robert W., Jr., and Wilkes-Weiss, D., 449, 456, 462
Hurwitz, Samuel, and Wolff, E., 467

I

Ileus, meconium, intestinal obstruction due to, in newborn infant, 486
Immunization, active artificial, in diphtheria, 641
Infants, eczema in, influence of breast and artificial feeding on, 223
Infants—Cont'd
  linear growth in, effect of vitamin D on, 1
  meconium specimens from, bacterial flora of, 624
  neurologic conditions in children and (critical review), 797
  newborn (critical review), 96
    anemia of, 427
    cyanosis in (panel discussion), 262
    intestinal obstruction due to meconium ileus in, 486
    intravascular clotting in abandoned fetal channels in, 318
    isolated peripheral radial nerve paralysis in, 483
    omphalitis in, 215
    pneumothorax, traumatic, in, 620
  prematurely born, 11
      angiomas in, 744
      mortality among, 17
      study of, 244, 717
  stillborn, intestinal contents of, bacterial flora of, 633
  technics for measuring, 187
  transfusion, citrated, in children and, 795
  vomiting in, its relief by x-ray, 81
Insulin, protamine, in children, 417
Intestine, contents of, bacterial flora of, of twenty-seven stillborn infants, 633
  obstruction of, due to meconium ileus in newborn infant, 486

J

Jaundice, congenital obstructive, 91
Jeans, P. C., Stearns, G., and Vandecar, V., 1
Jenss, Rachel M., Eliot, M. M., Nelson, E. M., Barnes, D. J., and Browne, F. A., 355
Johnston, Joseph A., 350

K

Kass, I. H., and Osgood, F. P., 91
Kato, Katsuji, and Steiner, P. E., 433
Koota, Jacob, and Greenwald, H. M., 472
Krafka, Joseph, Jr., and Mulherin, W. A., 318
Krakower, Cecil A., 728
—, Fothergill, L. D., and Freeman, D., 23

L

Landon, John F., and Deuell, W. D., 75
Lennarson, Vernon E., Swanson, W. W., and Adair, F. L., 11
Leopold, Jerome S., and Castrovinci, F., 620
Limper, Margaret A., and Hieronymus, E. E., 240
Liswood, Rebecca, and Rosenson, W., 751
Little, A. A., Jr., 62
Liver, atrophic changes in, edema associated with, and hypogenesis of serum protein, 604
  rupture, spontaneous, of, in child with complete recovery, 776
Lymphosarcoma, mediastinal, in childhood, 331

M

Marriott, W. McKim, 861
Martin, Alexander T., and Ellenberg, S. L., 234
Mastitis, puberty, 758
Mazel, M. S., and Halpern, L. J., 771
McAlenney, Paul F., Jr., and Dunham, E. C., 717
McCrackin, Robert H., 173
McQuarrie, Irvine, Thompson, W. H., and Bell, E. T., 604
Measurements, technics of, for infants, 187
Meconium, bacterial flora of, collected from sixty-four infants within four hours after delivery, 624
Mediterranean disease (*see* Anemia, erythroblastic)
Meningitis due to Morgan bacillus, 791
  influenzal, 449
    onset of, association of otitis media and pneumonia with, 456
    treatment of, with immune serum, 462
  tuberculous, spinal fluid sugar in, significance of diminution of, 763
Meningococcus, bactericidal property of blood against, 328
  presence of, in nasopharynx of normal individuals, 328
Mental hygiene, outline of pediatrist's relation to, 323
Milk, vitamin D, comparative value of cod liver oil, viosterol, and, in prevention of rickets, and of certain basic factors influencing their efficacy, 355
Mishulow, Lucy, Mowry, I., and Orange, R., 492
Mitchell, Reginald H., 791
Montgomery, Albert H., 249
Morgan, bacillus of, meningitis due to, 791
Mortality rate among prematurely born infants, 17
Mowry, Isabelle, Mishulow, L., and Orange, R., 492
Mulherin, W. A., and Krafka, J., Jr., 318

N

Nasopharynx, meningococcus, presence of, in, 328
Nelson, E. M., Eliot, M. M., Barnes, D. J., Browne, F. A., and Jenss, R. M., 355
Nerve, radial, isolated peripheral paralysis of, in newborn, 483
Neurology in infants and children (critical review), 797
Newborn (*see* Infants, newborn)
News and notes, 146, 278, 567, 712, 862
Nicholson, Percival, 647
Nutrition, recent advances in (round table discussion), 689

O

Omphalitis (*see* Umbilicus, infection)
Orange, Ruth, Mishulow, L., and Mowry, I., 492
Osgood, F. P., and Kass, I. H., 91
Otitis media, association of, with onset of influenzal meningitis, 456

P

Panel discussion on cyanosis in newborn, 262
Pediatrics, surgical, 513
Pediatrist's relation to mental hygiene, 323
Pertussis (*see* Whooping cough)
Pharynx, deep infection of, hemorrhage complicating, 68
Phosphorus and calcium, metabolism of, in case of intractable rickets, 56
Photometric test (Birch-Hirschfeld) for vitamin A deficiency, 655
Pneumonia, association of, with onset of influenzal meningitis, 456
Pneumothorax, traumatic, in newborn, 620
Poisoning, carbon tetrachloride, 662
Psychiatry, childhood (round table discussion), 549
Puberty mastitis, 758

R

Rambar, Alwin C., 744
Rheumatic fever, involvement of appendix in, 234
Rickets, effect of irradiated cholesterol and cod liver oil on, 421
  intractable, case of, calcium and phosphorus metabolism in, 56
  prevention of, comparative value of cod liver oil, viosterol, and vitamin D milk in, and of certain basic factors influencing their efficacy, 355
Roentgen ray, relief of infantile vomiting by, 81
Rosenblum, Philip, 758
Rosenson, William, and Liswood, R., 751
Rothman, Phillip E., 167
Round table discussion, allergy in children, 804
    appendicitis, 249
    childhood psychiatry, 549
    prophylaxis and discussion of whooping cough, 116
    recent advances in nutrition, 689

S

Sanford, Heyworth N., and Grulee, C. G., 223
Sclerodactylia, scleroderma with, and hemiatrophy, 173
Scleroderma with sclerodactylia and hemiatrophy, 173
Sclerosis, tuberous, encephalographic interpretation of, 203
Sella turcica, roentgenographic studies of, in abnormal children, 781
Serum administration, intravenous, continuous method of, 755
  protein of, hypogenesis of, edema associated with, and atrophic changes in liver, 604
Shorr, Eli Y., 49
Silverthorne, Nelles, 328, 755
Slesinger, H. A., 42
Snelling, Charles E., 655
Snyder, Marshall L., 624, 633
Sodium chloride in treatment of nocturnal enuresis in children, 751
Spinal fluid sugar, significance of diminution of, in tuberculous meningitis, 763
Stearns, Genevieve, Jeans, P. C., and Vandecar, V., 1
Steiner, Paul E., and Kato, K., 433
Swanson, William W., Lennarson, V. E., and Adair, F. L., 11
Syphilis, congenital, 569

T

Thalassemia (*see* Anemia, erythroblastic)
Thompson, W. H., McQuarrie, I., and Bell, E. T., 604
Tisdall, Frederick F., Drake, T. G. H., and Brown, A., 421
Transfusion, immuno-, nonspecific, importance of, in typhoid fever in children, 149
Tuberculosis, adult type, evolution of, from childhood type, 350
  ambulatory children with, follow-up study of, 467
  in children (critical review), 672
  reinfection, endogenous, evidence in favor of, 350
Typhoid fever, treatment of 19 cases of, in children, 149

U

Umbilicus, infection of, in newborn, 215

V

Vaginitis (*see* Gonorrheal vaginitis)
Vandecar, Verva, Stearns, G., and Jeans, P. C., 1
Veeder, Borden S., and Aldrich, C. A., 323
Viosterol, cod liver oil, and vitamin D milk, comparative value of, in prevention of rickets, and of certain basic factors influencing their efficacy, 355
Vitamin A, deficiency of, Birch-Hirschfeld photometric test for, 655
  C, capillary resistance test and its relation to, 226
  D, capillary resistance test and its relation to, 226
    effect of, on linear growth in infancy, 1
Vomiting, epidemic, and diarrhea, 87
  infantile, its relief by x-ray, 81
Von Gierke's disease (*see* Glycogen storage disease)
Vulvitis, gangrenous, case of, with associated mouth and rectal lesions in child, 75

W

Weichsel, Manfred, and Herzger, G., 763
Weld, C. B., 226
West, Theodora, Higgons, R. A., and Duryee, M., 81
Whipple, G. H., and Bradford, W. L., 279
Whooping cough, agglutinin response after vaccination with Sauer vaccine, 492

Whooping cough, agglutinin—Cont'd
response of, to vaccination with toxin vaccine, 492
response in untreated clinical pertussis, 492
prophylactic immunization, 49
prophylaxis and treatment of (round table discussion), 116
Whooping cough—Cont'd
treatment of, with intranasal antigen, 42
Wiglesworth, F. W., Childe, A. E., and Goldbloom, A., 331
Wilkes-Weiss, Dorothy, and Huntington, R. W., 449, 456, 462
Wolff, Ernest, and Hurwitz, S., 467